# NIDOVIRUSES

# NIDOVIRUSES

EDITED BY

## Stanley Perlman
Department of Microbiology
University of Iowa
Iowa City, Iowa

## Thomas Gallagher
Department of Microbiology and Immunology
Loyola University Medical Center
Maywood, Illinois

## Eric J. Snijder
Molecular Virology Laboratory
Department of Medical Microbiology
Leiden University Medical Center
Leiden, The Netherlands

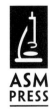

ASM
PRESS

WASHINGTON, DC

Address editorial correspondence to ASM Press, 1752 N St. NW, Washington, DC 20036-2904, USA

Send orders to ASM Press, P.O. Box 605, Herndon, VA 20172, USA
Phone: (800) 546-2416 or (703) 661-1593
Fax: (703) 661-1501
E-mail: books@asmusa.org
Online: estore.asm.org

**Library of Congress Cataloging-in-Publication Data**

Nidoviruses / edited by Stanley Perlman, Thomas Gallagher, Eric J. Snijder.
     p. ; cm.
  Includes bibliographical references and index.
  ISBN 978-1-55581-455-7 (hardcover)
  1. Nidoviruses. I. Perlman, Stanley. II. Gallagher, Thomas, 1956-  III. Snijder, Eric J.
  [DNLM: 1. Nidovirales.  QW 168 N664 2008]
  QR403.N53 2008
  579.2′5—dc22

                                                                              2007030717

10  9  8  7  6  5  4  3  2  1

ISBN 978-1-55581-455-7

*Cover design:* Ed Atkeson, Berg Design

*Cover illustration:* Schematic structures of particles of the major types of nidoviruses. Courtesy of Eric J. Snijder; adapted from Fig. 20.1 (p. 391) of E. J. Snijder, S. G. Siddell, and A. E. Gorbalenya, p. 390–404, *in* B. W. J. Mahy and V. ter Meulen (ed.)., *Topley & Wilson's Microbiology and Microbial Infections,* 10th ed., vol. 1, *Virology* (Hodder Arnold, London, United Kingdom, 2005). See also Color Plate 1.

# CONTENTS

# CONTRIBUTORS

**Enrique Alvarez**
Centro Nacional de Biotecnología (CNB), CSIC,
Campus Universidad Autónoma, Cantoblanco,
Darwin 3, 28049 Madrid, Spain

**Susan C. Baker**
Department of Microbiology and Immunology,
Loyola University Chicago Stritch School of
Medicine, Maywood, IL 60153

**Udeni B. Balasuriya**
Department of Veterinary Science, Gluck Equine
Research Center, University of Kentucky, Lexington,
KY 40456

**Ralph S. Baric**
Department of Epidemiology, School of Public
Health, University of North Carolina, 802 Mary
Ellen Jones Building, Chapel Hill, NC 27599

**Stephen W. Barthold**
Department of Pathology, Microbiology and
Immunology, School of Veterinary Medicine,
University of California, Davis, Davis,
CA 95616

**Cornelia C. Bergmann**
Department of Neurosciences, Cleveland Clinic,
Cleveland, OH 44195

**Berend Jan Bosch**
Virology Division, Faculty of Veterinary Medicine,
Utrecht University, Yalelaan 1, 3584 CL Utrecht,
The Netherlands

**Paul Britton**
Division of Microbiology, Institute for Animal
Health, Compton, Newbury, United
Kingdom

**Carmen Capiscol**
Centro Nacional de Biotecnología (CNB), CSIC,
Campus Universidad Autónoma, Cantoblanco,
Darwin 3, 28049 Madrid, Spain

**Dave Cavanagh**
Division of Microbiology, Institute for Animal
Health, Compton, Newbury, United Kingdom

**Hyeryun Choe**
Department of Pediatrics, Harvard Medical School,
Boston, MA 02215

**Jeff A. Cowley**
CSIRO Livestock Industries, Queensland Bioscience
Precinct, St. Lucia, Queensland 4067, Australia

**Marta L. DeDiego**
Centro Nacional de Biotecnología (CNB), CSIC,
Campus Universidad Autónoma, Cantoblanco,
Darwin 3, 28049 Madrid, Spain

**Raoul J. de Groot**
Virology Division, Department of Infectious
Diseases and Immunology, Faculty of Veterinary
Sciences, Utrecht University, Utrecht, The
Netherlands

**Damon J. Deming**
Department of Microbiology and Immunology,
School of Medicine, University of North Carolina,
Chapel Hill, NC 27599

**Mark R. Denison**
Department of Pediatrics, Department of
Microbiology and Immunology, and Elizabeth B.
Lamb Center for Pediatric Research, Vanderbilt
University Medical Center, Nashville,
TN 37232

**Marc Desforges**
Laboratoire de neuroimmunovirologie, INRS-Institut
Armand-Frappier, Laval, Québec H7V 1B7, Canada

**Luis Enjuanes**
Centro Nacional de Biotecnología (CNB), CSIC,
Campus Universidad Autónoma, Cantoblanco,
Darwin 3, 28049 Madrid, Spain

**Kay S. Faaberg**
Department of Veterinary and Biomedical Sciences,
College of Veterinary Medicine, University of
Minnesota, St. Paul, MN 55108

**Michael Farzan**
Department of Microbiology and Molecular
Genetics, Harvard Medical School, Southborough,
MA 01772

**Alexander E. Gorbalenya**
Molecular Virology Laboratory, Department of
Medical Microbiology, Leiden University Medical
Center, P.O. Box 9600, 2300 RC Leiden, The
Netherlands

**Armando E. Hoet**
Department of Veterinary Preventive Medicine,
College of Veterinary Medicine, The Ohio State
University, Columbus, OH 43210

**Brenda G. Hogue**
Biodesign Institute, School of Life Sciences, Arizona
State University, Tempe, AZ 85257-5401

**Cheng Huang**
Department of Microbiology and Immunology, The
University of Texas Medical Branch at Galveston,
Galveston, TX 77555-1019

**Hélène Jacomy**
Laboratoire de neuroimmunovirologie, INRS-Institut
Armand-Frappier, Laval, Québec H7V 1B7, Canada

**Thomas E. Lane**
Department of Molecular Biology and Biochemistry,
University of California, Irvine, CA 92697

**Julian L. Leibowitz**
Department of Microbial and Molecular Pathogenesis,
Texas A&M University System College of Medicine,
College Station, TX 77843-1114

**Wenhui Li**
Department of Microbiology and Molecular Genetics,
Harvard Medical School, Southborough, MA 01772

**Linda J. Lowenstine**
Department of Pathology, Microbiology and
Immunology, School of Veterinary Medicine,
University of California, Davis, CA 95616

**Carolyn E. Machamer**
Department of Cell Biology, Johns Hopkins University
School of Medicine, Baltimore, MD 21205-2196

**N. James MacLachlan**
Department of Pathology, Microbiology and
Immunology, School of Veterinary Medicine,
University of California, Davis, CA 95616

**Shinji Makino**
Department of Microbiology and Immunology, The
University of Texas Medical Branch at Galveston,
Galveston, TX 77555-1019

**Michael P. Murtaugh**
Department of Veterinary and Biomedical Sciences,
University of Minnesota, St. Paul, MN 55108

**Krishna Narayanan**
Department of Microbiology and Immunology, The
University of Texas Medical Branch at Galveston,
Galveston, TX 77555-1019

**Benjamin W. Neuman**
Department of Molecular and Integrative
Neurosciences, The Scripps Research Institute,
10550 N. Torrey Pines Rd., La Jolla, CA 92037

**John Nicholls**
Department of Pathology, The University of Hong
Kong, Hong Kong Special Administrative Region,
China

**J. S. Malik Peiris**
Department of Microbiology, The University of
Hong Kong, Hong Kong Special Administrative
Region, China

**Stanley Perlman**
Department of Microbiology, University of Iowa,
Iowa City, IA 52242

**Leo L. M. Poon**
Department of Microbiology, The University of
Hong Kong, Hong Kong SAR, China

**Peter J. M. Rottier**
Virology Division, Faculty of Veterinary Medicine,
Utrecht University, Yalelaan 1, 3584 CL Utrecht,
The Netherlands

*Linda J. Saif*
Food Animal Health Research Program, Ohio
Agricultural Research and Development Center, and
Department of Veterinary Preventive Medicine,
College of Veterinary Medicine, The Ohio State
University, Wooster, OH 44691

*Stuart Siddell*
Department of Cellular and Molecular Medicine,
Medical and Veterinary Sciences, University of Bristol,
University Walk, Bristol BS8 1TD, United Kingdom

*Eric J. Snijder*
Molecular Virology Laboratory, Department of
Medical Microbiology, Leiden University Medical
Center, P.O. Box 9600, 2300 RC Leiden, The
Netherlands

*Willy J. M. Spaan*
Molecular Virology Laboratory, Department of
Medical Microbiology, Leiden University Medical
Center, P.O. Box 9600, 2300 RC Leiden, The
Netherlands

*Stephen A. Stohlman*
Department of Neurosciences, Cleveland Clinic,
Cleveland, OH 44195

*Pierre J. Talbot*
Laboratoire de neuroimmunovirologie, INRS-Institut
Armand-Frappier, Laval, Québec H7V 1B7, Canada

*Erwin van den Born*
Department of Molecular Biosciences, University
of Oslo, P.O. Box 1041 Blindern, 0316 Oslo,
Norway

*Martijn J. van Hemert*
Molecular Virology Laboratory, Department
of Medical Microbiology, Leiden University
Medical Center, P.O. Box 9600, 2300 RC Leiden,
The Netherlands

*Gijs A. Versteeg*
Molecular Virology Laboratory, Department
of Medical Microbiology, Leiden University
Medical Center, P.O. Box 9600, 2300 RC Leiden,
The Netherlands

*Peter J. Walker*
CSIRO Livestock Industries, Australian Animal
Health Laboratory, Geelong, Victoria 3220,
Australia

*Susan R. Weiss*
Department of Microbiology, University of
Pennsylvania School of Medicine, Philadelphia,
PA 19104-6076

*John Ziebuhr*
Centre for Cancer Research and Cell Biology, School
of Biomedical Sciences, The Queen's University of
Belfast, Belfast, United Kingdom

# PREFACE

Viruses are remarkable for their diversity. This diversity is clearly evident in the nidoviruses, particularly with respect to their influence on host organisms. Viruses now known to be in this order were first recognized by their severe pathogenic effects in chickens and domesticated livestock, but as additional nidoviruses were identified and evaluated, it became clear that many of them had far more temperate relationships with their hosts. Notably, nidovirus infections in humans were considered to be relatively insignificant. The unexpected and fulminant severe acute respiratory syndrome (SARS) outbreak in 2002 and 2003 showed that a nidovirus infection of humans could be at least as severe as those previously identified in animals, and it greatly increased interest in this set of viruses, both in the scientific community and in the general population. The emergence of this disease also changed the focus of nidovirus research and enticed many new investigators into this field of research. These new investigations run the gamut of virology, (bio)chemistry, cell biology, immunology, and pathogenesis, and they also probe into the natural history of nidovirus infections. With ongoing research, we will be better positioned to recognize future nidovirus outbreaks and will be better able to take appropriate quarantine, vaccination, and therapeutic antiviral measures. This new knowledge, much of which is reviewed in this book, has already mitigated public concern over nidovirus outbreaks, and it will surely be used to save human and animal lives in the event of future epidemics.

Notably, there have been increased efforts to understand nidovirus replication. The coronavirus, torovirus, and ronivirus RNA genomes are the largest of any RNA viruses, and the genomes of the other nidovirus group, the arteriviruses, are also larger than those of most of the plus-strand RNA viruses. An outstanding question is why so much genetic information is required for a process that in other plus-strand RNA viruses is apparently performed more efficiently. Part of this requirement for additional genetic information may reflect the unique replicative strategy of nidoviruses. Transcription, in each case, yields a 3′ nested ("nido") set of subgenomic mRNAs, with all subgenomic RNAs of coronaviruses and arteriviruses also containing a common 5′ leader sequence. The joining of sequences that are noncontiguous in the genome RNA, in the absence of splicing, is unique and must be directed by specialized viral proteins, possibly aided by host cell factors. Understanding this process and the RNA signals and enzymes involved in genome replication and transcription is a major focus of nidovirus research. These investigations have been facilitated by the development of robust reverse genetics systems for many of the coronaviruses and arteriviruses. These genetic systems are combining with efforts to discern the crystal structures of virus-encoded enzymes, evaluate their in vitro biochemical functions, and study the membrane-associated replication/transcription complex in the context of the living infected cell. Nidovirus research is poised to make considerable advances in the understanding of RNA virus amplification.

Another important goal is to understand the mechanisms of virus entry, assembly, and exit from the infected cell. Enveloped nidoviruses enter cells through endosomes by a membrane fusion process, and new viruses assemble near the endoplasmic reticulum by a membrane fission process. Research into these events has focused on probing interactions between viral and host cell proteins. Studies of the interaction of the coronavirus surface glycoprotein and its host cell receptor have assumed special prominence because this entry stage profoundly influences virus tropism and is also amenable to therapeutic intervention with neutralizing antibodies. There is considerable potential for antiviral drugs targeting this entry stage as well. The details of the assembly and exit stages are beginning to be unraveled with new assays creating virus-like particles and recombinant viruses with specific defects in completing this unique intracellular assembly process. Research efforts into both of these areas will clearly advance as the structure of the nidovirus virion is revealed with increasingly greater resolution.

A characteristic feature of coronavirus genomes is that many so-called group-specific genes are interspersed with those encoding major virion proteins at the 3' end of the genome. The encoded group-specific proteins are not related to any known host cell or viral proteins and are not even shared among different coronavirus subgroups. Their functions are unknown, and paradoxically, while they are maintained in each virus, some can be deleted without any obvious effect on growth in tissue culture cells or in animals. Further, one unexpected finding is that several of these accessory proteins, which had been classified as nonstructural, are in fact present in the virion. These findings raise the possibility that at least some of the group-specific proteins operate at virus entry or assembly stages. Research on these "accessory" group-specific proteins, their role in the coronavirus growth cycle, and their possible influences on disease is being actively pursued.

A third area of nidovirus research is focused on virus-host interactions within infected humans or animals. The use of mice in which single genes are rendered nonfunctional by mutation (knockout mice) and of tools to identify virus-specific T and B cells has assisted our understanding of the T- and B-cell responses to the virus. Progress in pathogen-host interactions in general has shown the great importance of the innate immune response in controlling infections, and nidovirus infections are no exception to this rule. The host must respond rapidly and effectively to the infecting virus, but not excessively, as an overexuberant response will result in immunopathologic disease and a potentially lethal outcome for the host. The virus must be able to suppress this appropriate innate host response, at least enough to permit its amplification. Nidoviruses have developed mechanisms to counter the innate immune responses at the level of inhibition both of type I interferon induction and of signaling, mechanisms which are beginning to be understood.

All these research efforts are directed to increase our understanding of how nidoviruses replicate within the infected cell and animal host and also to form the basis for developing nidovirus vaccines and antiviral therapies. Several live attenuated animal nidovirus vaccines have been available for years. These vaccines exhibit varying efficacy, but most importantly, they show that live vaccines for human diseases must be very carefully designed. Some animal nidovirus vaccines have the clearly unintended effect of enhancing disease upon subsequent virus exposure, making appropriate selection of the vaccine immunogen a primary consideration. Nidoviruses exhibit a high recombination rate and readily mutate; as a consequence, vaccine strains have the potential to regain virulence via mutation and also to recombine with other vaccine strains as well as with wild-type virus, with the consequent development of new substrains. Since live attenuated vaccines are usually most effective in preventing disease upon subsequent challenge with wild-type virus, efforts to circumvent these problems are being made. Additionally, antiviral therapies for SARS coronavirus (SARS-CoV) and nidoviruses that infect farm or companion animals are being developed on the basis of recent advances in understanding the structure and function of individual nidovirus proteins.

One commonly asked question is whether SARS-CoV will reemerge as an important human pathogen. Thoughtful responses to this question require appreciation for zoonotic coronavirus transmissions and demand that we identify the most proximal nonhuman hosts for this virus. If the virus is typically endemic in bats, as is commonly believed at present, transmission to humans may not easily occur, since the bat viruses would likely need to mutate extensively, possibly requiring involvement of intermediate hosts (palm civets, raccoon dogs, etc.), before infecting humans. Even within human populations, extensive adaptation was required before the virus could be efficiently transmitted from person to person and cause severe disease. However, the SARS epidemic, as well as previous examples of nidovirus infections that crossed species barriers, shows that these viruses can relatively easily adapt to new hosts. In response to the SARS epidemic, investigators have identified a variety of novel coronaviruses in other animal species. Nidoviruses have to be viewed as common, ubiquitous infectious agents, with the recent isolation of a torovirus relative from fish (tentatively assigned to a new genus, *Bafinivirus*) underlining the amazing diversity of this virus cluster. Thus, even if SARS does not return, other animal or human nidoviruses may be infecting species that may associate with humans, raising the possibility of potentially severe new disease outbreaks. Increased understanding of nidoviruses is the best way to deal with this potential threat to health. The chapters in this book show that much exciting progress has been made in understanding nidovirus replication and pathogenesis. They also show that there is much more essential knowledge that can be rapidly generated now that there are facile approaches in place to identify these viruses in humans and animals, dissect their functions, and evaluate their pathogenic potential.

This book could not have been produced without the help of many individuals. In particular, we thank Gregory Payne of ASM Press for guidance and encouragement during the development of this book. Most importantly, we thank the authors of the chapters, as their collective efforts have created this book.

**Stanley Perlman**
**Thomas Gallagher**
**Eric J. Snijder**

# ABBREVIATIONS

| | | | |
|---|---|---|---|
| ACE2 | angiotensin converting enzyme 2 | FECV | feline enteric coronavirus |
| ADRP | ADP-ribose 1″-phosphatase | FIPV | feline infectious peritonitis virus |
| APC | antigen presenting cell | GAV | gill-associated virus |
| APN | aminopeptidase N | GP | glycoprotein |
| ARDS | acute respiratory disease syndrome | gRNA | genomic RNA |
| BAC | bacterial artificial chromosome | HCoV | human coronavirus |
| BCoV | bovine coronavirus | HE | hemagglutinin-esterase |
| BEV | Berne virus | HEL | helicase |
| BHK | baby hamster kidney | HR | heptad repeat |
| BRDC | bovine respiratory disease complex | HVR | hypervariable region |
| BRV | Breda virus | IBV | infectious bronchitis virus |
| BToV | bovine torovirus | ICTV | International Committee on Taxonomy of Viruses |
| CCoV | canine coronavirus | | |
| CEACAM1 | Carcinoembryonic antigen adhesion molecule 1 | IFN | interferon |
| | | IL | interleukin |
| $3CL^{pro}$ | 3C-like protease | LCMV | lymphocytic choriomeningitis virus |
| 3CLSP | 3C-like serine protease | LDV | lactate dehydrogenase-elevating virus |
| CMV | cytomegalovirus | | |
| CPD | cyclic phosphodiesterase | LV | Lelystad virus |
| CTL | cytotoxic T lymphocyte | MAb | monoclonal antibody |
| DI | defective interfering | MCMV | murine cytomegalovirus |
| DMV | double membrane vesicle | MEF | murine embryonic fibroblast |
| EAE | experimental allergic encephalomyelitis | MHV | mouse hepatitis virus |
| EAV | equine arteritis virus | MLV | modified live virus |
| EM | electron microscopy | MMP | matrix metalloproteinase |
| E protein | envelope protein | $M^{pro}$ | main protease |
| ER | endoplasmic reticulum | M protein | membrane protein |
| ERGIC | endoplasmic reticulum-Golgi intermediate compartment | MRCA | most recent common ancestor |
| | | MS | multiple sclerosis |
| EToV | equine torovirus | MT | methyltransferase |
| EVA | equine viral arteritis | NendoU | nidovirus uridylate-specific endoribonuclease |
| ExoN | exonuclease N | | |
| FCoV | feline coronavirus | N protein | nucleocapsid protein |

| | |
|---|---|
| nsp | nonstructural protein |
| ORF | open reading frame |
| PCA | procoagulant activity |
| PCP | papain-like cysteine protease |
| PD | Parkinson's disease |
| PEDV | porcine epidemic diarrhea virus |
| PhCoV | pheasant coronavirus |
| PHEV | porcine hemagglutinating encephalomyelitis virus |
| PL$^{pro}$ | papain-like protease |
| pp1a | polyprotein 1a |
| pp1ab | polyprotein 1ab |
| PRCV | porcine respiratory coronavirus |
| PRRSV | porcine reproductive and respiratory syndrome virus |
| PToV | porcine torovirus |
| RAG | recombination activation gene |
| RBD | receptor-binding domain |
| RdRp | RNA-dependent RNA polymerase |
| RFS | ribosomal frameshift signal (or site) |
| RTC | replication/transcription complex |
| SARS | severe acute respiratory syndrome |
| SARS-CoV | severe acute respiratory syndrome coronavirus |
| SHFV | simian hemorrhagic fever virus |
| sg | subgenomic |
| SIV | swine influenza A virus |
| S protein | spike glycoprotein |
| TCoV | turkey coronavirus |
| TGEV | transmissible gastroenteritis virus |
| TIMP | inhibitor of MMP |
| TMEV | Theiler's murine encephalomyelitis virus |
| TMRCA | time of most recent common ancestor |
| TNF | tumor necrosis factor |
| TRE | transcription-regulating element |
| TRS | transcription-regulating sequence |
| UTR | untranslated region |
| VNA | virus neutralization assay |
| WBV | white bream virus |
| WD | winter dysentery |
| YHV | yellow head virus |
| ZBD | zinc-binding domain |

Chapter 1

# An Introduction to Nidoviruses

STUART SIDDELL AND ERIC J. SNIJDER

Nidoviruses excite interest for two main reasons. First, nidovirus infections are often associated with severe disease. For example, human severe acute respiratory syndrome (SARS) is caused by a zoonotic coronavirus infection. Nidoviruses can also be associated with fatal diseases of companion animals (e.g., feline infectious peritonitis) and economically important diseases of livestock (e.g., infectious bronchitis of chickens or yellow head disease of penaeid prawns). As this volume demonstrates, we now understand, at least in outline, the principles governing the organization and expression of the nidovirus genome. A major challenge for the future will be to focus our attention on the pathogenesis of nidovirus infections and the development of novel, and more effective, intervention strategies.

Second, among the RNA viruses, the nidoviruses exhibit extraordinary genetic complexity. Even the smallest nidovirus genomes are relatively large (ca. 13,000 nucleotides), and the largest are roughly three to four times the size of a typical RNA virus genome. One reason for this complexity is that the replication and transcription of nidoviral RNA involve a complex array of virus-encoded proteins that are associated with a variety of unexpected enzymatic activities. The structure and function of these proteins, and their role in virus replication, constitute a particularly exciting aspect of contemporary nidovirus research. Furthermore, one group of nidoviruses, the coronaviruses, are unusual in that many encode a number of niche-specific proteins that are nonessential for virus replication in cell culture but appear to confer a selective advantage in vivo. Unraveling the mystery of how these proteins benefit the virus is also very exciting. Clearly, the evolution of nidoviruses is a tale of genome expansion. Understanding how this process has taken place and how the acquisition of novel functions relates to the ability of these viruses to expand their host range and adapt

rapidly to changing environmental conditions, while maintaining genomic stability, is a fascinating intellectual challenge for future generations of nidovirologists.

## HISTORICAL NOTES

Until very recently, nidovirologists were mainly concerned with viruses that are associated with overt disease. In many cases, the disease was recognized long before a virus etiology was established or the causative agent isolated and characterized. For example, feline infectious peritonitis was probably documented as early as 1914 (23), infectious bronchitis of chickens was described in 1931 (43), and yellow head disease was recognized in Thailand in 1950 (33). In some cases, however, the emergence of a new disease provoked the isolation and identification of a nidovirus. For example, outbreaks of "mystery swine disease" in the United States and Europe in the late 1980s (25) led to the discovery of *Porcine reproductive and respiratory syndrome virus* (PRRSV) (51) and the outbreak of SARS in 2002 led to the identification of *Severe acute respiratory syndrome coronavirus* (SARS-CoV) (12, 28, 39). Within the last few years, it has also become apparent that many animal species are likely to be infected with nidoviruses without overt disease, and the characterization of these orphan viruses will be of great interest in the future.

Despite this focus on nidovirus-associated diseases, many people would argue that our understanding of nidoviruses has been driven forward not by "clinical" imperatives but by the opportunities that arose from developments in the fields of molecular biology and recombinant DNA technology. Even today, many nidoviruses are considered difficult to isolate and propagate. For example, the isolation of the equine torovirus (*Berne virus*) in cell culture remains

**Stuart Siddell** • Department of Cellular and Molecular Medicine, Medical and Veterinary Sciences, University of Bristol, University Walk, Bristol BS8 1TD, United Kingdom. **Eric J. Snijder** • Molecular Virology Laboratory, Department of Medical Microbiology, Leiden University Medical Center, P.O. Box 9600, 2300 RC Leiden, The Netherlands.

Table 1. Some landmarks of nidovirus molecular biology

| Event | Yr | | | |
|---|---|---|---|---|
| | Coronavirus | Torovirus | Arterivirus | Ronivirus |
| First isolation of virus | 1937 | 1972 | 1953 | 1993 |
| Structural proteins identified | 1975 | 1984 | 1973 | 1997 |
| Infectivity of genomic RNA shown | 1977 | 1988 | 1975 | |
| Nested set of subgenomic mRNAs identified | 1980 | 1988 | 1982 | 2002 |
| Discovery of discontinuous transcription | 1983 | 2002 | 1990 | |
| Discovery of continuous transcription | | 2002 | | 2002 |
| First gene sequenced | 1983 | 1989 | 1989 | 2000 |
| First full-length genome sequenced | 1987 | 2005 | 1991 | 2002 |
| Subgenome-length minus-strand RNAs identified | 1989 | | 1996 | |
| ORF1a-ORF1b ribosomal frameshifting described | 1989 | 1990 | 1991 | 2000 |
| Identification of virus receptor | 1991 | | 2003 | |
| Reverse genetics: targeted recombination | 1992 | | | |
| Reverse genetics: infectious cDNA | 2000 | | 1997 | |
| First crystal structure of a virus protein | 2002 | | 2002 | |

a unique event and the roniviruses, *Gill-associated virus* (GAV) and *Yellow head virus* (YHV), can be propagated only in animals. But there are exceptions. Several coronaviruses and arteriviruses, such as *Murine hepatitis virus* (MHV), SARS-CoV, and *Equine arteritis virus* (EAV), can be propagated to relatively high titers in cell culture, and by focusing on these viruses it has been possible to elucidate the principles governing nidovirus replication. Tables 1 and 2 list some landmarks in studying the molecular biology of nidoviruses. We hope that after reading this book, the reader might wish to extend these tables and produce similar tables relating to the cellular biology and pathogenesis of nidovirus infections.

## TAXONOMY, CLASSIFICATION, AND NOMENCLATURE

The genome organization and the relatedness of the proteins involved in their RNA replication and transcription single the nidoviruses out as a distinct evolutionary lineage among the positive-strand RNA viruses. The most recent phylogenetic analysis (15), which is based essentially upon the virus RNA-dependent RNA polymerase (RdRp), divides the order *Nidovirales* into three families, the *Coronaviridae*, the *Arteriviridae*, and the *Roniviridae*. Of these, the *Coronaviridae* family is divided into the genera *Coronavirus* and *Torovirus*. It seems clear that the coronaviruses and toroviruses are the youngest members of the nidovirus order, but there is not enough information to decide whether it was the arteriviruses or the roniviruses that were the first to branch off from the nidovirus ancestral trunk. The recent discovery and sequence analysis of the first fish nidovirus, *White bream virus* (17, 44), suggest that there may be a much greater diversity of nidoviruses, particularly among nonmammalian hosts, than has previously been recognized. The reader is referred to chapter 2 for a more detailed account of the evolution of nidoviruses, and, undoubtedly, further taxonomic revisions of the order *Nidovirales* will be forthcoming.

Table 2. Additional landmarks of nidovirus molecular biology

| Yr | Event |
|---|---|
| 1990 | Evolutionary relationship between the replicase proteins of coronaviruses and toroviruses shown |
| 1991 | Evolutionary relationship between the replicase proteins of coronaviruses, toroviruses, and arteriviruses shown |
| 1995 | Model of nidovirus discontinuous extension during minus-strand RNA synthesis proposed |
| 1996 | Order *Nidovirales* established by the International Committee on the Taxonomy of Viruses |
| 2000 | Evolutionary relationship between the replicase proteins of coronaviruses, toroviruses, arteriviruses, and roniviruses shown |
| 2000 | Unified description of coronavirus and arterivirus replicase polyprotein processing |
| 2000 | Chimeric coronaviruses that cross species barrier in vitro constructed |
| 2003 | Unified description of the nidovirus replicase/transcriptase and its enzymatic activities |
| 2004 | Description of arterivirus-like particles consisting of RNA and the three major structural proteins |
| 2005 | Generic main protease inhibitors of coronaviruses described |
| 2007 | Coronavirus interferon antagonist proteins identified |

**Table 3.** List of species in the order *Nidovirales*

| Name | Abbreviation |
| --- | --- |
| *Coronaviridae* | |
|   *Coronavirus* | |
|     Group 1 species | |
|      *Canine coronavirus* | |
|       Canine coronavirus . . . . . . . . . . . . . . | CCoV |
|      *Feline coronavirus* | |
|       Feline coronavirus . . . . . . . . . . . . . . | FCoV |
|       Feline infectious peritonitis virus | |
|        (NC_007025) . . . . . . . . . . . . . . . . | FIPV |
|      *Human coronavirus 229E* | |
|       Human coronavirus 229E | |
|        (NC_002645) . . . . . . . . . . . . . . . . | HCoV-229E |
|       Human coronavirus NL-63 | |
|        (NC_005831) . . . . . . . . . . . . . . . . | HCoV-NL63 |
|      *Porcine epidemic diarrhea virus* | |
|       Porcine epidemic diarrhea virus | |
|        (NC_003436) . . . . . . . . . . . . . . . . | PEDV |
|      *Transmissible gastroenteritis virus* | |
|       Transmissible gastroenteritis virus | |
|        (NC_002306) . . . . . . . . . . . . . . . . | TGEV |
|       Porcine respiratory coronavirus . . . . . . | PRCoV |
|      *Bat coronavirus* | |
|       Bat coronavirus . . . . . . . . . . . . . . . . | BtCoV |
|      *Rabbit coronavirus* | |
|       Rabbit coronavirus . . . . . . . . . . . . . . | RbCoV |
|     Group 2 species | |
|      *Canine respiratory coronavirus* | |
|       Canine respiratory coronavirus 4182 . . | CRCoV-4182 |
|      *Bovine coronavirus* | |
|       Bovine coronavirus (NC_003045) . . . . | BCoV |
|      *Human coronavirus OC43* | |
|       Human coronavirus OC43 | |
|        (NC_005147) . . . . . . . . . . . . . . . . | HCoV-OC43 |
|       Human coronavirus HKU1 | |
|        (NC_006577) . . . . . . . . . . . . . . . . | HCoV-HKU1 |
|      *Human enteric coronavirus* | |
|       Human enteric coronavirus . . . . . . . . | HECoV |
|      *Murine hepatitis virus* | |
|       Murine hepatitis virus JHM | |
|        (NC_006852) . . . . . . . . . . . . . . . . | MHV-JHM |
|       Murine hepatitis virus A59 | |
|        (NC_001846) . . . . . . . . . . . . . . . . | MHV-A59 |
|      *Porcine hemagglutinating encephalomyelitis virus* | |
|       Porcine hemagglutinating encephalomyelitis | |
|        virus (NC_007732) . . . . . . . . . . . . | HEV |
|      *Puffinosis coronavirus* | |
|       Puffinosis coronavirus . . . . . . . . . . . . | PCoV |
|      *Rat coronavirus* | |
|       Rat coronavirus . . . . . . . . . . . . . . . . | RtCoV |
|       Sialodacryoadenitis virus . . . . . . . . . . | SDAV |
|      *Severe acute respiratory syndrome coronavirus* | |
|       Severe acute respiratory syndrome | |
|        coronavirus (NC_004718) . . . . . . . . | SARS-CoV |
|      *Bat coronavirus* | |
|       Bat coronavirus 133/2005 | |
|        (NC_008315) . . . . . . . . . . . . . . . . | BtCoV-133/2005 |
|     Group 3 species | |
|      *Infectious bronchitis virus* | |
|       Infectious bronchitis virus | |
|        (NC_001451) . . . . . . . . . . . . . . . . | IBV |
|      *Pheasant coronavirus* | |
|       Pheasant coronavirus . . . . . . . . . . . . | PhCoV |

**Table 3.** *Continued*

| Name | Abbreviation |
| --- | --- |
|      *Turkey coronavirus* | |
|       Turkey coronavirus . . . . . . . . . . . . . . | TCoV |
|   *Torovirus* | |
|      *Bovine torovirus* | |
|       Bovine torovirus . . . . . . . . . . . . . . . . | BToV |
|       Breda virus (NC_007447) . . . . . . . . . . | BRV |
|      *Equine torovirus* | |
|       Berne virus . . . . . . . . . . . . . . . . . . . | BEV |
|       Equine torovirus . . . . . . . . . . . . . . . . | EToV |
|      *Human torovirus* | |
|       Human torovirus . . . . . . . . . . . . . . . . | HToV |
|      *Porcine torovirus* | |
|       Porcine torovirus . . . . . . . . . . . . . . . . | PToV |
| *Arteriviridae* | |
|   *Arterivirus* | |
|      *Equine arteritis virus* | |
|       Equine arteritis virus strain Bucyrus | |
|        (NC_002532) . . . . . . . . . . . . . . . . | EAV |
|      *Lactate dehydrogenase-elevating virus* | |
|       Lactate dehydrogenase-elevating virus strain | |
|        Plagemann (NC_001639) . . . . . . . . . . | LDV |
|      *Porcine reproductive and respiratory syndrome virus* | |
|       Porcine reproductive and respiratory syndrome | |
|        virus, European genotype, strain Lelystad | |
|        (M96262), and North American genotype, | |
|        strain VR-2332 (U87392) . . . . . . . . . . | PRRSV |
|      *Simian hemorrhagic fever virus* | |
|       Simian hemorrhagic fever virus strain | |
|        LVR 42-0 (NC_003092) . . . . . . . . . . | SHFV |
| *Roniviridae* | |
|   *Okavirus* | |
|      *Gill-associated virus* | |
|       Gill-associated virus . . . . . . . . . . . . . . | GAV |
|      *Yellow head virus* | |
|       Yellow head virus . . . . . . . . . . . . . . . . | YHV |

A list of the viruses that are currently accepted as species of the order *Nidovirales* is shown in Table 3. In some cases, the literature also refers to strains or biotypes of a species (and these are sometimes given different names), and these are shown in nonitalic script. Genome sequence accession numbers and assigned abbreviations are also listed. The division of the coronavirus genus into three groups, groups 1, 2, and 3, was originally based upon a combination of virion antigenicity (as defined by serological cross-reactivity) and the genomic position and variety of open reading frames (ORFs) encoding niche-specific proteins. Subsequently, this grouping, which does not have taxonomic status, has been supported by genetic (nucleic and amino acid) similarity analysis. It is now also generally accepted that SARS-CoV (and some bat coronaviruses) comprise a group of coronaviruses that fall within group 2 but are sufficiently different to be considered as a distinct subgroup, subgroup 2b (16).

## MORPHOLOGY

If it is true that the nidoviruses are united by similarities in the replication and transcription of their RNAs, and the replicase proteins involved, it is almost as true that they are distinguished by differences in their structural proteins and the morphology of the virus particles. This is illustrated in Color Plate 1 (see color insert), which shows schematic representations of four different types of nidovirus particle. Coronaviruses and toroviruses are quite similar morphologically and appear to be enveloped particles 120 to 160 nm in diameter, with a prominent fringe of 15- to 20-nm surface projections. In some group 2 coronaviruses and some toroviruses, a second, inner fringe of shorter surface projections is also seen. Coronaviruses are described as roughly spherical, while toroviruses can be disk or rod shaped. The nucleocapsids of both corona- and toroviruses are elongated, tubular structures with a helical symmetry when relaxed. However, they may assume different geometrical forms (normally spheres in the case of coronaviruses and rods or toroids in the case of toroviruses) when constrained in the virus particle. In contrast, arteriviruses are described as spherical particles 50 to 70 nm in diameter with a surface pattern of indistinct projections. The arterivirus genome is surrounded by an icosahedral core shell 25 to 35 nm in diameter. Finally, roniviruses are bacilliform (approximately 170 by 50 nm) and have prominent structures extending about 11 nm from the surface. The ronivirus nucleocapsids have helical symmetry with a diameter of 13 to 18 nm, apparently consisting, in the virus particle, of coiled tubular structures arranged perpendicular to the ventral axis.

## GENOME STRUCTURE AND VIRION PROTEINS

The nidovirus genome is an infectious, single, positive-stranded, linear RNA that is polyadenylated. The coronavirus and arterivirus genomes have modified bases at their 5′ ends and are presumed to be capped. A number of sequence motifs and structural RNA elements that have important roles in the replication and transcription of the genome have been identified, and some of these are discussed below (see also chapters 3 and 8). Additionally, sequence analysis has shown that the nidoviruses share a broadly similar arrangement of genes. Basically, approximately two-thirds of each genome contains two large, 5′-proximal ORFs, designated ORF1a and ORF1b, that encode nonstructural proteins that are mainly involved in viral RNA synthesis. The remaining 3′-proximal third of the genome contains genes encoding the structural proteins of the virus, and in the case of coronaviruses, the structural protein genes are also interspersed with a variable number and arrangement of genes encoding accessory or niche-specific proteins.

The proteins that typically comprise the different nidovirus particles are listed in Table 4. The spike proteins (S proteins) of coronaviruses and toroviruses (see also chapters 9, 13, and 14) have a highly exposed globular domain and a stem portion containing heptad repeats, indicative of a coiled-coil structure. Recently, more detailed interpretations of the S protein structure of a coronavirus have been obtained by electron (cryo)microscopy (5, 36) and the structure of two coronavirus S protein domains, the fusion core and the receptor-binding domain, have been solved to atomic resolution (19, 54, 55). The membrane

**Table 4.** Components of the nidovirus particle

| Component | Abbreviation | Size | | | |
|---|---|---|---|---|---|
| | | Coronavirus[c] | Torovirus | Arterivirus | Ronivirus |
| Genomic RNA[a] | | 27.3–31.5 | 28.5 | 12.7–15.7 | 26.2 |
| Structural proteins[b] | | | | | |
| Spike glycoprotein | S | 180–220 | 200 | | |
| Major surface glycoprotein | GP5 | | | 30–45 | |
| Minor surface glycoprotein | GP2 | | | 25 | |
| | GP3 | | | 36–42 | |
| | GP4 | | | 15–28 | |
| Large spike glycoprotein | GP116 | | | | 110–135 |
| Small spike glycoprotein | GP64 | | | | 60–65 |
| Membrane protein | M | 23–35 | 27 | 16 | |
| Nucleocapsid protein | N | 50–60 | 19 | 12 | 20–22 |
| Small envelope protein | E | 9–12 | | 9 | |
| Hemagglutinin-esterase | HE | 65 | 65 | | |

[a]Sizes are in kilobases.
[b]Sizes are apparent molecular masses (in kilodaltons) estimated by sodium dodecyl sulfate-polyacrylamide gel electrophoresis.
[c]The niche-specific SARS-CoV proteins 3a and 7a are reported to be virus structural proteins, but they are also nonessential for replication in cell cultures and mice (20, 22, 59).

proteins (M proteins) of coronaviruses and toroviruses are different in sequence but alike in size, structure, and function. The M proteins have a similar triple- or quadruple-spanning membrane topology. In addition, coronaviruses have a small structural protein (E) within the envelope. The E protein is important but not absolutely essential for virus assembly (29, 30). Toroviruses seem to lack a homolog for the E protein. Some coronaviruses of group 2 and toroviruses contain an additional protein with hemagglutinin-esterase (HE) activity. Finally, the coronavirus and torovirus nucleocapsid proteins (N proteins) both serve to encapsidate the genomic RNA, but they are dissimilar in size and structure. The coronavirus N protein is phosphorylated and comprised of three conserved domains separated by variable spacer regions. The amino-proximal domains 1 and 2 are typical of other N proteins and are rich in basic residues. The carboxyl-proximal domain 3 has an excess of acidic residues and is referred to as the dimerization domain (32). Recently, X-ray crystallography has been used to elucidate the structures of coronavirus N protein domains 1 and 3 (13, 24, 60). The torovirus N protein is also basic and phosphorylated but is significantly smaller than its coronavirus homolog. Interestingly, it has been shown recently that the N proteins of SARS-CoV and MHV are able to inhibit the synthesis of type I interferons in human cells (27, 57).

The structural proteins of arteriviruses (see also chapter 15) are apparently unrelated to those of the other members of the order *Nidovirales*. There are seven proteins that have been identified in EAV and PRRSV virions, and these may be common to all arteriviruses: a 16- to 20-kDa nonglycosylated M protein is thought to transverse the membrane three times and thus structurally resembles the M protein of corona- and toroviruses. The heterogeneously N-glycosylated, putative triple-spanning major glycoprotein (GP5 for EAV, lactate dehydrogenase-elevating virus, and PRRSV) of variable size forms a disulfide-linked heterodimer with the M protein. Recently, a trimeric complex consisting of the three remaining viral glycoproteins (GP2, GP3, and GP4), which are all minor virion components, was described for EAV. The sixth structural protein of arteriviruses is a small, nonglycosylated, hydrophobic protein designated E protein that is believed to interact with the minor glycoprotein complex. And finally, the arterivirus N protein is phosphorylated and similar in size to the torovirus N protein. The X-ray crystal structure of the carboxyl-terminal 65 amino acids of the PRRSV N protein suggests a structural similarity to domain 3 of the SARS-CoV N protein (11).

Ronivirus structural proteins (see also chapter 25) have been studied mainly for YHV. YHV virions

contain three major structural proteins (110 to 135, 63 to 67, and 20 to 22 kDa). The 110- to 135-kDa protein (GP116) and the 63- to 67-kDa protein (GP64) are glycosylated and appear to be surface proteins that form the prominent peplomers of the virion. Mature GP116 and GP64 are generated by posttranslational processing of a precursor glyco-polyprotein. GP116 and GP64 are not linked by intramolecular disulfide bonds, but each is anchored in the virion by C-terminal hydrophobic transmembrane domains. The 20- to 22-kDa protein (p20) is associated with nucleocapsids and appears to function as the N protein.

## NIDOVIRUS REPLICATION

### Entry and Receptors

A number of different molecules are involved in nidovirus attachment to and entry into target cells. These include primary receptors, which have been shown to be necessary for infection in vivo, cell attachment molecules, which facilitate but are not sufficient to initiate infection, and alternative receptors that may be used by nidoviruses that have undergone adaptation, normally in cell culture. These molecules are listed in Table 5. Recognition of the receptor is mediated by a surface glycoprotein of the virus, which subsequently leads to the fusion of viral and cellular membranes, disassembly of the nucleocapsid, and translation of the genomic RNA. The reader is referred to chapters 9 to 12 for a more detailed account of nidovirus, and in particular coronavirus, entry.

### The RTC

The nidovirus genomic RNA functions as the mRNA for the two 5′-proximal ORFs encoding nonstructural proteins involved in viral RNA synthesis. The translation of ORF1a yields the pp1a polyprotein. Alternatively, in approximately 20 to 30% of cases, ribosomes undergo a programmed (−1) ribosomal frameshift at a specific "slippery" sequence within the overlap between the ORF1a and ORF1b regions and continue to translate ORF1b to produce polyprotein 1ab (pp1ab) (discussed in detail in chapter 3). The slippery sequence together with a downstream pseudoknot structure constitutes the ribosomal frameshifting signal. pp1a and pp1ab are co- and posttranslationally processed by virus-encoded proteases to produce, at least for corona-, toro-, and arteriviruses, between 12 and 16 mature proteins and an unknown number of intermediate products (see chapters 5 to 7 and 9). At present, there is no nidovirus-wide nomenclature for these nonstructural proteins, and they are numbered in

**Table 5.** Coronavirus and arterivirus receptors

| Receptor | Species | Virus(es)[a] | Type |
|---|---|---|---|
| *Coronavirus* | | | |
| Aminopeptidase N | Porcine | TGEV, PRCV | Primary |
| Aminopeptidase N | Feline | FIPV, FCoV | Primary |
| Aminopeptidase N | Canine | CCoV | Primary |
| Aminopeptidase N | Human | HCoV-229E | Primary |
| Carcinoembryonic antigen adhesion molecule 1 | Murine | MHV | Primary |
| Sialic acid | Bovine, murine, avian | BCoV, MHV, IBV | Attachment? |
| Heparin sulfate | Murine | MHV | Adaptive |
| Angiotensin-converting enzyme 2 | Human | SARS-CoV, HCoV-NL63 | Primary |
| CD209L (L-SIGN) | Human | SARS-CoV | Primary? |
| DC-SIGN | Human | SARS-CoV | Attachment |
| *Arterivirus* | | | |
| Sialoadhesin | Porcine | PRRSV | Primary |
| Sialic acid | Porcine | PRRSV | Attachment |

[a]For virus abbreviations, see Table 3.

the order in which they are encoded in pp1ab (e.g., nonstructural protein 1 [nsp1], nsp2, nsp3, etc.), or named according to their (putative) function (e.g., RdRp, helicase [HEL], etc.). The majority of these nonstructural proteins, together with other viral proteins, and possibly cellular proteins, assemble into a membrane-bound replication/transcription complex (RTC) (discussed in chapter 7), which accumulates in the perinuclear region of the infected cell and is associated with infection-induced, double-membrane vesicles (38, 40, 45, 46). Hydrophobic transmembrane domains are present in a number of the nonstructural proteins, and they likely serve to anchor the nascent polyproteins to membranes in the first step of forming an RTC. In arteriviruses and coronaviruses, from one to three (and possibly four) papain-like proteases (PL$^{pro}$s) control processing of the N-terminal part of pp1a/pp1ab, and a chymotrypsin-like protease is responsible for processing the remainder of pp1a/pp1ab polyproteins at 8 to 11 conserved cleavage sites.

Irrespective of the details of proteolytic processing, all nidoviruses are distinguished by a common backbone of conserved functional domains in their nonstructural proteins. This conservation, which implies that there has been continuous evolution from a common nidovirus ancestor, can be identified as the linear arrangement (in an amino-to-carboxyl direction) of (i) a chymotrypsin-like protease with a substrate specificity resembling that of picornavirus 3C proteases (M$^{pro}$) that is flanked by two hydrophobic transmembrane domains, (ii) a large RdRp, (iii) a protein including putative multinuclear Zn finger-like nucleoside triphosphate-binding and 5'-to-3' HEL domains, and (iv) a uridylate-specific endoribonuclease (NendoU). Depending upon the specific nidovirus family, this

backbone may then be adorned by additional functions, including one or more PL$^{pro}$s, ADP-ribose 1''-phosphatase (ADRP), RNA primase, 5'-to-3' exonuclease, 2'-O-methyltransferase, and cyclic phosphodiesterase (Table 6). Clearly, most of these enzymatic functions are concerned with viral RNA synthesis, although they may not necessarily be essential. The elucidation of their structure and function is an area of intense research at the moment (see chapters 2, 5, 6, and 9 for more information). Also, it should be noted that some of the nonstructural proteins encoded by ORF1a and -1b may have relevance to cellular processes. For example, the coronavirus PL$^{pro}$ activity of nsp3 has recently been shown to be a deubiquitinating enzyme (3, 31). Also, the ADRP activity of coronavirus nsp3 may act to influence the levels of ADP-ribose, a key regulatory molecule in the cell.

## RNA Synthesis: Replication and Transcription

The hallmark of nidovirus transcription is the production of multiple subgenome-length mRNAs in the infected cell. These mRNAs are 3' coterminal with respect to the genomic RNA and extend for various lengths in a 5' direction. It is now accepted that these subgenome-length mRNAs are transcribed from a corresponding set of 5'-coterminal subgenome-length minus-strand templates that have been copied from the genomic RNA. Formally, the amplification of mRNA1, which involves a genome-length minus-strand template, is equivalent to replication of the genome.

For many nidoviruses, i.e., coronavirus and arteriviruses, the basic blueprint described above is complicated by the fact that all of the subgenome-length

**Table 6.** Enyzmatic activities associated with nidovirus nonstructural protein domains

| Enzymatic activity | *Coronavirus* (MHV) | *Torovirus* (equine) | *Arterivirus* (EAV) | *Ronivirus* (GAV) |
|---|---|---|---|---|
| PL$^{pro}$ | Present | Present | Present | Unknown |
| ADRP | Present | Present | Absent | Absent |
| Chymotrypsin-like proteinase (M$^{pro}$) | Present | Present | Present | Present |
| RNA primase | Present | Unknown | Unknown | Unknown |
| RdRp | Present | Present | Present | Present |
| 5′-to-3′ HEL | Present | Present | Present | Present |
| 5′-to-3′ exonuclease | Present | Present | Absent | Present |
| NendoU | Present | Present | Present | Present |
| 2′-O-Methyltransferase | Present | Present | Absent | Present |
| Cyclic phosphodiesterase[a] | Present in subgroup 2a | Present | Absent | Absent |

[a] Encoded in ORF2.1 in coronaviruses.

mRNAs contain sequences derived from both ends of the genome. Thus, the generation of these subgenome-length mRNAs involves a process of discontinuous transcription. Each subgenome-length mRNA contains a short 5′ leader sequence, which corresponds to the 5′ end of the genome, joined to a so-called mRNA "body," which represents sequences from the 3′-poly(A) stretch to a position that is upstream of the ORF which will be expressed from that specific subgenome-length mRNA. Importantly, the junction of the leader and body elements can be identified in each mRNA by a characteristic, short, AU-rich motif of about 10 nucleotides that is known as the transcription-regulating sequence (TRS) (see chapter 8 for more details). In the genome, functional TRS motifs are found at the 3′ end of the leader (leader TRS) and in front of each ORF that is destined to become 5′ proximal in one of the subgenome-length mRNAs (body TRSs).

The current model used to explain the generation of coronavirus and arterivirus mRNAs is known as "discontinuous extension during subgenome-length minus strand synthesis" (Color Plate 2 [see color insert]). The basic tenets of this model are that the process of discontinuous transcription occurs during the synthesis of minus-strand subgenome-length templates and resembles the mechanism of similarity-assisted or high-frequency copy choice RNA recombination. Basically, the process can be viewed as a number of consecutive events: (i) the components of a functional RTC are recruited and minus-strand synthesis is initiated at the 3′ end of a genomic RNA, (ii) elongation of nascent minus-strand RNA continues until the first functional body TRS motif is encountered, (iii) a fixed proportion of RTCs will disregard the TRS motif and continue to elongate the nascent strand, or (iv) a fixed proportion of RTCs will stop synthesis of the nascent minus strand and will relocate on the template to a position at the 3′ end of the leader sequence. This relocation will be guided by complementarity between the 3′ end of the nascent minus strand and the leader TRS

motif, and (v) the translocated minus strand will be extended to copy the 3′ end of the template. The completed minus-strand RNA would then serve as a template for mRNA synthesis.

Although the process of discontinuous transcription during minus-strand synthesis is typical of nidoviruses, it is not a defining feature. Recent studies have shown that ronivirus and, with one exception to date, torovirus subgenome-length mRNAs do not have a 5′ leader sequence that corresponds to the 5′ end of the genome. Instead, the 5′ end of each mRNA, including mRNA1, corresponds to a related sequence found immediately upstream of each genomic ORF. The current interpretation of this observation is that in these viruses, transcriptional attenuation occurs at the 3′ end of nascent minus-strand templates but there is no equivalent to the process of discontinuous extension (Color Plate 2). This interpretation also implies that these viruses possess intragenomic elements necessary for the promotion of mRNA synthesis. This contrasts with the situation for coronaviruses and arteriviruses, where the promoters for both negative- and positive-strand RNA synthesis are thought to reside at the ends of the genome. The reader is referred to chapters 8, 9, and 25 and recent reviews (37, 41) for more information on the details of nidovirus transcription and replication. There is clearly a lot more to be learned.

### Translation of Subgenome-Length mRNA

The subgenome-length mRNAs synthesized in the nidovirus-infected cell are, in general, structurally polycistronic but functionally monocistronic. The majority are thought to be translated by cap-dependent initiation, with only the 5′-proximal ORF expressed as protein. This is certainly the case for most of the mRNAs encoding nidovirus structural proteins, with the exception of one or two mRNAs encoding minor glycoproteins of arteriviruses. In contrast, several of the niche-specific coronavirus proteins appear to be translated in a cap-independent manner from functionally polycistronic subgenome-length mRNAs. The exact mechanisms of translational initiation remain to be clarified but may include the internal initiation of protein synthesis and "leaky" ribosomal scanning. The reader is referred to chapter 3 for more details.

### Niche-Specific Proteins

Among the nidoviruses, the coronaviruses are unusual in that they encode a number of proteins that do not seem to be directly related to viral RNA synthesis, nor do they belong to the canonical set of coronavirus structural proteins. These proteins are referred to as accessory or niche-specific proteins, and they are the focus of attention in many laboratories. The current view is that although these proteins are dispensable for replication in cell culture, they act to increase virus fitness in vivo. In some cases, this conclusion seems obvious. For example, two of the SARS-CoV niche-specific proteins (encoded by ORF3b and ORF6) have been shown to be specific and potent antagonists of the innate immune response (27). In other cases, the role of these proteins is less obvious. For example, abrogation of the coronavirus protein encoded by the I ORF, an internal ORF that overlaps with the N protein gene in the +1 reading frame, is not associated with an easily detectable phenotype in vivo (14). Nevertheless, it seems reasonable to conclude that coronaviruses have acquired and, at least in vivo, conserved genes encoding proteins that increase virus fitness, for example, by facilitating the expansion of host range or the rapid adaptation to changing selective pressures. For more information, the reader is referred to chapter 16.

### Virion Assembly and Exit

The very different nature of the nidovirus structural proteins precludes a general description of their interactions during virion assembly and exit. The assembly of coronavirus particles (see chapters 13 and 14) starts with the formation of a ribonucleoprotein (RNP) in the cytoplasm. Virions mature by budding of the RNP through the endoplasmic reticulum and other pre-Golgi membranes, within which the S, M, and E proteins and, if present, HE are located. The M protein is central to the budding process and interacts with itself and with the other structural proteins to direct the assembly of the virion. The assembled virions are transported out of the cell via the exocytic secretory pathway. During exodus, the M and S proteins and HE are modified by glycosylation and the S protein may be proteolytically cleaved. The S protein and HE are not necessary for virus particle formation, though the S protein is essential for infectivity.

The assembly of arteriviruses (see chapter 15) bears some similarities to that of coronaviruses. For example, arterivirus nucleocapids bud into the lumen of smooth intracellular membranes of the exocytic pathway, probably including those of the Golgi complex. Also, arterivirus particles are released from infected cells via exocytosis. However, the interactions between arterivirus structural components during virus assembly must be fundamentally different from those in coronaviruses. First, it is clear that the formation of the icosahedral arterivirus RNP must differ from the assembly of the coronavirus RNP. Second, although it has been shown that both of the major arterivirus glycoproteins, GP5 and M protein, are essential for virus particle formation, while the minor (glyco)proteins, E protein, GP2, GP3, and GP4, are dispensable, it has not been possible to produce virus-like particles in cells that express N protein, GP5, and M protein. Thus, it appears that arterivirus particle assembly involves interactions, possibly RNA-protein interactions, that are not needed for the budding of coronavirus particles. It is also noteworthy that arterivirus particles that lack the minor glycoprotein-E protein complex are noninfectious, which implies a role for this complex in virus entry (52, 53).

## NIDOVIRUS GENETICS

### Classical Genetics

The classical approach to the genetic analysis of nidovirus replication, i.e., the characterization of conditionally lethal, usually temperature-sensitive, virus mutants that are unable to replicate when the infection is initiated and maintained at the nonpermissive temperature, has not been widely adopted. This is disappointing because a detailed characterization of the genotype and phenotype of such mutants should provide insights into almost every aspect of the replication cycle. For example, a recent analysis of coronavirus mutants that are unable to synthesize RNA when the infection is initiated and maintained at the nonpermissive temperature has provided new information on the functions of individual viral replicase proteins and the processing pathways that the replicase polyproteins must travel to assume functional configurations (42). Taken together, the results of this analysis are consistent with the idea that nsp4 to nsp10 of pp1a act together as a complex, multidomain structure or scaffold onto which *trans*-acting nonstructural proteins (e.g., nsp12, nsp14, and nsp16) and viral RNA associate. It is clear that this type of approach should be extended to other nidovirus mutants, including those with defects in functions associated with both structural and niche-specific proteins.

## Reverse Genetics

The development of reverse genetics has been one of the most important advances made in the field of nidovirus research in the last 10 to 15 years. This approach was pioneered by Paul Masters and colleagues, who developed the technique of targeted recombination in coronaviruses (26), and was followed by the development of infectious cDNA systems, initially for arteriviruses (35, 50) and then for coronaviruses (1, 48, 58). The ability to introduce specific mutations into the nidovirus genome has allowed the analysis of almost every aspect of nidovirus replication, ranging from the role of cis-acting RNA elements that regulate nidovirus replication to the structural protein interactions necessary for virion assembly and release. There is no doubt that this approach will be a major platform for many of the studies into the molecular and cellular biology of nidovirus replication and the pathogenesis of nidovirus infections for many years to come. It is also clear that reverse genetics of nidoviruses will be the method of choice for the generation of attenuated, live vaccines, biosafe replicons, and gene delivery vectors.

## IMMUNE RESPONSES

It is convenient, although clearly arbitrary, to consider the immune response to nidovirus infections in three categories: the innate response, the humoral response, and the cell-mediated response.

### Innate Responses

As would be expected, nidovirus infection induces a complex network of innate immune responses. At one level, these can be monitored by measuring the amounts of various cytokines and chemokines in clinical samples (e.g., plasma) from infected patients or animal models, or by expression profiling of immune response genes in cells from infected patients (e.g., peripheral blood mononuclear cells), animal models, or in vitro culture. However, each of these approaches has major limitations, and the interpretation of the data is often difficult. Also, each nidovirus infection is unique and it is impossible to make generalizations. The complexity of the problem can be illustrated by just one example. Thus, it is now clear that macrophages, conventional dendritic cells, fibroblasts, and lung epithelial cells are not able to mount a significant type I interferon response against SARS-CoV (62), which would correlate with the interferon antagonist function of the SARS-CoV N protein and the proteins encoded by ORF3b and ORF6 described above. However, plasmacytoid dendritic cells, which constitutively express interferon-regulatory factor 7 and facilitate alpha interferon expression independent of a beta interferon-mediated feedback loop, do produce type I interferon in response to SARS-CoV infection. Moreover, in an animal model, this response is sufficient to control infection of mice by MHV (9). Clearly, the innate immune response plays a critical role in the pathogenesis of nidovirus disease, but to evaluate this role, we need to have more specific information on, for example, the primary target cells of natural infection, the kinetics of infection and host responses in these cells, and the ability of individual nidoviruses to ablate or modify these responses in a cell-specific manner. The reader is referred to chapters 17 and 22 to 24, which address some of these issues.

### Humoral Responses

The surface glycoprotein (coronaviruses and toroviruses) and the major glycoprotein GP5 (arteriviruses) are the predominant inducers of neutralizing antibody during natural infection. The antigenic structure of the coronavirus S protein has been studied, and the picture that emerges is complex. Essentially, the majority of virus neutralization epitopes seem to be located in the amino-terminal half of the S protein, and they are conformational. The neutralization epitopes are clustered into domains, one of which is usually immunodominant, although two or three domains may carry neutralization epitopes. Glycosylation seems to be an important component of neutralization epitope structure. Although many neutralization epitopes have been defined, the mechanisms of virus neutralization are largely unknown. In the case of SARS-CoV, however, the crystal structure of the receptor-binding domain in complex with a neutralizing antibody shows that the antibody and receptor binding sites overlap very closely (21). This provides a rationale for the strong binding and broad neutralizing ability of the antibody. Although the S protein and GP5 are the prime inducers of humoral immunity, antibody responses to other structural proteins may also have a role in protection.

### Cell-Mediated Responses

As for most other viruses, the cell-mediated immune responses to nidovirus infection are less well characterized than the humoral immune responses. There is good evidence that the cell-mediated response is important in a variety of natural infections (7, 10) and the coronavirus S and N proteins (e.g., for SARS-CoV) (49, 61), as well as the arterivirus M protein (4), are predominant targets for cellular immune recognition. In a few cases, specific T-cell epitopes have been defined and helper or cytotoxic functions have been attributed to T-cell subpopulations. However, many important questions remain to be answered. For example, how important is the T-cell-mediated response in protection during the early stages of nidovirus infections, which antigens are important at the different stages of infection, and how important is the genetic background of the infected individual? The reader should see chapter 23 for further details.

## CLINICAL ASPECTS

The spectrum of disease caused by nidoviruses is summarized in Table 7. As is the case with many viruses, the majority of infections are asymptomatic, perhaps reflecting the pathogenic equilibrium reached during the coevolution of host and pathogen. Many of the clinical diseases listed in Table 7 are, in fact, manifested only in immunodeficient animals (e.g., neonates or pregnant animals). In contrast, when a nonnatural host is infected, or when the natural host is infected by an unusual route or virus variant, fulminant disease can also ensue. As there are no effective vaccines or antivirals that are able to successfully control nidovirus infections (see below), the majority of infections are controlled by management procedures. Thus, for example, the SARS outbreak was controlled by a combination of quarantine, isolation, contact tracing, and restrictions on movement. Similarly, environmental controls, which include good hygiene,

**Table 7.** Pathogenic nidovirus infections in natural hosts

| Virus[a] | Host | Infection[b] Respiratory | Enteric | Reproductive | Neurologic | MPS[c] | Other | Clinical disease |
|---|---|---|---|---|---|---|---|---|
| **Coronaviruses** | | | | | | | | |
| IBV | Chicken | ++ | — | + | — | — | +[d] | Infectious bronchitis |
| BCoV | Cattle | — | ++ | — | — | — | — | Neonatal calf diarrhea, winter dysentery |
| CCoV | Dog | — | ++ | — | — | — | — | Enteritis |
| CRCoV | Dog | ++ | — | — | — | — | — | ? |
| FCoV | Cat | + | ++ | — | + | — | +[e] | Enteritis, infectious peritonitis |
| HCoV-229E | Human | ++ | — | — | — | — | — | Common cold |
| HCoV-NL63 | Human | ++ | — | — | — | — | — | Common cold, laryngotracheitis |
| HCoV-OC43 | Human | ++ | — | — | — | — | — | Common cold |
| HCoV-HKU1 | Human | ++ | + | — | — | — | — | Common cold, bronchiolitis |
| SARS-CoV | Human | ++ | + | — | — | — | — | SARS |
| MHV | Mouse | + | ++ | — | + | — | +[f] | Enteritis, rhinitis, hepatitis |
| RtCoV | Rat | ++ | — | — | — | — | +[g] | Pneumonitis |
| PEDV | Pig | — | ++ | — | — | — | — | Epidemic diarrhea |
| TGEV | Pig | + | ++ | — | — | — | — | Transmissible gastroenteritis |
| HEV | Pig | + | — | — | ++ | — | — | Vomiting and wasting disease |
| TCoV | Turkey | — | ++ | — | — | — | — | Transmissible enteritis |
| **Toroviruses** | | | | | | | | |
| EToV | Horse | — | — | — | — | — | — | ? |
| BToV | Cattle | + | ++ | — | — | — | — | Gastroenteritis |
| HToV | Human | — | ++ | — | — | — | — | Gastroenteritis |
| PToV | Pig | — | ++ | — | — | — | — | Gastroenteritis |
| **Arteriviruses** | | | | | | | | |
| EAV | Horse | + | — | + | — | ++ | +[h] | Rhinitis, abortion |
| LDV | Mouse | — | — | — | + | ++ | — | Generally asymptomatic |
| SHFV | Monkey | — | — | — | — | ++ | — | Generally asymptomatic |
| PRRSV | Pig | + | — | + | + | ++ | — | Pneumonia, abortion |
| **Roniviruses** | | | | | | | | |
| GAV | Prawn | Roniviruses target tissues of ectodermal and mesodermal origin, including lymphoid organ, hemocytes, hematopoietic tissue, gill lamellae, and spongy connective tissue of the subcutis, gut, antenal gland, gonads, nerve tracts, and ganglia | | | | | | |
| YHV | Prawn | | | | | | | |

[a]For virus abbreviations, see Table 3.
[b]++, main target for infection; +, secondary target for infection; ?, circumstantial evidence of infection or disease; —, no evidence of involvement.
[c]MPS, mononuclear phagocyte system.
[d]Kidneys.
[e]Serous membranes.
[f]Liver.
[g]Salivary and lacrimal glands.
[h]Arteries.

isolation, and early weaning, are currently the most powerful and widely used tools for the control of feline coronavirus infection. In the case of the arterivirus PRRSV, despite the development of live attenuated and killed vaccines, the most effective control measures still, essentially, consist of the eradication of infected herds and restrictions on the movement of pigs from areas where the virus is enzootic. And finally, the current recommended procedures for the control of yellow head disease include the destruction of all infected and exposed shrimp by incineration or burial. Clearly, there is a need for a more rational approach to the control of many nidovirus infections, and research in the area of nidovirus antivirals and vaccines is a current focus for many laboratories.

## ANTIVIRALS AND VACCINES

### Antivirals

Although the complexity of the nidovirus genome and, in particular, the large number of virus-encoded proteins involved in RNA synthesis have sometimes frustrated research, they can also be viewed as a blessing. In addition to the usual replicative nonstructural proteins (proteinases, RdRp, and HEL), the nidoviruses offer a number of unusual activities (for example, NendoU) that could be viewed as potential targets for the development of antiviral drugs. However, at present, the nidovirus main proteinase still appears to be the most promising target. For example, it has recently been shown that optimized forms of a specific class of cysteine-proteinase inhibitors (the so-called Michael inhibitors) are able to inhibit the replication of a number of coronavirus species, at least in cell culture (56). Of course, this is a far cry from a safe, efficacious, and affordable pan-coronavirus antiviral drug, but at least the signs are promising.

In addition to antiviral drugs that target proteins involved in RNA synthesis, there is also the potential to develop drugs that target other phases of the replication cycle. For example, there has been considerable interest in the design of peptides that are able to inhibit the formation of a fusogenic form of the coronavirus surface glycoprotein, which is a prerequisite for the initiation of infection (6, 47). This approach is based upon using peptides to interfere with the conformational rearrangement of heptad repeat structures in the carboxy-proximal region of the S protein and is analogous to the strategy used to inhibit human immunodeficiency virus replication with the fusion inhibitor enfuvirtide. Finally, it should be noted that there is also considerable potential for the development of nucleic acid-based strategies for the control of nidovirus infections, but these are clearly at a very early stage.

### Vaccines

If one of the main reasons for studying nidoviruses is that they are associated with disease, then one of the major goals of nidovirus research has to be the development of effective vaccines. At present, there are vaccines available for a number of nidoviruses, including avian, bovine, canine, feline, and porcine coronaviruses, as well as PRRSV and EAV. However, there are many problems associated with the use of these vaccines. For example, even now, IBV vaccines are compromised by the diversity and emergence of new serotypes (8). Similarly, genetic and antigenic variants of PRRSV arise rapidly, precluding the development of an effective vaccine for this nidovirus (34). In the case of EAV, both attenuated and killed virus vaccines are available and the live vaccines induce long-lasting protection against clinical disease. However, they do not prevent reinfection with wild-type virus, nor do they prevent temporary virus shedding, which perpetuates the circulation of virus in the field and the potential for the emergence of novel viruses (2).

Clearly, the advent of nidovirus reverse genetics holds out the promise of a new generation of recombinant viruses in which defined mutations can be engineered to produce vaccines with the optimal properties of attenuation, immunogenicity, and stability (18). However, even if the technology to produce recombinant viruses is available, our understanding of the immune responses to different nidovirus infections and the correlates of protective immunity remains rudimentary. The same is true of the relationship between viral virulence, tropism, and pathogenesis, and the emphasis in this area of nidovirus research now has to shift to the cellular biology and immunobiology of infection in animal models and in the natural host. These studies will be more challenging, and more expensive, than the study of virus replication in cell culture, but they are a necessity if we wish to address the present and future burden of nidovirus-associated disease.

### REFERENCES

1. **Almazan, F., J. M. Gonzalez, Z. Penzes, A. Izeta, E. Calvo, J. Plana-Duran, and L. Enjuanes.** 2000. Engineering the largest RNA virus genome as an infectious bacterial artificial chromosome. *Proc. Natl. Acad. Sci. USA* **97:**5516–5521.
2. **Balasuriya, U. B., and N. J. MacLachlan.** 2004. The immune response to equine arteritis virus: potential lessons for other arteriviruses. *Vet. Immunol. Immunopathol.* **102:**107–129.
3. **Barretto, N., D. Jukneliene, K. Ratia, Z. Chen, A. D. Mesecar, and S. C. Baker.** 2005. The papain-like protease of severe acute respiratory syndrome coronavirus has deubiquitinating activity. *J. Virol.* **79:**15189–15198.
4. **Bautista, E. M., P. Suarez, and T. W. Molitor.** 1999. T cell responses to the structural polypeptides of porcine reproductive and respiratory syndrome virus. *Arch. Virol.* **144:**117–134.

5. Beniac, D. R., A. Andonov, E. Grudeski, and T. F. Booth. 2006. Architecture of the SARS coronavirus prefusion spike. *Nat. Struct. Mol. Biol.* **13**:751–752.

6. Bosch, B. J., B. E. Martina, R. Van Der Zee, J. Lepault, B. J. Haijema, C. Versluis, A. J. Heck, A. D. Osterhaus, and P. J. Rottier. 2004. Severe acute respiratory syndrome coronavirus (SARS-CoV) infection inhibition using spike protein heptad repeat-derived peptides. *Proc. Natl. Acad. Sci. USA* **101**:8455–8460.

7. Castillo-Olivares, J., J. P. Tearle, F. Montesso, D. Westcott, J. H. Kydd, N. J. Davis-Poynter, and D. Hannant. 2003. Detection of equine arteritis virus (EAV)-specific cytotoxic CD8+ T lymphocyte precursors from EAV-infected ponies. *J. Gen. Virol.* **84**:2745–2753.

8. Cavanagh, D. 2003. Severe acute respiratory syndrome vaccine development: experiences of vaccination against avian infectious bronchitis coronavirus. *Avian Pathol.* **32**:567–582.

9. Cervantes-Barragan, L., R. Zust, F. Weber, M. Spiegel, K. S. Lang, S. Akira, V. Thiel, and B. Ludewig. 2007. Control of coronavirus infection through plasmacytoid dendritic-cell-derived type I interferon. *Blood* **109**:1131–1137.

10. de Groot-Mijnes, J. D., J. M. van Dun, R. G. van der Most, and R. J. de Groot. 2005. Natural history of a recurrent feline coronavirus infection and the role of cellular immunity in survival and disease. *J. Virol.* **79**:1036–1044.

11. Doan, D. N., and T. Dokland. 2003. Structure of the nucleocapsid protein of porcine reproductive and respiratory syndrome virus. *Structure* **11**:1445–1451.

12. Drosten, C., S. Gunther, W. Preiser, S. van der Werf, H. R. Brodt, S. Becker, H. Rabenau, M. Panning, L. Kolesnikova, R. A. Fouchier, A. Berger, A. M. Burguiere, J. Cinatl, M. Eickmann, N. Escriou, K. Grywna, S. Kramme, J. C. Manuguerra, S. Muller, V. Rickerts, M. Sturmer, S. Vieth, H. D. Klenk, A. D. Osterhaus, H. Schmitz, and H. W. Doerr. 2003. Identification of a novel coronavirus in patients with severe acute respiratory syndrome. *N. Engl. J. Med.* **348**:1967–1976.

13. Fan, H., A. Ooi, Y. W. Tan, S. Wang, S. Fang, D. X. Liu, and J. Lescar. 2005. The nucleocapsid protein of coronavirus infectious bronchitis virus: crystal structure of its N-terminal domain and multimerization properties. *Structure* **13**:1859–1868.

14. Fischer, F., D. Peng, S. T. Hingley, S. R. Weiss, and P. S. Masters. 1997. The internal open reading frame within the nucleocapsid gene of mouse hepatitis virus encodes a structural protein that is not essential for viral replication. *J. Virol.* **71**:996–1003.

15. Gorbalenya, A. E., L. Enjuanes, J. Ziebuhr, and E. J. Snijder. 2006. Nidovirales: evolving the largest RNA virus genome. *Virus Res.* **117**:17–37.

16. Gorbalenya, A. E., E. J. Snijder, and W. J. Spaan. 2004. Severe acute respiratory syndrome coronavirus phylogeny: toward consensus. *J. Virol.* **78**:7863–7866.

17. Granzow, H., F. Weiland, D. Fichtner, H. Schutze, A. Karger, E. Mundt, B. Dresenkamp, P. Martin, and T. C. Mettenleiter. 2001. Identification and ultrastructural characterization of a novel virus from fish. *J. Gen. Virol.* **82**:2849–2859.

18. Haijema, B. J., H. Volders, and P. J. Rottier. 2004. Live, attenuated coronavirus vaccines through the directed deletion of group-specific genes provide protection against feline infectious peritonitis. *J. Virol.* **78**:3863–3871.

19. Hakansson-McReynolds, S., S. Jiang, L. Rong, and M. Caffrey. 2006. Solution structure of the severe acute respiratory syndrome-coronavirus heptad repeat 2 domain in the prefusion state. *J. Biol. Chem.* **281**:11965–11971.

20. Huang, C., N. Ito, C. T. Tseng, and S. Makino. 2006. Severe acute respiratory syndrome coronavirus 7a accessory protein is a viral structural protein. *J. Virol.* **80**:7287–7294.

21. Hwang, W. C., Y. Lin, E. Santelli, J. Sui, L. Jaroszewski, B. Stec, M. Farzan, W. A. Marasco, and R. C. Liddington. 2006. Structural basis of neutralization by a human anti-severe acute respiratory syndrome spike protein antibody, 80R. *J. Biol. Chem.* **281**:34610–34616.

22. Ito, N., E. C. Mossel, K. Narayanan, V. L. Popov, C. Huang, T. Inoue, C. J. Peters, and S. Makino. 2005. Severe acute respiratory syndrome coronavirus 3a protein is a viral structural protein. *J. Virol.* **79**:3182–3186.

23. Jakob, H. 1914. Therapeutische, kasuistische und statistische Mitteilung aus der Klinik fuer kleine Haustiere an der Reichstierarzneischule in Utrecht (Holland). Jahrgang 1912/13. *Z. Tiermed.* **18**:193.

24. Jayaram, H., H. Fan, B. R. Bowman, A. Ooi, J. Jayaram, E. W. Collisson, J. Lescar, and B. V. Prasad. 2006. X-ray structures of the N- and C-terminal domains of a coronavirus nucleocapsid protein: implications for nucleocapsid formation. *J. Virol.* **80**:6612–6620.

25. Keffaber, K. K. 1989. Reproductive failure of unknown etiology. *Am. Assoc. Swine Pract. Newsl.* **1**:1–9.

26. Koetzner, C. A., M. M. Parker, C. S. Ricard, L. S. Sturman, and P. S. Masters. 1992. Repair and mutagenesis of the genome of a deletion mutant of the coronavirus mouse hepatitis virus by targeted RNA recombination. *J. Virol.* **66**:1841–1848.

27. Kopecky-Bromberg, S. A., L. Martinez-Sobrido, M. Frieman, R. A. Baric, and P. Palese. 2007. Severe acute respiratory syndrome coronavirus open reading frame (ORF) 3b, ORF 6, and nucleocapsid proteins function as interferon antagonists. *J. Virol.* **81**:548–557.

28. Ksiazek, T. G., D. Erdman, C. S. Goldsmith, S. R. Zaki, T. Peret, S. Emery, S. Tong, C. Urbani, J. A. Comer, W. Lim, P. E. Rollin, S. F. Dowell, A. E. Ling, C. D. Humphrey, W. J. Shieh, J. Guarner, C. D. Paddock, P. Rota, B. Fields, J. DeRisi, J. Y. Yang, N. Cox, J. M. Hughes, J. W. LeDuc, W. J. Bellini, and L. J. Anderson. 2003. A novel coronavirus associated with severe acute respiratory syndrome. *N. Engl. J. Med.* **348**:1953–1966.

29. Kuo, L., K. R. Hurst, and P. S. Masters. 2007. Exceptional flexibility in the sequence requirements for coronavirus small envelope protein function. *J. Virol.* **81**:2249–2262.

30. Kuo, L., and P. S. Masters. 2003. The small envelope protein E is not essential for murine coronavirus replication. *J. Virol.* **77**:4597–4608.

31. Lindner, H. A., N. Fotouhi-Ardakani, V. Lytvyn, P. Lachance, T. Sulea, and R. Menard. 2005. The papain-like protease from the severe acute respiratory syndrome coronavirus is a deubiquitinating enzyme. *J. Virol.* **79**:15199–15208.

32. Masters, P. S. 2006. The molecular biology of coronaviruses. *Adv. Virus Res.* **66**:193–292.

33. Menasveta, P. 1990. The present status of aquaculture in Thailand and the potential use of biotechnology to increase coastal aquaculture production. National Center for Genetic Engineering and Biotechnology, Ministry of Science, Technology and Environment, Bangkok, Thailand.

34. Meng, X. J. 2000. Heterogeneity of porcine reproductive and respiratory syndrome virus: implications for current vaccine efficacy and future vaccine development. *Vet. Microbiol.* **74**:309–329.

35. Meulenberg, J. J., J. N. Bos-de Ruijter, G. Wensvoort, and R. J. Moormann. 1998. An infectious cDNA clone of porcine reproductive and respiratory syndrome virus. *Adv. Exp. Med. Biol.* **440**:199–206.

36. Neuman, B. W., B. D. Adair, C. Yoshioka, J. D. Quispe, G. Orca, P. Kuhn, R. A. Milligan, M. Yeager, and M. J. Buchmeier.

2006. Supramolecular architecture of severe acute respiratory syndrome coronavirus revealed by electron cryomicroscopy. *J. Virol.* **80:**7918–7928.

37. **Pasternak, A. O., W. J. Spaan, and E. J. Snijder.** 2006. Nidovirus transcription: how to make sense...? *J. Gen. Virol.* **87:**1403–1421.

38. **Pedersen, K. W., Y. van der Meer, N. Roos, and E. J. Snijder.** 1999. Open reading frame 1a-encoded subunits of the arterivirus replicase induce endoplasmic reticulum-derived double-membrane vesicles which carry the viral replication complex. *J. Virol.* **73:**2016–2026.

39. **Peiris, J. S., S. T. Lai, L. L. Poon, Y. Guan, L. Y. Yam, W. Lim, J. Nicholls, W. K. Yee, W. W. Yan, M. T. Cheung, V. C. Cheng, K. H. Chan, D. N. Tsang, R. W. Yung, T. K. Ng, and K. Y. Yuen.** 2003. Coronavirus as a possible cause of severe acute respiratory syndrome. *Lancet* **361:**1319–1325.

40. **Prentice, E., W. G. Jerome, T. Yoshimori, N. Mizushima, and M. R. Denison.** 2004. Coronavirus replication complex formation utilizes components of cellular autophagy. *J. Biol. Chem.* **279:**10136–10141.

41. **Sawicki, S. G., D. L. Sawicki, and S. G. Siddell.** 2007. A contemporary view of coronavirus transcription. *J. Virol.* **81:**20–29.

42. **Sawicki, S. G., D. L. Sawicki, D. Younker, Y. Meyer, V. Thiel, H. Stokes, and S. G. Siddell.** 2005. Functional and genetic analysis of coronavirus replicase-transcriptase proteins. *PLoS Pathog.* **1:**e39.

43. **Schalk, A. F., and M. C. Hawn.** 1931. An apparently new disease of chicks. *J. Am. Vet. Med. Assoc.* **78:**413–422.

44. **Schutze, H., R. Ulferts, B. Schelle, S. Bayer, H. Granzow, B. Hoffmann, T. C. Mettenleiter, and J. Ziebuhr.** 2006. Characterization of white bream virus reveals a novel genetic cluster of nidoviruses. *J. Virol.* **80:**11598–11609.

44a. **Snijder, E. J., S. G. Siddell, and A. E. Gorbalenya.** 2005. The order *Nidovirales*, p. 390–404. *In* B. W. J. Mahy and V. ter Meulen (ed.), *Topley & Wilson's Microbiology and Microbial Infections*, 10th ed., vol. 1. *Virology.* Hodder Arnold, London, United Kingdom.

45. **Snijder, E. J., Y. van der Meer, J. Zevenhoven-Dobbe, J. J. Onderwater, J. van der Meulen, H. K. Koerten, and A. M. Mommaas.** 2006. Ultrastructure and origin of membrane vesicles associated with the severe acute respiratory syndrome coronavirus replication complex. *J. Virol.* **80:**5927–5940.

46. **Stertz, S., M. Reichelt, M. Spiegel, T. Kuri, L. Martinez-Sobrido, A. Garcia-Sastre, F. Weber, and G. Kochs.** 2007. The intracellular sites of early replication and budding of SARS-coronavirus. *Virology* **361:**304–315.

47. **Supekar, V. M., C. Bruckmann, P. Ingallinella, E. Bianchi, A. Pessi, and A. Carfi.** 2004. Structure of a proteolytically resistant core from the severe acute respiratory syndrome coronavirus S2 fusion protein. *Proc. Natl. Acad. Sci. USA* **101:**17958–17963.

48. **Thiel, V., J. Herold, B. Schelle, and S. G. Siddell.** 2001. Infectious RNA transcribed in vitro from a cDNA copy of the human coronavirus genome cloned in vaccinia virus. *J. Gen. Virol.* **82:**1273–1281.

49. **Tsao, Y. P., J. Y. Lin, J. T. Jan, C. H. Leng, C. C. Chu, Y. C. Yang, and S. L. Chen.** 2006. HLA-A*0201 T-cell epitopes in severe acute respiratory syndrome (SARS) coronavirus nucleocapsid and spike proteins. *Biochem. Biophys. Res. Commun.* **344:**63–71.

50. **van Dinten, L. C., J. A. den Boon, A. L. Wassenaar, W. J. Spaan, and E. J. Snijder.** 1997. An infectious arterivirus cDNA clone: identification of a replicase point mutation that abolishes discontinuous mRNA transcription. *Proc. Natl. Acad. Sci. USA* **94:**991–996.

51. **Wensvoort, G., C. Terpstra, J. M. Pol, E. A. ter Laak, M. Bloemraad, E. P. de Kluyver, C. Kragten, L. van Buiten, A. den Besten, F. Wagenaar, et al.** 1991. Mystery swine disease in The Netherlands: the isolation of Lelystad virus. *Vet. Q.* **13:**121–130.

52. **Wieringa, R., A. A. de Vries, J. van der Meulen, G. J. Godeke, J. J. Onderwater, H. van Tol, H. K. Koerten, A. M. Mommaas, E. J. Snijder, and P. J. Rottier.** 2004. Structural protein requirements in equine arteritis virus assembly. *J. Virol.* **78:**13019–13027.

53. **Wissink, E. H., M. V. Kroese, H. A. van Wijk, F. A. Rijsewijk, J. J. Meulenberg, and P. J. Rottier.** 2005. Envelope protein requirements for the assembly of infectious virions of porcine reproductive and respiratory syndrome virus. *J. Virol.* **79:**12495–12506.

54. **Xu, Y., Y. Liu, Z. Lou, L. Qin, X. Li, Z. Bai, H. Pang, P. Tien, G. F. Gao, and Z. Rao.** 2004. Structural basis for coronavirus-mediated membrane fusion. Crystal structure of mouse hepatitis virus spike protein fusion core. *J. Biol. Chem.* **279:**30514–30522.

55. **Xu, Y., Z. Lou, Y. Liu, H. Pang, P. Tien, G. F. Gao, and Z. Rao.** 2004. Crystal structure of severe acute respiratory syndrome coronavirus spike protein fusion core. *J. Biol. Chem.* **279:**49414–49419.

56. **Yang, H., W. Xie, X. Xue, K. Yang, J. Ma, W. Liang, Q. Zhao, Z. Zhou, D. Pei, J. Ziebuhr, R. Hilgenfeld, K. Y. Yuen, L. Wong, G. Gao, S. Chen, Z. Chen, D. Ma, M. Bartlam, and Z. Rao.** 2005. Design of wide-spectrum inhibitors targeting coronavirus main proteases. *PLoS Biol.* **3:**e324.

57. **Ye, Y., K. Hauns, J. O. Langland, B. L. Jacobs, and B. G. Hogue.** 2007. Mouse hepatitis coronavirus A59 nucleocapsid protein is a type I interferon antagonist. *J. Virol.* **81:**2554–2563.

58. **Yount, B., M. R. Denison, S. R. Weiss, and R. S. Baric.** 2002. Systematic assembly of a full-length infectious cDNA of mouse hepatitis virus strain A59. *J. Virol.* **76:**11065–11078.

59. **Yount, B., R. S. Roberts, A. C. Sims, D. Deming, M. B. Frieman, J. Sparks, M. R. Denison, N. Davis, and R. S. Baric.** 2005. Severe acute respiratory syndrome coronavirus group-specific open reading frames encode nonessential functions for replication in cell cultures and mice. *J. Virol.* **79:**14909–14922.

60. **Yu, I. M., M. L. Oldham, J. Zhang, and J. Chen.** 2006. Crystal structure of the severe acute respiratory syndrome (SARS) coronavirus nucleocapsid protein dimerization domain reveals evolutionary linkage between corona- and arteriviridae. *J. Biol. Chem.* **281:**17134–17139.

61. **Zhou, M., D. Xu, X. Li, H. Li, M. Shan, J. Tang, M. Wang, F. S. Wang, X. Zhu, H. Tao, W. He, P. Tien, and G. F. Gao.** 2006. Screening and identification of severe acute respiratory syndrome-associated coronavirus-specific CTL epitopes. *J. Immunol.* **177:**2138–2145.

62. **Ziegler, T., S. Matikainen, E. Ronkko, P. Osterlund, M. Sillanpaa, J. Siren, R. Fagerlund, M. Immonen, K. Melen, and I. Julkunen.** 2005. Severe acute respiratory syndrome coronavirus fails to activate cytokine-mediated innate immune responses in cultured human monocyte-derived dendritic cells. *J. Virol.* **79:**13800–13805.

*Nidoviruses*
Edited by S. Perlman, T. Gallagher, and E. J. Snijder
© 2008 ASM Press, Washington, DC

Chapter 2

# Genomics and Evolution of the *Nidovirales*

ALEXANDER E. GORBALENYA

## NIDOVIRUSES AS A DISTINCT GROUP OF ssRNA+ VIRUSES

With genome sizes of 26 to 32 kb, coronaviruses, toroviruses, and roniviruses are found at the upper end of the genome size scale of viruses with single-stranded genomes of positive (mRNA) polarity (ssRNA+) (Fig. 1). Together with their much smaller arterivirus cousins (genome size of "only" 13 to 16 kb) they form a phylogenetically compact but diverse cluster with the taxonomic rank of order called *Nidovirales* (11, 20, 83, 87). The International Committee on Taxonomy of Viruses (27) recognized roniviruses (104) and arteriviruses (81) as distinct families, while the current taxonomic position of coronaviruses and toroviruses as two genera of the *Coronaviridae* family is being revised by elevating these virus groups to a higher taxonomic rank, that of either subfamily or family (30, 86). The order may include another high-rank group, provisionally called bafiniviruses, that is linked to toroviruses (74). Hereafter, I refer to coronaviruses, toroviruses, and roniviruses as "large" nidoviruses and to arteriviruses as "small" nidoviruses (32) to stress the clear genome size difference.

Nidovirus genomes contain a 5′ cap structure and a 3′ poly(A) tail. The genomes of nidoviruses include untranslated regions at their 5′ and 3′ genome termini. These flank an array of multiple genes whose number may vary in and among the families of the order *Nidovirales*. Roniviruses have only 4 ORFs, a bafinivirus has 5 ORFs, toroviruses have 6 ORFs, arteriviruses may have between 9 and 12 ORFs, and coronaviruses may contain 9 to 14 ORFs. In all nidoviruses, the two most 5′ and largest ORFs, ORF1a and ORF1b, occupy between two-thirds and three-quarters of the genome. They overlap in a small area containing a −1 ribosomal frameshift signal that directs translation of ORF1b by a fraction of ribosomes that have started protein synthesis at the ORF1a initiator AUG (for more details, see chapter 3). These two ORFs encode the subunits of the replicase machinery, which are produced by autoproteolytic processing of polyproteins 1a and 1ab, encoded by ORF1a and ORF1ab, respectively. The majority of the autoproteolytic reactions is mediated by a chymotrypsin-like protease (3CL$^{pro}$, main protease), and RNA synthesis is mediated by a poorly characterized replication complex including the cognate RNA-dependent RNA polymerase (RdRp) (77, 83) (see chapters 5 to 7 for more details).

The ORFs located downstream of ORF1b encode nucleocapsid and envelope protein(s), the numbers of which differ among the major nidovirus branches but which always include a major surface glycoprotein called S protein in coronaviruses. Family- and group-specific ORFs in this region may encode additional virion and nonstructural ("accessory") proteins. These ORFs located in the 3′ part of the genome are expressed from a nested set of subgenomic RNAs (sgRNAs), a property that was reflected in the name of the virus order (*nidus* in Latin means nest) (11). In the genomes of large nidoviruses, compared to small nidoviruses, both the region occupied by the replicase ORFs and that occupied by the 3′-proximal ORFs have been expanded proportionally.

In this chapter, I briefly overview some of the recent advancements and challenges in nidovirus research concerning the genetic diversity of nidoviruses and selected aspects of nidovirus classification and evolution. Although being nidovirus-wide in scope, most of the discussion concerns coronaviruses, which have been characterized most extensively. This chapter has benefited from a recently published review (32) to which the reader is referred, especially for details concerning protein domains and the

**Alexander E. Gorbalenya** • Molecular Virology Laboratory, Department of Medical Microbiology, Leiden University Medical Center, P.O. Box 9600, 2300 RC Leiden, The Netherlands.

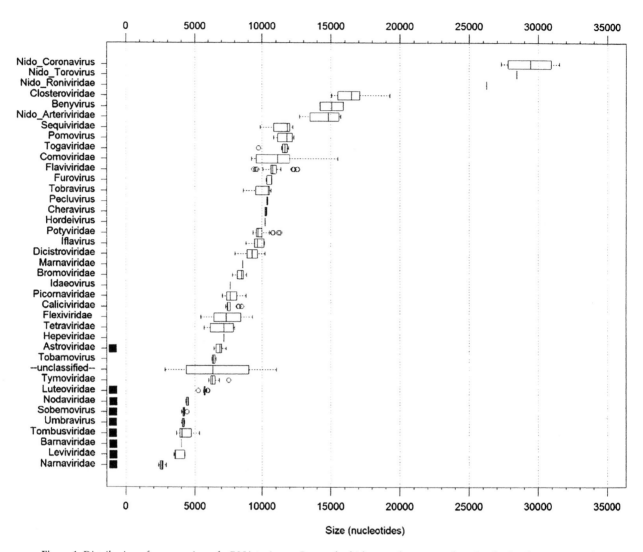

**Figure 1.** Distribution of genome sizes of ssRNA+ viruses. Box-and-whisker graphs were used to plot the family/group-specific distribution of genome sizes of all ssRNA+ viruses whose genome sequences have been placed in the NCBI Viral Genome Resource (2) by 7 December 2005 (J. Faase and A. E. Gorbalenya, unpublished data). The four major groups of nidoviruses are highlighted with the Nido- prefix, and the family *Coronaviridae* is split into the Nido-Coronavirus and Nido-Torovirus groups. The box spans from the first to the third quartiles and includes the median, indicated by the bold line. The whiskers extend to the extreme values that are distant from the box at most 1.5 times the interquartile range. Values beyond this distance are indicated by circles (outliers). Viruses that do not encode a helicase are indicated by black squares. Adapted from reference 32.

molecular biology of nidoviruses. Comparative genomics of nidoviruses and relationships of nidoviruses with cellular and other viral systems were previously reviewed in reference 31.

## NIDOVIRUS GENOME DIVERSITY AND PHYLOGENY

The first nidovirus genome completely sequenced was that of the coronavirus avian infectious bronchitis virus (IBV) in 1987 (6). When the genome sequence of equine arteritis virus, the arterivirus prototype,

was published 4 years later (19), it led to the realization that coronaviruses and arteriviruses must be united into a single higher ranking taxon, known now as *Nidovirales*. Instrumental in this advancement and the subsequent exploration of the nidovirus genomic space was the use of bioinformatics methods for comparative genome analysis that, particularly, unraveled the nidovirus-characteristic domain organization of the replicase polyproteins, drafted first for IBV (33).

Twenty years after publication of the first complete nidovirus genome sequence, public databases include almost 200 full-length and over 1,000 partial nidovirus genome sequences. The most extensive sequencing effort started very recently, after the 2003 severe acute respiratory syndrome coronavirus (SARS-CoV) outbreak (62, 71). Since then, our knowledge about nidovirus genome diversity, although it remains biased, has expanded roughly twice. The majority of genome sequences have been reported for mammalian coronaviruses, with arteriviruses being a distant second group. Among the recently completed coronavirus genome sequences are those of viruses that have been known for a long time, like feline coronavirus (FCoV) (25), human coronavirus OC43 (HCoV-OC43) (91, 102) and porcine hemagglutinating encephalomyelitis virus (PHEV) (100), as well as newly identified coronaviruses, including HCoV-NL63 (28, 99) and HCoV-HKU1 (107), and numerous coronaviruses that infect a wide range of species belonging to three bat families (see below). All these viruses belong to groups 1 and 2 (Fig. 2; see below), which each include more than a dozen known virus species with a completely sequenced genome. In contrast, IBV has remained the single group 3 species with a fully sequenced genome, although other coronavirus species appear to infect turkeys and wild birds, according to analyses of partial genome sequences of these viruses (50, 58).

The available information on the genetic variability of other nidovirus taxa is extremely limited, but it is critical, as it provides a window on the grand scale of nidovirus and host diversity. Only the genomes of prototype viruses, respectively, gill-associated virus (16) and white bream virus (WBV) (74), have been fully sequenced for the invertebrate roniviruses (104) and the bafiniviruses (74), which infect fish; the latter group remains to be formally recognized by the International Committee on Taxonomy of Viruses. The much more extensively studied mammalian toroviruses include two closely related viruses, equine torovirus and bovine torovirus, with fully sequenced genomes (24, 79).

Phylogenetically, the nidoviruses identified thus far form a large domain in the RNA virus tree with four profoundly separated and unevenly populated clusters: corona-, toro-, roni-, and arteriviruses (Fig. 2) (35). The evolutionary relationships among these clusters have been only partially resolved (30, 32). Toroviruses and the most recently identified WBV appear to have originated from an immediate common ancestor and split early in evolution (74). Numerous analyses involving the most conserved proteins and complete genomes strongly indicate that among the four nidovirus clusters, coronaviruses and toroviruses/WBV must have a monophyletic origin (7, 15, 19, 24, 31, 33, 35, 80) (Fig. 2).

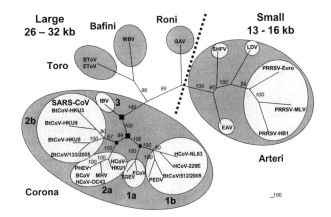

**Figure 2.** *Nidovirales* phylogeny. A tree depicting the evolutionary relationships between the five major groups of nidoviruses (coronaviruses, toroviruses, bafiniviruses, roniviruses, and arteriviruses) is shown. The dotted line separates large and small nidoviruses as defined in the text. This unrooted maximum parsimonious tree was inferred by using multiple nucleotide alignments of the RdRp-HEL region of a representative set of nidoviruses with the help of the PAUP* v.4.0b10 software (92a; A. E. Gorbalenya, unpublished data). Support for all bifurcations from 100 bootstraps is indicated. The coronaviruses analyzed were HCoV-229E, -HKU1, -OC43, and -NL63; transmissible gastroenteritis virus (TGEV); feline coronavirus (FCoV); porcine epidemic diarrhea virus (PEDV); mouse hepatitis virus (MHV); bovine coronavirus (BCoV); bat coronaviruses (BtCoV) HKU3, HKU5, HKU9, 133, and 512 (the last two isolated in 2005); PHEV; IBV; and SARS-CoV. The toroviruses analyzed were equine torovirus (EToV) and bovine torovirus (BToV). The bafinivirus analyzed was WBV. The arteriviruses analyzed were equine arteritis virus (EAV); simian hemorrhagic fever virus (SHFV); lactate dehydrogenase-elevating virus (LDV); and three porcine reproductive and respiratory syndrome viruses (PRRSV), Euro, HB1, and MLV. The ronivirus analyzed was gill-associated virus (GAV). SARS-CoV is highlighted with larger type than the other viruses. Due to the very large scale of the tree, three pairs of nodes formed by very closely related viruses (SARS-CoV and BtCoV-HKU3, BCoV and HCoV-OC43, and BToV and EToV) were collapsed. For coronaviruses, major groups and subgroups are highlighted and labeled (36); internal nodes defining group and subgroup bifurcations are indicated with black squares and circles, respectively. Subgroup 2b viruses may have been classified differently by other researchers (see the text and references 95, 108, and 110). For arteriviruses, four major clusters, prototyped by EAV, SHFV, LDV, and PRRSV, are highlighted.

In contrast, the relative phylogenetic position of arteriviruses and roniviruses is yet to be defined. Based on a comparison of replicase polyproteins, it was argued that roniviruses may group with coronaviruses and toroviruses/WBV to form a supercluster of nidoviruses with relatively large genomes (>26 kb; large nidoviruses), with the smaller arteriviruses being the first to split from the nidovirus trunk (32). Although this clustering is yet to be rigorously verified, in this review I consider the large and small nidoviruses as two separate phylogenetic clusters.

## CORONAVIRUS GROUPS

Comparative sequence analysis and other studies revealed three major genetic groups in coronaviruses, called groups 1, 2, and 3, and four comparably distant genetic clusters in arteriviruses (Fig. 2) (30, 36, 81, 86). It is apparent from these and other analyses that different regions of the genome coevolve, although likely at their own pace. Practically, it means that phylogenetic analysis of any sufficiently long region of genome produces essentially the same tree topology that may differ, due to homologous recombination, only in the branching of the most closely related viruses (see below). Obviously, not all regions of the nidovirus genome are equally qualified for being proper to be used in this type of analysis. Particularly, analysis of any accessory gene may be insightful only for the lineage that employs this gene. Because of a restricted phyletic distribution, some accessory genes were (and still are [for example, see reference 95]) considered to be group specific. However, with the steady expansion of our knowledge about the genome diversity among viruses of groups 1 and 2 over the last few years, this perception needs to be revised (36). It is now emerging that many of the known accessory genes are specific for either virus species or clusters that are (much) smaller than group lineages and, because of this, they may not serve as reliable group markers (32). In contrast, the replicase nsp1 gene was recognized recently to be an excellent genetic and evolutionary marker for coronavirus groups (36).

Since the three genetic clusters of coronaviruses were originally recognized as antigenic groups (76), some confusion seems to persist about the biological implications of placing a coronavirus into a (phylo)-genetic group (36). Only a few coronaviruses have been extensively characterized regarding antigenic cross-reactivity. When these data are analyzed in a phylogenetic context, it is apparent that each genetic cluster of coronaviruses may include more than one antigenic group, each likely forming a compact sub-cluster (30). To bridge the antigenic and (phylo)genetic classifications and to more precisely describe the position of coronaviruses in a constantly growing family, it was proposed to split groups into subgroups (Fig. 2). Thus, group 1 was the first to be split into subgroups, with subgroup 1a containing FCoV and porcine transmissible gastroenteritis virus and subgroup 1b containing HCoV-229E and porcine epidemic diarrhea virus (30); subsequently, SARS-CoV was proposed to be the prototype of subgroup 2b, with mouse hepatitis virus (MHV), bovine coronavirus (BCoV), and HCoV-OC43 being subgroup 2a viruses (80).

Unfortunately, rules governing criteria for demarcation between groups and subgroups have not been explicitly defined, partially due to the current informal status of the group classification. As a result, when a new relatively distant coronavirus is identified, it is left up to the individual researcher to decide what this new virus must prototype—a group or a subgroup. This uncertainty was one of major elements that effectively divided the coronavirus research community about the classification of SARS-CoV, which was distantly related to all coronaviruses known at the time: whether it should be the founding member of either subgroup 2b or group 4 (36). The recent explosion in the number of available coronavirus genome sequences, owing mostly to the identification (66) and further characterization (14, 55, 57, 69, 95, 108, 110) of the genetic diversity of bat coronaviruses, spectacularly revealed that the problem is not limited to the classification of a single virus. As of January 2007, genome sequences for more than 20 bat coronaviruses have been reported by three groups of researchers who adopted different criteria to classify these viruses. It is apparent from these publications that the currently known bat coronaviruses may form up to 10 species (and possibly more), some of which are profoundly separated from previously established coronaviruses. One team proposed to accommodate these viruses in four groups: the originally established groups 1 and 2, a fourth group prototyped by SARS-CoV, and a new fifth group (95). Another team placed the bat viruses in subgroups 1b and 2b and two new subgroups, 2c and 2d, the latter including a bat virus not described by others (108, 110). As before with SARS-CoV, it is obvious that the lack of a consensus on coronavirus classification hampers the exchange and dissemination of knowledge, and complicates the progress of fundamental and applied coronavirus research.

In this respect, rooted phylogenetic trees of coronaviruses may provide guidance, if not criteria, on how to demarcate groups and subgroups. According to my analysis, the group 3 lineage split off the coronavirus trunk before the bifurcation of groups 1 and 2 (80). This last bifurcation could be chosen as the defining boundary for viruses monophyletic with the founding viruses of either group 1 or 2. With this criterion, previously applied to SARS-CoV, all described bat coronaviruses must be recognized as belonging to either group 1 or 2 (Fig. 2). A similar logic could be applied to define subgroups, although a reasonable lower limit for subgroup divergence must also be observed. (Another common approach is to analyze pairwise virus distances [30]).

Consequently, to be recognized as belonging to a new group, a coronavirus must split off from the coronavirus tree *before* the group 1 and 2 bifurcation or be close to the group 3 root if the virus in question is monophyletic with group 3 viruses (Fig. 2). Interestingly, such a coronavirus may have indeed been identified. The sequence of the most conserved 66 amino acids of the RdRp domain of a coronavirus isolated from green-cheeked Amazon parrots was shown to be equidistant to those of other coronaviruses representing three established groups (37). Sequencing of the genome of this remarkable coronavirus is anticipated to resolve its phylogenetic position with great confidence.

## MECHANISMS OF EVOLUTION

As in other organisms, two evolutionary mechanisms—mutation and recombination—have been implicated in the generation of nidovirus genome diversity and the maintenance of genome stability. Both processes are believed to be replication mediated. Mutations are fixed as a result of neutral, positive, and negative (purifying) selection. It was argued that recombination could be effective in removing deleterious mutations and promoting advantageous mutations (12, 111). Also, major innovations introduced in the genome must have been accomplished using recombination. My colleagues and I also proposed that large nidoviruses may have uniquely evolved an oligonucleotide-directed *repair* mechanism(s) involving the diverse virus-encoded RNA-processing enzymes to improve the fidelity of RNA copying critical for the maintenance of their big genomes (32). Based on a homology-based parallel with two cellular intron-processing pathways, it was suggested that in large nidoviruses the genetically segregated and down-regulated superfamily 1 helicase (HEL1) (75), exonuclease (ExoN) (63), endonuclease (NendoU) (5, 46), and putative methyltransferase (O-MT) domains may provide RNA specificity, whereas the relatively abundant ADP-ribose 1″-phosphatase (ADRP) (67) and putative cyclic phosphodiesterase (CPD), when available, may modulate the pace of a reaction in a common pathway (80) (Fig. 3). This pathway could be part of the oligonucleotide-directed repair mechanism.

## MUTATION

Early studies of coronaviruses (73) and arteriviruses (47) estimated the mutation rate to be $10^{-3}$ to $10^{-4}$ substitutions per site per year, the range that is typical for other RNA viruses, with (much) smaller genomes, whose replicase fidelity is known to be low (10, 22, 23). Most recently, these numbers were

confirmed for SARS-CoV (72, 103, 114), HCoV-OC43 (101–103), PHEV (100), and HCoV-NL63 (68). Using this rate and a (relaxed) molecular clock model, Vijgen et al. estimated the time of the most recent common ancestors of BCoV and HCoV-OC43 and of PHEV, BCoV, and HCoV-OC43 to be in the late 19th century and not earlier than in the middle of the 16th century, respectively (100, 102). Under a strict molecular clock model, the time of the most recent common ancestors of HCoV-229E and HCoV-NL63 was estimated to be in the 11th century (68).

However, and in contrast to the numbers cited above, it was also reported that SARS-CoV may have evolved with a lower mutation rate, approximating 0.1 replacement per genome per replication (112), and an unusually high genome stability was claimed for an isolate of HCoV-OC43 (90) (however, see reference 103), corresponding to a mutation rate of $5.7 \times 10^{-6}$ substitutions per site per year (103). Also, an extensive heterogeneity in the mutation rate among sites was reported for SARS-CoV (72). Besides these reports, a general concern was raised that variations in the mutation rate might be greatly underestimated and the employed evolutionary models might be not adequate since the virus sampling currently available for analysis is limited to the most recent decades and our understanding of the mechanisms governing RNA virus evolution is rather poor (44). Thus, the reliability of the time estimates for the emergence of diverse coronaviruses is likely to deteriorate proportionally with the time difference separating contemporary viruses from the ancestral event.

It is common that the number of synonymous substitutions per synonymous site (dS) exceeds the number of nonsynonymous ones (dN), and an especially high and poorly understood dS/dN ratio was reported for the S protein gene of PHEV (100). Nonsynonymous substitutions are also accepted at an uneven rate across the nidovirus genome, with the structural protein genes, especially those encoding envelope glycoproteins, and the 5′-proximal half of ORF1a evolving relatively fast and the ORF1b-encoded replicase enzymes evolving relatively slowly (13, 56, 65, 101). The observed differences must be linked to the roles played by the respective products of these genome regions in the nidovirus life cycle.

In the most conserved parts of the genome, nonsynonymous substitutions start to accumulate significantly only between the major nidovirus groups separated by relatively large evolutionary distances. In these viruses, replacements have sometimes been accepted at places of extraordinary conservation, e.g., in the active site of the 3CL^pro, which are not known to have been mutated in their DNA-encoded homologs

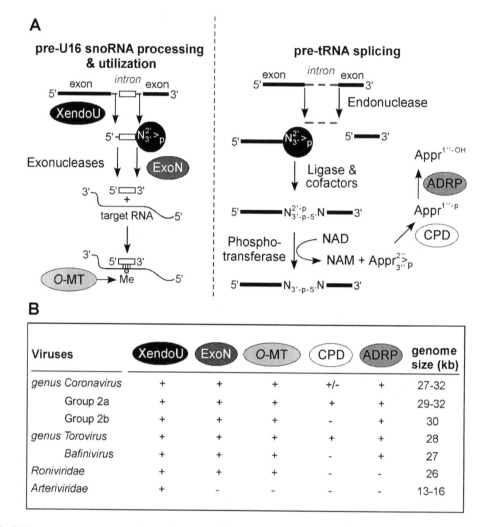

**Figure 3.** RNA-processing enzymes of nidoviruses: possible cooperation and virus distribution. (A) Cellular pathways for processing of pre-U16 small nucleolar RNA (snoRNA) and pre-tRNA splicing in which homologs of five nidovirus RNA-processing enzymes are involved. Note that both pathways produce intermediates with the 2′-3′-cyclic phosphate termini (black circles), indicating the structural basis for possible cooperation of the nidovirus homologs in a single pathway (80). XendoU is a cellular homolog of NendoU discussed with other enzymes in the text. (B) Table summarizing the conservation of five (putative) RNA-processing enzymes among representatives of large and small nidoviruses. This figure, updated from reference 32, is based on Fig. 5 in reference 80.

(74, 79, 84, 115). Although little is known about the absolute time scale of nidovirus evolution, it could have taken many millions of years to generate the diversity observed in the most conserved enzymes (51).

## RECOMBINATION

Recombination can be either homologous or heterologous. There is plenty of evidence for recombination between nidoviruses, especially corona- (41, 61) and toroviruses (78), either in the field or in experimental settings (for reviews, see references 8 and 54). This recombination commonly involves closely related viruses, either isolates of the same species or members of the same group of coronaviruses, and is believed to be mediated by replicase-driven template switching in a homologous genome region (homologous recombination) during genome replication. Its frequency may even approach 25% for the entire MHV genome (3). As a result, chimeric progeny genomes are produced with a collinear mosaic relationship to their parental templates.

The incongruency of trees inferred for different genome regions serves as a strong indicator of possible recombination and may in fact be the only evidence for recombination, unless parents are known or can otherwise be tracked. Commonly, the analyses of field isolates that invoke recombination are limited to several regions of the genome, in the replicase

ORF1ab and downstream of ORF1b (41). Therefore, a recent analysis using the complete genome sequences of 22 HCoV-HKU1 isolates obtained from March 2003 to February 2005 was unusually insightful as it allowed, for the first time, mapping of recombination sites in the entire genome (109). Using phylogenetic analysis, three genetic clusters (A to C) were identified in HCoV-HKU1. Although only two out of three clusters may represent genotypes (Gorbalenya, unpublished), the presented evidence for recombination is compelling and recombination was found to occur unevenly across the genome. Using bootscan analysis, the most plausible recombination points were identified in the nsp6–7 and nsp16-hemagglutinin-esterase (nsp16-HE) regions. Also, there may be numerous recombination crossover sites upstream of the nsp6-coding region; recombination seems to have erased differences between genotypes in this large and relatively fast-evolving region. Thus, the major crossover sites separate three major genome regions, ORF1a, ORF1b, and the region including ORFs expressed from sgRNAs. Since other recombination points have been identified in studies of other coronaviruses (41, 68), it would be interesting to see an extension of this genome-wide analysis to a larger HCoV-HKU1 data set and to other coronaviruses.

Among the known coronaviruses, the feline infectious peritonitis virus KU-2 strain, an isolate of FCoV, may have originated by homologous recombination between a pair of coronaviruses that have diverged most profoundly while belonging to the same group, subgroup 1a (64). It would be insightful to sequence the genomes of this virus and its parents. Most recently, homologous recombination between coronaviruses that belong to different groups was proposed to be involved in the origin of SARS-CoV (70, 88, 89). These analyses found incongruencies between phylogenetic trees generated for different regions of the replicase gene, most reproducibly between different parts of the RdRp domain. However, when these tree deviations were independently evaluated using a likelihood ratio test, a common statistical test, they were found to be not significant (44). An uneven site-specific mutation rate for coronaviruses belonging to different groups and/or recombination between coronavirus group ancestors before they diverged considerably might have left footprints in sequences of contemporary coronaviruses that can mislead when analyzing a highly biased data set, including deeply rooted and poorly sampled lineages like SARS-CoV at the time (44, 60). Another source of potentially significant complications in some of the conducted studies was the nonoptimal selection of outgroup viruses, e.g., arteriviruses and roniviruses in

the case of SARS-CoV, whose sequences may not be aligned with coronaviruses as well as those of toroviruses.

It was also due to the prior identification in the 3′ end of the SARS-CoV genome (52, 62, 105) of a group 3-specific RNA element, known as s2m (49, 50), that the involvement of intergroup recombination in the origin of SARS-CoV seemed a plausible idea. When the likelihood of this hypothesis is assessed, it is important to take into account that constraints governing the evolution of the genomic 3′-proximal region and replicase ORF1b appear to be different: coronaviruses easily tolerate many artificial and natural innovations in the former region (see, for example, references 39, 59, and 113), but the latter region has a uniform domain organization and is most strongly conserved (86). Thus, what is true for evolution of the s2m region may not be applicable to evolution of the ORF1b-encoded replicase region. Furthermore, although the observed phyletic distribution of s2m in coronaviruses would indeed be compatible with the involvement of intergroup recombination, no firm evidence to support this mechanism has been presented and other mechanisms, such as selective loss of the s2m element in other coronavirus lineages or recombination between a coronavirus and another ssRNA+ virus, remain plausible (49). Thus, none of the claims for intergroup homologous recombination among coronaviruses has been rigorously validated, regardless of the observed high frequency of intragroup homologous recombination. This experience calls for caution in interpreting phylogenetic analyses, especially those involving distant and lonely coronavirus lineages.

An aberrant variant of homologous recombination (53) may have also been involved in the expansion and shrinking of the nidovirus genome. Arteri- and coronaviruses have multiple (possibly up to four) copies of a papain-like protease (papain-like cysteine protease and papain-like protease [PL$^{pro}$], respectively) (18, 34, 117), which are likely to have arisen from duplication of a locus (see also chapters 5 and 6). Coronaviruses of group 1 and subgroup 2a have two PL$^{pro}$s, while those of subgroup 2b and group 3 encode one PL$^{pro}$ that is orthologous to PL2$^{pro}$ (80, 117). This pattern may have evolved by either independent duplication or loss of PL$^{pro}$ domains (117). Also, PL$^{pro}$ duplications may have occurred independently in arteri- and coronaviruses, since the PL$^{pro}$s of these two nidovirus branches do not seem to interleave with each other (116, 117). Duplications were also documented in a region immediately upstream of PL1$^{pro}$ in HCoV-HKU1 (107) and in the 3′-proximal region of the arterivirus simian hemorrhagic fever virus (29). Also, coronavirus nsp8 and nsp9 were proposed to have originated from ancient duplications of the catalytic domains of RdRp (45) and 3CL^{pro} (92), respectively, accompanied by subsequent extensive divergence and change of functions. PL^{pro} domains may also have been used as building blocks to develop new functional domains (98), which would explain the relative abundance of these domains in the nidoviruses.

Heterologous recombination, directed by template switching in nonhomologous regions, might have promoted the relocation of the CPD and HE genes in an ancestor of either toroviruses or group 2a coronaviruses. Under the alternative scenario, the CPD and HE genes must have been acquired independently by these ancestors from other viruses or the host (82). Heterologous RNA recombination may have generated the diverse gross changes in the nidovirus genome accounting for differences between large and small nidoviruses, and the major lineages of large nidoviruses. Almost nothing is known about the parameters of heterologous recombination in nidoviruses, including the origin of parental (donor) sequences which must account for (a part of) the replicase domains. This complete lack of information on the origin of specific sequences extends from the accessory protein genes in the 3′ part of the coronavirus genome to the nonessential, lineage-specific replicative domains and also includes the essential ExoN and putative methyltransferase domains that are specific for large nidoviruses.

## COEVOLUTION OF VIRUS AND HOST

Phylogenetic analysis of coronaviruses provides ample evidence for the lack of coronavirus-host cospeciation, an observation that may not yet have been corroborated for other nidoviruses, due to a less extensive virus sampling. Particularly, the four human coronaviruses, HCoV-229E, -OC43, -NL63, and -HKU1, do not form a compact genetic group but rather interleave with coronaviruses of two major genetic lineages, 1a and 2a, infecting other hosts (99, 102, 107). Likewise, four pairs of coronaviruses infecting either dogs or one of three bat species (Chinese horseshoe bats, Leschenault's rousette bats, and greater horseshoe bats) are considerably separated in the coronavirus tree and intertwine with coronaviruses infecting other hosts (26, 95, 108). This phylogenetic pattern is highly suggestive for (some of) these viruses having originated from other coronaviruses crossing a species barrier. Indeed, HCoV-OC43 may have emerged from BCoV adapted to humans approximately 100 years ago (102), and these viruses seem to have retained the ability to infect the other

host. Also, variants of the same coronavirus were isolated from different bat species, indicating a high likelihood of crossing the host species barrier in their recent evolution (95, 108). It is noteworthy that SARS-CoVs isolated from humans and palm civets, and an FCoV-like agent that devastated cheetah colonies, have all crossed the host species barrier but, for different reasons, were unable to found a new coronavirus species (38, 55, 57, 85, 106, 112).

## SELECTION FORCES OF EVOLUTION

Little is known about the selection forces that have *actually* driven the evolution of nidoviruses. This is not surprising given our limited understanding of the functions of practically all proteins and RNA elements encoded by the nidovirus genome. Prior studies showed a strong correlation between a few changes in the receptor-binding S protein that could be achieved by site-directed mutagenesis, recombination, or experimentally enforced selection and coronavirus cell tissue tropism (1, 4, 96). Consequently, coronaviruses can evolve new receptor specificities with relative ease, a property that might facilitate their fast adaptation to a new host environment. In good agreement with this conclusion, the SARS-CoV S protein gene was shown to be one of the few that has been under a selection pressure to change during animal-to-human and human-to-human transmissions (85, 112).

Also, a meaningful interpretation was provided for the evolution of other proteins encoded in the 3′ region of the genome, most notably accessory ORFs. Extensive comparative analysis of PCR-generated genome sequences of SARS-CoVs isolated from humans and palm civets revealed large deletions in the 3′ region of the genome of some but not other isolates (38, 40, 55, 57, 94). These deletions affect the region including ORF7a, -7b, -8a, and -8b (alternatively known as ORF8 to -11), and they are typical for human but not civet cat isolates. Two deletions, 82 and 415 nucleotides (nt) long, either disrupted or eliminated ORF7a. A 29-nt deletion effectively fused ORF8a and -8b into a single ORF (known also as ORF8ab), while a 386-nt deletion affected ORF8a and -8b. The presence of some deletions correlates with a specific phase of the 2003 SARS-CoV epidemic. All proteins affected are unique to the SARS-CoV phylogenetic lineage and nonessential for growth in cell culture. Like other unique proteins from this region (93), they may mediate virus-host interactions. Consequently, it was proposed that the deletions may have been fixed as a result of adaptation of SARS-CoV to a new human host.

Also, these unique ORFs could be affected upon propagation of SARS-CoV in tissue culture: the 45-nt in-frame deletion in ORF7b was fixed in a SARS-CoV variant adapted to grow in Vero cells (97). Likewise, cell culture adaptation of two human coronaviruses, HCoV-229E and HCoV-OC43, may have driven, respectively, the inactivation of ORF4 by a 2-nt deletion (21) and the interruption of the I gene by a stop codon (101). From these and other studies, involving, e.g., IBV (9, 43) and MHV and FCoV (17, 42), it could be concluded that the origin and evolution of unique ORFs in the genomic 3′-proximal region has been driven by the benefits of spreading into new niches and improving control of coronavirus-host interactions. The rapid advancement of our knowledge about the functions of the proteins encoded by these ORFs will contribute to defining these selection forces in molecular detail.

## ORIGINS OF THE *NIDOVIRALES* AND NIDOVIRUS FAMILIES

The complex genetic plan and replicase gene of nidoviruses must have evolved from simpler ones. Recently, a speculative scenario of major events in nidovirus evolution has been offered (32). This scenario assumes that, generally, RNA viruses expand rather than shrink their genomes, which may not be true at any given time point.

It was speculated that the most recent common ancestor (MRCA) of the *Nidovirales* may have had a genome size close to that of the contemporary arteriviruses. In this scenario, the transition from this arterivirus-like nidovirus MRCA to the MRCA of the large nidoviruses may have been accompanied by the acquisition of the otherwise unique ExoN domain (80) and a genome size increase of about 14 kb (Fig. 4). The correlation between these two events perfectly fits the relationship between the quality of genome copying and genome size, as observed in various biological systems. In this context, the ExoN domain may have been acquired to improve the low fidelity of RdRp-mediated RNA replication through its 3′→5′ exonuclease activity (63) (see above).

The ExoN function likely was acquired by an ancestral virus that already had a multisubunit replicase complex whose fidelity was good enough to copy a larger-than-average-size RNA genome. At the stage at which (presumably) the nidovirus MRCA emerged, the two genetic marker domains, the zinc-binding domain (ZBD) and NendoU, may have been acquired (Fig. 4). They may have been used to build a prototype repair mechanism sufficient to copy an ~14-kb genome that later, following the acquisition

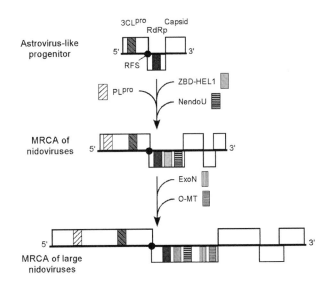

**Figure 4.** Origin and evolution of the nidovirus genome plan. A tentative evolutionary scenario leading to the origin of the MRCAs of nidoviruses and large nidoviruses from a progenitor with an astrovirus-like genome organization is illustrated. The three shown genomes are fictitious, although they are drawn to a relative common size scale and include major replicative domains found in genomes of respective contemporary viruses, as discussed in the text. Adapted from reference 32.

of ExoN, evolved into a more advanced system that was subsequently used in the *Coronaviridae/Roniviridae* branch. It is likely that extensive evolution producing a number of major virus lineages, which may either have become extinct or eluded identification thus far, preceded the emergence of the nidovirus MRCA.

Among contemporary viruses, the *Astroviridae* (48), which have relatively small genomes (Fig. 1), may most strongly resemble the reconstructed nidovirus MRCA in two major respects (Fig. 4). First, they have a nidovirus-like genetic plan with overlapping ORF1a/1b encoding replicase polyproteins and a downstream ORF for their capsid protein that is expressed from an sgRNA. Second, the backbone of the astrovirus replicase gene, which is composed of three domains, 3CL$^{pro}$-ribosomal frameshift signal-RdRp, matches the central part of the nidovirus-specific replicase domain arrangement. These three domains are key elements in the control of genome expression and replication, and therefore an ancestral relationship of *Astroviridae* and *Nidovirales* would also be in agreement with functional considerations.

An ancestral virus with the genome and replicase gene organization of astroviruses, already featuring the largest genomes among viruses lacking a helicase gene (Fig. 1), may have acquired a HEL1 domain from a virus of the alphavirus-like supergroup or another source. HEL1 evolved its 5′→3′ polarity and was, in association with the ZBD, inserted downstream of the RdRp domain, three novelties among RNA viruses that may have been essential for genome expansion. The acquisition of other replicase domains may have ensued, also through duplication and subsequent divergence of the original set of genes (see above). Particularly, the acquisition of the PL$^{pro}$ domain may have been an early milestone driven by the necessity to diversify the control of expression of gradually growing replicase polyproteins and virus-host interactions. The growth of the replicase gene might have made possible the expansion of the 3'-proximal genome region, encoding structural proteins that have evolved to form enveloped virions, eventually resulting in the MRCA of nidoviruses (Fig. 4).

## FUTURE DIRECTIONS

The progression of our understanding of nidovirus evolution depends on advancements in many research areas, including studies on nidovirus-specific RNA and protein synthesis, interactions of these viruses with their hosts, virus sampling in the field, and diverse evolutionary analyses. These advancements may help to dissect the molecular mechanisms that nidoviruses have evolved to synthesize and express their giant genomes and maintain the necessary balance between fast adaptation to changing environmental conditions on the one hand and genome stability on the other. To better understand this aspect, information on how nidoviruses make use of the unprecedented complexity and special features of their replicase machinery will be of prime interest, particularly with respect to controlling mutation frequencies that need to be measured for different nidoviruses. Furthermore, a comprehensive understanding of the parameters of nidovirus adaptability may result in the identification of the driving forces that have shaped nidovirus evolution. In this context, it will be essential to continue the sampling of the natural diversity of nidoviruses, also to see whether the genome size gap between the small and large nidoviruses will be filled with viruses with intermediate-size genomes, and whether nidoviruses infecting other phyla, e.g., plants and insects, can be identified. Ultimately, we may hope to learn whether the large nidoviruses (particularly, coronaviruses) have reached the theoretical genome size limit that nature may have set for RNA viruses. Finally, and more practically, our progress in understanding the fundamental aspects of RNA virus genome expansion may help to monitor and control infections caused by (known and potentially emerging) nidoviruses.

**Acknowledgments.** I am indebted to Luis Enjuanes, Eric Snijder, and John Ziebuhr for collaboration in preparing a review (32) that was used as a basis for this work. The kind help of Johan Faase in preparing Fig. 1 is gratefully acknowledged.

## REFERENCES

1. **Ballesteros, M. L., C. M. Sanchez, and L. Enjuanes.** 1997. Two amino acid changes at the N-terminus of transmissible gastroenteritis coronavirus spike protein result in the loss of enteric tropism. *Virology* **227:**378–388.
2. **Bao, Y., S. Federhen, D. Leipe, V. Pham, S. Resenchuk, M. Rozanov, R. Tatusov, and T. Tatusova.** 2004. National Center for Biotechnology Information Viral Genomes Project. *J. Virol.* **78:**7291–7298.
3. **Baric, R. S., K. Fu, M. C. Schaad, and S. A. Stohlman.** 1990. Establishing a genetic-recombination map for murine coronavirus strain A59 complementation groups. *Virology* **177:**646–656.
4. **Baric, R. S., B. Yount, L. Hensley, S. A. Peel, and W. Chen.** 1997. Episodic evolution mediates interspecies transfer of a murine coronavirus. *J. Virol.* **71:**1946–1955.
5. **Bhardwaj, K., L. Guarino, and C. C. Kao.** 2004. The severe acute respiratory syndrome coronavirus Nsp15 protein is an endoribonuclease that prefers manganese as a cofactor. *J. Virol.* **78:**12218–12224.
6. **Boursnell, M. E. G., T. D. K. Brown, I. J. Foulds, P. F. Green, F. M. Tomley, and M. M. Binns.** 1987. Completion of the sequence of the genome of the coronavirus avian infectious bronchitis virus. *J. Gen. Virol.* **68:**57–77.
7. **Bredenbeek, P. J., E. J. Snijder, F. H. Noten, J. A. den Boon, W. M. Schaaper, M. C. Horzinek, and W. J. Spaan.** 1990. The polymerase gene of corona- and toroviruses: evidence for an evolutionary relationship. *Adv. Exp. Med. Biol.* **276:**307–316.
8. **Brian, D. A., and W. J. M. Spaan.** 1997. Recombination and coronavirus defective interfering RNAs. *Semin. Virol.* **8:**101–111.
9. **Casais, R., M. Davies, D. Cavanagh, and P. Britton.** 2005. Gene 5 of the avian coronavirus infectious bronchitis virus is not essential for replication. *J. Virol.* **79:**8065–8078.
10. **Castro, C., J. J. Arnold, and C. E. Cameron.** 2005. Incorporation fidelity of the viral RNA-dependent RNA polymerase: a kinetic, thermodynamic and structural perspective. *Virus Res.* **107:**141–149.
11. **Cavanagh, D.** 1997. Nidovirales: a new order comprising Coronaviridae and Arteriviridae. *Arch. Virol.* **142:**629–633.
12. **Chao, L.** 1988. Evolution of sex in RNA viruses. *J. Theor. Biol.* **133:**99–112.
13. **Chouljenko, V. N., X. Q. Lin, J. Storz, K. G. Kousoulas, and A. E. Gorbalenya.** 2001. Comparison of genomic and predicted amino acid sequences of respiratory and enteric bovine coronaviruses isolated from the same animal with fatal shipping pneumonia. *J. Gen. Virol.* **82:**2927–2933.
14. **Chu, D. K. W., L. L. M. Poon, K. H. Chan, H. Chen, Y. Guan, K. Y. Yuen, and J. S. M. Peiris.** 2006. Coronaviruses in bent-winged bats (Miniopterus spp.). *J. Gen. Virol.* **87:**2461–2466.
15. **Cowley, J. A., C. M. Dimmock, K. M. Spann, and P. J. Walker.** 2000. Gill-associated virus of Penaeus monodon prawns: an invertebrate virus with ORF1a and ORF1b genes related to arteri- and coronaviruses. *J. Gen. Virol.* **81:**1473–1484.
16. **Cowley, J. A., and P. J. Walker.** 2002. The complete genome sequence of gill-associated virus of Penaeus monodon prawns indicates a gene organization unique among nidoviruses. *Arch. Virol.* **147:**1977–1987.

17. de Haan, C. A. M., P. S. Masters, X. L. Shen, S. Weiss, and P. J. M. Rottier. 2002. The group-specific murine coronavirus genes are not essential, but their deletion, by reverse genetics, is attenuating in the natural host. *Virology* **296:**177–189.

18. den Boon, J. A., K. S. Faaberg, J. J. Meulenberg, A. L. Wassenaar, P. G. Plagemann, A. E. Gorbalenya, and E. J. Snijder. 1995. Processing and evolution of the N-terminal region of the arterivirus replicase ORF1a protein: identification of two papainlike cysteine proteases. *J. Virol.* **69:**4500–4505.

19. den Boon, J. A., E. J. Snijder, E. D. Chirnside, A. A. de Vries, M. C. Horzinek, and W. J. Spaan. 1991. Equine arteritis virus is not a togavirus but belongs to the coronaviruslike superfamily. *J. Virol.* **65:**2910–2920.

20. de Vries, A. A. F., M. C. Horzinek, P. J. M. Rottier, and R. J. de Groot. 1997. The genome organization of the Nidovirales: similarities and differences between Arteri-, Toro-, and Coronaviruses. *Semin. Virol.* **8:**33–47.

21. Dijkman, R., M. F. Jebbink, B. Wilbrink, K. Pyrc, H. L. Zaaijer, P. D. Minor, S. Franklin, B. Berkhout, V. Thiel, and L. van der Hoek. 2006. Human coronavirus 229E encodes a single ORF4 protein between spike and the envelope genes. *Virol. J.* **3:**106.

22. Domingo, E., and J. J. Holland. 1997. RNA virus mutations and fitness for survival. *Annu. Rev. Microbiol.* **51:**151–178.

23. Drake, J. W., and J. J. Holland. 1999. Mutation rates among RNA viruses. *Proc. Natl. Acad. Sci. USA* **96:**13910–13913.

24. Draker, R., R. L. Roper, M. Petric, and R. Tellier. 2006. The complete sequence of the bovine torovirus genome. *Virus Res.* **115:**56–68.

25. Dye, C., and S. G. Siddell. 2005. Genomic RNA sequence of feline coronavirus strain FIPVWSU-79/1146. *J. Gen. Virol.* **86:**2249–2253.

26. Erles, K., C. Toomey, H. W. Brooks, and J. Brownlie. 2003. Detection of a group 2 coronavirus in dogs with canine infectious respiratory disease. *Virology* **310:**216–223.

27. Fauquet, C. M., M. A. Mayo, J. Maniloff, U. Desselberger, and L. A. Ball (ed.). 2005. *Virus Taxonomy: Eighth Report of the International Committee on Taxonomy of Viruses*. Elsevier Academic Press, San Diego, CA.

28. Fouchier, R. A. M., N. G. Hartwig, T. M. Bestebroer, B. Niemeyer, J. C. de Jong, J. H. Simon, and A. D. M. E. Osterhaus. 2004. A previously undescribed coronavirus associated with respiratory disease in humans. *Proc. Natl. Acad. Sci. USA* **101:**6212–6216.

29. Godeny, E. K., A. A. de Vries, X. C. Wang, S. L. Smith, and R. J. de Groot. 1998. Identification of the leader-body junctions for the viral subgenomic mRNAs and organization of the simian hemorrhagic fever virus genome: evidence for gene duplication during arterivirus evolution. *J. Virol.* **72:**862–867.

30. González, J. M., P. Gomez-Puertas, D. Cavanagh, A. E. Gorbalenya, and L. Enjuanes. 2003. A comparative sequence analysis to revise the current taxonomy of the family Coronaviridae. *Arch. Virol.* **148:**2207–2235.

31. Gorbalenya, A. E. 2001. Big Nidovirus genome: when count and order of domains matter. *Adv. Exp. Med. Biol.* **494:**1–17.

32. Gorbalenya, A. E., L. Enjuanes, J. Ziebuhr, and E. J. Snijder. 2006. Nidovirales: evolving the largest RNA virus genome. *Virus Res.* **117:**17–37.

33. Gorbalenya, A. E., E. V. Koonin, A. P. Donchenko, and V. M. Blinov. 1989. Coronavirus genome: prediction of putative functional domains in the nonstructural polyprotein by comparative amino acid sequence analysis. *Nucleic Acids Res.* **17:**4847–4861.

34. Gorbalenya, A. E., E. V. Koonin, and M. M. C. Lai. 1991. Putative papain-related thiol proteases of positive-strand RNA viruses. *FEBS Lett.* **288:**201–205.

35. Gorbalenya, A. E., F. M. Pringle, J. L. Zeddam, B. T. Luke, C. E. Cameron, J. Kalmakoff, T. N. Hanzlik, K. H. Gordon, and V. K. Ward. 2002. The palm subdomain-based active site is internally permuted in viral RNA-dependent RNA polymerases of an ancient lineage. *J. Mol. Biol.* **324:**47–62.

36. Gorbalenya, A. E., E. J. Snijder, and W. J. Spaan. 2004. Severe acute respiratory syndrome coronavirus phylogeny: toward consensus. *J. Virol.* **78:**7863–7866.

37. Gough, R. E., S. E. Drury, F. Culver, P. Britton, and D. Cavanagh. 2006. Isolation of a coronavirus from a green-cheeked Amazon parrot (Amazon viridigenalis Cassin). *Avian Pathol.* **35:**122–126.

38. Guan, Y., B. J. Zheng, Y. Q. He, X. L. Liu, Z. X. Zhuang, C. L. Cheung, S. W. Luo, P. H. Li, L. J. Zhang, Y. J. Guan, K. M. Butt, K. L. Wong, K. W. Chan, W. Lim, K. F. Shortridge, K. Y. Yuen, J. S. M. Peiris, and L. L. M. Poon. 2003. Isolation and characterization of viruses related to the SARS coronavirus from animals in Southern China. *Science* **302:**276–278.

39. Haijema, B. J., H. Volders, and P. J. M. Rottier. 2004. Live, attenuated coronavirus vaccines through the directed deletion of group-specific genes provide protection against feline infectious peritonitis. *J. Virol.* **78:**3863–3871.

40. He, J. F., G. W. Peng, J. Min, D. W. Yu, W. J. Liang, S. Y. Zhang, R. H. Xu, H. Y. Zheng, X. W. Wu, J. Xu, Z. H. Wang, L. Fang, X. Zhang, H. Li, X. G. Yan, J. H. Lu, Z. H. Hu, J. C. Huang, Z. Y. Wan, J. L. Hou, J. Y. Lin, H. D. Song, S. Y. Wang, X. J. Zhou, G. W. Zhang, B. W. Gu, H. J. Zheng, X. L. Zhang, M. He, K. Zheng, B. F. Wang, G. Fu, X. N. Wang, S. J. Chen, Z. Chen, P. Hao, H. Tang, S. X. Ren, Y. Zhong, Z. M. Guo, Q. Liu, Y. G. Miao, X. Y. Kong, W. Z. He, Y. X. Li, C. I. Wu, G. P. Zhao, R. W. K. Chiu, S. S. C. Chim, Y. K. Tong, P. K. S. Chan, J. S. Tam, and Y. M. D. Lo. 2004. Molecular evolution of the SARS coronavirus during the course of the SARS epidemic in China. *Science* **303:**1666–1669.

41. Herrewegh, A. A. P. M., I. Smeenk, M. C. Horzinek, P. J. M. Rottier, and R. J. de Groot. 1998. Feline coronavirus type II strains 79-1683 and 79-1146 originate from a double recombination between feline coronavirus type I and canine coronavirus. *J. Virol.* **72:**4508–4514.

42. Herrewegh, A. A. P. M., H. Vennema, M. C. Horzinek, P. J. M. Rottier, and R. J. Degroot. 1995. The molecular genetics of feline coronaviruses—comparative sequence analysis of the Orf7A/7B transcription unit of different biotypes. *Virology* **212:**622–631.

43. Hodgson, T., P. Britton, and D. Cavanagh. 2006. Neither the RNA nor the proteins of open reading frames 3a and 3b of the coronavirus infectious bronchitis virus are essential for replication. *J. Virol.* **80:**296–305.

44. Holmes, E. C., and A. Rambaut. 2004. Viral evolution and the emergence of SARS coronavirus. *Philos. Trans. R. Soc. Lond. B* **359:**1059–1065.

45. Imbert, I., J. C. Guillemot, J. M. Bourhis, C. Bussetta, B. Coutard, M. P. Egloff, F. Ferron, A. E. Gorbalenya, and B. Canard. 2006. A second, non-canonical RNA-dependent RNA polymerase in SARS coronavirus. *EMBO J.* **25:**4933–4942.

46. Ivanov, K. A., T. Hertzig, M. Rozanov, S. Bayer, V. Thiel, A. E. Gorbalenya, and J. Ziebuhr. 2004. Major genetic marker of nidoviruses encodes a replicative endoribonuclease. *Proc. Natl. Acad. Sci. USA* **101:**12694–12699.

47. Jenkins, G. M., M. Worobey, C. H. Woelk, and E. C. Holmes. 2001. Nonquasispecies evidence for the evolution of RNA viruses. *Mol. Biol. Evol.* **18:**987–994.

48. Jiang, B. M., S. S. Monroe, E. V. Koonin, S. E. Stine, and R. I. Glass. 1993. RNA sequence of astrovirus—distinctive genomic organization and a putative retrovirus-like ribosomal frame-shifting signal that directs the viral replicase synthesis. *Proc. Natl. Acad. Sci. USA* **90:**10539–10543.

49. Jonassen, C. M., T. O. Jonassen, and B. Grinde. 1998. A common RNA motif in the 3′ end of the genomes of astroviruses, avian infectious bronchitis virus and an equine rhinovirus. *J. Gen. Virol.* **79**:715–718.

50. Jonassen, C. M., T. Kofstad, I. L. Larsen, A. Lovland, K. Handeland, A. Follestad, and A. Lillehaug. 2005. Molecular identification and characterization of novel coronaviruses infecting graylag geese (Anser anser), feral pigeons (Columbia livia) and mallards (Anas platyrhynchos). *J. Gen. Virol.* **86**:1597–1607.

51. Koonin, E. V., and A. E. Gorbalenya. 1989. Evolution of RNA genomes—does the high mutation rate necessitate high rate of evolution of viral proteins? *J. Mol. Evol.* **28**:524–527.

52. Ksiazek, T. G., D. Erdman, C. S. Goldsmith, S. R. Zaki, T. Peret, S. Emery, S. X. Tong, C. Urbani, J. A. Comer, W. Lim, P. E. Rollin, S. F. Dowell, A. E. Ling, C. D. Humphrey, W. J. Shieh, J. Guarner, C. D. Paddock, P. Rota, B. Fields, J. DeRisi, J. Y. Yang, N. Cox, J. M. Hughes, J. W. Leduc, W. J. Bellini, and L. J. Anderson. 2003. A novel coronavirus associated with severe acute respiratory syndrome. *N. Engl. J. Med.* **348**:1953–1966.

53. Lai, M. M. C. 1992. RNA recombination in animal and plant viruses. *Microbiol. Rev.* **56**:61–79.

54. Lai, M. M. C. 1996. Recombination in large RNA viruses: coronaviruses. *Semin. Virol.* **7**:381–388.

55. Lau, S. K. P., P. C. Y. Woo, K. S. M. Li, Y. Huang, H. W. Tsoi, B. H. L. Wong, S. S. Y. Wong, S. Y. Leung, K. H. Chan, and K. Y. Yuen. 2005. Severe acute respiratory syndrome coronavirus-like virus in Chinese horseshoe bats. *Proc. Natl. Acad. Sci. USA* **102**:14040–14045.

56. Lee, H. J., C. K. Shieh, A. E. Gorbalenya, E. V. Koonin, N. La Monica, J. Tuler, A. Bagdzhadzhyan, and M. M. Lai. 1991. The complete sequence (22 kilobases) of murine coronavirus gene 1 encoding the putative proteases and RNA polymerase. *Virology* **180**:567–582.

57. Li, W. D., Z. L. Shi, M. Yu, W. Z. Ren, C. Smith, J. H. Epstein, H. Z. Wang, G. Crameri, Z. H. Hu, H. J. Zhang, J. H. Zhang, J. McEachern, H. Field, P. Daszak, B. T. Eaton, S. Y. Zhang, and L. F. Wang. 2005. Bats are natural reservoirs of SARS-like coronaviruses. *Science* **310**:676–679.

58. Lin, T. L., C. C. Loa, and C. C. Wu. 2004. Complete sequences of 3′ end coding region for structural protein genes of turkey coronavirus. *Virus Res.* **106**:61–70.

59. Lissenberg, A., M. M. Vrolijk, A. L. W. van Vliet, M. A. Langereis, J. D. F. Groot-Mijnes, P. J. M. Rottier, and R. J. de Groot. 2005. Luxury at a cost? Recombinant mouse hepatitis viruses expressing the accessory hemagglutinin esterase protein display reduced fitness in vitro. *J. Virol.* **79**:15054–15063.

60. Magiorkinis, G., E. Magiorkinis, D. Paraskevis, A. M. Vandamme, M. Van Ranst, V. Moulton, and A. Hatzakis. 2004. Phylogenetic analysis of the full-length SARS-CoV sequences: evidence for phylogenetic discordance in three genomic regions. *J. Med. Virol.* **74**:369–372.

61. Makino, S., J. G. Keck, S. T. Stohlman, and M. M. C. Lai. 1986. High-frequency RNA recombination of murine coronaviruses. *J. Virol.* **57**:729–737.

62. Marra, M. A., S. J. M. Jones, C. R. Astell, R. A. Holt, A. Brooks-Wilson, Y. S. N. Butterfield, J. Khattra, J. K. Asano, S. A. Barber, S. Y. Chan, A. Cloutier, S. M. Coughlin, D. Freeman, N. Girn, O. L. Griffin, S. R. Leach, M. Mayo, H. McDonald, S. B. Montgomery, P. K. Pandoh, A. S. Petrescu, A. G. Robertson, J. E. Schein, A. Siddiqui, D. E. Smailus, J. E. Stott, G. S. Yang, F. Plummer, A. Andonov, H. Artsob, N. Bastien, K. Bernard, T. F. Booth, D. Bowness, M. Czub, M. Drebot, L. Fernando, R. Flick, M. Garbutt, M. Gray, A. Grolla, S. Jones, H. Feldmann, A. Meyers, A. Kabani, Y. Li, S. Normand, U. Stroher, G. A. Tipples, S. Tyler, R. Vogrig, D. Ward, B. Watson, R. C. Brunham, M. Krajden, M. Petric, D. M. Skowronski, C. Upton, and R. L. Roper. 2003. The genome sequence of the SARS-associated coronavirus. *Science* **300**:1399–1404.

63. Minskaia, E., T. Hertzig, A. E. Gorbalenya, V. Campanacci, C. Cambillau, B. Canard, and J. Ziebuhr. 2006. Discovery of an RNA virus 3′→5′ exoribonuclease that is critically involved in coronavirus RNA synthesis. *Proc. Natl. Acad. Sci. USA* **103**:5108–5113.

64. Motokawa, K., T. Hohdatsu, C. Aizawa, H. Koyama, and H. Hashimoto. 1995. Molecular cloning and sequence determination of the peplomer protein gene of feline infectious peritonitis virus type I. *Arch. Virol.* **140**:469–480.

65. Nelsen, C. J., M. P. Murtaugh, and K. S. Faaberg. 1999. Porcine reproductive and respiratory syndrome virus comparison: divergent evolution on two continents. *J. Virol.* **73**:270–280.

66. Poon, L. L. M., D. K. W. Chu, K. H. Chan, O. K. Wong, T. M. Ellis, Y. H. C. Leung, S. K. P. Lau, P. C. Y. Woo, K. Y. Suen, K. Y. Yuen, Y. Guan, and J. S. M. Peiris. 2005. Identification of a novel coronavirus in bats. *J. Virol.* **79**:2001–2009.

67. Putics, A., W. Filipowicz, J. Hall, A. E. Gorbalenya, and J. Ziebuhr. 2005. ADP-ribose-1″-monophosphatase: a conserved coronavirus enzyme that is dispensable for viral replication in tissue culture. *J. Virol.* **79**:12721–12731.

68. Pyrc, K., R. Dijkman, L. Deng, M. F. Jebbink, H. A. Ross, B. Berkhout, and L. van der Hoek. 2006. Mosaic structure of human coronavirus NL63, one thousand years of evolution. *J. Mol. Biol.* **364**:964–973.

69. Ren, W., W. D. Li, M. Yu, P. Hao, Y. Zhang, P. Zhou, S. Y. Zhang, G. P. Zhao, Y. Zhong, S. Y. Wang, L. F. Wang, and Z. Shi. 2006. Full-length genome sequences of two SARS-like coronaviruses in horseshoe bats and genetic variation analysis. *J. Gen. Virol.* **87**:3355–3359.

70. Rest, J. S., and D. P. Mindell. 2003. SARS associated coronavirus has a recombinant polymerase and coronaviruses have a history of host-shifting. *Infection, Genet. Evol.* **3**:219–225.

71. Rota, P. A., M. S. Oberste, S. S. Monroe, W. A. Nix, R. Campagnoli, J. P. Icenogle, S. Penaranda, B. Bankamp, K. Maher, M. H. Chen, S. X. Tong, A. Tamin, L. Lowe, M. Frace, J. L. Derisi, Q. Chen, D. Wang, D. D. Erdman, T. C. T. Peret, C. Burns, T. G. Ksiazek, P. E. Rollin, A. Sanchez, S. Liffick, B. Holloway, J. Limor, K. McCaustland, M. Olsen-Rasmussen, R. Fouchier, S. Gunther, A. D. M. E. Osterhaus, C. Drosten, M. A. Pallansch, L. J. Anderson, and W. J. Bellini. 2003. Characterization of a novel coronavirus associated with severe acute respiratory syndrome. *Science* **300**:1394–1399.

72. Salemi, M., W. M. Fitch, M. Ciccozzi, M. J. Ruiz-Alvarez, G. Rezza, and M. J. Lewis. 2004. Severe acute respiratory syndrome coronavirus sequence characteristics and evolutionary rate estimate from maximum likelihood analysis. *J. Virol.* **78**:1602–1603.

73. Sanchez, C. M., F. Gebauer, C. Sune, A. Mendez, J. Dopazo, and L. Enjuanes. 1992. Genetic evolution and tropism of transmissible gastroenteritis coronaviruses. *Virology* **190**:92–105.

74. Schutze, H., R. Ulferts, B. Schelle, S. Bayer, H. Granzow, B. Hoffmann, T. C. Mettenleiter, and J. Ziebuhr. 2006. Characterization of white bream virus reveals a novel genetic cluster of nidoviruses. *J. Virol.* **80**:11598–11609.

75. Seybert, A., A. Hegyi, S. G. Siddell, and J. Ziebuhr. 2000. The human coronavirus 229E superfamily 1 helicase has RNA and DNA duplex-unwinding activities with 5′-to-3′ polarity. *RNA* **6**:1056–1068.

76. Siddell, S. 1995. *The Coronaviridae.* Plenum Press, New York, NY.

77. Siddell, S. G., J. Ziebuhr, and E. J. Snijder. 2005. Coronaviruses, toroviruses and arteriviruses, p. 823–856. *In* B. W. J. Mahy and V. ter Meulen (ed.), *Topley & Wilson's Microbiology and Microbial Infections. Virology*. Hodder Arnold, London, United Kingdom.

78. Smits, S. L., A. Lavazza, K. Matiz, M. C. Horzinek, M. P. Koopmans, and R. J. de Groot. 2003. Phylogenetic and evolutionary relationship among torovirus field variants: evidence for multiple intertypic recombination events. *J. Virol.* **77:**9567–9577.

79. Smits, S. L., E. J. Snijder, and R. J. de Groot. 2006. Characterization of a torovirus main proteinase. *J. Virol.* **80:**4157–4167.

80. Snijder, E. J., P. J. Bredenbeek, J. C. Dobbe, V. Thiel, J. Ziebuhr, L. L. M. Poon, Y. Guan, M. Rozanov, W. J. M. Spaan, and A. E. Gorbalenya. 2003. Unique and conserved features of genome and proteome of SARS-coronavirus, an early split-off from the coronavirus group 2 lineage. *J. Mol. Biol.* **331:**991–1004.

81. Snijder, E. J., M. A. Brinton, K. S. Faaberg, E. K. Godeny, A. E. Gorbalenya, N. J. MacLachlan, W. L. Mengeling, and P. G. Plagemann. 2005. Family *Arteriviridae*, p. 965–974. *In* C. M. Fauquet, M. A. Mayo, J. Maniloff, U. Desselberger, and L. A. Ball (ed.), *Virus Taxonomy. Eighth Report of the International Committee on Taxonomy of Viruses*. Elsevier, Academic Press, Amsterdam, The Netherlands.

82. Snijder, E. J., J. A. den Boon, M. C. Horzinek, and W. J. Spaan. 1991. Comparison of the genome organization of toro- and coronaviruses: evidence for two nonhomologous RNA recombination events during Berne virus evolution. *Virology* **180:**448–452.

83. Snijder, E. J., S. G. Siddell, and A. E. Gorbalenya. 2005. The order Nidovirales, p. 390–404. *In* B. W. J. Mahy and V. ter Meulen (ed.), *Topley & Wilson's Microbiology and Microbial Infections. Virology*, vol. 1. Hodder Arnold, London, United Kingdom.

84. Snijder, E. J., A. L. Wassenaar, L. C. van Dinten, W. J. Spaan, and A. E. Gorbalenya. 1996. The arterivirus nsp4 protease is the prototype of a novel group of chymotrypsin-like enzymes, the 3C-like serine proteases. *J. Biol. Chem.* **271:**4864–4871.

85. Song, H. D., C. C. Tu, G. W. Zhang, S. Y. Wang, K. Zheng, L. C. Lei, Q. X. Chen, Y. W. Gao, H. Q. Zhou, H. Xiang, H. J. Zheng, S. W. W. Chern, F. Cheng, C. M. Pan, H. Xuan, S. J. Chen, H. M. Luo, D. H. Zhou, Y. F. Liu, J. F. He, P. Z. Qin, L. H. Li, Y. Q. Ren, W. J. Liang, Y. D. Yu, L. Anderson, M. Wang, R. H. Xu, X. W. Wu, H. Y. Zheng, J. D. Chen, G. D. Liang, Y. Gao, M. Liao, L. Fang, L. Y. Jiang, H. Li, F. Chen, B. Di, L. J. He, J. Y. Lin, S. X. Tong, X. G. Kong, L. Du, P. Hao, H. Tang, A. Bernini, X. J. Yu, O. Spiga, Z. M. Guo, H. Y. Pan, W. Z. He, J. C. Manuguerra, A. Fontanet, A. Danchin, N. Niccolai, Y. X. Li, C. I. Wu, and G. P. Zhao. 2005. Cross-host evolution of severe acute respiratory syndrome coronavirus in palm civet and human. *Proc. Natl. Acad. Sci. USA* **102:**2430–2435.

86. Spaan, W. J. M., D. Brian, D. Cavanagh, R. J. de Groot, L. Enjuanes, A. E. Gorbalenya, K. V. Holmes, P. S. Masters, P. Rottier, F. Taguchi, and P. Talbot. 2005. Family Coronaviridae, p. 947–964. *In* C. M. Fauquet, M. A. Mayo, J. Maniloff, U. Desselberger, and L. A. Ball (ed.), *Virus Taxonomy. Eighth Report of the International Committee on Taxonomy of Viruses*. Elsevier Academic Press, San Diego, CA.

87. Spaan, W. J. M., D. Cavanagh, R. J. de Groot, L. Enjuanes, A. E. Gorbalenya, E. J. Snijder, and P. J. Walker. 2005. Order Nidovirales, p. 937–945. *In* C. M. Fauquet, M. A. Mayo, J. Maniloff, U. Desselberger, and L. A. Ball (ed.), *Virus Taxonomy. Eighth Report of the International Committee on Taxonomy of Viruses*. Elsevier Academic Press, San Diego, CA.

88. Stanhope, M. J., J. R. Brown, and H. Amrine-Madsen. 2004. Evidence from the evolutionary analysis of nucleotide sequences for a recombinant history of SARS-CoV. *Infect. Genet. Evol.* **4:**15–19.

89. Stavrinides, J., and D. S. Guttman. 2004. Mosaic evolution of the severe acute respiratory syndrome coronavirus. *J. Virol.* **78:**76–82.

90. St-Jean, J. R., H. Jacomy, M. Desforges, and P. J. Talbot. 2005. Genetic variability of human respiratory coronavirus OC43. *J. Virol.* **79:**3224–3225. (Authors' reply to letter to the editor.)

91. St-Jean, J. R., H. Jacomy, M. Desforges, A. Vabret, F. Freymuth, and P. J. Talbot. 2004. Human respiratory coronavirus OC43: genetic stability and neuroinvasion. *J. Virol.* **78:**8824–8834.

92. Sutton, G., E. Fry, L. Carter, S. Sainsbury, T. Walter, J. Nettleship, N. Berrow, R. Owens, R. Gilbert, A. Davidson, S. Siddell, L. L. M. Poon, J. Diprose, D. Alderton, M. Walsh, J. M. Grimes, and D. I. Stuart. 2004. The nsp9 replicase protein of SARS-coronavirus, structure and functional insights. *Structure* **12:**341–353.

92a. Swofford, D. L. 2000. PAUP*: phylogenetic analysis using parsimony (*and other methods), version 4. Sinauer Associates, Sunderland, MA.

93. Tan, Y. J., E. Teng, S. Shen, T. H. P. Tan, P. Y. Goh, B. C. Fielding, E. E. Ooi, H. C. Tan, S. G. Lim, and W. Hong. 2004. A novel severe acute respiratory syndrome coronavirus protein, U274, is transported to the cell surface and undergoes endocytosis. *J. Virol.* **78:**6723–6734.

94. Tang, J. W., J. L. K. Cheung, I. M. T. Chu, J. J. Y. Sung, M. Peiris, and P. K. S. Chan. 2006. The large 386-nt deletion in SARS-associated coronavirus: evidence for quasispecies? *J. Infect. Dis.* **194:**808–813.

95. Tang, X. C., J. X. Zhang, S. Y. Zhang, P. Wang, X. H. Fan, L. F. Li, G. Li, B. Q. Dong, W. Liu, C. L. Cheung, K. M. Xu, W. J. Song, D. Vijaykrishna, L. L. M. Poon, J. S. M. Peiris, G. J. D. Smith, H. Chen, and Y. Guan. 2006. Prevalence and genetic diversity of coronaviruses in bats from China. *J. Virol.* **80:**7481–7490.

96. Thackray, L. B., and K. V. Holmes. 2004. Amino acid substitutions and an insertion in the spike glycoprotein extend the host range of the murine coronavirus MHV-A59. *Virology* **324:**510–524.

97. Thiel, V., K. A. Ivanov, A. Putics, T. Hertzig, B. Schelle, S. Bayer, B. Weissbrich, E. J. Snijder, H. Rabenau, H. W. Doerr, A. E. Gorbalenya, and J. Ziebuhr. 2003. Mechanisms and enzymes involved in SARS coronavirus genome expression. *J. Gen. Virol.* **84:**2305–2315.

98. Tijms, M. A., L. C. van Dinten, A. E. Gorbalenya, and E. J. Snijder. 2001. A zinc finger-containing papain-like protease couples subgenomic mRNA synthesis to genome translation in a positive-stranded RNA virus. *Proc. Natl. Acad. Sci. USA* **98:**1889–1894.

99. van der Hoek, L., K. Pyrc, M. F. Jebbink, W. Vermeulen-Oost, R. J. M. Berkhout, K. C. Wolthers, P. M. E. Wertheim-van Dillen, J. Kaandorp, J. Spaargaren, and B. Berkhout. 2004. Identification of a new human coronavirus. *Nat. Med.* **10:**368–373.

100. Vijgen, L., E. Keyaerts, P. Lemey, P. Maes, K. Van Reeth, H. Nauwynck, M. Pensaert, and M. Van Ranst. 2006. Evolutionary history of the closely related group 2 coronaviruses: porcine hemagglutinating encephalomyelitis virus, bovine coronavirus, and human coronavirus OC43. *J. Virol.* **80:**7270–7274.

101. Vijgen, L., E. Keyaerts, P. Lemey, E. Moes, S. Li, A. M. Vandamme, and M. Van Ranst. 2005. Circulation of

genetically distinct contemporary human coronavirus OC43 strains. *Virology* 337:85–92.

102. Vijgen, L., E. Keyaerts, E. Moes, I. Thoelen, E. Wollants, P. Lemey, A. M. Vandamme, and M. Van Ranst. 2005. Complete genomic sequence of human coronavirus OC43: molecular clock analysis suggests a relatively recent zoonotic coronavirus transmission event. *J. Virol.* 79:1595–1604.

103. Vijgen, L., P. Lemey, E. Keyaerts, and M. Van Ranst. 2005. Genetic variability of human respiratory coronavirus OC43. *J. Virol.* 79:3223–3224. (Letter to the editor.)

104. Walker, P. J., J. R. Bonami, V. Boonsaeng, P. S. Chang, J. A. Cowley, L. Enjuanes, T. W. Flegel, D. V. Lightner, P. C. Loh, E. J. Snijder, and K. Tang. 2005. Family Roniviridae, p. 975–979. *In* C. M. Fauquet, M. A. Mayo, J. Maniloff, U. Desselberger, and L. A. Ball (ed.), *Virus Taxonomy. Eighth Report of the International Committee on Taxonomy of Viruses.* Elsevier, Academic Press, Amsterdam, The Netherlands.

105. Wang, D., A. Urisman, Y. T. Liu, M. Springer, T. G. Ksiazek, D. D. Erdman, E. R. Mardis, M. Hickenbotham, V. Magrini, J. Eldred, J. P. Latreille, R. K. Wilson, D. Ganem, and J. L. Derisi. 2003. Viral discovery and sequence recovery using DNA microarrays. *PLoS Biol.* 1:257–260.

106. Wilkerson, A. J. P., E. C. Teeling, J. L. Troyer, G. K. Bar-Gal, M. Roelke, L. Marker, J. Pecon-Slattery, and S. J. O'Brien. 2004. Coronavirus outbreak in cheetahs: lessons for SARS. *Curr. Biol.* 14:R227–R228.

107. Woo, P. C. Y., S. K. P. Lau, C. M. Chu, K. H. Chan, H. W. Tsoi, Y. Huang, B. H. L. Wong, H. L. Wong, R. W. S. Poon, J. J. Cai, W. K. Luk, L. L. M. Poon, S. S. Y. Wong, Y. Guan, J. S. M. Peiris, and K. Y. Yuen. 2005. Characterization and complete genome sequence of a novel coronavirus, coronavirus HKU1, from patients with pneumonia. *J. Virol.* 79:884–895.

108. Woo, P. C. Y., S. K. P. Lau, K. S. M. Li, R. W. S. Poon, B. H. L. Wong, H. W. Tsoi, B. C. K. Yip, Y. Huang, K. H. Chan, and K. Y. Yuen. 2006. Molecular diversity of coronaviruses in bats. *Virology* 351:180–187.

109. Woo, P. C. Y., S. K. P. Lau, C. C. Y. Yip, Y. Huang, H. W. Tsoi, K. H. Chan, and K. Y. Yuen. 2006. Comparative analysis of 22 coronavirus HKU1 genomes reveals a novel geno-type and evidence of natural recombination in coronavirus HKU1. *J. Virol.* 80:7136–7145.

110. Woo, P. C. Y., M. Wang, S. K. P. Lau, H. Xu, R. W. S. Poon, R. Guo, B. H. L. Wong, K. Gao, H.-W. Tsoi, Y. Huang, K. S. M. Li, C. S. F. Lam, K.-H. Chan, B.-J. Zheng, and K.-Y. Yuen. 2007. Comparative analysis of twelve genomes of three novel group 2c and group 2d coronaviruses reveals unique group and subgroup features. *J. Virol.* 81:1574–1585.

111. Worobey, M., and E. C. Holmes. 1999. Evolutionary aspects of recombination in RNA viruses. *J. Gen. Virol.* 80:2535–2543.

112. Yeh, S. H., H. Y. Wang, C. Y. Tsai, C. L. Kao, J. Y. Yang, H. W. Liu, I. J. Su, S. F. Tsai, D. S. Chen, and P. J. Chen. 2004. Characterization of severe acute respiratory syndrome coronavirus genomes in Taiwan: molecular epidemiology and genome evolution. *Proc. Natl. Acad. Sci. USA* 101:2542–2547.

113. Yount, B., R. S. Roberts, A. C. Sims, D. Deming, M. B. Frieman, J. Sparks, M. R. Denison, N. Davis, and R. S. Baric. 2005. Severe acute respiratory syndrome coronavirus group-specific open reading frames encode nonessential functions for replication in cell cultures and mice. *J. Virol.* 79:14909–14922.

114. Zhao, Z., H. Li, X. Wu, Y. Zhong, K. Zhang, Y.-P. Zhang, E. Boerwinkle, and Y.-X. Fu. 2004. Moderate mutation rate in the SARS coronavirus genome and its implications. *BMC Evol. Biol.* 4:21.

115. Ziebuhr, J., S. Bayer, J. A. Cowley, and A. E. Gorbalenya. 2003. The 3C-like proteinase of an invertebrate nidovirus links coronavirus and potyvirus homologs. *J. Virol.* 77:1415–1426.

116. Ziebuhr, J., E. J. Snijder, and A. E. Gorbalenya. 2000. Virus-encoded proteinases and proteolytic processing in the Nidovirales. *J. Gen. Virol.* 81:853–879.

117. Ziebuhr, J., V. Thiel, and A. E. Gorbalenya. 2001. The auto-catalytic release of a putative RNA virus transcription factor from its polyprotein precursor involves two paralogous papain-like proteases that cleave the same peptide bond. *J. Biol. Chem.* 276:33220–33232.

*Nidoviruses*
Edited by S. Perlman, T. Gallagher, and E. J. Snijder
© 2008 ASM Press, Washington, DC

Chapter 3

# Nidovirus Genome Organization and Expression Mechanisms

PAUL BRITTON AND DAVE CAVANAGH

The order *Nidovirales* comprises three families of viruses with linear single-stranded RNA genomes of positive polarity: the *Coronaviridae,* comprising the two genera *Coronavirus* and *Torovirus,* together with *Arteriviridae* and *Roniviridae.* The nidovirus members have some common features with respect to genome organization, replication, transcription, and translation of gene products. The name *Nidovirales,* derived from the Latin *nidus* for nest, reflects the nested-set arrangement of the subgenomic mRNAs (sg mRNAs) produced by this order of viruses during their replication cycle. The coronaviruses, toroviruses, and roniviruses possess the longest known RNA genomes, ranging from 26 to 32 kb (7, 9, 27, 28, 49, 77, 79), and are related by some common features to the arteriviruses, which have smaller genomes, ranging from 13 to 16 kb (37, 49) (Fig. 1). The coronaviruses are presently divided into three groups. The groupings were based initially on cross-reactivity in neutralization and immunofluorescence assays but more recently on phylogenetic relationships and genome organization. The features of the various coronavirus subgroups are summarized in greater detail in chapters 2, 12, and 15. Nidoviruses replicate in the cytoplasm of an infected cell, although one of the structural proteins, the nucleocapsid (N) protein, for some viruses has been found to be located within the nucleolar region of the nucleus in virus infected cells (25, 56, 111, 113, 142, 153, 156). For general reviews, please see references 42, 43, 77, 90, 125, 126, and 137.

This chapter covers the genome organization and expression mechanisms of the nidoviruses as outlined in the five parts numbered in Fig. 2. Following infection of a susceptible cell by a nidovirus and uncoating of the RNA genome, the first step in a successful replication cycle is the production of the replicase proteins. The nidovirus genomic RNA (gRNA) initially acts as a eukaryotic mRNA for the translation of the replicase proteins. Following synthesis of the replicase proteins, the positive-sense gRNA is copied into negative-sense counterparts which act as templates for the synthesis of new gRNAs. In addition to a negative-sense gRNA, nidoviruses produce a series of negative-sense counterparts of the sg mRNAs. The synthesis of both full-length and subgenome-length negative-sense RNAs is initiated at the 3' end of the gRNA. Synthesis of negative-sense RNAs may terminate at different points along the gRNA template, yielding subgenome-length minus-strand RNAs. Attenuation of minus-strand RNA synthesis occurs at sequences, known as transcription regulatory sequences (TRSs), which are well conserved in a virus type but differ between groups, genera, and families of viruses. Failure to terminate at any of the TRSs results in the synthesis of a full-length negative-sense RNA (or "antigenome"). The negative-sense sgRNAs of coronaviruses and arteriviruses acquire a leader sequence of 65 to 100 nucleotides for coronaviruses but 150 to 210 nucleotides for arteriviruses, copied from the 5' end of the gRNA, as part of the process of discontinuous minus-strand RNA synthesis. The negative-sense sgRNAs act as templates for the synthesis of the positive-sense sgRNAs, which are usually generated in a large excess compared to their negative-sense counterparts. The mechanism for the synthesis of nidovirus sgRNAs is called discontinuous extension of minus-strand RNA (115–118; reviewed in chapter 8 and reference 119).

Toroviruses have two transcription strategies involved in their production of the sg mRNAs. Only the largest sg mRNA, RNA2, contains a leader sequence that is derived from the 5' end of the gRNA and is thought to be added by a mechanism involving discontinuous RNA synthesis, according to the current model, analogous to the method used for sgRNA synthesis for corona- and arteriviruses (148). The other three torovirus sg mRNAs are colinear with the 3' end of the genome and do not contain a 5' leader sequence

**Paul Britton and Dave Cavanagh**  •  Division of Microbiology, Institute for Animal Health, Compton, Newbury, United Kingdom.

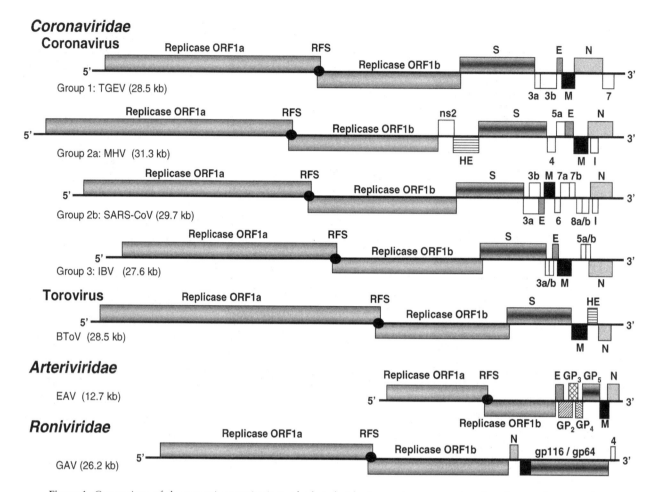

**Figure 1.** Comparison of the genomic organizations of selected nidoviruses. A representative virus from each coronavirus group is included. The genomes are drawn to scale to emphasize that the first two-thirds of most nidovirus genomes consist of the replicase genes, ORF1a and ORF1b. The −1 frameshift site (RFS) for each virus is indicated. The drawings are derived from complete genome sequences of the representative viruses: porcine TGEV, MHV, SARS-CoV, avian IBV, bovine torovirus (BToV), EAV, and GAV. All the nonreplicase nonstructural protein genes are indicated with open boxes. The structural genes are those encoding S, M, E, N, HE, and GP proteins; I is an internal ORF identified in the N protein genes of some group 2 coronaviruses. S is shown as a double-shaded box, with the GP116/GP64 region of GAV having some structural similarities to an S gene. E is indicated as a dark gray box, M as a black box, and N as light gray box. The 5′ end of the GAV GP116/GP64 is colored black, as this part of the gene product is predicted to have triple membrane-spanning motifs that are reminiscent of the M protein. The arterivirus GP5 gene has a function equivalent to that of the S gene in coronaviruses and toroviruses.

derived from the gRNA (128). Analysis of RNA isolated from the lymphoid organ of prawns *(Penaeus monodon)* infected with the ronivirus gill-associated virus (GAV), identified two sg mRNAs, neither of which contained a leader sequence (29). The nidovirus sg mRNAs, with or without a leader sequence, are used for the expression of all viral genes with the exception of the replicase gene products.

## GENOME ORGANIZATION

All nidoviruses have a positive-sense single-stranded RNA genome of 26,200 to 31,500 nucleotides for roniviruses, toroviruses, and coronaviruses

and 12,700 to 15,700 nucleotides for arteriviruses. The genomes are capped at the 5′ end and polyadenylated at the 3′ end (49, 125). In addition, the genomes contain untranslated regions (UTRs) at their 5′ and 3′ termini that play a role in both genome replication and synthesis of sgRNAs.

The overall genomic organization of nidoviruses is 5′-UTR-replicase open reading frame 1a (ORF1a)-replicase ORF1b-nonreplicase genes-3′-UTR-poly(A). However, as illustrated in Fig. 1, apart from the sizes of the various regions, the major differences between the nidovirus genomes involve the type and organization of the nonreplicase genes, with greater differences occurring between the different families of viruses. For example, the coronaviruses and

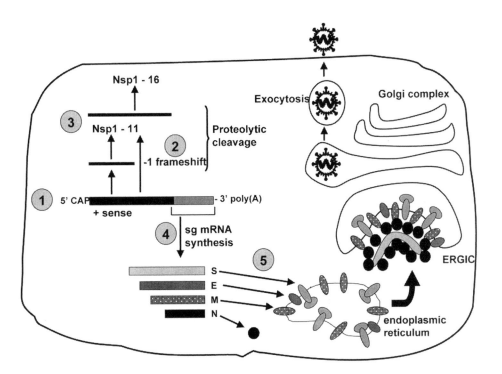

**Figure 2.** Schematic diagram representing the replication cycle of a nidovirus following infection of a susceptible cell. The diagram has five numbered regions that represent the topics discussed in this chapter: (1) gRNA, released from a virus particle that has infected the cell, to highlight that it initially acts as an mRNA for the translation of the replicase proteins; (2) programmed −1 frameshifting event, common to all nidoviruses, for the translation of the replicase polyproteins, pp1a and pp1ab, in differing amounts; (3) another common feature of nidoviruses, proteolytic cleavage of the replicase polyproteins by virus-encoded proteinases; (4) another feature of nidoviruses, the generation of sg mRNAs (mainly polycistronic but functionally monocistronic) for the expression of the other virus-derived proteins; (5) expression strategies used for the translation of the sg mRNAs into virus proteins. Only the sg mRNAs encoding the structural proteins are shown. The rest of the diagram represents the interaction of the virus proteins for assembly and release of virus particles. ERGIC, endoplasmic reticulum-Golgi intermediate compartment.

toroviruses have the general genome organization 5′-UTR-ORF1a-ORF1b-S-E-M-N-3′-UTR-poly(A) (S is spike protein, E is envelope protein, and M is integral membrane protein); it should be noted that no sequence for a protein equivalent to the coronavirus E protein has been identified in a torovirus genome. As can be seen from Fig. 1, the organization and type of genes in the 3′-proximal region of arterivirus and ronivirus genomes are very different.

Nidovirus genomes can be divided into two regions, which vary within and between the different virus families within the order *Nidovirales*. The first region, gene 1, represents approximately two-thirds of the genome (20 kb for coronaviruses, toroviruses, and roniviruses) and encodes the replicase/transcriptase functions of the viruses. Two large polyproteins are expressed from gene 1, polyprotein 1a (pp1a) and pp1ab; pp1ab is expressed in smaller amounts as a C-terminal extension of pp1a following a −1 frameshift event (11–13), as discussed later in this chapter. The second region of a nidovirus genome encodes the structural and accessory proteins. The structure and function of the nidovirus replicase genes are two of

the features that distinguish this family of viruses from other positive-sense RNA viruses. The two replicase polyproteins, pp1a and pp1ab, are cleaved during de novo synthesis by two types of virus-encoded proteinases. There are common motifs within the replicase gene that are shared between the different members of the nidoviruses, characteristic of proteinase, polymerase, helicase, and endoribonuclease activities that are located at specific regions of the replicase gene. The ORF1b region of the replicase encodes two proteins or domains that have not been identified in other RNA virus families, a zinc-binding domain (ZBD) (27, 50, 124, 130, 146) and a uridylate-specific endoribonuclease (NendoU) (6, 60, 104, 129), which can be considered genetic markers for nidoviruses (49).

## 5′ and 3′ UTRs

The 5′ UTR is between 200 and 800 nucleotides long for coronaviruses and toroviruses, 150 and 220 nucleotides for arteriviruses, and 34 nucleotides for the ronivirus GAV. The very 5′ end of the coronavirus and arterivirus UTR is the so-called leader sequence that is attached to all coronavirus and arterivirus sg mRNAs. The sg mRNAs from roniviruses do not contain a leader sequence, possibly reflected in the fact that roniviruses have very short 5′ UTRs. The 3′ UTR is between 200 and 500 nucleotides long for coroviruses and toroviruses, 60 and 150 nucleotides for arteriviruses, and 129 nucleotides for the ronivirus GAV. The nidovirus 3′ UTR occurs after the last functional gene, mainly the N protein gene, except for some group 1 coronaviruses, i.e., transmissible gastroenteritis virus (TGEV), canine coronavirus, and feline coronavirus, which have one or two genes following the N protein gene, and the roniviruses that have a predicted ORF (ORF4) as the last ORF preceding the poly(A) tract (Fig. 1). In addition, some coronaviruses that may be similar to infectious bronchitis virus (IBV) have recently been isolated from a variety of avian species (geese, mallards, and pigeons) that also have one or two ORFs following the N protein gene (17, 65). The IBV 3′ UTR can be divided into two regions; the first is immediately downstream of the N protein gene, is hypervariable among IBV strains, and is deleted from some strains (e.g., M41), whereas the second region is highly conserved (17).

A number of RNA secondary structures have been either predicted or identified within the 5′ and 3′ UTRs of various nidoviruses and play a role in both genome replication and synthesis of sgRNAs. Coronavirus replication signals within the 5′ and 3′ ends of the genomes were initially investigated using defective RNA (D-RNA) genomes; the minimal lengths of these regions necessary for replication of D-RNAs in the presence of helper virus are summarized in Table 1 and include both the UTRs and 5′ and 3′ regions of the genomes containing parts of the replicase and N protein genes, respectively. Three stem-loop structures were predicted in the first 100 nucleotides of the 5′ UTR of the group 3 coronavirus IBV, of which the 5′-proximal stem-loop (I)

showed a high degree of covariance among different IBV strains, providing phylogenetic support for this structure (136). Similar stem-loop structures were predicted in the first 106 nucleotides of the 5′ UTR of the group 2 coronavirus mouse hepatitis virus (MHV), although analysis of a further 120 nucleotides identified two more stem-loop structures (151). Analysis of the first 210 nucleotides of the 5′ UTR of another group 2 coronavirus, bovine coronavirus (BCoV), predicted four stem-loop structures, of which stem-loops III and IV showed phylogenetic conservation and whose structures were supported by enzymatic analysis of a BCoV D-RNA (109, 110). Analysis of the 5′ UTR of the arterivirus equine arteritis virus (EAV) has also led to the prediction of secondary RNA structures, most of which were supported by phylogenetic conservation and by enzymatic and chemical analyses (145).

The nidovirus 3′ UTRs have also been predicted to contain secondary and even tertiary RNA structures that have been implicated in RNA synthesis during the nidovirus replication cycle. A 68-nucleotide stem-loop was identified immediately downstream of the MHV N protein gene (59). A similar structure has been found in the 3′ UTR of the group 3 coronaviruses, IBV (Fig. 3) and turkey coronavirus (TCoV). There is a high degree of covariance among different IBV strains, providing phylogenetic support for this structure (31). Interestingly, in most IBV strains the stem-loop structure is found not adjacent to the end of the N protein gene but at the junction of the hypervariable and conserved regions of the IBV 3′ UTR. However, in IBV strains lacking the hypervariable region, the stem-loop structure is adjacent to the end of the N protein gene. It is possible that the hypervariable region of the IBV 3′ UTR may be the remnants of ORFs that have been lost during evolution of the virus. In addition to the 3′ UTR stem-loop structures, an RNA pseudoknot structure was identified downstream of the stem-loop structure,

Table 1. Minimal lengths of nidovirus terminal 5′ and 3′ regions involved in replication

| Family | Group | Virus | Minimum length (nucleotides) | |
| --- | --- | --- | --- | --- |
| | | | 5′ end | 3′ end |
| Coronaviridae | Coronavirus | | | |
| | 1 | TGEV | 649 | 492 |
| | 2 | MHV | 466 | 436 |
| | 3 | IBV | 544 | 338 |
| | Torovirus | EToV | 607 | 242 |
| Arteriviridae | Arterivirus | EAV | 296 | 354 |
| Roniviridae | Okavirus | GAV | ND[a] | ND |

[a]ND, not determined.

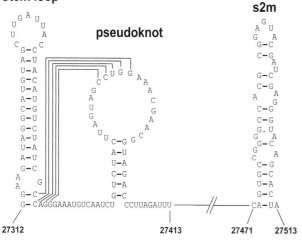

**Figure 3.** RNA structural elements in the 3′ UTR of the avian coronavirus IBV. The IBV 3′ UTR contains three predicted RNA structures, a stem-loop associated with a pseudoknot structure and a second stem-loop structure, s2m. Similar stem-loop and associated pseudoknot RNA structures have been identified in the 3′ UTRs of other coronaviruses. The s2m structure in the IBV 3′ UTR also occurs in the 3′ UTRs of various astroviruses and a human rhinovirus as well as in 3′ UTR of TCoV, another group 3 coronavirus related to IBV. Neither the s2m structure nor its composite sequence was identified in the 3′ UTR of any other non-group 3 coronavirus, until the isolation of SARS-CoV. The numbers represent the IBV genomic nucleotide positions.

initially in the 3′ UTR of BCoV (152). The authors postulated that the pseudoknot functions in the plus strand as a regulatory control element in coronavirus RNA replication. Similar structures were predicted to be present in the 3′ UTRs of other coronaviruses. An example of a coronavirus 3′ UTR stem-loop and pseudoknot structure is shown in Fig. 3. Further analysis of the MHV stem-loop/pseudoknot structures indicated that they may be involved in an RNA switch governing a transition between different steps of virus replication (47, 58). Analysis of the 3′ UTR of the severe acute respiratory syndrome coronavirus (SARS-CoV) identified both a stem-loop and a pseudoknot structure that overlapped in a manner similar to that identified for MHV and BCoV, potentially reflecting some shared common ancestry between the viruses (47). Further work demonstrated that the SARS-CoV 3′ UTR could functionally replace the MHV 3′ UTR, whereas 3′ UTRs from group 1 and 3 coronaviruses could not replace the MHV 3′ UTR, providing more evidence that SARS-CoV shares some common ancestry with group 2 coronaviruses (48). A second stem-loop structure, s2m (Fig. 3), was identified in the 3′ UTR of all IBV strains to date, with remarkable similarity in both sequence and structure to stem-loop structures identified in the genomic 3′ ends of astroviruses isolated from humans, pigs,

sheep, and turkeys and of the picornavirus equine rhinovirus serotype 2 (64). The sequence representing the s2m stem-loop structure was also identified in the 3′ UTR of the coronaviruses isolated from geese, pigeons, and mallard ducks (65). Remarkably, an almost identical sequence and predicted s2m structure was identified in the 3′ UTR of SARS-CoV (89). A 2.7-Å resolution three-dimensional crystal structure of the SARS-CoV s2m RNA element has been determined (112). In addition to the RNA structures identified in the 3′ UTRs of coronaviruses, an octanucleotide motif, 5′-GGAAGAGC-3′, of unknown function has been identified 70 to 80 nucleotides proximal to the poly(A) tract in all coronavirus genomes examined to date.

Analysis of the nidovirus 3′ UTR has been mainly restricted to coronaviruses. However, a kissing-loop interaction has been proposed for the arterivirus porcine reproductive and respiratory virus (PRRSV), between the loops of stem-loop structures in the 3′ UTR and N protein gene, to be crucial for minus-strand RNA synthesis (149). A stem-loop structure in the 3′ UTR of the arterivirus simian hemorrhagic fever virus (SHFV) was identified that contains binding sites for two cellular proteins (88). A stem-loop structure that may act as a recognition sequence for the initiation of minus-strand RNA synthesis has been identified at the 3′-terminal end of the arterivirus EAV 3′ UTR (5). The identification of potential RNA structures involved in RNA synthesis for torovirus or roniviruses has not been published.

## Replicase Gene Region

The overall organization of the nidovirus replicase gene motifs is TM1-TM2-3CL^pro-TM3-RFS-RdRp-ZBD-HEL-NendoU, in which TM represents hydrophobic transmembrane domains, 3CL^pro is a chymotrypsin-like proteinase (so called because it has substrate specificities similar to those of picornavirus 3C proteinases), RFS is the ribosomal frameshift site required for the expression of the ORF1b-encoded proteins, RdRp is the RNA-dependent RNA polymerase, and HEL is a helicase (49). The three hydrophobic TMs have been postulated to be involved in anchoring the replicase proteins to membrane compartments, forming the so-called replication/transcription complexes. In addition, other motifs, representing other replicase gene functions but more related to RNA processing, have been identified in the replicase genes of coronaviruses, toroviruses, and roniviruses, with one (NendoU) also occurring in arteriviruses (129). Although the in vitro functions of some of these gene products have been confirmed, their roles in replication/transcription have yet to be determined. The proteins include a 3′-to-5′ exonucle-ase, a 2′-O-ribose methyl transferase, and a cyclic phosphodiesterase (CPD). The CPD motif (ns2; Fig. 1) was initially identified in the group 2 corona-virus MHV, not as a part of the replicase gene but as ORF2a in sg mRNA2. The CPD motif is present within the replicase gene of toroviruses. A domain corre-sponding to an ADP-ribose 1″-phosphatase (ADRP) has been identified in coronaviruses (nsp3) (129) and toroviruses (38). The activity of bacterially expressed ADRP domains from SARS-CoV (114), human coro-navirus 229E (HCoV-229E [106]), and TGEV (107) has been verified in vitro, and the structure of the SARS-CoV ADRP has been solved (114). The func-tion of the nidovirus replicase proteins is discussed in more detail in chapters 5 and 6.

The replicase polyproteins, pp1a and pp1ab, are proteolytically processed during translation by two types of virus-encoded proteinases, a papain-like pro-teinase (PL^pro) and a chymotrypsin-like viral main proteinase, 3CL^pro, into 16 nonstructural proteins (nsp1 to nsp16) for most coronaviruses, except the avian coronavirus IBV, which lacks nsp1 and encodes 15 (nsp2 to nsp16) replicase gene-derived proteins. Most coronavirus genomes contain two PL^pro domains; however, IBV and SARS-CoV only encode one copy of PL^pro. The arterivirus replicase polypro-teins are cleaved by similar enzymes and may encode up to three PL^pro domains, resulting in 13 or 14 prod-ucts (nsp1 to nsp12), including the products of a recently described internal cleavage of nsp7 (144). Expression of the torovirus replicase gene has been postulated to result in 12 proteins (128). The ronivi-rus replicase gene appears to encode only one pro-teinase, equivalent to 3CL^pro, and potentially gives rise to at least four proteins (27, 49).

## Structural and Accessory Protein Gene Regions

In contrast to the first (replicase) region of the genome, the structural and accessory protein gene products are expressed from a series of sg mRNAs. The sg mRNAs are produced as a "nested" set of RNAs that have different 5′ end regions but common 3′ extensions, often referred to as a 3′-coterminal nested set of sg mRNAs; synthesis of nidovirus sgRNAs is discussed in chapter 8. The sg mRNAs encode the virion structural proteins and, though only for coro-naviruses, a set of small nonstructural proteins, of unknown function, that are referred to as accessory proteins. Synthesis of the coronavirus and arterivirus sgRNAs is via a discontinuous process, as indicated in the introduction. Negative-sense counterparts of the sg mRNAs are synthesized from the full-length gRNA as a result of being attenuated or terminated at

conserved nucleotide sequences, the TRSs, upstream of almost every virus gene. The consequence of the polymerase terminating at TRSs is that the sgRNAs can be produced in unequal amounts, in effect con-trolling the amounts of the gene products. The fac-tors and/or sequences that regulate whether or how the polymerase terminates at a TRS have been an area of considerable interest. Sequences flanking the TRSs have been postulated to play a role in control-ling the levels of sgRNA, as the lengths of identical nucleotides in flanking regions of a TRS and those at the leader junction vary (55). The roles of the flank-ing regions have been investigated for both coronavi-ruses (2, 55, 133, 158) and arteriviruses (35, 98–100, 147). These are discussed in chapter 8.

All of the sg mRNAs, except the smallest RNA, are structurally polycistronic, but they are usually functionally monocistronic. The coronaviruses syn-thesize between five (IBV) and eight (SARS-CoV) sg mRNAs encoding four structural proteins, S, E, M, and N proteins, and various numbers of nonstruc-tural accessory proteins (Fig. 1). The overall gene arrangement of the coronavirus structural proteins is highly conserved, following the pattern hemaggluti-nin-esterase (HE)-S-E-M-N (Fig. 1). Some group 2 coronaviruses, BCoV, HCoV-OC43, and MHV, encode a fifth structural protein, HE (67). Interest-ingly, it has been demonstrated that rearrangement of this gene order is not deleterious to MHV replication (34). Coronaviruses differ with respect to both the number and location of the accessory protein genes (Fig. 1; reviewed in reference 77) and, in some cases, in the mode of translation of the proteins, which is discussed later. The toroviruses synthesize four sg mRNAs and have the gene order S-M-HE-N (Fig. 1), where the HE gene is intact in bovine torovirus but a pseudogene in equine torovirus (37). The arterivi-ruses EAV, PRRSV, and lactate dehydrogenase-elevat-ing virus (LDV) synthesize six sg mRNAs all encoding structural proteins, all of which, apart from the N protein, are M proteins (Fig. 1). The arteriviruses express proteins equivalent to the coronavirus E, M, and N proteins, with either four extra membrane gly-coproteins for EAV/PRRSV/LDV and possibly up to seven extra M proteins for SHFV, of which three may have arisen by a putative triple gene duplication event. Only two viruses, GAV and yellow head virus, which infect prawns, have been assigned to the family *Roniviridae,* and on the basis of sequence analysis their replicase genes have been shown to be related to those of coronaviruses, toroviruses, and arteriviruses. The roniviruses produce two sg mRNAs; both the gene order and the format of the structural proteins are very different from those identified in the genomes of coronaviruses, toroviruses, and arteriviruses. A gene equivalent to the N protein gene of other nidoviruses is found immediately downstream of ORF1b (Fig. 1).

In addition to the structural protein genes, the coronavirus genomes contain a variety of accessory protein genes, which are interspersed among the structural protein genes and which in some group 1 and 3 coronaviruses are found downstream of the N protein gene (Fig. 1). A number of laboratories have shown that the accessory protein genes are not essential for virus replication in vitro, in vivo, or ex vivo (21, 30, 33, 51, 57, 97, 132).

## RIBOSOMAL FRAMESHIFTING

One of the main characteristic features of nidovirus genomes is the large replicase gene region, of which approximately two-thirds of the genome encodes the proteins involved in replication and synthesis of sgRNAs. The replicase polyproteins, pp1a and pp1ab, are produced from the same initiation codon; pp1ab is a C-terminally extended form of pp1a as a result of a programmed −1 ribosomal frameshifting event occurring in the region where ORF1a and ORF1b briefly overlap. As a result, the ORF1b-derived replicase proteins are produced in smaller amounts (approximately 60 to 80% less) than the ORF1a-derived replicase proteins. The ORF1b-encoded proteins include proteins with key replicative functions, like RdRp and HEL activities, indicating that the conserved frameshift mechanism is a way of down-regulating the expression of these enzymes, which must be an important control system in the nidovirus life cycle. Programmed −1 ribosomal frameshifting has been reported to occur during the translation of other viral genes, including those in the animal virus families *Retroviridae* (61), *Astroviridae* (63), *Totiviridae* (150), and *Flaviviridae* (26, 154) and various plant viruses (68, 105).

Completion of the first coronavirus genome sequence, for IBV (7), raised the question of the mechanism for expression of ORF1b. Sequence analysis showed that ORF1a terminated at genome nucleotide 12382 and that ORF1b, which overlapped ORF1a by 42 nucleotides, was in a −1 reading frame with respect to ORF1a (Fig. 4). No sg mRNA equivalent to a size required for the expression of ORF1b had been detected in IBV-infected cells, and no IBV TRS, CUUAACAA, had been identified upstream of ORF1b. Nucleotide comparisons of the IBV ORF1a/1b junction with the *gag-pol* overlap region of Rous sarcoma virus, a region suspected to elicit a frameshifting event (62), showed significant sequence identity. As a result of the conundrum of how ORF1b

is expressed and the above observations, ribosomal frameshifting, as a mechanism for translating ORF1b of the nidovirus replicase genes, was confirmed for IBV (10–12).

The potential for ribosomal frameshifting within the IBV replicase gene was shown by the insertion of the IBV ORF1a/1b overlap region into a reporter gene and testing of the construct for any frameshifting ability in vitro using a transcription and translation system (11). Results indicated that the region mediated a −1 frameshift event, with about 30% of the ribosomes changing frame within the ORF1a/1b overlap region. Subsequently, similar experiments were used to demonstrate ORF1a/1b frameshifting for other coronaviruses (8, 15, 41, 54, 140), a torovirus (equine torovirus) (130), an arterivirus (EAV) (36), and a ronivirus (GAV) (27), with putative frameshift sites identified in other sequenced nidovirus genomes.

Following the demonstration that frameshifting could occur in IBV, potential signals involved in directing the frameshifting events were investigated (12, 14, 16, 134). Potential signals were located within the ORF1a/1b junction (Fig. 4) and comprised two *cis*-acting RNA elements, the first representing the heptameric slippery sequence, UUUAAAC, conforming to the predicted slippery sequence motif XXXYYYN, the site of the actual −1 frameshift (Fig. 4). In vitro experiments showed that 30% of the ribosomes that entered the sequence in the ORF1a frame, U-UUA-AAC, left in the ORF1b frame representing the codons UUU-AAA-C (Fig. 5). Interestingly, all the coronavirus, torovirus, and arterivirus genomes sequenced to date have the same UUUAAAC slippery sequence, apart from EAV, which has the sequence GUUAAAC (Fig. 6). The two ronivirus replicase sequences available, those for GAV and yellow head virus, have AAAUUUU as their slippery sequence. Experiments showed that the slippery sequence was not in itself sufficient to result in the ribosomes' changing frame. A second element required for frameshifting to occur was identified as an RNA pseudoknot (Fig. 4 and 7), an RNA structure composed of two base-paired regions stacked coaxially and connected by two single-stranded loop regions (19, 103). No particular nucleotide sequences were identified as playing an essential role, although the overall shape and predicted stabilities of the structure had to be maintained for efficient frameshifting. The primary role of the RNA pseudoknot is believed to involve slowing down or stalling of the ribosome as it translates through the slippery sequence (Fig. 7), to allow realignment of the decoding tRNA on the mRNA in a new frame (Fig. 5). The RNA pseudoknot has to be positioned within 5 to 7 nucleotides downstream of

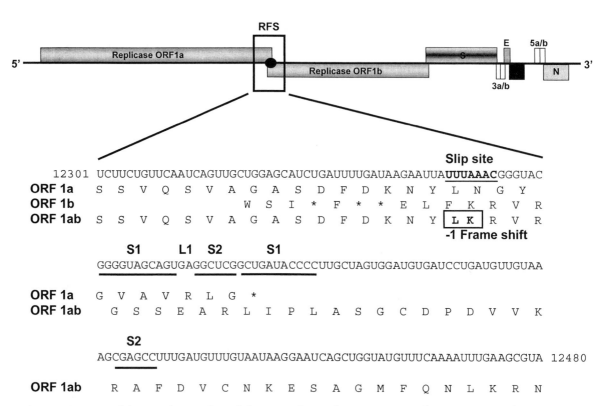

**Figure 4.** Sequence of the IBV ribosome frameshifting site. The top drawing represents the IBV gRNA, as shown in Fig. 1 and 3. The sequence representing the junction of ORF1a and ORF1b, corresponding to the RFS site, is expanded below the gRNA drawing. The numbers represent the IBV genomic nucleotide positions. The positions of the heptameric UUUAAC slip site sequences (in bold) are shown; the nucleotides forming the stem and loop structures of the pseudoknot (shown in Fig. 6) are underlined. The amino acid sequences corresponding to ORF1a, -1b, and -1ab are shown below the IBV genomic nucleotide sequence. ORF1a terminates at nucleotide 12382. There is no initiation codon for ORF1b, but a contiguous amino acid-encoding sequence starts at nucleotide 12342 and terminates at nucleotide 20417. The −1 frameshift site, highlighted in bold, takes place within the coding context of the slip site in which an asparagine residue, encoded by ORF1a, is replaced by a lysine residue, encoded by ORF1b, due to the ribosome moving the RNA back one nucleotide (shown in Fig. 5). As a result of the −1 frameshift event, ORF1a is extended by the ORF1b coding sequence and terminates as an ORF1ab fusion protein at nucleotide 20415. Translation termination codons are marked with asterisks.

the slip site (Fig. 7) for efficient frameshifting (14). The actual mechanism of frameshifting is thought to occur by the simultaneous slippage, into the −1 frame, of two ribosome-bound tRNAs within the aminoacyl and peptidyl sites of the ribosome during the translation of the slippery sequence (44, 52, 86). For the coronavirus IBV the incorporation of the amino acid lysine, derived from the ORF1b sequence, into pp1a, instead of the amino acid asparagine (Fig. 5), results in the generation of pp1ab.

Although the pseudoknot structures cause the ribosome to pause, resulting in the ribosomal aminoacyl and peptidyl sites being placed over the slippery sequence (70), the pausing is insufficient for −1 frameshifting to occur (143); the duration of the pausing does not necessarily correlate with the level of frameshifting observed (70, 101). Crystallographic studies, in concert with molecular studies, indicate that the pseudoknot restricts movement of the RNA during

the tRNA accommodation step of elongation by filling the entrance of the ribosomal mRNA tunnel (40, 102). The restriction on the movement of the RNA can be eased in two ways: (i) unwinding or melting of the pseudoknot, which allows the RNA to move forward, or (ii) movement or slippage of the RNA one nucleotide backwards, resulting in the −1 frameshift (reviewed in reference 52). Cryoelectron microscopy of mammalian 80S ribosomes paused at a coronavirus pseudoknot revealed an intermediate of frameshifting in which it was possible to determine how the pseudoknot interacts with the ribosome (96).

## REGULATION AND EXPRESSION STRATEGIES

The nidovirus gRNAs, like the genomes of other positive-strand RNA viruses, such as the *Flaviviridae* and *Togaviridae*, contain an $m^7GpppN$ cap structure

## Simultaneous Slippage Model

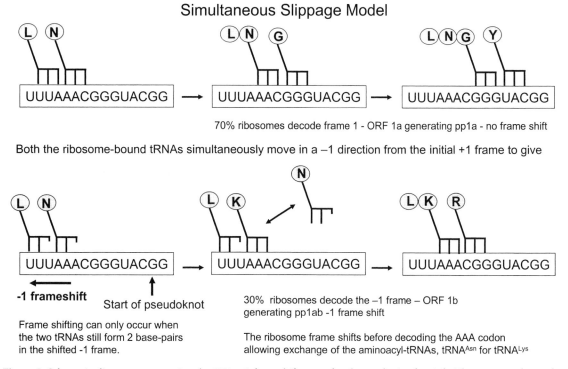

70% ribosomes decode frame 1 - ORF 1a generating pp1a - no frame shift

Both the ribosome-bound tRNAs simultaneously move in a −1 direction from the initial +1 frame to give

**-1 frameshift**   Start of pseudoknot

Frame shifting can only occur when
the two tRNAs still form 2 base-pairs
in the shifted -1 frame.

30% ribosomes decode the −1 frame − ORF 1b
generating pp1ab -1 frame shift

The ribosome frame shifts before decoding the AAA codon
allowing exchange of the aminoacyl-tRNAs, tRNA$^{Asn}$ for tRNA$^{Lys}$

**Figure 5.** Schematic diagram representing the IBV −1 frameshift event for the synthesis of pp1ab. The top part shows the progression of a ribosome along the IBV gRNA over the UUUAAAC slip site. Shown are the positions of the aminoacyl-tRNAs decoding the ORF1a codons, elongation of the polypeptide chain, and decoding of the next codon, resulting in the synthesis of pp1a. The lower part represents a −1 frameshift event as proposed by the simultaneous-slippage model, in which the ribosome-bound aminoacyl-tRNAs are proposed to slip simultaneously one nucleotide to a −1 frame position from their initial frame. Frameshifting can only occur when the anticodons of the two aminoacyl-tRNAs associated with the ribosome and mRNA can still form two base pairs with the RNA in the shifted −1 frame, indicated by the first and second anticodon-codon base pairings, but with disruption of base pairing at the third position. Following the −1 slippage event, aminoacyl-tRNA$^{Asn}$ dissociates from the ribosome complex, before decoding the mRNA, allowing the next aminoacyl-tRNA, aminoacyl-tRNA$^{Lys}$, to move into the aminoacyl site of the ribosome, in which there is full complementarity between the anticodon of the tRNA and codon on the mRNA in the ORF1b frame. The mRNA is then decoded at this position, allowing elongation and movement of the ribosome to the next codon. The IBV replicase gene is now decoded in the ORF1b frame, resulting in translation of pp1ab.

at the 5′ end. This essentially makes the gRNAs into mRNAs, imparting a dual role in which the gRNAs can act as a template for the synthesis of negative-sense RNAs (replication) and for the translation of the replicase polyproteins. As nidovirus gRNAs and sg mRNAs contain a 5′ cap structure, ribosomes are able to initiate translation in a cap-dependent manner.

There is evidence from the analysis of some coronaviruses that translation can be regulated by both viral and host cell factors acting in *trans* or by *cis*-acting sequences within the virus 5′ UTR (122). An interaction of the MHV N protein with the leader sequence has been proposed to stimulate translation of viral mRNAs (138, 139). Interestingly, the IBV N protein was found to be essential for the rescue of IBV from intracellular T7 polymerase-generated infectious RNA in IBV reverse genetics systems (22, 157). N protein was not required for the rescue of infectious viruses in reverse genetics systems for the

coronaviruses HCoV-229E and MHV (141), although the presence of N protein was later shown to increase the efficiency of rescue and replication of HCoV-229E (120) and TGEV (1) replicons. This indicates that the N protein has some effect on coronavirus replication, possibly by protecting the viral RNAs, or involvement in translation of the viral RNAs; however, N protein is dispensable for synthesis of arterivirus RNA (95).

Nidovirus RNAs are very similar to host cell mRNAs and therefore dependent on the availability and activities of host cellular factors, although, as indicated above, various viral RNA elements or virus-encoded products (N protein) may increase the efficiency of translation. Cellular initiation factors bind to the m$^7$GpppN cap structure at the 5′ end of the viral RNAs for recruitment of the 43S ribosomal complex and formation of the 48S ribosomal complex, which scans the mRNA for AUG initiation codons. On encountering the AUG codon, GTP is

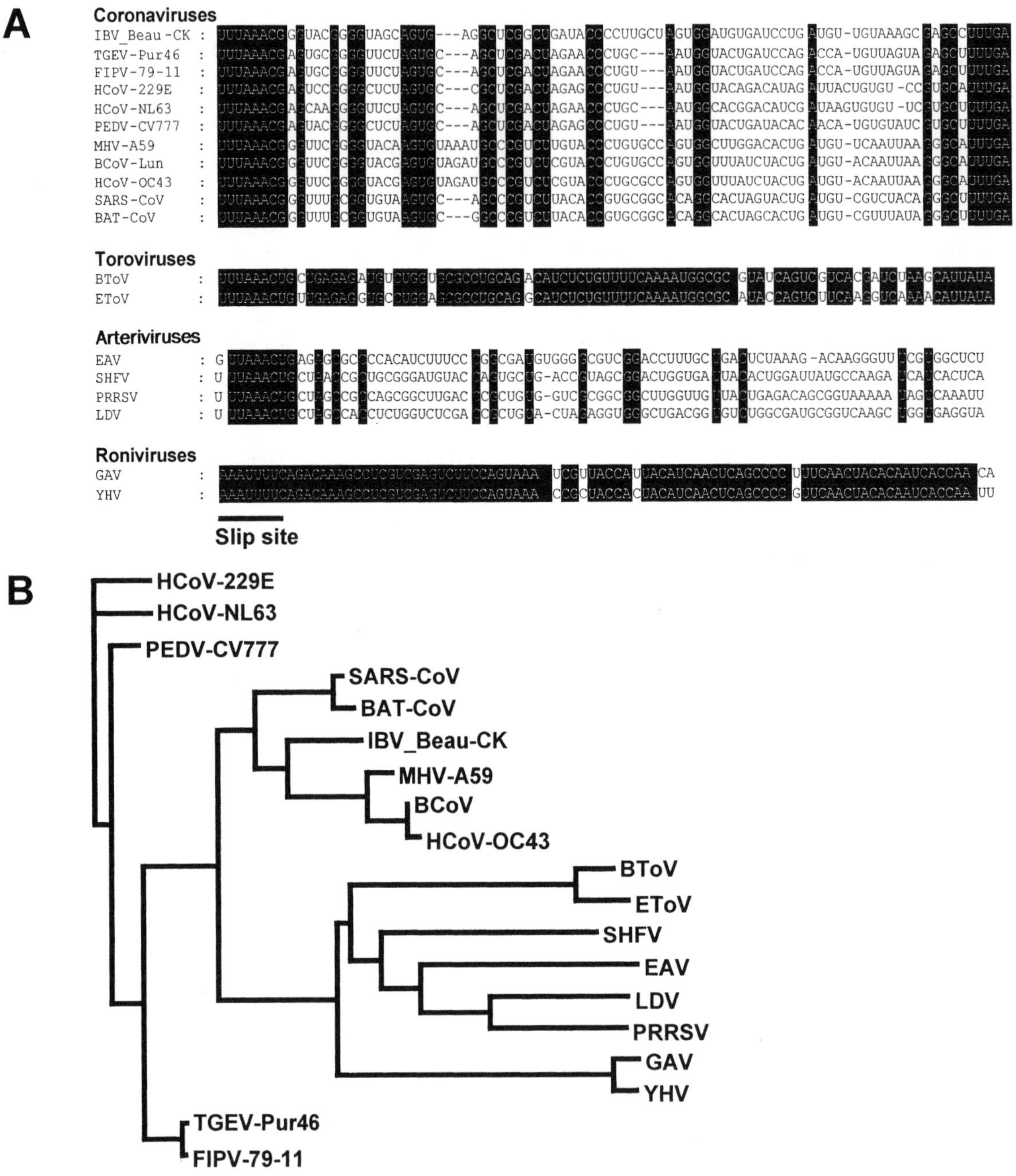

**Figure 6.** Comparison of the nidovirus replicase gene frameshifting sites. (A) Independent alignment of the gRNA sequences, from the slip site, over the pseudoknot sequences of various coronavirus, torovirus, arterivirus, and ronivirus sequences. Nucleotides common within the grouped sequences are highlighted in black. The RFS slip site is underlined. (B) Phylogenetic groupings of all the aligned nidovirus sequences from panel A to demonstrate that as well as falling within their genus groupings, the coronavirus-derived sequences also fall within their groups, indicating that the viruses are related through their RFSs. FIPV, feline infectious peritonitis virus; PEDV, porcine epidemic diarrhea virus; BToV, bovine torovirus; YHV, yellow head virus.

hydrolyzed, initiation factors are released, and the 60S ribosomal subunit binds to the preinitiation complex for formation of the 80S ribosome for translation and elongation of the virus product (reviewed in reference 39). One initiation factor, eukaryotic initiation factor 4E (eIF-4E), the cap-binding protein involved in binding of the initiation complex, can be phosphorylated, which increases its binding to the $m^7$GpppN cap structure at the 5' end of eukaryotic mRNAs and to eIF-G4, usually enhancing translation rates (46). The phosphorylation of eIF-4E plays a regulatory role in translation initiation, and viruses

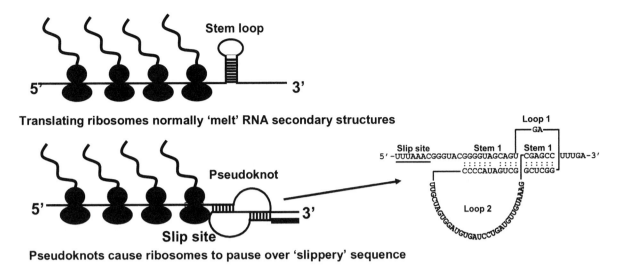

**Figure 7.** Schematic diagram indicating the pausing of ribosomes by a pseudoknot structure. The top part represents ribosomes encountering a stem-loop structure on an mRNA being decoded. The ribosomes may be slowed down by such a structure, but they are able to melt the structure and decode the mRNA. The lower part represents ribosomes encountering a pseudoknot structure with an upstream slip site. Provided the slip site and pseudoknot are separated by no more than 5 to 7 nucleotides, the pausing effect of the pseudoknot can cause a −1 frameshift as illustrated in Fig. 6. The predicted RNA structure of the IBV pseudoknot is shown as an example to highlight the nucleotides forming the slip site and the stem and loop structures.

have utilized this process for controlling host protein synthesis (reviewed in reference 93). Increased phosphorylation of eIF-4E has been observed in cells infected with the coronaviruses MHV (4) and SARS-CoV (92) as a result of the activation of p38 mitogen-activated protein kinase.

## Regulation and Expression of the Replicase Gene

A complexity for the translation of RNAs from viruses with a positive-sense RNA genome is associated with the gRNA, which can act either as an mRNA or as a template for replication. The signals for replication can be in either the 5′ or 3′ UTR or both. Interactions between the 5′ and 3′ ends of the gRNA of some positive-sense RNA viruses have been shown to control the switch between translation and replication (39). As discussed above, the 5′ and 3′ UTRs of the nidovirus genomes contain a variety of RNA structures that may be involved in interactions with viral and cellular proteins. Most studies have involved interactions of proteins with the 3′ UTR of group 2 coronaviruses. For example, the poly(A) tail of MHV and BCoV was found to be an important *cis*-acting signal for replication and was found to bind poly(A)-binding protein (135). Studies using MHV D-RNAs indicated that 466 nucleotides from the 5′ end and 436 nucleotides from the 3′ end of the genome are required for D-RNA replication (69, 81) (Table 1). In addition, both ends of the MHV genome are required for positive-strand synthesis, but only the last 55 nucleotides

are required for synthesis of negative-strand RNA (82). Evidence for interactions between the 5′ and 3′ ends of nidovirus genomes has not been documented. As indicated in the introduction, the 5′ UTRs of the gRNA are between 200 and 800 nucleotides long for coronaviruses and toroviruses and 150 and 220 nucleotides for arteriviruses. Although the 5′ UTRs of coronaviruses and arteriviruses are relatively devoid of initiation codons, a small ORF, the intraleader ORF, coding for 3 to 11 amino acids, is found in the coronavirus 5′ UTRs. These include ORFs of 24 nucleotides, beginning at position 99 in the 209-nucleotide 5′ UTR of MHV-A59 (80); 24 nucleotides, beginning at position 101 in the 210-nucleotide 5′ UTR of BCoV (109); 33 nucleotides, beginning at position 81 in the 293-nucleotide 5′ UTR of HCoV-229E (53); 9 nucleotides, beginning at position 117 in the 313-nucleotide 5′ UTR of TGEV (41); and 33 nucleotides, beginning at position 131 in the 528-nucleotide 5′ UTR of IBV (7). A slightly larger intraleader ORF, of 111 nucleotides, is found beginning at position 14 in the 211-nucleotide 5′ UTR of the arterivirus EAV (66). The intraleader ORF initiation codon was identified as forming part of the stem structure of stem-loop III of the group 2 coronavirus BCoV. The authors indicated that such ORFs may be part of stem-loop structures identified in the 5′ UTRs of other coronaviruses (109). The identification of such ORFs led to the proposal that they may play a role in regulation of translation of the replicase gene from the gRNA (122). Recombinant EAVs in which either the Kozak sequence of the intraleader ORF was optimized or the initiation codon was incapacitated exhibited similar phenotypes but showed reduced replication kinetics, plaque size, and viral yields compared to those of the parental virus (3). It should be noted that inactivation of the EAV intraleader ORF by Molenkamp et al. (94) did not have an effect on virus growth, indicating that the results obtained by Archambault et al. (3) could be due to changes in RNA structure rather than intraleader ORF expression.

## Regulation and Expression of Genes Encoding Structural and Accessory Proteins

The nidovirus nonreplicase proteins, the structural and accessory proteins, are not produced as polyproteins but are expressed from the sg mRNAs. In most cases the cap-dependent mechanism directs translation of the 5′-most ORF from an sg mRNA, which apart from the smallest species are structurally polycistronic but functionally monocistronic. The synthesis of the sg mRNAs is not equimolar, although in most cases the smallest sg mRNA, usually producing the N protein, is produced in the largest amounts. Although the group 1 coronaviruses and some newly identified group 3 coronaviruses have ORFs downstream of the N protein sequence, these smaller sg mRNAs are often produced in much smaller amounts than other sg mRNAs. In effect, a control on the amount of sg mRNA determines the amount of protein produced. Nevertheless, some coronaviruses have more than one ORF translated from a particular sg mRNA. The majority of these are bicistronic, though the group 3 coronavirus IBV and the related TCoV and pheasant coronavirus (PhCoV) express a tricistronic sg mRNA (23, 24, 83, 85).

All coronaviruses identified to date contain at least one functionally bicistronic sg mRNA, some of which are summarized in Table 2. The number and position of the genes expressed from such sg mRNAs vary with the different types and groups of coronaviruses. The group 1 coronaviruses include viruses that have only one functionally bicistronic sg mRNA, for example, TGEV, in which the 3a and 3b genes are expressed from sg mRNA3 (18), and HCoV-229E, in which the 4a and 4b genes are expressed from sg mRNA4 (108). Other group 1 coronaviruses have more than one functionally bi- or tricistronic sg mRNA, for example, feline coronavirus, in which sg mRNA3 has the capacity to express three genes (3a, 3b, and 3c [51, 155]) and sg mRNA7 produces two genes (7a and 7b [32]). In general, the group 2 coronaviruses have only one functionally bicistronic sg mRNA, e.g., sg mRNA5 of MHV, which expresses two genes, 5a and 5b, the latter encoding the E protein (20, 127). SARS-CoV yields three functionally bicistronic sg mRNAs, sg mRNA3, -7, and -8, which produce the 3a and 3b, 7a and 7b, and 8a and 8b proteins, respectively (140). In all the cases described above, the functionally bi- or tricistronic sg mRNAs express two or three ORFs from the 5′ end of the mRNA. However, some type 2 coronaviruses, MHV (45), BCoV (123), and SARS-CoV (140), have a different type of functionally bicistronic sg mRNA to express an I ORF within the N protein gene. The I ORF is in a +1 reading frame located downstream of the N protein gene initiation codon. Recent studies of the structure of the SARS-CoV I ORF (ORF9b) indicated that the protein has a dimeric tent-like β structure with an amphipathic surface and a central hydrophobic cavity that binds lipid molecules (91). The authors indicated that the hydrophobic cavity was likely to be involved in membrane attachment and showed the ORF9b protein to associate with intracellular vesicles.

The group 3 coronaviruses IBV, TCoV, and PhCoV produce a functionally tricistronic sg mRNA3, which encodes the 3a, 3b, and 3c proteins, where the ORF3c product is the E protein (23, 24, 83, 85), and a bicistronic sg mRNA5, which produces the 5a and 5b proteins (23, 24, 84). Arteriviruses also contain a functional bicistronic sg mRNA; the EAV E and glycoprotein 2 (GP2) structural proteins are encoded by two overlapping ORFs, ORF2a and ORF2b, which are both expressed from sg mRNA2 (131).

**Table 2.** Coronavirus sg mRNAs expressing more than one product

| Coronavirus | Group | No. | sg mRNA | Products[a] |
|---|---|---|---|---|
| TGEV | 1 | 1 | 3 | 3a, 3b |
| HCoV-229E | 1 | 1 | 4 | 4a, 4b |
| FCoV | 1 | 2 | 3 and 7 | 3a, 3b, 3c, 7a, 7b |
| MHV | 2a | 2 | 5 and 8 | 5a, 5b (E), N, I |
| SARS-CoV | 2b | 4 | 3, 7, 8, and 9 | 3a, 3b, 7a, 7b, 8a, 8b, N, I |
| IBV | 3 | 2 | 3 and 5 | 3a, 3b, 3c (E), 5a, 5b |
| TCoV | 3 | 2 | 3 and 5 | 3a, 3b, 3c (E), 5a, 5b |
| PhCoV | 3 | 2 | 3 and 5 | 3a, 3b, 3c (E), 5a, 5b |

[a]It should be noted that the nidovirus gRNA is a functionally bicistronic mRNA for the replicase gene (gene 1), but structurally a polycistronic mRNA.

Homologous genes in other arteriviruses, PRRSV, LDV, and SHFV, are also postulated to be expressed from functionally bicistronic sg mRNAs.

The second and third ORFs expressed from the functionally bicistronic and tricistronic sg mRNAs are expressed as independent proteins. The simplest mechanism for the expression of a downstream ORF is leaky scanning (71, 72, 74). The ribosome-scanning model predicts that the efficiency with which a particular ORF is translated depends on its location in the mRNA and the sequence context of the AUG initiation codon (71, 73, 75, 76). In this mechanism, pre-initiation complexes, on encountering the first AUG initiation codon, either form an active 80S ribosome for de novo synthesis of the associated protein or bypass the first AUG codon and continue to scan down the mRNA until they encounter another AUG codon. For leaky scanning to occur, the first AUG codon ideally should have an unfavorable sequence context, allowing a proportion of ribosomes to bypass the first initiation codon and have the opportunity to initiate protein synthesis at a second or third AUG codon with a more favorable sequence context (76). Most of the coronavirus and arterivirus sg mRNAs that are capable of expressing two gene products are believed to do so as a result of leaky scanning. The sequence context of the initiation codons may control the amounts of the proteins produced. In some cases the second ORF may play an important role in the replication cycle of the virus; e.g., MHV ORF5b yields the E protein, a structural protein required for budding of virus particles. The I ORF within the N protein gene of BCoV (121) or MHV (45) is also thought to be produced as the result of leaky scanning. Thus, expression of the MHV E and I proteins as the second products of their sg mRNAs indicates that bicistronic sg mRNAs contribute to controlling the expression of these genes.

Another translation strategy for the control of expression of virus gene products adopted by some viruses, like picornaviruses, is the initiation of the translation of an internal ORF using an internal ribosome entry site (IRES). An IRES element is usually part of a complex RNA structure for cap-independent translation. Its use allows viruses the opportunity to interfere with cap-dependent translation, effectively inhibiting cellular protein synthesis without affecting translation of virus-derived mRNAs. However, as indicated above, coronaviruses, like all members of the nidovirus order, employ the normal eukaryotic cap-dependent strategy for the translation of most virus-derived RNAs.

sg mRNA3 of the avian coronavirus IBV is a tricistronic mRNA, for the 3a, 3b, and 3c proteins; 3c is the E protein. Studies have shown that 3a and 3b are in fact accessory proteins and not required for growth of IBV in cell culture (57). A series of experiments using in vitro-generated RNA transcripts modifying either the Kozak context sequences for the three gene 3 ORFs, expression in the absence of the 5′ cap analog 7-methyl-GTP, introduction of 5′ structures to prevent expression of ORF3a and ORF3b, or expression of the three ORFs downstream of the influenza A virus N protein gene showed that ORF3c was still expressed when the expression of ORF3a and ORF3b had been prevented (85). These observations led the authors to propose that the expression of 3c was being directed by a cap-independent method involving internal initiation that is dependent on the 3ab sequence and that the 3b protein was expressed as the result of leaky scanning using cap-dependent translation. An RNA structure was predicted and proposed to play a role in the internal entry of ribosomes for the translation of ORF3c by Le et al. (78). The proposed coronavirus IRES elements are very different from those identified for picornaviruses; this is not surprising, as the picornavirus IRES elements are for cap-independent translation, whereas coronaviruses must function in concert with cap-dependent translation. If proteins are produced from coronavirus IRES-like elements, there remains the possibility that these may also be expressed from other virus RNAs, gRNA and larger sg mRNAs, which also contain these IRES-like elements and downstream ORFs.

Most of the coronavirus products, apart from the E proteins of MHV and IBV, expressed from the functionally bicistronic or tricistronic sg mRNAs represent small nonstructural genes of unknown function (for reviews, see references 19, 77, and 87). As outlined under "Structural and Accessory Protein Gene Regions," recent work has confirmed that these are accessory proteins and are not required for replication per se. The observation that the synthesis of these products involves a variety of expression "tricks" raises the possibility that they play an important role in the viral replication cycle.

### REFERENCES

1. **Almazan, F., C. Galan, and L. Enjuanes.** 2004. The nucleoprotein is required for efficient coronavirus genome replication. *J. Virol.* **78:**12683–12688.
2. **Alonso, S., A. Izeta, I. Sola, and L. Enjuanes.** 2002. Transcription regulatory sequences and mRNA expression levels in the coronavirus transmissible gastroenteritis virus. *J. Virol.* **76:**1293–1308.
3. **Archambault, D., A. Kheyar, A. A. de Vries, and P. J. Rottier.** 2006. The intraleader AUG nucleotide sequence context is important for equine arteritis virus replication. *Virus Genes* **33:**59–68.
4. **Banerjee, S., K. Narayanan, T. Mizutani, and S. Makino.** 2002. Murine coronavirus replication-induced p38 mitogen-activated protein kinase activation promotes interleukin-6

production and virus replication in cultured cells. *J. Virol.* **76:**5937–5948.

5. Beerens, N., and E. J. Snijder. 2006. RNA signals in the 3′ terminus of the genome of equine arteritis virus are required for viral RNA synthesis. *J. Gen. Virol.* **87:**1977–1983.

6. Bhardwaj, K., L. Guarino, and C. C. Kao. 2004. The severe acute respiratory syndrome coronavirus nsp15 protein is an endoribonuclease that prefers manganese as a cofactor. *J. Virol.* **78:**12218–12224.

7. Boursnell, M. E. G., T. D. K. Brown, I. J. Foulds, P. F. Green, F. M. Tomley, and M. M. Binns. 1987. Completion of the sequence of the genome of the coronavirus avian infectious bronchitis virus. *J. Gen. Virol.* **68:**57–77.

8. Bredenbeek, P. J., C. J. Pachuk, A. F. H. Noten, J. Charite, W. Luytjes, S. R. Weiss, and W. J. M. Spaan. 1990. The primary structure and expression of the second open reading frame of the polymerase gene of the coronavirus MHV-A59—a highly conserved polymerase is expressed by an efficient ribosomal frameshifting mechanism. *Nucleic Acids Res.* **18:**1825–1832.

9. Brian, D. A., and R. S. Baric. 2005. Coronavirus genome structure and replication. *Curr. Top. Microbiol. Immunol.* **287:**1–30.

10. Brierley, I. 1995. Ribosomal frameshifting on viral RNAs. *J. Gen. Virol.* **76:**1885–1892.

11. Brierley, I., M. E. G. Boursnell, M. M. Binns, B. Bilimoria, V. C. Blok, T. D. K. Brown, and S. C. Inglis. 1987. An efficient ribosomal frame-shifting signal in the polymerase encoding region of the coronavirus IBV. *EMBO J.* **6:**3779–3785.

12. Brierley, I., P. Digard, and S. C. Inglis. 1989. Characterization of an efficient coronavirus ribosomal frameshifting signal—requirement for an RNA pseudoknot. *Cell* **57:**537–547.

13. Brierley, I., and F. J. Dos Ramos. 2006. Programmed ribosomal frameshifting in HIV-1 and the SARS-CoV. *Virus Res.* **119:**29–42.

14. Brierley, I., A. J. Jenner, and S. C. Inglis. 1992. Mutational analysis of the "slippery-sequence" component of a coronavirus ribosomal frameshifting signal. *J. Mol. Biol.* **227:**463–479.

15. Brierley, I., and S. Pennell. 2001. Structure and function of the stimulatory RNAs involved in programmed eukaryotic −1 ribosomal frameshifting. *Cold Spring Harbor Symp. Quant. Biol.* **66:**233–248.

16. Brierley, I., N. J. Rolley, A. J. Jenner, and S. C. Inglis. 1991. Mutational analysis of the RNA pseudoknot component of a coronavirus ribosomal frameshifting signal. *J. Mol. Biol.* **220:**889–902.

17. Britton, P., and D. Cavanagh. 2007. Avian coronavirus diseases and infectious bronchitis vaccine development. *In* V. Thiel (ed.), *Coronaviruses: Molecular and Cellular Biology and Diseases.* Caister Academic Press, Norwich, United Kingdom.

18. Britton, P., C. L. Otin, J. M. M. Alonso, and F. Para. 1989. Sequence of the coding regions from the 3.0Kb and 3.9Kb mRNA subgenomic species from a virulent isolate of transmissible gastroenteritis virus. *Arch. Virol.* **105:**165–178.

19. Brown, T. D. K., and I. Brierly. 1995. The coronavirus nonstructural proteins, p. 191–217. *In* S. G. Siddell (ed.), *The Coronaviridae.* Plenum Press, New York, NY.

20. Budzilowicz, C. J., and S. R. Weiss. 1987. In vitro synthesis of two polypeptides from a nonstructural gene of coronavirus mouse hepatitis virus strain A59. *Virology* **157:**509–515.

21. Casais, R., M. Davies, D. Cavanagh, and P. Britton. 2005. Gene 5 of the avian coronavirus infectious bronchitis virus is not essential for replication. *J. Virol.* **79:**8065–8078.

22. Casais, R., V. Thiel, S. G. Siddell, D. Cavanagh, and P. Britton. 2001. Reverse genetics system for the avian coronavirus infectious bronchitis virus. *J. Virol.* **75:**12359–12369.

23. Cavanagh, D., K. Mawditt, M. Sharma, S. E. Drury, H. L. Ainsworth, P. Britton, and R. E. Gough. 2001. Detection of a coronavirus from turkey poults in Europe genetically related to infectious bronchitis virus of chickens. *Avian Pathol.* **30:**355–368.

24. Cavanagh, D., K. Mawditt, D. D. B. Welchman, P. Britton, and R. E. Gough. 2002. Coronaviruses from pheasants *(Phasianus colchicus)* are genetically closely related to coronaviruses of domestic fowl (infectious bronchitis virus) and turkeys. *Avian Pathol.* **31:**81–93.

25. Chen, H., T. Wurm, P. Britton, G. Brooks, and J. A. Hiscox. 2002. Interaction of the coronavirus nucleoprotein with nucleolar antigens and the host cell. *J. Virol.* **76:**5233–5250.

26. Choi, J., Z. Xu, and J.-H. Ou. 2003. Triple decoding of hepatitis C virus RNA by programmed translational frameshifting. *Mol. Cell. Biol.* **23:**1489–1497.

27. Cowley, J. A., C. M. Dimmock, K. M. Spann, and P. J. Walker. 2000. Gill-associated virus of Penaeus monodon prawns: an invertebrate virus with ORF1a and ORF1b genes related to arteri- and coronaviruses. *J. Gen. Virol.* **81:**1473–1484.

28. Cowley, J. A., C. M. Dimmock, K. M. Spann, and P. J. Walker. 2001. Gill-associated virus of Penaeus monodon prawns. Molecular evidence for the first invertebrate nidovirus. *Adv. Exp. Med. Biol.* **494:**43–48.

29. Cowley, J. A., C. M. Dimmock, and P. J. Walker. 2002. Gill-associated nidovirus of Penaeus monodon prawns transcribes 3′-coterminal subgenomic mRNAs that do not possess 5′-leader sequences. *J. Gen. Virol.* **83:**927–935.

30. Curtis, K. M., B. Yount, and R. S. Baric. 2002. Heterologous gene expression from transmissible gastroenteritis virus replicon particles. *J. Virol.* **76:**1422–1434.

31. Dalton, K., R. Casais, K. Shaw, K. Stirrups, S. Evans, P. Britton, T. D. Brown, and D. Cavanagh. 2001. *cis*-Acting sequences required for coronavirus infectious bronchitis virus defective-RNA replication and packaging. *J. Virol.* **75:**125–133.

32. De Groot, R. J., A. C. Andeweg, M. C. Horzinek, and W. J. M. Spaan. 1988. Sequence analysis of the 3′ end of the feline coronavirus FIPV 79-1146 genome: comparison with the genome of porcine coronavirus TGEV reveals large insertions. *Virology* **167:**370–376.

33. de Haan, C. A., P. S. Masters, X. Shen, S. Weiss, and P. J. Rottier. 2002. The group-specific murine coronavirus genes are not essential, but their deletion, by reverse genetics, is attenuating in the natural host. *Virology* **296:**177–189.

34. de Haan, C. A., H. Volders, C. A. Koetzner, P. S. Masters, and P. J. Rottier. 2002. Coronaviruses maintain viability despite dramatic rearrangements of the strictly conserved genome organization. *J. Virol.* **76:**12491–12502.

35. den Boon, J. A., M. F. Kleijnen, W. J. Spaan, and E. J. Snijder. 1996. Equine arteritis virus subgenomic mRNA synthesis: analysis of leader-body junctions and replicative-form RNAs. *J. Virol.* **70:**4291–4298.

36. den Boon, J. A., E. J. Snijder, E. D. Chirnside, A. A. de Vries, M. C. Horzinek, and W. J. Spaan. 1991. Equine arteritis virus is not a togavirus but belongs to the coronavirus like superfamily. *J. Virol.* **65:**2910–2920.

37. de Vries, A. A. F., M. C. Horzinek, P. J. M. Rottier, and R. J. de Groot. 1997. The genome organisation of the Nidovirales: similarities and differences between Arteri-, Toro- and Coronaviruses. *Semin. Virol.* **8:**33–47.

38. Draker, R., R. L. Roper, M. Petric, and R. Tellier. 2006. The complete sequence of the bovine torovirus genome. *Virus Res.* **115:**56–68.

39. Edgil, D., and E. Harris. 2006. End-to-end communication in the modulation of translation by mammalian RNA viruses. *Virus Res.* **119:**43–51.

40. Egli, M., S. Sarkhel, G. Minasov, and A. Rich. 2003. Structure and function of the ribosomal frameshifting pseudoknot RNA from beet western yellow virus. *Helv. Chim. Acta* **86:**1709–1727.

41. Eleouet, J. F., D. Rasschaert, P. Lambert, L. Levy, P. Vende, and H. Laude. 1995. Complete sequence (20 kilobases) of the polyprotein-encoding gene 1 of transmissible gastroenteritis virus. *Virology* **206:**817–822.

42. Enjuanes, L. (ed.). 2005. *Current Topics in Microbiology and Immunology,* vol. 287. *Coronavirus Replication and Reverse Genetics.* Springer, New York, NY.

43. Enjuanes, L., F. Almazan, I. Sola, and S. Zuniga. 2006. Biochemical aspects of coronavirus replication and virus-host interaction. *Annu. Rev. Microbiol.* **60:**211–230.

44. Farabaugh, P. J. 1996. Programmed translational frameshifting. *Microbiol. Rev.* **60:**103–134.

45. Fischer, F., D. Peng, S. T. Hingley, S. R. Weiss, and P. S. Masters. 1997. The internal open reading frame within the nucleocapsid gene of mouse hepatitis virus encodes a structural protein that is not essential for viral replication. *J. Virol.* **71:**996–1003.

46. Gingras, A. C., B. Raught, and N. Sonenberg. 1999. eIF4 initiation factors: effectors of mRNA recruitment to ribosomes and regulators of translation. *Annu. Rev. Biochem.* **68:**913–963.

47. Goebel, S. J., B. Hsue, T. F. Dombrowski, and P. S. Masters. 2004. Characterization of the RNA components of a putative molecular switch in the 3' untranslated region of the murine coronavirus genome. *J. Virol.* **78:**669–682.

48. Goebel, S. J., J. Taylor, and P. S. Masters. 2004. The 3' cis-acting genomic replication element of the severe acute respiratory syndrome coronavirus can function in the murine coronavirus genome. *J. Virol.* **78:**7846–7851.

49. Gorbalenya, A. E., L. Enjuanes, J. Ziebuhr, and E. J. Snijder. 2006. Nidovirales: evolving the largest RNA virus genome. *Virus Res.* **117:**17–37.

50. Gorbalenya, A. E., and E. V. Koonin. 1989. Viral proteins containing the purine NTP-binding sequence pattern. *Nucleic Acids Res.* **17:**8413–8440.

51. Haijema, B. J., H. Volders, and P. J. Rottier. 2004. Live, attenuated coronavirus vaccines through the directed deletion of group-specific genes provide protection against feline infectious peritonitis. *J. Virol.* **78:**3863–3871.

52. Harger, J. W., A. Meskauskas, and J. D. Dinman. 2002. An 'integrated model' of programmed ribosomal frameshifting. *Trends Biochem. Sci.* **27:**448–454.

53. Herold, J., T. Raabe, B. Schelle-Prinz, and S. G. Siddell. 1993. Nucleotide sequence of the human coronavirus 229E RNA polymerase locus. *Virology* **195:**680–691.

54. Herold, J., and S. G. Siddell. 1993. An 'elaborated' pseudoknot is required for high frequency frameshifting during translation of HCV 229E polymerase mRNA. *Nucleic Acids Res.* **21:**5838–5842.

55. Hiscox, J. A., K. L. Mawditt, D. Cavanagh, and P. Britton. 1995. Investigation of the control of coronavirus subgenomic mRNA transcription by using T7-generated negative-sense RNA transcripts. *J. Virol.* **69:**6219–6227.

56. Hiscox, J. A., T. Wurm, L. Wilson, P. Britton, D. Cavanagh, and G. Brooks. 2001. The coronavirus infectious bronchitis virus nucleoprotein localizes to the nucleolus. *J. Virol.* **75:**506–512.

57. Hodgson, T., P. Britton, and D. Cavanagh. 2006. Neither the RNA nor the proteins of open reading frames 3a and 3b of the coronavirus infectious bronchitis virus are essential for replication. *J. Virol.* **80:**296–305.

58. Hsue, B., T. Hartshorne, and P. S. Masters. 2000. Characterization of an essential RNA secondary structure in the 3' untranslated region of the murine coronavirus genome. *J. Virol.* **74:**6911–6921.

59. Hsue, B., and P. S. Masters. 1997. A bulged stem-loop structure in the 3' untranslated region of the genome of the coronavirus mouse hepatitis virus is essential for replication. *J. Virol.* **71:**7567–7578.

60. Ivanov, K. A., T. Hertzig, M. Rozanov, S. Bayer, V. Thiel, A. E. Gorbalenya, and J. Ziebuhr. 2004. Major genetic marker of nidoviruses encodes a replicative endoribonuclease. *Proc. Natl. Acad. Sci. USA* **101:**12694–12699.

61. Jacks, T., H. D. Madhani, F. R. Masiarz, and H. E. Varmus. 1988. Signals for ribosomal frameshifting in the Rous sarcoma virus gag-pol region. *Cell* **55:**447–458.

62. Jacks, T., and H. E. Varmus. 1985. Expression of the Rous sarcoma virus pol gene by ribosomal frameshifting. *Science* **230:**1237–1242.

63. Jiang, B., S. S. Monroe, E. V. Koonin, S. E. Stine, and R. I. Glass. 1993. RNA sequence of astrovirus: distinctive genomic organization and a putative retrovirus-like ribosomal frameshifting signal that directs the viral replicase synthesis. *Proc. Natl. Acad. Sci. USA* **90:**10539–10543.

64. Jonassen, C. M., T. O. Jonassen, and B. Grinde. 1998. A common RNA motif in the 3' end of the genomes of astroviruses, avian infectious bronchitis virus and an equine rhinovirus. *J. Gen. Virol.* **79:**715–718.

65. Jonassen, C. M., T. Kofstad, I. L. Larsen, A. Lovland, K. Handeland, A. Follestad, and A. Lillehaug. 2005. Molecular identification and characterization of novel coronaviruses infecting graylag geese (Anser anser), feral pigeons (Columbia livia) and mallards (Anas platyrhynchos). *J. Gen. Virol.* **86:**1597–1607.

66. Kheyar, A., G. St-Laurent, and D. Archambault. 1996. Sequence determination of the extreme 5' end of equine arteritis virus leader region. *Virus Genes* **12:**291–295.

67. Kienzle, T. E., S. Abraham, B. G. Hogue, and D. A. Brian. 1990. Structure and orientation of expressed bovine coronavirus hemagglutinin-esterase protein. *J. Virol.* **64:**1834–1838.

68. Kim, K. H., and S. A. Lommel. 1994. Identification and analysis of the site of −1 ribosomal frameshifting in red clover necrotic mosaic virus. *Virology* **200:**574–582.

69. Kim, Y.-N., Y. S. Jeong, and S. Makino. 1993. Analysis of cis-acting sequences essential for coronavirus defective interfering RNA replication. *Virology* **197:**53–63.

70. Kontos, H., S. Napthine, and I. Brierley. 2001. Ribosomal pausing at a frameshifter RNA pseudoknot is sensitive to reading phase but shows little correlation with frameshift efficiency. *Mol. Cell. Biol.* **21:**8657–8670.

71. Kozak, M. 1981. Mechanism of mRNA recognition by eukaryotic ribosomes during initiation of protein synthesis. *Curr. Top. Microbiol. Immunol.* **93:**81–123.

72. Kozak, M. 1981. Possible role of flanking nucleotides in recognition of the AUG initiator codon by eukaryotic ribosomes. *Nucleic Acids Res.* **9:**5233–5252.

73. Kozak, M. 1986. Regulation of protein synthesis in virus-infected animal cells. *Adv. Virus Res.* **31:**229–292.

74. Kozak, M. 1986. Bifunctional messenger RNAs in eukaryotes. *Cell* **47:**481–483.

75. Kozak, M. 1987. At least six nucleotides preceding the AUG initiator codon enhance translation in mammalian cells. *J. Mol. Biol.* **196:**947–950.

76. Kozak, M. 1989. The scanning model for translation: an update. *J. Cell Biol.* **108:**229–241.

77. Lai, M. M., and D. Cavanagh. 1997. The molecular biology of coronaviruses. *Adv. Virus Res.* **48:**1–100.

78. Le, S. Y., N. Sonenberg, and J. V. Maizel, Jr. 1994. Distinct structural elements and internal entry of ribosomes in mRNA3

encoded by infectious bronchitis virus. *Virology* **198**:405–411.

79. **Lee, H.-J., C.-K. Shieh, A. E. Gorbalenya, E. V. Koonin, N. La Monica, J. Tuler, A. Bagdzhadzhyan, and M. M. C. Lai.** 1991. The complete sequence (22 kilobases) of murine coronavirus gene 1 encoding the putative proteases and RNA polymerase. *Virology* **180**:567–582.

80. **Leparc-Goffart, I., S. T. Hingley, M. M. Chua, X. Jiang, E. Lavi, and S. R. Weiss.** 1997. Altered pathogenesis of a mutant of the murine coronavirus MHV-A59 is associated with a Q159L amino acid substitution in the spike protein. *Virology* **239**:1–10.

81. **Lin, Y. J., and M. M. C. Lai.** 1993. Deletion mapping of a mouse hepatitis virus defective interfering RNA reveals the requirement of an internal and discontiguous sequence for replication. *J. Virol.* **67**:6110–6118.

82. **Lin, Y. J., C. L. Liao, and M. M. Lai.** 1994. Identification of the *cis*-acting signal for minus-strand RNA synthesis of a murine coronavirus: implications for the role of minus-strand RNA in RNA replication and transcription. *J. Virol.* **68**:8131–8140.

83. **Liu, D. X., D. Cavanagh, P. Green, and S. C. Inglis.** 1991. A polycistronic mRNA specified by the coronavirus infectious bronchitis virus. *Virology* **184**:531–544.

84. **Liu, D. X., and S. C. Inglis.** 1992. Identification of two new polypeptides encoded by mRNA5 of the coronavirus infectious bronchitis virus. *Virology* **186**:342–347.

85. **Liu, D. X., and S. C. Inglis.** 1992. Internal entry of ribosomes on a tricistronic mRNA encoded by infectious bronchitis virus. *J. Virol.* **66**:6143–6154.

86. **Lopinski, J. D., J. D. Dinman, and J. A. Bruenn.** 2000. Kinetics of ribosomal pausing during programmed −1 translational frameshifting. *Mol. Cell. Biol.* **20**:1095–1103.

87. **Luytjes, W.** 1995. Coronavirus gene expression: genome organisation and protein synthesis, p. 33–54. *In* S. G. Siddell (ed.), *The Coronaviridae.* Plenum Press, New York, NY.

88. **Maines, T. R., M. Young, N. N. Dinh, and M. A. Brinton.** 2005. Two cellular proteins that interact with a stem loop in the simian hemorrhagic fever virus 3′ (+)NCR RNA. *Virus Res.* **109**:109–124.

89. **Marra, M. A., S. J. Jones, C. R. Astell, R. A. Holt, A. Brooks-Wilson, Y. S. Butterfield, J. Khattra, J. K. Asano, S. A. Barber, S. Y. Chan, A. Cloutier, S. M. Coughlin, D. Freeman, N. Girn, O. L. Griffith, S. R. Leach, M. Mayo, H. McDonald, S. B. Montgomery, P. K. Pandoh, A. S. Petrescu, A. G. Robertson, J. E. Schein, A. Siddiqui, D. E. Smailus, J. M. Stott, G. S. Yang, F. Plummer, A. Andonov, H. Artsob, N. Bastien, K. Bernard, T. F. Booth, D. Bowness, M. Czub, M. Drebot, L. Fernando, R. Flick, M. Garbutt, M. Gray, A. Grolla, S. Jones, H. Feldmann, A. Meyers, A. Kabani, Y. Li, S. Normand, U. Stroher, G. A. Tipples, S. Tyler, R. Vogrig, D. Ward, B. Watson, R. C. Brunham, M. Krajden, M. Petric, D. M. Skowronski, C. Upton, and R. L. Roper.** 2003. The genome sequence of the SARS-associated coronavirus. *Science* **300**:1399–1404.

90. **Masters, P. S.** 2006. The molecular biology of coronaviruses. *Adv. Virus Res.* **66**:193–292.

91. **Meier, C., A. R. Aricescu, R. Assenberg, R. T. Aplin, R. J. C. Gilbert, J. M. Grimes, and D. I. Stuart.** 2006. The crystal structure of ORF-9b, a lipid binding protein from the SARS coronavirus. *Structure* **14**:1157–1165.

92. **Mizutani, T., S. Fukushi, M. Saijo, I. Kurane, and S. Morikawa.** 2004. Phosphorylation of p38 MAPK and its downstream targets in SARS coronavirus-infected cells. *Biochem. Biophys. Res. Commun.* **319**:1228–1234.

93. **Mohr, I.** 2006. Phosphorylation and dephosphorylation events that regulate viral mRNA translation. *Virus Res.* **119**:89–99.

94. **Molenkamp, R., S. Greve, W. J. Spaan, and E. J. Snijder.** 2000. Efficient homologous RNA recombination and requirement for an open reading frame during replication of equine arteritis virus defective interfering RNAs. *J. Virol.* **74**:9062–9070.

95. **Molenkamp, R., H. van Tol, B. C. Rozier, Y. van Der Meer, W. J. Spaan, and E. J. Snijder.** 2000. The arterivirus replicase is the only viral protein required for genome replication and subgenomic mRNA transcription. *J. Gen. Virol.* **81**:2491–2496.

96. **Namy, O., S. J. Moran, D. I. Stuart, R. J. Gilbert, and I. Brierley.** 2006. A mechanical explanation of RNA pseudoknot function in programmed ribosomal frameshifting. *Nature* **441**:244–247.

97. **Ortego, J., I. Sola, F. Almazan, J. E. Ceriani, C. Riquelme, M. Balasch, J. Plana, and L. Enjuanes.** 2003. Transmissible gastroenteritis coronavirus gene 7 is not essential but influences in vivo virus replication and virulence. *Virology* **308**:13–22.

98. **Pasternak, A. O., A. P. Gultyaev, W. J. Spaan, and E. J. Snijder.** 2000. Genetic manipulation of arterivirus alternative mRNA leader-body junction sites reveals tight regulation of structural protein expression. *J. Virol.* **74**:11642–11653.

99. **Pasternak, A. O., W. J. Spaan, and E. J. Snijder.** 2004. Regulation of relative abundance of arterivirus subgenomic mRNAs. *J. Virol.* **78**:8102–8113.

100. **Pasternak, A. O., E. van den Born, W. J. M. Spaan, and E. J. Snijder.** 2003. The stability of the duplex between sense and antisense transcription-regulating sequences is a crucial factor in arterivirus subgenomic mRNA synthesis. *J. Virol.* **77**:1175–1183.

101. **Plant, E. P., and J. D. Dinman.** 2006. Comparative study of the effects of heptameric slippery site composition on −1 frameshifting among different eukaryotic systems. *RNA* **12**:666–673.

102. **Plant, E. P., K. L. M. Jacobs, J. W. Harger, A. Meskauskas, J. L. Jacobs, J. L. Baxter, A. N. Petrov, and J. D. Dinman.** 2003. The 9-Å solution: how mRNA pseudoknots promote efficient programmed −1 ribosomal frameshifting. *RNA* **9**:168–174.

103. **Pleij, C. W. A., and L. Bosch.** 1989. RNA pseudoknots: structure, detection and prediction. *Methods Enzymol.* **180**:289–303.

104. **Posthuma, C. C., D. D. Nedialkova, J. C. Zevenhoven-Dobbe, J. H. Blokhuis, A. E. Gorbalenya, and E. J. Snijder.** 2006. Site-directed mutagenesis of the nidovirus replicative endoribonuclease NendoU exerts pleiotropic effects on the arterivirus life cycle. *J. Virol.* **80**:1653–1661.

105. **Prufer, D., E. Tacke, J. Schmitz, B. Kull, A. Kaufmann, and W. Rohde.** 1992. Ribosomal frameshifting in plants: a novel signal directs the −1 frameshift in the synthesis of the putative viral replicase of potato leafroll luteovirus. *EMBO J.* **11**:1111–1117.

106. **Putics, A., W. Filipowicz, J. Hall, A. E. Gorbalenya, and J. Ziebuhr.** 2005. ADP-ribose-1″-monophosphatase: a conserved coronavirus enzyme that is dispensable for viral replication in tissue culture. *J. Virol.* **79**:12721–12731.

107. **Putics, A., A. E. Gorbalenya, and J. Ziebuhr.** 2006. Identification of protease and ADP-ribose 1″-monophosphatase activities associated with transmissible gastroenteritis virus non-structural protein 3. *J. Gen. Virol.* **87**:651–656.

108. **Raabe, T., and S. Siddell.** 1989. Nucleotide sequence of the human coronavirus HCV 229E mRNA 4 and mRNA 5 unique regions. *Nucleic Acids Res.* **17**:6387.

109. **Raman, S., P. Bouma, G. D. Williams, and D. A. Brian.** 2003. Stem-loop III in the 5′ untranslated region is a *cis*-acting element in bovine coronavirus defective interfering RNA replication. *J. Virol.* **77**:6720–6730.

110. **Raman, S., and D. A. Brian.** 2005. Stem-loop IV in the 5′ untranslated region is a *cis*-acting element in bovine coronavirus defective interfering RNA replication. *J. Virol.* **79:** 12434–12446.

111. **Reed, M. L., B. K. Dove, R. M. Jackson, R. Collins, G. Brooks, and J. A. Hiscox.** 2006. Delineation and modelling of a nucleolar retention signal in the coronavirus nucleocapsid protein. *Traffic* **7:**1–16.

112. **Robertson, M. P., H. Igel, R. Baertsch, D. Haussler, M. Ares, and W. G. Scott.** 2005. The structure of a rigorously conserved RNA element within the SARS virus genome. *PLoS Biol.* **3:**e5.

113. **Rowland, R. R., R. Kerwin, C. Kuckleburg, A. Sperlich, and D. A. Benfield.** 1999. The localisation of porcine reproductive and respiratory syndrome virus nucleocapsid protein to the nucleolus of infected cells and identification of a potential nucleolar localisation signal sequence. *Virus Res.* **64:** 1–12.

114. **Saikatendu, K. S., J. S. Joseph, V. Subramanian, T. Clayton, M. Griffith, K. Moy, J. Velasquez, B. W. Neuman, M. J. Buchmeier, R. C. Stevens, and P. Kuhn.** 2005. Structural basis of severe acute respiratory syndrome coronavirus ADP-ribose-1″-phosphate dephosphorylation by a conserved domain of nsP3. *Structure* **13:**1665–1675.

115. **Sawicki, D., T. Wang, and S. Sawicki.** 2001. The RNA structures engaged in replication and transcription of the A59 strain of mouse hepatitis virus. *J. Gen. Virol.* **82:**385–396.

116. **Sawicki, S. G., and D. L. Sawicki.** 1995. Coronaviruses use discontinuous extension for synthesis of subgenome-length negative strands. *Adv. Exp. Med. Biol.* **380:**499–506.

117. **Sawicki, S. G., and D. L. Sawicki.** 1998. A new model for coronavirus transcription. *Adv. Exp. Med. Biol.* **440:**215–219.

118. **Sawicki, S. G., and D. L. Sawicki.** 2005. Coronavirus transcription: a perspective. *Curr. Top. Microbiol. Immunol.* **287:** 31–55.

119. **Sawicki, S. G., D. L. Sawicki, and S. G. Siddell.** 2007. A contemporary view of coronavirus transcription. *J. Virol.* **81:** 20–29.

120. **Schelle, B., N. Karl, B. Ludewig, S. G. Siddell, and V. Thiel.** 2005. Selective replication of coronavirus genomes that express nucleocapsid protein. *J. Virol.* **79:**6620–6630.

121. **Senanayake, S. D., and D. A. Brian.** 1997. Bovine coronavirus I protein synthesis follows ribosomal scanning on the bicistronic N mRNA. *Virus Res.* **48:**101–105.

122. **Senanayake, S. D., and D. A. Brian.** 1999. Translation from the 5′ untranslated region (UTR) of mRNA 1 is repressed, but that from the 5′ UTR of mRNA 7 is stimulated in coronavirus-infected cells. *J. Virol.* **73:**8003–8009.

123. **Senanayake, S. D., M. A. Hofmann, J. L. Maki, and D. A. Brian.** 1992. The nucleocapsid protein gene of bovine coronavirus is bicistronic. *J. Virol.* **66:**5277–5283.

124. **Seybert, A., C. C. Posthuma, L. C. van Dinten, E. J. Snijder, A. E. Gorbalenya, and J. Ziebuhr.** 2005. A complex zinc finger controls the enzymatic activities of nidovirus helicases. *J. Virol.* **79:**696–704.

125. **Siddell, S., J. Ziebuhr, and E. J. Snijder.** 2005. Coronaviruses, toroviruses and arteriviruses, p. 823–856. *In* B. W. J. Mahy and V. ter Meulen (ed.), *Topley and Wilson's Microbiology and Microbial Infections: Virology.* Hodder Arnold, London, United Kingdom.

126. **Siddell, S. G. (ed.).** 1995. *The Coronaviridae.* Plenum, New York, NY.

127. **Skinner, M. A., D. Ebner, and S. G. Siddell.** 1985. Coronavirus MHV-JHM mRNA 5 has a sequence arrangement which potentially allows translation of a second, downstream open reading frame. *J. Gen. Virol.* **66:**581–592.

128. **Smits, S. L., E. J. Snijder, and R. J. de Groot.** 2006. Characterization of a torovirus main proteinase. *J. Virol.* **80:**4157–4167.

129. **Snijder, E. J., P. J. Bredenbeek, J. C. Dobbe, V. Thiel, J. Ziebuhr, L. L. Poon, Y. Guan, M. Rozanov, W. J. Spaan, and A. E. Gorbalenya.** 2003. Unique and conserved features of genome and proteome of SARS-coronavirus, an early split-off from the coronavirus group 2 lineage. *J. Mol. Biol.* **331:**991–1004.

130. **Snijder, E. J., J. A. den Boon, P. J. Bredenbeek, M. C. Horzinek, R. Rijnbrand, and W. Spaan.** 1990. The carboxyl-terminal part of the putative Berne virus polymerase is expressed by ribosomal frameshifting and contains sequence motifs which indicate that toro- and coronaviruses are evolutionarily related. *Nucleic Acids Res.* **18:**4535–4542.

131. **Snijder, E. J., H. van Tol, K. W. Pedersen, M. J. Raamsman, and A. A. de Vries.** 1999. Identification of a novel structural protein of arteriviruses. *J. Virol.* **73:**6335–6345.

132. **Sola, I., S. Alonso, S. Zuniga, M. Balasch, J. Plana-Duran, and L. Enjuanes.** 2003. Engineering the transmissible gastroenteritis virus genome as an expression vector inducing lactogenic immunity. *J. Virol.* **77:**4357–4369.

133. **Sola, I., J. L. Moreno, S. Zuniga, S. Alonso, and L. Enjuanes.** 2005. Role of nucleotides immediately flanking the transcription-regulating sequence core in coronavirus subgenomic mRNA synthesis. *J. Virol.* **79:**2506–2516.

134. **Somogyi, P., A. J. Jenner, I. Brierley, and S. C. Inglis.** 1993. Ribosomal pausing during translation of an RNA pseudoknot. *Mol. Cell. Biol.* **13:**6931–6940.

135. **Spagnolo, J. F., and B. G. Hogue.** 2000. Host protein interactions with the 3′ end of bovine coronavirus RNA and the requirement of the poly(A) tail for coronavirus defective genome replication. *J. Virol.* **74:**5053–5065.

136. **Stirrups, K., K. Shaw, S. Evans, K. Dalton, D. Cavanagh, and P. Britton.** 2000. Leader switching occurs during the rescue of defective RNAs by heterologous strains of the coronavirus infectious bronchitis virus. *J. Gen. Virol.* **81:** 791–801.

137. **Sturman, L. S., and K. V. Holmes.** 1983. The molecular biology of coronaviruses. *Adv. Virus Res.* **28:**35–112.

138. **Tahara, S. M., T. A. Dietlin, C. C. Bergmann, G. W. Nelson, S. Kyuwa, R. P. Anthony, and S. A. Stohlman.** 1994. Coronavirus translational regulation: leader affects mRNA efficiency. *Virology* **202:**621–630.

139. **Tahara, S. M., T. A. Dietlin, G. W. Nelson, S. A. Stohlman, and D. J. Manno.** 1998. Mouse hepatitis virus nucleocapsid protein as a translational effector of viral mRNAs. *Adv. Exp. Med. Biol.* **440:**313–318.

140. **Thiel, V., K. A. Ivanov, A. Putics, T. Hertzig, B. Schelle, S. Bayer, B. Weissbrich, E. J. Snijder, H. Rabenau, H. W. Doerr, A. E. Gorbalenya, and J. Ziebuhr.** 2003. Mechanisms and enzymes involved in SARS coronavirus genome expression. *J. Gen. Virol.* **84:**2305–2315.

141. **Thiel, V., and S. G. Siddell.** 2005. Reverse genetics of coronaviruses using vaccinia virus vectors. *Curr. Top. Microbiol. Immunol.* **287:**199–227.

142. **Tijms, M. A., Y. van der Meer, and E. J. Snijder.** 2002. Nuclear localization of nonstructural protein 1 and nucleocapsid protein of equine arteritis virus. *J. Gen. Virol.* **83:** 795–800.

143. **Tu, C., T. H. Tzeng, and J. A. Bruenn.** 1992. Ribosomal frameshifting impeded at a pseudoknot required for frameshifting. *Proc. Natl. Acad. Sci. USA* **89:**8636–8640.

144. **van Aken, D., J. Zevenhoven-Dobbe, A. E. Gorbalenya, and E. J. Snijder.** 2006. Proteolytic maturation of replicase polyprotein pp1a by the nsp4 main proteinase is essential for

equine arteritis virus replication and includes internal cleavage of nsp7. *J. Gen. Virol.* **87**:3473–3482.

145. **van den Born, E., A. P. Gultyaev, and E. J. Snijder.** 2004. Secondary structure and function of the 5'-proximal region of the equine arteritis virus RNA genome. *RNA* **10**:424–437.

146. **van Dinten, L. C., H. van Tol, A. E. Gorbalenya, and E. J. Snijder.** 2000. The predicted metal-binding region of the arterivirus helicase protein is involved in subgenomic mRNA synthesis, genome replication, and virion biogenesis. *J. Virol.* **74**:5213–5223.

147. **van Marle, G., L. C. van Dinten, W. J. Spaan, W. Luytjes, and E. J. Snijder.** 1999. Characterization of an equine arteritis virus replicase mutant defective in subgenomic mRNA synthesis. *J. Virol.* **73**:5274–5281.

148. **van Vliet, A. L. W., S. L. Smits, P. J. M. Rottier, and R. J. de Groot.** 2002. Discontinuous and non-discontinuous subgenomic RNA transcription in a nidovirus. *EMBO J.* **21**:6571–6580.

149. **Verheije, M. H., R. C. Olsthoorn, M. V. Kroese, P. J. Rottier, and J. J. Meulenberg.** 2002. Kissing interaction between 3' noncoding and coding sequences is essential for porcine arterivirus RNA replication. *J. Virol.* **76**:1521–1526.

150. **Wang, A. L., H. M. Yang, K. A. Shen, and C. C. Wang.** 1993. Giardiavirus double-stranded RNA genome encodes a capsid polypeptide and a gag-pol-like fusion protein by a translation frameshift. *Proc. Natl. Acad. Sci. USA* **90**:8595–8599.

151. **Wang, Y., and X. Zhang.** 2000. The leader RNA of coronavirus mouse hepatitis virus contains an enhancer-like element for subgenomic mRNA transcription. *J. Virol.* **74**:10571–10580.

152. **Williams, G. D., R. Y. Chang, and D. A. Brian.** 1999. A phylogenetically conserved hairpin-type 3' untranslated region pseudoknot functions in coronavirus RNA replication. *J. Virol.* **73**:8349–8355.

153. **Wurm, T., H. Chen, T. Hodgson, P. Britton, G. Brooks, and J. A. Hiscox.** 2001. Localization to the nucleolus is a common feature of coronavirus nucleoproteins, and the protein may disrupt host cell division. *J. Virol.* **75**:9345–9356.

154. **Xu, Z., J. Choi, T. S. Yen, W. Lu, A. Strohecker, S. Govindarajan, D. Chien, M. J. Selby, and J. Ou.** 2001. Synthesis of a novel hepatitis C virus protein by ribosomal frameshift. *EMBO J.* **20**:3840–3848.

155. **Yamanaka, M., T. Crisp, R. Brown, and B. Dale.** 1998. Nucleotide sequence of the inter-structural gene region of feline infectious peritonitis virus. *Virus Genes* **16**:317–318.

156. **You, J., B. K. Dove, L. Enjuanes, M. L. DeDiego, E. Alvarez, G. Howell, P. Heinen, M. Zambon, and J. A. Hiscox.** 2005. Subcellular localization of the severe acute respiratory syndrome coronavirus nucleocapsid protein. *J. Gen. Virol.* **86**:3303–3310.

157. **Youn, S., J. L. Leibowitz, and E. W. Collisson.** 2005. In vitro assembled, recombinant infectious bronchitis viruses demonstrate that the 5a open reading frame is not essential for replication. *Virology* **332**:206–215.

158. **Zúñiga, S., I. Sola, S. Alonso, and L. Enjuanes.** 2004. Sequence motifs involved in the regulation of discontinuous coronavirus subgenomic RNA synthesis. *J. Virol.* **78**:980–994.

Chapter 4

# Genetics and Reverse Genetics of Nidoviruses

Damon J. Deming and Ralph S. Baric

The order *Nidovirales* includes a broad group of mammalian, avian, and crustacean viruses grouped among the families *Coronaviridae, Arteriviridae,* and *Roniviridae.* The family *Coronaviridae* is further divided into the genera *Coronavirus* and *Torovirus.* Although nidoviruses differ significantly in genome size, sequence, virion morphology, and host range specificity, they are grouped within the same order due to several shared traits (reviewed in reference 38). All nidoviruses are positive-stranded RNA viruses with large replicase domains (designated open reading frame 1a [ORF1a] and ORF1b) which are functionally conserved and carried at the 5′ end of the genome. Translation of the replicase polyprotein is regulated by a ribosomal frameshift event which directs the expression of either an ORF1a or an ORF1a/b full-length polyprotein and is, in turn, proteolytically processed by virally encoded proteases. Another characteristic unique to nidoviruses is that several structural and nonstructural ORFs are encoded downstream of the replicase polyprotein and expression of these ORFs is mediated by a 3′ coterminal nested set of subgenomic RNAs which are generated by a unique strategy of discontinuous transcription. There are significant differences between the genome sizes of nidoviruses, which range from the smallest arterivirus genomes of ~13 kb to the largest coronavirus genomes of ~31 kb. The genomes of nidoviruses are infectious, and virus replication is initiated as the genome is delivered to the cytoplasm and the replicase is translated by the host cell ribosomes. For many nidoviruses, a typically narrow host range is dictated by the highly specific interaction between the glycoprotein spike displayed on the virion and a particular receptor on permissive cells. However, characteristic high mutation and recombination rates allow these viruses to evolve to infect new cells and expand beyond their normal tissue tropisms and host range limitations.

The desire to improve our understanding of nidovirus biology is largely motivated by the fact that several of these viruses present a direct threat to the health of humans or economically valuable species. Several coronaviruses are associated with human respiratory diseases with pathologies ranging in severity from relatively benign cold-like illnesses to fatal pneumonia. Human coronavirus 229E (HCoV-229E) and HCoV-OC43 were identified in the 1960s and have been attributed as the cause of ~15% of common colds in the winter (42, 74). In 2003, a new coronavirus was identified (26, 54) which emerged from its animal reservoir (40, 80), most likely bats (60, 65, 83), and was associated with the severe acute respiratory syndrome (SARS) epidemic that resulted in approximately 8,000 confirmed infections and nearly 800 deaths (44). Since then, two new coronaviruses have been isolated from humans exhibiting lower respiratory infections, NL63 (31, 32, 106) and HKU1 (117). Significant agricultural losses are also associated with all three families of nidoviruses. These infections are usually respiratory or enteric in nature, and the economic loss associated with them is the result of lower animal weights, neonatal mortality, or abortion in infected animals. Transmissible gastroenteritis virus (TGEV) (87), porcine epidemic diarrhea virus (81), infectious bronchitis virus (IBV) (12), and bovine coronavirus (BCoV) (67) are some of the coronaviruses effecting loss in the swine, poultry, and bovine industries, respectively. Arteriviruses, including equine arteritis virus (EAV) and porcine reproductive and respiratory syndrome virus (PRRSV) (77), and bovine torovirus (119), porcine torovirus (53), and equine torovirus (115) similarly afflict their respective livestock. Disease is not limited to mammals

**Damon J. Deming** • Department of Microbiology and Immunology, School of Medicine, University of North Carolina, Chapel Hill, NC 27599. **Ralph S. Baric** • Department of Epidemiology, School of Public Health, University of North Carolina, Chapel Hill, NC 27599.

and avians, with the roniviruses gill-associated virus and yellow head virus linked to outbreaks and mortality in prawn farms (22, 23).

Nidovirus reverse-genetics systems are needed to better understand aspects of their complex replication strategy, pathogenesis, and mechanisms of host range expansion, and for the generation of safe and effective antiviral therapies. Among nidoviruses, the small size of the arterivirus genome, ranging from 13 to 16 kb, allowed for the rapid development of molecular clones as early as 1997 (107). In contrast, the large size of the coronavirus genome and *Escherichia coli*-associated toxicity of regions within the polymerase gene delayed the construction of stable full-length cDNA templates until 2000 (2, 124). Fortunately for coronavirus research, several independent strategies were successfully employed to overcome these limitations and develop viable reverse-genetics systems.

## NIDOVIRUSES AS EMERGING AND REEMERGING INFECTIOUS AGENTS

It is estimated that 73% of human emerging and reemerging infectious diseases—caused by pathogens rapidly increasing in incidence, expanding in geographic range, or extending infection into new host species—are due to zoonotic pathogens that have bridged the species barrier (55, 120). Accounting for approximately 37% of all emerging and reemerging pathogens, RNA viruses are well represented (120). In order for a virus to expand outside of its normal host range, the virus must evolve the capacity to interact with novel cellular factors and adapt to evade or usurp mechanisms which normally function to ablate virus entry, replication, or transmission in a new host species. An emerging virus requires the opportunity to interact with a new prospective host and must possess molecular mechanisms with which to adapt and replicate efficiently within the hostile cellular environment. Coronaviruses, with a very broad distribution among several different animal species, many of which maintain close contact to humans, and its replication, characterized by high mutation and recombination rates, exemplify the nidovirus' ability to exploit opportunities to interact with a new potential host by rapidly evolving to changing cellular environments and selective pressures. As the majority of existing research into the mechanisms of nidovirus host range expansion has been completed in coronavirus models, this section is devoted to coronaviruses.

With established reservoirs in humans and wild and domesticated animals, nidoviruses have ample

opportunity to make contact with species normally outside of their restricted host range. Many animals hosting coronaviruses are maintained close to other animals or humans, including equine, swine, bovine, canine, feline, and avian species. Several examples of emergent viruses illustrate the coronaviruses' ability to expand their host range. For instance, porcine epidemic diarrhea virus, an economically significant cause of severe swine gastroenteritis in Europe and Asia, is closely related to HCoV-229E and is believed to be the result of transmission from humans to swine (8, 28, 81). BCoV is believed to have passed into dogs (30) and several species of ruminants, including elk (69), waterbuck, sambar deer, and white-tailed deer populations (104), and has been associated with at least one enteric infection in humans (43, 128). Close genetic and antigenic similarities between the group 2 coronaviruses BCoV, HCoV-OC43, and porcine hemagglutinating encephalomyelitits virus suggest that they may have only recently diverged from a common ancestor (112).

A recent, and certainly the most extensively studied, example of an emerging coronavirus is SARS coronavirus (SARS-CoV) (26, 54). The epidemic strains of SARS-CoV likely evolved from a zoonotic strain (40, 80) naturally maintained in bats (60, 65, 83). It is believed that the virus crossed into humans through use of a liaison species such as the palm civet or raccoon dog infected while maintained in live-animal markets and housed close to several other species, including bats (40, 66, 91, 105). Seropositivity in wet-market animal handlers who were asymptomatic for signs of SARS suggests that a SARS-CoV-like progenitor virus was also transmitted to humans during their contact with animals in live-animal markets (14, 40, 84). Indeed, antibody detected in a low percentage (1.8%) of people in Hong Kong 2 years prior to the epidemic suggests that a coronavirus antigenically similar to SARS-CoV had infringed into human populations at least 2 years before the virus evolved to efficiently replicate within a human host, cause disease, and spread from human to human (130).

Although nidoviruses have the opportunity to expand their host ranges, they must be able to exploit such opportunities by rapidly adapting to fit their new host. The potential for a virus to successfully adapt to a new host and cross the species barrier involves its ability to adapt to new or changing cellular environments and find new ecological niches via genetic variation (68). Nidoviruses can explore the range of viable genetic variation through two mechanisms, mutation and recombination. As viruses dependent upon a polymerase lacking a proofreading mechanism, nidovirus replication introduces approximately $10^{-3}$ to $10^{-5}$ errors per replication cycle (71), or, on average, three mutations per newly synthesized coronavirus genome. This high rate of error, common for RNA viruses, leads to the generation of genetically variable quasispecies and contributes to their genetic plasticity and ability to rapidly evolve in response to changes in selective pressure (7, 47, 111). Comparing the sequences of SARS-CoV isolated from live-market animals and early human cases to those of the late epidemic virus illustrates the rapid adaptation and high mutation rate, estimated at approximately two mutations per human passage (between $1.8 \times 10^{-6}$ and $8.3 \times 10^{-6}$ nucleotide substitutions per site per day or ~0.17 mutation per genome per day) (17, 108, 122).

There is reason to believe that at least one other strain of SARS-CoV-like coronavirus emerged independently in the human population, although not as successfully as the Urbani and related epidemic strains. Between 16 December 2003 and 8 January 2004, four patients were independently hospitalized in Guangdong Province, China, and confirmed to have SARS. The patients did not have contact with each other or other SARS patients, presented with mild symptoms, and likely contacted SARS-CoV through contact with infected animals from live markets. Analysis of these isolates showed sequence similarity closer to zoonotic strains than that of the initial epidemic strain (17, 49, 78, 91). Given the facts that they were found relatively late in the epidemic and their sequences did not appear to derive from the epidemic strain, these viruses likely represent an independent reemergence of SARS-CoV in human populations. Spread within human populations was limited at least in part due to the rapid response of the Chinese government to quarantine infected individuals and cull animals suspected of harboring the virus.

A second aspect of nidovirus biology that contributes to remarkably high adaptability to new hosts is a high rate of recombination. In 1995, the high recombination rates of coronaviruses were recognized as an aspect of replication that would likely contribute to these viruses' becoming significant threats as emerging pathogens (3). Coronaviruses, along with arteriviruses and toroviruses, rely on homologous recombination as part of their replication strategy to generate subgenomic RNAs from which to express their downstream genes. Using complementation of temperature-sensitive mutants, the homologous recombination frequency for the entire genome of the coronavirus mouse hepatitis virus (MHV) was found to approach 20% or more (4, 58). Increasingly higher recombination rates progressing from the 5' to 3' end have been observed in coronaviruses (33, 34) and arteriviruses (76) and likely

reflect the increasing number of subgenomic RNA strands formed during replication with which recombination can occur (33, 70). Indeed, the highly successful targeted RNA recombination system described below relies upon frequent recombination between these RNA templates.

New strains of nidoviruses have been generated by recombination in the lab and in the wild. For example, recombination resulting in viable viruses has been illustrated in experimentally infected animals with murine coronaviruses (50) and in eggs infected with IBV (52). Evidence of homologous recombination between coronaviruses in the wild has also been found in novel strains of IBV (13, 48, 57, 62), including recombination involving vaccine strains (63, 90, 113). Several examples of recombination within feline coronaviruses (FCoVs) are also known. A novel serotype of FCoV, serotype II, is the result of a double-recombination event with canine coronavirus (46). Four FCoV type II strains have been isolated and shown to be the result of independent recombination events (109), suggesting that such events are not rare. SARS-CoV has been postulated to have derived from multiple recombination events among progenitor coronaviruses of all three groups, although these analyses are more tenuous (85, 92, 93, 129). Critics of the recombinatory-origin hypothesis for SARS-CoV point out that these studies assume that there is ample opportunity for recombination events to occur between divergent groups, which often exhibit distinctly different host ranges, and that there are few data supporting extensive recombination of this sort (36, 72). Evidence of recombination between genotypes of the recently identified HKU-1 may be the first demonstration of coronavirus recombination in humans (118).

Nidoviruses have the opportunity and ability to quickly adapt to new cellular environments, and ongoing studies are devoted to understanding the molecular changes mapping to expanded tropisms. Coronavirus specificity is primarily mediated at binding and entry by the interaction of the spike glycoprotein (S glycoprotein) with specific cellular receptors (10, 21, 24), as transfection of genomic RNA (64, 75) or expression of the appropriate receptor (24, 29, 101, 121) allows infection of otherwise nonpermissive cells. Not surprisingly, many of the mutations critical for extended host ranges are the result of mutations within the S glycoprotein.

Several in vitro models have been developed for studying the molecular determinants of coronavirus cross-species expansion. Persistent cell models were developed to identify the genetic alterations that arise in coronaviruses that occur as the viruses and their host cells coevolve in response to long-term persistent

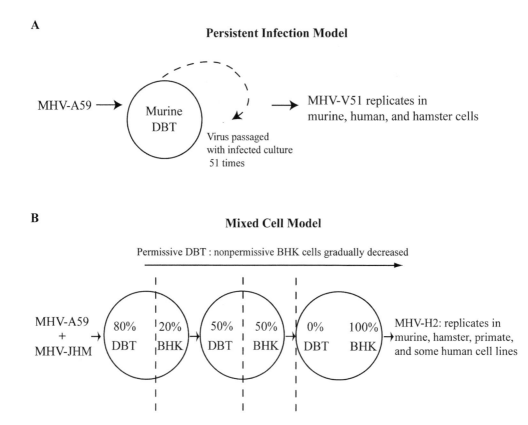

**Figure 1.** In vitro models for studying the mechanisms of coronavirus host range expansion. (A) Persistent-infection model. DBT cells were persistently infected with MHV-A59. After 51 passages, the mutant MHV-V51 was isolated and shown to have expanded its tropism from murine cells to include human and hamster cultures. (B) Mixed-cell model. Mixed cultures of DBT and BHK cells were coinfected with the A59 and JHM strains of MHV. Over successive passages, the ratio of the permissive DBT cells was diminished relative to the nonpermissive BHK cells until the culture consisted only of BHK cells. The MHV-H2 isolate was shown to have adapted to the changing selective pressures and evolved an extended host range tropism.

infections (5, 15). In one such model, murine astrocytoma cells (DBT cells) were infected with MHV-A59 and serially passaged 51 times for 210 days (Fig. 1A). Persistent infection of these cultures by MHV establishes a selective pressure whereby the DBT host cells decrease their ability to be infected by down-regulating expression of the MHV receptor, carcinoembryonic antigen adhesion molecule (CEACAM) (15, 21). In response, the virus adapts by changing the S protein gene to alter receptor specificity (15). After 51 passages, changes within the mutant MHV-V51's S glycoprotein significantly enhanced the susceptibility of hamster and human cells to viral infection (15) by increasing the protein's ability to bind the nonmurine CEACAM orthologues that are poorly recognized by wild-type MHV S protein (21). A similar persistent-infection model using MHV and murine 17Cl1 cells resulted in an extended-host-range mutant with affinity for hamster, feline, bovine, rat, monkey, and human cells (88, 89, 97, 98). Such changes occurring over the course of a persistent infection could account for the altered tropism of viruses such as FCoV. The

lethal form of FCoV, feline infectious peritonitis virus (FIPV), likely arises from accumulated mutations within the S protein gene which alter the tropism of the persistent low-virulence feline enteric coronavirus from cells of the enteric tract to macrophages (86, 110).

A second in vitro model of coronavirus host range expansion uses persistently infected mixed cell cultures (Fig.1B). A culture containing two cell lines, MHV-permissive DBT cells and the resistant Syrian baby hamster kidney (BHK) cells, were infected with MHV-A59, MHV-JHM, or a combination of the two strains. Although both MHV strains are unable to infect BHK cells, MHV-JHM causes receptor-independent fusion between DBT and BHK cells in vitro and was included in the study for its potential to enhance virus evolution and adaptation to the BHK cells (6, 35). The ratio of permissive DBT cells to resistant BHK cells was changed with passage, with the relative amount of DBT cells decreased. This pressure for the virus to adapt to infect the normally nonpermissive cells produced an extended-host-range mutant in the case of the coinfected cultures. After more than 200 days of serial passage in cultures with an ever-diminishing ratio of DBT cells, virus derived from the dually infected MHV-A59–MHV-JHM cultures was able to efficiently infect BHK cells. The relaxation in tropism specificity also gave the virus the ability to infect primate and some human cultures while it retained efficient replication in murine cell lines, further emphasizing the plasticity of the coronavirus genome and demonstrating the ability of these viruses to rapidly evolve new and expanded tropisms.

Although the models used to examine host range expansion emphasize the importance of the S glycoprotein-receptor interaction as determinants for host range expansion, there is evidence that mutation of other regions of the genome can also be critical for the successful adaptation of a coronavirus to a new host. In an attempt to develop a mouse model for HCoV-229E, mice were genetically engineered to express the viral receptor human aminopeptidase N (hAPN) (101, 116). Although primary cell cultures established from the animals were permissive to infection, the mice from which the cultures had been derived were not (116). However, mice expressing hAPN and deficient in *Stat1* were highly susceptible to infection with a strain of HCoV-229E that was passaged in *hAPN*$^{+/+}$ cells (59), indicating that the virus was not able to replicate within an immunocompetent animal despite successful binding and entry. A second example showing that other viral factors can affect virulence independently of S protein-mediated binding and entry was reported when SARS-CoV accessory protein 6 was expressed from MHV-JHM. Expression of SARS-CoV protein 6 from an attenuated MHV-JHM genome increased the virulence in mice and resulted in a lethal disease. SARS-CoV protein 6 was not associated with the virion of the chimeric virus, had no effect upon the expression or processing of S protein, and did not alter virion assembly, maturation, or release. Instead, the enhanced replication was due to a direct increase in RNA replication and, subsequently, protein synthesis (82, 96).

## NIDOVIRUS REVERSE-GENETICS SYSTEMS

Reverse-genetics systems allow viral genomes to be directly manipulated and linked to a given phenotype. The development of reverse-genetics systems sparked a revolution in nidovirus research, significantly contributing to the understanding of gene function and factors that regulate transcription, replication, pathogenesis, assembly, and release. The first

nidovirus reverse-genetics system was developed by Paul Masters in 1992 based on a targeted recombination system that matured to allow for the ready manipulation of the 3′ most ~10 kb of the genome. However, this system did not allow modification to most of the replicase gene, which makes up nearly two-thirds of the viral genome. Modification of the replicase genes required the development of a full-length-cDNA-based infectious clone. An infectious clone provides a cDNA template which can be manipulated by standard molecular biological techniques to alter the viral genome sequence. Virus is generated from the full-length cDNA copy of the viral genome by either a "DNA launch" or "RNA launch" (Fig. 2). In the DNA launch, a cytomegalovirus (CMV) promoter is engineered at the 5′ end of the full-length cDNA genome, which is then transfected into the host cell. RNA is transcribed by the host cell and the infectious RNA genome is exported into the cytoplasm, where viral replication occurs normally. The RNA launch is achieved through use of an in vitro transcription reaction using T7 or SP6 RNA polymerases which begin transcription at an engineered promoter sequence at the 5′ end of the viral sequence. The synthesized RNA is then electroporated into the host cell, where infection begins in the cytoplasm.

Although an infectious DNA clone for EAV was reported in 1997, attempts to develop a system for coronaviruses were complicated by the large genome size and cDNA instability when amplified in bacterial vectors. Eventually, stable coronavirus infectious cDNA systems were developed by overcoming the amplification difficulties by one of three different approaches. One strategy, and the first to yield the successful generation of infectious virus from a full-length infectious clone, made use of highly stable bacterial artificial chromosomes. The second strategy disrupted toxic regions encoded within the cDNA copy of the viral genome by separating the clone into contiguous fragments in multiple bacterial plasmids. The full-length cDNA clone was then reconstructed by excising the viral cDNA from the bacterial plasmids and ligating them together in vitro. A more recently described approach cloned the full-length genome into poxvirus vectors. All three of these systems, targeted RNA recombination, full-length infectious cDNA expressed in stable amplification systems, and infectious clones amplified as multicomponent cDNAs, are currently used in research and have relative strengths.

### Targeted RNA Recombination

The first nidovirus genetics approach was developed for MHV, the prototypic coronavirus (reviewed

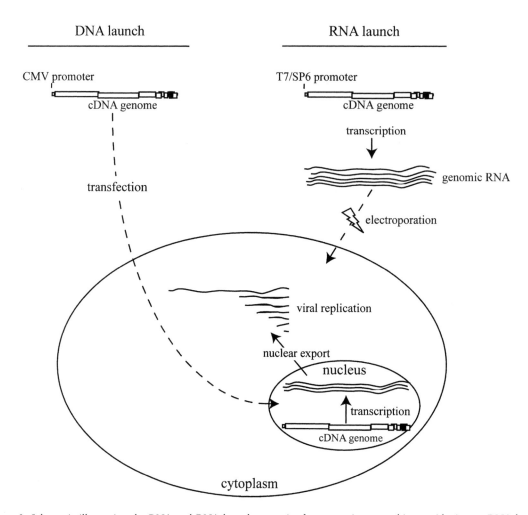

**DNA launch**

**RNA launch**

**Figure 2.** Schematic illustrating the DNA and RNA launch strategies for generating recombinant nidoviruses. DNA launch requires that the full-length cDNA copy of the viral genome be delivered to the nucleus of the cell by transfection. Once there, the host cell's transcriptional machinery drives infectious transcripts from a CMV promoter engineered at the 5′ end of the nidovirus genome cDNA. The viral RNA is exported from the nucleus to the cytoplasm, where replication occurs. RNA launches begin with an in vitro transcription of infectious synthetic RNA using T7 or SP6 RNA polymerase. The RNA is electroporated into the cytoplasm of the cell, where infection begins.

in reference 73). Recognizing the difficulty in developing full-length 30-kb molecular clones, the targeted RNA recombination approach takes advantage of the high rate of recombination which occurs during coronavirus replication. The system relied upon a recombination event to transfer genes from a donor construct to a recipient viral genome, followed by selection conditions which efficiently promoted and amplified the replication of recombinants over the parent genome (Fig. 3). The earliest version of the system relied upon a temperature-sensitive mutant genome recipient, Alb4, which contained a mutation in the nucleocapsid protein (N protein) gene that allows normal replication at permissive temperatures (<34°C) but becomes severely attenuated at higher, or nonpermissive, temperatures (~39°C). Donor RNA encoded wild-type N protein. Successful recombination transferred donor

RNA lacking the thermolabile mutation to the host genome, and the resulting recombinants were capable of efficient growth, and plaqued efficiently, at the nonpermissive temperature. Recombinant viruses were selected on the basis of plaque size when grown at the nonpermissive temperature.

Several improvements have been made to the system since its original conception over a decade ago. The original iteration of the targeted RNA recombination system was limited to the production of robust viruses, since selection was based on the comparison of growth fitness at the nonpermissive temperature. In the case of genetic manipulations resulting in viruses attenuated at the nonpermissive temperature, whether due to their own temperature sensitivity or simply to a loss of growth fitness in general, selection was lost. The target size of the portion

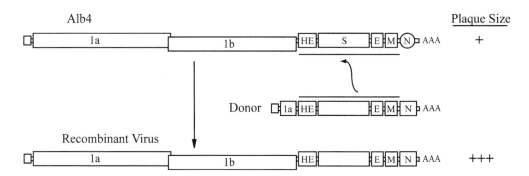

**Figure 3.** Initial version of the targeted recombination reverse-genetics system for coronaviruses. Alb4, which contains a mutation in the N protein gene (circle), produced a limited number of small plaques at the nonpermissive temperature. Following transfection of subgenomic RNA7 and infection of Alb4, RNA recombinants are generated that result in wild-type plaque phenotypes. This process requires the integration of the wild-type N protein gene (square) and is evidenced by large plaques that can easily be distinguished from Alb4. HE, hemagglutinin-esterase; E, envelope protein; M, membrane protein; AAA, poly-A tail.

of the genome amenable to mutagenesis was mostly limited to the N protein gene located at the 3' end of the genome. These limitations were overcome by taking advantage of the narrow host ranges of certain coronaviruses. A chimeric donor virus was engineered which expressed the ectodomain of the S glycoprotein, which determines receptor specificity, of FIPV fused with the C-terminal membrane-spanning domain of the MHV S glycoprotein, encoded within the MHV genetic background (56) (Fig. 4). The chimeric feline MHV (fMHV) was able to grow on feline cell lines, while wild-type MHV could not, confirming previous data that argued that the S glycoprotein was a principal determinant of coronavirus host range. More importantly, fMHV was unable to infect cells derived from mice which are permissive to MHV. However, following successful recombination with a

donor construct containing the MHV S protein gene, the recombinant virus simultaneously lost the ability to infect feline cells and gained the ability to infect murine cells. This system provided a powerful positive selection step (i.e., growth on murine cells) which readily allowed for the isolation of attenuated mutant viruses. Later improvements to the targeted recombinant system include a mechanism for limiting multiple recombination events, especially at the 3' end of the genome. Although successful recombination required that a functional copy of the MHV S protein gene be selected, there was the possibility of further recombination events occurring (Fig. 5). These are particularly likely when an introduced mutation at the 3' end of the genome is debilitating. The likelihood of multiple recombination events occurring was reduced by moving the N protein gene of the recipient

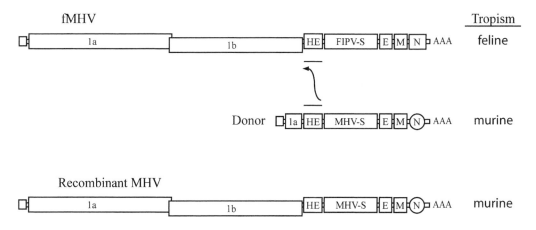

**Figure 4.** Improved targeted recombination system using cell specificity for selection of successful recombinants. A chimeric virus of MHV, fMHV, expressing the S protein gene of FIPV infects feline cells transfected with RNA from a donor molecule, pMH54, bearing a mutated MHV N protein gene (circle). Successfully recombined virus is screened by growth on murine cells, which requires the incorporation of the MHV S protein gene from the donor molecule. HE, hemagglutinin-esterase; E, envelope protein; M, membrane protein; AAA, poly-A tail.

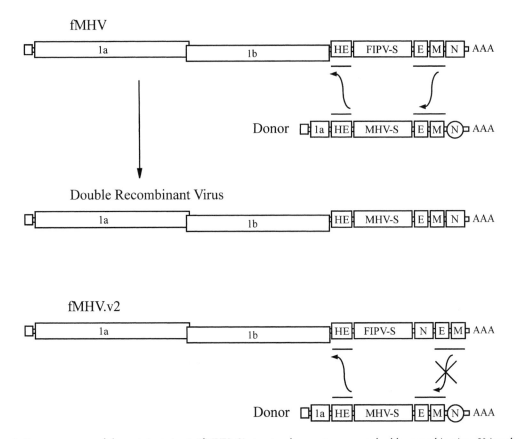

**Figure 5.** Rearrangement of the recipient virus's (fMHV.v2) structural genes to prevent double recombination. Using the targeted recombination system, it is possible to get a double recombinant which results in the exclusion of the desired mutation (in the N protein gene [circle]) while integrating the MHV S protein gene needed for replicating on murine cells. By rearranging the position of the MHV N and membrane protein (M protein) genes on the recipient chimeric virus, the opportunity for double recombination is reduced since a second event is likely to exclude at least part of one of the major structural genes encoding a protein critical for replication. HE, hemagglutinin-esterase; E, envelope protein; AAA, poly-A tail.

virus immediately downstream of the S protein gene. In the event of a second recombination event downstream of the S protein gene, the resulting virus would lack the essential N protein gene and would be unviable. The targeted recombination system has been extended to MHV-JHM (79), TGEV, and FIPV and remains a powerful technology for altering genes and sequence motifs at the 3′-most 10 kb of the genome (41).

### Infectious cDNA Clones

#### Arterivirus

In 1997, a full-length cDNA clone of EAV from which infectious RNA was transcribed was developed (107). The development of the cDNA infectious clone allowed manipulation of any part of the 12.7-kb genome. In contrast to the difficulties experienced with developing cDNA copies of other nidoviruses, the full-length EAV clone is stable in bacterial

vectors and can be amplified and purified by standard laboratory techniques. Recombinant EAV was generated by RNA launch (Fig. 2): a T7 RNA polymerase promoter was cloned upstream of the cDNA of the viral genome which was used to synthesize infectious RNA in vitro. RNA is then transfected or electroporated into permissive cells, and progeny virus is generated.

Infectious clones of other arteriviruses, including the 15.2-kb Lelystad virus (LV) isolate (75), the highly virulent PRRSV isolate p129 (61), and PRRSV isolate VNSL 97-7895 (103), were constructed using a similar strategy. Like the EAV infectious clone, these arterivirus clones are stable in bacteria, although the LV cDNA clone made use of a low-copy-number bacterial vector to overcome reported stability issues. Another PRRSV infectious clone was also expressed in the low-copy-number bacterial artificial chromosome (BAC) system (18), although it is not clear if the choice to use the highly stable BAC system was based on a lack of stability in other bacterial amplification vectors.

## CORONAVIRUS INFECTIOUS CLONES

### BAC System

The first full-length cDNA infectious clone of a coronavirus was that of TGEV and was accomplished by the stepwise reconstruction of the full genomic cDNA from a defective interfering (DI) minigenome (2). The final missing fragment of the TGEV genome, which caused instability in standard bacterial vectors, was added in the last step. The full-length cDNA was transferred to a BAC, which attains a high degree of stability by maintaining a very low plasmid copy number (no more than two copies per cell) (2). Recombinant viruses were generated via DNA launch. That is, the full-length genomic cDNA was transfected directly into cells and RNA was transcribed from within the nucleus of a cell from a CMV promoter located upstream of the viral sequence. Notably, the majority of viral RNA does not undergo deleterious mRNA splicing as it is exported from the nucleus of transfected cells into the cytoplasm, where the virus replicates normally. After detection of some level of cDNA instability in the TGEV BAC system upon extensive passage in *Escherichia coli,* the system was further stabilized by inserting an intron into the regions of the ORF1 gene responsible for the toxicity in bacteria (37). The introns, which disrupt the viral sequence, were excised as the RNA transcripts were transported from the nucleus. Expression of full-length infectious cDNA clones of HCoV-OC43 (94) and SARS-CoV (1) have also used this approach. The full-length cDNA copies of these two clones, however, were not constructed by rebuilding an incomplete DI genome but were pieced together using unique restriction sites either present within the genome or added with the introduction of silent mutations.

A second strategy for producing full-length cDNA infectious clones of coronaviruses was also presented in 2000. The development of molecular clones for coronaviruses, especially those belonging to group 2, had been complicated by the presence of several toxic regions within the cDNA copy of the viral genome. These regions were identified by systematically removing viral sequence until plasmid stability had been achieved and then engineering nuclease restriction sites such as BsmBI or BglI to allow reassembly between adjacent fragments (Fig. 6). Use of these enzymes allows for a high degree of variability among different BglI digests, unique complementation, and high specificity between contiguous fragments. As a result, regions of the genomic cDNA that were toxic in bacteria were specifically disrupted by separating the toxic domain into two genomic segments and stably propagated in *E. coli.* Following restriction enzyme digestion, cDNA fragments were seamlessly ligated to generate a full-length cDNA

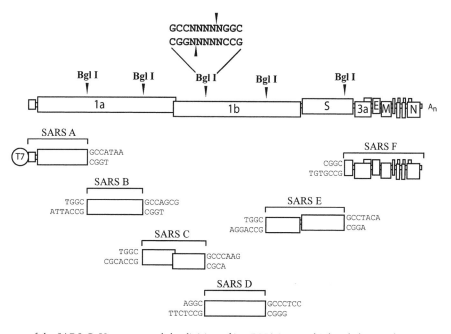

**Figure 6.** Diagram of the SARS-CoV genome and the division of its cDNA into multiple subclones. The SARS-CoV genome is amplified using a six-component system, with each fragment maintained separately in its own plasmid. Reassembly makes use of BglI, which cleaves at highly variable sequences. Since this variability includes those nucleotides involved in the resulting overhang, the entire coronavirus genome fragments can be excised from their bacterial amplification plasmids by BglI digestion and fragment purification and then seamlessly religated in the correct order and orientation. The T7 promoter sequence at the 5′ end of the genomic cDNA is used to drive transcripts in vitro for an RNA launch of recombinant SARS-CoV. E, envelope protein; M, membrane protein.

copy of the viral genome from which RNA was transcribed and electroporated into cells to form virus. Unlike the BAC reverse-genetics system, the multicomponent system relies upon an RNA launch for generating recombinant virus using T7 RNA polymerase (Fig. 2). This assembly strategy was first applied to the development of a six-component TGEV infectious clone (124). The first full-length infectious clones of MHV-A59 (126), SARS-CoV (125), and IBV (123) were generated using this approach.

### Vaccinia Virus Expression System

After reporting difficulty in maintaining cDNA stability in bacterial systems, including the BAC, Thiel and associates described a technique by which full-length cDNA of HCoV-229E was amplified in a vaccinia virus eukaryotic cloning vector (99; reviewed in reference 100) (Fig. 7). The full-length coronavirus genome cDNA was systematically assembled and cloned into a vaccinia virus vector. The recombinant vector was then packaged into infectious vaccinia virus particles following transfection into cells previously infected with a helper poxvirus, isolated, and screened. Following verification that the coronavirus genome had been successfully integrated, the recombinant vaccinia virus was amplified in tissue culture and vector DNA was isolated and purified. The coronavirus cDNA was excised from the vector and used as a transcription template for an RNA launch. Avian IBV (11) was derived from a full-length cDNA by an alternative strategy using poxvirus vectors. Following transfection of the vaccinia virus vector containing the IBV cDNA, cells were infected with fowlpox virus expressing T7 RNA polymerase. A T7 promoter was engineered before the IBV cDNA, and viral RNA was transcribed within the cell, initiating viral replication. More recently, another MHV infectious clone was

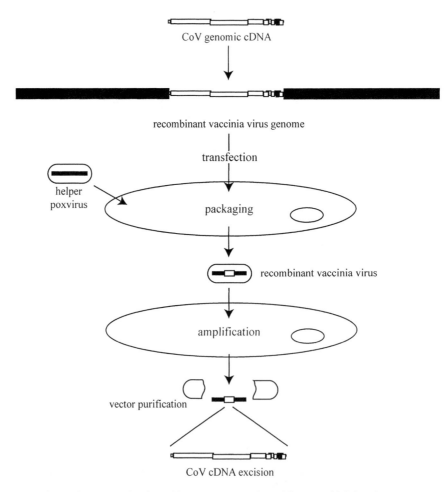

**Figure 7.** Diagram outlining the strategy for the stable propagation and amplification of full-length coronavirus cDNA in a vaccinia virus vector. The coronavirus cDNA is incorporated into a recombinant vaccinia virus genome which is then transfected into a cell infected with a helper poxvirus. The recombinant genome containing the coronavirus genome is then packaged in a vaccinia virus virion, which is itself infectious and can be amplified in subsequent rounds of infection. The coronavirus cDNA can be excised from the purified genome of the recombinant vaccinia virus and used as a template for DNA or RNA launch.

developed in the vaccinia virus vector (20). One benefit to the vaccinia virus system is the ability to introduce changes into the cDNA clone by taking advantage of the high-frequency homologous recombination that occurs within vaccinia viruses (9, 20). This allows mutation of the coronavirus genome without the need to reconstruct modified full-length infectious clones by standard molecular biological techniques.

The EAV infectious clone is nearly the ideal paradigm of a reverse-genetics system. Its stability in *E. coli* plasmid amplification vectors facilitates ease of use and allows researchers to alter any region of the genome. Although other arterivirus infectious clones, such as LV, may not enjoy quite the same level of plasmid stability, use of the BAC system, while slightly more labor-intensive, restores its facility. Coronavirus researchers have not been quite as fortunate as their arterivirus counterparts. When comparing the coronavirus reverse-genetics systems, it becomes apparent that each boasts its own strengths while enduring specific weaknesses. The targeted recombination system has the distinction of being the first to allow modification of a coronavirus genome, and a tremendous amount of work has been and continues to be accomplished with it. Exploiting the high recombination rate of coronaviruses, the targeted recombination system employs a powerful means of selecting successful recombinants. However, the primary limitation of this powerful tool is that modification of the sequence encoding the replicase, nearly two-thirds of the genome, is beyond reach.

The infectious clone systems overcame the limitation of the targeted recombination system and allowed modification of any part of the coronavirus genome. The first coronavirus infectious cDNA clone was of TGEV and retained cDNA stability using the BAC system, although two regions of the viral template of TGEV had to be disrupted with introns in order to achieve long-term stability. This required that the regions responsible for toxicity be identified and specifically and adequately disrupted with an introduced intron, and that the intron be efficiently excised upon transport from the nucleus. Relative to the multicomponent and some vaccinia virus-based infectious clones, the DNA launch utilized by this model has the advantage of not relying on expensive in vitro transcription reagents in order to produce virus. In the years since its introduction, the BAC-based coronavirus infectious clones have proven functionally robust in their application to a number of strains.

Rather than achieving plasmid stability of the entire cDNA copy of the coronavirus genome, the multicomponent infectious clone fragments the genome over several contiguous plasmids which are amplified separately. This system provides unique benefits, including the more rapid introduction of mutations and a higher degree of safety when working with genomes of infectious human agents. Since the genome is divided into several smaller fragments, specific genetic alterations can be introduced by working only with the relevant plasmids. This often increases the availability of convenient nuclease restriction sites. A higher degree of safety is also attained during these manipulations, as only nonreplicating fragments of the viral genome are manipulated. Potential drawbacks of the multicomponent system include the time needed for establishing an infectious clone for each virus as well as the need for stringent purity of individual fragments. When generating an infectious clone of a virus, regions of instability, which vary in number and degree of toxicity for each virus, must be systematically located and disrupted. When introducing highly attenuating mutations into a cDNA fragment, care must be taken that the corresponding wild-type fragment is not present at even low levels within the preparations of any fragment included in the ligation reaction.

The vaccinia virus vector system provides an alternative to bacterial amplification of genomic cDNA. Like the other infectious-clone strategies, the poxvirus cloning vehicle has been used to generate infectious clones of coronaviruses from all three groups of the family. Virus has successfully been generated by both DNA and RNA launch, and there have not been any reports of even low levels of cDNA instability over time. An additional benefit to the vaccinia virus vector is that it allows the incorporation of mutations by homologous recombination, eliminating the need to clone the genetically modified fragment into the full-length construct by more conventional techniques. There are potential safety concerns with this system with regard to particularly pathogenic strains of coronaviruses, such as SARS-CoV. The vector contains the entire genome of the virus, is itself replication competent and infectious, and is amplified in cells which may themselves be amenable to coronavirus replication. The potential for the unexpected activation of the coronavirus genome, rearrangement of DNA to generate a viable poxvirus/coronavirus chimera, or simple exposure events must be considered, even if such occurrences are improbable.

## SYNTHETIC GENOMES AND REVERSE GENETIC RESURRECTION OF RARE SARS-CoV

Along with the creation of reverse-genetics systems, recent advances in the rapid, affordable, and accurate synthesis of DNA provide many new opportunities for nidovirus research. The ability to generate DNA

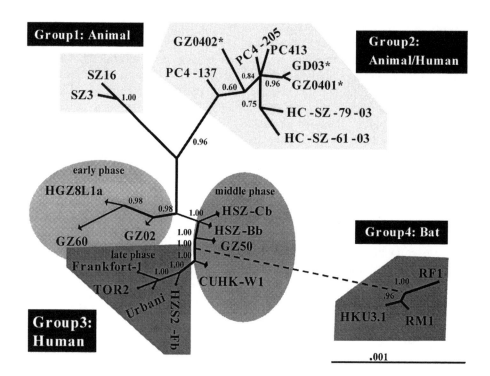

**Figure 8.** Phylogenetic analysis of human, bat, and civet/raccoon dog virus S protein sequences. Shown is an unrooted Bayesian phylogenetic gene tree of 24 SARS-CoVs divided into four groups. Group 1 includes viruses isolated from animals in southern China in 2003. Group 2 is a cluster of viruses isolated from animals and humans (asterisks) in 2003. Group 3 includes viruses from all three phases (early, middle, and late) of the human SARS epidemic of 2002-2003. Group 4 represents a cluster of viruses isolated from bats in 2005-2006. A multiple-sequence alignment of the S protein gene of each virus was created using ClustalX 1.83 with default settings. Bayesian inference was conducted with Mr. Bayes, with Markov chain Monte Carlo sampling of four chains for 500,000 generations, and a consensus tree was generated using the 50% majority rule with a burn-in of 1,000. Branch confidence values are shown as posterior probabilities. The three human isolates that fall within the animal cluster (GZ0402, GD03, and GZ0401) may represent infections where a human acquired the virus from animals. The dashed line between group 3 and group 4 is used to represent a much longer line in the tree (~10 times longer); thus, the distance of the line is not representative of the distance between bat and human SARS-CoVs.

sequences de novo without biological samples will undoubtedly prove a powerful method for advancing our understanding of the evolution and mechanisms of virus-host interactions. These new technologies are also extremely useful for the development and application of antiviral therapies. One example is the generation of a new challenge model of SARS-CoV for the efficacy study of candidate vaccines.

Although a tremendous amount of work has been put into the development of an effective SARS-CoV vaccine, nearly all existing challenge studies rely upon the use of the Urbani epidemic strain, or one of its close genetic relatives, for testing vaccine effectiveness. The Urbani and other epidemic strains represent viruses that have adapted to human hosts. However, a reemergent SARS-CoV-like virus will likely expand from its animal reservoir, and little work has been done to test the effectiveness of vaccines against strains more closely related to their zoonotic progenitors. Through the use of synthetic biology and the

multicomponent SARS-CoV reverse-genetics system, a recent study has created a novel challenge strain of virus expressing the S glycoprotein of GD03 (25), a SARS-CoV strain that emerged independently in the human population and has an S protein which bears amino acid similarity to zoonotic strains (Fig. 8) (17). Relative to the Urbani S protein, the GD03 glycoprotein contains 17 amino acid changes, many falling within known neutralization sites (Fig. 9A) (16, 19, 27, 39, 45, 51, 95, 102, 114). A chimeric SARS-Cov virus, icGD03-S ("ic" denotes infectious clone derived), was constructed by replacing the Urbani S protein gene with a synthetic GD03 S protein gene derived only from a publicly available sequence database, a necessity given that the virus was never successfully propagated in tissue culture. Antibody specific for the Urbani S protein was reduced in its ability to neutralize icGD03-S, providing a stringent challenge virus for testing the effectiveness of a potential vaccine against a newly emergent strain (Fig. 9B).

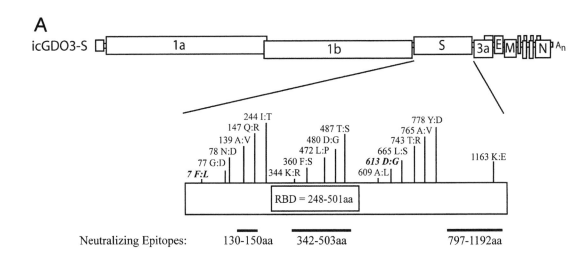

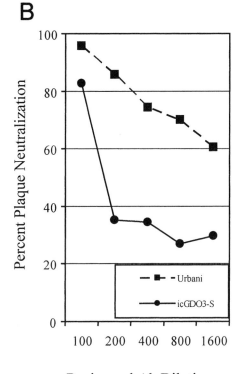

Figure 9. The novel challenge SARS-CoV strain icGDO3-S. (A) A novel challenge strain of SARS-CoV was generated by replacing the Urbani S protein gene with a synthetic S protein gene of GDO3. Amino acid changes unique to GDO3 relative to Urbani are indicated, with the GDO3 S protein amino acid listed on the left of the colon and the corresponding Urbani amino acid on the right. The amino acid changes are shown in relation to the receptor-binding domain (RBD) and known neutralizing epitopes. Two mutations which arose during tissue culture passage of the chimeric icGDO3-S are shown in bold italics. (B). Urbani or icGDO3-S was treated with the indicated dilution of anti-Urbani S protein sera and the number of resulting plaques was compared to the average number of plaques formed after treatment with control antibody and expressed as a percentage. Relative to Urbani, icGDO3-S was more resistant to neutralization.

## CONCLUSION

The biology of nidoviruses makes them significant threats as existing, emerging, and reemerging pathogens. With their broad distribution across many species of animals and the ability to rapidly adapt to changing selective pressures, nidoviruses have a history of causing damage to human health and interests, and it is very likely that the nature of this threat will remain unchanged for the near future. The recent advent of nidovirus reverse-genetics systems demarcates the beginning of the golden age in nidovirus research. These systems provide powerful instruments for dissecting the mechanisms of nidovirus replication and pathogenesis. Use of the nidovirus reverse-genetics systems is only beginning to define the wealth of functions encoded within the nidovirus genome, including novel functions required for RNA replication and a series of interferon antagonists that contribute to pathogenesis. Significant gains are also being made in the development of antinidovirus therapies as new therapies are developed. For instance, alteration of the conserved transcriptional regulatory sequences found at the beginning of each ORF significantly reduces the opportunity for discontinuous recombination between otherwise-identical strains of virus, making them an attractive framework from which to design attenuated vaccine strains (127). The existence of effective reverse-genetics systems nearly ensures an exciting and productive future in nidovirus research.

## REFERENCES

1. **Almazan, F., M. L. Dediego, C. Galan, D. Escors, E. Alvarez, J. Ortego, I. Sola, S. Zuniga, S. Alonso, J. L. Moreno, A. Nogales, C. Capiscol, and L. Enjuanes.** 2006. Construction of a severe acute respiratory syndrome coronavirus infectious cDNA clone and a replicon to study coronavirus RNA synthesis. *J. Virol.* 80:10900–10906.

2. **Almazan, F., J. M. Gonzalez, Z. Penzes, A. Izeta, E. Calvo, J. Plana-Duran, and L. Enjuanes.** 2000. Engineering the largest RNA virus genome as an infectious bacterial artificial chromosome. *Proc. Natl. Acad. Sci. USA* 97:5516–5521.

3. **Baric, R. S., K. Fu, W. Chen, and B. Yount.** 1995. High recombination and mutation rates in mouse hepatitis virus suggest that coronaviruses may be potentially important emerging viruses. *Adv. Exp. Med. Biol.* 380:571–576.

4. **Baric, R. S., K. Fu, M. C. Schaad, and S. A. Stohlman.** 1990. Establishing a genetic recombination map for murine coronavirus strain A59 complementation groups. *Virology* 177:646–656.

5. **Baric, R. S., E. Sullivan, L. Hensley, B. Yount, and W. Chen.** 1999. Persistent infection promotes cross-species transmissibility of mouse hepatitis virus. *J. Virol.* 73:638–649.

6. **Baric, R. S., B. Yount, L. Hensley, S. A. Peel, and W. Chen.** 1997. Episodic evolution mediates interspecies transfer of a murine coronavirus. *J. Virol.* 71:1946–1955.

7. **Biebricher, C. K., and M. Eigen.** 2006. What is a quasispecies? *Curr. Top. Microbiol. Immunol.* 299:1–31.

8. **Bridgen, A., M. Duarte, K. Tobler, H. Laude, and M. Ackermann.** 1993. Sequence determination of the nucleocapsid protein gene of the porcine epidemic diarrhoea virus confirms that this virus is a coronavirus related to human coronavirus 229E and porcine transmissible gastroenteritis virus. *J. Gen. Virol.* 74(Pt. 9):1795–1804.

9. **Britton, P., S. Evans, B. Dove, M. Davies, R. Casais, and D. Cavanagh.** 2005. Generation of a recombinant avian coronavirus infectious bronchitis virus using transient dominant selection. *J. Virol. Methods* 123:203–211.

10. **Casais, R., B. Dove, D. Cavanagh, and P. Britton.** 2003. Recombinant avian infectious bronchitis virus expressing a heterologous spike gene demonstrates that the spike protein is a determinant of cell tropism. *J. Virol.* 77:9084–9089.

11. **Casais, R., V. Thiel, S. G. Siddell, D. Cavanagh, and P. Britton.** 2001. Reverse genetics system for the avian coronavirus infectious bronchitis virus. *J. Virol.* 75:12359–12369.

12. **Cavanagh, D.** 2005. Coronaviruses in poultry and other birds. *Avian Pathol.* 34:439–448.

13. **Cavanagh, D., P. Davis, J. Cook, and D. Li.** 1990. Molecular basis of the variation exhibited by avian infectious bronchitis coronavirus (IBV). *Adv. Exp. Med. Biol.* 276:369–372.

14. **Centers for Disease Control and Prevention.** 2003. Prevalence of IgG antibody to SARS-associated coronavirus in animal traders—Guangdong Province, China, 2003. *Morb. Mortal. Wkly. Rep.* 52:986–987.

15. **Chen, W., and R. S. Baric.** 1996. Molecular anatomy of mouse hepatitis virus persistence: coevolution of increased host cell resistance and virus virulence. *J. Virol.* 70:3947–3960.

16. **Chen, Z., L. Zhang, C. Qin, L. Ba, C. E. Yi, F. Zhang, Q. Wei, T. He, W. Yu, J. Yu, H. Gao, X. Tu, A. Gettie, M. Farzan, K. Y. Yuen, and D. D. Ho.** 2005. Recombinant modified vaccinia virus Ankara expressing the spike glycoprotein of severe acute respiratory syndrome coronavirus induces protective neutralizing antibodies primarily targeting the receptor binding region. *J. Virol.* 79:2678–2688.

17. **The Chinese SARS Molecular Epidemiology Consortium.** 2004. Molecular evolution of the SARS coronavirus during the course of the SARS epidemic in China. *Science* 303:1666–1669.

18. **Choi, Y. J., S. I. Yun, S. Y. Kang, and Y. M. Lee.** 2006. Identification of 5′ and 3′ *cis*-acting elements of the porcine reproductive and respiratory syndrome virus: acquisition of novel 5′ AU-rich sequences restored replication of a 5′-proximal 7-nucleotide deletion mutant. *J. Virol.* 80:723–736.

19. **Chou, T. H., S. Wang, P. V. Sakhatskyy, I. Mboudoudjeck, J. M. Lawrence, S. Huang, S. Coley, B. Yang, J. Li, Q. Zhu, and S. Lu.** 2005. Epitope mapping and biological function analysis of antibodies produced by immunization of mice with an inactivated Chinese isolate of severe acute respiratory syndrome-associated coronavirus (SARS-CoV). *Virology* 334:134–143.

20. **Coley, S. E., E. Lavi, S. G. Sawicki, L. Fu, B. Schelle, N. Karl, S. G. Siddell, and V. Thiel.** 2005. Recombinant mouse hepatitis virus strain A59 from cloned, full-length cDNA replicates to high titers in vitro and is fully pathogenic in vivo. *J. Virol.* 79:3097–3106.

21. **Compton, S. R., C. B. Stephensen, S. W. Snyder, D. G. Weismiller, and K. V. Holmes.** 1992. Coronavirus species specificity: murine coronavirus binds to a mouse-specific epitope on its carcinoembryonic antigen-related receptor glycoprotein. *J. Virol.* 66:7420–7428.

22. **Cowley, J. A., C. M. Dimmock, K. M. Spann, and P. J. Walker.** 2000. Gill-associated virus of Penaeus monodon prawns: an invertebrate virus with ORF1a and ORF1b genes related to arteri- and coronaviruses. *J. Gen. Virol.* 81:1473–1484.

23. **Cowley, J. A., C. M. Dimmock, C. Wongteerasupaya, V. Boonsaeng, S. Panyim, and P. J. Walker.** 1999. Yellow head virus from Thailand and gill-associated virus from Australia are closely related but distinct prawn viruses. *Dis. Aquat. Org.* 36:153–157.

24. **Delmas, B., J. Gelfi, R. L'Haridon, L. K. Vogel, H. Sjostrom, O. Noren, and H. Laude.** 1992. Aminopeptidase N is a major receptor for the entero-pathogenic coronavirus TGEV. *Nature* 357:417–420.

25. **Deming, D., T. Sheahan, M. Heise, B. Yount, N. Davis, A. Sims, M. Suthar, J. Harkema, A. Whitmore, R. Pickles, A. West, E. Donaldson, K. Curtis, R. Johnston, and R. Baric.** 2006. Vaccine efficacy in senescent mice challenged with recombinant SARS-CoV bearing epidemic and zoonotic spike variants. *PLoS Med.* 3:e525.

26. **Drosten, C., S. Gunther, W. Preiser, S. van der Werf, H. R. Brodt, S. Becker, H. Rabenau, M. Panning, L. Kolesnikova, R. A. Fouchier, A. Berger, A. M. Burguiere, J. Cinatl, M. Eickmann, N. Escriou, K. Grywna, S. Kramme, J. C. Manuguerra, S. Muller, V. Rickerts, M. Sturmer, S. Vieth, H. D. Klenk, A. D. Osterhaus, H. Schmitz, and H. W. Doerr.** 2003. Identification of a novel coronavirus in patients with severe acute respiratory syndrome. *N. Engl. J. Med.* 348:1967–1976.

27. **Duan, J., X. Yan, X. Guo, W. Cao, W. Han, C. Qi, J. Feng, D. Yang, G. Gao, and G. Jin.** 2005. A human SARS-CoV neutralizing antibody against epitope on S2 protein. *Biochemi. Biophys. Res. Commun.* 333:186–193.

28. **Duarte, M., and H. Laude.** 1994. Sequence of the spike protein of the porcine epidemic diarrhoea virus. *J. Gen. Virol.* 75(Pt 5):1195–1200.

29. Dveksler, G. S., M. N. Pensiero, C. B. Cardellichio, R. K. Williams, G. S. Jiang, K. V. Holmes, and C. W. Dieffenbach. 1991. Cloning of the mouse hepatitis virus (MHV) receptor: expression in human and hamster cell lines confers susceptibility to MHV. *J. Virol.* **65**:6881–6891.

30. Erles, K., C. Toomey, H. W. Brooks, and J. Brownlie. 2003. Detection of a group 2 coronavirus in dogs with canine infectious respiratory disease. *Virology* **310**:216–223.

31. Esper, F., C. Weibel, D. Ferguson, M. L. Landry, and J. S. Kahn. 2005. Evidence of a novel human coronavirus that is associated with respiratory tract disease in infants and young children. *J. Infect. Dis.* **191**:492–498.

32. Fouchier, R. A., N. G. Hartwig, T. M. Bestebroer, B. Niemeyer, J. C. de Jong, J. H. Simon, and A. D. Osterhaus. 2004. A previously undescribed coronavirus associated with respiratory disease in humans. *Proc. Natl. Acad. Sci. USA* **101**:6212–6216.

33. Fu, K., and R. S. Baric. 1992. Evidence for variable rates of recombination in the MHV genome. *Virology* **189**:88–102.

34. Fu, K., and R. S. Baric. 1994. Map locations of mouse hepatitis virus temperature-sensitive mutants: confirmation of variable rates of recombination. *J. Virol.* **68**:7458–7466.

35. Gallagher, T. M., M. J. Buchmeier, and S. Perlman. 1992. Cell receptor-independent infection by a neurotropic murine coronavirus. *Virology* **191**:517–522.

36. Goebel, S. J., J. Taylor, and P. S. Masters. 2004. The 3′ cis-acting genomic replication element of the severe acute respiratory syndrome coronavirus can function in the murine coronavirus genome. *J. Virol.* **78**:7846–7851.

37. Gonzalez, J. M., Z. Penzes, F. Almazan, E. Calvo, and L. Enjuanes. 2002. Stabilization of a full-length infectious cDNA clone of transmissible gastroenteritis coronavirus by insertion of an intron. *J. Virol.* **76**:4655–4661.

38. Gorbalenya, A. E., L. Enjuanes, J. Ziebuhr, and E. J. Snijder. 2006. Nidovirales: evolving the largest RNA virus genome. *Virus Res.* **117**:17–37.

39. Greenough, T. C., G. J. Babcock, A. Roberts, H. J. Hernandez, W. D. Thomas, Jr., J. A. Coccia, R. F. Graziano, M. Srinivasan, I. Lowy, R. W. Finberg, K. Subbarao, L. Vogel, M. Somasundaran, K. Luzuriaga, J. L. Sullivan, and D. M. Ambrosino. 2005. Development and characterization of a severe acute respiratory syndrome-associated coronavirus-neutralizing human monoclonal antibody that provides effective immunoprophylaxis in mice. *J. Infect. Dis.* **191**:507–514.

40. Guan, Y., B. J. Zheng, Y. Q. He, X. L. Liu, Z. X. Zhuang, C. L. Cheung, S. W. Luo, P. H. Li, L. J. Zhang, Y. J. Guan, K. M. Butt, K. L. Wong, K. W. Chan, W. Lim, K. F. Shortridge, K. Y. Yuen, J. S. Peiris, and L. L. Poon. 2003. Isolation and characterization of viruses related to the SARS coronavirus from animals in southern China. *Science* **302**:276–278.

41. Haijema, B. J., H. Volders, and P. J. Rottier. 2003. Switching species tropism: an effective way to manipulate the feline coronavirus genome. *J. Virol.* **77**:4528–4538.

42. Hamre, D. and J. J. Procknow. 1966. A new virus isolated from the human respiratory tract. *Proc. Soc. Exp. Biol. Med.* **121**:190–193.

43. Han, M. G., D. S. Cheon, X. Zhang, and L. J. Saif. 2006. Cross-protection in gnotobiotic calves between a human enteric coronavirus and a virulent bovine enteric coronavirus. *J. Virol.* **80**:12350–12356.

44. Han, Y., H. Geng, W. Feng, X. Tang, A. Ou, Y. Lao, Y. Xu, H. Lin, H. Liu, and Y. Li. 2003. A follow-up study of 69 discharged SARS patients. *J. Tradit. Chin. Med.* **23**:214–217.

45. He, Y., Q. Zhu, S. Liu, Y. Zhou, B. Yang, J. Li, and S. Jiang. 2005. Identification of a critical neutralization determinant of severe acute respiratory syndrome (SARS)-associated coronavirus: importance for designing SARS vaccines. *Virology* **334**:74–82.

46. Herrewegh, A. A., I. Smeenk, M. C. Horzinek, P. J. Rottier, and R. J. de Groot. 1998. Feline coronavirus type II strains 79-1683 and 79-1146 originate from a double recombination between feline coronavirus type I and canine coronavirus. *J. Virol.* **72**:4508–4514.

47. Holland, J. J. 2006. Transitions in understanding of RNA viruses: a historical perspective. *Curr. Top. Microbiol. Immunol.* **299**:371–401.

48. Jia, W., K. Karaca, C. R. Parrish, and S. A. Naqi. 1995. A novel variant of avian infectious bronchitis virus resulting from recombination among three different strains. *Arch. Virol.* **140**:259–271.

49. Kan, B., M. Wang, H. Jing, H. Xu, X. Jiang, M. Yan, W. Liang, H. Zheng, K. Wan, Q. Liu, B. Cui, Y. Xu, E. Zhang, H. Wang, J. Ye, G. Li, M. Li, Z. Cui, X. Qi, K. Chen, L. Du, K. Gao, Y. T. Zhao, X. Z. Zou, Y. J. Feng, Y. F. Gao, R. Hai, D. Yu, Y. Guan, and J. Xu. 2005. Molecular evolution analysis and geographic investigation of severe acute respiratory syndrome coronavirus-like virus in palm civets at an animal market and on farms. *J. Virol.* **79**:11892–11900.

50. Keck, J. G., G. K. Matsushima, S. Makino, J. O. Fleming, D. M. Vannier, S. A. Stohlman, and M. M. Lai. 1988. In vivo RNA-RNA recombination of coronavirus in mouse brain. *J. Virol.* **62**:1810–1813.

51. Keng, C.-T., A. Zhang, S. Shen, K.-M. Lip, B. C. Fielding, T. H. P. Tan, C.-F. Chou, C. B. Loh, S. Wang, J. Fu, X. Yang, S. G. Lim, W. Hong, and Y.-J. Tan. 2005. Amino acids 1055 to 1192 in the S2 region of severe acute respiratory syndrome coronavirus S protein induce neutralizing antibodies: implications for the development of vaccines and antiviral agents. *J. Virol.* **79**:3289–3296.

52. Kottier, S. A., D. Cavanagh, and P. Britton. 1995. Experimental evidence of recombination in coronavirus infectious bronchitis virus. *Virology* **213**:569–580.

53. Kroneman, A., L. A. Cornelissen, M. C. Horzinek, R. J. de Groot, and H. F. Egberink. 1998. Identification and characterization of a porcine torovirus. *J. Virol.* **72**:3507–3511.

54. Ksiazek, T. G., D. Erdman, C. S. Goldsmith, S. R. Zaki, T. Peret, S. Emery, S. Tong, C. Urbani, J. A. Comer, W. Lim, P. E. Rollin, S. F. Dowell, A. E. Ling, C. D. Humphrey, W. J. Shieh, J. Guarner, C. D. Paddock, P. Rota, B. Fields, J. DeRisi, J. Y. Yang, N. Cox, J. M. Hughes, J. W. LeDuc, W. J. Bellini, and L. J. Anderson. 2003. A novel coronavirus associated with severe acute respiratory syndrome. *N. Engl. J. Med.* **348**:1953–1966.

55. Kuiken, T., R. Fouchier, G. Rimmelzwaan, and A. Osterhaus. 2003. Emerging viral infections in a rapidly changing world. *Curr. Opin. Biotechnol.* **14**:641–646.

56. Kuo, L., G. J. Godeke, M. J. Raamsman, P. S. Masters, and P. J. Rottier. 2000. Retargeting of coronavirus by substitution of the spike glycoprotein ectodomain: crossing the host cell species barrier. *J. Virol.* **74**:1393–1406.

57. Kusters, J. G., E. J. Jager, H. G. Niesters, and B. A. van der Zeijst. 1990. Sequence evidence for RNA recombination in field isolates of avian coronavirus infectious bronchitis virus. *Vaccine* **8**:605–608.

58. Lai, M. M., R. S. Baric, S. Makino, J. G. Keck, J. Egbert, J. L. Leibowitz, and S. A. Stohlman. 1985. Recombination between nonsegmented RNA genomes of murine coronaviruses. *J. Virol.* **56**:449–456.

59. Lassnig, C., A. Kolb, B. Strobl, L. Enjuanes, and M. Muller. 2005. Studying human pathogens in animal models: fine tuning the humanized mouse. *Transgenic Res.* **14**:803–806.

60. Lau, S. K., P. C. Woo, K. S. Li, Y. Huang, H. W. Tsoi, B. H. Wong, S. S. Wong, S. Y. Leung, K. H. Chan, and K. Y. Yuen. 2005. Severe

acute respiratory syndrome coronavirus-like virus in Chinese horseshoe bats. *Proc. Natl. Acad. Sci. USA* **102**:14040–14045.

61. Lee, C., J. G. Calvert, S. K. Welch, and D. Yoo. 2005. A DNA-launched reverse genetics system for porcine reproductive and respiratory syndrome virus reveals that homodimerization of the nucleocapsid protein is essential for virus infectivity. *Virology* **331**:47–62.

62. Lee, C. W., and M. W. Jackwood. 2000. Evidence of genetic diversity generated by recombination among avian coronavirus IBV. *Arch. Virol.* **145**:2135–2148.

63. Lee, C. W., and M. W. Jackwood. 2001. Spike gene analysis of the DE072 strain of infectious bronchitis virus: origin and evolution. *Virus Genes* **22**:85–91.

64. Levis, R., C. B. Cardellichio, C. A. Scanga, S. R. Compton, and K. V. Holmes. 1995. Multiple receptor-dependent steps determine the species specificity of HCV-229E infection. *Adv. Exp. Med. Biol.* **380**:337–343.

65. Li, W., Z. Shi, M. Yu, W. Ren, C. Smith, J. H. Epstein, H. Wang, G. Crameri, Z. Hu, H. Zhang, J. Zhang, J. McEachern, H. Field, P. Daszak, B. T. Eaton, S. Zhang, and L. F. Wang. 2005. Bats are natural reservoirs of SARS-like coronaviruses. *Science* **310**:676–679.

66. Li, W., C. Zhang, J. Sui, J. H. Kuhn, M. J. Moore, S. Luo, S. K. Wong, I. C. Huang, K. Xu, N. Vasilieva, A. Murakami, Y. He, W. A. Marasco, Y. Guan, H. Choe, and M. Farzan. 2005. Receptor and viral determinants of SARS-coronavirus adaptation to human ACE2. *EMBO J.* **24**:1634–1643.

67. Liu, L., S. Hagglund, M. Hakhverdyan, S. Alenius, L. E. Larsen, and S. Belak. 2006. Molecular epidemiology of bovine coronavirus on the basis of comparative analyses of the S gene. *J. Clin. Microbiol.* **44**:957–960.

68. Louz, D., H. E. Bergmans, B. P. Loos, and R. C. Hoeben. 2005. Cross-species transfer of viruses: implications for the use of viral vectors in biomedical research, gene therapy and as live-virus vaccines. *J. Gene Med.* **7**:1263–1274.

69. Majhdi, F., H. C. Minocha, and S. Kapil. 1997. Isolation and characterization of a coronavirus from elk calves with diarrhea. *J. Clin. Microbiol.* **35**:2937–2942.

70. Makino, S., J. G. Keck, S. A. Stohlman, and M. M. Lai. 1986. High-frequency RNA recombination of murine coronaviruses. *J. Virol.* **57**:729–737.

71. Manrubia, S. C., C. Escarmis, E. Domingo, and E. Lazaro. 2005. High mutation rates, bottlenecks, and robustness of RNA viral quasispecies. *Gene* **347**:273–282.

72. Masters, P. S. 2006. The molecular biology of coronaviruses. *Adv. Virus. Res.* **66**:193–292.

73. Masters, P. S., and P. J. Rottier. 2005. Coronavirus reverse genetics by targeted RNA recombination. *Curr. Top. Microbiol. Immunol.* **287**:133–159.

74. McIntosh, K., J. H. Dees, W. B. Becker, A. Z. Kapikian, and R. M. Chanock. 1967. Recovery in tracheal organ cultures of novel viruses from patients with respiratory disease. *Proc. Natl. Acad. Sci. USA* **57**:933–940.

75. Meulenberg, J. J., J. N. Bos-de Ruijter, R. van de Graaf, G. Wensvoort, and R. J. Moormann. 1998. Infectious transcripts from cloned genome-length cDNA of porcine reproductive and respiratory syndrome virus. *J. Virol.* **72**:380–387.

76. Molenkamp, R., S. Greve, W. J. Spaan, and E. J. Snijder. 2000. Efficient homologous RNA recombination and requirement for an open reading frame during replication of equine arteritis virus defective interfering RNAs. *J. Virol.* **74**:9062–9070.

77. Neumann, E. J., J. B. Kliebenstein, C. D. Johnson, J. W. Mabry, E. J. Bush, A. H. Seitzinger, A. L. Green, and J. J. Zimmerman. 2005. Assessment of the economic impact of porcine reproductive and respiratory syndrome on swine production in the United States. *J. Am. Vet. Med. Assoc.* **227**:385–392.

78. Normile, D. 2004. Infectious diseases. Viral DNA match spurs China's civet roundup. *Science* **303**:292.

79. Ontiveros, E., L. Kuo, P. S. Masters, and S. Perlman. 2001. Inactivation of expression of gene 4 of mouse hepatitis virus strain JHM does not affect virulence in the murine CNS. *Virology* **289**:230–238.

80. Peiris, J. S., C. M. Chu, V. C. Cheng, K. S. Chan, I. F. Hung, L. L. Poon, K. I. Law, B. S. Tang, T. Y. Hon, C. S. Chan, K. H. Chan, J. S. Ng, B. J. Zheng, W. L. Ng, R. W. Lai, Y. Guan, and K. Y. Yuen. 2003. Clinical progression and viral load in a community outbreak of coronavirus-associated SARS pneumonia: a prospective study. *Lancet* **361**:1767–1772.

81. Pensaert, M. B., and P. de Bouck. 1978. A new coronavirus-like particle associated with diarrhea in swine. *Arch. Virol.* **58**:243–247.

82. Pewe, L., H. Zhou, J. Netland, C. Tangudu, H. Olivares, L. Shi, D. Look, T. Gallagher, and S. Perlman. 2005. A severe acute respiratory syndrome-associated coronavirus-specific protein enhances virulence of an attenuated murine coronavirus. *J. Virol.* **79**:11335–11342.

83. Poon, L. L., D. K. Chu, K. H. Chan, O. K. Wong, T. M. Ellis, Y. H. Leung, S. K. Lau, P. C. Woo, K. Y. Suen, K. Y. Yuen, Y. Guan, and J. S. Peiris. 2005. Identification of a novel coronavirus in bats. *J. Virol.* **79**:2001–2009.

84. Poon, L. L., Y. Guan, J. M. Nicholls, K. Y. Yuen, and J. S. Peiris. 2004. The aetiology, origins, and diagnosis of severe acute respiratory syndrome. *Lancet Infect. Dis.* **4**:663–671.

85. Rest, J. S., and D. P. Mindell. 2003. SARS associated coronavirus has a recombinant polymerase and coronaviruses have a history of host-shifting. *Infect. Genet. Evol.* **3**:219–225.

86. Rottier, P. J., K. Nakamura, P. Schellen, H. Volders, and B. J. Haijema. 2005. Acquisition of macrophage tropism during the pathogenesis of feline infectious peritonitis is determined by mutations in the feline coronavirus spike protein. *J. Virol.* **79**:14122–14130.

87. Saif, L. J. 1996. Mucosal immunity: an overview and studies of enteric and respiratory coronavirus infections in a swine model of enteric disease. *Vet. Immunol. Immunopathol.* **54**:163–169.

88. Schickli, J. H., L. B. Thackray, S. G. Sawicki, and K. V. Holmes. 2004. The N-terminal region of the murine coronavirus spike glycoprotein is associated with the extended host range of viruses from persistently infected murine cells. *J. Virol.* **78**:9073–9083.

89. Schickli, J. H., B. D. Zelus, D. E. Wentworth, S. G. Sawicki, and K. V. Holmes. 1997. The murine coronavirus mouse hepatitis virus strain A59 from persistently infected murine cells exhibits an extended host range. *J. Virol.* **71**:9499–9507.

90. Smati, R., A. Silim, C. Guertin, M. Henrichon, M. Marandi, M. Arella, and A. Merzouki. 2002. Molecular characterization of three new avian infectious bronchitis virus (IBV) strains isolated in Quebec. *Virus Genes* **25**:85–93.

91. Song, H. D., C. C. Tu, G. W. Zhang, S. Y. Wang, K. Zheng, L. C. Lei, Q. X. Chen, Y. W. Gao, H. Q. Zhou, H. Xiang, H. J. Zheng, S. W. Chern, F. Cheng, C. M. Pan, H. Xuan, S. J. Chen, H. M. Luo, D. H. Zhou, Y. F. Liu, J. F. He, P. Z. Qin, L. H. Li, Y. Q. Ren, W. J. Liang, Y. D. Yu, L. Anderson, M. Wang, R. H. Xu, X. W. Wu, H. Y. Zheng, J. D. Chen, G. Liang, Y. Gao, M. Liao, L. Fang, L. Y. Jiang, H. Li, F. Chen, B. Di, L. J. He, J. Y. Lin, S. Tong, X. Kong, L. Du, P. Hao, H. Tang, A. Bernini, X. J. Yu, O. Spiga, Z. M. Guo, H. Y. Pan, W. Z. He, J. C. Manuguerra, A. Fontanet, A. Danchin, N. Niccolai, Y. X. Li, C. I. Wu, and G. P. Zhao. 2005. Cross-host evolution of severe acute respiratory syndrome coronavirus in palm civet and human. *Proc. Natl. Acad. Sci. USA* **102**:2430–2435.

92. **Stanhope, M. J., J. R. Brown, and H. Amrine-Madsen.** 2004. Evidence from the evolutionary analysis of nucleotide sequences for a recombinant history of SARS-CoV. *Infect. Genet. Evol.* **4:**15–19.

93. **Stavrinides, J., and D. S. Guttman.** 2004. Mosaic evolution of the severe acute respiratory syndrome coronavirus. *J. Virol.* **78:**76–82.

94. **St-Jean, J. R., M. Desforges, F. Almazan, H. Jacomy, L. Enjuanes, and P. J. Talbot.** 2006. Recovery of a neurovirulent human coronavirus OC43 from an infectious cDNA clone. *J. Virol.* **80:**3670–3674.

95. **Sui, J., W. Li, A. Murakami, A. Tamin, L. J. Matthews, S. K. Wong, M. J. Moore, A. S. Tallarico, M. Olurinde, H. Choe, L. J. Anderson, W. J. Bellini, M. Farzan, and W. A. Marasco.** 2004. Potent neutralization of severe acute respiratory syndrome (SARS) coronavirus by a human mAb to S1 protein that blocks receptor association. *Proc. Natl. Acad. Sci. USA* **101:**2536–2541.

96. **Tangudu, C., H. Olivares, J. Netland, S. Perlman, and T. Gallagher.** 2006. 7. Severe acute respiratory syndrome coronavirus protein 6 accelerates murine coronavirus infections. *J. Virol.* **81:**1220–1229.

97. **Thackray, L. B., and K. V. Holmes.** 2004. Amino acid substitutions and an insertion in the spike glycoprotein extend the host range of the murine coronavirus MHV-A59. *Virology* **324:**510–524.

98. **Thackray, L. B., B. C. Turner, and K. V. Holmes.** 2005. Substitutions of conserved amino acids in the receptor-binding domain of the spike glycoprotein affect utilization of murine CEACAM1a by the murine coronavirus MHV-A59. *Virology* **334:**98–110.

99. **Thiel, V., J. Herold, B. Schelle, and S. G. Siddell.** 2001. Infectious RNA transcribed in vitro from a cDNA copy of the human coronavirus genome cloned in vaccinia virus. *J. Gen. Virol.* **82:**1273–1281.

100. **Thiel, V., and S. G. Siddell.** 2005. Reverse genetics of coronaviruses using vaccinia virus vectors. *Curr. Top. Microbiol. Immunol.* **287:**199–227.

101. **Tresnan, D. B., R. Levis, and K. V. Holmes.** 1996. Feline aminopeptidase N serves as a receptor for feline, canine, porcine, and human coronaviruses in serogroup I. *J. Virol.* **70:**8669–8674.

102. **Tripp, R. A., L. M. Haynes, D. Moore, B. Anderson, A. Tamin, B. H. Harcourt, L. P. Jones, M. Yilla, G. J. Babcock, T. Greenough, et al.** 2005. Monoclonal antibodies to SARS-associated coronavirus (SARS-CoV): identification of neutralizing and antibodies reactive to S, N, M and E viral proteins. *J. Virol. Methods* **128:**21–28.

103. **Truong, H. M., Z. Lu, G. F. Kutish, J. Galeota, F. A. Osorio, and A. K. Pattnaik.** 2004. A highly pathogenic porcine reproductive and respiratory syndrome virus generated from an infectious cDNA clone retains the in vivo virulence and transmissibility properties of the parental virus. *Virology* **325:**308–319.

104. **Tsunemitsu, H., Z. R. el-Kanawati, D. R. Smith, H. H. Reed, and L. J. Saif.** 1995. Isolation of coronaviruses antigenically indistinguishable from bovine coronavirus from wild ruminants with diarrhea. *J. Clin. Microbiol.* **33:**3264–3269.

105. **Tu, C., G. Crameri, X. Kong, J. Chen, Y. Sun, M. Yu, H. Xiang, X. Xia, S. Liu, T. Ren, Y. Yu, B. T. Eaton, H. Xuan, and L. F. Wang.** 2004. Antibodies to SARS coronavirus in civets. *Emerg. Infect. Dis.* **10:**2244–2248.

106. **van der Hoek, L., K. Pyrc, M. F. Jebbink, W. Vermeulen-Oost, R. J. Berkhout, K. C. Wolthers, P. M. Wertheim-van Dillen, J. Kaandorp, J. Spaargaren, and B. Berkhout.** 2004. Identification of a new human coronavirus. *Nat. Med.* **10:**368–373.

107. **van Dinten, L. C., J. A. den Boon, A. L. Wassenaar, W. J. Spaan, and E. J. Snijder.** 1997. An infectious arterivirus cDNA clone: identification of a replicase point mutation that abolishes discontinuous mRNA transcription. *Proc. Natl. Acad. Sci. USA* **94:**991–996.

108. **Vega, V. B., Y. Ruan, J. Liu, W. H. Lee, C. L. Wei, S. Y. Se-Thoe, K. F. Tang, T. Zhang, P. R. Kolatkar, E. E. Ooi, A. E. Ling, L. W. Stanton, P. M. Long, and E. T. Liu.** 2004. Mutational dynamics of the SARS coronavirus in cell culture and human populations isolated in 2003. *BMC Infect. Dis.* **4:**32.

109. **Vennema, H.** 1999. Genetic drift and genetic shift during feline coronavirus evolution. *Vet. Microbiol.* **69:**139–141.

110. **Vennema, H., A. Poland, J. Foley, and N. C. Pedersen.** 1998. Feline infectious peritonitis viruses arise by mutation from endemic feline enteric coronaviruses. *Virology* **243:**150–157.

111. **Vignuzzi, M., J. K. Stone, J. J. Arnold, C. E. Cameron, and R. Andino.** 2006. Quasispecies diversity determines pathogenesis through cooperative interactions in a viral population. *Nature* **439:**344–348.

112. **Vijgen, L., E. Keyaerts, P. Lemey, P. Maes, K. Van Reeth, H. Nauwynck, M. Pensaert, and M. Van Ranst.** 2006. Evolutionary history of the closely related group 2 coronaviruses: porcine hemagglutinating encephalomyelitis virus, bovine coronavirus, and human coronavirus OC43. *J. Virol.* **80:**7270–7274.

113. **Wang, L., D. Junker, and E. W. Collisson.** 1993. Evidence of natural recombination within the S1 gene of infectious bronchitis virus. *Virology* **192:**710–716.

114. **Wang, S., T. H. Chou, P. V. Sakhatskyy, S. Huang, J. M. Lawrence, H. Cao, X. Huang, and S. Lu.** 2005. Identification of two neutralizing regions on the severe acute respiratory syndrome coronavirus spike glycoprotein produced from the mammalian expression system. *J. Virol.* **79:**1906–1910.

115. **Weiss, M., F. Steck, and M. C. Horzinek.** 1983. Purification and partial characterization of a new enveloped RNA virus (Berne virus). *J. Gen. Virol.* **64(Pt 9):**1849–1858.

116. **Wentworth, D. E., D. B. Tresnan, B. C. Turner, I. R. Lerman, B. Bullis, E. M. Hemmila, R. Levis, L. H. Shapiro, and K. V. Holmes.** 2005. Cells of human aminopeptidase N (CD13) transgenic mice are infected by human coronavirus-229E in vitro, but not in vivo. *Virology* **335:**185–197.

117. **Woo, P. C., S. K. Lau, C. M. Chu, K. H. Chan, H. W. Tsoi, Y. Huang, B. H. Wong, R. W. Poon, J. J. Cai, W. K. Luk, L. L. Poon, S. S. Wong, Y. Guan, J. S. Peiris, and K. Y. Yuen.** 2005. Characterization and complete genome sequence of a novel coronavirus, coronavirus HKU1, from patients with pneumonia. *J. Virol.* **79:**884–895.

118. **Woo, P. C., S. K. Lau, C. C. Yip, Y. Huang, H. W. Tsoi, K. H. Chan, and K. Y. Yuen.** 2006. Comparative analysis of 22 coronavirus HKU1 genomes reveals a novel genotype and evidence of natural recombination in coronavirus HKU1. *J. Virol.* **80:**7136–7145.

119. **Woode, G. N., D. E. Reed, P. L. Runnels, M. A. Herrig, and H. T. Hill.** 1982. Studies with an unclassified virus isolated from diarrheic calves. *Vet. Microbiol.* **7:**221–240.

120. **Woolhouse, M. E., and S. Gowtage-Sequeria.** 2005. Host range and emerging and reemerging pathogens. *Emerg. Infect. Dis.* **11:**1842–1847.

121. **Yeager, C. L., R. A. Ashmun, R. K. Williams, C. B. Cardellichio, L. H. Shapiro, A. T. Look, and K. V. Holmes.** 1992. Human aminopeptidase N is a receptor for human coronavirus 229E. *Nature* **357:**420–422.

122. **Yeh, S. H., H. Y. Wang, C. Y. Tsai, C. L. Kao, J. Y. Yang, H. W. Liu, I. J. Su, S. F. Tsai, D. S. Chen, and P. J. Chen.** 2004.

Characterization of severe acute respiratory syndrome coronavirus genomes in Taiwan: molecular epidemiology and genome evolution. *Proc. Natl. Acad. Sci. USA* **101:**2542–2547.

123. **Youn, S., J. L. Leibowitz, and E. W. Collisson.** 2005. In vitro assembled, recombinant infectious bronchitis viruses demonstrate that the 5a open reading frame is not essential for replication. *Virology* **332:**206–215.

124. **Yount, B., K. M. Curtis, and R. S. Baric.** 2000. Strategy for systematic assembly of large RNA and DNA genomes: transmissible gastroenteritis virus model. *J. Virol.* **74:**10600–10611.

125. **Yount, B., K. M. Curtis, E. A. Fritz, L. E. Hensley, P. B. Jahrling, E. Prentice, M. R. Denison, T. W. Geisbert, and R. S. Baric.** 2003. Reverse genetics with a full-length infectious cDNA of severe acute respiratory syndrome coronavirus. *Proc. Natl. Acad. Sci. USA* **100:**12995–13000.

126. **Yount, B., M. R. Denison, S. R. Weiss, and R. S. Baric.** 2002. Systematic assembly of a full-length infectious cDNA of mouse hepatitis virus strain A59. *J. Virol.* **76:**11065–11078.

127. **Yount, B., R. S. Roberts, L. Lindesmith, and R. S. Baric.** 2006. Rewiring the severe acute respiratory syndrome coronavirus (SARS-CoV) transcription circuit: engineering a recombination-resistant genome. *Proc. Natl. Acad. Sci. USA* **103:**12546–12551.

128. **Zhang, X. M., W. Herbst, K. G. Kousoulas, and J. Storz.** 1994. Biological and genetic characterization of a hemagglutinating coronavirus isolated from a diarrhoeic child. *J. Med. Virol.* **44:**152–161.

129. **Zhang, X. W., Y. L. Yap, and A. Danchin.** 2005. Testing the hypothesis of a recombinant origin of the SARS-associated coronavirus. *Arch. Virol.* **150:**1–20.

130. **Zheng, B. J., K. H. Wong, J. Zhou, K. L. Wong, B. W. Young, L. W. Lu, and S. S. Lee.** 2004. SARS-related virus predating SARS outbreak, Hong Kong. *Emerg. Infect. Dis.* **10:**176–178.

*Nidoviruses*
Edited by S. Perlman, T. Gallagher, and E. J. Snijder
© 2008 ASM Press, Washington, DC

Chapter 5

# Coronavirus Replicative Proteins

John Ziebuhr

## ORGANIZATION AND EXPRESSION OF THE CORONAVIRUS REPLICASE GENE

The coronavirus replicase is a multisubunit protein complex that mediates genome replication and transcription and probably is involved in virus-host interactions (82, 147). Its core components are encoded by the viral replicase gene, which occupies the 5′-terminal two-thirds of the coronavirus genome (113, 142). Furthermore, this protein complex contains the nucleocapsid protein (4, 16, 101, 130) and, probably, a number of cellular proteins (111). The replicase gene is comprised of two large open reading frames, ORF1a and ORF1b, whose expression is regulated at both the translational and posttranslational levels. ORF1b translation requires a programmed ribosomal frameshift into the −1 reading frame which occurs just upstream of the ORF1a translation stop codon (18). Direct data on the frameshift rate in coronavirus-infected cells are not available, but there is ample evidence from in vitro studies to suggest that more than one-third of the ribosomes shift their reading frame when they encounter the frameshift signal near the ORF1a/1b junction (17, 30, 55, 88). The signal involves a "slippery" heptanucleotide sequence which is followed by an RNA pseudoknot structure (see also chapter 3). The use of ribosomal frameshifting for ORF1b expression ensures that the proteins specified by ORF1b are produced in smaller amounts than are ORF1a-encoded proteins. The frameshifting mechanism is conserved in coronaviruses and other nidoviruses, suggesting that differential gene expression of ORF1a versus ORF1b products is biologically relevant or even essential for coronavirus (nidovirus) replication. Expression of the replicase ORFs, ORF1a and ORF1b, gives rise to two large polyproteins with partly overlapping sequences (Fig. 1). The ORF1a

translation product is called polyprotein 1a (pp1a), whereas the term pp1ab refers to a carboxy-terminally-extended version of pp1a. As its name suggests, pp1ab is encoded by ORF1a and ORF1b.

Both co- and posttranslationally, pp1a and pp1ab are subject to extensive proteolytic processing by two (in infectious bronchitis virus [IBV] and severe acute respiratory syndrome coronavirus [SARS-CoV]) or three (in all other coronaviruses) ORF1a-encoded proteases (148). While the amino-terminal pp1a/pp1ab regions are cleaved at two or three sites by one or two papain-like cysteine proteases (8, 51, 54, 67, 78, 94, 128, 149), the central and carboxy-terminal pp1a/pp1ab regions, which also include the conserved key replicative enzymes, are processed by a chymotrypsin-like protease which, because of its relationship to picornavirus 3C proteases, is often called 3C-like protease (3CL$^{pro}$) (43). More recently, the enzyme has generally been referred to as the coronavirus main protease, M$^{pro}$, to stress its dominant role in coronavirus polyprotein processing—as opposed to the less critical, accessory role of papain-like proteases (PL$^{pro}$s) (148). Inter- and intramolecular autoprocessing of pp1a and pp1ab results in 15 (in IBV) or 16 (in all other coronaviruses) mature proteins, called nonstructural proteins (nsp1 to -16), and a large number of processing intermediates, with some of them being relatively stable over extended periods (67, 102, 148). Likewise, peptide cleavage data revealed that specific protease cleavage sites are processed less efficiently than others (37, 53). The coronavirus-wide conservation of very efficiently versus less efficiently cleaved sites strongly suggests that differential processing kinetics of specific sites may be biologically relevant (37, 53). Both the available evidence for coronaviruses and a large body of information on polyprotein processing in other plus-strand

**John Ziebuhr** • Centre for Cancer Research and Cell Biology, School of Biomedical Sciences, The Queen's University of Belfast, Belfast, United Kingdom.

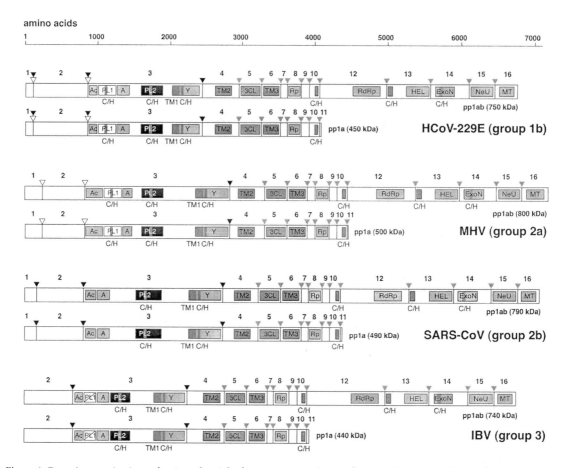

**Figure 1.** Domain organizations of pp1a and pp1ab of representative viruses of coronavirus groups 1b, 2a, 2b, and 3 (46). Arrowheads indicate sites in pp1a and pp1ab that are cleaved by PL1$^{pro}$ and PL2$^{pro}$ (white and black, respectively) or the 3C-like main protease (gray). The proteolytic cleavage products (nsps) are numbered, and conserved domains are highlighted. Abbreviations: C/H, domains with conserved cysteine and histidine residues; Ac, acidic domain; A, ADRP; Y, Y domain; Rp, noncanonical RNA polymerase (potential primase); HEL, helicase; NeU, NendoU. Note that the IBV PL1 domain is proteolytically inactive.

RNA viruses support the idea that coronavirus pp1a/pp1ab processing is temporally regulated and that the coordinated release of individual processing intermediates and end products controls the various activities of the replicase (120, 127, 148). In line with this idea, coronavirus protease inhibitors can be used to block viral replication (137). Furthermore, mouse hepatitis virus (MHV) and human coronavirus 229E (HCoV-229E) pp1a/pp1ab cleavage site mutants, although being viable in a number of cases, were shown to have defects in viral replication (28, 32, 48, 145), demonstrating that controlled processing of the conserved replicase cleavage sites is an important (if not essential) regulatory factor of coronavirus replicase functions.

Coronaviruses form one genus in the family *Coronaviridae,* which also contains the genus *Torovirus* and the tentative genus *Bafinivirus.* The family *Coronaviridae* has been grouped with the families *Arteriviridae* and *Roniviridae* in the virus order *Nidovirales* (22, 41, 42, 103, 115, 117, 118). Apart from similar genome structures and expression strategies, the phylogenetic relationship of corona-, toro-, bafini-, roni-, and arteriviruses (see chapters 1 to 3) is evident from the conserved array of replicase gene-encoded protein functions (42, 115, 118), which includes (i) a chymotrypsin-like protease (3CL$^{pro}$/M$^{pro}$) that is flanked by membrane-spanning domains, (ii) a superfamily 1 RNA-dependent RNA polymerase (RdRp), (iii) a superfamily 1 helicase that has an amino-terminal Zn-binding domain (ZBD), and (iv) a uridylate-specific endoribonuclease (NendoU). Furthermore, coronaviruses encode 3′-to-5′ exoribonuclease (ExoN), putative ribose-2′-O-methyltransferase (MT), PL$^{pro}$, and ADP-ribose 1″-phosphatase (ADRP) activities, whereas putative cyclic nucleotide phosphodiesterase domains have been identified only in group 2a coronaviruses (42, 114, 115, 118, 142). A second, "noncanonical"

**Table 1.** Characteristics of coronavirus replicase gene-encoded nsps

| Protein | Protein size (kDa)[a] | Features[b] |
|---|---|---|
| nsp1 | 12–27 | Conserved within but not between coronavirus genetic groups; potential regulatory functions in the host cell |
| nsp2 | 65–87 | Dispensable for MHV and SARS-CoV replication in tissue culture |
| nsp3 | 177–222 | Acidic domain; macro domain with ADRP and poly(ADP-ribose)-binding activities; one or two ZBD-containing PL$^{pro}$s; Y domain |
| nsp4 | 54–56 | TM2 |
| nsp5 | 33–34 | 3C-like main protease, homodimer |
| nsp6 | 32–34 | TM3 |
| nsp7 | 9–10 | Interacts with nsp8 to form a hexadecameric complex |
| nsp8 | 22–23 | Noncanonical RNA polymerase (primase); interacts with nsp7 to form a hexadecameric complex |
| nsp9 | 12 | ssRNA-binding protein, dimer |
| nsp10 | 14–15 | RNA-binding protein, homododecamer, ZBD |
| nsp11 | 1–2 | ND |
| nsp12 | 105–108 | RdRp |
| nsp13 | 66–67 | ZBD, NTPase, dNTPase, 5′-to-3′ RNA and DNA helicase, RNA 5′-triphosphatase |
| nsp14 | 58–60 | 3′-to-5′ exoribonuclease, ZBD |
| nsp15 | 38–42 | NendoU, homohexamer |
| nsp16 | 33–34 | Putative MT |

[a] Protein sizes were calculated for four representative viruses from three genetic groups: HCoV-229E (group 1b), MHV-A59 (group 2a), SARS-CoV (group 2b), and IBV (group 3).
[b] Listed are key features of the nsps and/or their subdomains. See text for further details. ND, no data.

polymerase activity has recently been identified in coronaviruses, which may act as a primase, thus further adding to the amazing complexity of the enzymology involved in coronavirus RNA synthesis (60). The functional domains and enzymatic activities associated with coronavirus nsp1 to nsp16 are summarized in Fig. 1 and Table 1.

## ENZYMATIC ACTIVITIES

### PL$^{pro}$s

The amino-proximal regions of the coronavirus replicase polyproteins are processed by one or two PL$^{pro}$s, called PL1$^{pro}$ and PL2$^{pro}$, that are part of nsp3 (Fig. 1). There is evidence that some coronavirus PL$^{pro}$s may also act as deubiquitinating enzymes (79, 122). Thus, the SARS-CoV PL$^{pro}$ has been reported to deconjugate ubiquitin and ubiquitin-like modifiers from fusion proteins and to disassemble branched polyubiquitin chains (79). The deubiquitination activity has been speculated to play a role in interactions with the host, for example, in evading the host's innate immune defense (122).

The structure of the SARS-CoV PL$^{pro}$ catalytic domain has recently been determined by X-ray crystallography (95). The catalytic core domain was found to form an extended right-hand structure with palm, thumb, and finger subdomains. At its amino

terminus, the crystallized protein features another, ubiquitin-like domain (95). The finger domain is formed by a four-stranded, twisted β-sheet which in its fingertip region contains four cysteine residues that coordinate a zinc ion (95, 123). The structure of the zinc-binding site has been classified as belonging to the group of circularly permutated, zinc ribbon folds. In both HCoV-229E PL1$^{pro}$ and SARS-CoV PL$^{pro}$, the zinc-binding ability appears to be required for the proteolytic activity and structural integrity of the protein (9, 56). Coronavirus PL$^{pro}$s employ a classic catalytic cysteine-histidine-aspartic acid triad as found in other papain-like cysteine proteases (9, 95, 122). In the SARS-CoV PL$^{pro}$ crystal structure, the catalytic cysteine was located 3.7 Å from the catalytic histidine which, in turn, was located within hydrogen-bonding distance (2.7 Å) of the catalytic aspartic acid residue. In the case of the SARS-CoV PL$^{pro}$, the "oxyanion hole" that typically stabilizes the developing negative charge on tetrahedral transition state intermediates during serine and cysteine protease catalysis is suggested to be formed by a tryptophan and, possibly, an asparagine residue. Whereas the asparagine is well conserved in coronavirus PL$^{pro}$s, the tryptophan is not, suggesting that other residues (e.g., glutamine) fulfill this role in other coronavirus PL$^{pro}$s.

With only a few exceptions (see below), coronavirus PL$^{pro}$s require small residues, glycine or alanine, at both the P1 and P2 positions of the cleavage sites

(15, 29, 148). The SARS-CoV PL$^{pro}$ structure revealed the structural basis for this restricted specificity (95). It shows that the access to the S1 and S2 specificity sites is restricted by several loops whose spatial orientations are stabilized by a number of interacting residues, thus preventing the collapse of the loops into the active site. In contrast to most other coronavirus PL$^{pro}$s, the PL1$^{pro}$s of MHV and several other group 2a coronaviruses cleave sequences that have significantly larger residues (arginine and cysteine) at the P2 position and basic residues at the P4 and P2′ positions (29, 148). On the basis of these differences in coronavirus PL$^{pro}$ substrate specificities, and supported by sequence comparisons and modeling studies, Sulea et al. (123) proposed a binding site-based classification of coronavirus PL$^{pro}$s into two major groups, called the R group and the O group (123). The R group encompasses all coronavirus PL2$^{pro}$s (including the active PL$^{pro}$s of SARS-CoV and IBV) and the PL1$^{pro}$s of group 1 coronaviruses (HCoV-229E, porcine epidemic diarrhea virus, transmissible gastroenteritis virus, and HCoV-NL63). R-group enzymes were suggested to have a catalytic core domain resembling that of HAUSP (59) and other ubiquitin-specific proteases, which was largely confirmed by the SARS-CoV PL$^{pro}$ crystal structure. It was further proposed that the restricted (R) binding site of R-group proteases may involve (i) a conserved signature of critical substrate-binding residues and (ii) occluded S1 and S2 subsites that are suitable to accommodate a P1-P2 diglycine but no side chains larger than that of alanine. By contrast, coronaviral O-group PL$^{pro}$s were predicted to share an open (O) S2 subsite that allows for binding of larger P2 side chains. The model also receives support from the differential inhibitor profiles reported for MHV PL1$^{pro}$ and PL2$^{pro}$ (67). Further structural studies will be needed to obtain a more detailed understanding of the structure-specificity relationships of coronavirus PL$^{pro}$s.

If coronaviruses are grouped on the basis of nsp1 sequence relationships and the number and specificities of their PL$^{pro}$s, the resulting groups perfectly mirror the current classification of coronaviruses into four major lineages (46, 145). This strongly suggests that the profoundly divergent evolution of the amino-terminal pp1a/pp1ab region, including its PL$^{pro}$ domain(s), was a key event in the evolution of coronaviruses, which probably occurred relatively early. Since PL2$^{pro}$ (but not PL1$^{pro}$) is absolutely conserved, it seems reasonable to postulate that coronaviruses first evolved PL2$^{pro}$ and later acquired PL1$^{pro}$, probably by gene duplication in one of the coronavirus ancestors and subsequent loss of PL1$^{pro}$ in some lineages (e.g., the SARS-CoV lineage). But clearly, other scenarios,

including the repeated loss and gain of PL1$^{pro}$ domains in different lineages, are also conceivable (145, 149). Consistent with the universal conservation of PL2$^{pro}$ in coronaviruses, HCoV-229E reverse-genetics studies revealed that PL2$^{pro}$ is essential for viral replication, whereas PL1$^{pro}$ is not (145). HCoV-229E biochemical and reverse-genetics data further suggest that the expression of the nsp1-to-nsp4 region is tightly regulated and involves PL$^{pro}$ paralogs with similar (but not identical) specificities (145, 149). Unlike HCoV-229E, MHV employs PL$^{pro}$ domains with nonoverlapping specificities. Consequently, inactivation of PL1$^{pro}$ in MHV resulted in viruses with growth defects that were much more severe than in HCoV-229E, most probably because in the latter case the lack of PL1$^{pro}$ activity at the nsp1–2 site could be partially compensated by the activity of PL2$^{pro}$ (48, 145). Interestingly, the replication defects seen in PL1$^{pro}$-deficient MHV mutants turned out to be less severe if the active-site mutation was combined with cleavage site deletions, suggesting that unproductive protease-substrate interactions adversely affected the functionality of the nsp1–3 region (48). The data indicate that specific steps involved in proteolytic processing, such as substrate binding, cleavage, and product release, may induce significant conformational changes in specific subdomains of the polyprotein precursor and/or its processing products.

## M$^{pro}$

Coronavirus M$^{pro}$ (or 3CL$^{pro}$) is a protein of slightly more than 300 residues. It resides in nsp5 and releases itself from the flanking hydrophobic proteins (nsp4 and nsp6) by autoproteolytic cleavage. The enzyme cleaves as many as 11 sites in pp1a/pp1ab to release a total of 13 processing products (Fig. 1) (148). Besides having a central role in the formation of an active replicase complex, 3CL$^{pro}$ has more specific functions, for example, in controlling the switch from negative-strand to efficient plus-strand RNA synthesis (100).

Coronavirus M$^{pro}$s are comprised of an amino-terminal chymotrypsin-like fold (β-domains I and II) and a C-terminal α-helical domain (domain III) (6, 7, 138). The active site is located in the center of the cleft between domains I and II. Coronavirus 3CL$^{pro}$s form homodimers, which are thought to be the active form of the protease (6, 26, 57, 110). In the dimer, the two protomers are oriented almost perpendicular to each other. Dimerization mainly occurs through interactions between the carboxy-terminal domains (6, 110, 138). Furthermore, hydrogen-bonding interactions between the protein's amino terminus ("N finger") and residues near the S1 subsite of the other monomer have been suggested to stabilize the homodimer (6, 58). It has been generally accepted that 3CL[pro] dimerization and protease activity are interconnected (24, 50, 58, 109, 141). Molecular dynamics simulations combined with mutational studies have suggested that the appropriate conformation for catalysis in one protomer can be induced by dimer formation and that only one protomer in the dimer is active at one time (24). The precise details of how homodimerization activates 3CL[pro] are presently not clear but appear to be complex (10, 109). The N finger may be one of the factors involved. Besides its role in dimerization (see above), the N finger has been proposed to stabilize the active site of the other monomer in the dimer in a catalytically competent conformation (6, 37, 58, 125, 138, 141).

The mechanisms involved in the release of 3CL[pro] from larger precursors also remain to be elucidated. The majority of structural studies have been performed using fully processed 3CL[pro]s (6, 7, 11, 137, 138), which obviously have limitations in their predictive value regarding structures of relevant precursor molecules. Structure information has also been obtained for a 3CL[pro] carrying heterologous amino- and carboxy-terminal sequences (57). However, given that the neighboring membrane-spanning regions (nsp4 and nsp6) are known to affect the structure and/or function of the 3CL[pro] (90, 129), it remains to be seen whether the structure of 3CL[pro] fused to heterologous sequences really reflects the structure of a precursor in which 3CL[pro] is flanked by authentic viral sequences. Structural studies using larger 3CL[pro]-containing precursors are desirable to address this question.

It appears that 3CL[pro] domains are able to dimerize (albeit not efficiently) when still part of the polyprotein (57). On the basis of structures of 3CL[pro] active-site mutants carrying amino- and/or carboxy-terminal extensions, a four-step release and maturation process has been proposed (57). The process starts with two unprocessed polyproteins that interact with each other and proceeds through several processing intermediates to finally yield the fully processed and dimeric form of the 3CL[pro], which is seen in crystal structures and thought to be required for *trans*-cleavage activity. The model further predicts that the release of 3CL[pro] is a relatively slow process, which is consistent with the presence of long-lived 3CL[pro]-containing precursors in coronavirus-infected cells, which have been suggested to be biologically relevant (100, 102). It remains to be addressed if, prior to its release from pp1a/pp1ab, the 3CL[pro] domain is able to cleave in *cis* or *trans* at a limited number of sites in the polyproteins.

The distant relationship between coronavirus M[pro]s and picornavirus 3C proteases (3C[pro]s) inspired the name 3C-like for this type of coronavirus proteases (43). However, despite their similar substrate specificities (see below) and the conservation of a two-β-barrel fold, the two groups of proteases differ from each other in many structural details and even their catalytic residues. While 3C[pro]s employ a cysteine-histidine-aspartic (glutamic) acid catalytic triad (1, 84, 87, 105, 139), the coronavirus homologs employ a cysteine-histidine catalytic dyad (6, 7, 52, 80, 81, 125, 138, 143, 144). A stable water molecule that occupies the position of the usual third member of the triad has been suggested to stabilize the protonated histidine in the intermediate state during proteolytic cleavage (6, 7), which may compensate for the lack of an acidic catalytic residue in coronavirus M[pro]s.

Despite moderate sequence conservation, the substrate specificities are extremely well conserved among coronavirus M[pro]s (53, 128). Glutamine is invariably present at the P1 position, whereas small residues (e.g., alanine, serine, and glycine) are conserved at the P1′ position of the cleavage sites (148). The presence of larger residues, such as asparagine and leucine, at the P1′ position has detrimental effects on cleavage efficiency (36, 37, 53). At the P2 position, leucine is typically conserved, but also bulkier hydrophobic residues, such as phenylalanine, may be accommodated in the S2 site (138). Furthermore, the S4 subsite contributes to the enzyme's specificity by accommodating valine, threonine, alanine, or serine residues (36, 128, 148). This well-conserved specificity correlates with a highly conservative substrate recognition pocket, as revealed by crystal structure analyses of representative 3CL[pro]s from all three genetic groups of coronaviruses (137). The enzyme is considered an attractive target for antiviral therapy, and a variety of selective inhibitors have been developed (76, 136).

## RNA Polymerase Activities

The coronavirus RdRp domain occupies the carboxy-terminal part of nsp12 and has been classified as an outgroup of superfamily 1 RdRps (71). On the basis of structural information available for other viral RNA polymerases, a model has been developed for the coronavirus RdRp catalytic domain which shows the typical right-hand topology formed by the fingers, palm, and thumb subdomains, and also the conserved sequence motifs that are predicted to be involved in polymerase activity were identified in the model (134). The predicted polymerase activity has been demonstrated for a bacterially expressed form of SARS-CoV nsp12 (25). Both the carboxy-terminal catalytic domain and a 110-residue amino-terminal domain were found to be required for polymerase activity. nsp12 likely interacts with other replicase subunits, including a number of ORF1a-encoded proteins (19).

A second RdRp activity has recently been reported to be associated with nsp8 (60). The activity is sequence specific but has relatively low fidelity and processivity. It produces short oligonucleotides, of less than 6 nucleotides, in a metal ion-dependent reaction. The enzyme prefers 5'-(G/U)CCNN-3' as a template, and RNA synthesis always starts by incorporation of an initiating (+1) GTP nucleotide. nsp8 has been proposed to act as a primase to synthesize the oligonucleotide primer required by the nsp12-associated RdRp activity. Based on the SARS-CoV nsp8 crystal structure and mutagenesis data, three conserved residues that are essential for activity, Lys-58, Lys-82, and Ser-85 (SARS-CoV nsp8 numbering), were proposed to be part of the catalytic center mediating the phosphoryl transfer reaction (60). Further details of the nsp8 structure are discussed below.

### Helicase

The coronavirus helicase domain resides in the carboxy-terminal half of nsp13 and has been classified as belonging to superfamily 1 of helicases (43, 44) (Fig. 1). Coronavirus helicases share at their amino terminus a complex ZBD that includes 12 conserved cysteine and histidine residues predicted to form a binuclear cluster (12, 43, 131). The ZBD is critically involved in the enzymatic activities of coronavirus helicases (107), and conservative mutations of zinc-coordinating residues abolish coronavirus RNA synthesis (T. Hertzig and J. Ziebuhr, unpublished data), demonstrating the essential function of this nidovirus-wide conserved domain. Biochemical studies have revealed multiple enzymatic activities for coronavirus helicases, including nucleic acid-stimulated NTPase and dNTPase as well as RNA and DNA duplex-unwinding activities (62, 63, 106, 108, 126, 128). Furthermore, nsp13 was demonstrated to have RNA 5'-triphosphatase activity which has been proposed to be involved in the 5'-capping reaction of coronavirus RNAs (62, 63).

Fueled by ribonucleotide or nucleotide hydrolysis, coronavirus helicases move in a 5'-to-3' direction along RNA and require a 5' single-stranded "tail" to initiate strand separation of double-stranded RNA (dsRNA) substrates. The 5'-to-3' polarity in the unwinding reaction is a conserved feature of nidovirus helicases. This is of note because other plus-strand RNA virus helicases generally operate with 3'-to-5' polarity (65, 106). The biological meaning of the differential polarity of plus-strand RNA virus helicases is currently not clear. Besides their activity on dsRNA, coronavirus helicases are able to separate

dsDNA substrates with high efficiency (62, 63, 106, 128). The dual specificity for both RNA and DNA is a feature that is rarely found in cellular helicases. However, given that coronaviruses replicate in the cytoplasm and nsp13 is not transported to the nucleus (16, 62, 116), the DNA helicase activity of coronavirus helicases is unlikely to be of biological relevance.

### RNases

Coronaviruses and other nidoviruses with large genomes (i.e., toroviruses, bafiniviruses, and roniviruses) encode a 3'-to-5' exoribonuclease (ExoN) that resides in the amino-terminal part of nsp14 (85, 114) (Fig. 1). ExoN is related to the DEDD superfamily of exonucleases (86, 150), which also includes enzymes involved in DNA-replication-associated proofreading mechanisms. Both the relationship with these cellular enzymes and the fact that arteriviruses, featuring significantly smaller genomes than other nidoviruses, lack an ExoN homolog has led to the speculation that the ExoN activities conserved in large nidoviruses might be involved in pathways related to proofreading and repair (42, 114; see also chapter 2). However, there is currently no evidence for superior fidelities of coronavirus RNA polymerase activities (compared to other RNA virus polymerases) to support this idea.

SARS-CoV ExoN has been demonstrated to have metal ion-dependent 3'-to-5' exoribonuclease activity that acts on both single-stranded RNA (ssRNA) and dsRNA (85), but not on DNA and ribose-2'-O-methylated RNA. Although the precise specificity of the enzyme remains to be determined, it seems clear that RNA structure is an important factor in substrate binding and/or activity. ExoN has been shown to be essential for coronavirus replication (85). Substitutions of putative ExoN active-site residues engineered into the HCoV-229E genome resulted in severe defects in viral RNA synthesis (85). Besides drastically reduced genome replication, distinct defects in subgenome-length RNA synthesis were observed, including aberrant sizes of two subgenomic RNAs (sgRNAs) and altered molar ratios between specific sgRNAs. A deletion of the entire nsp14-coding sequence from a SARS-CoV replicon RNA was shown to reduce sgRNA levels below the detection threshold, whereas an ExoN active-site mutation resulted in significantly reduced but still detectable sgRNA synthesis (3). The molecular mechanisms underlying the diverse defects in RNA synthesis remain to be identified, but based on the available data, it seems reasonable to suggest that an ExoN-mediated 3'-to-5' exonuclease ("trimming") activity may be required at some stage of genomic RNA and/or sgRNA synthesis, for example, to remove nucleotide misincorporations during RNA synthesis or nucleotide mismatches at leader-body junctions during minus-strand RNA synthesis (85).

Coronaviruses encode a second RNase activity that is called NendoU (<u>n</u>idoviral <u>endo</u>ribonuclease, specific for <u>U</u>). NendoU is conserved in all nidoviruses (but no other RNA virus), making it one of the unique genetic markers of the order *Nidovirales* (42, 61, 114). NendoU is related to a family of cellular proteins that is prototyped by the poly(U)-specific endoribonuclease, XendoU, which is involved in the processing of a small nucleolar RNA (snoRNA) derived from an intron of a *Xenopus laevis* ribosomal protein gene (40, 77). Reverse-genetics data obtained for both corona- and arteriviruses have implicated NendoU in a critical (but currently unknown) function in the viral life cycle (61, 91). Whereas substitutions of several conserved aspartic acid codons proved to be lethal when introduced in the arterivirus equine arteritis virus (see chapter 6) and coronavirus HCoV-229E genomes (61, 91), other substitutions, including those replacing presumed active-site His residues, caused only moderate defects in viral RNA synthesis (91; Hertzig and Ziebuhr, unpublished). By contrast, the replacement of one of the active-site histidine residues in the SARS-CoV replicon caused a more than 100-fold decrease in sg mRNA synthesis (3). Interestingly, the production of infectious virus was shown to be affected much more profoundly than viral RNA synthesis in equine arteritis virus and HCoV-229E (91; Hertzig and Ziebuhr, unpublished), suggesting that NendoU may also have functions at a later stage of the viral replication cycle. For example, NendoU could be involved in the processing of specific viral and/or cellular RNAs in order to promote the production of fully infectious viral genomes. Alternatively, NendoU may modulate specific cellular pathways in order to promote the efficient production and release of infectious virus particles. It has been suggested (114) that the coexpression of endoribonuclease, exoribonuclease, and MT activities in coronaviruses may be functionally related to (or interfere with) pathways of cellular snoRNA processing and site-specific RNA methylation, which employs a similar set of enzyme activities (39, 70; see also chapter 2). Thus far, however, this possibility has not been explored experimentally.

nsp15-associated NendoU activities have been reported for SARS-CoV, HCoV-229E, MHV, and IBV (13, 61, 135). The activities were consistently reported to be significantly enhanced by $Mn^{2+}$ ions (13, 61, 135), and there was little activity in the presence of $Mg^{2+}$ or $Ca^{2+}$ (61). The precise role of $Mn^{2+}$ in NendoU activity and the residues involved in metal ion coordination have not been identified conclusively

(13, 61, 97, 135). It has been suggested that metal ions may enhance RNA binding (14), whereas a role in catalysis seems less likely (97, 135). NendoU cleaves at the 3' side of uridylate residues in both ssRNA and dsRNA (14, 61). Both the local RNA structure and the sequence context of the uridylate residue appear to be critically involved in substrate binding and cleavage (14). The biologically relevant substrate(s) of coronavirus NendoUs remains to be identified. The nucleolytic activity of NendoU produces molecules with 2'-3' cyclic phosphate ends (61), causing an aberrant migration of NendoU cleavage products in polyacrylamide gels that led to erroneous conclusions on the precise site of cleavage in initial studies (13). The generation of 2'-3' cyclic phosphates in the cleavage reaction suggests that the 2' hydroxyl group is involved in the NendoU-catalyzed hydrolysis reaction, which is in agreement with data showing that ribose-2'-O-methylated RNA is resistant to cleavage by NendoU (61). Crystal structure analyses of the SARS-CoV and MHV NendoU homologs show that coronavirus NendoUs form hexamers, which are thought to be the active form of the enzyme (97, 135). The hexameric form of the MHV nsp15 was reported to have a slightly lower $K_m$ than the monomer, indicating that hexamer formation may promote substrate binding (135), a conclusion that is also supported by a model of an nsp15-RNA complex derived from a cryoelectron microscopy study (14). However, the relatively minor differences in $K_m$ and virtually identical $k_{cat}$ values determined for the monomeric and hexameric nsp15, together with the fact that maltose-binding protein–nsp15 fusion proteins that do not form hexameric structures possess nucleolytic activity (61), indicate that hexamer formation is not essential for NendoU activity.

The NendoU monomer has a unique fold that, with the exception of XendoU (96), is not related to other nucleases, providing further, strong support for the phylogenetic relationship between the nsp15 carboxy-terminal domain and a family of cellular proteins prototyped by XendoU (61, 114). The available structural information and mutagenesis data (40, 61, 97, 135) suggest that NendoU employs a catalytic center that involves two histidines and one lysine residue (97). The structural basis of the pronounced uridylate specificity has not been fully resolved but may involve stacking interactions between the pyrimidine ring and the phenol ring of a conserved tyrosine as well as a conserved serine/threonine residue (97).

## ADP-Ribose-1″-Phosphatase

The ADRP domain is located upstream of PL2$^{pro}$ in coronavirus nsp3 and was originally identified as a conserved domain (called X domain) in coronaviruses and viruses of the alphavirus-like supergroup (45, 72). It is also conserved in toroviruses and bafiniviruses (31, 103), but not in arteri- or roniviruses (114). The domain is related to a large family of macro domain proteins that are named after the nonhistone domain of macroH2A histones. Macro domain proteins are known to be associated with ADP-ribose binding and processing of ADP-ribose derivatives, such as ADP-ribose 1″-phosphate (69).

Characterization of the HCoV-229E ADRP revealed that the protein dephosphorylates ADP-ribose 1″-phosphate to ADP-ribose in a very specific manner (93). Similar data were subsequently reported for ADRPs from SARS-CoV and transmissible gastroenteritis virus (94, 98). Structures of SARS-CoV ADRP have been determined both for the unliganded form and in complex with ADP-ribose (34, 98). The protein was revealed to have a three-layered α/β/α core that is similar to the fold of cellular macro domains, although there is significant structural diversity among these proteins with respect to (i) the loops connecting the core secondary structure elements and (ii) amino- and carboxy-terminal extensions flanking the ADRP core structure (2, 34, 74, 98). The ADP-ribose molecule was found to be bound in a slightly bent conformation in an uncharged cleft located at the carboxy-terminal part of the central β-sheet. Mutagenesis and structural data implicate residues from four conserved regions of ADRP in the ADP-ribose binding site, and key residues involved in the binding to adenine, the α and β phosphates and the two ribose moieties, were identified (34). At present, the catalytic mechanism employed by ADRP to dephosphorylate ADP-ribose 1″-phosphate is not entirely clear. Modeling of a complex of the SARS-CoV ADRP domain with ADP-ribose 1″-phosphate and site-directed mutagenesis data imply a strictly conserved asparagine residue in activity (34). The oxygen of the side chain of this asparagine interacts with three main chain NH groups, and as a result, the amino group of the asparagine side chain is suitably positioned to interact with (i) the 2′ and 3′ hydroxyl groups of the (second) ribose moiety, (ii) two main chain oxygens, and (iii) a water molecule, the last being maintained in its position by hydrogen bonds with several main chain atoms. The water molecule is conserved in all macro domain structures, and it interacts with the 2′ and 3′ hydroxyl residues of the ribose, suggesting that it may promote a nucleophilic attack on the phosphorus of the ADP-ribose 1″-monophosphate.

Site-directed mutagenesis of the strictly conserved asparagine in the HCoV-229E full-length infectious clone revealed no significant effect on viral replication in tissue culture (93), suggesting that the ADRP activity may have functions in the infected host (rather than in viral RNA synthesis and production of infectious virus progeny). Alternatively, the ADRP activity may not represent the biologically relevant activity of the protein or may represent only one (minor) function among other more important functions in the viral life cycle. It has been noted, in this context, that cellular and viral macro domains have suspiciously low ADP-ribose 1″-monophosphatase activities but that some of them bind poly(ADP-ribose) very efficiently (34, 69, 74, 93, 112). Similarly, the poly(ADP-ribose)-binding activities determined for several coronavirus and togavirus macro domains did not correlate with their ADP-ribose 1″-monophosphatase activities, suggesting that in some cases, macro domain proteins may have evolved divergent specificities and/or activities (34). A possible functional link between macro domains and poly(ADP-ribose)-regulated pathways was further corroborated by a structure model developed for the SARS-CoV macro domain in complex with di-ADP-ribose (34). The model showed that a second ADP-ribose molecule could be readily accommodated in a groove formed by partially conserved residues adjacent to the ADP-ribose-binding crevice described above.

The remarkable diversity of the macro domain family, and the conservation of macro domains in organisms representing all kingdoms of life, suggests that members of this family may be involved in diverse biological processes that are controlled by binding to and/or processing of ADP-ribose or structurally related molecules (69, 75). Similarly, the conservation of macro domains in different RNA virus families and all virus species of the family *Coronaviridae*, which infect a broad range of animals, including mammals, birds, and fish, suggests a universal and important regulatory role for these domains in diverse hosts. Future studies on macro domains of cellular and viral systems can therefore be expected to provide interesting new insights into the functional significance of this diverse group of proteins.

## Other Predicted Enzyme Activities

Group 2a coronaviruses (e.g., MHV and bovine coronavirus) have been reported to encode a putative nucleotide cyclic phosphodiesterase (CPD). The domain is also conserved in the genomes of bovine and equine toroviruses (31, 114; see also chapter 9). The predicted enzymatic activity remains to be characterized, and it is known that the CPD domain is dispensable for MHV replication in cell culture (104). CPD has been suggested to operate in conjunction with ADRP in the same metabolic pathway (114), where it is predicted to convert ADP-ribose 1″,2″-cyclic phosphate, a side product of tRNA splicing (27), to ADP-ribose 1″-phosphate, which may then be further processed by ADRP. Both the pattern of conservation in the *Coronaviridae* and the available reverse-genetics information suggest that the ADRP and CPD activities may provide a selective advantage in vivo (93, 119). As discussed above for ADRP, the substrates of CPD and the biologically relevant metabolic pathways remain to be characterized.

nsp16 has been predicted to mediate MT activity (38, 114, 132), and reverse-genetics experiments have shown that the MT domain is essential for viral RNA synthesis in HCoV-229E and SARS-CoV (3; T. Hertzig, B. Schelle, and J. Ziebuhr, unpublished data). The enzyme is probably involved in the production of the cap 1 structures of coronaviral RNAs (132), but it is also conceivable that it cooperates with NendoU and ExoN in other RNA processing pathways (see above). Thus, for example, endonucleolytic cleavage of specific viral and/or cellular RNAs by NendoU could generate small RNAs that subsequently act as cofactors for site-specific RNA ribose-2′-O methylation reactions mediated by MT (similar to the cellular snoRNA processing pathways discussed above). Alternatively, MT might methylate specific RNAs to protect them from NendoU-mediated cleavage (61). At present, however, there is no direct proof to support this hypothesis.

## OTHER REPLICASE GENE-ENCODED PROTEINS

### nsp1 to nsp4

Apart from the nsp3-associated protease and ADRP activities discussed above, the functions associated with the highly divergent amino-terminal pp1a/pp1ab regions have not been very well characterized. nsp1 is not conserved in avian (group 3) coronaviruses, and the nsp1s of group 1 and 2 coronaviruses are not evidently related to one another. However, there is evidence for a common ancestry of the nsp1s from coronaviruses belonging to the same group (114). The homology between the nsp1 sequences of SARS-CoV and several group 2 coronaviruses was an important piece of evidence supporting the proposed common ancestry of SARS-CoV-like viruses and group 2 coronaviruses (46, 114). In all group 1 and 2 coronaviruses, nsp1 is liberated from pp1a/pp1ab by nsp3-associated PL$^{pro}$s, even though the proteases involved may vary among different groups and subgroups (8, 51, 54, 145). The nsp1s of MHV and SARS-CoV have been implicated in virus-host interactions. Overexpression of MHV nsp1 was shown to cause cell cycle arrest in the $G_0/G_1$ phase, and SARS-CoV nsp1 was

implicated in mRNA (but not rRNA) degradation (23, 66). The biological significance and implications of both these observations remain to be elucidated in detail. The MHV nsp1 carboxy-terminal domain was shown to be dispensable for MHV replication in tissue culture but proved to be important for efficient cleavage of the nsp1–2 site and optimal viral replication (20). MHV mutants containing deletions of the amino-terminal or central nsp1 domains (residues 1 to 123 and 87 to 164, respectively) were not viable, and several single-residue substitutions in nsp1 resulted in nonviable viruses, suggesting that nsp1 has critical functions in viral replication (20). However, possible deleterious effects of the mutations and deletions on viral RNA structure or the folding of the amino-terminal pp1a/pp1ab region cannot be fully excluded as possible causes of the observed defects. However, the proposed role of nsp1 in viral replication receives independent support by the documented colocalization of nsp1 with viral replication complexes and interactions between nsp1 and two other replication complex-associated proteins (nsp7 and nsp10) (21).

Despite the recent progress in the characterization of nsp1 homologs from group 2 coronaviruses, the biological functions of this protein remain obscure. Also, the recently reported nuclear magnetic resonance structure of the SARS-CoV nsp1 segment from residues 13 to 128 does not provide definitive clues to the function of this protein (5). The structure revealed an α/β fold with no statistically significant structural similarity to any other protein described to date. The amino-terminal and carboxy-terminal domains (residues 1 to 12 and 129 to 179, respectively) were found to be flexibly disordered. The central globular domain adopted a mixed parallel/antiparallel six-stranded β-barrel, where the spatial arrangement of the β-strands was β1-β2-β5-β3-β4-β6, and β1 made contact with β6. An α-helix (α1) was located across one opening of the barrel, and one $3_{10}$-helix was located alongside the barrel. It has been speculated that the exceptionally irregular fold of the nsp1 β-barrel domain may be linked to a novel (currently unknown) physiological function of nsp1 (5).

Coronavirus nsp2 sequences are profoundly divergent, and there is little information on possible functions of these proteins. It has been shown that nsp2 is not required for viral replication of either MHV or SARS-CoV (49). Mutant viruses lacking the entire nsp2 coding sequence had only minor reductions in peak titers (0.5 to 1 $\log_{10}$) and an ~50% reduction of viral RNA synthesis, with all RNA species being equally affected. The data suggest that both nsp2 and the relatively stable nsp2–3 processing intermediate are dispensable for MHV and SARS-CoV replication in tissue culture.

Sequence comparisons of coronavirus nsp3s revealed a conserved subdomain structure (149). The sequential order of conserved domains in nsp3 is as follows (from amino terminus to carboxy terminus): acidic domain-PL1$^{pro}$-ADRP-PL2$^{pro}$-Y domain. Despite these similarities in the nsp3 subdomain organization, there are important differences, which, for example, relate to the number and activities/specificities of PL$^{pro}$s (see above) and the presence of additional protein domains with currently unknown functions in several viruses (114, 149). The available information on the structures and functions of the PL$^{pro}$ and ADRP domains has been summarized above. The function of the amino-terminal acidic domain is not known, and there is limited information on the physiological role of the Y domain. The latter domain contains a number of conserved cysteine residues and a putative transmembrane (TM) domain. The TM domain was reported to be required for PL2$^{pro}$-mediated processing of the nsp3–4 site in both SARS-CoV and MHV (51, 68). Furthermore, the TM domain was revealed to be inserted into membranes, and its luminal domain was shown to be glycosylated at two (in SARS-CoV) or one (in MHV) asparagine residue. A more detailed characterization of the MHV nsp3-associated TM domain revealed that the domain has four membrane-spanning helices. When fused to a cytosolic protein, the domain was able to confer membrane association to a cytosolic protein, strongly supporting the previously suggested role of the domain in mediating membrane association of nsp3 (149). nsp4, which in pp1a/pp1ab is located immediately downstream of the nsp3 Y domain, may be another TM protein involved in anchoring the viral replicase to intracellular membranes (43) (Fig. 1). Furthermore, nsp4 appears to have a specific role in RNA synthesis, as shown by experiments using MHV temperature-sensitive *(ts)* mutants (100).

## nsp6 to nsp11

Crystal structures have recently been reported for SARS-CoV nsp7, -8, -9, and -10 (33, 64, 89, 121, 124, 140). They provide a wealth of structural information that, along with biochemical data, provides interesting new insight into the quaternary structure and assembly of the coronavirus replication complex as well as possible functions of these ORF1a-encoded proteins (Fig. 1). Three of the proteins, nsp8, nsp9, and nsp10, were shown to have RNA-binding activities, and all four proteins (nsp7 to nsp10) appear to be involved in homo- and/or heterotypic interactions with other proteins from the pp1a/pp1ab region (33, 64, 83, 121, 124).

nsp7 and nsp8 form a hexadecameric supercomplex comprised of eight copies each of nsp7 and nsp8 (140). The complex has a cylinder-like structure with an inner diameter of approximately 30 Å. On the basis of (i) the diameter of the cylinder, (ii) the positively charged inner surface, and (iii) RNA-binding data obtained for nsp8, it has been proposed that the complex may encircle dsRNA and act as a processivity factor of the RdRp (140). More recently, however, it has been found that nsp8 itself is an(other) RdRp. The protein has template-dependent, oligonucleotide-synthesizing polymerase activity that may produce the RNA primers required for the primer-dependent RdRp activity associated with nsp12 (60).

The structure of nsp7 is comprised of three α-helices that form an amino-terminal triple-stranded antiparallel coiled coil ("helical bundle") and a fourth carboxy-terminal α-helix (89, 140). nsp8, by contrast, folds into a "golf club"-like structure with amino-terminal "shaft" and carboxy-terminal "head" domains. The golf club-like structure adopts two different conformations (featuring either a straight or a bent shaft) that were called nsp8I and nsp8II, respectively (140). The bent shaft in nsp8II becomes possible because the long α-helix NH3 found in nsp8I bends into two helices, NH3α and NH3β. The two different conformations of nsp8 are essential to form the octameric and, ultimately, hexadecameric supercomplex structures seen in the crystal structure (140). Whereas nsp8I and nsp8II form the framework of this supercomplex, the eight nsp7 molecules further stabilize it by filling some of the remaining space. This unique subunit arrangement in the supercomplex has been compared with the roles of bricks (nsp8) and mortar (nsp7) (140). Imbert et al. (60) identified a structural similarity of the nsp8 head domain with members of a family of RNA-binding domains prototyped by heterogeneous nuclear ribonucleoprotein D (35), and they used molecular modeling, sequence comparisons, and mutagenesis data to develop a model for a quaternary initiation complex involving two nsp8 monomers, an ssRNA template, and the first two complementary nucleotides incorporated (GTP and CTP). In this model, the ssRNA is stacked by the hydrophobic surface provided by the nsp8 head domains and points towards the inner part of the hexadecamer channel (60). One nsp8 molecule binds the ssRNA template, and the second molecule binds the nascent RNA. The two first NTPs incorporated are bound to two strictly conserved basic residues, Arg-75 and Lys-82. All the conserved residues required for polymerase activity are part of the long α-helix called α2 (60) or NH3 (140), and two of the conserved residues, Lys-58 and Arg-75, are also close to the central channel. The identification of a primase activity in coronaviruses is an important step towards understanding the mechanisms involved in the initiation of coronaviral RNA synthesis, but further studies will be required to understand this process in its molecular details.

The nsp7-nsp8 supercomplex is thought to interact with other replicase subunits, and one of them has been confirmed to be nsp9, a dimeric, ssRNA-binding protein that has been reported to interact with nsp8 (33, 124). Crystal structures have been determined by two laboratories for SARS-CoV nsp9 (33, 124). The structures revealed an open six-stranded β-barrel fold that is related to the β-barrel domains of viral and cellular chymotrypsin-like proteases (124). Interestingly, both laboratories noticed a distant similarity (but no structural homology) of the nsp9 structure with the oligosaccharide/oligonucleotide-binding fold. The β-barrel core of nsp9 is flanked by an amino-terminal extension and a carboxy-terminal helix.

Crystal structures have also been elucidated for the SARS-CoV nsp10 (64, 121). nsp10 adopts a novel α/β fold comprised of five α-helices, one $3_{10}$-helix, and three β-strands. In one of the structures, the protein forms trimers which, in turn, are assembled into a dodecameric structure in which the trimers are related by a tetrahedral symmetry (121). Two zinc-binding sites were identified that are formed by conserved cysteine residues and one histidine residue (Cys-74/Cys-77/His-83/Cys-90; Cys-117/Cys-120/Cys-128/Cys-130). The amino-terminal zinc finger coordinates the $Zn^{2+}$ ion in a unique conformation and is located on the inner surface of the dodecamer. The carboxy-terminal zinc finger is located on the outer surface and belongs to the polymerase "gag-knuckle" family of zinc fingers (64, 73, 121). The protein was confirmed to bind single-stranded and double-stranded RNA and DNA without obvious specificity (64, 83). nsp10 can be cross-linked with nsp9, suggesting the existence of a complex network of protein-protein interactions involving nsp7, -8, -9, and -10. An MHV *ts* mutant encoding a substitution of a conserved glutamine, Gln-65, with glutamate in nsp10 was shown to cause a defect in minus-strand synthesis. The structures suggest that the substitution responsible for the observed functional defect may have affected the conformational stability of the α4-helix, which forms part of the amino-terminal zinc finger, thereby possibly perturbing the folding of nsp10 (or, more generally, that of pp1a/pp1ab) into a conformation that is not active in minus-strand synthesis (121). Alternatively, the additional negative charge on the molecule's surface may have altered a critical binding interface involved in protein and/or RNA binding (64).

The large multimeric complexes seen in the crystal structures of nsp7, nsp8, and nsp10 may provide an explanation for the conservation of a ribosomal frameshifting mechanism in coronaviruses. This mechanism might ensure that ORF1a- and ORF1b-encoded proteins are expressed in a specific molar ratio, and the relative overexpression of ORF1a proteins might provide an abundant supply of the protomers required for the assembly of functional multimers. However, the fact that also nsp15, which is encoded by ORF1b, assembles into hexamers (97) suggests that yet other evolutionary driving forces may have shaped the evolution of the frameshift mechanism. Thus, for example, it is tempting to speculate that the relative down-regulation of ORF1b expression improves the specificity of viral RNA synthesis, which would be jeopardized if there was an overproduction of catalytic activities (mainly encoded by ORF1b) in relation to specificity-determining factors (suggested to be mainly encoded by ORF1a). Clearly, a lack of specificity for the appropriate viral templates would be detrimental to both viral replication and host cell viability. Although potentially existing specificity-determining functions of ORF1a proteins need to be substantiated in further studies, several of the activities associated with ORF1a-encoded proteins (e.g., protease activities, membrane association, primase activity, RNA-binding activity, and potential RdRp cofactors) would be consistent with this idea. For example, ORF1a-encoded proteins may act to (i) create a structural scaffold for viral RNA synthesis, (ii) recruit appropriate templates, (iii) ensure specific initiation of RNA synthesis, and (iv) control the processivity of the polymerase. In other words, the ribosomal frameshift would provide a mechanism that maintains a postulated functional balance between specificity-determining factors (including sequence-specific primase activity) and "core replicative enzymes."

Interesting functional differences between ORF1a- and ORF1b-encoded proteins were also revealed by studies of MHV *ts* mutants (100). It was found that most ORF1a gene products are *cis* active, and ORF1a mutants form a single complementation group encompassing the entire nsp4–10 region. By contrast, most (if not all) ORF1b mutants were revealed to belong to different complementation groups, suggesting that ORF1b-encoded proteins are *trans* active and "diffusible" between replication/transcription complexes. In agreement with these genetic data, MHV nsp12 was reported to assemble with the viral replicase when expressed as a green fluorescent protein-tagged fusion protein in virus-infected cells (19), providing additional evidence that nsp12 and possibly other ORF1b-encoded proteins are diffusible and can be exchanged between different replication/transcription complexes.

It seems reasonable to suggest that the complex homo- and heteromultimers described above are functionally relevant and that they are assembled from mature nsps. This, however, leaves us with the question of how polymerase activity can be attained early in infection when polyprotein processing is not complete and the required processing end products are either in short supply or not available. We also have to consider that, most probably, the release of the active (that is, dimeric) form of 3CL$^{pro}$ from pp1a/pp1ab is a slow process which has been proposed to require intermolecular cleavages between different polyprotein molecules (57). High pp1a/pp1ab concentrations, which would promote such intermolecular cleavages, are unlikely to exist early in the infection cycle, which may delay the release and, thus, activation of 3CL$^{pro}$. Similarly, the observed longevity of 3CL$^{pro}$-containing precursors in MHV-infected cells (67) argues against an efficient and early release of 3CL$^{pro}$ from pp1a/p1ab. If the currently held belief that 3CL$^{pro}$ operates only in *trans* and not in *cis* was proved to be correct, then the slow release of 3CL$^{pro}$ from pp1a/pp1ab would cause a significant delay in the production of fully processed nsp7, -8, -9, and -10, which are the protomers required for assembling functional di- or multimers. This apparent discrepancy between incomplete processing early in infection and the identification of functional multimers produced from processing end products could be resolved if we postulate different protein requirements for specific steps in viral RNA synthesis. For example, it seems reasonable to think that minus-strand synthesis, which obviously is an early step in viral replication, does not depend on fully processed polyproteins. In this context, it is important to remember that minus-strand synthesis strictly depends on ongoing protein synthesis (99). This suggests, but does not prove, that (largely) unprocessed replicase polyproteins are active in, and required for, minus-strand synthesis. As these polyproteins undergo proteolytic autoprocessing, they need to be replenished in order to keep minus-strand synthesis going, which is in agreement with the observation that minus-strand polymerases are unstable (133). Also, the decline of minus-strand synthesis later in infection may be explained by the accumulation of fully activated 3CL$^{pro}$, which, later in infection, may cause a drastic reduction of the half-lives of replicase precursors required for minus-strand polymerases activity. By contrast, plus-strand synthesis may proceed initially at a relatively low level but become more efficient later in infection when fully processed subunits become available, which assemble into multimeric complexes active in plus-strand synthesis. This model is supported by genetic data showing that the 3CL$^{pro}$ has a role in the production of efficient plus-strand polymerases (100). In conclusion, it is tempting to speculate that the multimeric complexes generated in vitro from bacterially expressed proteins have functional counterparts in the infected cell, but only at a later stage of infection when the presence of high concentrations of dimeric 3CL$^{pro}$ allows the replicase polyproteins to be cleaved highly efficiently, thereby generating the processing end products required for a structural and functional reorganization of the replication complex (92, 146). In other words, the complex multimers seen in the crystal structures of nsp7, -8, and -10 might represent protein structures that act later in infection, for example, at a time when plus-strand RNA synthesis reaches its maximum.

nsp6 is a hydrophobic protein featuring several membrane-spanning domains. The protein has not been studied in any detail, but similar to the TM domains in nsp3 and nsp4, it is believed to help anchor the replication complex to intracellular membranes derived from the endoplasmic reticulum (47, 116).

nsp11 is a small peptide of generally less than 20 residues (Table 1) that shares its amino-terminal residues (upstream of the frameshift site) with nsp12. The short nsp11 coding sequence overlaps with important sequence and structure elements involved in ribosomal frameshifting. It therefore seems unlikely that the ORF1a 3′ end would have a second role as a coding sequence for a nonconserved oligopeptide sequence. The peptide has also not been detected in coronavirus-infected cells.

## CONCLUDING REMARKS

Over the past few years, impressive progress into the functions and structures of coronavirus replicative proteins has been made (11, 82, 147). Nevertheless, our understanding of the molecular mechanisms that coronaviruses have evolved to synthesize, express, and maintain their unusually large RNA genomes is still far from being complete. Research efforts in the areas of bioinformatics, structural biology, biochemistry, and cell biology as well as forward- and reverse-genetics approaches will be needed to elucidate the molecular mechanisms, enzymatic reactions, and structures of the protein complexes involved in the initiation of coronavirus RNA synthesis, in continuous/discontinuous synthesis, and in termination of coronavirus RNA synthesis and the further processing and turnover of these RNAs. Further studies can also be expected to identify replicase gene-encoded functions involved in critical interactions with the host. Obviously, all these studies will provide a continuously increasing knowledge base for antiviral drug design which, in the long run, may allow us to combat these important human and animal pathogens more effectively.

Coronaviruses and, more generally, nidoviruses occupy a unique position among plus-strand RNA viruses (see chapter 2). It therefore seems likely that further systematic studies into the molecular biology of coronaviruses will continue to reveal spectacular and unexpected findings without parallels in other viral and cellular systems. In view of their special molecular biology and medical importance, coronaviruses clearly deserve further study and will probably continue to be a challenging and exciting field of research in the years to come.

## REFERENCES

1. Allaire, M., M. M. Chernaia, B.A. Malcolm, and M. N. James. 1994. Picornaviral 3C cysteine proteinases have a fold similar to chymotrypsin-like serine proteinases. *Nature* 369:72–76.

2. Allen, M. D., A. M. Buckle, S. C. Cordell, J. Löwe, and M. Bycroft. 2003. The crystal structure of AF1521 a protein from Archaeoglobus fulgidus with homology to the non-histone domain of macroH2A. *J. Mol. Biol.* 330:503–511.

3. Almazán, F., M. L. Dediego, C. Galán, D. Escors, E. Álvarez, J. Ortego, I. Sola, S. Zuñiga, S. Alonso, J. L. Moreno, A. Nogales, C. Capiscol, and L. Enjuanes. 2006. Construction of a severe acute respiratory syndrome coronavirus infectious cDNA clone and a replicon to study coronavirus RNA synthesis. *J. Virol.* 80:10900–10906.

4. Almazán, F., C. Galán, and L. Enjuanes. 2004. The nucleoprotein is required for efficient coronavirus genome replication. *J. Virol.* 78:12683–12688.

5. Almeida, M. S., M. A. Johnson, T. Herrmann, M. Geralt, and K. Wüthrich. 2007. Novel β-barrel fold in the nuclear magnetic resonance structure of the replicase nonstructural protein 1 from the severe acute respiratory syndrome coronavirus. *J. Virol.* 81:3151–3161.

6. Anand, K., G. J. Palm, J. R. Mesters, S. G. Siddell, J. Ziebuhr, and R. Hilgenfeld. 2002. Structure of coronavirus main proteinase reveals combination of a chymotrypsin fold with an extra alpha-helical domain. *EMBO J.* 21:3213–3224.

7. Anand, K., J. Ziebuhr, P. Wadhwani, J. R. Mesters, and R. Hilgenfeld. 2003. Coronavirus main proteinase (3CL^pro) structure: basis for design of anti-SARS drugs. *Science* 300:1763–1767.

8. Baker, S. C., C. K. Shieh, L. H. Soe, M. F. Chang, D. M. Vannier, and M. M. Lai. 1989. Identification of a domain required for autoproteolytic cleavage of murine coronavirus gene A polyprotein. *J. Virol.* 63:3693–3699.

9. Barretto, N., D. Jukneliene, K. Ratia, Z. Chen, A. D. Mesecar, and S. C. Baker. 2005. The papain-like protease of severe acute respiratory syndrome coronavirus has deubiquitinating activity. *J. Virol.* 79:15189–15198.

10. Barrila, J., U. Bacha, and E. Freire. 2006. Long-range cooperative interactions modulate dimerization in SARS 3CL^pro. *Biochemistry* 45:14908–14916.

11. Bartlam, M., H. Yang, and Z. Rao. 2005. Structural insights into SARS coronavirus proteins. *Curr. Opin. Struct. Biol.* 15:664–672.

12. Bernini, A., O. Spiga, V. Venditti, F. Prischi, L. Bracci, J. Huang, J. A. Tanner, and N. Niccolai. 2006. Tertiary structure prediction of SARS coronavirus helicase. *Biochem. Biophys. Res. Commun.* 343:1101–1104.

13. Bhardwaj, K., L. Guarino, and C. C. Kao. 2004. The severe acute respiratory syndrome coronavirus Nsp15 protein is an endoribonuclease that prefers manganese as a cofactor. *J. Virol.* 78:12218–12224.

14. Bhardwaj, K., J. Sun, A. Holzenburg, L. A. Guarino, and C. C. Kao. 2006. RNA recognition and cleavage by the SARS coronavirus endoribonuclease. *J. Mol. Biol.* 361:243–256.

15. Bonilla, P. J., S. A. Hughes, and S. R. Weiss. 1997. Characterization of a second cleavage site and demonstration of activity in *trans* by the papain-like proteinase of the murine coronavirus mouse hepatitis virus strain A59. *J. Virol.* 71:900–909.

16. Bost, A. G., E. Prentice, and M. R. Denison. 2001. Mouse hepatitis virus replicase protein complexes are translocated to sites of M protein accumulation in the ERGIC at late times of infection. *Virology* 285:21–29.

17. Brierley, I. 1995. Ribosomal frameshifting viral RNAs. *J. Gen. Virol.* 76:1885–1892.

18 Brierley, I., M. E. Boursnell, M. M. Binns, B. Bilimoria, V. C. Blok, T. D. Brown, and S. C. Inglis. 1987. An efficient ribosomal frame-shifting signal in the polymerase-encoding region of the coronavirus IBV. *EMBO J.* 6:3779–3785.

19. Brockway, S. M., C. T. Clay, X. T. Lu, and M. R. Denison. 2003. Characterization of the expression, intracellular localization, and replication complex association of the putative mouse hepatitis virus RNA-dependent RNA polymerase. *J. Virol.* 77:10515–10527.

20. Brockway, S. M., and M. R. Denison. 2005. Mutagenesis of the murine hepatitis virus nsp1-coding region identifies residues important for protein processing, viral RNA synthesis, and viral replication. *Virology* 340:209–223.

21. Brockway, S. M., X. T. Lu, T. R. Peters, T. S. Dermody and M. R. Denison. 2004. Intracellular localization and protein interactions of the gene 1 protein p28 during mouse hepatitis virus replication. *J. Virol.* 78:11551–11562.

22. Cavanagh, D. 1997. *Nidovirales*: a new order comprising *Coronaviridae* and *Arteriviridae*. *Arch. Virol.* 142:629–633.

23. Chen, C.-J., K. Sugiyama, H. Kubo, C. Huang, and S. Makino. 2004. Murine coronavirus nonstructural protein p28 arrests cell cycle in $G_0/G_1$ phase. *J. Virol.* 78:10410–10419.

24. Chen, H., P. Wei, C. Huang, L. Tan, Y. Liu, and L. Lai. 2006. Only one protomer is active in the dimer of SARS 3C-like proteinase. *J. Biol. Chem.* 281:13894–13898.

25. Cheng, A., W. Zhang, Y. Xie, W. Jiang, E. Arnold, S. G. Sarafianos, and J. Ding. 2005. Expression, purification, and characterization of SARS coronavirus RNA polymerase. *Virology* 335:165–176.

26. Chou, C. Y., H. C. Chang, W. C. Hsu, T. Z. Lin, C. H. Lin, and G. G. Chang. 2004. Quaternary structure of the severe acute respiratory syndrome (SARS) coronavirus main protease. *Biochemistry* 43:14958–14970.

27. Culver, G. M., S. A. Consaul, K. T. Tycowski, W. Filipowicz, and E. M. Phizicky. 1994. tRNA splicing in yeast and wheat germ. A cyclic phosphodiesterase implicated in the metabolism of ADP-ribose 1″,2″-cyclic phosphate. *J. Biol. Chem.* 269:24928–24934.

28. Denison, M. R., B. Yount, S. M. Brockway, R. L. Graham, A. C. Sims, X. Lu, and R. S. Baric. 2004. Cleavage between

replicase proteins p28 and p65 of mouse hepatitis virus is not required for virus replication. *J. Virol.* **78**:5957–5965.

29. **Dong, S., and S. C. Baker.** 1994. Determinants of the p28 cleavage site recognized by the first papain-like cysteine proteinase of murine coronavirus. *Virology* **204**:541–549.

30. **Dos Ramos, F., M. Carrasco, T. Doyle, and I. Brierley.** 2004. Programmed −1 ribosomal frameshifting in the SARS coronavirus. *Biochem. Soc. Trans.* **32**:1081–1083.

31. **Draker, R., R. L. Roper, M. Petric, and R. Tellier.** 2006. The complete sequence of the bovine torovirus genome. *Virus Res.* **115**:56–68.

32. **Eckerle, L. D., S. M. Brockway, S. M. Sperry, X. Lu, and M. R. Denison.** 2006. Effects of mutagenesis of murine hepatitis virus nsp1 and nsp14 on replication in culture. *Adv. Exp. Med. Biol.* **581**:55–60.

33. **Egloff, M. P., F. Ferron, V. Campanacci, S. Longhi, C. H. Rancurel, H. Dutartre, E. J. Snijder, A. E. Gorbalenya, C. Cambillau, and B. Canard.** 2004. The severe acute respiratory syndrome-coronavirus replicative protein nsp9 is a single-stranded RNA-binding subunit unique in the RNA virus world. *Proc. Natl. Acad. Sci. USA* **101**:3792–3796.

34. **Egloff, M. P., H. Malet, Á. Putics, M. Heinonen, H. Dutartre, A. Frangeul, A. Gruez, V. Campanacci, C. Cambillau, J. Ziebuhr, T. Ahola, and B. Canard.** 2006. Structural and functional basis for ADP-ribose and poly(ADP-ribose) binding by viral macro domains. *J. Virol.* **80**:8493–8502.

35. **Enokizono, Y., Y. Konishi, K. Nagata, K. Ouhashi, S. Uesugi, F. Ishikawa, and M. Katahira.** 2005. Structure of hnRNP D complexed with single-stranded telomere DNA and unfolding of the quadruplex by heterogeneous nuclear ribonucleoprotein D. *J. Biol. Chem.* **280**:18862–18870.

36. **Fan, K., L. Ma, X. Han, H. Liang, P. Wei, Y. Liu, and L. Lai.** 2005. The substrate specificity of SARS coronavirus 3C-like proteinase. *Biochem. Biophys. Res. Commun.* **329**:934–940.

37. **Fan, K., P. Wei, Q. Feng, S. Chen, C. Huang, L. Ma, B. Lai, J. Pei, Y. Liu, J. Chen, and L. Lai.** 2004. Biosynthesis, purification, and substrate specificity of severe acute respiratory syndrome coronavirus 3C-like proteinase. *J. Biol. Chem.* **279**:1637–1642.

38. **Feder, M., J. Pas, L. S. Wyrwicz, and J. M. Bujnicki.** 2003. Molecular phylogenetics of the RrmJ/fibrillarin superfamily of ribose 2′-O-methyltransferases. *Gene* **302**:129–138.

39. **Filipowicz, W., and V. Pogačić.** 2002. Biogenesis of small nucleolar ribonucleoproteins. *Curr. Opin. Cell Biol.* **14**:319–327.

40. **Gioia, U., P. Laneve, M. Dlakić, M. Arceci, I. Bozzoni, and E. Caffarelli.** 2005. Functional characterization of XendoU, the endoribonuclease involved in small nucleolar RNA biosynthesis. *J. Biol. Chem.* **280**:18996–19002.

41. **González, J. M., P. Gomez-Puertas, D. Cavanagh, A. E. Gorbalenya, and L. Enjuanes.** 2003. A comparative sequence analysis to revise the current taxonomy of the family Coronaviridae. *Arch. Virol.* **148**:2207–2235.

42. **Gorbalenya, A. E., L. Enjuanes, J. Ziebuhr, and E. J. Snijder.** 2006. Nidovirales: evolving the largest RNA virus genome. *Virus Res.* **117**:17–37.

43. **Gorbalenya, A. E., E. V. Koonin, A. P. Donchenko, and V. M. Blinov.** 1989. Coronavirus genome: prediction of putative functional domains in the non-structural polyprotein by comparative amino acid sequence analysis. *Nucleic Acids Res.* **17**:4847–4861.

44 **Gorbalenya, A. E., E. V. Koonin, A. P. Donchenko, and V. M. Blinov.** 1989. Two related superfamilies of putative helicases involved in replication, recombination, repair and expression of DNA and RNA genomes. *Nucleic Acids Res.* **17**:4713–4730.

45. **Gorbalenya, A. E., E. V. Koonin, and M. M. Lai.** 1991. Putative papain-related thiol proteases of positive-strand RNA viruses.

Identification of rubi- and aphthovirus proteases and delineation of a novel conserved domain associated with proteases of rubi-, alpha- and coronaviruses. *FEBS Lett.* **288**:201–205.

46. **Gorbalenya, A. E., E. J. Snijder, and W. J. Spaan.** 2004. Severe acute respiratory syndrome coronavirus phylogeny: toward consensus. *J. Virol.* **78**:7863–7866.

47. **Gosert, R., A. Kanjanahaluethai, D. Egger, K. Bienz, and S. C. Baker.** 2002. RNA replication of mouse hepatitis virus takes place at double-membrane vesicles. *J. Virol.* **76**:3697–3708.

48. **Graham, R. L., and M. R. Denison.** 2006. Replication of murine hepatitis virus is regulated by papain-like proteinase 1 processing of nonstructural proteins 1, 2, and 3. *J. Virol.* **80**:11610–11620.

49. **Graham, R. L., A. C. Sims, S. M. Brockway, R. S. Baric, and M. R. Denison.** 2005. The nsp2 replicase proteins of murine hepatitis virus and severe acute respiratory syndrome coronavirus are dispensable for viral replication. *J. Virol.* **79**:13399–13411.

50. **Graziano, V., W. J. McGrath, L. Yang, and W. F. Mangel.** 2006. SARS CoV main proteinase: the monomer-dimer equilibrium dissociation constant. *Biochemistry* **45**:14632–14641.

51. **Harcourt, B. H., D. Jukneliene, A. Kanjanahaluethai, J. Bechill, K. M. Severson, C. M. Smith, P. A. Rota, and S. C. Baker.** 2004. Identification of severe acute respiratory syndrome coronavirus replicase products and characterization of papain-like protease activity. *J. Virol.* **78**:13600–13612.

52. **Hegyi, A., A. Friebe, A. E. Gorbalenya, and J. Ziebuhr.** 2002. Mutational analysis of the active centre of coronavirus 3C-like proteases. *J. Gen. Virol.* **83**:581–593.

53. **Hegyi, A., and J. Ziebuhr.** 2002. Conservation of substrate specificities among coronavirus main proteases. *J. Gen. Virol.* **83**:595–599.

54. **Herold, J., A. E. Gorbalenya, V. Thiel, B. Schelle, and S. G. Siddell.** 1998. Proteolytic processing at the amino terminus of human coronavirus 229E gene 1-encoded polyproteins: identification of a papain-like proteinase and its substrate. *J. Virol.* **72**:910–918.

55. **Herold, J., and S. G. Siddell.** 1993. An 'elaborated' pseudoknot is required for high frequency frameshifting during translation of HCV 229E polymerase mRNA. *Nucleic Acids Res.* **21**:5838–5842.

56. **Herold, J., S. G. Siddell, and A. E. Gorbalenya.** 1999. A human RNA viral cysteine proteinase that depends upon a unique $Zn^{2+}$-binding finger connecting the two domains of a papain-like fold. *J. Biol. Chem.* **274**:14918–14925.

57. **Hsu, M. F., C. J. Kuo, K. T. Chang, H. C. Chang, C. C. Chou, T. P. Ko, H. L. Shr, G. G. Chang, A. H. Wang, and P. H. Liang.** 2005. Mechanism of the maturation process of SARS-CoV 3CL protease. *J. Biol. Chem.* **280**:31257–31266.

58. **Hsu, W. C., H. C. Chang, C. Y. Chou, P. J. Tsai, P. I. Lin, and G. G. Chang.** 2005. Critical assessment of important regions in the subunit association and catalytic action of the severe acute respiratory syndrome coronavirus main protease. *J. Biol. Chem.* **280**:22741–22748.

59. **Hu, M., P. Li, M. Li, W. Li, T. Yao, J. W. Wu, W. Gu, R. E. Cohen, and Y. Shi.** 2002. Crystal structure of a UBP-family deubiquitinating enzyme in isolation and in complex with ubiquitin aldehyde. *Cell* **111**:1041–1054.

60. **Imbert, I., J. C. Guillemot, J. M. Bourhis, C. Bussetta, B. Coutard, M. P. Egloff, F. Ferron, A. E. Gorbalenya, and B. Canard.** 2006. A second, non-canonical RNA-dependent RNA polymerase in SARS coronavirus. *EMBO J.* **25**:4933–4942.

61. **Ivanov, K. A., T. Hertzig, M. Rozanov, S. Bayer, V. Thiel, A. E. Gorbalenya, and J. Ziebuhr.** 2004. Major genetic marker of nidoviruses encodes a replicative endoribonuclease. *Proc. Natl. Acad. Sci. USA* **101**:12694–12699.

62. Ivanov, K. A., V. Thiel, J. C. Dobbe, Y. van der Meer, E. J. Snijder, and J. Ziebuhr. 2004. Multiple enzymatic activities associated with severe acute respiratory syndrome coronavirus helicase. *J. Virol.* 78:5619–5632.

63. Ivanov, K. A., and J. Ziebuhr. 2004. Human coronavirus 229E nonstructural protein 13: characterization of duplex-unwinding, nucleoside triphosphatase, and RNA 5′-triphosphatase activities. *J. Virol.* 78:7833–7838.

64. Joseph, J. S., K. S. Saikatendu, V. Subramanian, B. W. Neuman, A. Brooun, M. Griffith, K. Moy, M. K. Yadav, J. Velasquez, M. J. Buchmeier, R. C. Stevens, and P. Kuhn. 2006. Crystal structure of nonstructural protein 10 from the severe acute respiratory syndrome coronavirus reveals a novel fold with two zinc-binding motifs. *J. Virol.* 80:7894–7901.

65. Kadaré, G., and A. L. Haenni. 1997. Virus-encoded RNA helicases. *J. Virol.* 71:2583–2590.

66. Kamitani, W., K. Narayanan, C. Huang, K. Lokugamage, T. Ikegami, N. Ito, H. Kubo, and S. Makino. 2006. Severe acute respiratory syndrome coronavirus nsp1 protein suppresses host gene expression by promoting host mRNA degradation. *Proc. Natl. Acad. Sci. USA* 103:12885–12890.

67. Kanjanahaluethai, A., and S. C. Baker. 2000. Identification of mouse hepatitis virus papain-like proteinase 2 activity. *J. Virol.* 74:7911–7921.

68. Kanjanahaluethai, A., Z. Chen, D. Jukneliene, and S. C. Baker. 2007. Membrane topology of murine coronavirus replicase nonstructural protein 3. *Virology* 361:391–401.

69. Karras, G. I., G. Kustatscher, H. R. Buhecha, M. D. Allen, C. Pugieux, F. Sait, M. Bycroft, and A. G. Ladurner. 2005. The macro domain is an ADP-ribose binding module. *EMBO J.* 24:1911–1920.

70. Kiss, T. 2001. Small nucleolar RNA-guided post-transcriptional modification of cellular RNAs. *EMBO J.* 20:3617–3622.

71. Koonin, E. V. 1991. The phylogeny of RNA-dependent RNA polymerases of positive-strand RNA viruses. *J. Gen. Virol.* 72:2197–2206.

72. Koonin, E. V., A. E. Gorbalenya, M. A. Purdy, M. N. Rozanov, G. R. Reyes, and D. W. Bradley. 1992. Computer-assisted assignment of functional domains in the nonstructural polyprotein of hepatitis E virus: delineation of an additional group of positive-strand RNA plant and animal viruses. *Proc. Natl. Acad. Sci. USA* 89:8259–8263.

73. Krishna, S. S., I. Majumdar, and N. V. Grishin. 2003. Structural classification of zinc fingers: survey and summary. *Nucleic Acids Res.* 31:532–550.

74. Kumaran, D., S. Eswaramoorthy, F. W. Studier, and S. Swaminathan. 2005. Structure and mechanism of ADP-ribose-1″-monophosphatase (Appr-1″-pase), a ubiquitous cellular processing enzyme. *Protein Sci.* 14:719–726.

75. Kustatscher, G., M. Hothorn, C. Pugieux, K. Scheffzek, and A. G. Ladurner. 2005. Splicing regulates NAD metabolite binding to histone macroH2A. *Nat. Struct. Mol. Biol.* 12:624–625.

76. Lai, L., X. Han, H. Chen, P. Wei, C. Huang, S. Liu, K. Fan, L. Zhou, Z. Liu, J. Pei, and Y. Liu. 2006. Quaternary structure, substrate selectivity and inhibitor design for SARS 3C-like proteinase. *Curr. Pharm. Des.* 12:4555–4564.

77. Laneve, P., F. Altieri, M. E. Fiori, A. Scaloni, I. Bozzoni, and E. Caffarelli. 2003. Purification, cloning, and characterization of XendoU, a novel endoribonuclease involved in processing of intron-encoded small nucleolar RNAs in Xenopus laevis. *J. Biol. Chem.* 278:13026–13032.

78. Lim, K. P., L. F. Ng, and D. X. Liu. 2000. Identification of a novel cleavage activity of the first papain-like proteinase domain encoded by open reading frame 1a of the coronavirus avian infectious bronchitis virus and characterization of the cleavage products. *J. Virol.* 74:1674–1685.

79. Lindner, H. A., N. Fotouhi-Ardakani, V. Lytvyn, P. Lachance, T. Sulea, and R. Menard. 2005. The papain-like protease from the severe acute respiratory syndrome coronavirus is a deubiquitinating enzyme. *J. Virol.* 79:15199–15208.

80. Liu, D. X., and T. D. Brown. 1995. Characterisation and mutational analysis of an ORF 1a-encoding proteinase domain responsible for proteolytic processing of the infectious bronchitis virus 1a/1b polyprotein. *Virology* 209:420–427.

81. Lu, Y., X. Lu, and M. R. Denison. 1995. Identification and characterization of a serine-like proteinase of the murine coronavirus MHV-A59. *J. Virol.* 69:3554–3559.

82. Masters, P. S. 2006. The molecular biology of coronaviruses. *Adv. Virus Res.* 66:193–292.

83. Matthes, N., J. R. Mesters, B. Coutard, B. Canard, E. J. Snijder, R. Moll, and R. Hilgenfeld. 2006. The non-structural protein Nsp10 of mouse hepatitis virus binds zinc ions and nucleic acids. *FEBS Lett.* 580:4143–4149.

84. Matthews, D. A., W. W. Smith, R. A. Ferre, B. Condon, G. Budahazi, W. Sisson, J. E. Villafranca, C. A. Janson, H. E. McElroy, C. L. Gribskov, et al. 1994. Structure of human rhinovirus 3C protease reveals a trypsin-like polypeptide fold, RNA-binding site, and means for cleaving precursor polyprotein. *Cell* 77:761–771.

85. Minskaia, E., T. Hertzig, A. E. Gorbalenya, V. Campanacci, C. Cambillau, B. Canard, and J. Ziebuhr. 2006. Discovery of an RNA virus 3′→5′ exoribonuclease that is critically involved in coronavirus RNA synthesis. *Proc. Natl. Acad. Sci. USA* 103:5108–5113.

86. Moser, M. J., W. R. Holley, A. Chatterjee, and I. S. Mian. 1997. The proofreading domain of Escherichia coli DNA polymerase I and other DNA and/or RNA exonuclease domains. *Nucleic Acids Res.* 25:5110–5118.

87. Mosimann, S. C., M. M. Cherney, S. Sia, S. Plotch, and M. N. James. 1997. Refined X-ray crystallographic structure of the poliovirus 3C gene product. *J. Mol. Biol.* 273:1032–1047.

88. Namy, O., S. J. Moran, D. I. Stuart, R. J. Gilbert, and I. Brierley. 2006. A mechanical explanation of RNA pseudoknot function in programmed ribosomal frameshifting. *Nature* 441:244–247.

89. Peti, W., M. A. Johnson, T. Herrmann, B. W. Neuman, M. J. Buchmeier, M. Nelson, J. Joseph, R. Page, R. C. Stevens, P. Kuhn, and K. Wüthrich. 2005. Structural genomics of the severe acute respiratory syndrome coronavirus: nuclear magnetic resonance structure of the protein nsP7. *J. Virol.* 79:12905–12913.

90. Piñon, J. D., R. R. Mayreddy, J. D. Turner, F. S. Khan, P. J. Bonilla, and S. R. Weiss. 1997. Efficient autoproteolytic processing of the MHV-A59 3C-like proteinase from the flanking hydrophobic domains requires membranes. *Virology* 230:309–322.

91. Posthuma, C. C., D. D. Nedialkova, J. C. Zevenhoven-Dobbe, J. H. Blokhuis, A. E. Gorbalenya, and E. J. Snijder. 2006. Site-directed mutagenesis of the nidovirus replicative endoribonuclease NendoU exerts pleiotropic effects on the arterivirus life cycle. *J. Virol.* 80:1653–1661.

92. Prentice, E., J. McAuliffe, X. Lu, K. Subbarao, and M. R. Denison. 2004. Identification and characterization of severe acute respiratory syndrome coronavirus replicase proteins. *J. Virol.* 78:9977–9986.

93. Putics, Á., W. Filipowicz, J. Hall, A. E. Gorbalenya, and J. Ziebuhr. 2005. ADP-ribose-1″-monophosphatase: a conserved coronavirus enzyme that is dispensable for viral replication in tissue culture. *J. Virol.* 79:12721–12731.

94. Putics, Á., A. E. Gorbalenya, and J. Ziebuhr. 2006. Identification of protease and ADP-ribose 1″-monophosphatase activities associated with transmissible gastroenteritis virus non-structural protein 3. *J. Gen. Virol.* 87:651–656.

95. Ratia, K., K. S. Saikatendu, B. D. Santarsiero, N. Barretto, S. C. Baker, R. C. Stevens, and A. D. Mesecar. 2006. Severe acute respiratory syndrome coronavirus papain-like protease: structure of a viral deubiquitinating enzyme. *Proc. Natl. Acad. Sci. USA* **103:**5717–5722.

96. Renzi, F., E. Caffarelli, P. Laneve, I. Bozzoni, M. Brunori, and B. Vallone. 2006. The structure of the endoribonuclease XendoU: from small nucleolar RNA processing to severe acute respiratory syndrome coronavirus replication. *Proc. Natl. Acad. Sci. USA* **103:**12365–12370.

97. Ricagno, S., M. P. Egloff, R. Ulferts, B. Coutard, D. Nurizzo, V. Campanacci, C. Cambillau, J. Ziebuhr, and B. Canard. 2006. Crystal structure and mechanistic determinants of SARS coronavirus nonstructural protein 15 define an endoribonuclease family. *Proc. Natl. Acad. Sci. USA* **103:**11892–11897.

98. Saikatendu, K. S., J. S. Joseph, V. Subramanian, T. Clayton, M. Griffith, K. Moy, J. Velasquez, B. W. Neuman, M. J. Buchmeier, R. C. Stevens, and P. Kuhn. 2005. Structural basis of severe acute respiratory syndrome coronavirus ADP-ribose-1″-phosphate dephosphorylation by a conserved domain of nsP3. *Structure* **13:**1665–1675.

99. Sawicki, S. G., and D. L. Sawicki. 1986. Coronavirus minus-strand RNA synthesis and effect of cycloheximide on coronavirus RNA synthesis. *J. Virol.* **57:**328–334.

100. Sawicki, S. G., D. L. Sawicki, D. Younker, Y. Meyer, V. Thiel, H. Stokes, and S. G. Siddell. 2005. Functional and genetic analysis of coronavirus replicase-transcriptase proteins. *PLoS Pathog.* **1:**e39.

101. Schelle, B., N. Karl, B. Ludewig, S. G. Siddell, and V. Thiel. 2005. Selective replication of coronavirus genomes that express nucleocapsid protein. *J. Virol.* **79:**6620–6630.

102. Schiller, J. J., A. Kanjanahaluethai, and S. C. Baker. 1998. Processing of the coronavirus MHV-JHM polymerase polyprotein: identification of precursors and proteolytic products spanning 400 kilodaltons of ORF1a. *Virology* **242:**288–302.

103. Schütze, H., R. Ulferts, B. Schelle, S. Bayer, H. Granzow, B. Hoffmann, T. C. Mettenleiter, and J. Ziebuhr. 2006. Characterization of *White bream virus* reveals a novel genetic cluster of nidoviruses. *J. Virol.* **80:**11598–11609.

104. Schwarz, B., E. Routledge, and S. G. Siddell. 1990. Murine coronavirus nonstructural protein ns2 is not essential for virus replication in transformed cells. *J. Virol.* **64:**4784–4791.

105. Seipelt, J., A. Guarné, E. Bergmann, M. James, W. Sommergruber, I. Fita, and T. Skern. 1999. The structures of picornaviral proteinases. *Virus Res.* **62:**159–168.

106. Seybert, A., A. Hegyi, S. G. Siddell, and J. Ziebuhr. 2000. The human coronavirus 229E superfamily 1 helicase has RNA and DNA duplex-unwinding activities with 5′-to-3′ polarity. *RNA* **6:**1056–1068.

107. Seybert, A., C. C. Posthuma, L. C. van Dinten, E. J. Snijder, A. E. Gorbalenya, and J. Ziebuhr. 2005. A complex zinc finger controls the enzymatic activities of nidovirus helicases. *J. Virol.* **79:**696–704.

108. Seybert, A., L. C. van Dinten, E. J. Snijder, and J. Ziebuhr. 2000. Biochemical characterization of the equine arteritis virus helicase suggests a close functional relationship between arterivirus and coronavirus helicases. *J. Virol.* **74:**9586–9593.

109. Shi, J., and J. Song. 2006. The catalysis of the SARS 3C-like protease is under extensive regulation by its extra domain. *FEBS J.* **273:**1035–1045.

110. Shi, J., Z. Wei, and J. Song. 2004. Dissection study on the SARS 3C-like protease reveals the critical role of the extra domain in dimerization of the enzyme: defining the extra domain as a new target for design of highly-specific protease inhibitors. *J. Biol. Chem.* **279:**24765–24773.

111. Shi, S. T., and M. M. Lai. 2005. Viral and cellular proteins involved in coronavirus replication. *Curr. Top. Microbiol. Immunol.* **287:**95–131.

112. Shull, N. P., S. L. Spinelli, and E. M. Phizicky. 2005. A highly specific phosphatase that acts on ADP-ribose 1″-phosphate, a metabolite of tRNA splicing in Saccharomyces cerevisiae. *Nucleic Acids Res.* **33:**650–660.

113. Siddell, S. G., J. Ziebuhr, and E. J. Snijder. 2005. Coronaviruses, toroviruses, and arteriviruses, p. 823–856. *In* B. W. J. Mahy and V. ter Meulen (ed.), *Topley & Wilson's Microbiology and Microbial Infections*, 10th ed., *Virology*, vol. 1. Hodder Arnold, London, United Kingdom.

114. Snijder, E. J., P. J. Bredenbeek, J. C. Dobbe, V. Thiel, J. Ziebuhr, L. L. Poon, Y. Guan, M. Rozanov, W. J. Spaan, and A. E. Gorbalenya. 2003. Unique and conserved features of genome and proteome of SARS-coronavirus, an early split-off from the coronavirus group 2 lineage. *J. Mol. Biol.* **331:**991–1004.

115. Snijder, E. J., S. G. Siddell, and A. E. Gorbalenya. 2005. The order *Nidovirales*, p. 390–404. *In* B. W. J. Mahy and V. ter Meulen (ed.), *Topley & Wilson's Microbiology and Microbial Infections*, 10th ed., *Virology*, vol. 1. Hodder Arnold, London, United Kingdom.

116. Snijder, E. J., Y. van der Meer, J. Zevenhoven-Dobbe, J. J. Onderwater, J. van der Meulen, H. K. Koerten, and A. M. Mommaas. 2006. Ultrastructure and origin of membrane vesicles associated with the severe acute respiratory syndrome coronavirus replication complex. *J. Virol.* **80:**5927–5940.

117. Spaan, W. J. M., D. Brian, D. Cavanagh, R. J. de Groot, L. Enjuanes, A. E. Gorbalenya, K. V. Holmes, P. S. Masters, P. Rottier, F. Taguchi, and P. Talbot. 2005. Family *Coronaviridae*, p. 947–964. *In* C. M. Fauquet, M. A. Mayo, J. Maniloff, U. Desselberger, and L. A. Ball (ed.), *Virus Taxonomy. Eighth Report of the International Committee on Taxonomy of Viruses.* Elsevier Academic Press, San Diego, CA.

118. Spaan, W. J. M., D. Cavanagh, R. J. de Groot, L. Enjuanes, A. E. Gorbalenya, E. J. Snijder, and P. J. Walker. 2005. Order *Nidovirales*, p. 937–945. *In* C. M. Fauquet, M. A. Mayo, J. Maniloff, U. Desselberger, and L. A. Ball (ed.), *Virus Taxonomy. Eighth Report of the International Committee on Taxonomy of Viruses.* Elsevier Academic Press, San Diego, CA.

119. Sperry, S. M., L. Kazi, R. L. Graham, R. S. Baric, S. R. Weiss, and M. R. Denison. 2005. Single-amino-acid substitutions in open reading frame (ORF) 1b-nsp14 and ORF 2a proteins of the coronavirus mouse hepatitis virus are attenuating in mice. *J. Virol.* **79:**3391–3400.

120. Strauss, J. H., and E. G. Strauss. 1994. The alphaviruses: gene expression, replication, and evolution. *Microbiol. Rev.* **58:**491–562.

121. Su, D., Z. Lou, F. Sun, Y. Zhai, H. Yang, R. Zhang, A. Joachimiak, X. C. Zhang, M. Bartlam, and Z. Rao. 2006. Dodecamer structure of severe acute respiratory syndrome coronavirus nonstructural protein nsp10. *J. Virol.* **80:**7902–7908.

122. Sulea, T., H. A. Lindner, E. O. Purisima, and R. Ménard. 2005. Deubiquitination, a new function of the severe acute respiratory syndrome coronavirus papain-like protease? *J. Virol.* **79:**4550–4551.

123. Sulea, T., H. A. Lindner, E. O. Purisima, and R. Ménard. 2006. Binding site-based classification of coronaviral papain-like proteases. *Proteins* **62:**760–775.

124. Sutton, G., E. Fry, L. Carter, S. Sainsbury, T. Walter, J. Nettleship, N. Berrow, R. Owens, R. Gilbert, A. Davidson, S. Siddell, L. L. Poon, J. Diprose, D. Alderton, M. Walsh, J. M. Grimes, and D. I. Stuart. 2004. The nsp9 replicase protein of

SARS-coronavirus, structure and functional insights. *Structure* **12**:341–353.

125. Tan, J., K. H. Verschueren, K. Anand, J. Shen, M. Yang, Y. Xu, Z. Rao, J. Bigalke, B. Heisen, J. R. Mesters, K. Chen, X. Shen, H. Jiang, and R. Hilgenfeld. 2005. pH-dependent conformational flexibility of the SARS-CoV main proteinase (M$^{pro}$) dimer: molecular dynamics simulations and multiple X-ray structure analyses. *J. Mol. Biol.* **354**:25–40.

126. Tanner, J. A., R. M. Watt, Y. B. Chai, L. Y. Lu, M. C. Lin, J. S. Peiris, L. L. Poon, H. F. Kung, and J. D. Huang. 2003. The severe acute respiratory syndrome (SARS) coronavirus NTPase/helicase belongs to a distinct class of 5′ to 3′ viral helicases. *J. Biol. Chem.* **278**:39578–39582.

127. ten Dam, E., M. Flint, and M. D. Ryan. 1999. Virus-encoded proteinases of the *Togaviridae*. *J. Gen. Virol.* **80**:1879–1888.

128. Thiel, V., K. A. Ivanov, Á. Putics, T. Hertzig, B. Schelle, S. Bayer, B. Weissbrich, E. J. Snijder, H. Rabenau, H. W. Doerr, A. E. Gorbalenya, and J. Ziebuhr. 2003. Mechanisms and enzymes involved in SARS coronavirus genome expression. *J. Gen. Virol.* **84**:2305–2315.

129. Tibbles, K. W., I. Brierley, D. Cavanagh, and T. D. Brown. 1996. Characterization in vitro of an autocatalytic processing activity associated with the predicted 3C-like proteinase domain of the coronavirus avian infectious bronchitis virus. *J. Virol.* **70**:1923–1930.

130. van der Meer, Y., E. J. Snijder, J. C. Dobbe, S. Schleich, M. R. Denison, W. J. Spaan, and J. Krijnse Locker. 1999. Localization of mouse hepatitis virus nonstructural proteins and RNA synthesis indicates a role for late endosomes in viral replication. *J. Virol.* **73**:7641–7657.

131. van Dinten, L. C., H. van Tol, A. E. Gorbalenya, and E. J. Snijder. 2000. The predicted metal-binding region of the arterivirus helicase protein is involved in subgenomic mRNA synthesis, genome replication, and virion biogenesis. *J. Virol.* **74**:5213–5223.

132. von Grotthuss, M., L. S. Wyrwicz, and L. Rychlewski. 2003. mRNA cap-1 methyltransferase in the SARS genome. *Cell* **113**:701–702.

133. Wang, T., and S. G. Sawicki. 2001. Mouse hepatitis virus minus-strand templates are unstable and turnover [sic] during viral replication. *Adv. Exp. Med. Biol.* **494**:491–497.

134. Xu, X., Y. Liu, S. Weiss, E. Arnold, S. G. Sarafianos, and J. Ding. 2003. Molecular model of SARS coronavirus polymerase: implications for biochemical functions and drug design. *Nucleic Acids Res.* **31**:7117–7130.

135. Xu, X., Y. Zhai, F. Sun, Z. Lou, D. Su, Y. Xu, R. Zhang, A. Joachimiak, X. C. Zhang, M. Bartlam, and Z. Rao. 2006. New antiviral target revealed by the hexameric structure of mouse hepatitis virus nonstructural protein nsp15. *J. Virol.* **80**:7909–7917.

136. Yang, H., M. Bartlam, and Z. Rao. 2006. Drug design targeting the main protease, the Achilles' heel of coronaviruses. *Curr. Pharm. Des.* **12**:4573–4590.

137. Yang, H., W. Xie, X. Xue, K. Yang, J. Ma, W. Liang, Q. Zhao, Z. Zhou, D. Pei, J. Ziebuhr, R. Hilgenfeld, K. Y. Yuen, L. Wong, G. Gao, S. Chen, Z. Chen, D. Ma, M. Bartlam, and Z. Rao. 2005. Design of wide-spectrum inhibitors targeting coronavirus main proteases. *PLoS Biol.* **3**:e324.

138. Yang, H., M. Yang, Y. Ding, Y. Liu, Z. Lou, Z. Zhou, L. Sun, L. Mo, S. Ye, H. Pang, G. F. Gao, K. Anand, M. Bartlam, R. Hilgenfeld, and Z. Rao. 2003. The crystal structures of severe acute respiratory syndrome virus main protease and its complex with an inhibitor. *Proc. Natl. Acad. Sci. USA* **100**:13190–13195.

139. Yin, J., E. M. Bergmann, M. M. Cherney, M. S. Lall, R. P. Jain, J. C. Vederas, and M. N. James. 2005. Dual modes of modification of hepatitis A virus 3C protease by a serine-derived beta-lactone: selective crystallization and formation of a functional catalytic triad in the active site. *J. Mol. Biol.* **354**:854–871.

140. Zhai, Y., F. Sun, X. Li, H. Pang, X. Xu, M. Bartlam, and Z. Rao. 2005. Insights into SARS-CoV transcription and replication from the structure of the nsp7-nsp8 hexadecamer. *Nat. Struct. Mol. Biol.* **12**:980–986.

141. Zheng, K., G. Ma, J. Zhou, M. Zen, W. Zhao, Y. Jiang, Q. Yu, and J. Feng. 2007. Insight into the activity of SARS main protease: molecular dynamics study of dimeric and monomeric form of enzyme. *Proteins* **66**:467–479.

142. Ziebuhr, J. 2005. The coronavirus replicase. *Curr. Top. Microbiol. Immunol.* **287**:57–94.

143. Ziebuhr, J., J. Herold, and S. G. Siddell. 1995. Characterization of a human coronavirus (strain 229E) 3C-like proteinase activity. *J. Virol.* **69**:4331–4338.

144. Ziebuhr, J., G. Heusipp, and S. G. Siddell. 1997. Biosynthesis, purification, and characterization of the human coronavirus 229E 3C-like proteinase. *J. Virol.* **71**:3992–3997.

145. Ziebuhr, J., B. Schelle, N. Karl, E. Minskaia, S. Bayer, S. G. Siddell, A. E. Gorbalenya, and V. Thiel. 2007. Human coronavirus 229E papain-like proteases have overlapping specificities but distinct functions in viral replication. *J. Virol.* **81**:3922–3932.

146. Ziebuhr, J., and S. G. Siddell. 1999. Processing of the human coronavirus 229E replicase polyproteins by the virus-encoded 3C-like proteinase: identification of proteolytic products and cleavage sites common to pp1a and pp1ab. *J. Virol.* **73**:177–185.

147. Ziebuhr, J., and E. J. Snijder. 2007. The coronavirus replicase gene: special enzymes for special viruses. *In* V. Thiel (ed.), *Coronaviruses: Molecular Biology and Diseases.* Horizon Scientific Press, Norwich, United Kingdom.

148. Ziebuhr, J., E. J. Snijder, and A. E. Gorbalenya. 2000. Virus-encoded proteinases and proteolytic processing in the Nidovirales. *J. Gen. Virol.* **81**:853–879.

149. Ziebuhr, J., V. Thiel, and A. E. Gorbalenya. 2001. The autocatalytic release of a putative RNA virus transcription factor from its polyprotein precursor involves two paralogous papain-like proteases that cleave the same peptide bond. *J. Biol. Chem.* **276**:33220–33232.

150. Zuo, Y., and M. P. Deutscher. 2001. Exoribonuclease superfamilies: structural analysis and phylogenetic distribution. *Nucleic Acids Res.* **29**:1017–1026.

*Nidoviruses*
Edited by S. Perlman, T. Gallagher, and E. J. Snijder
© 2008 ASM Press, Washington, DC

Chapter 6

# The Arterivirus Replicase

MARTIJN J. VAN HEMERT AND ERIC J. SNIJDER

This chapter focuses on the arterivirus proteins that are involved in genome replication and subgenomic RNA (sgRNA) synthesis. These proteins, which are collectively referred to as "replicase/transcriptase" or—for simplicity—just "replicase," are encoded by open reading frames 1a and 1b (ORF1a and ORF1b) of the arterivirus genome. In contrast to coronavirus replication, for which the nucleocapsid protein is thought to be required (2, 47), for arteriviruses the replicase polyprotein is the only viral protein required for genome replication and transcription (34). Furthermore, the replicase of arteriviruses and other nidoviruses includes multiple proteinases that are involved in processing of the large replicase precursor polyproteins into smaller functional subunits.

After infection of a susceptible host cell and uncoating of the genome, the arterivirus replication cycle is initiated with the translation of the large replicase gene at the 5' end of the genomic RNA (which is also referred to as RNA1). The gene consists of two large ORFs, ORF1a and ORF1b, which partially overlap near the 3' end of ORF1a. Translation of ORF1a yields a polyprotein (pp1a) that ranges in size from 1,727 to 2,503 amino acids (aa), depending on the virus (Table 1). ORF1b is in the −1 reading frame with respect to ORF1a and is translated after a ribosomal frameshift that occurs immediately upstream of the ORF1a termination codon, which results in the synthesis of a 3,175- to 3,960-aa ORF1ab-encoded polypeptide (pp1ab). Subsequently, pp1a and pp1ab undergo extensive autoproteolytic processing, theoretically yielding at least 13 end products, named nsp1 to nsp12 (with processing of a recently described, conserved internal cleavage site in equine arteritis virus [EAV] nsp7 yielding nsp7α and nsp7β [66]). The processed replicase subunits, and probably some processing intermediates as well, become associated

with intracellular membranes and form the replication/transcription complex (RTC) that is responsible for viral RNA synthesis. The ORF1b-encoded replicase subunits are presumed to contain the core enzymatic activities for viral RNA synthesis, such as the RNA-dependent RNA polymerase (RdRp) and helicase (HEL), while ORF1a contains the proteinases involved in polyprotein processing and several hydrophobic domains that presumably anchor the RTC to modified intracellular membranes (see also chapter 7).

Expression of the arterivirus/nidovirus replicase is regulated at multiple levels. The extent of genome replication controls the abundance of the replicase mRNA, the translation of which is under the control of regulatory signals in its 5' end. The ORF1a/1b ribosomal frameshift regulates the balance between ORF1a- and ORF1b-encoded subunits. Finally, the proteolytic processing of the replicase polyproteins controls expression (in time and space) of the various replicase processing intermediates and end products.

## COMPARATIVE SEQUENCE ANALYSIS OF ARTERIVIRUS REPLICASES

Comparative sequence analysis of the various prototypic arterivirus genomes (16, 18, 33, 35, 38), and comparison with more distantly related nidoviruses (see also chapters 1 to 3), led to the identification of a number of conserved domains within the replicase (Fig. 1). The arterivirus replicase gene covers approximately 75% of the genome (Table 1). An arterivirus-wide comparison reveals a similar general organization based on the same array of conserved domains, even though the genes vary considerably in

**Martijn J. van Hemert and Eric J. Snijder** • Molecular Virology Laboratory, Department of Medical Microbiology, Leiden University Medical Center, P.O. Box 9600, Leiden, The Netherlands.

Table 1. Comparison of arterivirus replicase gene features

| Virus | GenBank accession no. | Genome size (nt) | Replicase gene (start–end nt) | Space occupied by replicase gene (%) | pp1a size (aa) | pp1ab size (aa) |
|---|---|---|---|---|---|---|
| EAV | X53459.3 | 12,704 | 225–9751 | 75 | 1,727 | 3,175 |
| SHFV | AF180391 | 15,717 | 210–10996 | 69 | 2,105 | 3,596 |
| LDV-P | U15146.1 | 14,104 | 157–11006 | 77 | 2,206 | 3,616 |
| PRRSV-LV | M96262.2 | 15,111 | 222–11785 | 77 | 2,396 | 3,854 |
| PRRSV-VR | U87392.3 | 15,451 | 191–12072 | 77 | 2,503 | 3,960 |

length. The largest variation in terms of size (1,727 to 2,503 aa) and amino acid composition is found in pp1a. Most of these variable regions are located in the N-terminal half of the polypeptide, especially in the nsp2 region (Fig. 1). Compared to the other arteriviruses, EAV has a large (>50-aa) deletion of the region just upstream of the PCPβ domain of nsp1 (see below). Compared to EAV, simian hemorrhagic fever virus (SHFV) and lactate dehydrogenase-elevating virus (LDV) have large insertions in the nsp2 region. This insertion is even larger in porcine respiratory and reproductive syndrome virus (PRRSV) (Fig. 1). The vast amount of sequence data available for various PRRSV isolates reveal substantial amino acid variation

in pp1a. The pp1a proteins of European and American PRRSV isolates share only 47% amino acid identity and exhibit the greatest divergence (32% identity) in the nsp2 region (1). In addition, the nsp2 protein of virulent strain MN184 has deletions of aa 324 to 434, 486, and 505 to 523 compared to the North American prototype strain VR-2332 (24).

The ORF1b-encoded part of the replicase is much more conserved in terms of size (1,411 to 1,491 aa) and sequence. The variability in the N-terminal region of pp1a/pp1ab suggests that in the course of evolution, species-specific functions have been added to a conserved "core replicase" that is encoded by the 3′ part of ORF1a and ORF1b (nsp3–12).

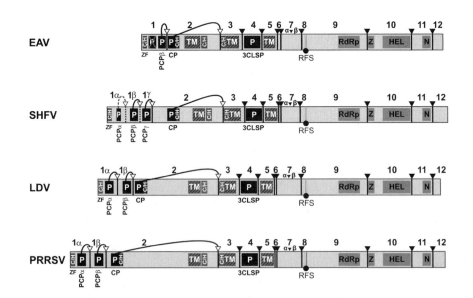

Figure 1. Schematic representation of the replicases of the arteriviruses EAV, SHFV, LDV, and PRRSV. Sequences are aligned on the ribosomal frameshift site (RFS), and nsp numbers are shown above each sequence. The (putative) PCPα, PCPβ, PCPγ, and CP cleavage sites are indicated with open triangles, and the 3CLSP cleavage sites are indicated with black triangles. Conserved domains are indicated with black and gray boxes. ZF, putative zinc finger; C/H, cysteine/histidine-rich clusters; TM, predicted transmembrane regions; P, protease domain; Z, ZBD; N, NendoU. The diagram was based on the EAV Bucyrus strain (Swiss-Prot accession no. P19811) (16), SHFV strain LVR 42-0 (Q68772), the LDV P strain (Q83017) (38), and PRRSV strain VR-2332 (Q9WJB2) (35).

## OVERVIEW OF ORF1a-ENCODED CONSERVED DOMAINS

### Protease PCPα

The most N-terminal protease domain of PRRSV and LDV, a papain-like cysteine proteinase (PCP) that has been named PCPα (MEROPS family C31), resides in the N-terminal ~170 aa of the replicase. Its putative catalytic dyad is formed by Cys-76 and His-146 (PRRSV) or His-147 (LDV), and it catalyzes the rapid release of an approximately 20-kDa N-terminal cleavage product (nsp1α) from the replicase of these viruses (15). In the case of EAV, PCPα has become inactivated due to the loss of its active-site cysteine. Consequently, nsp1α remains attached to the downstream subunit (called nsp1β in PRRSV and LDV), and this protein is referred to as nsp1 (53). For SHFV, experimental data on the processing of the nsp1 region have not been published, but sequence analysis predicts yet an alternative arrangement of PCP domains and cleavage sites (see below).

### Protease PCPβ

den Boon et al. predicted the presence of a PCP domain in the N-terminal region of the EAV replicase (16), of which the activity was confirmed in in vitro assays (53). This domain (Asp-157 to Gly-261 of EAV pp1a/pp1ab) was later termed PCPβ (MEROPS family C32). The presumed Cys and His residues of the catalytic dyad (Cys-164 and His-230 in EAV) are conserved in all arteriviruses (15, 54), and like PCPα, PCPβ contains a Trp immediately downstream of its catalytic cysteine, a residue that is often found at this position in positive-strand RNA virus PCPs (23).

### The nsp2 CP

A third cysteine protease (CP) domain (MEROPS family C33) was identified in the N-terminal domain of EAV nsp2 by comparative sequence analysis and mutagenesis studies (55). Although substantial size differences and sequence variation are observed in the nsp2s of arteriviruses, the CP domain is highly conserved. In EAV, Cys-270 and His-332 form its putative active site (55). The CP domain (Gly-261 to Ser-360 in EAV) is most similar to other viral PCPs, although the catalytic cysteine is not followed by a Trp residue.

### The nsp4 3CLSP or "Main" Protease

By comparative sequence analysis a 3C-like serine protease (3CLSP) consensus sequence, with a predicted catalytic triad formed by His-1103, Asp-1129, and Ser-1184, was identified between aa 1080 and 1220 of the EAV replicase (16). The proteolytic activity of this domain (MEROPS family S32), which resides in nsp4, was confirmed by expression and mutagenesis studies (54, 56). The protease adopts a chymotrypsin-like fold (3) and has a substrate specificity similar to that of the picornavirus 3C CPs, even though its active-site nucleophile is a serine. The nsp4 protease is highly conserved among all arteriviruses, in terms of amino acid sequence and location within the replicase, and in view of its role in the processing of the core of the arterivirus replicase, it has also been coined "main protease."

### Hydrophobic Domains

Three extensive hydrophobic regions are present in nsp2, nsp3, and nsp5 (EAV aa 530 to 645, 829 to 997, and 1291 to 1405). They are assumed to be involved in targeting the arterivirus RTC to intracellular membranes (17, 54, 67). Each of these regions is predicted to contain several transmembrane helices, although experimental data on their exact membrane topology remain to be obtained.

### Cysteine/Histidine-Rich Clusters

The ORF1a-encoded protein sequence contains several clusters of conserved cysteine and histidine residues. These are found in the extreme N terminus of the nsp1 region (a putative zinc finger between Cys-25 and Cys-44; see below), overlapping with the nsp2 CP domain (residues 319, 349, 354, and 356 in EAV), in the conserved C-terminal domain (CTD) of nsp2 (EAV residues 650, 653, 657, 683, 703, and 746), and in nsp3 (EAV residues 855, 864, 879, and 884) (16, 54). Some of these residues might be involved in metal binding and/or zinc finger formation, although experimental data to support this are currently lacking.

## OVERVIEW OF ORF1b-ENCODED CONSERVED DOMAINS

### RdRp

A typical RdRp motif was identified in nsp9 between aa Gly-2104 and Arg-2300 in the ORF1b-encoded part of EAV pp1ab (16, 29, 41). The GDD signature, which includes the two catalytic Asp residues in all positive-strand RNA virus RdRps (27, 41) has been replaced with the sequence SDD in all nidoviruses known to date.

### ZBD

A cysteine/histidine-rich domain in the N terminus of nsp10 (between Cys-2374 and Cys-2426 in EAV) was predicted to bind metal ions and adopt a zinc finger-like conformation (16, 18). Therefore, and for reasons described below, this domain is referred to as the zinc-binding domain (ZBD). In fact, a homologous domain is found at this position in all nidovirus HEL proteins, and therefore, the ZBD is considered a genetic marker of the order *Nidovirales* (21).

## HEL

A type 1 superfamily HEL motif was identified in EAV nsp10, between Val-2525 and Ile-2758 (16), and its functionality was later confirmed in biochemical studies (50). This domain is the most conserved region of the arterivirus replicase and includes a typical NTP-binding motif (EAV Gly-2528 to Thr-2535) (19, 26). The location of the HEL domain downstream of the RdRp is a unique feature of nidoviruses, as in other positive-strand RNA virus replicases the HEL domain resides upstream of the RdRp (22).

## NendoU

A highly conserved domain located between His-2961 and Phe-3039 in the CTD of the EAV replicase (nsp11) was originally described as a "nidovirus-specific conserved domain" of unknown function (16). Based on its homology to the endoribonuclease XendoU of *Xenopus laevis* (31), it was later proposed

to be a nidovirus uridylate-specific endoribonuclease (NendoU) (51), an activity that was subsequently verified for the coronavirus NendoU (25, 44). NendoU has no known homologs in other RNA viruses and can therefore be considered to be another nidovirus-specific genetic marker (21).

## THE ORF1a/1b RIBOSOMAL FRAMESHIFT

Translation of ORF1b requires a −1 ribosomal frameshift in the region just upstream of the ORF1a termination codon, resulting in the C-terminal extension of pp1a to give pp1ab. The ORF1a/ORF1b overlap region contains two sequence elements that are assumed to direct this ribosomal frameshift: the slippery sequence UUUAAAC (or GUUAAC in EAV), which is the actual frameshift site, and an RNA pseudoknot structure downstream of the slippery sequence (16, 18, 33, 35) (Fig. 2; see also chapter 3).

Experimental data obtained with EAV reporter gene constructs (16) and analysis of the LDV-P replicase in an in vitro translation system (17) confirmed the functionality of the frameshift signal. For EAV a frameshifting efficiency of 15 to 20% was observed (16), which—if representative for the in vivo situation—would imply that ORF1b-encoded proteins would have about five times lower expression levels than ORF1a-encoded replicase subunits.

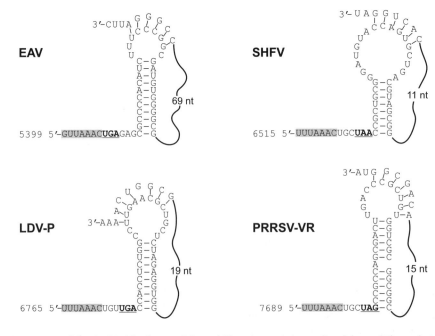

**Figure 2.** RNA sequence of the ORF1a/1b ribosomal frameshift region and the predicted frameshift-regulating RNA pseudoknot structure. The proposed slippery sequence is indicated with a gray box; the ORF1a stop codon (bold) is underlined. The structures were adapted from or modeled based on references 16, 18, and 33. The SHFV structure was modeled using sequence data from GenBank accession no. AF180391.

The first nucleotide (G) of the EAV slippery sequence differs from that of other nidoviruses (U). This difference is probably not the cause of the lower frameshifting efficiency of EAV compared to that reported for other nidoviruses (7, 8, 16), since mutating the EAV slippery sequence to UUUAAAC did not increase frameshifing efficiency in vitro (14). Sequences upstream or downstream of the slippery sequence might influence the frameshift efficiency, as was found for, e.g., infectious bronchitis virus and severe acute respiratory syndrome coronavirus (SARS-CoV) (57).

The putative RNA pseudoknot structure just downstream of the slippery sequence was predicted to be generally similar in terms of size and stability in all arteriviruses (Fig. 2), although the sequence identity is found to be merely 45 to 60% when arteriviruses are compared (18). For EAV, a domain containing the sequence 5'-CCGGGA-3', 69 nucleotides (nt) downstream of the predicted stem-loop structure, was shown to be essential for frameshifting (16). The spacing between the stem-loop structure and the downstream domain varies considerably (11 to 69 nt) among arteriviruses (Fig. 2), but its influence on frameshifting efficiency is unknown.

## PROTEOLYTIC PROCESSING OF THE REPLICASE

Proteolytic processing plays an important role during the arterivirus life cycle and presumably is a way to control the temporal and spatial release of replicase subunits. The maturation of a subunit can be influenced by factors like its location within the polyprotein and—obviously—the rate at which the flanking cleavage sites are processed, which might depend on their amino acid sequence and conformation and/or the presence of cofactors.

Arterivirus pp1a and pp1ab are proteolytically processed by three or four ORF1a-encoded proteases, located in nsp1 (α and β), nsp2, and nsp4. The pp1ab polyprotein is now thought to be cleaved 11 times in the case of EAV and 12 times for PRRSV, LDV, and SHFV (Fig. 3). Together with the ribosomal frameshift, complete processing of the EAV replicase thus yields 13 processing end products (including nsp7α and nsp7β [66]). In the case of PRRSV and LDV, an extra cleavage occurs within nsp1, yielding nsp1α and nsp1β. Several of the processing intermediates have considerable half-lives and therefore may have a specific function during the viral life cycle.

Most of the experimental data on proteolytic processing have been obtained for the EAV replicase (15, 54–56, 65, 70, 72, 74), which has thus been the

basis for the description in the following sections. However, the absolute conservation of protease domains and their cognate cleavage sites in the replicases of all known arteriviruses strongly suggests that their processing schemes will be comparable, if not identical.

### PCPα/PCPβ-Mediated Processing

The activity of a previously predicted PCP domain in the N-terminal (nsp1) region of the EAV replicase was experimentally confirmed by in vitro translation and mutagenesis studies (53). This domain (PCPβ) was shown to catalyze cleavage of the nsp1/2 junction, thus releasing the approximately 29-kDa nsp1 subunit (53) (Fig. 4). N-terminal sequencing of nsp2 and mutagenesis studies indicated that cleavage occurs between Gly-260 and Gly-261 (53) (Fig. 3). Pulse-chase experiments revealed that the nsp1/2 site was processed quickly (within ~15 min, probably even cotranslationally) and that consequently nsp1 is the first protein released from the replicase polyproteins (54). nsp1 was found to be very stable throughout the viral life cycle (54).

PRRSV and LDV both contain an active PCPα domain upstream of PCPβ (18, 33), which cleaves the nsp1α/β junction and catalyzes the rapid release of the approximately 20-kDa nsp1α from the N terminus of the PRRSV and LDV replicase (15). The exact nsp1α/1β cleavage site could not be predicted by sequence alignment, but experimental data suggest it resides around aa 170 (15). Based on sequence comparison and the size of cleavage products, the nsp1β/2 cleavage was predicted to occur at Tyr-384/Gly-385 for PRRSV and Tyr-380/Gly-381 for LDV (15). SHFV contains a PCPα, a PCPβ, and probably also a PCPγ domain in its nsp1 region (Fig. 5; see below). However, as in EAV, PCPα may have become inactivated since it contains a large deletion between the putative active-site Cys and His residues. Which of these SHFV PCP domains are proteolytically active remains to be experimentally determined.

### CP-Mediated Processing

The CP that is present in the N-terminal domain of nsp2 was shown to cleave the nsp2/3 junction (55). Like nsp1, nsp2 is almost instantaneously released from the replicase polyproteins, and protein levels remain virtually unchanged throughout the course of infection (54). Mutagenesis studies suggested that EAV nsp2 cleaves at or close to the Gly-831/Gly-832 site (56). Mutations that inactivate nsp2 CP activity or the nsp2/3 cleavage site also affect the processing

| nsp | virus | position in pp1a / pp1ab | length (aa) | C-terminal cleavage site P1 and P1′ | cleaved by |
|-----|-------|--------------------------|-------------|-------------------------------------|------------|
| 1 | EAV | Met1 - Gly260 | 260 | GG | PCPß |
| 1α? | SHFV | Met1 - ? | ? | ? | PCPα? |
| 1α | PRRSV | Met1 - ? | ? | ? | PCPα |
| 1α | LDV | Met1 - ? | ? | ? | PCPα |
| 1β | SHFV | ? - ? | ? | ? | PCPβ |
| 1β | PRRSV | ? - Tyr384 | ? | YG | PCPβ |
| 1β | LDV | ? - Tyr380 | ? | YG | PCPβ |
| 1γ | SHFV | ? - Tyr479 | ? | YG | PCPγ? |
| 2 | EAV | Gly261 - Gly831 | 571 | GG | CP |
| 2 | SHFV | Gly480 - Gly1236 | 757 | GG | CP |
| 2 | PRRSV | Gly385 - Gly1462 | 1078 | GG | CP |
| 2 | LDV | Gly381 - Gly1286 | 906 | GG | CP |
| 3 | EAV | Gly832 - Glu1064 | 233 | EG | 3CLSP |
| 3 | SHFV | Gly1237 - Glu1463 | 227 | EG | 3CLSP |
| 3 | PRRSV | Gly1463 - Glu1693 | 231 | EG | 3CLSP |
| 3 | LDV | Gly1287 - Glu1512 | 226 | EG | 3CLSP |
| 4 | EAV | Gly1065 - Glu1268 | 204 | ES | 3CLSP |
| 4 | SHFV | Gly1464 - Glu1664 | 201 | EG | 3CLSP |
| 4 | PRRSV | Gly1694 - Glu1896 | 203 | EG | 3CLSP |
| 4 | LDV | Gly1513 - Glu1708 | 196 | EG | 3CLSP |
| 5 | EAV | *Ser1269 - Glu1430* | *162* | *EG* | *3CLSP* |
| 5 | SHFV | *Gly1665 - Glu1830* | *166* | *EG* | *3CLSP* |
| 5 | PRRSV | *Gly1463 - Glu2066* | *170* | *EG* | *3CLSP* |
| 5 | LDV | *Gly1709 - Glu1878* | *170* | *EG* | *3CLSP* |
| 6 | EAV | *Gly1431 - Glu1452* | *22* | *ES* | *3CLSP* |
| 6 | SHFV | *Gly1831 - Glu1843* | *13* | *ES* | *3CLSP* |
| 6 | PRRSV | *Gly2067 - Glu2082* | *16* | *ES* | *3CLSP* |
| 6 | LDV | *Gly1879 - Glu1894* | *16* | *EG* | *3CLSP* |
| 7α | EAV | Ser1453 - Glu1575 | 123 | EA | 3CLSP |
| 7α | SHFV | Ser1844 - Glu1974 | 131 | EG | 3CLSP |
| 7α | PRRSV | Ser2083 - Glu2231 | 149 | EN | 3CLSP |
| 7α | LDV | Gly1895 - Glu2026 | 132 | EN | 3CLSP |
| 7β | EAV | Ala1576 - Glu1677 | 102 | EG | 3CLSP |
| 7β | SHFV | Gly1975 - Glu2055 | 81 | ES | 3CLSP |
| 7β | PRRSV | Asn2232 - Glu2351 | 120 | EA | 3CLSP |
| 7β | LDV | Asn2027 - Glu2161 | 135 | EG | 3CLSP |
| 8 | EAV | Gly1678 - Asn1727 | 50 | - | 3CLSP |
| 8 | SHFV | Ser2056 - Cys2105 | 50 | - | 3CLSP |
| 8 | PRRSV | Ala2352 - Cys2397 | 46 | - | 3CLSP |
| 8 | LDV | Gly2162 - Cys2206 | 45 | - | 3CLSP |
| 9 | EAV | Gly1678 - Glu2370 | 693 | ES | 3CLSP |
| 9 | SHFV | Ser2056 - Glu2746 | 691 | EG | 3CLSP |
| 9 | PRRSV | Ala2352 - Glu3036 | 685 | EG | 3CLSP |
| 9 | LDV | Gly2162 - Glu2843 | 682 | EK | 3CLSP |
| 10 | EAV | Ser2371 - Gln2837 | 467 | QS | 3CLSP |
| 10 | SHFV | Gly2747 - Glu3196 | 450 | ES | 3CLSP |
| 10 | PRRSV | Gly3037 - Glu3478 | 442 | EG | 3CLSP |
| 10 | LDV | Lys2844 - Glu3272 | 429 | EG | 3CLSP |
| 11 | EAV | Ser2838 - Glu3056 | 219 | EG | 3CLSP |
| 11 | SHFV | Ser3197 - Glu3419 | 223 | EG | 3CLSP |
| 11 | PRRSV | Gly3479 - Glu3702 | 224 | EG | 3CLSP |
| 11 | LDV | Gly3273 - Glu3494 | 222 | EG | 3CLSP |
| 12 | EAV | Gly3057 - Val3175 | 119 | - | 3CLSP |
| 12 | SHFV | Gly3420 - Pro3596 | 177 | - | 3CLSP |
| 12 | PRRSV | Gly3703 - Pro3854 | 152 | - | 3CLSP |
| 12 | LDV | Gly3495 - Lys3616 | 122 | - | 3CLSP |

**Figure 3.** Proteolytic processing of arterivirus pp1ab polyproteins. Cleavages that only occur as part of the minor pathway (74) are indicated in italics. The P1 and P1′ residues of the C-terminal cleavage site of each nsp are indicated in single-letter amino acid code; for SHFV, PRRSV, and LDV, these are predicted sites based on comparative sequence analysis. Cleavage sites for various nsp1 PCP domains are unknown and therefore indicated with a question mark. The data and numbering relate to the EAV Bucyrus strain (Swiss-Prot accession no. P19811), SHFV (Q68772), the PRRSV Lelystad strain (Q04561), and the LDV P strain (Q83017).

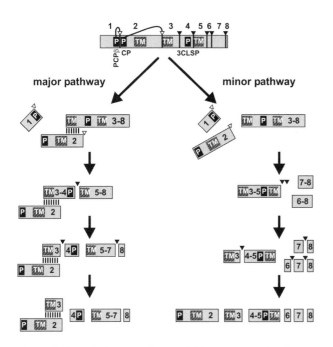

**Figure 4.** Proteolytic processing of EAV replicase pp1a via the major and minor pathways, of which the former depends on an interaction between nsp2 and nsp3–8 (74). The proteases involved in processing are indicated with a white P in a black box. Sites cleaved by PCPβ and by CP are indicated by open triangles. Cleavages mediated by the 3CLSP nsp4 are indicated by black triangles. TM indicates predicted transmembrane domains.

of the downstream nsp3–8 region by the nsp4 main proteinase (56).

### 3CLSP-Mediated Processing

The arterivirus main protease, which is involved in the processing of the remaining cleavage sites, was shown to reside in nsp4 (54). Based on comparative sequence analysis and the (predicted) characteristics of 3CLSP, its putative cleavage sites were predicted to have the signature (Glu and Asp)/(Gly, Ser, and Ala) (18, 56). EAV 3CLSP-mediated cleavage of nine predicted sites was experimentally supported by mutagenesis and expression studies (56, 70, 74).

Originally, the 187-kDa EAV pp1a was assumed to be subject to only five proteolytic cleavages (54). The identification of two additional nsp4 cleavage sites, Glu-1430/Gly-1431 (now known as the nsp5/6 site) and Glu-1452/Ser-1453 (nsp6/7 site), through a combination of experimental and theoretical approaches (74) indicated that (theoretically) pp1a is cleaved into at least eight end products. This fact, not recognized in the literature before 1997, led to a renumbering of the ORF1a-encoded subunits into nsp1 to nsp8. Recently, yet another "low frequency" internal cleavage was detected in the EAV nsp6–8 region, which gives rise to two small proteins that are produced from nsp7: nsp7α and nsp7β (66).

The predicted and experimentally supported EAV 3CSLP cleavage sites (56) in pp1a are shown in Fig. 3. The nsp5/6 and nsp6/7 cleavage sites were shown to be cleaved as part of a minor processing pathway (explained below) (74). Mutagenesis studies initially suggested that replacement of Glu-1430 had no effect on processing, but probably this effect was obscured by the cleavage after the nearby Glu-1452 (56, 74). Expression of a hexahistidine-tagged nsp2–7 protein from a Sindbis virus-based vector, followed by radiosequencing of the nsp5 and nsp7 N termini, confirmed Glu/Ser as a genuine EAV 3CLSP cleavage site (74).

The ORF1b-encoded part of the EAV replicase was predicted to be cleaved three times by the 3CSLP, which was supported by the identification of cleavage products of 80, 50, 26, and 12 kDa (nsp9 to nsp12, respectively) in EAV-infected cells (72). The predicted cleavage sites (Fig. 3) were experimentally probed by mutagenesis studies (70). ORF1ab expression constructs encoding polyproteins with either wild-type 3CLSP or an active-site mutant confirmed that this protease is indeed responsible for processing of the ORF1b-encoded part of pp1ab (70). Although the sizes of the experimentally identified end products are in agreement with the positions of the predicted cleavage sites, the existence of small or low-abundance additional cleavage products cannot be formally excluded, as exemplified by the recent discovery of an additional cleavage within nsp7 (66).

The Gln at the P1 position of the EAV nsp10/11 cleavage site (Gln-2837/Ser-2838) is unique among arteriviruses (Fig. 3), but it still matches the substrate specificity of 3C-like proteases. Replacement of the P1 residue of the EAV nsp10/11 site with other amino acids with similar properties (Asp and Asn) did not significantly affect cleavage, and substitution with Glu (the 3CLSP consensus residue) even stimulated cleavage (70). During evolution EAV may have acquired the Glu-to-Gln substitution at the P1 position of the nsp10/11 junction as a means to modulate processing and expression levels of certain end products or intermediates. Remarkably, however, Gln was not tolerated as the P1 residue of the nsp7/8 cleavage site when introduced using the reverse-genetics system (66).

The kinetics of replicase processing were studied by pulse-chase experiments in combination with immunoprecipitation. No significant differences were observed in the order and kinetics of replicase processing at early (4 h postinfection) and later (8 h postinfection) time points during the EAV replication cycle (54). After rapid processing of the nsp1/2 and nsp2/3 cleavage sites, the remaining nsp3–8 precursor is first cleaved by the nsp4 3CLSP at the nsp4/5

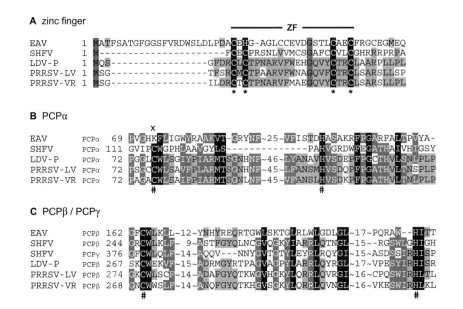

**Figure 5.** Alignment of the putative nsp1 zinc finger and PCP domains of arteriviruses. Conserved residues are shown in black. Residues 75 and 50% conserved are indicated in dark and light gray, respectively. Numbers refer to the amino acid position in the pp1ab sequence. (A) Conserved Cys (or His) residues in the putative zinc finger domain that might be involved in metal ion coordination are indicated with asterisks. Active-site Cys and His residues in the PCPα (B) and PCPβ (C) domains are indicated with pound signs. The missing catalytic Cys in EAV PCPα is indicated with an "X" above the sequence. SHFV contains an additional PCPγ domain, which could be aligned with the PCPβ domains of the other arteriviruses. Alignments were generated and edited with MAFFT (28) and the GeneDoc software, using sequence data from the PRRSV Lelystad strain (Swiss-Prot accession no. Q04561) and the sequences of other arteriviruses as indicated in the legend to Fig. 1.

site, after which slow processing (requiring more than 3 h to be complete) of the nsp3–4 and nsp5–8 intermediates takes place (54). Two alternative, mutually exclusive pathways exist for the processing of the nsp3–8 precursor (74) (Fig. 4). When the major pathway is followed, the nsp4/5 cleavage site is processed first, yielding nsp3–4 and nsp5–8 (74). Subsequently, the nsp3/4 site is cleaved and the nsp5–8 precursor is cleaved at the nsp7/8 site, but not at the nsp5/6 and nsp6/7 sites, which appear to be inaccessible (74). When the minor pathway is followed, the nsp5/6 and nsp6/7 sites are processed first and the nsp4/5 site remains uncleaved (74). The association of cleaved nsp2 with the nsp3–8 precursor appears to determine whether the major pathway is followed and whether the 3CSLP can cleave the nsp4/5 site at its own C terminus (74). In the absence of nsp2, in an expression system, the nsp4/5 site is not cleaved, leading to processing of nsp3–8 via the minor pathway. The presence of nsp1 had no effect on either of these pathways (74). Cleavage of the nsp4/5 site is abolished in pp1a mutants containing an inactive nsp2 protease or an inactivating mutation at the nsp2/3 cleavage site (56, 74). nsp2 appears to be able to exert its cofactor role in *trans,* and nsp2 protease activity is not required for nsp4/5 cleavage by the 3CSLP (74). The fact that

nsp2 appears to function as a cofactor for the nsp4/5 cleavage only, and does not affect other nsp4-mediated cleavages, suggests that it influences the properties or conformation of the nsp4/5 junction rather than the activity of the nsp4 3CLSP domain. Cleavage of the nsp4/5 site might depend on a specific conformation or on the membrane association of the polypeptide. The minor processing pathway might be considered to merely generate dead end products resulting from the failure of a small proportion of the nsp3–8 molecules to associate with (membrane-bound) nsp2. However, the full conservation of the two minor pathway cleavage sites among arteriviruses suggests a specific function in the viral life cycle as well. This notion was recently supported by reverse-genetics analysis of nsp5/6 and nsp6/7 cleavage site mutants, which revealed that cleavage at these sites is essential for viral RNA synthesis (66). The existence of two alternative proteolytic pathways leads to the generation of an extensive set of different polyprotein processing intermediates. In particular, the minor pathway produces several intermediates in which the nsp4 3CLSP is linked to one or more hydrophobic domains, which therefore might be membrane associated. Fully cleaved nsp4 is probably cytoplasmic and was shown to be able to cleave the replicase in *trans* (70).

Processing of the ORF1b-encoded part of the replicase is relatively slow compared to pp1a processing, and cleavages do not appear to occur in a specific order (72). When mutations that block processing of nsp9–12 were introduced in an infectious cDNA clone, the EAV life cycle was affected at different stages (70). Blocking of nsp9/10 or nsp11/12 cleavage abolished replication and sgRNA synthesis (70). Blocking of nsp10/11 cleavage led to a low level of replication and transcription, but no infectious virus was produced (70). Additional experiments indicated that this was unlikely due to an effect at the level of RNA structure or genome packaging (70).

In conclusion, the arterivirus replicase can be cleaved by the nsp4 main protease at nine conserved sites, six in pp1a and three in the ORF1b-encoded part of the replicase. These cleavage sites are conserved in all arteriviruses (Fig. 3). Reverse-genetics studies support the view that each of these processing steps is crucial for EAV viability and that inactivation of cleavage sites abolishes viral RNA synthesis or prevents the production of infectious virus (66, 70).

## PROPERTIES OF REPLICASE SUBUNITS

### nsp1 (nsp1α, nsp1β, and nsp1γ)

In vitro translation and mutagenesis studies revealed that a previously postulated papain-like cysteine protease (16) was responsible for the release of an ~29-kDa N-terminal replicase subunit (nsp1) in EAV (53). The identification of the putative active-site residues of this PCPβ domain was supported by mutagenesis, in vitro translation studies, and in vivo analysis of cleavage products in infected and transfected cells (53, 54). For EAV, the putative catalytic dyad is formed by Cys-164 and His-230 (53). Replacement of Cys-164 with Gly or Ser and His-230 with Ala, Gly, or Val abolished activity, while replacing another His in this region (His-219) had no effect (53). This Cys-His catalytic dyad is conserved in all arteriviruses (Fig. 5). Mutagenesis and in vitro translation studies identified Cys-276 and His-345 as the probable PRRSV PCPβ catalytic dyad and Cys-269 and His-340 as the likely LDV active-site residues (15).

Determination of the EAV PCPβ cleavage site by N-terminal sequencing of the C-terminal cleavage product indicated that cleavage occurs between Gly-260 (P1) and Gly-261 (P1′) (53). Sequence requirements were further probed by mutating the P1 and P1′ positions of the cleavage site (nomenclature of Schechter and Berger [46]). Mutation of Gly-260 or Gly-261 to Ala was largely tolerated, while a change of Gly-260 or Gly-261 to Val abolished or strongly reduced cleavage (53). The PCPβ domain only catalyzes cleavage in *cis*,

as was shown by *trans*-cleavage assays in which radio-labeled substrates containing the nsp1/2 cleavage site were mixed with in vitro-translated PCPβ (53). This property might be due to a mechanism in which the C terminus of the enzyme folds back into and seals its active site, analogous to what was observed for the chymotrypsin-like serine proteinases of Sindbis virus (13).

As described earlier, the nsp1 region of PRRSV and LDV contains a PCPα domain in addition to the downstream PCPβ domain. This PCPα catalyzes the rapid release of the 20- to 22-kDa nsp1α protein from the N terminus of the PRRSV and LDV replicase (15). The subsequent PCPβ-mediated cleavage of the nsp1β/2 junction releases the ~27-kDa nsp1β protein (15). Cys-76 and His-146 for PRRSV and Cys-76 and His-147 for LDV were experimentally identified as likely PCPα active-site residues (15). Inactivation of PCPβ by mutagenesis blocked processing of the nsp1β/2 cleavage site, indicating that also PCPα only functions in *cis* and is not able to cleave the downstream nsp1β/2 junction (15). The PCPα domain in EAV nsp1, which lacks the active-site Cys, is inactive (Fig. 5). However, the sequence surrounding EAV His-122 still exhibits significant similarity to the region near the active-site His-147 and His-146 residues of the PRRSV and LDV PCPα domains (15). The SHFV PCPα domain may be inactive as well, since, compared to the other arteriviruses, it contains a substantial deletion between the active-site Cys and His (see the alignment in Fig. 5). However, also in this domain the region directly downstream of the putative active-site His is clearly conserved. A unique feature of the SHFV nsp1 region is the apparent presence of a third PCP, PCPγ, which is likely responsible for the liberation of the nsp2 N terminus (Fig. 5).

The nsp1 PCP domains of arteriviruses are considered to be so-called leader proteases, enzymes that catalyze a single cleavage in the N terminus of the replicase, in contrast to the main protease, which is responsible for extensive processing of the replicase through multiple cleavages (23, 78). Accessory proteases have also been found in other nidoviruses and many positive-strand RNA viruses and are predominantly of the papain-like type (78).

EAV nsp1 is considered to be a multifunctional protein. Besides its role in replicase proteolysis, it also plays an essential role in sgRNA synthesis (61). Deletion of the nsp1-coding sequence from the infectious cDNA clone abolished sgRNA synthesis, while genome replication was not affected (61). Expression of nsp1 from an internal ribosomal entry site inserted into the 3′ end of the genome, separated from the rest of the replicase, complemented the transcription defect of a Δnsp1 mutant replicon, suggesting that nsp1 can activate transcription in *trans* (61).

A putative zinc finger, containing four conserved Cys and His residues, was predicted near the N terminus of nsp1 (Fig. 5). Zinc fingers are present in many cellular transcription factors and can play a role in protein-DNA, protein-RNA, and protein-protein interactions (for a review, see reference 30). Metal chelate affinity chromatography with phage display expression constructs containing the EAV nsp1 zinc finger domain suggest that it is able to interact with metal ions (36). However, verification of the predicted zinc binding in the context of the full-length (native) protein and determination of the structure of this domain would require the purification, crystallization, and biochemical characterization of nsp1.

Analysis of a set of nsp1 truncation mutants suggested that an intact nsp1 protein is required for its function in transcription. Therefore, using the RNA replicon (DITRAC) that expresses nsp1 from its 3' part, the different domains of nsp1 were probed by mutagenesis of conserved residues (61). Replacing the putative zinc-coordinating residue Cys-25 or Cys-44 with Ala completely abolished transcription, while mutagenesis of PCPα (His-122) or PCPβ (Cys-164, inactivation) had no effect on transcription (61). This indicated that the zinc finger domain is involved in transcription, while an active protease domain is not required.

nsp1 mainly localizes to the cytoplasm and, in line with its role in transcription, partly colocalizes with other replicase subunits to the perinuclear region of the EAV-infected cell, which contains the viral RTCs (60). nsp1 also partly localizes to the nucleus, especially early in infection (60) (Fig. 6). Nuclear import of nsp1 was suggested to be an active process, and a deletion mutant lacking the C-terminal PCPβ domain (aa 157 to 260) was no longer imported into the nucleus (60). This could be due to loss of either a nuclear import signal or a domain responsible for an interaction with a cellular protein that cotransports nsp1 to the nucleus. Nuclear localization also

appeared to depend on host cell properties, e.g., the stage in the cell cycle (60). The nuclear function of nsp1 currently remains unclear. It might influence host cell transcription or modulate host processes that are beneficial or detrimental for (early stages of) replication and/or sgRNA synthesis. Alternatively, it might recruit nuclear proteins to the viral replication complex.

Yeast two-hybrid assays suggested that nsp1 forms dimers or multimers (59). Screening of a HeLa cell cDNA library in the two-hybrid system with nsp1 as bait identified a number of potential interaction partners (59). Although most of these interactions remain to be confirmed in independent systems (preferably in vivo), the interaction between nsp1 and the p100 protein was also observed by coimmunoprecipitation when the two proteins were coexpressed (59).

The ubiquitously expressed p100 is a protein that has been shown to be a coactivator of the Epstein-Barr virus-encoded transcription factor EBNA-2, as well as of the interleukin 4-dependent cellular Stat6 and Stat5 transcription factors (9, 39, 62, 63, 77). In addition, Caudy et al. discovered that p100 is a component of the RNA-induced silencing complex (RISC) and demonstrated that it exhibits nuclease activity (11). The p100 protein contains four staphylococcal nuclease domains and a Tudor domain (10). Tudor domains are conserved protein modules of unknown function that might mediate protein-protein interactions and are often present in proteins that associate with RNA (48). Although p100 contains noncanonical active-site residues in its staphylococcal nuclease domains, it does exhibit nuclease activity in vitro (11). nsp1 interacts with the 229 C-terminal residues of p100, which contain the Tudor domain (59). The nsp1 domain responsible for interaction with p100 has not been determined yet, although it was shown that point mutations in the putative zinc finger of nsp1, which abolish sgRNA synthesis, did not affect its interaction with p100 (59).

Considering the properties and cellular functions of p100, it is tempting to speculate it might be involved in EAV transcription (sgRNA synthesis) as well, through its interaction with nsp1. On the other hand, nsp1 could also play a role in protecting viral double-stranded RNA (dsRNA) by interfering with RISC-mediated RNA degradation through its interaction with p100. Nevertheless, the presence of p100 and its interaction with nsp1 in EAV-permissive cells and in the natural host remain to be confirmed.

In summary, EAV nsp1 appears to be a key regulator of the viral life cycle, as it links genome expression and replicase processing to transcription (structural protein expression). The mechanism by

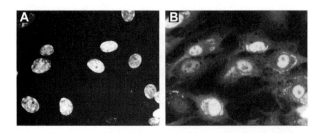

**Figure 6.** Nuclear and perinuclear localization of nsp1 in EAV-infected cells. Shown is immunofluorescence staining of EAV-infected BHK-21 cells, 8 h after infection. Nuclei were stained with Hoechst 33528 (A), and nsp1 was detected using a rabbit polyclonal antiserum (B).

which nsp1 regulates transcription remains unclear. The protein might interact with RNA sequences (e.g., transcription-regulatory sequences) or the RdRp or other replicase subunits involved in RNA synthesis, or it could recruit host factors essential for transcription to the RTC.

## nsp2

Although nsp2 is the most divergent arterivirus replicase subunit—its length varies from 571 to 1,196 aa—several features have been conserved in all arteriviruses. The N-terminal CP domain and overlapping cysteine-rich region are well conserved (Fig. 7). In contrast, the central region is highly variable in amino acid sequence and size; e.g., it is ~250 aa in EAV, ~600 aa in LDV and SHFV, and ~730 aa in PRRSV. Despite this divergence, all arteriviruses have retained an extensive hydrophobic region in this part of nsp2. The ~200-aa C-terminal part of nsp2 exhibits less sequence variation and contains a cluster of conserved cysteines.

EAV nsp2 was identified as a CP responsible for processing of the nsp2/3 junction (55). The nsp2 CP domain exhibits similarity to viral PCPs, although its active site lacks a characteristic Cys-Trp (Tyr) dipeptide and contains a Cys-Gly instead (Fig. 7). Interestingly, when the Gly-271 sequence was mutated to the canonical Trp, proteolytic activity was lost (55). Another striking difference with PCPs is the ability of the nsp2 CP to cleave in *trans*. Therefore, the CP was concluded to be a somewhat unusual CP (55), which was subsequently proposed to belong to a new superfamily of CPs including members from a wide variety of sources (32). Interestingly, several members of this "OTU superfamily" have been implicated in deubiquitination (for a review, see reference 58).

Mutagenesis and expression studies identified Cys-270 and His-332 as putative active-site residues (55). However, other domains, conserved cysteines, and the integrity of nsp2 were also shown to be required for cleavage, as (small) deletions in the region between the CP and the nsp2/3 junction were not tolerated and mutation of conserved Cys-319, Cys-349, or Cys-354 also abolished proteolytic activity (55).

Even some mutations of nonconserved cysteines, Cys-344 and Cys-356, reduced activity of nsp2 (55).

EAV nsp2 is able to cleave the nsp2/3 junction in *trans*, and prior cleavage of the nsp1/2 site is not required (54, 55). Like nsp1, nsp2 is almost instantaneously released from the replicase polyprotein, as indicated by the fact that hardly any nsp2-containing precursors are observed in immunoprecipitation experiments (54). Pulse-chase experiments indicated that EAV nsp2 is a stable protein, as no significant degradation occurred over a 3-h period (54).

Based on the substrate specificity of other PCPs, comparative sequence analysis, and the observed size of cleavage products, EAV nsp2-mediated cleavage was predicted to occur at or close to Gly-831 and Gly-832 (56). A change of Gly-831 to Pro blocked cleavage, in support of the predicted cleavage site (56).

EAV nsp2 interacts with a number of other replicase subunits. It functions as a cofactor for nsp4-mediated cleavage of the nsp3–8 precursor at the nsp4/5 junction (74). Furthermore, coimmunoprecipitation experiments (under stringent conditions) with EAV-infected cell lysates revealed that nsp2 strongly interacts with nsp3 (54).

In Vero cells, but not in BHK-21 or RK-13 cells, EAV nsp2 is subject to an additional cleavage, probably by a host protease that is absent in the other cell types (52). This cleavage leads to the generation of an 18-kDa N-terminal and 44-kDa C-terminal part, which was shown to interact with nsp3 (52).

nsp2 colocalizes with several other nsps to the perinuclear region of EAV-infected cells (67), where it is associated with typical double-membrane vesicles (DMVs) (40) (see also chapter 7). nsp2 and nsp3 have been implicated in the formation of these structures, since their coexpression (in an alphavirus expression system) suffices to induce DMV-like structures (52). Biochemical analysis suggested that nsp2 is associated with intracellular membranes (67).

## nsp3

nsp3 is the most hydrophobic subunit of the arterivirus replicase, and the distribution of hydrophobic domains and predicted membrane topology

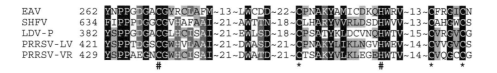

| EAV | 262 | YNPEGDGACGYRCLAFM~13~LWCDD~22~CPNAKYAMICDKQHWRV~13~CFRGICN |
| SHFV | 634 | FIPPPDGGCGVHAFAAI~21~AWTTN~18~CLHARYVVRLDSDHWVV~13~CAHGWCS |
| LDV-P | 382 | YSPPGDGACGLHCISAI~21~EWLSD~18~CPSATYKLDCVNQHWTV~15~CVRGVCG |
| PRRSV-LV | 421 | YSPPTDGSCGWHVLAAI~21~DWASD~21~CPNAKYIKLNGVHWTV~14~CVVGVCS |
| PRRSV-VR | 429 | YSPPAEGNCGWHCISAI~21~DWATD~21~CTSAKYVLKLEGEHWTV~14~CVQGCCG |

**Figure 7.** Multiple alignment of the arterivirus nsp2 CP domain. The Cys and His residues of the catalytic dyad are indicated with pound signs. Conserved Cys residues that are required for activity in EAV are indicated with asterisks. Numbers refer to the amino acid position in the pp1ab sequence. For further details, see the legend to Fig. 5.

are conserved among all arteriviruses. The first (predicted) luminal domain of nsp3 contains a cluster of four conserved cysteines (aa 855, 864, 879, and 884 in EAV pp1a). Cell fractionation experiments and biochemical analysis indicated that EAV nsp3 is an integral membrane protein (67). However, these experiments do not formally exclude the possibility that nsp3 membrane association is due to its strong interaction with nsp2 (54), although the hydrophobicity and predicted transmembrane helices in nsp3 make this a less likely scenario. EAV nsp3 strongly interacts with the C-terminal part of nsp2 (52, 54). It is currently unknown whether the hydrophobic regions or the cysteine-rich clusters that are present in both proteins play a role in this interaction.

nsp3 localizes to DMVs in the perinuclear region of EAV-infected cells (40). Formation of DMV-like structures is observed when nsp3 is coexpressed with nsp2 (52), indicating that these are the only viral proteins required for this process. Therefore, nsp3 and nsp2 could be considered structural components of the DMVs with which the viral RTC is associated (see also chapter 7).

## nsp4

By comparative sequence analysis, a chymotrypsin-like serine protease was predicted in the nsp4 region of all arterivirus replicases (16, 18, 54). These proteins were concluded to represent a novel subgroup of proteases that combine the classical His-Asp-Ser catalytic triad of chymotrypsin with the substrate specificity of picornavirus 3C CPs and related enzymes (20, 56). Therefore, the term 3CLSP was chosen to refer to the similarity with 3C-like enzymes, while also highlighting that the enzyme uses Ser instead of Cys as its active-site nucleophile (56, 78).

The proteolytic activity of the EAV 3CSLP was demonstrated using a vaccinia virus expression system (56), and using this system His-1103, Asp-1129, and Ser-1184 were confirmed as the likely catalytic triad of EAV nsp4. Remarkably, a change of Asp-1129 to Glu abolished processing of the nsp3/4 and nsp5/6 junction, while the nsp4/5 site was still processed with wild-type efficiency (56). Mutagenesis of Thr-1179

and His-1199, which were predicted to be involved in substrate recognition, also affected cleavage (56), depending on the replacement and the cleavage site monitored. For example, in some mutants the nsp4/5 site was still processed (with reduced efficiency), while processing of the nsp5/6 site was completely abolished (56). All catalytic triad residues and predicted substrate-binding residues are invariant in arteriviruses (Fig. 8). nsp4 processes (at least) nine cleavage sites in the replicase, six in pp1a and three in the ORF1b-encoded part of pp1ab (Fig. 3), and is therefore regarded as the arterivirus main protease (56, 70, 74).

In contrast to their cellular counterparts, 3C-like proteases have a strict substrate specificity and mainly cleave the sequence (Gln and Glu)/(Gly, Ala, and Ser) (5, 20). This property was used to predict a number of cleavage sites by alignment of arterivirus pp1ab sequences (18). For EAV the nsp4 cleavage sites were experimentally confirmed by mutagenesis and expression studies (56, 70, 74). Most cleavages occur at Glu/Gly and Glu/Ser sites (Fig. 3), but the predicted Gln/Ser, Glu/Ala, and Glu/Lys sites are notable exceptions. Except for Glu/Lys, all these sites match the canonical 3C-like cleavage site. Mutagenesis data for the region of the EAV replicase from Glu-2835 to Ser-2838 indicated that the P3′ position might influence cleavage as well (70). Recently, an in vitro assay with bacterially expressed recombinant nsp4 was developed, which might be used for further characterization of the enzyme and its cleavage sites and, e.g., for the identification of protease inhibitors (64).

Besides nsp4, EAV-infected cells also contain nsp3–4 and nsp4–5 processing intermediates in which a hydrophobic domain is associated with the main proteinase (54). Thus, membrane-associated and cytoplasmic nsp4 might play different roles in the viral life cycle and replicase processing.

The three-dimensional structure of bacterially expressed EAV nsp4 was determined at 2.0-Å resolution (3). The protein was shown to adopt a chymotrypsin-like fold, and the catalytic triad consisting of His-1103, Asp-1129, and Ser-1184 was confirmed (Fig. 9). nsp4 consists of two β-barrels, each consisting of six β-strands, with cores that contain conserved hydrophobic residues (3). The oxyanion hole was

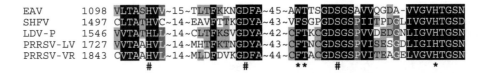

```
EAV      1098  VLTASHVV~15~TLTFKKNGDFA~45~AWTTSGDSGSAVVQGDA~VVGVHTGSN
SHFV     1497  CLTATHVC~14~EAVFTTKGDYA~43~VFSGPGDSGSPIITPDCLIVGVHTGSD
LDV-P    1546  VVTATHLL~14~CLTFKSVGDYA~42~CFTKCGDSGSPVVDEDCNLIGVHTGSN
PRRSV-LV 1727  VVTAAHVL~14~MHTFKTNGDYA~43~CFTNCGDSGSPVISESCDLIGIHTGSN
PRRSV-VR 1843  CVTAAHVL~14~MLDFDVKGDFA~44~CFTACGDSGSPVITEACELVGVHTGSN
               #              #              **    #              *
```

**Figure 8.** Multiple alignment of the 3CSLP (main protease) domain of arterivirus nsp4 proteins. The conserved residues of the catalytic triad are indicated with pound signs. Residues predicted to be involved in substrate recognition are indicated with asterisks. Numbers refer to the amino acid position in the pp1ab sequence. For further details, see the legend to Fig. 5.

C-terminal extension   C-terminal ß-barrel   N-terminal ß-barrel

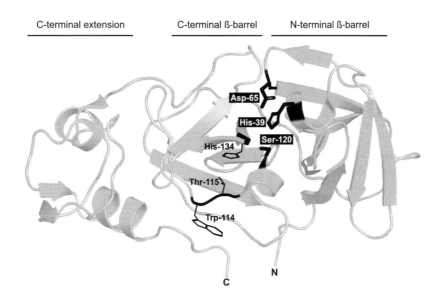

**Figure 9.** Structural model of EAV nsp4, the main protease. The N- and C-terminal β-barrels and the C-terminal extension are indicated above the model. Catalytic triad residues (thick black sticks) are indicated with white text in a black box. Residues involved in substrate recognition (thin black sticks) are indicated by black text. Numbers refer to the amino acid position in the nsp4 subunit. The ribbon model was prepared with Pymol (Delano Scientific) and PDB entry 1MBM.

found to exist both in a collapsed inactive conformation and in the standard active confirmation, which might be a mechanism for regulating proteolytic activity. The substrate-binding groove is lined with conserved residues and contains the solvent-exposed conserved Trp-1178 as well as the neighboring Thr-1179, which was suggested to be involved in substrate recognition as well (3, 56). His-1198 and Thr-1179 are at the base and wall, respectively, of the substrate specificity pocket and are probably involved in hydrogen bonding the side chain of the P1 residue of the substrate (3). The nsp4 CTD contains an α/β extension domain that might be involved in protein-protein interactions (3) and is absent in most other chymotrypsin-like enzymes, but a similar extension is also found in the 3C-like proteases of other nidoviruses.

The nsp4 CTD can adopt different conformations with respect to the rest of the protein, which might influence substrate binding and proteolysis (Fig. 9). This movement might be facilitated by a proposed hinge region (aa 1218 to 1225), which connects the CTD to the main β-barrel structure (65). Thr-1221 or Ser-1225 could act as a hinge, and mutations in this region affected replicase processing and virus viability to various extents (65). Deletion of the CTD and mutations affecting the flexibility of the proposed hinge region had the strongest negative effect on processing and were lethal when introduced in an infectious cDNA clone. Nevertheless, the same study made it clear that the CTD is not required for

nsp4 proteolytic activity per se (65). The production of nsp7–8 seems to be relatively resistant to mutations in the CTD, which again demonstrated that EAV has the capacity to differentially process cleavage sites that have identical P1 and P1′ residues.

The nsp4 crystal structure revealed a conformation in which the N- and C-terminal ends of the protein are not in or near the substrate-binding pocket, thus preventing self-inhibition and supporting *trans* cleavage (3). However, the presence of disordered regions in the N and C termini suggested the protein to be able to undergo the conformational rearrangements that would be required for *cis* cleavage of the flanking nsp3/4 and nsp4/5 sites as well (3).

EAV nsp4 colocalizes with most other nsps to the perinuclear region of the infected cell (67), where it is associated with DMVs (40). It is unknown whether this localization is due to hydrophobic domains in the nsp4-containing precursors or whether nsp4 interacts with other nsps that are part of membrane-associated replication complexes.

## nsp5–8

The arterivirus nsp5–7 protein is a 391- to 445-aa end product of the major pp1a processing pathway, in which the nsp5/6 and nsp6/7 junctions remain uncleaved (Fig. 4) (74). The nsp5 part of this protein is highly hydrophobic and is predicted to contain four transmembrane helices. The function of the protein remains to be elucidated, and it has no significant similarity to any other protein of known function. It might be involved in targeting other replicase subunits to intracellular membranes, as biochemical experiments indicated that nsp5 targets the nsp5–12 precursor to a membrane fraction (67). nsp5 is not required for the formation of DMV-like structures in an expression system (52).

nsp6 and nsp7 are end products of the minor pathway (74). The 13- to 22-aa nsp6 polypeptide is probably too small to adopt a stable functional conformation by itself, but it might modulate the functions of the nsp5 and/or nsp7 subunits, to which it is attached in a variety of processing intermediates (66). The 212- to 269-aa nsp7 exhibits no similarities to other proteins, and it remains to be determined which role it plays in the viral life cycle. Recently, an internal cleavage site was discovered within nsp7. Processing of this site by nsp4 yields an ~14-kDa nsp7α and an ~11-kDa nsp7β (66).

The 45- to 50-aa nsp8 is not very conserved between arteriviruses. It might be functional on its own, but the nsp7/8 cleavage might merely serve to release the ORF1b-encoded subunits of pp1ab, after which nsp8 forms the N-terminal domain of nsp9, the RdRp-containing subunit.

### nsp9

The 682- to 693-aa nsp9 contains a number of consensus motifs (between Gly-2104 and Arg-2300 in EAV) that have been identified in the RdRps of all RNA viruses (16, 29, 41). The hallmark GDD motif that includes two catalytic Asp residues in all positive-strand RNA virus RdRps (27, 41) is changed into SDD in all known nidoviruses. This motif is indispensable for RdRp function, as mutation of the GDD motif to SGA (EAV aa 2236 to 2238) was lethal when tested using the infectious cDNA clone of EAV (73). All viral RdRps probably adapt a similar basic "right hand shape" with fingers and palm and thumb domains (37). This conformation provides the correct spatial arrangement for interacting with the template, incoming NTPs, and metal ions at the active site and for transferring the products out of the catalytic cavity (68). The SARS-CoV ortholog of nsp9 (nsp12) exhibited RNA polymerase activity on homopolymeric templates in an in vitro system, using a recombinant bacterially expressed protein domain (12). Recently, bacterially expressed and purified EAV nsp9 was found to be catalytically active in an in vitro RdRp assay as well (5a).

EAV nsp9 localizes to the perinuclear region of infected cells (72) and is associated with DMVs (40), which is in line with its role in viral RNA synthesis.

### nsp10

The arterivirus HEL, the 429- to 467-aa nsp10, is the most conserved nidovirus replicase subunit. It contains a putative zinc-binding, cysteine-rich domain at its N terminus and a HEL/NTPase domain in its C-terminal part (16) (Fig. 10). The combination of a

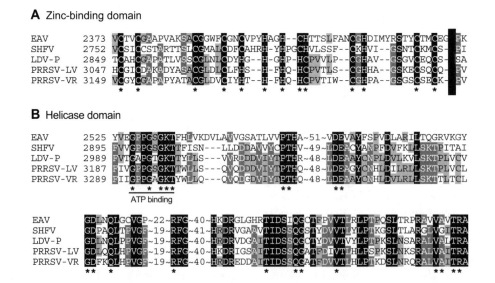

**Figure 10.** Multiple alignment of arterivirus nsp10 domains. (A) Putative ZBD. Conserved Cys and His residues are indicated with asterisks. The Ser in the putative hinge region is boxed (hatched) (B) The NTPase/HEL domain. The NTP-binding motif is underlined, and residues that are conserved in type 1 superfamily HELs are indicated with asterisks. For further details, see the legend to Fig. 5.

ZBD and HEL domain appears to be a unique nido-virus-specific feature (21).

A superfamily 1 HEL motif is present between Val-2525 and Ile-2758 of EAV pp1ab (16, 26). This domain is the most conserved region of the arterivirus replicase and includes the typical NTP-binding motif (EAV Gly-2528 to Thr-2535) present in the replicases of all positive-strand RNA viruses (19, 26). EAV nsp10, expressed as a recombinant maltose-binding fusion protein, has $Mg^{2+}$-dependent ATPase (and GTPase) activity (50). The protein has a 5'-to-3' duplex-unwinding activity on both dsRNA and dsDNA (50). A similar NTPase and polynucleotide-stimulated nucleotide unwinding activity was found for PRRSV nsp10, of which kinetic properties and optimal reaction conditions were analyzed in detail (4). The enzyme required divalent cations and was extremely sensitive to temperatures above 37.5°C and a pH below 7. Replacement of the Walker A box residue Lys-2534 with Gln abolished ATPase activity and rendered the EAV cDNA clone noninfectious (50). Mutations that abolish NTPase or HEL activity block replication and transcription in EAV (49).

The ZBD (between Cys-2374 and Cys-2426 in EAV pp1ab) was predicted to bind metal ions and adapt a zinc finger-like conformation (16, 18), a notion supported by protein-refolding experiments that identified $Zn^{2+}$ as an essential factor for enzymatic activity (49). The EAV ZBD was characterized by site-directed mutagenesis in the EAV infectious cDNA clone (71). Replacement of 11 of the 13 conserved Cys and His residues (including conservative Cys→His and His→Cys replacements) completely abolished RNA synthesis. The ATPase and HEL activities of bacterially expressed recombinant nsp10 with mutations in the conserved Cys and His of the ZBD were determined in an in vitro assay (49). Most mutations in the ZBD abolished both activities, suggesting that the ZBD influences the activity of the HEL domain and plays a vital role in RNA synthesis (49).

A noninfectious EAV cDNA clone, obtained during the construction of an EAV reverse-genetics system, was found to contain a serendipitous point mutation leading to a Ser-2429→Pro substitution in nsp10 (69). Remarkably, the RNA derived from this clone was replication competent, but it was severely impaired in sgRNA synthesis (69, 73). Ser-2429 is located just downstream of the ZBD and might be part of a flexible hinge region that connects the ZBD and HEL domain. Several other mutations of Ser-2429 and/or Pro-2430 were later shown to specifically affect transcription (71). HEL and ATPase activities of these mutants were not affected (49), suggesting that nsp10 has an additional, HEL-independent function in sgRNA synthesis. Replacement of Ser-2429

with Pro might disturb the protein conformation or the orientation of the two nsp10 domains with respect to each other, leading to the observed phenotype. For transcription, a specific nsp10 conformation, influenced by Ser-2429, might be required for proper interaction(s) with RNA or components of the transcription machinery.

Surprisingly, trans-complementation of the mutation of Ser-2429 to Pro by expression of wild-type nsp10 was impossible (71). Opposite to the normal localization of nsp10 to the RTC (72), immunofluorescence microscopy showed a mainly diffuse cytoplasmic localization for the separately expressed nsp10, suggesting that it did not properly associate with the RTC (71). Thus, expression as part of the replicase polyprotein, including the hydrophobic domains, may be vital for the correct targeting of nsp10.

A remarkable ZBD mutant, with a change of His-2414 to Cys, was both replication and transcription competent but not able to produce infectious virus (71). Whether this implies a direct role for nsp10 in virion biogenesis or whether this defect is caused indirectly (e.g., by a subtle disturbance of sgRNA levels resulting in an imbalance in the structural protein ratios) remains to be determined.

## nsp11

The 219- to 224-aa arterivirus nsp11 contains the highly conserved NendoU domain (between His-2961 and Phe-3039 in EAV pp1ab) (43, 51), a nidovirus-specific domain with homology to the Xenopus laevis endoribonuclease XendoU (31). XendoU is a $Mn^{2+}$-dependent endonuclease that cleaves at stretches of Us and is involved in the processing of small nucleolar RNAs (31). For multiple coronavirus NendoU-containing proteins (nsp15) in vitro endoribonuclease activity was confirmed (6, 25). Like XendoU, coronavirus nsp15 is $Mn^{2+}$ dependent and produces 2',3'-cyclic phosphate ends (6, 25, 31). The enzyme was reported to cleave upstream and downstream of the U in the sequence GU or GUU, and both single-stranded RNA and dsRNA were cleaved (6, 25). The crystal structure of SARS-CoV nsp15 revealed that it has a unique fold and forms a toric hexamer (44). The tunnel traversing the hexamer is too small to accommodate an RNA substrate, and therefore the active site should be located elsewhere (44). The conserved His-234, His-249, and Lys-289 of SARS-CoV nsp15, the equivalents of EAV pp1ab His-2963, His-2978, and Lys-3007 (43, 51), were found to be located close together and were proposed to be in the active site, lying in a positively charged groove on the outside of the toric structure (44). The structure of mouse hepatitis virus nsp15 was solved as well, also revealing a hexameric conformation consisting of two back-to-back trimers with the two conserved histidines and the lysine in the active site (76).

It is currently unknown whether the arterivirus nsp11 protein has similar structural properties and/or in vitro endonuclease activity. Deletion of the NendoU domain and mutagenesis of two conserved Asp residues (EAV Asp-3014 and Asp-3038) in the C-terminal part of NendoU, which abolished coronavirus NendoU activity (25), rendered an EAV cDNA clone noninfectious (43). Surprisingly, however, replacement of His-2963, His-2978, and Lys-3007 was not lethal, although virus titers and plaque sizes were severely reduced. All mutants had a moderate but specific defect in sgRNA synthesis, while genome replication was only moderately affected (43).

## nsp12

Arterivirus nsp12 is highly variable in terms of size (119 to 177 aa), sequence, and physical properties. No experimental data are available on nsp12, and it contains no known motifs or significant similarity to other viral or cellular proteins of known function.

## THE ARTERIVIRUS REPLICATION/ TRANSCRIPTION COMPLEX

In immunofluorescence microscopy, many EAV replicase subunits, including the nsp9-RdRp and nsp10-HEL, produce a punctuate staining pattern and colocalize in the perinuclear region of the infected cell. This area also contains de novo-made viral RNA and therefore is the apparent location of the viral RTC (54, 67, 72) (see also chapter 7). Several EAV nsps were shown to colocalize with the endoplasmic reticulum marker PDI, suggesting that the replication complex is associated with membrane structures derived from this organelle (40, 67).

Arterivirus-infected cells were shown to contain typical virus-induced DMVs with a reported diameter of 80 to 300 nm (40, 42, 45, 75). For EAV, using immunoelectron microscopy, these structures were shown to contain several nsps and de novo-made viral RNA and were therefore proposed to carry the RTC (40). EAV nsp2 and nsp3 are likely responsible for DMV formation, since coexpression of just nsp2 and nsp3 suffices to induce formation of paired membranes and DMV-like structures (52). The third hydrophobic protein, nsp5, appears to be dispensable for DMV formation.

Cell fractionation and biochemical analysis suggested that hydrophobic domains in nsp2, nsp3, and nsp5 are responsible for targeting replicase subunits to intracellular membranes (67). For LDV it was shown that the hydrophobic nsp3–5 region was responsible for membrane association of in vitro translation products (17). Carbonate treatment and protease protection assays suggested that these proteins contain transmembrane domains (17).

Replicase subunits that lack hydrophobic domains (e.g., nsp4 and all ORF1b-encoded proteins) might be targeted to the membrane-associated replication complex by their association with the hydrophobic subunits. Indeed, strong interactions between several replicase subunits and precursors were discovered in immunoprecipitation experiments (67, 72). Temporal regulation of polyprotein processing, e.g., the slow processing of certain cleavage sites, might also be responsible for correct localization of subunits lacking their own hydrophobic domain, through hydrophobic domains present in larger precursors. Future research on the structure, morphogenesis, and function of DMVs and the associated RTC should provide more insight into the working environment of the arterivirus replicase and the reasons for the formation of these intriguing and unusual membrane structures.

Acknowledgments. For pleasant contacts and collaborations, and helpful discussions through the years, we thank our past and present colleagues at the Leiden University Medical Center, and many colleagues from the nidovirus field.

This work was supported in part by grants from the Council for Chemical Sciences of the Netherlands Organization for Scientific Research (NWO-CW grant 700.52.306) and the European Union (FP6 IP VIZIER LSHG-CT-2004-511960).

## REFERENCES

1. Allende, R., T. L. Lewis, Z. Lu, D. L. Rock, G. F. Kutish, A. Ali, A. R. Doster, and F. A. Osorio. 1999. North American and European porcine reproductive and respiratory syndrome viruses differ in non-structural protein coding regions. *J. Gen. Virol.* 80:307–315.

2. Almazan, F., C. Galan, and L. Enjuanes. 2004. The nucleoprotein is required for efficient coronavirus genome replication. *J. Virol.* 78:12683–12688.

3. Barrette-Ng, I. H., K. K. Ng, B. L. Mark, D. Van Aken, M. M. Cherney, C. Garen, Y. Kolodenko, A. E. Gorbalenya, E. J. Snijder, and M. N. James. 2002. Structure of arterivirus nsp4. The smallest chymotrypsin-like proteinase with an alpha/beta C-terminal extension and alternate conformations of the oxyanion hole. *J. Biol. Chem.* 277:39960–39966.

4. Bautista, E. M., K. S. Faaberg, D. Mickelson, and E. D. McGruder. 2002. Functional properties of the predicted helicase of porcine reproductive and respiratory syndrome virus. *Virology* 298:258–270.

5. Bazan, J. F., and R. J. Fletterick. 1988. Viral cysteine proteases are homologous to the trypsin-like family of serine proteases: structural and functional implications. *Proc. Natl. Acad. Sci. USA* 85:7872–7876.

5a. Beerens, N., B. Selisko, S. Ricagno, I. Imbert, A. L. van der Zanden, E. J. Snijder, and B. Canard. 2007. De novo initiation of RNA synthesis by the arterivirus RNA-dependent RNA polymerase. *J. Virol.* 81:8384–8395.

6. Bhardwaj, K., L. Guarino, and C. C. Kao. 2004. The severe acute respiratory syndrome coronavirus Nsp15 protein is an endoribonuclease that prefers manganese as a cofactor. *J. Virol.* **78:**12218–12224.

7. Bredenbeek, P. J., C. J. Pachuk, A. F. Noten, J. Charite, W. Luytjes, S. R. Weiss, and W. J. Spaan. 1990. The primary structure and expression of the second open reading frame of the polymerase gene of the coronavirus MHV-A59; a highly conserved polymerase is expressed by an efficient ribosomal frameshifting mechanism. *Nucleic Acids Res.* **18:**1825–1832.

8. Brierley, I., M. E. Boursnell, M. M. Binns, B. Bilimoria, V. C. Blok, T. D. Brown, and S. C. Inglis. 1987. An efficient ribosomal frame-shifting signal in the polymerase-encoding region of the coronavirus IBV. *EMBO J.* **6:**3779–3785.

9. Broadhurst, M. K., R. S. Lee, S. Hawkins, and T. T. Wheeler. 2005. The p100 EBNA-2 coactivator: a highly conserved protein found in a range of exocrine and endocrine cells and tissues in cattle. *Biochim. Biophys. Acta* **1681:**126–133.

10. Callebaut, I., and J. P. Mornon. 1997. The human EBNA-2 coactivator p100: multidomain organization and relationship to the staphylococcal nuclease fold and to the tudor protein involved in Drosophila melanogaster development. *Biochem. J.* **321:**125–132.

11. Caudy, A. A., R. F. Ketting, S. M. Hammond, A. M. Denli, A. M. Bathoorn, B. B. Tops, J. M. Silva, M. M. Myers, G. J. Hannon, and R. H. Plasterk. 2003. A micrococcal nuclease homologue in RNAi effector complexes. *Nature* **425:**411–414.

12. Cheng, A., W. Zhang, Y. Xie, W. Jiang, E. Arnold, S. G. Sarafianos, and J. Ding. 2005. Expression, purification, and characterization of SARS coronavirus RNA polymerase. *Virology* **335:**165–176.

13. Choi, H. K., L. Tong, W. Minor, P. Dumas, U. Boege, M. G. Rossmann, and G. Wengler. 1991. Structure of Sindbis virus core protein reveals a chymotrypsin-like serine proteinase and the organization of the virion. *Nature* **354:**37–43.

14. den Boon, J. A. 1996. *Equine Arteritis Virus. Replication and Transcription of a Coronaviruslike Virus.* Ph.D. Thesis. Leiden University, Leiden, The Netherlands.

15. den Boon, J. A., K. S. Faaberg, J. J. Meulenberg, A. L. Wassenaar, P. G. Plagemann, A. E. Gorbalenya, and E. J. Snijder. 1995. Processing and evolution of the N-terminal region of the arterivirus replicase ORF1a protein: identification of two papainlike cysteine proteases. *J. Virol.* **69:**4500–4505.

16. den Boon, J. A., E. J. Snijder, E. D. Chirnside, A. A. de Vries, M. C. Horzinek, and W. J. Spaan. 1991. Equine arteritis virus is not a togavirus but belongs to the coronaviruslike superfamily. *J. Virol.* **65:**2910–2920.

17. Faaberg, K. S., and P. G. Plagemann. 1996. Membrane association of the C-terminal half of the open reading frame 1a protein of lactate dehydrogenase-elevating virus. *Arch. Virol.* **141:**1337–1348.

18. Godeny, E. K., L. Chen, S. N. Kumar, S. L. Methven, E. V. Koonin, and M. A. Brinton. 1993. Complete genomic sequence and phylogenetic analysis of the lactate dehydrogenase-elevating virus (LDV). *Virology* **194:**585–596.

19. Gorbalenya, A. E., V. M. Blinov, A. P. Donchenko, and E. V. Koonin. 1989. An NTP-binding motif is the most conserved sequence in a highly diverged monophyletic group of proteins involved in positive strand RNA viral replication. *J. Mol. Evol.* **28:**256–268.

20. Gorbalenya, A. E., A. P. Donchenko, V. M. Blinov, and E. V. Koonin. 1989. Cysteine proteases of positive strand RNA viruses and chymotrypsin-like serine proteases. A distinct protein superfamily with a common structural fold. *FEBS Lett.* **243:**103–114.

21. Gorbalenya, A. E., L. Enjuanes, J. Ziebuhr, and E. J. Snijder. 2006. Nidovirales: evolving the largest RNA virus genome. *Virus Res.* **117:**17–37.

22. Gorbalenya, A. E., E. V. Koonin, A. P. Donchenko, and V. M. Blinov. 1989. Coronavirus genome: prediction of putative functional domains in the non-structural polyprotein by comparative amino acid sequence analysis. *Nucleic Acids Res.* **17:**4847–4861.

23. Gorbalenya, A. E., E. V. Koonin, and M. M. Lai. 1991. Putative papain-related thiol proteases of positive-strand RNA viruses. Identification of rubi- and aphthovirus proteases and delineation of a novel conserved domain associated with proteases of rubi-, alpha- and coronaviruses. *FEBS Lett.* **288:**201–205.

24. Han, J., Y. Wang, and K. S. Faaberg. 2006. Complete genome analysis of RFLP 184 isolates of porcine reproductive and respiratory syndrome virus. *Virus Res.* **122:**175–182.

25. Ivanov, K. A., T. Hertzig, M. Rozanov, S. Bayer, V. Thiel, A. E. Gorbalenya, and J. Ziebuhr. 2004. Major genetic marker of nidoviruses encodes a replicative endoribonuclease. *Proc. Natl. Acad. Sci. USA* **101:**12694–12699.

26. Kadare, G., and A. L. Haenni. 1997. Virus-encoded RNA helicases. *J. Virol.* **71:**2583–2590.

27. Kamer, G., and P. Argos. 1984. Primary structural comparison of RNA-dependent polymerases from plant, animal and bacterial viruses. *Nucleic Acids Res.* **12:**7269–7282.

28. Katoh, K., K. Misawa, K. Kuma, and T. Miyata. 2002. MAFFT: a novel method for rapid multiple sequence alignment based on fast Fourier transform. *Nucleic Acids Res.* **30:**3059–3066.

29. Koonin, E. V. 1991. The phylogeny of RNA-dependent RNA polymerases of positive-strand RNA viruses. *J. Gen. Virol.* **72**(Pt. 9):2197–2206.

30. Laity, J. H., B. M. Lee, and P. E. Wright. 2001. Zinc finger proteins: new insights into structural and functional diversity. *Curr. Opin. Struct. Biol.* **11:**39–46.

31. Laneve, P., F. Altieri, M. E. Fiori, A. Scaloni, I. Bozzoni, and E. Caffarelli. 2003. Purification, cloning, and characterization of XendoU, a novel endoribonuclease involved in processing of intron-encoded small nucleolar RNAs in Xenopus laevis. *J. Biol. Chem.* **278:**13026–13032.

32. Makarova, K. S., L. Aravind, and E. V. Koonin. 2000. A novel superfamily of predicted cysteine proteases from eukaryotes, viruses and Chlamydia pneumoniae. *Trends Biochem. Sci.* **25:**50–52.

33. Meulenberg, J. J., M. M. Hulst, E. J. de Meijer, P. L. Moonen, A. den Besten, E. P. De Kluyver, G. Wensvoort, and R. J. Moormann. 1993. Lelystad virus, the causative agent of porcine epidemic abortion and respiratory syndrome (PEARS), is related to LDV and EAV. *Virology* **192:**62–72.

34. Molenkamp, R., H. van Tol, B. C. Rozier, Y. van der Meer, W. J. Spaan, and E. J. Snijder. 2000. The arterivirus replicase is the only viral protein required for genome replication and subgenomic mRNA transcription. *J. Gen. Virol.* **81:**2491–2496.

35. Nelsen, C. J., M. P. Murtaugh, and K. S. Faaberg. 1999. Porcine reproductive and respiratory syndrome virus comparison: divergent evolution on two continents. *J. Virol.* **73:**270–280.

36. Oleksiewicz, M. B., E. J. Snijder, and P. Normann. 2004. Phage display of the equine arteritis virus nsp1 ZF domain and examination of its metal interactions. *J. Virol. Methods* **119:**159–169.

37. O'Reilly, E. K., and C. C. Kao. 1998. Analysis of RNA-dependent RNA polymerase structure and function as guided by known polymerase structures and computer predictions of secondary structure. *Virology* **252:**287–303.

38. Palmer, G. A., L. Kuo, Z. Chen, K. S. Faaberg, and P. G. Plagemann. 1995. Sequence of the genome of lactate dehydrogenase-elevating virus: heterogenicity between strains P and C. *Virology* **209**:637–642.

39. Paukku, K., J. Yang, and O. Silvennoinen. 2003. Tudor and nuclease-like domains containing protein p100 function as coactivators for signal transducer and activator of transcription 5. *Mol. Endocrinol.* **17**:1805–1814.

40. Pedersen, K. W., Y. van der Meer, N. Roos, and E. J. Snijder. 1999. Open reading frame 1a-encoded subunits of the arterivirus replicase induce endoplasmic reticulum-derived double-membrane vesicles which carry the viral replication complex. *J. Virol.* **73**:2016–2026.

41. Poch, O., I. Sauvaget, M. Delarue, and N. Tordo. 1989. Identification of four conserved motifs among the RNA-dependent polymerase encoding elements. *EMBO J.* **8**:3867–3874.

42. Pol, J. M., F. Wagenaar, and J. E. Reus. 1997. Comparative morphogenesis of three PRRS virus strains. *Vet. Microbiol.* **55**:203–208.

43. Posthuma, C. C., D. D. Nedialkova, J. C. Zevenhoven-Dobbe, J. H. Blokhuis, A. E. Gorbalenya, and E. J. Snijder. 2006. Site-directed mutagenesis of the nidovirus replicative endoribonuclease NendoU exerts pleiotropic effects on the arterivirus life cycle. *J. Virol.* **80**:1653–1661.

44. Ricagno, S., M. P. Egloff, R. Ulferts, B. Coutard, D. Nurizzo, V. Campanacci, C. Cambillau, J. Ziebuhr, and B. Canard. 2006. Crystal structure and mechanistic determinants of SARS coronavirus nonstructural protein 15 define an endoribonuclease family. *Proc. Natl. Acad. Sci. USA* **103**:11892–11897.

45. Ritzi, D. M., M. Holth, M. S. Smith, W. J. Swart, W. A. Cafruny, G. W. Plagemann, and J. A. Stueckemann. 1982. Replication of lactate dehydrogenase-elevating virus in macrophages. 1. Evidence for cytocidal replication. *J. Gen. Virol.* **59**:245–262.

46. Schechter, I., and A. Berger. 1967. On the size of the active site in proteases. I. Papain. *Biochem. Biophys. Res. Commun.* **27**:157–162.

47. Schelle, B., N. Karl, B. Ludewig, S. G. Siddell, and V. Thiel. 2005. Selective replication of coronavirus genomes that express nucleocapsid protein. *J. Virol.* **79**:6620–6630.

48. Selenko, P., R. Sprangers, G. Stier, D. Buhler, U. Fischer, and M. Sattler. 2001. SMN tudor domain structure and its interaction with the Sm proteins. *Nat. Struct. Biol.* **8**:27–31.

49. Seybert, A., C. C. Posthuma, L. C. van Dinten, E. J. Snijder, A. E. Gorbalenya, and J. Ziebuhr. 2005. A complex zinc finger controls the enzymatic activities of nidovirus helicases. *J. Virol.* **79**:696–704.

50. Seybert, A., L. C. van Dinten, E. J. Snijder, and J. Ziebuhr. 2000. Biochemical characterization of the equine arteritis virus helicase suggests a close functional relationship between arterivirus and coronavirus helicases. *J. Virol.* **74**:9586–9593.

51. Snijder, E. J., P. J. Bredenbeek, J. C. Dobbe, V. Thiel, J. Ziebuhr, L. L. Poon, Y. Guan, M. Rozanov, W. J. Spaan, and A. E. Gorbalenya. 2003. Unique and conserved features of genome and proteome of SARS-coronavirus, an early split-off from the coronavirus group 2 lineage. *J. Mol. Biol.* **331**:991–1004.

52. Snijder, E. J., H. van Tol, N. Roos, and K. W. Pedersen. 2001. Non-structural proteins 2 and 3 interact to modify host cell membranes during the formation of the arterivirus replication complex. *J. Gen. Virol.* **82**:985–994.

53. Snijder, E. J., A. L. Wassenaar, and W. J. Spaan. 1992. The 5′ end of the equine arteritis virus replicase gene encodes a papain-like cysteine protease. *J. Virol.* **66**:7040–7048.

54. Snijder, E. J., A. L. Wassenaar, and W. J. Spaan. 1994. Proteolytic processing of the replicase ORF1a protein of equine arteritis virus. *J. Virol.* **68**:5755–5764.

55. Snijder, E. J., A. L. Wassenaar, W. J. Spaan, and A. E. Gorbalenya. 1995. The arterivirus Nsp2 protease. An unusual cysteine protease with primary structure similarities to both papain-like and chymotrypsin-like proteases. *J. Biol. Chem.* **270**:16671–16676.

56. Snijder, E. J., A. L. Wassenaar, L. C. van Dinten, W. J. Spaan, and A. E. Gorbalenya. 1996. The arterivirus nsp4 protease is the prototype of a novel group of chymotrypsin-like enzymes, the 3C-like serine proteases. *J. Biol. Chem.* **271**:4864–4871.

57. Su, M. C., C. T. Chang, C. H. Chu, C. H. Tsai, and K. Y. Chang. 2005. An atypical RNA pseudoknot stimulator and an upstream attenuation signal for −1 ribosomal frameshifting of SARS coronavirus. *Nucleic Acids Res.* **33**:4265–4275.

58. Sulea, T., H. A. Lindner, and R. Menard. 2006. Structural aspects of recently discovered viral deubiquitinating activities. *Biol. Chem.* **387**:853–862.

59. Tijms, M. A., and E. J. Snijder. 2003. Equine arteritis virus non-structural protein 1, an essential factor for viral subgenomic mRNA synthesis, interacts with the cellular transcription co-factor p100. *J. Gen. Virol.* **84**:2317–2322.

60. Tijms, M. A., Y. van der Meer, and E. J. Snijder. 2002. Nuclear localization of non-structural protein 1 and nucleocapsid protein of equine arteritis virus. *J. Gen. Virol.* **83**:795–800.

61. Tijms, M. A., L. C. van Dinten, A. E. Gorbalenya, and E. J. Snijder. 2001. A zinc finger-containing papain-like protease couples subgenomic mRNA synthesis to genome translation in a positive-stranded RNA virus. *Proc. Natl. Acad. Sci. USA* **98**:1889–1894.

62. Tong, X., R. Drapkin, R. Yalamanchili, G. Mosialos, and E. Kieff. 1995. The Epstein-Barr virus nuclear protein 2 acidic domain forms a complex with a novel cellular coactivator that can interact with TFIIE. *Mol. Cell. Biol.* **15**:4735–4744.

63. Valineva, T., J. Yang, R. Palovuori, and O. Silvennoinen. 2005. The transcriptional co-activator protein p100 recruits histone acetyltransferase activity to STAT6 and mediates interaction between the CREB-binding protein and STAT6. *J. Biol. Chem.* **280**:14989–14996.

64. Van Aken, D., W. E. Benckhuijsen, J. W. Drijfhout, A. L. Wassenaar, A. E. Gorbalenya, and E. J. Snijder. 2006. Expression, purification, and in vitro activity of an arterivirus main proteinase. *Virus Res.* **120**:97–106.

65. Van Aken, D., E. J. Snijder, and A. E. Gorbalenya. 2006. Mutagenesis analysis of the nsp4 main proteinase reveals determinants of arterivirus replicase polyprotein autoprocessing. *J. Virol.* **80**:3428–3437.

66. Van Aken, D., J. Zevenhoven-Dobbe, A. E. Gorbalenya, and E. J. Snijder. 2006. Proteolytic maturation of replicase polyprotein pp1a by the nsp4 main proteinase is essential for equine arteritis virus replication and includes internal cleavage of nsp7. *J. Gen. Virol.* **87**:3473–3482.

67. van der Meer, Y., H. van Tol, J. K. Locker, and E. J. Snijder. 1998. ORF1a-encoded replicase subunits are involved in the membrane association of the arterivirus replication complex. *J. Virol.* **72**:6689–6698.

68. van Dijk, A. A., E. V. Makeyev, and D. H. Bamford. 2004. Initiation of viral RNA-dependent RNA polymerization. *J. Gen. Virol.* **85**:1077–1093.

69. van Dinten, L. C., J. A. den Boon, A. L. Wassenaar, W. J. Spaan, and E. J. Snijder. 1997. An infectious arterivirus cDNA clone: identification of a replicase point mutation that abolishes discontinuous mRNA transcription. *Proc. Natl. Acad. Sci. USA* **94**:991–996.

70. van Dinten, L. C., S. Rensen, A. E. Gorbalenya, and E. J. Snijder. 1999. Proteolytic processing of the open reading frame 1b-encoded part of arterivirus replicase is mediated by nsp4

serine protease and is essential for virus replication. *J. Virol.* 73:2027–2037.

71. **van Dinten, L. C., H. van Tol, A. E. Gorbalenya, and E. J. Snijder.** 2000. The predicted metal-binding region of the arterivirus helicase protein is involved in subgenomic mRNA synthesis, genome replication, and virion biogenesis. *J. Virol.* 74:5213–5223.

72. **van Dinten, L. C., A. L. Wassenaar, A. E. Gorbalenya, W. J. Spaan, and E. J. Snijder.** 1996. Processing of the equine arteritis virus replicase ORF1b protein: identification of cleavage products containing the putative viral polymerase and helicase domains. *J. Virol.* 70:6625–6633.

73. **van Marle, G., L. C. van Dinten, W. J. Spaan, W. Luytjes, and E. J. Snijder.** 1999. Characterization of an equine arteritis virus replicase mutant defective in subgenomic mRNA synthesis. *J. Virol.* 73:5274–5281.

74. **Wassenaar, A. L., W. J. Spaan, A. E. Gorbalenya, and E. J. Snijder.** 1997. Alternative proteolytic processing of the arterivirus replicase ORF1a polyprotein: evidence that NSP2 acts as a cofactor for the NSP4 serine protease. *J. Virol.* 71:9313–9322.

75. **Wood, O., N. Tauraso, and H. Liebhaber.** 1970. Electron microscopic study of tissue cultures infected with simian haemorrhagic fever virus. *J. Gen. Virol.* 7:129–136.

76. **Xu, X., Y. Zhai, F. Sun, Z. Lou, D. Su, Y. Xu, R. Zhang, A. Joachimiak, X. C. Zhang, M. Bartlam, and Z. Rao.** 2006. New antiviral target revealed by the hexameric structure of mouse hepatitis virus nonstructural protein nsp15. *J. Virol.* 80:7909–7917.

77. **Yang, J., S. Aittomaki, M. Pesu, K. Carter, J. Saarinen, N. Kalkkinen, E. Kieff, and O. Silvennoinen.** 2002. Identification of p100 as a coactivator for STAT6 that bridges STAT6 with RNA polymerase II. *EMBO J.* 21:4950–4958.

78. **Ziebuhr, J., E. J. Snijder, and A. E. Gorbalenya.** 2000. Virus-encoded proteinases and proteolytic processing in the Nidovirales. *J. Gen. Virol.* 81:853–879.

*Nidoviruses*
Edited by S. Perlman, T. Gallagher, and E. J. Snijder
© 2008 ASM Press, Washington, DC

Chapter 7

# Cell Biology of Nidovirus Replication Complexes

SUSAN C. BAKER AND MARK R. DENISON

Viruses are obligate intracellular parasites that modify the host cell to generate an environment for optimal production of progeny virus. Positive-strand RNA viruses modify intracellular membranes to generate "factories" for viral RNA synthesis. These factories are made up of viral replicase proteins and host cell membranes that assemble to form novel structures, which can be visualized by electron microscopy (EM). For example, the replication complex of brome mosaic virus, a positive-strand RNA virus of plants, induces invaginations and spherule formation in the endoplasmic reticulum (ER) (56). These spherules sequester the viral genomic RNA and polymerase together and allow for the efficient synthesis of viral genomic and subgenomic mRNAs. The replication complexes of hepatitis C virus form a membranous web in the cytoplasm of hepatoma cells (21). This membranous web may provide an environment for persistence of viral RNA during chronic infection. For nidoviruses, a striking feature is that viral replicase proteins induce the formation of double-membrane vesicles (DMVs), which are the sites of viral RNA synthesis. Here, we review the current literature on the visualization and assembly of nidovirus DMVs and describe recent studies that provide insight into the possible host cell pathways subverted by the viral replication complexes to help generate these factories for nidovirus RNA synthesis.

## GENERATING THE NIDOVIRUS REPLICATION COMPLEX

The order *Nidovirales* is made up of the families *Coronaviridae*, *Arteriviridae*, *Toroviridae*, and *Roniviridae*. These viruses are grouped in the order *Nido-*

*virales* because of their common replication strategy: they all generate a "nested set" of mRNAs (*nido* means "nest" in Latin). The proposed mechanisms for generating the nested set of viral mRNAs have been recently reviewed (36, 40) (chapter 10). The viral replication/transcription complex (RTC) is the factory that drives the synthesis of the nested set of mRNAs and the replication of the viral genomic RNA. Therefore, elucidating the structure and assembly of the nidovirus RTC is of great interest. Three model systems that have been used extensively for studies of the nidovirus RTCs are the arterivirus equine arteritis virus (EAV), the murine coronavirus mouse hepatitis virus (MHV), and the coronavirus responsible for severe acute respiratory syndrome (SARS-CoV). The genomes of these viruses share a common structure but vary considerably in size. The genomic RNA of EAV is 12.7 kb, whereas that of MHV is 31.5 kb, the largest viral RNA genome identified so far. The 5′-most gene of the nidovirus genomic RNA, gene 1, encodes the viral RNA-dependent RNA polymerase and is therefore termed the replicase gene. Gene 1 encompasses two-thirds of the genome and contains two large open reading frames (ORFs), ORF1a and ORF1b, which are joined by a ribosomal frameshifting sequence. Translation of gene 1 generates two polyproteins, pp1a and pp1ab, which are extensively processed by virus-specific proteases to generate from 13 to 16 mature products, termed nonstructural proteins. The domain organization of the nidovirus replicases is outlined in Fig. 1. The details of proteolytic processing of EAV (reviewed in chapter 6) and several coronaviruses (reviewed in chapter 5) have been well documented, whereas the details of the processing of the torovirus (60) and ronivirus (87) replicase polyproteins are incomplete but active areas of research. Briefly, the amino-terminal part of the replicase polyproteins is

Susan C. Baker • Department of Microbiology and Immunology, Loyola University Chicago Stritch School of Medicine, Maywood, IL 60153. Mark R. Denison • Department of Pediatrics, Department of Microbiology and Immunology, and Elizabeth B. Lamb Center for Pediatric Research, Vanderbilt University Medical Center, Nashville, TN 37232.

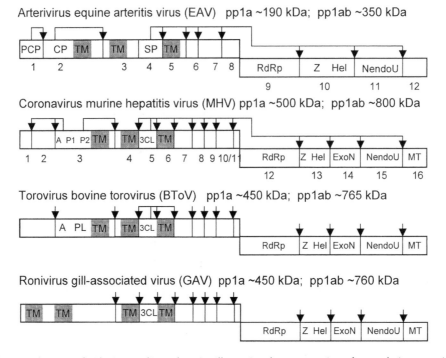

**Figure 1.** Schematic diagram of nidovirus replicase domains illustrating the conservation of proteolytic processing and enzymatic activity in arteri-, corona-, toro-, and ronivirus families. Connected arrows indicate confirmed cleavage sites processed by the indicated protease. Arrowheads indicate predicted sites for proteolytic processing. Abbreviations: PCP/P1/P2/PL, papain-like cysteine proteases; CP, cysteine protease; A, ADP-ribose- 1″-phosphatase; SP, serine protease; 3CL, 3C-like protease (also termed M^pro); RdRp, RNA-dependent RNA polymerase; Z, zinc-binding domain; Hel, helicase; NendoU, nidovirus uridylate-specific endoribonuclease; ExoN, exonuclease; MT, methyltransferase.

processed by viral cysteine proteases (termed PCPs and CP for EAV; either one or two papain-like proteases [PL^pro] for coronaviruses [Fig. 1]). The remaining processing is mediated by the protease activity of the viral 3C-like protease (termed 3CL^pro, for its picornavirus 3C-like protease specificity; also termed main protease [M^pro]), nsp4 in arteriviruses, and nsp5 in coronaviruses, which is either a cysteine or a serine protease belonging to the chymotrypsin-like family. An outline of one example of the cascade of proteolytic processing events that eventually leads to the generation of 16 mature coronavirus replicase products is depicted in Fig. 2. Further work is needed to delineate the entire coronavirus processing cascade and compare it to the more detailed understanding of the regulated processing of the EAV replicase (reviewed in chapter 6). Processing of the replicase polyproteins by viral proteases is essential for generating an active RTC. Inhibition of processing by protease inhibitors has been shown to block coronavirus replication (30, 78). Therefore, these viral proteases are attractive targets for the development of antiviral drugs that would block the formation of the replication complex and therefore inhibit viral RNA synthesis.

Structural information is now available for multiple nidovirus replicase domains, including EAV (4)

and coronavirus 3CL^pro (2, 3, 80), SARS-CoV PL^pro (47), SARS-CoV ADP-1-ribose 1″-phosphatase (51), the novel hexadecamer formed by nsp7–nsp8 (26, 85), the nsp9 RNA-binding domain (19, 66), and MHV nsp15 (79). This structural information has provided new insights into nidovirus replicase function. For example, the initial bioinformatics prediction of SARS-CoV PL^pro deubiquitinating activity (65) has been verified using biochemical assays (5, 34) and by structural studies (47). The role of this viral deubiquitinating activity is unclear, but it may alter protein stability, localization, or activation of innate immune responses. Resolution of the structure of SARS-CoV nsp7–nsp8 revealed that these proteins assemble into a complex that is likely to function as either a primase or processivity factor for the viral RNA-dependent RNA polymerase (26, 85). Thus, analysis of individual domains of the replicase is providing important new information on the enzymatic activity of each product. However, ultimately these replicase components must assemble to generate the complex machine that synthesizes nidovirus RNA. Investigation of this assembly process will provide new information on virus-host cell interaction and potentially reveal new targets for antiviral drug development.

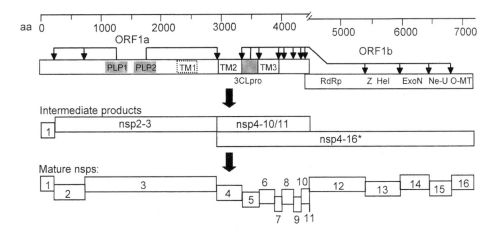

**Figure 2.** Cascade of proteolytic processing for murine coronavirus replicase polyprotein. Processing by papain-like proteases (PLP1 and PLP2) and 3CL$^{pro}$ is indicated by the arrows. Intermediates nsp2–3 (22) and nsp4–10 (28) have been detected in pulse-chase studies. nsp4–16 is proposed based on a protein band of >450 kDa. Ne-U, nidovirus uridylate-specific endoribonuclease; for other abbreviations, see legend to Fig. 1.

Another conserved feature of the nidovirus replicase is the transmembrane (TM) domains present in ORF1a (indicated in Fig. 1 and 2). These domains are predicted to be essential for association of the replicase with host cell membranes and possibly for subversion of cellular membranes to generate the modified vesicular structures. Recent studies revealed that the coronavirus nsp3 TM domain is glycosylated and contains multiple membrane-spanning domains (25, 29). Understanding how these TM domains direct the replicase complex to host cell membranes and induce formation of DMVs is important, and these domains may provide additional novel targets for antiviral drugs.

## VISUALIZING NIDOVIRUS RTCs

Novel structures generated by viral replicase protein of the arterivirus EAV and coronaviruses MHV and SARS-CoV have been visualized by immunofluorescence microscopy and transmission EM. Initially, replicase-specific antisera were generated and used to identify replicase products from virus-infected cells (Color Plate 3 [see color insert]). Immunofluorescence studies revealed punctate, perinuclear staining for replicase products of EAV (70, 74), MHV (7, 10, 15, 54, 59), and SARS-CoV (25, 46, 61) in infected cells. Viral replicase products were further characterized by biochemical fractionation to determine membrane association, and by pulse-chase radiolabeling experiments to determine precursor-product relationships. Studies of EAV revealed major and minor replicase-processing pathways (and showed that nsp2, nsp3, and nsp5 are integral

membrane proteins [70, 76]; reviewed in chapter 6). Studies using replicase-specific antisera to MHV replicase products revealed replicase intermediates nsp2–3 (22) and nsp4–11 (28) and that replicase products colocalized with newly synthesized viral RNA (15, 59). Biochemical fractionation studies indicated that all replicase products coprecipitated with intracellular membranes and that MHV replicase products nsp3 and nsp4 were integral membrane proteins (22). Nidovirus replicase integral membrane proteins may serve as the scaffold for assembly of the replication complex. Most recently, anti-replicase antibodies were generated to SARS-CoV replicase products and the characteristic punctate, perinuclear staining that colocalized with newly synthesized viral RNA was detected in SARS-CoV-infected cells (25, 46, 61). Overall, the biochemical fractionation studies and immunofluorescence studies of EAV, MHV, and SARS-CoV are consistent with the model of a multi-subunit, membrane-bound RTC.

The most striking structural feature associated with nidovirus RTCs was revealed by EM studies. EM analysis of EAV-infected (41), MHV-infected (22), and SARS-CoV-infected (20, 61) cells revealed virus-induced DMVs as the site of viral RNA synthesis (Fig. 3). These DMVs accumulate over the course of virus infection and are not present in uninfected cells. The EAV-induced DMVs are approximately 80 to 100 nm in diameter, whereas the DMVs induced by MHV and SARS-CoV infection are generally larger, from 200 to 400 nm in diameter. The DMVs in SARS-CoV-infected cells are sometimes detected as single-membrane vesicles within a larger vesicle (20). The DMVs were detected both in SARS-CoV-infected Vero-E6 cells and in

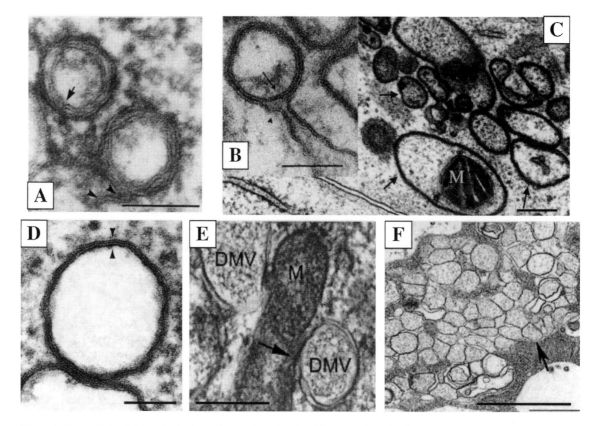

**Figure 3.** Transmission EM analysis of membrane alterations in nidovirus-infected cells. (A and B) DMV formation in EAV-infected BHK-21 cells at 4 postinfection. Bar, 100 nm. (C) Formation of DMVs from paired ER membranes upon EAV nsp2–3 expression in BHK-21 cells at 8 h posttransfection. Bar, 100 nm. (D) DMVs seen in MHV-A59-infected 17cl-1 cells at 7 postinfection. The double membrane is fused into a trilayer (arrowheads). Bar, 100 nm. (E) Analysis of SARS-CoV-infected Vero-E6 cells cryofixed by high-speed plunge freezing in liquid ethane, a step followed by freeze substitution with 1% osmium tetroxide and 0.5% uranyl acetate in acetone and embedment in epoxy LX-112 resin. The arrow indicates apparent continuity between the other membrane of a DMV and a mitochondrion (M), which was occasionally observed. Bar, 250 nm. (F) Ultrastructural characteristics of a broncho alveolar lavage specimen from a patient with SARS. DMVs (arrow) are shown to contain diffuse, granular material. Bar, 1 μm. Reproduced with permission from Pedersen et al., 1999 (A); Snijder et al., 2001 (B and C); Gosert et al., 2002 (D); Snijder et al., 2006 (E); and Goldsmith et al., 2004 (public access) (F).

bronchoalveolar lavage (BAL) specimens isolated from patients suffering from SARS (20) (Fig. 3). Snijder and coworkers found that SARS-CoV-induced DMVs were somewhat fragile and difficult to preserve using standard EM procedures for fixation and embedding of infected cells. However, using cryofixation and embedment in epoxy LX-112 resin, the SARS-CoV DMVs were well preserved and the apposed double membranes could be visualized (Fig. 3E) (61). Classical EM studies had previously identified virus-induced vesicular structures in arterivirus- and coronavirus-infected cells, but the function of the vesicles was unclear (11, 17, 43, 63, 77; F. Weiland, H. Granzow, M. Wieczorek-Krohmer, and E. Weiland, presented at the 3rd Congress of the European Society of Veterinary Virology, 1995). More recent studies using immuno-EM and in situ hybridization experiments found evidence that the DMVs were indeed the site of viral RNA

synthesis. Immuno-EM analysis showed that viral replicase proteins colocalize with the DMVs and that newly synthesized viral RNA is associated with the DMVs (20, 22, 41, 61). The experiments demonstrating association of de novo-made viral RNA with DMVs involved metabolic labeling RNA with bromouridine triphosphate (BrUTP). To label viral RNA, BrUTP is transfected into virus-infected cells in the presence of actinomycin D. Only newly synthesized viral RNA is labeled with BrUTP under these conditions, since the synthesis of cellular mRNA is inhibited by actinomycin D (59). A monoclonal antibody specific to BrdU that is conjugated with gold beads is used to detect the labeled RNA. The results of the immuno-EM experiments showed that newly synthesized viral RNA is detected in association with DMVs (22, 41). In addition, in situ hybridization with riboprobes that detect viral RNA revealed colocalization with DMVs (20, 22). Thus, the DMVs are the factories that drive nidovirus RNA synthesis.

## PATHWAYS TO NIDOVIRUS DMVs: ER, AUTOPHAGY, OR BOTH?

The source of the intracellular membranes used to generate nidovirus DMVs is currently under investigation. Studies of EAV replication indicate that ER membranes are the likely source for assembly of EAV DMVs. Double-labeling immunofluorescence microscopy experiments showed that EAV replicase proteins colocalized with ER markers such as protein disulfide isomerase (70, 74). EM studies of serial sections of EAV-infected cells revealed that EAV DMVs were predominantly perinuclear and present in only two or three serial sections, and therefore unlikely to be long, tubular structures. Some EAV DMVs appeared to arise by protrusion of paired ER membranes (see Fig. 3A and B). In some cases, a "neck-like" connection to the ER was detected. Currently, it is unclear if the EAV DMV is eventually pinched off from the ER or if the EAV DMVs remain contiguous with ER membranes.

For coronavirus DMVs, several possible membrane sources have been suggested. Colocalization studies indicated that MHV replicase proteins colocalize with ER marker GRP-78 in mouse 17cl-1 fibroblasts, but with a Golgi marker in BHK and HeLa cells that express the MHV receptor (7, 59). Alternatively, coronaviruses may utilize components of the host cell autophagy pathway for the assembly of DMVs. Autophagy is a stress response pathway that functions to recycle proteins and organelles (48). This recycling process is mediated by the formation of characteristic double-membrane autophagic vesicles that surround the material to be recycled and deliver it to lysosomes for degradation. Recent studies indicate that bacteria and viruses may subvert this stress response pathway to avoid immune surveillance and perhaps to promote their own replication (31). A role for cellular autophagy in the formation of MHV RTC-associated membrane structures has been proposed by Prentice et al. based on immunofluorescence, biochemical, and EM experiments (45). In that study, MHV infection was reported to up-regulate autophagy by an unknown mechanism that was resistant to 3-methyladenine, a nucleoside analog that inhibits the phosphatidylinositol 3-kinase signaling pathways required for stress- or rapamycin-induced autophagy. MHV replicase proteins were found to colocalize quantitatively at cytoplasmic foci with each other and with LC3, the murine homolog of ATG8, a marker for intact autophagosomes, but not with markers for

lysosomes. In addition, MHV infection of murine embryonic stem cells that were lacking ATG5, a critical protein in autophagosome formation, resulted in a >3-log reduction in virus replication. This growth defect was complemented by stable expression of ATG5 in the ATG5$^{-/-}$ cells. In addition, while DMVs were observed in the MHV-infected ATG5$^{+/+}$ cells, in the ATG$^{-/-}$ cells DMVs were rare but there was dramatic derangement and proliferation of the membranes that had the appearance of ER based on contiguity with nuclear membranes and EM evidence for ribosomes decorating the altered membranes. Based on these data, the authors concluded that components of the autophagy pathway, specifically ATG5, were involved in and required for MHV RTC formation and function. However, the lack of impairment of MHV-induced autophagy by 3-methyladenine, and the lack of colocalization of endosome or lysosome markers with replication complexes, indicates that the process is not identical to stress-induced autophagy. DMVs may result from direct modification of cellular membranes, likely ER membranes, by MHV proteins that interact with proteins of the autophagy pathways. In a separate study of SARS-CoV replicase protein localization, nsp8 was shown to colocalize with LC3 in SARS-CoV-infected Vero-E6 cells. The result suggested that SARS-CoV may interact with pathways similar to those used by MHV to generate viral replication complexes (46).

In contrast to these results, Snijder and coworkers reported no detectable colocalization of SARS-CoV replicase proteins with LC3, either by antibodies or LC3-green fluorescent protein expression (61). Instead, EM analysis of DMVs (Fig. 3) and colocalization of SARS-CoV nsp13 and protein disulfide isomerase, an ER marker, were the basis for the conclusion that ER membranes, not autophagic membranes, were the origin of SARS-CoV DMVs in Vero-E6 cells. This is more similar to the results observed for EAV, which also suggested an ER origin for DMV membranes.

While both studies clearly demonstrate similar immunofluorescence assay characteristics of SARS-CoV RTCs in Vero-E6 cells, and colocalization of multiple replicase proteins to the complexes, the LC3 localization results are just as clearly different. It is possible to propose biological or technical differences in the studies to account for the disparate results, but until additional studies are performed the data cannot be directly reconciled. However, an important question is raised in these studies. Does coronavirus RTC formation require targeting of a specific cellular membrane biosynthesis or degradation pathway? More precisely, do the coronavirus replicase proteins have to choose between the ER, autophagosomes, or some other membrane pathway? Autophagy is a response to stress, notably starvation, in all eukaryotic cells that degrades and recycles organelles and cytoplasmic contents. Several recent studies in yeasts have established a clear link between ER membranes and autophagy in eukaryotic cells. ER and Golgi membranes have been shown to be sources of membranes for autophagosomes during starvation-induced stress (27, 49). Recent studies from three different labs reported that ER stress, independent of starvation, induces autophagy and that autophagy regulates ER expansion and recycling of ER contents in coordination with the unfolded-protein response (6, 39, 81). While these studies remain to be replicated in mammalian cells, there is an increasingly recognized interaction of ER biogenesis/function and autophagy in eukaryotic cells. It is intriguing to speculate that nidovirus replication may induce ER stress and up-regulation of autophagy in virus-infected cells. However, the autophagy process must also be regulated in such a way as to prevent degradation of viral RTCs. Investigating this area will provide new information on virus-host cell interaction and potential subversion of host cell stress response pathways.

Interestingly, recent studies indicate that some viruses may be able to use multiple membrane sources or even different membrane arrangements for the formation of their replication complexes. Schwartz and coworkers showed that for brome mosaic virus, the complex could be redirected from the ER to the mitochondrial membranes without impeding viral RNA synthesis (57). These results indicate that some viral replicase proteins are able to utilize whatever membrane source they are directed to for the assembly of the RNA-synthesizing machinery. For some viruses, there is controversy concerning the cellular processes or membrane sources that are utilized to generate replication complexes. For poliovirus, Bienz and coworkers, using immuno-EM studies, identified single-membrane vesicles that coalesce into "rosette-like" structures as the site of RNA synthesis (8, 9). Three-dimensional reconstruction imaging studies indicated that host cell COPII vesicles are subverted by poliovirus replicase proteins, in a mechanism homologous to vesicle formation of the anterograde membrane transport pathway, to generate the single-membrane structures (50). In contrast, Kirkegaard and coworkers provide evidence that poliovirus induces formation of DMVs that are likely derived by subversion of the cellular autophagy pathway (55, 64). For both picornaviruses and nidoviruses, further studies will be needed to determine if only one host cell membrane source is utilized to generate replication complexes, if multiple cellular membrane sources can be subverted during virus replication, or if virus

infection induces or mimicks pathways such as autophagy to generate specific physical and functional structures essential for replication.

## NIDOVIRUS DMVs AND THE "SURFACE" OF VIRAL RNA SYNTHESIS

Colocalization and immuno-EM studies indicate that DMVs are the site of nidovirus RNA synthesis. However, does nidovirus RNA synthesis take place inside the vesicles or on the outside surface? Two possible scenarios are illustrated in Fig. 4. The first possibility is modeled from studies of the BMV replicase in which it has been shown that viral RNA is sequestered inside the replicase-induced spherules (57). In this scenario, the nidovirus replicase proteins may initially cluster on the ER membranes, with an associated copy of viral positive-strand RNA. The clustering of the replicase proteins may induce membrane curvature, resulting in an invagination of the ER membrane and trapping of the template RNA with the replicase. Once sequestered inside the membrane, the RNA may be copied to generate double-stranded RNA (dsRNA) and subsequently generate progeny mRNA. The progeny RNA could be released from the "neck" of the vesicle or through hypothetical "transport channels" generated by replicase membrane-spanning products

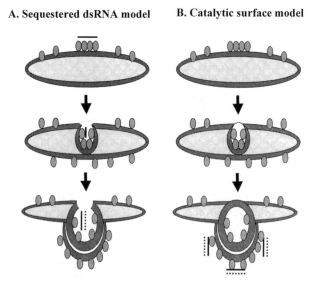

**A. Sequestered dsRNA model**    **B. Catalytic surface model**

**Figure 4.** Models of nidovirus replicase proteins driving formation of DMVs and replication of viral RNA. Nidovirus replicase complexes are depicted as gray circles; viral positive-strand RNA is depicted as a solid line, and negative-strand RNA is depicted as a dotted line. (A) DMV formation sequesters viral genomic RNA for transcription and replication. (B) DMV formation generates a catalytic surface area competent for transcription and replication of viral RNA.

such as coronavirus nsp6. In this model, the template dsRNA could be subjected to many rounds of transcription and/or replication inside the protected environment of the DMV. The critical, testable features of this model are that the template is protected inside the DMV and that necks or channels exist for the exit of newly synthesized mRNA. Support for this model comes from a study by Sethna and Brian that demonstrates distinct buoyant-density populations of membranes containing transmissible gastroenteritis virus RNA protected from nuclease digestion in the absence of detergent (58).

The second model is based on evidence of an "RNA polymerase lattice" structure which has been visualized for poliovirus (35). In this model, viral RNA polymerases are concentrated in the surface of vesicles, where they can efficiently elongate newly synthesized RNA. For nidoviruses, replicase proteins may induce membrane curvature and DMV formation. However, since the replicase proteins are detected in copious amounts on the cytosolic surface of the host cell membranes, they may assemble to form a surface area where viral RNA can be efficiently replicated. Such a "catalytic surface" could be an efficient mechanism for copying large quantities of viral mRNA and genomic RNA. One advantage of this model is the ready access of the RTC to cytoplasmic sources of energy and nucleotides for viral mRNA synthesis. A potential disadvantage is that the viral dsRNA may be detected in the cytoplasm and trigger innate immune mechanisms that sense dsRNA. These models depict two possible scenarios for the assembly of the DMV factories that drive nidovirus replication. A better understanding of the replicase components that induce DMV formation and mediate viral RNA synthesis will contribute to improved models and generate testable hypotheses for factory assembly, and ultimately lead to new ways to block DMV factory assembly and reduce nidovirus-associated disease.

## USING REVERSE GENETICS TO PROBE NIDOVIRUS REPLICATION COMPLEX FORMATION AND FUNCTION

The development of reverse-genetics systems for several arteri- and coronaviruses, including EAV (71), porcine reproductive and respiratory syndrome virus (PRRSV) (32, 38), MHV (14, 84), transmissible gastroenteritis virus (1, 82), human coronavirus 229E (67), avian infectious bronchitis virus (13), and SARS-CoV (83), has allowed rapid progress in defining replication requirements and protein functions. In addition, the use of reverse genetics provides the

promise of addressing fundamental questions in how nidovirus replicase proteins interact with the host cell to form the active RTCs.

The first reverse genetics system for any nidovirus arose from the development of a full-length cDNA clone of the arterivirus EAV (71). The authors cloned the entire EAV cDNA into a plasmid, synthesized full-length RNA in vitro, and electroporated the RNA into BHK cells, which allowed for translation and replication of the viral genomic RNA and production of progeny infectious virus particles. In the initial study, the authors identified a point mutation in EAV replicase nsp10 (Ser-2429→Pro) that allowed for viral RNA replication but no production of subgenomic RNA, which provided experimental evidence that the requirements for replication and transcription of subgenomic mRNAs may be separated. This study opened the door for the analysis of the role of proteolytic processing and specific enzymatic activity of replicase products, and the investigation of the role of transcription-regulating sequences in EAV replication. Regarding replicase processing and function, van Dinten and coworkers showed that processing by EAV nsp4 (the 3CL^pro serine protease) is essential for generating a fully functional RTC (72), and van Aken et al. recently identified an additional nsp4 processing site within nsp7 (69). These studies provide experimental evidence for the importance of regulated processing of the replicase polyprotein by the viral proteases. Furthermore, mutagenesis of sequences in individual replicase products revealed the essential role of the metal binding domain in nsp10 (73, 75), the zinc finger domain in nsp1 (68), and the nidovirus uridylate-specific endoribonuclease domain in nsp11 (44) in EAV replication.

For coronaviruses, reverse-genetics studies have focused on the role of the amino-terminal replicase proteins (nsp1, nsp2, and nsp3) and papain-like protease-mediated proteolytic processing in coronavirus replication. For MHV and SARS-CoV, an in-frame deletion of the nsp2 protein domain is tolerated, with only modest consequences to growth fitness (24). This result was surprising in that it showed that at least one replicase product was not essential for assembly of a functional replication complex. MHV also tolerates deletion of the carboxy-terminal half of nsp1 (12), as well as deletion of cleavage sites between nsp1–nsp2 (16) and nsp2–nsp3 (23). The deletion of the cleavage sites revealed that polyprotein intermediates could assemble and function as part of the replication complex. Thus, proteolytic processing may facilitate rapid assembly of the replication complex, but processing at cleavage sites one and two is not required for MHV replication complex function. More recently, it has been demonstrated that PLP1 of

MHV can be inactivated in viable mutants, albeit with extreme impairment of replication in the absence of adaptive passage (23). This is the first example of generating a viable recombinant coronavirus with mutation of a catalytic residue in the protease domain. This study illustrates the full potential of using the reverse-genetics system to identify mutations that debilitate but do not obliterate virus replication. Ongoing studies in the Denison lab also show the ability of viable engineered mutants of MHV to tolerate deletion of cleavage sites flanking nsp5 and nsp14 (J. S. Sparks, L. D. Eckerle, and M. R. Denison, unpublished data). For the ORF1b proteins, a substitution mutation in the carboxy-half of MHV nsp14 (Tyr-414→His) has been shown to have no effect on replication in culture while attenuating virulence in mice (62). In contrast, mutations in the exonuclease N active residues of nsp14 have been reported to be lethal for virus recovery (37).

With regard to replication complex formation and membrane interactions, the coronavirus nsp3, nsp4, and nsp6 proteins are the most likely candidates for membrane modification or nucleation of replication complexes on membranes. They were first predicted to be replicase anchors based on the prominent stretches of hydrophobic amino acids (33). Subsequently, nsp4 and nsp6 were shown to confer a membrane requirement on nsp5 ($3CL^{pro}$) processing activity when expressed as a polyprotein in vitro (42, 54). More recent bioinformatics analyses indicate that all of the putative membrane-spanning motifs lie within coronavirus nsp3, nsp4, and nsp6 (86). This prediction is supported by data demonstrating the integral membrane character of nsp3 and nsp4 during virus infection (22), including N-linked glycosylation of luminal domains in nsp3 (25, 29) and nsp4 (A. Kanjanahaluethai and S. C. Baker, unpublished data). So far, there have been no reports of nsp6 localization, presumably due to the fact that it has not been possible to establish useful reagents that detect this hydrophobic protein.

The evidence to date suggests that the formation of a membrane-associated RTC is a critical step in the replication of nidoviruses. Therefore, targeting the replicase TM domains by site-directed mutagenesis and deletion analysis may reveal components essential for localization and function. However, this targeting of replicase integral membrane proteins may be lethal for replication and not allow recovery of viable mutants for study. The use of complementing cell lines expressing combinations of nsp3, nsp4, and nsp6 could be considered to rescue mutant genomes, but this approach has not yet been possible, at least in the MHV system, due to toxicity of the cloned and expressed protein. In addition, for poliovirus, expression of viral replicase membrane proteins led to membrane alterations that reduced virus replication and did not support replication complex formation in *trans* (18). If RTC formation is an obligatory *cis* function of nidovirus replicase proteins, then expression complementation studies may be challenging.

Alternatively, the use of "classical" temperature-sensitive (ts) mutants combined with verification of specific mutations using reverse genetics is likely to yield important new information on the function and assembly of the nidovirus RTC. Previous studies using coronavirus ts mutants identified cistrons within the replicase polyprotein that affected positive- and negative-strand RNA synthesis (53). Recently, Sawicki and colleagues sequenced a series of MHV ts mutants and identified mutations within nsp4 (Alb ts6), nsp5 (Alb ts16), nsp10 (LA ts6), nsp12 (Alb ts22), nsp14 (Wu ts38 and Alb ts17), and nsp16 (Wu ts36 and Wu ts18) that are likely responsible for specific ts phenotypes (52). Interestingly, these ts mutants are defective in different steps in RNA synthesis. For example, LA ts6 is defective in continuing negative-strand viral RNA synthesis, whereas Alb ts16 appeared to be defective in positive-strand RNA synthesis. By using reverse genetics to test the effect of specific mutations of viral RNA synthesis, researchers will be able to identify the replicase products that are required for each step in viral RNA synthesis. These studies will provide a starting point for future detailed genetic studies of how replicase proteins interact to assemble the replication complex and how they must interact, and possibly alter conformation, to mediate positive-strand and negative-strand RNA synthesis.

## FUTURE DIRECTIONS

Understanding the process by which nidoviruses replicase proteins generate DMV-associated viral RTCs is in the early stages. To date, researchers have made significant progress in identifying the cascade of proteolytic processing steps and the mature replicase products that are required to generate a functional replication complex. EM studies have revealed the dramatic changes that take place to assemble the DMV factories required for efficient viral RNA synthesis. Genetic studies have identified both essential and dispensable regions of the replicase for replication in culture. The challenge for the future is to determine how viral replicase proteins coax the cell into generating these factories that will ultimately lead to rapid production of viral RNA and progeny viral particles. Understanding these early events in the assembly of the viral replication machinery may lead to new opportunities to block virus replication and ameliorate nidovirus-induced disease.

**Acknowledgments.** We thank members of our laboratories for helpful comments and suggestions during the preparation of this chapter.

We thank the National Institutes of Health for ongoing support for research (grants AI045798 and AI060915 to S.C.B. and AI50083, AI26603, and AI59943 to M.R.D.).

## REFERENCES

1. Almazan, F., J. M. Gonzalez, Z. Penzes, A. Izeta, E. Calvo, J. Plana-Duran, and L. Enjuanes. 2000. Engineering the largest RNA virus genome as an infectious bacterial artificial chromosome. *Proc. Natl. Acad. Sci. USA* 97:5516–5521.

2. Anand, K., G. J. Palm, J. R. Mesters, S. G. Siddell, J. Ziebuhr, and R. Hilgenfeld. 2002. Structure of coronavirus main proteinase reveals combination of a chymotrypsin fold with an extra alpha-helical domain. *EMBO J.* 21:3213–3224.

3. Anand, K., J. Ziebuhr, P. Wadhwani, J. R. Mesters, and R. Hilgenfeld. 2003. Coronavirus main proteinase (3CLpro) structure: basis for design of anti-SARS drugs. *Science* 300:1763–1767.

4. Barrette-Ng, I. H., K. K. Ng, B. L. Mark, D. Van Aken, M. M. Cherney, C. Garen, Y. Kolodenko, A. E. Gorbalenya, E. J. Snijder, and M. N. James. 2002. Structure of arterivirus nsp4. The smallest chymotrypsin-like proteinase with an alpha/beta C-terminal extension and alternate conformations of the oxyanion hole. *J. Biol. Chem.* 277:39960–39966.

5. Barretto, N., D. Jukneliene, K. Ratia, Z. Chen, A. D. Mesecar, and S. C. Baker. 2005. The papain-like protease of severe acute respiratory syndrome coronavirus has deubiquitinating activity. *J. Virol.* 79:15189–15198.

6. Bernales, S., K. L. McDonald, and P. Walter. 2006. Autophagy counterbalances endoplasmic reticulum expansion during the unfolded protein response. *PLoS Biol.* 4:e423.

7. Bi, W., J. D. Pinon, S. Hughes, P. J. Bonilla, K. V. Holmes, S. R. Weiss, and J. L. Leibowitz. 1998. Localization of mouse hepatitis virus open reading frame 1A derived proteins. *J. Neurovirol.* 4:594–605.

8. Bienz, K., D. Egger, T. Pfister, and M. Troxler. 1992. Structural and functional characterization of the poliovirus replication complex. *J. Virol.* 66:2740–2747.

9. Bienz, K., D. Egger, M. Troxler, and L. Pasamontes. 1990. Structural organization of poliovirus RNA replication is mediated by viral proteins of the P2 genomic region. *J. Virol.* 64:1156–1163.

10. Bost, A. G., R. H. Carnahan, X. T. Lu, and M. R. Denison. 2000. Four proteins processed from the replicase gene polyprotein of mouse hepatitis virus colocalize in the cell periphery and adjacent to sites of virion assembly. *J. Virol.* 74:3379–3387.

11. Breese, S. S., and W. H. McCollum. 1970. Electron microscopic characterization of equine arteritis virus, pp. 133–139. *In proceedings of the 2nd International Conference on Equine Infectious Diseases.*

12. Brockway, S. M., and M. R. Denison. 2005. Mutagenesis of the murine hepatitis virus nsp1-coding region identifies residues important for protein processing, viral RNA synthesis, and viral replication. *Virology* 340:209–223.

13. Casais, R., V. Thiel, S. G. Siddell, D. Cavanagh, and P. Britton. 2001. Reverse genetics system for the avian coronavirus infectious bronchitis virus. *J. Virol.* 75:12359–12369.

14. Coley, S. E., E. Lavi, S. G. Sawicki, L. Fu, B. Schelle, N. Karl, S. G. Siddell, and V. Thiel. 2005. Recombinant mouse hepatitis virus strain A59 from cloned, full-length cDNA replicates to high titers in vitro and is fully pathogenic in vivo. *J. Virol.* 79:3097–3106.

15. Denison, M. R., W. J. Spaan, Y. van der Meer, C. A. Gibson, A. C. Sims, E. Prentice, and X. T. Lu. 1999. The putative helicase of the coronavirus mouse hepatitis virus is processed from the replicase gene polyprotein and localizes in complexes that are active in viral RNA synthesis. *J. Virol.* 73:6862–6871.

16. Denison, M. R., B. Yount, S. M. Brockway, R. L. Graham, A. C. Sims, X. Lu, and R. S. Baric. 2004. Cleavage between replicase proteins p28 and p65 of mouse hepatitis virus is not required for virus replication. *J. Virol.* 78:5957–5965.

17. Dubois-Dalcq, M., B. Rentier, E. Hooghe-Peters, M. V. Haspel, R. L. Knobler, and K. Holmes. 1982. Acute and persistent viral infections of differentiated nerve cells. *Rev. Infect. Dis.* 4:999–1014.

18. Egger, D., N. Teterina, E. Ehrenfeld, and K. Bienz. 2000. Formation of the poliovirus replication complex requires coupled viral translation, vesicle production, and viral RNA synthesis. *J. Virol.* 74:6570–6580.

19. Egloff, M. P., F. Ferron, V. Campanacci, S. Longhi, C. Rancurel, H. Dutartre, E. J. Snijder, A. E. Gorbalenya, C. Cambillau, and B. Canard. 2004. The severe acute respiratory syndrome-coronavirus replicative protein nsp9 is a single-stranded RNA-binding subunit unique in the RNA virus world. *Proc. Natl. Acad. Sci. USA* 101:3792–3796.

20. Goldsmith, C. S., K. M. Tatti, T. G. Ksiazek, P. E. Rollin, J. A. Comer, W. W. Lee, P. A. Rota, B. Bankamp, W. J. Bellini, and S. R. Zaki. 2004. Ultrastructural characterization of SARS coronavirus. *Emerg. Infect. Dis.* 10:320–326.

21. Gosert, R., D. Egger, V. Lohmann, R. Bartenschlager, H. E. Blum, K. Bienz, and D. Moradpour. 2003. Identification of the hepatitis C virus RNA replication complex in Huh-7 cells harboring subgenomic replicons. *J. Virol.* 77:5487–5492.

22. Gosert, R., A. Kanjanahaluethai, D. Egger, K. Bienz, and S. C. Baker. 2002. RNA replication of mouse hepatitis virus takes place at double-membrane vesicles. *J. Virol.* 76:3697–3708.

23. Graham, R. L., and M. R. Denison. 2006. Replication of murine hepatitis virus is regulated by papain-like proteinase 1 processing of nonstructural proteins 1, 2, and 3. *J. Virol.* 80:11610–11620.

24. Graham, R. L., A. C. Sims, S. M. Brockway, R. S. Baric, and M. R. Denison. 2005. The nsp2 replicase proteins of murine hepatitis virus and severe acute respiratory syndrome coronavirus are dispensable for viral replication. *J. Virol.* 79:13399–13411.

25. Harcourt, B. H., D. Jukneliene, A. Kanjanahaluethai, J. Bechill, K. M. Severson, C. M. Smith, P. A. Rota, and S. C. Baker. 2004. Identification of severe acute respiratory syndrome coronavirus replicase products and characterization of papain-like protease activity. *J. Virol.* 78:13600–13612.

26. Imbert, I., J. C. Guillemot, J. M. Bourhis, C. Bussetta, B. Coutard, M. P. Egloff, F. Ferron, A. E. Gorbalenya, and B. Canard. 2006. A second, non-canonical RNA-dependent RNA polymerase in SARS coronavirus. *EMBO J.* 25:4933–4942.

27. Ishihara, N., M. Hamasaki, S. Yokota, K. Suzuki, Y. Kamada, A. Kihara, T. Yoshimori, T. Noda, and Y. Ohsumi. 2001. Autophagosome requires specific early Sec proteins for its formation and NSF/SNARE for vacuolar fusion. *Mol. Biol. Cell* 12:3690–3702.

28. Kanjanahaluethai, A., and S. C. Baker. 2000. Identification of mouse hepatitis virus papain-like proteinase 2 activity. *J. Virol.* 74:7911–7921.

29. Kanjanahaluethai, A., Chen, Z., D. Jukneliene, and S. C. Baker. 2007. Membrane topology of murine coronavirus replicase nonstructural protein 3. *Virology* **361**:391–401.

30. Kim, J. C., R. A. Spence, P. F. Currier, X. Lu, and M. R. Denison. 1995. Coronavirus protein processing and RNA synthesis is inhibited by the cysteine proteinase inhibitor E64d. *Virology* **208**:1–8.

31. Kirkegaard, K., M. P. Taylor, and W. T. Jackson. 2004. Cellular autophagy: surrender, avoidance and subversion by microorganisms. *Nat. Rev. Microbiol.* **2**:301–314.

32. Lee, C., J. G. Calvert, S. K. Welch, and D. Yoo. 2005. A DNA-launched reverse genetics system for porcine reproductive and respiratory syndrome virus reveals that homodimerization of the nucleocapsid protein is essential for virus infectivity. *Virology* **331**:47–62.

33. Lee, H. J., C. K. Shieh, A. E. Gorbalenya, E. V. Koonin, N. La Monica, J. Tuler, A. Bagdzhadzhyan, and M. M. Lai. 1991. The complete sequence (22 kilobases) of murine coronavirus gene 1 encoding the putative proteases and RNA polymerase. *Virology* **180**:567–582.

34. Lindner, H. A., N. Fotouhi-Ardakani, V. Lytvyn, P. Lachance, T. Sulea, and R. Menard. 2005. The papain-like protease from the severe acute respiratory syndrome coronavirus is a deubiquitinating enzyme. *J. Virol.* **79**:15199–15208.

35. Lyle, J. M., E. Bullitt, K. Bienz, and K. Kirkegaard. 2002. Visualization and functional analysis of RNA-dependent RNA polymerase lattices. *Science* **296**:2218–2222.

36. Masters, P. S. 2006. The molecular biology of coronaviruses. *Adv. Virus Res.* **66**:193–292.

37. Minskaia, E., T. Hertzig, A. E. Gorbalenya, V. Campanacci, C. Cambillau, B. Canard, and J. Ziebuhr. 2006. Discovery of an RNA virus 3′→5′ exoribonuclease that is critically involved in coronavirus RNA synthesis. *Proc. Natl. Acad. Sci. USA* **103**:5108–5113.

38. Nielsen, H. S., G. Liu, J. Nielsen, M. B. Oleksiewicz, A. Botner, T. Storgaard, and K. S. Faaberg. 2003. Generation of an infectious clone of VR-2332, a highly virulent North American-type isolate of porcine reproductive and respiratory syndrome virus. *J. Virol.* **77**:3702–3711.

39. Ogata, M., S. Hino, A. Saito, K. Morikawa, S. Kondo, S. Kanemoto, T. Murakami, M. Taniguchi, I. Tanii, K. Yoshinaga, S. Shiosaka, J. A. Hammarback, F. Urano, and K. Imaizumi. 2006. Autophagy is activated for cell survival after endoplasmic reticulum stress. *Mol. Cell. Biol.* **26**:9220–9231.

40. Pasternak, A. O., W. J. Spaan, and E. J. Snijder. 2006. Nidovirus transcription: how to make sense ...? *J. Gen. Virol.* **87**:1403–1421.

41. Pedersen, K. W., Y. van der Meer, N. Roos, and E. J. Snijder. 1999. Open reading frame 1a-encoded subunits of the arterivirus replicase induce endoplasmic reticulum-derived double-membrane vesicles which carry the viral replication complex. *J. Virol.* **73**:2016–2026.

42. Pinon, J. D., R. R. Mayreddy, J. D. Turner, F. S. Khan, P. J. Bonilla, and S. R. Weiss. 1997. Efficient autoproteolytic processing of the MHV-A59 3C-like proteinase from the flanking hydrophobic domains requires membranes. *Virology* **230**:309–322.

43. Pol, J. M., F. Wagenaar, and J. E. Reus. 1997. Comparative morphogenesis of three PRRS virus strains. *Vet. Microbiol.* **55**:203–208.

44. Posthuma, C. C., D. D. Nedialkova, J. C. Zevenhoven-Dobbe, J. H. Blokhuis, A. E. Gorbalenya, and E. J. Snijder. 2006. Site-directed mutagenesis of the nidovirus replicative endoribonuclease NendoU exerts pleiotropic effects on the arterivirus life cycle. *J. Virol.* **80**:1653–1661.

45. Prentice, E., W. G. Jerome, T. Yoshimori, N. Mizushima, and M. R. Denison. 2004. Coronavirus replication complex formation utilizes components of cellular autophagy. *J. Biol. Chem.* **279**:10136–10141.

46. Prentice, E., J. McAuliffe, X. Lu, K. Subbarao, and M. R. Denison. 2004. Identification and characterization of severe acute respiratory syndrome coronavirus replicase proteins. *J. Virol.* **78**:9977–9986.

47. Ratia, K., K. S. Saikatendu, B. D. Santarsiero, N. Barretto, S. C. Baker, R. C. Stevens, and A. D. Mesecar. 2006. Severe acute respiratory syndrome coronavirus papain-like protease: structure of a viral deubiquitinating enzyme. *Proc. Natl. Acad. Sci. USA* **103**:5717–5722.

48. Reggiori, F., and D. J. Klionsky. 2002. Autophagy in the eukaryotic cell. *Eukaryot. Cell* **1**:11–21.

49. Reggiori, F., C. W. Wang, U. Nair, T. Shintani, H. Abeliovich, and D. J. Klionsky. 2004. Early stages of the secretory pathway, but not endosomes, are required for Cvt vesicle and autophagosome assembly in Saccharomyces cerevisiae. *Mol. Biol. Cell.* **15**:2189–2204.

50. Rust, R. C., L. Landmann, R. Gosert, B. L. Tang, W. Hong, H. P. Hauri, D. Egger, and K. Bienz. 2001. Cellular COPII proteins are involved in production of the vesicles that form the poliovirus replication complex. *J. Virol.* **75**:9808–9818.

51. Saikatendu, K. S., J. S. Joseph, V. Subramanian, T. Clayton, M. Griffith, K. Moy, J. Velasquez, B. W. Neuman, M. J. Buchmeier, R. C. Stevens, and P. Kuhn. 2005. Structural basis of severe acute respiratory syndrome coronavirus ADP-ribose-1″-phosphate dephosphorylation by a conserved domain of nsP3. *Structure* (Cambridge) **13**:1665–1675.

52. Sawicki, S. G., D. L. Sawicki, D. Younker, Y. Meyer, V. Thiel, H. Stokes, and S. G. Siddell. 2005. Functional and genetic analysis of coronavirus replicase-transcriptase proteins. *PLoS Pathog.* **1**:e39.

53. Schaad, M. C., S. A. Stohlman, J. Egbert, K. Lum, K. Fu, T. Wei, Jr., and R. S. Baric. 1990. Genetics of mouse hepatitis virus transcription: identification of cistrons which may function in positive and negative strand RNA synthesis. *Virology* **177**:634–645.

54. Schiller, J. J., A. Kanjanahaluethai, and S. C. Baker. 1998. Processing of the coronavirus MHV-JHM polymerase polyprotein: identification of precursors and proteolytic products spanning 400 kilodaltons of ORF1a. *Virology* **242**:288–302.

55. Schlegel, A., T. H. Giddings, Jr., M. S. Ladinsky, and K. Kirkegaard. 1996. Cellular origin and ultrastructure of membranes induced during poliovirus infection. *J. Virol.* **70**:6576–6588.

56. Schwartz, M., J. Chen, M. Janda, M. Sullivan, J. den Boon, and P. Ahlquist. 2002. A positive-strand RNA virus replication complex parallels form and function of retrovirus capsids. *Mol. Cell* **9**:505–514.

57. Schwartz, M., J. Chen, W. M. Lee, M. Janda, and P. Ahlquist. 2004. Alternate, virus-induced membrane rearrangements support positive-strand RNA virus genome replication. *Proc. Natl. Acad. Sci. USA* **101**:11263–11268.

58. Sethna, P. B., and D. A. Brian. 1997. Coronavirus genomic and subgenomic minus-strand RNAs copartition in membrane-protected replication complexes. *J. Virol.* **71**:7744–7749.

59. Shi, S. T., J. J. Schiller, A. Kanjanahaluethai, S. C. Baker, J. W. Oh, and M. M. Lai. 1999. Colocalization and membrane association of murine hepatitis virus gene 1 products and de novo-synthesized viral RNA in infected cells. *J. Virol.* **73**:5957–5969.

60. Smits, S. L., E. J. Snijder, and R. J. de Groot. 2006. Characterization of a torovirus main proteinase. *J. Virol.* **80:** 4157–4167.

61. Snijder, E. J., Y. van der Meer, J. Zevenhoven-Dobbe, J. J. Onderwater, J. van der Meulen, H. K. Koerten, and A. M. Mommaas. 2006. Ultrastructure and origin of membrane vesicles associated with the severe acute respiratory syndrome coronavirus replication complex. *J. Virol.* **80:**5927–5940.

61a. Snijder, E. J., H. van Tol, N. Roos, and K. W. Pedersen. 2001. Non-structural proteins 2 and 3 interact to modify host cell membranes during the formation of the arterivirus replication complex. *J. Gen. Virol.* **82:**985–994.

62. Sperry, S. M., L. Kazi, R. L. Graham, R. S. Baric, S. R. Weiss, and M. R. Denison. 2005. Single-amino-acid substitutions in open reading frame (ORF) 1b-nsp14 and ORF 2a proteins of the coronavirus mouse hepatitis virus are attenuating in mice. *J. Virol.* **79:**3391–3400.

63. Stueckemann, J. A., M. Holth, W. J. Swart, K. Kowalchyk, M. S. Smith, A. J. Wolstenholme, W. A. Cafruny, and P. G. Plagemann. 1982. Replication of lactate dehydrogenase-elevating virus in macrophages. 2. Mechanism of persistent infection in mice and cell culture. *J. Gen. Virol.* **59:**263–272.

64. Suhy, D. A., T. H. Giddings, Jr., and K. Kirkegaard. 2000. Remodeling the endoplasmic reticulum by poliovirus infection and by individual viral proteins: an autophagy-like origin for virus-induced vesicles. *J. Virol.* **74:**8953–8965.

65. Sulea, T., H. A. Lindner, E. O. Purisima, and R. Ménard. 2005. Deubiquitination, a new function of the severe acute respiratory syndrome coronavirus papain-like protease? *J. Virol.* **79:**4550–4551.

66. Sutton, G., E. Fry, L. Carter, S. Sainsbury, T. Walter, J. Nettleship, N. Berrow, R. Owens, R. Gilbert, A. Davidson, S. Siddell, L. L. Poon, J. Diprose, D. Alderton, M. Walsh, J. M. Grimes, and D. I. Stuart. 2004. The nsp9 replicase protein of SARS-coronavirus, structure and functional insights. *Structure* **12:**341–353.

67. Thiel, V., J. Herold, B. Schelle, and S. G. Siddell. 2001. Infectious RNA transcribed in vitro from a cDNA copy of the human coronavirus genome cloned in vaccinia virus. *J. Gen. Virol.* **82:**1273–1281.

68. Tijms, M. A., L. C. van Dinten, A. E. Gorbalenya, and E. J. Snijder. 2001. A zinc finger-containing papain-like protease couples subgenomic mRNA synthesis to genome translation in a positive-stranded RNA virus. *Proc. Natl. Acad. Sci. USA* **98:**1889–1894.

69. van Aken, D., J. Zevenhoven-Dobbe, A. E. Gorbalenya, and E. J. Snijder. 2006. Proteolytic maturation of replicase polyprotein pp1a by the nsp4 main proteinase is essential for equine arteritis virus replication and includes internal cleavage of nsp7. *J. Gen. Virol.* **87:**3473–3482.

70. van der Meer, Y., H. van Tol, J. K. Locker, and E. J. Snijder. 1998. ORF1a-encoded replicase subunits are involved in the membrane association of the arterivirus replication complex. *J. Virol.* **72:**6689–6698.

71. van Dinten, L. C., J. A. den Boon, A. L. Wassenaar, W. J. Spaan, and E. J. Snijder. 1997. An infectious arterivirus cDNA clone: identification of a replicase point mutation that abolishes discontinuous mRNA transcription. *Proc. Natl. Acad. Sci. USA* **94:**991–996.

72. van Dinten, L. C., S. Rensen, A. E. Gorbalenya, and E. J. Snijder. 1999. Proteolytic processing of the open reading frame 1b-encoded part of arterivirus replicase is mediated by nsp4 serine protease and is essential for virus replication. *J. Virol.* **73:**2027–2037.

73. van Dinten, L. C., H. van Tol, A. E. Gorbalenya, and E. J. Snijder. 2000. The predicted metal-binding region of the arterivirus helicase protein is involved in subgenomic mRNA synthesis, genome replication, and virion biogenesis. *J. Virol.* **74:**5213–5223.

74. van Dinten, L. C., A. L. Wassenaar, A. E. Gorbalenya, W. J. Spaan, and E. J. Snijder. 1996. Processing of the equine arteritis virus replicase ORF1b protein: identification of cleavage products containing the putative viral polymerase and helicase domains. *J. Virol.* **70:**6625–6633.

75. van Marle, G., L. C. van Dinten, W. J. Spaan, W. Luytjes, and E. J. Snijder. 1999. Characterization of an equine arteritis virus replicase mutant defective in subgenomic mRNA synthesis. *J. Virol.* **73:**5274–5281.

76. Wassenaar, A. L., W. J. Spaan, A. E. Gorbalenya, and E. J. Snijder. 1997. Alternative proteolytic processing of the arterivirus replicase ORF1a polyprotein: evidence that NSP2 acts as a cofactor for the NSP4 serine protease. *J. Virol.* **71:**9313–9322.

77. Wood, O., N. Tauraso, and H. Liebhaber. 1970. Electron microscopic study of tissue cultures infected with simian haemorrhagic fever virus. *J. Gen. Virol.* **7:**129–136.

78. Wu, C. Y., J. T. Jan, S. H. Ma, C. J. Kuo, H. F. Juan, Y. S. Cheng, H. H. Hsu, H. C. Huang, D. Wu, A. Brik, F. S. Liang, R. S. Liu, J. M. Fang, S. T. Chen, P. H. Liang, and C. H. Wong. 2004. Small molecules targeting severe acute respiratory syndrome human coronavirus. *Proc. Natl. Acad. Sci. USA* **101:** 10012–10017.

79. Xu, X., Y. Zhai, F. Sun, Z. Lou, D. Su, Y. Xu, R. Zhang, A. Joachimiak, X. C. Zhang, M. Bartlam, and Z. Rao. 2006. New antiviral target revealed by the hexameric structure of mouse hepatitis virus nonstructural protein nsp15. *J. Virol.* **80:**7909–7917.

80. Yang, H., M. Yang, Y. Ding, Y. Liu, Z. Lou, Z. Zhou, L. Sun, L. Mo, S. Ye, H. Pang, G. F. Gao, K. Anand, M. Bartlam, R. Hilgenfeld, and Z. Rao. 2003. The crystal structures of severe acute respiratory syndrome virus main protease and its complex with an inhibitor. *Proc. Natl. Acad. Sci. USA* **100:** 13190–13195.

81. Yorimitsu, T., U. Nair, Z. Yang, and D. J. Klionsky. 2006. Endoplasmic reticulum stress triggers autophagy. *J. Biol. Chem.* **281:**30299–30304.

82. Yount, B., K. M. Curtis, and R. S. Baric. 2000. Strategy for systematic assembly of large RNA and DNA genomes: transmissible gastroenteritis virus model. *J. Virol.* **74:**10600–10611.

83. Yount, B., K. M. Curtis, E. A. Fritz, L. E. Hensley, P. B. Jahrling, E. Prentice, M. R. Denison, T. W. Geisbert, and R. S. Baric. 2003. Reverse genetics with a full-length infectious cDNA of severe acute respiratory syndrome coronavirus. *Proc. Natl. Acad. Sci. USA* **100:**12995–13000.

84. Yount, B., M. R. Denison, S. R. Weiss, and R. S. Baric. 2002. Systematic assembly of a full-length infectious cDNA of mouse hepatitis virus strain A59. *J. Virol.* **76:**11065–11078.

85. Zhai, Y., F. Sun, X. Li, H. Pang, X. Xu, M. Bartlam, and Z. Rao. 2005. Insights into SARS-CoV transcription and replication from the structure of the nsp7-nsp8 hexadecamer. *Nat. Struct. Mol. Biol.* **12:**980–986.

86. Ziebuhr, J. 2005. The coronavirus replicase. *Curr. Top. Microbiol. Immunol.* **287:**57–94.

87. Ziebuhr, J., S. Bayer, J. A. Cowley, and A. E. Gorbalenya. 2003. The 3C-like proteinase of an invertebrate nidovirus links coronavirus and potyvirus homologs. *J. Virol.* **77:**1415–1426.

*Nidoviruses*
Edited by S. Perlman, T. Gallagher, and E. J. Snijder
© 2008 ASM Press, Washington, DC

Chapter 8

# RNA Signals Regulating Nidovirus RNA Synthesis

Erwin van den Born and Eric J. Snijder

As discussed extensively in previous chapters (e.g., chapters 1 to 3), the order *Nidovirales* includes the virus groups with the largest known RNA genomes, with sizes ranging up to 31.5 kb. Maintaining the integrity of such very large RNA genomes probably requires a number of sophisticated mechanisms not known for other RNA viruses. As explained in chapter 2, the evolution of the nidovirus genome and its replication machinery is likely to have been a stepwise process during which a variety of novel replicase functions were acquired and tailored to serve one of the most complex RNA virus life cycles. In addition to the proposed common ancestry of key replicase domains, nidoviruses are united by having a polycistronic genome. Consequently, besides amplifying the genome RNA ("replication"), nidoviruses produce a set of up to 10 subgenomic mRNAs (sg mRNAs) to express the genes that are located downstream of the replicase gene (Fig. 1). It is now generally accepted that the latter process (which is referred to as "transcription" in this chapter) involves the generation of subgenome-length minus-strand templates, one for each sg mRNA.

Recognition by the RNA-dependent RNA polymerase (RdRp) complex of RNA signals near the 3′ end of the nidovirus genome precedes the initiation of full-length minus-strand RNA (or "antigenome") synthesis. This minus strand, in turn, serves as the template for the synthesis of new genome RNA and must therefore also carry recognition signals in its 3′ end. Viral RNA synthesis is asymmetric and produces much more plus- than minus-strand RNA (87). In addition to being replicated, the nidovirus genome is also assumed to be the template for the production of subgenome-length minus strands that are used as templates for transcription (see below). Elegant biochemical studies by Sawicki et al., using the

coronavirus mouse hepatitis virus (MHV) as a model, showed that both antigenome- and subgenome-length minus strands are produced very early in infection (87). Each sg mRNA is produced from a corresponding transcription intermediate that contains the subgenome-length minus-strand template. These complexes synthesize the various sg mRNAs in nonequimolar but relatively constant amounts. Also, the ratio of genome to sg mRNAs is constant throughout the MHV replication cycle (87, 90).

Nidovirus RNA synthesis has now been studied at the molecular level for almost three decades, but our understanding of the molecular interplay between RNA signals and protein functions that is the basis for replication and transcription is still in its infancy (8, 64, 79, 91). It is known that nidovirus RNA synthesis takes place in close association with cytoplasmic cellular membranes (reviewed in chapter 7), but the enzyme complexes responsible for full-length and subgenome-length plus- and minus-strand synthesis have not been defined in any detail, and their respective compositions are unknown. At the RNA level, in particular the multifunctionality of the genomic plus strand is intriguing, since it serves as a template for replicase gene translation and full-length and subgenome-length minus-strand RNA synthesis and ultimately needs to be packaged into progeny virions. In the past 15 years, the advent of nidovirus replicon systems and reverse genetics (chapter 4) has aided tremendously in identifying and characterizing *cis*-acting elements involved in the regulation of nidovirus RNA synthesis. In this chapter, we summarize what is known about these primary and higher-order RNA structures, in particular for coronaviruses and arteriviruses, and address various other aspects of nidovirus replication and transcription.

**Erwin van den Born** • Department of Molecular Biosciences, University of Oslo, P.O. Box 1041 Blindern, 0316 Oslo, Norway. **Eric J. Snijder** • Molecular Virology Laboratory, Department of Medical Microbiology, Leiden University Medical Center, P.O. Box 9600, 2300 RC Leiden, The Netherlands.

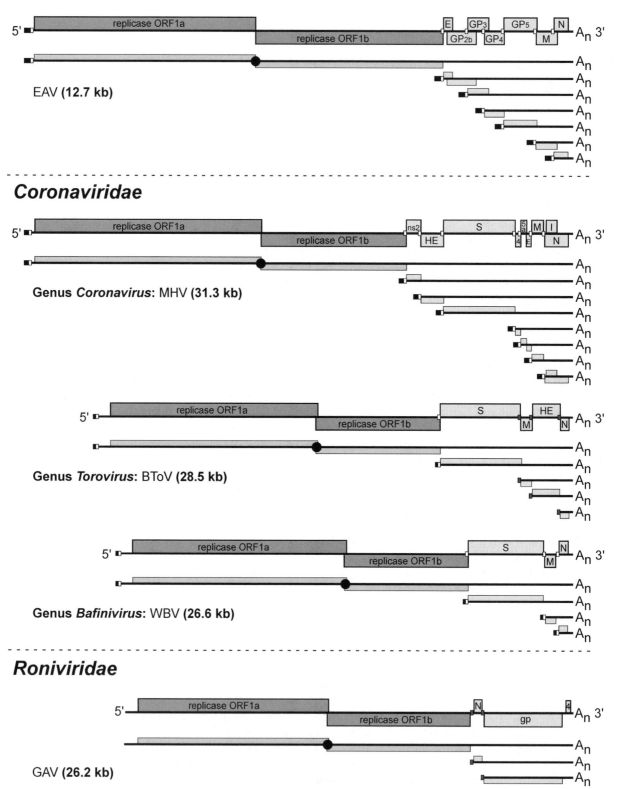

**Figure 1.** Nidoviruses produce a 3′-coterminal nested set of mRNAs. The genome organization and expression strategies of the arterivirus EAV, the coronavirus MHV, bovine torovirus (BToV), WBV (tentative genus, *Bafinivirus*), and the ronivirus gill-associated virus (GAV) are summarized. Shown are structural relationships of the genome-length and subgenome-length mRNAs. The leader sequence and leader TRS found at the genomic 5′ ends of EAV, MHV, and WBV are indicated as black and white boxes, respectively. The same color coding is used for the genome and largest sg mRNA of BToV. The TREs found at the 5′ ends of all other BToV and GAV sg mRNAs are indicated as dark gray boxes. The ribosomal frameshifting element found in genome-length mRNA is indicated as a black circle. Only the translated ORFs are indicated for each mRNA. E, envelope protein; M, membrane protein; GP, glycoprotein; S, spike glycoprotein; HE, hemagglutinin-esterase protein; ns2, nonstructural protein 2; I, internal gene product. Adapted from reference 98.

## RNA SIGNALS REGULATING NIDOVIRUS REPLICATION

### Replication Signals in *Coronaviridae* Genomes

Coronavirus defective interfering (DI) genomes have been useful tools to investigate RNA signals and elements involved in replication. DI RNAs are replication-competent RNA molecules that result from extensive deletions in the viral genome that are due to replication errors. They have retained the *cis*-acting sequence elements necessary for replication but depend on the presence of helper virus, with which DI RNAs compete for replicase proteins and other factors required for RNA synthesis. Cloned cDNA copies of DI RNA genomes have been subjected to mutagenesis to probe the importance of specific RNA sequences. In vitro-generated DI RNAs can be transfected into infected cells to study the consequences of mutations. The major disadvantage of the DI RNA-based systems is the inevitable risk of (homologous) recombination between the DI RNA replicon and the helper virus genome. The amplification step that is often required to analyze the phenotype of the DI RNA replicons, which is commonly achieved by (repeated) passaging of the DI RNA after the initial transfection experiment, is another disadvantage of the DI RNA system. DI RNAs that lack a functional packaging signal cannot be passaged and are therefore not always readily detected, but they may still be replication competent. The recent development of reverse-genetic systems based on cloned full-length cDNA copies of coronavirus genomes (reviewed in chapter 4) has now provided an alternative to the use of DI RNA systems and will further enhance our understanding of coronavirus replication signals.

### Group 1 coronaviruses

In an elegant study aimed at determining the minimal replication signals required for the group 1 coronavirus transmissible gastroenteritis virus (TGEV), a two-step amplification system was used that allowed for analysis of DI RNA replication without passaging

(38). A TGEV DI RNA was generated in the nucleus of transfected cells by cellular RNA polymerase II-mediated transcription and was further amplified, after export from the nucleus to the cytoplasm, by the viral replicase produced by the helper virus. In this system, the maximal sequences required for DI RNA replication were reduced to the 5′-terminal 1,348 nucleotides (nt) and the 3′-terminal 492 nt of the genome. The 5′-terminal region required for replication was further reduced to 649 nt by showing that an artificial viral mRNA was amplified when it contained at least this domain (Table 1) (24). More recently, computer-assisted analysis of the 275-nt 3′ untranslated region (UTR) of feline coronavirus, a close relative of TGEV, identified a hairpin structure located at the 5′ end of this region and a predicted downstream pseudoknot structure (Fig. 2) (23). These two RNA structure elements are conserved among group 2 coronaviruses and were shown to play an essential role in RNA synthesis (see below).

### Group 2 coronaviruses

The replication signals of MHV have been characterized quite extensively. The minimal *cis*-acting 5′-proximal region required for genome replication is approximately 466 nt (Table 1) and was determined using several DI RNA-based systems (18, 46, 59, 65, 115). Deletions within this domain were not tolerated, suggesting that the entire region is required for replication (55). This 5′-proximal region interacts with heterogeneous nuclear ribonucleoprotein A1 (hnRNP A1), and the complementary strand interacts with polypyrimidine tract-binding protein (PTB). It was demonstrated in vitro that both proteins are able to form an RNP complex with RNA fragments representing the 5′- and 3′-proximal regions of the MHV genome. These studies suggested that an interaction between hnRNP A1 and PTB may provide a molecular mechanism for cross talk between the 5′ and 3′ ends of the MHV genome, which may be important for translation, replication, and/or transcription (37, 48). The finding that overexpression of hnRNP A1

**Table 1.** Maximal *cis*-acting replication signals in nidovirus genomes

| Family | Subgroup | Virus | 5′-Proximal genome region (nt) | 3′-Proximal genome region (nt) |
|---|---|---|---|---|
| *Coronaviridae* | Group 1 coronavirus | TGEV | 649 | 492 |
| | Group 2 coronavirus | MHV | 466 | 436 |
| | | BCoV | 498 | ND[a](1,637) |
| | Group 3 coronavirus | IBV | 544 | 338 |
| | Torovirus | BEV | 607 | 242 |
| *Arteriviridae* | Arterivirus | EAV | 296 | 354 |

[a]ND, not determined in detail.

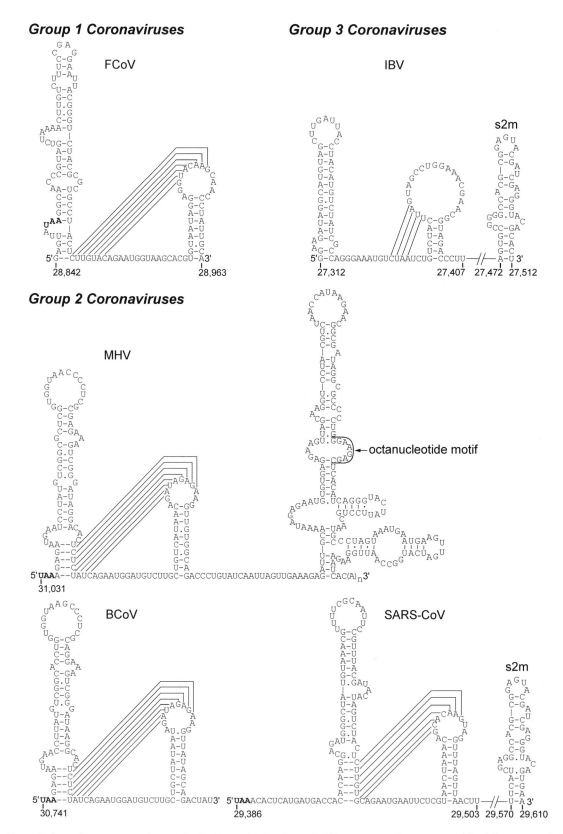

**Figure 2.** Secondary-structure elements in the 3'-proximal regions of different coronavirus genomes. The feline coronavirus (FCoV; feline infectious peritonitis virus WSU-79/1146 strain) structure was adapted from reference 23. The MHV (A59 strain) structure was combined and adapted from references 28 and 57. The conserved octanucleotide motif (GGAAGAGC) is indicated. The BCoV (Mebus strain) and SARS-CoV (Urbani strain) RNA structures are adapted from references 126 and 28, respectively. The IBV (strain Beaudette) and SARS-CoV s2m hairpins were taken from reference 86. The most 5'-positioned hairpin of the IBV structure and the pseudoknot were adapted from references 17 and 126, respectively. The translation stop codon (UAA) of the N protein ORF is indicated in bold.

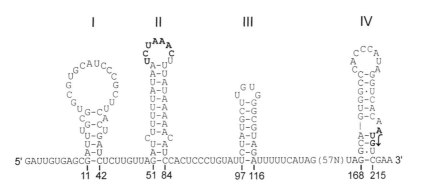

**Figure 3.** Secondary-structure model of the BCoV 5′ UTR. The BCoV (Mebus strain) structure model was adapted from reference 84. The replicase translation initiation codon is indicated in bold and is marked with an arrow. The core sequence of the leader TRS is also indicated in bold. Nucleotide numbers refer to positions in the BCoV genome.

accelerated the kinetics of viral RNA synthesis appeared to strengthen the case for an important role of hnRNP A1 in MHV replication, even more since a dominant negative hnRNP A1 mutant inhibited viral RNA synthesis (96). However, conflicting information was derived from a study using an hnRNP A1 knockout cell line, in which MHV replication was not affected at all, suggesting that the protein is nonessential for viral RNA synthesis (95). Whether functional redundancy of hnRNP A1 and its family members may explain this observation remains to be evaluated.

Similar to the case of MHV, the 5′-terminal 498 nt of the bovine coronavirus (BCoV) genome were found to be required for replication of a DI RNA-derived replicon (Table 1) (11). Computer-aided analysis and structure probing of the 210-nt 5′ UTR that is part of this region identified four stem-loop structures (Fig. 3), designated hairpins I to IV (12, 83, 84). Nucleotide substitutions that were designed to disrupt and then restore the conformation of hairpins I and II rapidly reverted back to the wild-type sequence, indicating that these mutations have an effect on BCoV DI RNA replication. Since deletion of hairpin I rendered the DI RNA replication incompetent, it was postulated that this structure is a *cis*-acting element in BCoV replication (11, 12). In subsequent studies, the integrity of hairpins III and IV was shown to be important for BCoV DI RNA replication, suggesting that also these structures are essential *cis*-acting RNA elements. Hairpins III and IV are conserved among group 2 coronaviruses, which supports their importance in the life cycle of this virus group. Potential hairpin III and IV homologs may also be present in the 5′ UTRs of the genomes of group 1 and group 3 coronaviruses (83, 84).

A combination of studies revealed that the 3′-terminal 436 nt of the MHV genome are required for DI RNA replication (Table 1) (18, 46, 55, 65, 115,

116). This suggested that the 3′ *cis*-acting replication signal must encompass the entire 301-nt 3′ UTR as well as a portion of the adjacent nucleocapsid (N) protein gene. However, the MHV N protein gene can be moved to a more distant position in the genome without affecting replication (19, 28), implying that the 3′ UTR essentially contains all 3′ *cis*-acting signals for RNA synthesis. Since initiation of MHV minus-strand synthesis requires only the 3′-terminal 55 nt plus a poly(A) tail, a major part of the 3′ *cis*-acting replication signals is thought to be necessary for the initiation of plus-strand synthesis (56, 105). Although there is no information about the minimal 3′-proximal region required for BCoV replication, a naturally occurring BCoV DI RNA was described that contains the 3′-terminal 1,637 nt (Table 1) (11).

Several RNA structures located within the genomic 3′ UTR of group 2 coronaviruses were identified as "replication mediators," and this has produced an elaborate picture of RNA elements involved. Initially a RNA pseudoknot structure was identified in the BCoV 3′ UTR (Fig. 2), and its existence was supported by enzymatic probing. This structure has a counterpart in all coronavirus subgroups and is conserved in terms of location and higher-order structure, but not at the sequence level. Mutagenesis experiments demonstrated that this RNA pseudoknot is involved in BCoV replication (125, 126). Secondly, a 68-nt bulged hairpin is located at the 5′ end of the 3′ UTR, directly upstream of the pseudoknot and directly downstream of the N protein gene (Fig. 2). This structure appeared to be essential for replication and was suggested to function during plus-strand RNA synthesis (34, 35). Because the base of this hairpin partly overlaps with the 5′ side of the pseudoknot, their formation is mutually exclusive. Therefore, it was speculated that these structures might constitute an RNA switch, i.e., one structure forming at the expense of the other (33). Support for this molecular switch came with the generation of a viable MHV mutant that contained a triple mutation involving both sides of the base stem region of the hairpin and the interacting loop of the pseudoknot, such that all base-pairing possibilities are maintained (28). Further downstream in the MHV 3′ UTR, a large hairpin was identified (57), which is not well conserved at the primary- or secondary-structure level (Fig. 2). Paradoxically, the hairpin contains an octanucleotide motif (GGAAGAGC) that is strictly conserved among coronaviruses (Fig. 2) (30, 34). Remarkably, extensive mutagenesis and deletion analysis of this octanucleotide and a large portion of the hairpin (between nt 46 and 156) of which it is part did not affect MHV replication in vitro but seriously influenced MHV pathogenicity in a mouse model (29). This finding differed considerably from the severe inhibition of DI RNA replication and transcription that was reported following small deletions or mutations in this motif and the hairpin (36, 37, 40, 58, 130), underlining that results obtained from mutagenesis in DI RNA-based systems need to be confirmed using full-length genomes.

In an attempt to identify RNA elements shared by the two viruses, the 3′ UTR of the MHV genome was successfully replaced with its BCoV counterpart, underlining the close relationship between these viruses (34). Moreover, it was demonstrated that MHV could serve as helper virus for the replication of a BCoV DI RNA. Thus, 5′-proximal as well as 3′-proximal cis-acting BCoV replication elements can be recognized by the MHV replication machinery (128). With the functional replacement of the MHV genomic 3′ UTR by the corresponding RNA element of severe acute respiratory syndrome coronavirus (SARS-CoV), additional biological support was provided for the classification of SARS-CoV in coronavirus group 2 (31). In contrast, the 3′ UTR of the group 1 coronavirus TGEV and the group 3 coronavirus infectious bronchitis virus (IBV) could not functionally replace the MHV 3′ UTR. Indeed, RNA secondary-structure analysis of the SARS-CoV 3′ UTR identified a hairpin structure that overlaps with a pseudoknot (Fig. 2) and is similar to the structures discovered in the corresponding regions of the MHV and BCoV genomes (30). An attempt to replace the MHV 5′ UTR with that of SARS-CoV was unsuccessful, even when the MHV genome was equipped with both the 5′ and 3′ UTRs of SARS-CoV. However, it was shown that three predicted RNA structures within the SARS-CoV 5′ UTR (SL1, SL2, and SL4) could support MHV replication when they replaced their putative MHV counterparts (45).

Besides replication elements located at the genome termini, an MHV-JHM-derived DI RNA required a 135-nt internal replication signal for its amplification by MHV-A59 helper virus (46, 55). A 55-nt hairpin structure, located around 3.2 kb from the 5′ end of the MHV genome, appeared to be involved, and its structure was supported by probing experiments. Mutagenesis studies suggested that this structure exerted its replicative function in the plus polarity only (47, 85). In contrast, for the closely related MHV-A59 strain, a similar internal replication signal was not required for replication of a DI RNA-derived replicon (18, 59, 65, 113). It was suggested that the cell types used might explain the observed difference (59).

## Group 3 coronaviruses

The minimal sequence requirements for replication of the group 3 coronavirus IBV were determined using a DI RNA system. The results indicated that the 5′-terminal 544 nt and 3′-terminal 338 nt contained the signals necessary for replication (Table 1). Secondary-structure analysis of the first 100 nt of this 5′-terminal region identified three hairpin structures. For the most 5′-proximal hairpin, a high degree of covariance among IBV strains provided phylogenetic support for its importance (106). Within the 3′-proximal region, which is part of the IBV 3′ UTR, a hairpin was identified that is highly conserved among group 3 coronaviruses. Moreover, deletion of this structure abolished DI RNA replication, suggesting that it has a function in replication (17). This coronavirus group 3-specific hairpin is located 10 nt upstream of the pseudoknot structure that is conserved throughout the coronavirus genus (Fig. 2). However, the predicted IBV pseudoknot is structurally not very convincing and displays only little resemblance to the group 1 and 2 coronavirus structures (126). It should be noted that group 3 coronaviruses contain a conserved so-called "s2m motif" in the 3′ UTRs of their genomes, which is also present in picorna- and astroviruses (41, 42). Remarkably, this RNA element is also found in the 3′ UTR of SARS-CoV, which is considered to occupy a position distant from group 3. The s2m motifs of both IBV and SARS-CoV may adopt similar hairpin structures (Fig. 2). The three-dimensional structure of the SARS-CoV s2m motif was determined by nuclear magnetic resonance studies (86).

## Toroviruses

Two DI RNA genomes of equine torovirus (strain Berne) of approximately 1.0 and 1.4 kb were isolated and characterized after serial undiluted passaging of this virus in cell culture. The smallest DI

RNA contained the 5′-terminal 607 nt fused to the 3′-terminal 242 nt (Table 1) (101).

### Replication Signals in Arterivirus Genomes

Although reverse-genetics systems using full-length genomes of the arteriviruses equine arteritis virus (EAV) and porcine reproductive and respiratory syndrome virus (PRRSV) were developed a few years before those for coronaviruses (67, 117), the functional dissection of arterivirus genome replication lags behind. A first idea of the signals required for EAV replication was obtained through deletion mutagenesis of a cloned cDNA copy of a DI RNA that had been obtained by serial undiluted passaging of EAV in cell culture. The maximal sequences required for DI RNA replication were reduced to the 5′-terminal 589 nt and the 3′-terminal 1,066 nt of the genome. Furthermore, a 583-nt sequence from the central part of replicase open reading frame 1b (ORF1b) (nt 8566 to 9149 in the EAV genome) was found to be essential for DI RNA replication (72). Unexpectedly, full-length genome replication required only 354 nt (Table 1), not 1,066 nt, of the 3′-terminal part of the genome (73). The 5′-terminal sequences required for replication were further reduced to 296 nt when an EAV RNA lacking nt 297 to 1004 was found to replicate to wild-type levels (Table 1) (109). For both EAV genome termini, RNA secondary-structure models (Fig. 4A and B) were developed using a combination of bioinformatics, phylogenetic analysis, RNA structure probing, and site-directed mutagenesis (7, 110). The two most 3′-proximal hairpins within the 3′-terminal region of the genome (Fig. 4B) contain key signals for viral RNA synthesis, whereas only a moderate role was attributed to the elaborate hairpin structure that is located upstream (7).

In another study, the presence of essential replication elements within the structural protein-coding region of the PRRSV genome was documented. Deletion analysis showed that a stretch of 34 nucleotides within ORF7, which encodes the N protein, is essential for replication. The 34-nt stretch is highly conserved among PRRSV isolates and is predicted to fold into a hairpin. Sequences within the loop of this structure were shown to base-pair with the loop of a hairpin located in the 3′ UTR, resulting in a so-called kissing loop interaction (Fig. 4C), which was confirmed to be required for replication (122).

### Role of N Protein in Nidovirus RNA Synthesis

Several (viral and cellular) proteins have been implicated in nidovirus replication and transcription (reviewed in, e.g., reference 97), and of these, the viral N protein is of particular interest. Arterivirus RNA synthesis does not require N protein, in spite of the fact that the protein partly colocalizes with the viral replication complex (73). Engineered EAV mutants that could not express N protein displayed normal levels of both replication and transcription (73, 80). In contrast, there are strong indications that N protein is involved in coronavirus RNA synthesis. Also, part of the coronavirus N protein colocalizes with replicative proteins at the sites of viral RNA synthesis early in infection (112). Most importantly, N protein has been found to enhance the efficiency of replication of transfected in vitro-engineered replicon or genome RNA (1, 10, 92, 107, 129). Although it has been proposed that N protein participates in sgRNA synthesis, due to its specific binding to transcription-regulating sequences (13, 74), its effect is probably not exhibited at the level of transcription, since an engineered human coronavirus 229E replicon RNA lacking all structural protein genes retained the ability to synthesize sg mRNAs (92, 108). So far, the exact role of N protein in corona-virus replication is not understood.

## RNA SIGNALS REGULATING NIDOVIRUS TRANSCRIPTION

### sgRNA Synthesis in the *Nidovirales*

The synthesis of one or multiple sg mRNAs is a mechanism that many positive-strand RNA viruses have evolved to selectively express structural and accessory proteins from ORFs other than those encoding the replicase (poly)proteins (69). Three different mechanisms have been proposed to explain sg mRNA production by positive-strand RNA viruses (69, 124). The most common mechanism is internal initiation of subgenomic plus-strand synthesis from the antigenome by the RdRp, which is recruited by promoter sequences in the viral minus-strand RNA, as was initially described for brome mosaic virus (68). The second model, premature termination of minus-strand RNA synthesis, proposes that minus-strand synthesis is terminated when the RdRp encounters a regulatory sequence in the plus-strand template. This attenuation step thus produces a subgenomic minus-strand molecule that serves as the template for sg mRNA synthesis. The third model, discontinuous extension of minus-strand RNA synthesis (Fig. 5A), is uniquely employed by most—but not all—nidoviruses (see below) and shares characteristics with the premature-termination model described above.

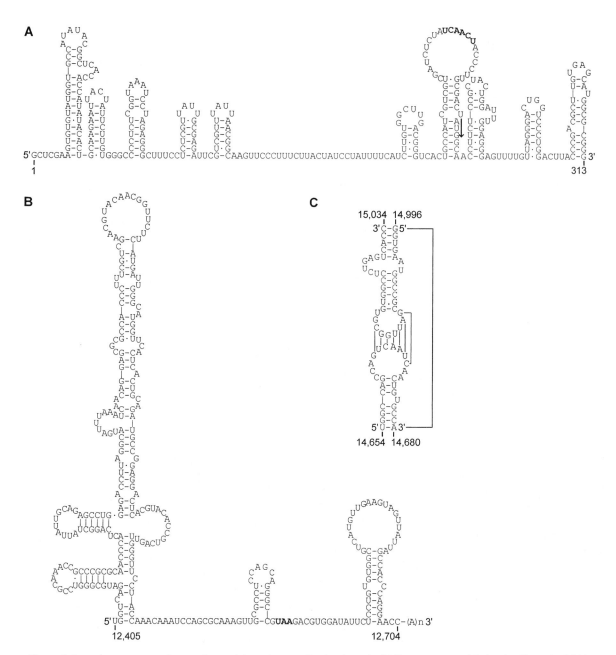

**Figure 4.** Secondary-structure elements in arterivirus genomes. Depicted are the RNA structure models for the 5′-terminal 313 nt (A) and the 3′-terminal 300 nt (B) of the EAV genome (Bucyrus strain). Adapted from references 110 and 7, respectively. The replicase translation initiation codon is indicated with an arrow. The leader TRS (UCAACU) and the translation stop codon of the N protein gene are indicated in bold. (C) Model of the kissing loop interaction identified in the 3′-proximal region of the PRRSV genome (Lelystad strain), adapted from reference 122.

Members of the *Coronavirus* and *Arterivirus* genera, and the recently identified torovirus-like white bream virus (WBV; proposed genus, *Bafinivirus*) (93), exclusively produce sg mRNAs that consist of a "leader" and a "body" segment, derived from sequences that are noncontiguous in the viral genome. Using a mechanism of discontinuous RNA synthesis (see below), the 5′ common leader is attached to the different sg mRNA bodies at a conserved sequence element, the transcription-regulating sequence (TRS) (Fig. 5A) (5, 22, 49, 104). Alternative designations for TRSs that have been used in the literature are "transcription-associated sequence," "intergenic sequence," and "leader-body junction site."

A leader TRS is located at the 3′ end of the genomic leader sequence, and body TRSs are found preceding each ORF in the 3′-terminal domain of the genome (118, 136). Transcription of the largest of the

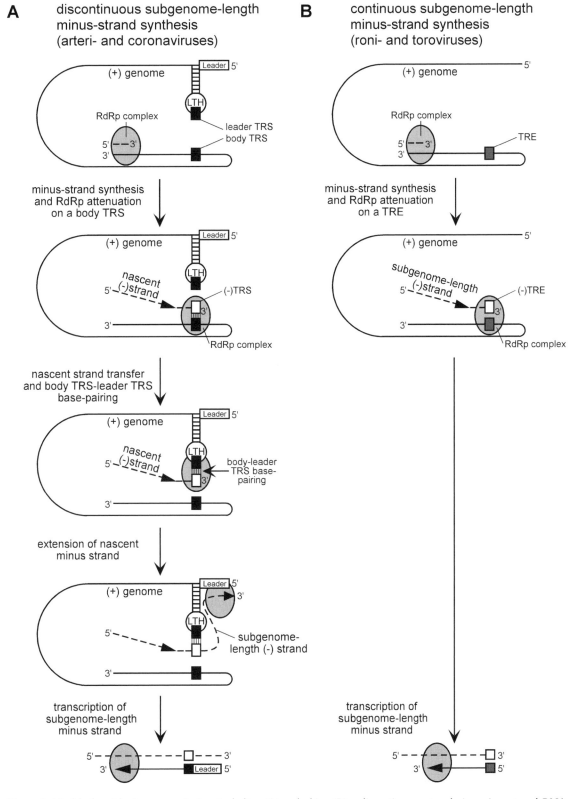

**Figure 5.** Models for nidovirus transcription, including (A) or lacking (B) a discontinuous step during minus-strand RNA synthesis. Plus- and minus-strand RNAs are represented by solid and dashed lines, respectively. See the text for details.

four torovirus sg mRNAs also involves a discontinuous step (see chapter 9 for details), but the other torovirus sg mRNAs and the ronivirus sg mRNAs do not carry a leader sequence that is derived from the 5′ end of the genome. Still, also in these viruses, conserved (presumably) regulatory sequences that correspond to body TRSs are found at the 5′ end of each of the genome segments that will be converted into an sg mRNA (see also chapters 9 and 25) (15, 121).

To avoid confusion, it should be noted that in most nidoviruses the "common leader" of the viral mRNAs is different from (but also part of) the translational leader (or 5′ UTR) of genome and sg mRNAs. The distance and sequence between the 3′ end of the common leader sequence and the translation initiation codon of the most 5′-proximal ORF are different in each of the sg mRNAs. Thus, in terms of translation, the leaders of mRNAs of nidoviruses that employ discontinuous RNA synthesis have different 3′ segments but share the same 5′ segment, which equals the transcriptional leader sequence.

Over the years, different models have been proposed to explain the discontinuous step in arteri-, corona-, and now also bafinivirus sgRNA synthesis (reviewed comprehensively in, e.g., references 64, 79, and 91). One of these, the discontinuous minus-strand extension model, originally proposed by Sawicki and Sawicki (89), has now gained considerable experimental support from both biochemical and genetic studies (90). This model postulates that the fusion of the sgRNA body to the common leader sequence occurs during minus-strand RNA synthesis. This process of discontinuous extension of nascent minus-strand RNAs is thought to yield subgenome-length minus-strand templates for sg mRNA production (Fig. 5A). Following "regular" initiation of minus-strand RNA synthesis at the 3′ end of the genome template, RNA synthesis is thought to be attenuated at one of the body TRSs to yield a minus-strand intermediate carrying the complement of a body TRS at its 3′ end. Guided by a base-pairing interaction with the leader TRS, the nascent minus strand is thought to be translocated to the 5′ end of the genome template. Subsequently, minus-strand synthesis is resumed to add the complement of the leader sequence ("antileader"), thus completing the subgenome-length minus-strand template. In a variant of this model, recently proposed for coronaviruses, a 5′-3′ interaction in the genomic template would promote the formation of a leader TRS-containing complex that may scan the nascent minus strand to identify the body TRS complement for base-pairing, whereafter the RdRp complex would switch to copy the leader sequence (103).

Since minus-strand RNA synthesis presumably terminates prior to strand transfer, the attenuation step in nidovirus discontinuous minus-strand extension is similar to that of the premature termination model of sgRNA synthesis mentioned above. Furthermore, in view of the crucial role of the base-pairing interaction between nascent RNA strand and "acceptor template," nidovirus discontinuous RNA synthesis mechanistically resembles similarity-assisted copy choice RNA recombination (9, 12, 80). As in the case of RNA recombination, the higher-order structure of the template (and possibly also of the nascent strand) may play an important role, in particular in the regions where the leader TRS and body TRSs reside. Many details of the mechanism that regulates the joining of sequences that are noncontiguous in the nidovirus genome remain to be elucidated.

## Attenuation of Minus-Strand RNA Synthesis

The proposed attenuation step during discontinuous sgRNA synthesis has been extensively studied using coronavirus DI RNA systems as well as full-length arteri- and coronavirus genomes. It was found that the most conserved part of the body TRS (or core TRS), without its flanking sequences, was sufficient to direct sgRNA synthesis when introduced into the 3′-proximal third of an MHV DI RNA (35), although the amount of sg mRNA produced from a core body TRS was larger when the entire 18-nt sgRNA7 TRS was introduced (60). Deletions or mutations within the body TRS influenced sg mRNA synthesis dramatically (43, 61, 114). Additional factors or structural elements must contribute to attenuation, because nidovirus genome sequences can contain multiple TRS-like sequences that are apparently not recognized as body TRSs (21, 43, 61, 77). This notion was highlighted by the finding, in several independent cases, that a body TRS is not even necessary for sgRNA production. Leader-to-body joining can occur either randomly, but with a low efficiency, within a defined region on the genome, generating multiple species of sg mRNA (25, 131), or at unique sequences that differ from the consensus TRS (20, 32, 135). Thus, the consensus body TRS is important, but it does not seem to be an absolute prerequisite for leader-to-body joining. The first evidence for a role of flanking sequences came from studies in which a body TRS was inserted at different locations in a coronavirus DI RNA replicon. This resulted in different levels of sgRNA synthesis from the DI RNA genome, which were determined by the flanking sequences and not by the location of this TRS in the DI RNA (39). Since then, the repressing or enhancing effect of downstream or upstream sequences was demonstrated or suggested in several studies (2, 3, 16, 75, 103, 119).

In general, the smallest sg mRNAs of nidoviruses are more abundant than the larger sg mRNAs, which could simply be explained (at least in part) by the fact that smaller RNA molecules can be amplified at a higher rate. However, there are clear indications that this polar effect is determined prior to subgenomic plus-strand synthesis, i.e., at the level of subgenome-length minus-strand RNA production. Downstream body TRSs have a negative effect on transcription levels from upstream body TRSs (19, 35, 44, 78, 119). In the model for discontinuous minus-strand extension, the number of transcription complexes reaching upstream body TRSs is obviously determined by the number of attenuation events occurring at downstream body TRSs. So, what determines RdRp stalling? It has been argued that the accessibility of the body TRS itself determines or influences attenuation. However, the general activity of a body TRS appears to be unrelated to the question of whether the TRS is part of a base-paired region or is present in an open conformation. Mutagenesis studies designed to open or close body TRS regions did not influence their activity (75–77). Other studies have proposed a role of (upstream) attenuating structures that may stall the RdRp when it encounters a body TRS (16).

Previously, a model was proposed to explain the termination of subgenomic minus-strand synthesis of red clover necrotic mosaic virus (99). It was demonstrated that a hairpin structure in the transactivator element of RNA1 base-paired with a region within the subgenomic promoter in RNA2, thereby physically blocking the progressing RdRp involved in RNA2 minus-strand synthesis. When in close proximity to a body TRS, the nidovirus leader TRS may be involved in a similar interaction to terminate or attenuate subgenome-length minus-strand synthesis. Such a long-distance RNA-RNA interaction is reminiscent of the "RNA network" identified in tombusviruses, which is involved in premature termination of minus-strand RNA synthesis to produce the template for sg mRNA production (54). However, in the case of arteriviruses and coronaviruses, a direct RNA-RNA interaction between the genomic leader TRS and body TRSs in the 3′-proximal part of the genome is not possible, since these sequences are identical and not complementary. Interacting proteins or additional regulatory RNA elements may therefore replace this type of interaction (see below).

## Strand Transfer and Completion of the Subgenome-Length Minus-Strand Template

How the attenuated nascent minus-strand intermediate of arteri- and coronaviruses would be transferred from the body TRS to the leader TRS is unknown. Circularization of the genome, or some kind of other higher-order structural feature, may bring leader TRS and body TRS in close proximity, an event that could be promoted by protein factors (48). Base-pairing between the leader TRS and a body TRS complement is an essential step during sgRNA synthesis, and the type and position of TRS nucleotides influence the efficiency of this process (43, 80, 118). In general, the relative amount of sg mRNA correlates with the calculated stability of the corresponding leader TRS-body TRS duplex (81, 136). In the past, experiments designed to unravel the function of the coronavirus leader in sgRNA synthesis were hampered by recombination between the helper virus RNA and the DI RNA replicons used for these studies. Nevertheless, deletion analysis of the leader region showed that at least the leader TRS and both its flanking sequences are required for the efficient generation of sg mRNAs (53, 56, 123, 133, 134). Subsequently, it was shown that both the arterivirus and coronavirus leader TRSs may be located in a hairpin structure (Fig. 6) (12, 110, 118). The existence of an arterivirus (EAV) leader TRS hairpin (LTH) was firmly supported by various lines of experimental evidence. The arterivirus LTH is thought to play an important role in sgRNA synthesis by acting as a platform that facilitates the leader TRS-body TRS interaction (Fig. 5A) (110, 111). For coronaviruses, the prediction of an LTH may depend on the approach used (45), and therefore it remains to be established whether the functional similarity between arteri- and coronaviruses indeed extends to this structural element near the 5′ end of the genome.

Following sense-antisense TRS base pairing, minus-strand synthesis must resume to complete the subgenome-length minus strand by adding the complement of the genomic leader sequence. Several studies support the model that the subgenome-length minus strands subsequently serve as templates for the synthesis of the positive-strand sgRNAs (6, 87, 88), although this finding was not confirmed in a few other studies (e.g., see reference 70). Opposite to what was originally proposed after the discovery of the subgenome-length minus strands (94), sgRNAs themselves appear to be unable to function as replicons, presumably because they cannot act as templates for minus-strand synthesis. This was concluded from experiments demonstrating that a synthetic sg mRNA7 (with a natural 65-nt leader) that was transfected into BCoV-infected cells did not replicate, whereas the same construct with the 5′-terminal replication signals of 498 nt (Table 1) could be amplified (11). The latter result showed that some RNA signals that are essential for genome replication are lacking

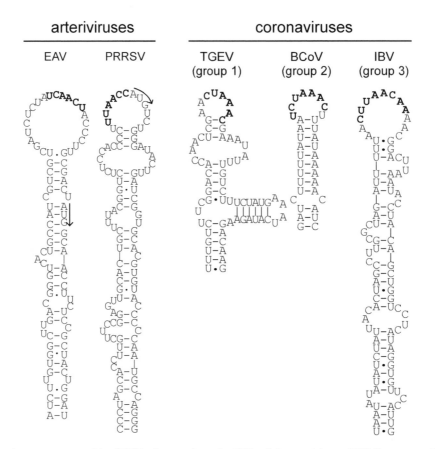

**Figure 6.** Secondary-structure models of LTHs. Presented are the LTHs of the arteriviruses EAV (Bucyrus strain) and PRRSV (VR-2332 strain), adapted from reference 111. The LTH of a representative of each of the three coronavirus subgroups is shown: TGEV (Purdue strain), BCoV (Quebec strain), and IBV (Beaudette strain), adapted from reference 110. The core sequence of the leader TRS is indicated in bold. The arterivirus replicase translation initiation codon is marked with an arrow.

in sg mRNAs, a finding that can probably be extended to the arterivirus system too (109–111). This would provide the genome with the exclusive possibility of being amplified through its antigenome intermediate, whereas sg mRNA production would depend on (and be determined at the level of) discontinuous subgenome-length minus-strand RNA synthesis.

### Protein Factors Involved in Transcription

In addition to RNA elements, other factors are likely involved in regulation of discontinuous sgRNA synthesis, such as proteins of cellular or viral origin. Three replicase proteins of EAV, nsp1, nsp10, and nsp11, have been implicated, to a variable degree, in arterivirus transcription (82, 109, 117, 120). Also, cellular factors may be involved in the generation of sg mRNAs. The consensus binding site of a cellular protein, hnRNP A1, is similar to the complement of the MHV TRS. A correlation was found between hnRNP A1 binding and sgRNA synthesis when body

TRS7 was mutated (27, 52, 132). Although this may indicate that hnRNP A1 regulates sgRNA synthesis, this role became less clear when the absence of the protein from infected cells was found not to affect MHV replication (95). Another cellular protein, PTB (also known as hnRNP I), was found to interact with the MHV leader TRS, and it was proposed that this interaction could regulate sgRNA synthesis (14, 27, 51). There are some indications that PTB can influence sgRNA synthesis by inducing a conformational change of a structure located in the complementary strand of the genomic 3′ UTR (36). However, the authors did not evaluate the effect of the PTB interaction on DI RNA replication.

### Nidovirus Transcription without Discontinuous RNA Synthesis: Toroviruses and Roniviruses

In contrast to arteri- and coronaviruses, viruses belonging to the genera *Ronivirus* and *Torovirus* produce sg mRNAs lacking a common leader sequence, with the exception of the largest sg mRNA (encoding the spike protein) of toroviruses (15, 101, 102, 121). Conserved transcription-regulating elements (TREs; see chapter 9) were identified preceding each ORF downstream of the roni- and torovirus replicase gene (15, 102, 121). It has been shown that the torovirus TREs are essential and sufficient to drive sg mRNA synthesis (100). Most likely, they play a dual role, with the sense version acting as a terminator of minus-strand RNA synthesis and its complement located at the 3′ end of the subgenome-length minus-strand template being an initiation signal for sg mRNA synthesis (Fig. 5B). The toro- and ronivirus TREs do not function as donor sites for similarity-assisted template switching, as was proposed for the arteri- and coronavirus body TRSs. The mechanism for sgRNA synthesis used by roni- and toroviruses appears to be similar to that of the closteroviruses, a family of plus-strand RNA viruses of plants that also has a polycistronic genome and produces an extensive set of 3′-coterminal sg mRNAs (4).

A TRE does not precede the torovirus spike protein gene, which is expressed from the single sg mRNA that appears to be produced via discontinuous synthesis of a subgenome-length minus-strand template. Notably, a hairpin structure just upstream of the crossover site, which appears to be conserved among toroviruses, was postulated to direct or promote the template switch. The combination of this hairpin and sequence identity between the region just downstream of it and a domain in the genomic 5′-proximal region are thought to form a crossover hot spot for discontinuous minus-strand RNA synthesis. Thus, toroviruses have been proposed to combine two different transcription strategies, discontinuous and continuous minus-strand RNA synthesis, placing them in an intermediate and interesting position in the evolution of nidovirus transcription (121).

### Recombination

Frequent homologous RNA recombination is a remarkable feature of coronaviruses and likely also other nidoviruses (for a review, see reference 50). Its occurrence has often been linked to genome size and the unique nidovirus transcription mechanism. Recombination is an evolutionary mechanism that may also account for the diversity in the genomic structure of nidoviruses (see also chapter 2). By using temperature-sensitive mutants for recombination assays, the recombination frequency for the entire MHV genome was estimated to be approximately 25% during one replication cycle (26). This high frequency was exploited in the development of a targeted recombination approach that enables the

introduction of specific mutations in the large coronavirus genome and has become an important tool for studying several aspects of coronavirus replication (66).

Coronaviruses exhibit the phenomenon of leader switching, which is presumably based on frequent RdRp template switching occurring near the 5′ end of the genome (12, 62, 106). In cells simultaneously infected with two different MHV strains, up to half of the mRNAs may carry a leader sequence from the coinfecting strain (63). Coronavirus and arterivirus RdRps may be especially prone to switch templates, since the synthesis of their subgenome-length minus-strand RNAs requires a template switch (79). It is unknown whether this mechanism is restricted to be exclusively intramolecular or may also occur in an intermolecular fashion using different donor and acceptor templates (127). It has been reported that recombination in both virus groups occurs more frequently near the 3′ end of the genome (26, 71), suggesting that body TRSs may promote recombination, which may thus in part be driven by factors and/or signals similar to those involved in transcription.

### CONCLUDING REMARKS

Despite almost three decades of research into the molecular details of nidovirus RNA synthesis, and despite the recent contributions of SARS-CoV-inspired research, many mechanistic details of nidovirus replication and transcription remain to be unraveled. The enzymatic activity of several replicase subunits has recently been demonstrated and a detailed picture of the RNA landscape of the genome is slowly emerging. On the other hand, little is known about the interplay between the identified RNA elements and nidoviral and host proteins. Reverse-genetics systems have significantly facilitated the functional dissection of RNA elements and proteins involved in nidovirus RNA synthesis, and will certainly continue to do so in the near future. However, reverse-genetics systems have their clear limitations, because intermediate steps in RNA synthesis are difficult to pinpoint and analyze. Consequently, for the systematic dissection of the mechanistic details of nidovirus RNA synthesis, the development of in vitro systems faithfully reproducing the various steps in RNA synthesis seems essential and inevitable.

**Acknowledgments.** For pleasant contacts and collaborations, and helpful discussions through the years, we thank our past and present colleagues at the Leiden University Medical Center, and many colleagues from the nidovirus field, in particular, Stanley Sawicki, Dorothea Sawicki, and Stuart Siddell.

This work was supported in part by a grant from the Council for Chemical Sciences of the Netherlands Organization for Scientific Research (NWO-CW grant 99-010).

## REFERENCES

1. **Almazan, F., C. Galan, and L. Enjuanes.** 2004. The nucleoprotein is required for efficient coronavirus genome replication. *J. Virol.* **78:**12683–12688.
2. **Alonso, S., A. Izeta, I. Sola, and L. Enjuanes.** 2002. Transcription regulatory sequences and mRNA expression levels in the coronavirus transmissible gastroenteritis virus. *J. Virol.* **76:**1293–1308.
3. **An, S. W., and S. Makino.** 1998. Characterizations of coronavirus cis-acting RNA elements and the transcription step affecting its transcription efficiency. *Virology* **243:**198–207.
4. **Ayllon, M. A., S. Gowda, T. Satyanarayana, and W. O. Dawson.** 2004. Cis-acting elements at opposite ends of the Citrus tristeza virus genome differ in initiation and termination of subgenomic RNAs. *Virology* **322:**41–50.
5. **Baric, R. S., S. A. Stohlman, and M. M. Lai.** 1983. Characterization of replicative intermediate RNA of mouse hepatitis virus: presence of leader RNA sequences on nascent chains. *J. Virol.* **48:**633–640.
6. **Baric, R. S., and B. Yount.** 2000. Subgenomic negative-strand RNA function during mouse hepatitis virus infection. *J. Virol.* **74:**4039–4046.
7. **Beerens, N., and E. J. Snijder.** 2006. RNA signals in the 3' terminus of the genome of Equine arteritis virus are required for viral RNA synthesis. *J. Gen. Virol.* **87:**1977–1983.
8. **Brian, D. A., and R. S. Baric.** 2005. Coronavirus genome structure and replication. *Curr. Top. Microbiol. Immunol.* **287:**1–30.
9. **Brian, D. A., and W. J. M. Spaan.** 1997. Recombination and coronavirus defective interfering RNAs. *Semin. Virol.* **8:**101–111.
10. **Casais, R., V. Thiel, S. G. Siddell, D. Cavanagh, and P. Britton.** 2001. Reverse genetics system for the avian coronavirus infectious bronchitis virus. *J. Virol.* **75:**12359–12369.
11. **Chang, R. Y., M. A. Hofmann, P. B. Sethna, and D. A. Brian.** 1994. A *cis*-acting function for the coronavirus leader in defective interfering RNA replication. *J. Virol.* **68:**8223–8231.
12. **Chang, R. Y., R. Krishnan, and D. A. Brian.** 1996. The UCUAAAC promoter motif is not required for high-frequency leader recombination in bovine coronavirus defective interfering RNA. *J. Virol.* **70:**2720–2729.
13. **Chen, H., A. Gill, B. K. Dove, S. R. Emmett, C. F. Kemp, M. A. Ritchie, M. Dee, and J. A. Hiscox.** 2005. Mass spectroscopic characterization of the coronavirus infectious bronchitis virus nucleoprotein and elucidation of the role of phosphorylation in RNA binding by using surface plasmon resonance. *J. Virol.* **79:**1164–1179.
14. **Choi, K. S., P. Huang, and M. M. Lai.** 2002. Polypyrimidine-tract-binding protein affects transcription but not translation of mouse hepatitis virus RNA. *Virology* **303:**58–68.
15. **Cowley, J. A., C. M. Dimmock, and P. J. Walker.** 2002. Gill-associated nidovirus of Penaeus monodon prawns transcribes 3'-coterminal subgenomic mRNAs that do not possess 5'-leader sequences. *J. Gen. Virol.* **83:**927–935.
16. **Curtis, K. M., B. Yount, A. C. Sims, and R. S. Baric.** 2004. Reverse genetic analysis of the transcription regulatory sequence of the coronavirus transmissible gastroenteritis virus. *J. Virol.* **78:**6061–6066.
17. **Dalton, K., R. Casais, K. Shaw, K. Stirrups, S. Evans, P. Britton, T. D. Brown, and D. Cavanagh.** 2001. *cis*-Acting sequences required for coronavirus infectious bronchitis virus defective-RNA replication and packaging. *J. Virol.* **75:**125–133.
18. **de Groot, R. J., R. G. van der Most, and W. J. M. Spaan.** 1992. The fitness of defective interfering murine coronavirus DI-a and its derivatives is decreased by nonsense and frameshift mutations. *J. Virol.* **66:**5898–5905.
19. **de Haan, C. A. M., H. Volders, C. A. Koetzner, P. S. Masters, and P. J. M. Rottier.** 2002. Coronaviruses maintain viability despite dramatic rearrangements of the strictly conserved genome organization. *J. Virol.* **76:**12491–12502.
20. **den Boon, J. A., M. F. Kleijnen, W. J. M. Spaan, and E. J. Snijder.** 1996. Equine arteritis virus subgenomic mRNA synthesis: analysis of leader-body junctions and replicative-form RNAs. *J. Virol.* **70:**4291–4298.
21. **den Boon, J. A., E. J. Snijder, E. D. Chirnside, A. A. de Vries, M. C. Horzinek, and W. J. M. Spaan.** 1991. Equine arteritis virus is not a togavirus but belongs to the coronaviruslike superfamily. *J. Virol.* **65:**2910–2920.
22. **de Vries, A. A., E. D. Chirnside, P. J. Bredenbeek, L. A. Gravestein, M. C. Horzinek, and W. J. M. Spaan.** 1990. All subgenomic mRNAs of equine arteritis virus contain a common leader sequence. *Nucleic Acids Res.* **18:**3241–3247.
23. **Dye, C., and S. G. Siddell.** 2005. Genomic RNA sequence of Feline coronavirus strain FIPV WSU-79/1146. *J. Gen. Virol.* **86:**2249–2253.
24. **Escors, D., A. Izeta, C. Capiscol, and L. Enjuanes.** 2003. Transmissible gastroenteritis coronavirus packaging signal is located at the 5' end of the virus genome. *J. Virol.* **77:**7890–7902.
25. **Fischer, F., C. F. Stegen, C. A. Koetzner, and P. S. Masters.** 1997. Analysis of a recombinant mouse hepatitis virus expressing a foreign gene reveals a novel aspect of coronavirus transcription. *J. Virol.* **71:**5148–5160.
26. **Fu, K., and R. S. Baric.** 1994. Map locations of mouse hepatitis virus temperature-sensitive mutants: confirmation of variable rates of recombination. *J. Virol.* **68:**7458–7466.
27. **Furuya, T., and M. M. Lai.** 1993. Three different cellular proteins bind to complementary sites on the 5'-end-positive and 3'-end-negative strands of mouse hepatitis virus RNA. *J. Virol.* **67:**7215–7222.
28. **Goebel, S. J., B. Hsue, T. F. Dombrowski, and P. S. Masters.** 2004. Characterization of the RNA components of a putative molecular switch in the 3' untranslated region of the murine coronavirus genome. *J. Virol.* **78:**669–682.
29. **Goebel, S. J., T. B. Miller, C. J. Bennett, K. A. Bernard, and P. S. Masters.** 2006. A hypervariable region within the 3' cis-acting element of the murine coronavirus genome is nonessential for RNA synthesis but affects pathogenesis. *J. Virol.* **81:**1274–1287.
30. **Goebel, S. J., J. Taylor, and P. S. Masters.** 2004. The 3' cis-acting genomic replication element of the severe acute respiratory syndrome coronavirus can function in the murine coronavirus genome. *J. Virol.* **78:**7846–7851.
31. **Gorbalenya, A. E., E. J. Snijder, and W. J. M. Spaan.** 2004. Severe acute respiratory syndrome coronavirus phylogeny: toward consensus. *J. Virol.* **78:**7863–7866.
32. **Hofmann, M. A., R. Y. Chang, S. Ku, and D. A. Brian.** 1993. Leader–mRNA junction sequences are unique for each subgenomic mRNA species in the bovine coronavirus and remain so throughout persistent infection. *Virology* **196:**163–171.
33. **Hsue, B., T. Hartshorne, and P. S. Masters.** 2000. Characterization of an essential RNA secondary structure in the 3' untranslated region of the murine coronavirus genome. *J. Virol.* **74:**6911–6921.
34. **Hsue, B., and P. S. Masters.** 1997. A bulged stem-loop structure in the 3' untranslated region of the genome of the

coronavirus mouse hepatitis virus is essential for replication. *J. Virol.* **71:**7567–7578.

35. **Hsue, B., and P. S. Masters.** 1999. Insertion of a new transcriptional unit into the genome of mouse hepatitis virus. *J. Virol.* **73:**6128–6135.

36. **Huang, P., and M. M. Lai.** 1999. Polypyrimidine tract-binding protein binds to the complementary strand of the mouse hepatitis virus 3′ untranslated region, thereby altering RNA conformation. *J. Virol.* **73:**9110–9116.

37. **Huang, P., and M. M. Lai.** 2001. Heterogeneous nuclear ribonucleoprotein a1 binds to the 3′-untranslated region and mediates potential 5′-3′-end cross talks of mouse hepatitis virus RNA. *J. Virol.* **75:**5009–5017.

38. **Izeta, A., C. Smerdou, S. Alonso, Z. Penzes, A. Mendez, J. Plana-Duran, and L. Enjuanes.** 1999. Replication and packaging of transmissible gastroenteritis coronavirus-derived synthetic minigenomes. *J. Virol.* **73:**1535–1545.

39. **Jeong, Y. S., J. F. Repass, Y. N. Kim, S. M. Hwang, and S. Makino.** 1996. Coronavirus transcription mediated by sequences flanking the transcription consensus sequence. *Virology* **217:**311–322.

40. **Johnson, R. F., M. Feng, P. Liu, J. J. Millership, B. Yount, R. S. Baric, and J. L. Leibowitz.** 2005. Effect of mutations in the mouse hepatitis virus 3′(+)42 protein binding element on RNA replication. *J. Virol.* **79:**14570–14585.

41. **Jonassen, C. M., T. O. Jonassen, and B. Grinde.** 1998. A common RNA motif in the 3′ end of the genomes of astroviruses, avian infectious bronchitis virus and an equine rhinovirus. *J. Gen. Virol.* **79:**715–718.

42. **Jonassen, C. M., T. Kofstad, I. L. Larsen, A. Lovland, K. Handeland, A. Follestad, and A. Lillehaug.** 2005. Molecular identification and characterization of novel coronaviruses infecting graylag geese (Anser anser), feral pigeons (Columbia livia) and mallards (Anas platyrhynchos). *J. Gen. Virol.* **86:**1597–1607.

43. **Joo, M., and S. Makino.** 1992. Mutagenic analysis of the coronavirus intergenic consensus sequence. *J. Virol.* **66:**6330–6337.

44. **Joo, M., and S. Makino.** 1995. The effect of two closely inserted transcription consensus sequences on coronavirus transcription. *J. Virol.* **69:**272–280.

45. **Kang, H., M. Feng, M. E. Schroeder, D. P. Giedroc, and J. L. Leibowitz.** 2006. Putative *cis*-acting stem-loops in the 5′ untranslated region of the severe acute respiratory syndrome coronavirus can substitute for their mouse hepatitis virus counterparts. *J. Virol.* **80:**10600–10614.

46. **Kim, Y. N., Y. S. Jeong, and S. Makino.** 1993. Analysis of cis-acting sequences essential for coronavirus defective interfering RNA replication. *Virology* **197:**53–63.

47. **Kim, Y. N., and S. Makino.** 1995. Characterization of a murine coronavirus defective interfering RNA internal *cis*-acting replication signal. *J. Virol.* **69:**4963–4971.

48. **Lai, M. M.** 1998. Cellular factors in the transcription and replication of viral RNA genomes: a parallel to DNA-dependent RNA transcription. *Virology* **244:**1–12.

49. **Lai, M. M., R. S. Baric, P. R. Brayton, and S. A. Stohlman.** 1984. Characterization of leader RNA sequences on the virion and mRNAs of mouse hepatitis virus, a cytoplasmic RNA virus. *Proc. Natl. Acad. Sci. USA* **81:**3626–3630.

50. **Lai, M. M. C.** 1996. Recombination in large RNA viruses: coronaviruses. *Semin. Virol.* **7:**381–388.

51. **Li, H. P., P. Huang, S. Park, and M. M. Lai.** 1999. Polypyrimidine tract-binding protein binds to the leader RNA of mouse hepatitis virus and serves as a regulator of viral transcription. *J. Virol.* **73:**772–777.

52. **Li, H. P., X. Zhang, R. Duncan, L. Comai, and M. M. Lai.** 1997. Heterogeneous nuclear ribonucleoprotein A1 binds to the transcription-regulatory region of mouse hepatitis virus RNA. *Proc. Natl. Acad. Sci. USA* **94:**9544–9549.

53. **Liao, C. L., and M. M. Lai.** 1994. Requirement of the 5′-end genomic sequence as an upstream *cis*-acting element for coronavirus subgenomic mRNA transcription. *J. Virol.* **68:**4727–4737.

54. **Lin, H. X., and K. A. White.** 2004. A complex network of RNA-RNA interactions controls subgenomic mRNA transcription in a tombusvirus. *EMBO J.* **23:**3365–3374.

55. **Lin, Y. J., and M. M. Lai.** 1993. Deletion mapping of a mouse hepatitis virus defective interfering RNA reveals the requirement of an internal and discontiguous sequence for replication. *J. Virol.* **67:**6110–6118.

56. **Lin, Y. J., C. L. Liao, and M. M. Lai.** 1994. Identification of the *cis*-acting signal for minus-strand RNA synthesis of a murine coronavirus: implications for the role of minus-strand RNA in RNA replication and transcription. *J. Virol.* **68:**8131–8140.

57. **Liu, Q., R. F. Johnson, and J. L. Leibowitz.** 2001. Secondary structural elements within the 3′ untranslated region of mouse hepatitis virus strain JHM genomic RNA. *J. Virol.* **75:**12105–12113.

58. **Liu, Q., W. Yu, and J. L. Leibowitz.** 1997. A specific host cellular protein binding element near the 3′ end of mouse hepatitis virus genomic RNA. *Virology* **232:**74–85.

59. **Luytjes, W., H. Gerritsma, and W. J. M. Spaan.** 1996. Replication of synthetic defective interfering RNAs derived from coronavirus mouse hepatitis virus-A59. *Virology* **216:**174–183.

60. **Makino, S., and M. Joo.** 1993. Effect of intergenic consensus sequence flanking sequences on coronavirus transcription. *J. Virol.* **67:**3304–3311.

61. **Makino, S., M. Joo, and J. K. Makino.** 1991. A system for study of coronavirus mRNA synthesis: a regulated, expressed subgenomic defective interfering RNA results from intergenic site insertion. *J. Virol.* **65:**6031–6041.

62. **Makino, S., and M. M. Lai.** 1989. High-frequency leader sequence switching during coronavirus defective interfering RNA replication. *J. Virol.* **63:**5285–5292.

63. **Makino, S., S. A. Stohlman, and M. M. Lai.** 1986. Leader sequences of murine coronavirus mRNAs can be freely reassorted: evidence for the role of free leader RNA in transcription. *Proc. Natl. Acad. Sci. USA* **83:**4204–4208.

64. **Masters, P. S.** 2006. The molecular biology of coronaviruses. *Adv. Virus Res.* **66:**193–292.

65. **Masters, P. S., C. A. Koetzner, C. A. Kerr, and Y. Heo.** 1994. Optimization of targeted RNA recombination and mapping of a novel nucleocapsid gene mutation in the coronavirus mouse hepatitis virus. *J. Virol.* **68:**328–337.

66. **Masters, P. S., and P. J. Rottier.** 2005. Coronavirus reverse genetics by targeted RNA recombination. *Curr. Top. Microbiol. Immunol.* **287:**133–159.

67. **Meulenberg, J. J. M., J. N. A. Bos-De Ruijter, R. van de Graaf, G. Wensvoort, and R. J. M. Moormann.** 1998. Infectious transcripts from cloned genome-length cDNA of porcine reproductive and respiratory syndrome virus. *J. Virol.* **72:**380–387.

68. **Miller, W. A., T. W. Dreher, and T. C. Hall.** 1985. Synthesis of brome mosaic virus subgenomic RNA in vitro by internal initiation on (−)-sense genomic RNA. *Nature* **313:**68–70.

69. **Miller, W. A., and G. Koev.** 2000. Synthesis of subgenomic RNAs by positive-strand RNA viruses. *Virology* **273:**1–8.

70. **Mizutani, T., J. F. Repass, and S. Makino.** 2000. Nascent synthesis of leader sequence-containing subgenomic mRNAs in

coronavirus genome-length replicative intermediate RNA. *Virology* **275**:238–243.

71. Molenkamp, R., S. Greve, W. J. M. Spaan, and E. J. Snijder. 2000. Efficient homologous RNA recombination and requirement for an open reading frame during replication of equine arteritis virus defective interfering RNAs. *J. Virol.* **74**:9062–9070.

72. Molenkamp, R., B. C. Rozier, S. Greve, W. J. M. Spaan, and E. J. Snijder. 2000. Isolation and characterization of an arterivirus defective interfering RNA genome. *J. Virol.* **74**:3156–3165.

73. Molenkamp, R., H. van Tol, B. C. Rozier, Y. van der Meer, W. J. M. Spaan, and E. J. Snijder. 2000. The arterivirus replicase is the only viral protein required for genome replication and subgenomic mRNA transcription. *J. Gen. Virol.* **81**:2491–2496.

74. Nelson, G. W., S. A. Stohlman, and S. M. Tahara. 2000. High affinity interaction between nucleocapsid protein and leader/intergenic sequence of mouse hepatitis virus RNA. *J. Gen. Virol.* **81**:181–188.

75. Ozdarendeli, A., S. Ku, S. Rochat, G. D. Williams, S. D. Senanayake, and D. A. Brian. 2001. Downstream sequences influence the choice between a naturally occurring noncanonical and closely positioned upstream canonical heptameric fusion motif during bovine coronavirus subgenomic mRNA synthesis. *J. Virol.* **75**:7362–7374.

76. Pasternak, A. O. 2003. *Nidovirus Transcription-Regulating Sequences*. Ph.D. thesis. Leiden University, Leiden, The Netherlands.

77. Pasternak, A. O., A. P. Gultyaev, W. J. M. Spaan, and E. J. Snijder. 2000. Genetic manipulation of arterivirus alternative mRNA leader-body junction sites reveals tight regulation of structural protein expression. *J. Virol.* **74**:11642–11653.

78. Pasternak, A. O., W. J. M. Spaan, and E. J. Snijder. 2004. Regulation of relative abundance of arterivirus subgenomic mRNAs. *J. Virol.* **78**:8102–8113.

79. Pasternak, A. O., W. J. M. Spaan, and E. J. Snijder. 2006. Nidovirus transcription: how to make sense . . . ? *J. Gen. Virol.* **87**:1403–1421.

80. Pasternak, A. O., E. van den Born, W. J. M. Spaan, and E. J. Snijder. 2001. Sequence requirements for RNA strand transfer during nidovirus discontinuous subgenomic RNA synthesis. *EMBO J.* **20**:7220–7228.

81. Pasternak, A. O., E. van den Born, W. J. M. Spaan, and E. J. Snijder. 2003. The stability of the duplex between sense and antisense transcription-regulating sequences is a crucial factor in arterivirus subgenomic mRNA synthesis. *J. Virol.* **77**:1175–1183.

82. Posthuma, C. C., D. D. Nedialkova, J. C. Zevenhoven-Dobbe, J. H. Blokhuis, A. E. Gorbalenya, and E. J. Snijder. 2006. Site-directed mutagenesis of the nidovirus replicative endoribonuclease NendoU exerts pleiotropic effects on the arterivirus life cycle. *J. Virol.* **80**:1653–1661.

83. Raman, S., P. Bouma, G. D. Williams, and D. A. Brian. 2003. Stem-loop III in the 5′ untranslated region is a *cis*-acting element in bovine coronavirus defective interfering RNA replication. *J. Virol.* **77**:6720–6730.

84. Raman, S., and D. A. Brian. 2005. Stem-loop IV in the 5′ untranslated region is a *cis*-acting element in bovine coronavirus defective interfering RNA replication. *J. Virol.* **79**:12434–12446.

85. Repass, J. F., and S. Makino. 1998. Importance of the positive-strand RNA secondary structure of a murine coronavirus defective interfering RNA internal replication signal in positive-strand RNA synthesis. *J. Virol.* **72**:7926–7933.

86. Robertson, M. P., H. Igel, R. Baertsch, D. Haussler, M. Ares, Jr., and W. G. Scott. 2005. The structure of a rigorously conserved RNA element within the SARS virus genome. *PLoS Biol.* **3**:e5.

87. Sawicki, D., T. Wang, and S. Sawicki. 2001. The RNA structures engaged in replication and transcription of the A59 strain of mouse hepatitis virus. *J. Gen. Virol.* **82**:385–396.

88. Sawicki, S. G., and D. L. Sawicki. 1990. Coronavirus transcription: subgenomic mouse hepatitis virus replicative intermediates function in RNA synthesis. *J. Virol.* **64**:1050–1056.

89. Sawicki, S. G., and D. L. Sawicki. 1995. Coronaviruses use discontinuous extension for synthesis of subgenome-length negative strands. *Adv. Exp. Med. Biol.* **380**:499–506.

90. Sawicki, S. G., and D. L. Sawicki. 2005. Coronavirus transcription: a perspective. *Curr. Top. Microbiol. Immunol.* **287**:31–55.

91. Sawicki, S. G., D. L. Sawicki, and S. G. Siddell. 2007. A contemporary view of coronavirus transcription. *J. Virol.* **81**:20–29.

92. Schelle, B., N. Karl, B. Ludewig, S. G. Siddell, and V. Thiel. 2005. Selective replication of coronavirus genomes that express nucleocapsid protein. *J. Virol.* **79**:6620–6630.

93. Schutze, H., R. Ulferts, B. Schelle, S. Bayer, H. Granzow, B. Hoffmann, T. C. Mettenleiter, and J. Ziebuhr. 2006. Characterization of white bream virus reveals a novel genetic cluster of nidoviruses. *J. Virol.* **80**:11598–11609.

94. Sethna, P. B., S. L. Hung, and D. A. Brian. 1989. Coronavirus subgenomic minus-strand RNAs and the potential for mRNA replicons. *Proc. Natl. Acad. Sci. USA* **86**:5626–5630.

95. Shen, X., and P. S. Masters. 2001. Evaluation of the role of heterogeneous nuclear ribonucleoprotein A1 as a host factor in murine coronavirus discontinuous transcription and genome replication. *Proc. Natl. Acad. Sci. USA* **98**:2717–2722.

96. Shi, S. T., P. Huang, H. P. Li, and M. M. Lai. 2000. Heterogeneous nuclear ribonucleoprotein A1 regulates RNA synthesis of a cytoplasmic virus. *EMBO J.* **19**:4701–4711.

97. Shi, S. T., and M. M. Lai. 2005. Viral and cellular proteins involved in coronavirus replication. *Curr. Top. Microbiol. Immunol.* **287**:95–131.

98. Siddell, S. G., J. Ziebuhr, and E. J. Snijder. 2005. Coronaviruses, toroviruses, and arteriviruses, p. 823–856. *In* B. W. J. Mahy and V. ter Meulen (ed.), *Topley and Wilson's Microbiology and Microbial Infections*, 10th ed. *Virology*. Hodder Arnold, London, United Kingdom.

99. Sit, T. L., A. A. Vaewhongs, and S. A. Lommel. 1998. RNA-mediated trans-activation of transcription from a viral RNA. *Science* **281**:829–832.

100. Smits, S. L., A. L. W. van Vliet, K. Segeren, H. el Azzouzi, M. van Essen, and R. J. de Groot. 2005. Torovirus nondiscontinuous transcription: mutational analysis of a subgenomic mRNA promoter. *J. Virol.* **79**:8275–8281.

101. Snijder, E. J., J. A. den Boon, M. C. Horzinek, and W. J. M. Spaan. 1991. Characterization of defective interfering RNAs of Berne virus. *J. Gen. Virol.* **72**:1635–1643.

102. Snijder, E. J., M. C. Horzinek, and W. J. M. Spaan. 1990. A 3′-coterminal nested set of independently transcribed mRNAs is generated during Berne virus replication. *J. Virol.* **64**:331–338.

103. Sola, I., J. L. Moreno, S. Zuniga, S. Alonso, and L. Enjuanes. 2005. Role of nucleotides immediately flanking the transcription-regulating sequence core in coronavirus subgenomic mRNA synthesis. *J. Virol.* **79**:2506–2516.

104. Spaan, W. J. M., H. Delius, M. Skinner, J. Armstrong, P. Rottier, S. Smeekens, B. A. van der Zeijst, and S. G. Siddell. 1983. Coronavirus mRNA synthesis involves fusion of noncontiguous sequences. *EMBO J.* **2**:1839–1844.

105. Spagnolo, J. F., and B. G. Hogue. 2000. Host protein interactions with the 3′ end of bovine coronavirus RNA and the

requirement of the poly(A) tail for coronavirus defective genome replication. *J. Virol.* **74:**5053–5065.

106. **Stirrups, K., K. Shaw, S. Evans, K. Dalton, D. Cavanagh, and P. Britton.** 2000. Leader switching occurs during the rescue of defective RNAs by heterologous strains of the coronavirus infectious bronchitis virus. *J. Gen. Virol.* **81:**791–801.

107. **Thiel, V., J. Herold, B. Schelle, and S. G. Siddell.** 2001. Infectious RNA transcribed in vitro from a cDNA copy of the human coronavirus genome cloned in vaccinia virus. *J. Gen. Virol.* **82:**1273–1281.

108. **Thiel, V., J. Herold, B. Schelle, and S. G. Siddell.** 2001. Viral replicase gene products suffice for coronavirus discontinuous transcription. *J. Virol.* **75:**6676–6681.

109. **Tijms, M. A., L. C. van Dinten, A. E. Gorbalenya, and E. J. Snijder.** 2001. A zinc finger-containing papain-like protease couples subgenomic mRNA synthesis to genome translation in a positive-stranded RNA virus. *Proc. Natl. Acad. Sci. USA* **98:**1889–1894.

110. **van den Born, E., A. P. Gultyaev, and E. J. Snijder.** 2004. Secondary structure and function of the 5′-proximal region of the equine arteritis virus RNA genome. *RNA* **10:**424–437.

111. **van den Born, E., C. C. Posthuma, A. P. Gultyaev, and E. J. Snijder.** 2005. Discontinuous subgenomic RNA synthesis in arteriviruses is guided by an RNA hairpin structure located in the genomic leader region. *J. Virol.* **79:**6312–6324.

112. **van der Meer, Y., E. J. Snijder, J. C. Dobbe, S. Schleich, M. R. Denison, W. J. M. Spaan, and J. Krijnse Locker.** 1999. Localization of mouse hepatitis virus nonstructural proteins and RNA synthesis indicates a role for late endosomes in viral replication. *J. Virol.* **73:**7641–7657.

113. **van der Most, R. G., P. J. Bredenbeek, and W. J. M. Spaan.** 1991. A domain at the 3′ end of the polymerase gene is essential for encapsidation of coronavirus defective interfering RNAs. *J. Virol.* **65:**3219–3226.

114. **van der Most, R. G., R. J. de Groot, and W. J. M. Spaan.** 1994. Subgenomic RNA synthesis directed by a synthetic defective interfering RNA of mouse hepatitis virus: a study of coronavirus transcription initiation. *J. Virol.* **68:**3656–3666.

115. **van der Most, R. G., L. Heijnen, W. J. M. Spaan, and R. J. de Groot.** 1992. Homologous RNA recombination allows efficient introduction of site-specific mutations into the genome of coronavirus MHV-A59 via synthetic co-replicating RNAs. *Nucleic Acids Res.* **20:**3375–3381.

116. **van der Most, R. G., W. Luytjes, S. Rutjes, and W. J. M. Spaan.** 1995. Translation but not the encoded sequence is essential for the efficient propagation of the defective interfering RNAs of the coronavirus mouse hepatitis virus. *J. Virol.* **69:**3744–3751.

117. **van Dinten, L. C., J. A. den Boon, A. L. M. Wassenaar, W. J. M. Spaan, and E. J. Snijder.** 1997. An infectious arterivirus cDNA clone: identification of a replicase point mutation that abolishes discontinuous mRNA transcription. *Proc. Natl. Acad. Sci. USA* **94:**991–996.

118. **van Marle, G., J. C. Dobbe, A. P. Gultyaev, W. Luytjes, W. J. M. Spaan, and E. J. Snijder.** 1999. Arterivirus discontinuous mRNA transcription is guided by base pairing between sense and antisense transcription-regulating sequences. *Proc. Natl. Acad. Sci. USA* **96:**12056–12061.

119. **van Marle, G., W. Luytjes, R. G. van der Most, T. van der Straaten, and W. J. Spaan.** 1995. Regulation of coronavirus mRNA transcription. *J. Virol.* **69:**7851–7856.

120. **van Marle, G., L. C. van Dinten, W. J. M. Spaan, W. Luytjes, and E. J. Snijder.** 1999. Characterization of an equine arteritis

121. **van Vliet, A. L., S. L. Smits, P. J. Rottier, and R. J. de Groot.** 2002. Discontinuous and non-discontinuous subgenomic RNA transcription in a nidovirus. *EMBO J.* **21:**6571–6580.

122. **Verheije, M. H., R. C. L. Olsthoorn, M. V. Kroese, P. J. M. Rottier, and J. J. M. Meulenberg.** 2002. Kissing interaction between 3′ noncoding and coding sequences is essential for porcine arterivirus RNA replication. *J. Virol.* **76:**1521–1526.

123. **Wang, Y., and X. Zhang.** 2000. The leader RNA of coronavirus mouse hepatitis virus contains an enhancer-like element for subgenomic mRNA transcription. *J. Virol.* **74:**10571–10580.

124. **White, K. A.** 2002. The premature termination model: a possible third mechanism for subgenomic mRNA transcription in (+)-strand RNA viruses. *Virology* **304:**147–154.

125. **Williams, G. D., R. Y. Chang, and D. A. Brian.** 1995. Evidence for a pseudoknot in the 3′ untranslated region of the bovine coronavirus genome. *Adv. Exp. Med. Biol.* **380:**511–514.

126. **Williams, G. D., R. Y. Chang, and D. A. Brian.** 1999. A phylogenetically conserved hairpin-type 3′ untranslated region pseudoknot functions in coronavirus RNA replication. *J. Virol.* **73:**8349–8355.

127. **Wu, H. Y., and D. A. Brian.** 2007. 5′-Proximal hotspot for an inducible positive-to-negative-strand template switch by coronavirus RNA-dependent RNA polymerase. *J. Virol.* **81:**3206–3215.

128. **Wu, H. Y., J. S. Guy, D. Yoo, R. Vlasak, E. Urbach, and D. A. Brian.** 2003. Common RNA replication signals exist among group 2 coronaviruses: evidence for in vivo recombination between animal and human coronavirus molecules. *Virology* **315:**174–183.

129. **Yount, B., M. R. Denison, S. R. Weiss, and R. S. Baric.** 2002. Systematic assembly of a full-length infectious cDNA of mouse hepatitis virus strain A59. *J. Virol.* **76:**11065–11078.

130. **Yu, W., and J. L. Leibowitz.** 1995. A conserved motif at the 3′ end of mouse hepatitis virus genomic RNA required for host protein binding and viral RNA replication. *Virology* **214:**128–138.

131. **Zhang, X., and M. M. Lai.** 1994. Unusual heterogeneity of leader-mRNA fusion in a murine coronavirus: implications for the mechanism of RNA transcription and recombination. *J. Virol.* **68:**6626–6633.

132. **Zhang, X., and M. M. Lai.** 1995. Interactions between the cytoplasmic proteins and the intergenic (promoter) sequence of mouse hepatitis virus RNA: correlation with the amounts of subgenomic mRNA transcribed. *J. Virol.* **69:**1637–1644.

133. **Zhang, X., and M. M. Lai.** 1996. A 5′-proximal RNA sequence of murine coronavirus as a potential initiation site for genomic-length mRNA transcription. *J. Virol.* **70:**705–711.

134. **Zhang, X., C. L. Liao, and M. M. Lai.** 1994. Coronavirus leader RNA regulates and initiates subgenomic mRNA transcription both in *trans* and in *cis. J. Virol.* **68:**4738–4746.

135. **Zhang, X., and R. Liu.** 2000. Identification of a noncanonical signal for transcription of a novel subgenomic mRNA of mouse hepatitis virus: implication for the mechanism of coronavirus RNA transcription. *Virology* **278:**75–85.

136. **Zuniga, S., I. Sola, S. Alonso, and L. Enjuanes.** 2004. Sequence motifs involved in the regulation of discontinuous coronavirus subgenomic RNA synthesis. *J. Virol.* **78:**980–994.

*Nidoviruses*
Edited by S. Perlman, T. Gallagher, and E. J. Snijder
© 2008 ASM Press, Washington, DC

Chapter 9

# Molecular Biology and Evolution of Toroviruses

RAOUL J. DE GROOT

*Unknown, unkissed and lost that is unsought*
Geoffrey Chaucer

This chapter is affectionately dedicated to Marian C. Horzinek, former head of the Virology Division, Faculty of Veterinary Sciences, Utrecht University, Utrecht, The Netherlands, on the occasion of his 70th birthday.

Toroviruses were discovered in 1972, but in comparison to their more glamorous nidovirus cousins, the corona- and arteriviruses, they have received precious little attention. Yet the early studies in particular, though limited in number, provide a wealth of information. Here, these observations are combined with more recent findings, yielding a rough but intriguing picture of the molecular biology, life cycle, and evolution of this fascinating group of viruses. For further reading, the reader is referred to excellent previous reviews (32, 37, 43, 69, 71) as well as to chapter 24.

## DISCOVERY, TAXONOMY, AND EPIDEMIOLOGY

### Torovirology: the Early Years

In 1972, during routine diagnostic work at the Surgery Clinic in Berne, Switzerland, Franz Steck isolated by chance the first torovirus. The source was a rectal swab taken from a *Salmonella* Lille-infected diarrheic horse. Cytopathic in cultured equine cells, "Berne virus" (BEV) was not neutralized by any diagnostic antiserum tested. Moreover, virions purified from tissue culture supernatant from infected cells had an unusual morphology, comprising a mixture of enveloped rod-, kidney-, and disk-shaped particles (76). Although in hindsight,

these observations would already have called for an immediate follow-up, further analysis was not pursued until after 1979, when Gerald Woode and coworkers identified another unclassified kidney-shaped virus as the etiological agent of severe neonatal gastroenteritis in cattle. The virus was named after the township where the initial outbreak occurred: Breda, Iowa (78). Marian Horzinek—at that time the head of the Virology Division of the Faculty of Veterinary Sciences, Utrecht University, and scientific coach of the Swiss team—noted the morphological resemblance between the "Breda agent" (Breda virus [BRV]) and BEV and realized that these viruses might be representatives of a new taxon of animal viruses. Profiting from the decisive advantage that BEV can be propagated in vitro, Horzinek, together with Marianne Weiss, Joke Ederveen, Eric Snijder, and many others, embarked on a series of elegant experiments, the results of which were seminal.

By virus neutralization assay (VNA) and enzyme-linked immunosorbent assay, BEV was swiftly established to be serologically related to BRV as well as to Lyon-4 virus (76), an agent which, in the meanwhile, had been isolated from diarrheic cattle in France (50). The presence of a lipid-containing envelope, as already indicated by electron microscopy (EM), was confirmed for BEV by demonstrating its sensitivity to organic solvents (chloroform and diethyl ether). As the propagation of BEV was not affected by iododeoxyuridine—an inhibitor of DNA virus replication—the virus was concluded to possess an RNA genome (76). Transfection of virion-extracted RNA into BEV-permissive cells showed it to be infectious and thus of positive polarity (68).

The remarkable structure of the discoidal BEV virions, which by thin-section EM were shown to

Raoul J. de Groot • Virology Division, Department of Infectious Diseases and Immunology, Faculty of Veterinary Sciences, Utrecht University, Utrecht, The Netherlands.

contain a rod-like nucleocapsid bent in an open ring, prompted Horzinek (on the basis of a suggestion by Fred Murphy) to coin the name torovirus (from the Latin *torus,* bulge, protuberance; also used to describe a particular architectural element in the form of a doughnut-shaped molding at the base of a column) (33, 37, 38). Initially, it was proposed—with ardor, one might add—that these unassigned viruses be placed in a new family of vertebrate RNA viruses, *Toroviridae* (33, 37, 38). In support, a paper was published provocatively entitled "Berne virus is not 'coronavirus-like,'" in which, indeed, major differences in viron composition between toro- and coronaviruses were reported (39). It therefore came as a bit of a blow—at least to torovirus aficionados—that BEV turned out to be coronavirus-like after all, not only with respect to the organization and expression of its genome but also genetically. Comparative sequence analysis of replicase genes revealed that toro- and coronaviruses were more closely related to each other than to any other positive-stranded RNA virus known at that time (34, 42, 63, 70, 71). As a consequence, toroviruses were assigned a mere genus and included together with the "true" coronaviruses in a bigeneric family, *Coronaviridae* (8, 9). However, related though toro- and coronaviruses may be, they are nonetheless separated by an evolutionary distance far greater than customary between genera in other virus families (26). Moreover, there really are salient differences between toro- and coronaviruses with respect to virion architecture and replication (see below). Finally, very recently, a new taxon of teleost nidoviruses was described, represented by white bream virus (proposed genus, *Bafinivirus,* bacilliform fish nidovirus). Phylogenetic analyses suggest that the "bafini-" and extant toroviruses evolved from a common ancestor that split off from the lineage that produced the present-day coronaviruses (55). All matters considered, a taxonomic reassessment of the order *Nidovirales* seems in order, a sentiment shared by the Nidovirus Study Group of the International Committee on the Taxonomy of Viruses (chapters 1 and 2). Chances are that toroviruses will soon acquire the family status after all, or at least make it to the subfamily level.

Table 1 lists the toroviruses that have been encountered so far, with names and abbreviations according to the recommendations of the Nidovirus Study Group. For historical reasons, the first equine and bovine isolates, BEV and BRV, are referred to in the text using their original names and abbreviations.

## Torovirus Host Range and Epidemiology

Torovirus-like particles are commonly seen in the feces of cattle and swine (20, 32, 47, 49, 50, 52,

**Table 1.** Torovirus species

| Species | Abbreviation | Isolate/variant | Reference(s) |
|---|---|---|---|
| Equine torovirus | EToV | *Berne virus* (BEV) | 76 |
| Bovine torovirus | BToV | | |
| Type 1 | BToV-1 | *Breda virus* (BRV) | 78 |
| Type 2 | BToV-2 | B6 | 59 |
| Type 3 | BToV-3 | B150 | 59 |
| Porcine torovirus | PToV | | |
| Type 1 | PToV-1 | P4[a] | 59 |
| Type 2 | PToV2 | P-Mar[a] | 47, 59 |
| Human torovirus | HToV | | 3, 17 |
| Ovine torovirus[b] | OToV | | 77 |
| Caprine torovirus[b] | CToV | | 77 |
| Rabbit torovirus[b] | RToV | | 77 |
| Murine torovirus[b] | MToV | | 77 |

[a]PToV-2 strains are of recombinant origin and have arisen from a genetic exchange between a PToV-1 strain and a hitherto-unidentified torovirus type. It is not clear which genotype, P4 or P-MAR, represents the PToV parent and which represents the recombinant offspring. P4, however, is the oldest PToV isolate characterized so far (59).
[b]These torovirus species have not yet been isolated and characterized; evidence for their existence is based solely upon reported detection of BEV-neutralizing antibodies in serum samples (77).

56, 57, 59, 78; L. J. Saif, D. R. Redman, K. W. Theil, P. D. Moorhead, and C. K. Smith, presented at the 62nd Annual Meeting Conference for Research Workers of Animal Diagnostics, Chicago, IL, 1981), but they have also been observed in fecal samples from cats (51) and dogs (24) as well as in human stools (2, 3, 17, 46). However, identification of toroviruses solely by EM (and even by immuno-EM) is fraught with error because of the common occurrence of noninfectious, pleomorphic fringed particles in feces and body fluids (3). Indirect but convincing evidence for torovirus infection in various mammalian host species was obtained by heterotypic VNA. BEV-neutralizing antibodies were detected not only in horses and cattle but also in swine, sheep, goats, rabbits, and mice (77). Toroviruses have a worldwide distribution, and seroprevalence in ungulates is very high; for instance, in epidemiological surveys in The Netherlands and Germany, 95% of cattle tested seropositive by BRV-ELISA (45), while >80% of swine were positive for torovirus antibody by VNA (47).

Genetic evidence for torovirus infections, based upon reverse transcriptase PCR amplification of torovirus sequences from fecal samples and/or nasal secretions, has been published for cattle (16, 27, 29–31, 49, 59), swine (47, 49, 59), and, notably, also for humans (17). Disconcertingly, however, the amplicons from human stool samples were essentially identical in sequence to the corresponding (3' untranslated) region of the BEV genome, with individual amplicons differing by single nucleotide changes from BEV, but also from each other. Puzzlingly, the amplicons were only 91 and 76% identical to the corresponding regions in bovine torovirus (BToV) and porcine torovirus (PToV), respectively (17, 44, 47). So, either human toroviruses and BEV are very closely related (at least in the 3′ ends of their genomes) or the findings must be ascribed to a PCR contamination with BEV sequences. The same authors later reported reverse transcriptase PCR amplification of a torovirus hemagglutinin-esterase (HE) gene from human stools (18). Interestingly, the sequence of this gene and its product are unique and quite divergent from the HE sequences of other toroviruses (59; see also below).

Early studies comparing BToV isolates from Iowa (strain BRV-1) (78) and Ohio (strain BRV-2) (Saif et al., presented previously) by hemagglutination inhibition assay suggested that these viruses represent different serotypes (79). Further evidence for the existence of multiple BToV types came from a more recent study of European field strains, revealing considerable sequence heterogeneity, apparently brought about by both genetic drift and shift (59). As detailed below, some BToV field strains have acquired

sequences via homologous RNA recombination from PToV and even from toroviruses that hitherto have not been identified and characterized. Similar events have occurred during PToV divergence. At present, we can distinguish three BToV and two PToV "genotypes" (in lieu of a better phrase [Table 1]).

## THE VIRION: MORPHOLOGY AND STRUCTURAL PROTEINS

### Virion Architecture

The most distinctive virion element is the core or nucleocapsid, a flexible rod ~100 nm in length and ~23 nm across (76), composed of the ~28-kb genome (15, 60) and multiple copies of the nucleocapsid (N) protein (36). Electron micrographs of purified BEV nucleocapsids showed a "conspicuous transverse striation" with a periodicity of ~4.5 nm (Fig. 1a) (36, 76), whereas cross sections revealed a translucent central channel (~10 nm in diameter [Fig. 1b]) (22, 74, 76). The combined data suggest the torovirus nucleocapsid to be tightly coiled into a hollow tube of helical symmetry (36, 76).

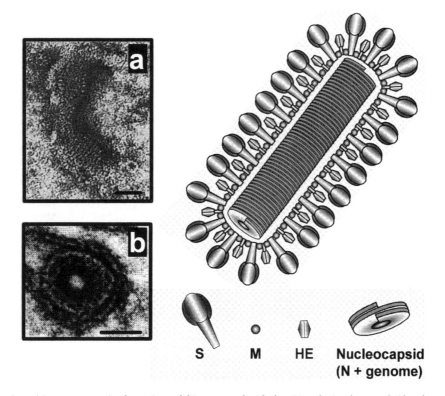

**Figure 1.** Torovirus virion structure. A schematic model is presented with the virion depicted as a rod. Also shown are electron micrographs reprinted from the *Journal of General Virology* (36, 74) with permission of the publisher. (a) A purified BEV nucleocapsid with the envelope removed by ethyl ether treatment; note the transverse striation. (b) Cross section through a BEV virion. The particle appears as three concentric circles of high electron density. Note the electron lucent center, thought to represent the hollow inner space of the tubular nucleocapsid, which itself appears as the electron-dense inner ring. Bar markers represent 25 nm.

The nucleocapsid is wrapped in an envelope with the integral membrane (M) protein as the main viral constituent. The virus particles are adorned with two types of surface projections: elongated petal-shaped peplomers of ~20 nm, comprised of the spike (S) protein, and smaller (~6- to 9-nm) protrusions, comprised of HE (11, 78). In BEV particles, HE spikes are lacking, as the BEV HE gene is largely deleted (65). Loss of HE expression must have occurred during virus propagation in tissue culture cells (see, for example, reference 48); all other toroviruses characterized to date carry an intact HE gene (10, 18, 59).

The disk-shaped particles abundant in electron micrographs of BEV (but notably less so in those of BToVs and PToVs [47, 52, 56, 76, 78) captured the imagination of the early researchers and inspired the name of the taxon. Ironically, however, the discoids likely represent damaged virions of which the membrane has detached from one side of the nucleocapsid and of which the core has been curved due to "shrink-wrapping" during EM preparation. Presumably, intact torovirus virions are rod-shaped, like those of roniviruses (72) and white bream virus (55), with rounded ends and measuring 100 to 140 by 35 to 42 nm (Fig. 1) (22, 25, 74, 76, 78; Saif et al., presented previously); the variation in morphology adopted by extracellular torovirions is likely the consequence of the flexibility of core and particle, i.e., the absence of a rigid structure (25).

## N Protein

With a molecular mass of ~18 kDa (159 to 167 residues), the torovirus N protein is only about one-third the size of its coronavirus equivalent (45 to 60 kDa). It binds single-stranded RNA, as can be demonstrated by North-Western blotting, in point of fact, a property that was key to its identification as an N protein in the first place (36). The N protein appears to be the main virion component, estimated to account for 80% of total protein mass (36).

The BEV N protein is a phosphoprotein (36). For each of the torovirus N protein sequences, multiple potential phosphorylation sites can be predicted (4), but only one of these (for protein kinase C) is strictly conserved (ATF<u>T</u>IKV, Thr-154 in BEV [Fig. 2]).

Among the most conspicuous features of the amino acid sequence of the N protein are two overlapping regions, one extremely rich in glutamine and asparagine and the other containing clusters of arginines. The latter region is reminiscent of the arginine-rich motifs (ARMs) that mediate sequence-specific RNA binding in various other proteins of viral and cellular origin (Fig. 2) (1). It is tempting to speculate that this part of the N protein is crucially involved in

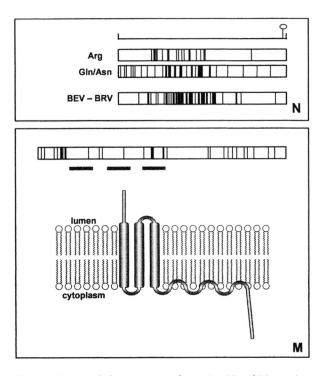

**Figure 2.** Structural characteristics of torovirus N and M proteins. (Upper panel) Linear representations of the N protein, depicted either as a horizontal bar (top) or as boxes (below), indicating the location of a conserved potential protein kinase C phosphorylation site (lollipop) and the distribution of arginine residues (vertical bars; top box), of glutamine/asparagine residues (middle), and of the amino acid differences between the N proteins of BEV and BRV (bottom). (Lower panel) Linear representation of the M protein depicted as a box, with vertical bars indicating the locations of amino acid differences among all known equine torovirus, BToV, and PToV M proteins. The locations of predicted transmembrane domains are indicated by horizontal black boxes underneath. A topological model of the torovirus M protein (adapted from reference 14) is presented at the bottom.

specific recognition of the viral genome and in RNA binding in general. Puzzlingly, however, it is also in the Arg- and Gln/Asn-rich regions that most sequence variation is seen (Fig. 2). In fact, sequence divergence is considerable; the N proteins of BRV and BEV, BRV and PToV-MAR, and BEV and PToV-MAR are identical for only 80, 67, and 65%, respectively (47). Remarkably, the N proteins of PToV field variants are highly similar to those of BToV type 2 and 3 strains (90 to 96% identity), a peculiarity ascribed to RNA recombination (59), as is explained in more detail below.

## M Protein

The torovirus M protein is a 26-kDa (233-residue) nonglycosylated class III integral M protein with a noncleavable internal signal sequence (14, 35). Its structural characteristics and membrane topology, as predicted by computer analysis and confirmed by biochemical analysis, are remarkably similar to those of its coronavirus equivalent, with a short hydrophilic N-terminal domain exposed on the outside of the virion, three successive transmembrane α-helices, and a long, mostly amphipathic C-terminal tail buried within the particle (14). In agreement with this model, antisera directed against the N terminus of the M protein decorate the virion surface in immunolabeling assays, whereas sera recognizing the C terminus do not (25).

Among the toroviruses studied so far, the sequence of the M protein is highly conserved. Maximum divergence is only 10%, the M proteins of BRV and BEV, BRV and PToV-MAR, and BEV and PToV-MAR sharing 93, 91, and 90% identity, respectively (59). Comparative sequence analysis shows that variation occurs throughout the protein but, as might be expected, prominently in the N-terminal ectodomain (Fig. 2).

The torovirus M protein is likely the key player in viral assembly. Presumably, it organizes the envelope, creating a well-ordered lattice through lateral homotypic interactions. Moreover, the M protein can be envisaged to recruit and position HE and S protein oligomers into this lattice through heterotypic interactions as well as to drive viral budding by binding via its C-terminal domain to preformed nucleocapsids (see below). One may even speculate that the exceptional physicochemical properties of BEV, i.e., its unusual stability against extremely low pH values (down to pH 2.5) and its resistance to deoxycholate (75), are adaptations to gastroenteric replication that are directly related to characteristics of the M protein.

## S Protein

The S protein is a large (1,562- to 1,584-residue) and excessively N-glycosylated class I membrane glycoprotein. Produced as a 180,000-molecular-weight (180K) precursor, the S protein is proteolytically cleaved, presumably by furin-like enzymes at a conserved RRXRR multibasic residue motif, to yield products of 82K and 95K; these polypeptides apparently correspond to the membrane-bound C-terminal (S2) and the remaining N-terminal portion of the molecule (S1), respectively (35, 67). Although the function of the S protein has not been studied in much detail and direct evidence is lacking, we may safely assume that the spikes mediate receptor binding and membrane fusion; in support, the S protein is a target for virus-neutralizing antibodies (40), and in its C-terminal half two heptad repeats are present (67), i.e., amino acid motifs that are indicative of α-helical domains that engage in coiled-coil

structures and that are a hallmark of type I viral fusion proteins (6, 21).

Although torovirus and coronavirus S proteins share no significant sequence identity whatsoever, there are obvious similarities in size and in the relative positions of particular sequence elements. As in the coronavirus S proteins (5, 6, 13), a short (~42-residue) heptad repeat (HR2) is located immediately adjacent to the transmembrane domain. A longer (~73-residue) heptad repeat (HR1) is located further upstream with, at its N terminus, a stretch of 22 hydrophobic residues that may function as an internal fusion peptide (Fig. 3) (67; see also chapters 12 and 13). It is not clear whether the similarities between the S proteins of toro- and coronaviruses, and those between their M proteins, result from convergent evolution, or—as proposed previously (14)—should be taken as yet another indication of the common ancestry of these viruses.

In order to determine the quaternary structure of the torovirus spike, Snijder et al. (67) performed sucrose gradient centrifugation analysis and concluded it to be a homodimer. However, the shape of the molecule (elongated rather than globular) must have affected its sedimentation behavior (in fact, a major caveat of this approach); from our current understanding of type I viral fusion proteins (41, 54), the torovirus spike is almost certainly a trimer in which the C-terminal S2 subunits form an elongated membrane-anchored stalk, constituting the fusion engine, and in which the N-terminal S1 subunits form the membrane-distal globular top part of the molecule involved in receptor binding and virion attachment.

Comparison of the S proteins of BToVs, PToVs, and BEV shows that the S1 subunits are least conserved (73, 66, and 62% identity between BRV and

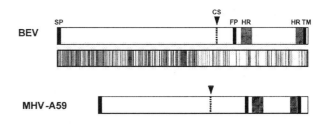

**Figure 3.** Structural characteristics of the torovirus S protein. Linear representations of S proteins of a torovirus (BEV) and a coronavirus (mouse hepatitis virus strain A59), depicted as boxes and on scale. The locations of signal peptides (SP), putative fusion peptides (FP), and transmembrane domains (TM) are indicated as black boxes. The locations of regions with heptad repeat periodicity (HR) are indicated by hatched boxes. Dashed vertical bars plus arrowheads indicate the positions of cleavage sites (CS) for furin-like cellular proteases. The middle box shows the distribution of amino acid differences (indicated by vertical bars) between the BEV and BRV S proteins.

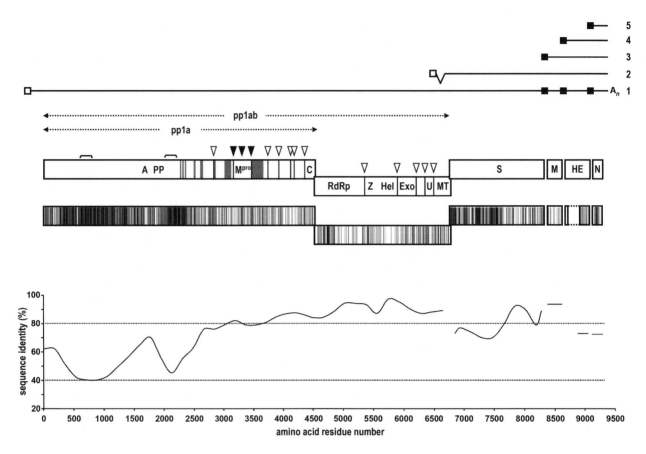

**Figure 4.** Organization and expression of the torovirus genome. The central portion shows a schematic representation of the torovirus genome (on scale), with the genes for the structural proteins (S, M, and N proteins and HE) and for the replicase polyproteins (pp1a and pp1ab) depicted as boxes. The various domains in the replicase polyproteins are indicated using the following abbreviations: A, ADP-ribose 1″-phosphatase; PP, papain-like proteinase; C, cyclic phosphodiesterase; Z, zinc-binding domain; Hel, helicase; Exo, 3′-to-5′ exoribonuclease domain; U, nidoviral uridylate-specific endoribonuclease; and MT, ribose-2′-O methyltransferase. Hydrophobic segments in pp1a are indicated by cross-hatching. Arrowheads and vertical bars indicate M$^{pro}$ cleavage sites, established by N-terminal sequence analysis (closed) or predicted on the basis of the cleavage site consensus sequence and comparative sequence analysis (open). Two hypervariable regions in pp1a are indicated by brackets (15, 60, 63). The lower set of boxes shows the amino acid sequence variation between the BEV and BRV proteomes, with amino acid differences indicated by vertical bars. The bottom graph shows the amino acid sequence identity between BEV and BRV. Sliding-window analysis of the BEV-BRV proteome alignment was performed for the replicase polyproteins and the S protein with a window size of 500 residues and a 250-residue step size; for the M (partial) and N proteins and HE, overall sequence identity is given. The upper panel shows the structure of the intracellular viral RNAs (1 through 5), with RNA1 representing the viral genome and RNA2 through -5 the sg mRNAs for the S and M proteins, HE, and N protein, respectively. Internal TREs, located upstream of the genes for the M and N proteins and HE, are indicated by black boxes. The genomic TRE, present at the 5′ ends of RNA1 and -2, is indicated by an open box. A$_n$, poly(A) tail.

BEV, BRV and P-Mar, and BEV and P-Mar, respectively, versus 89, 89, and 85%, respectively, in S2 [Fig. 4]). This may be explained by antigenic variation and immune selection primarily acting on S1, but it may also reflect differences in receptor specificity.

## HE

HE is perhaps the most elusive virion component. Remarkably, this 65K (416- to 430-residue) class I envelope glycoprotein is not even unique to toroviruses. Similar proteins, sharing 30% sequence

identity, also occur in group 2 coronaviruses and in influenza C virus (10, 65). A more distant relative, but a member of the HE family nonetheless, was found in infectious salmon anemia virus, an orthomyxovirus of teleosts (23, 28). It has been suggested that an ancestor of present-day toroviruses acquired its HE gene through heterologous RNA recombination, though from which source is not known (10, 65).

HE proteins possess two seemingly contradictory activities. They are lectins specific for particular O-acetylated sialic acids and serve as receptor-binding proteins. At the same time, they are sialate-O-acetyl esterases and act as receptor-destroying enzymes. As a net effect, HE proteins mediate reversible binding of virions to sialic acid receptor determinants (for a recent review, see reference 12).

The influenza C virus HE fusion protein (HEF) is a homotrimeric molecule with a three-domain structure. The monomer is synthesized as an 88-kDa precursor and is cleaved by a cellular protease to yield an N-terminal subunit, HEF1, and a C-terminal subunit, HEF2. In the trimer, the HEF2 subunits form an elongated, membrane-bound stalk involved in membrane fusion, whereas the HEF1 subunits form a globular headpiece, with the esterase domains located at its base and sialic acid-binding sites at the tip of the molecule (53). In torovirus HEs, the esterase domain, with its active site composed of a Ser-His-Asp catalytic triad, is highly conserved. However, the primary sequence of the region that would correspond to the lectin domain is quite different from that in HEF1, and the fusion domain is lacking completely (11, 12). Torovirus HE spikes as they appear on virions are almost certainly homo-oligomers, but whether they are trimers (as is HEF) or dimers (as seems to be the case for coronavirus HEs) or have another quaternary structure is not yet known.

In phylogenetic trees, the torovirus HE proteins form a monophyletic group, clustering separately from HEF and from the HEs of coronaviruses. Still, sequence variation among torovirus HEs is substantial, and at present, five distinct variants differing by 25 to 50% can be distinguished. Two of these originate from BToVs, and two others originate from PToV field strains (58, 59). The remaining one is an HE from—reportedly—a human torovirus (18). Like the influenza C virus HEF and the HEs of most coronaviruses, the PToV HEs prefer 9-O-acetylated sialic acid as a substrate. Remarkably, both types of BToV HEs showed a preference for 5-N-acetyl-7,9-di-O-acetylneuraminic acid (58). Under the assumption that substrate preference reflects lectin ligand specificity, it would appear that BToVs use 7,9-di-O-acetylated sialic acid as a (co)receptor/initial attachment factor.

As poignantly demonstrated by the in vitro growth properties of BEV, HE is not required for propagation in cell culture. The sequence variation in the HEs of PToV and BToV field strains suggests, however, that during natural infections this protein is an important target for the immune system and subject to both antigenic drift and shift (59). The fact that in the field, viral mutants are selected for that, rather than having lost, have altered or even swapped their HE genes (via homologous RNA recombination; see below) indicates that under natural conditions HE expression is highly advantageous, if not essential.

## THE TOROVIRUS GENOME

### Organization and Expression

For two toroviruses, BEV and BRV-1, the genome has now been sequenced to completion. With a genome size of ~28 kb, toroviruses are among the giants—at least in the RNA virus realm—equaling the coronaviruses with regard to genetic complexity. The genomic RNA is capped (73) and polyadenylated (68), with a 5' untranslated region (UTR) of more than 800 nucleotides (821 and 857 nucleotides for BEV and BRV, respectively) and a 3' UTR of 200 residues (15, 66, 73). Synthetic RNAs, comprised of only the 5'-most 604 nucleotides of the BEV genome fused to the 3' UTR, are coreplicated in BEV-infected cells and behave as defective interfering RNAs (61, 64); hence, the signals essential for genome replication, and presumably also those for encapsidation, reside within these sequences. The exceptional length of the 5' UTR, however, suggests that it may have additional functions not directly related to RNA synthesis and packaging, with a role in (the enhancement of) translation initiation as the most obvious possibility.

The torovirus genome organization (as based on data currently available for equine toroviruses, BToVs, and PToVs (10, 15, 19, 59, 60, 63–67) is depicted in Fig. 4. The largest part of the genome (73%) is taken up by the overlapping open reading frames 1a and 1b (ORF1a and ORF1b). The latter is expressed only upon ribosomal frameshifting, which occurs with an estimated efficiency of 20 to 30% at a pseudoknot structure at the 3' end of ORF1a (15, 63; see also chapter 3). Translation thus yields two huge polyproteins, polyprotein 1a (pp1a) and pp1ab, from which by proteolytic cleavage the various subunits of the viral replicase/transcriptase are derived as well as a number of accessory proteins of as-yet-unknown function. Downstream of ORF1b, there are the genes for the structural proteins (S protein, M protein, HE, and N protein as ordered from 5' to 3'); these are translated from four subgenomic mRNAs (sg mRNAs) numbered 2 through 5 (with the genomic RNA being RNA1), which—as is typical for the *Nidovirales*—form a 3'-coterminal nested set (70).

### RNA Recombination

The torovirus genome has been shaped and molded by heterologous and homologous RNA recombination. There is clear-cut evidence for two heterologous RNA recombination events that must have occurred relatively recently (65), that is, after the corona-"bafini"-torovirus split (55). One of these led to the acquisition of the HE gene; as already alluded to, an ancestral torovirus must have captured the HE gene from a cellular or viral donor. The other sequence acquired through heterologous recombination is located at the 3′-most end of ORF1a and encodes a (predicted) cyclic phosphodiesterase (Fig. 4). A related protein, 2A, occurs in group 2b coronaviruses, but here it is encoded by a separate gene, located immediately downstream of ORF1b and expressed from a subgenomic mRNA (62, 65).

Homologous RNA recombination may not affect overall genome organization, but it is a major factor contributing to torovirus survival and evolution (Fig. 5). Type 2 BToVs appear to have arisen from a BRV-like type I BToV parent that swapped its N protein gene for that of PToV. In turn, a type 2 BToV seems to have replaced its coding sequences for the HE ectodomain for those of an unknown torovirus, giving rise to the type 3 BToVs. Similarly, a so-far-unidentified torovirus must have served as a donor of HE sequences during PToV evolution, and as a result there are now at least two types of PToV; which of these represents the parental lineage and which represents the recombinant offspring cannot be determined from current data (59).

Toro- and coronaviruses differ in their coding strategy with respect to the number and nature of genes downstream of ORF1b. Coronaviruses possess, in addition to a common set of four structural protein genes, a variable set of up to seven group-specific (and sometimes even virus-specific) accessory genes that are expressed from specific sg mRNAs (see chapter 3). In contrast, in toroviruses the only genes located downstream of ORF1b and expressed from sg mRNAs are those for the structural proteins. With the—debatable—exception of the HE gene, accessory genes are curiously lacking, suggesting that toroviruses are less adept than coronaviruses are at accommodating foreign sequences as new transcription units into their genome.

## Torovirus Transcription

The genes for the M and N proteins and HE are preceded by short noncoding "intergenic" regions, containing a transcription-regulating element (TRE) conforming to the consensus 5′ (C)ACN$_{3-4}$CUUUAGA 3′ (61, 70). A copy of this sequence is also present at the extreme 5′ terminus of the genome (73). In contrast, the S protein gene overlaps with the replicase gene and the N-terminal 28 residues of the S protein are in fact encoded by an internal (−1) reading frame within ORF1b (63, 67); moreover, there is no TRE preceding the S protein gene (67, 73).

The significance of these observations became clear only when the exact 5′ end of each BEV sg mRNA was determined. As it turns out, toroviruses are unique among RNA viruses in that they employ a mixed transcription strategy combining continuous and discontinuous sgRNA synthesis (73). Like the sgRNAs of corona-, "bafini-," and arteriviruses (55; see chapter 8), the BEV mRNA for the S protein (RNA2) is chimeric and carries a 15- to 18-nucleotide (nt) leader derived from the 5′ end of the genome (73). Remarkably, however, the other BEV mRNAs

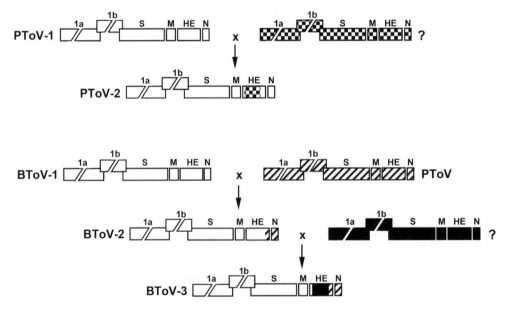

**Figure 5.** Genetic exchanges among PToV and BToV field variants. Torovirus genomes are depicted schematically, with the various genes represented by boxes. Types of PToVs and BToVs are indicated; question marks indicate parental toroviruses that have not been identified so far.

(RNA3 to RNA5) do not possess a leader. They are fully collinear with the genome, with transcription initiating at the 5'-most adenosines within their respective TREs (70, 73). A 16-nt sequence comprising the TRE and flanking sequences is sufficient to drive sgRNA synthesis, while substitution of the initiating adenylate or flanking conserved cytidylates in the element reduces transcription, in most cases to undetectable levels (61).

Like corona- and arteriviruses, toroviruses presumably employ subgenomic minus-strand RNAs as templates for sg mRNA synthesis. In support, subgenomic minus-strand RNA species corresponding to each of the sg mRNAs have been detected in BEV-infected cells by both Northern blot assay and rapid amplification of cDNA ends-PCR (A. L. van Vliet and R. J. de Groot, unpublished observations). In the current working model (Fig. 6), the TREs that direct continuous sgRNA synthesis have dual functions, acting as termination and initiation signals (promoters) during minus- and plus-strand production, respectively. Discontinuous RNA synthesis seems to be directed by a sequence also conserved in BToV and PToV, provisionally designated the discontinuous transcription element (DTE). It consists of a short hairpin and a homology region that shares sequence identity with nt 16 to 38 at the 5' end of the genome (Fig. 6). The fusion of leader and body sequences is thought to occur during minus-strand synthesis via a mechanism

similar to, yet distinct from, that in corona- and arteriviruses (see chapter 8). As fusion consistently occurs at the base of the stem-loop structure, the hairpin presumably acts as an attenuator of minus-strand synthesis. This would facilitate a subsequent similarity-assisted copy choice RNA recombination event, guided by sequence similarity and duplex formation between the antisense DTE homology region in the nascent minus chain and its complementary sequence at the 5' end of the genome. The resulting chimeric minus-strand RNA would carry a 3' anti-TRE and thus be transcription competent (73).

Why toroviruses use two different transcription strategies and how this came about is not known. However, the arrangement, with the S protein gene overlapping with ORF1b and the mRNA2 leader-body fusion site being located at a considerable distance (175 nt) of the S protein initiation codon, does give the impression of a makeshift solution to a recombination accident. A scenario can be envisaged in which, in an ancestral torovirus, the 5' end of the S protein gene, together with the intergenic region and TRE, was deleted and/or replaced by foreign sequences and in which the loss of the initiation codon was remedied by in-frame fusion of the remaining part of the S protein gene to an internal ORF in the replicase gene. Fortuitous low-frequency template switching at the present mRNA2 leader-body fusion site may already have occurred in the parental

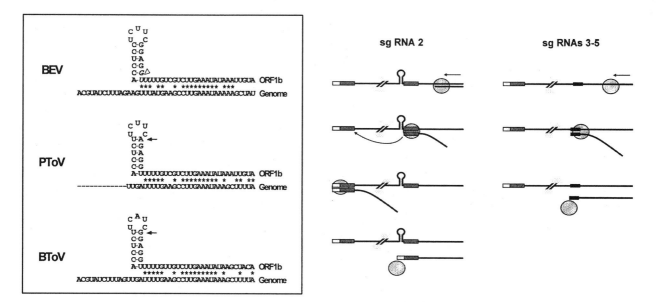

**Figure 6.** Torovirus transcription. (Left panel) Structure of the BEV DTE in ORF1b and corresponding sequences in the PToV and BToV genomes (15, 73). The DTE consists of a hairpin followed by a region sharing sequence similarity with the 5' end of the genome; ORF1b-genome alignments are shown, with asterisks indicating identical residues. The arrowhead indicates the mRNA2 leader-body fusion site; arrows indicate nucleotide substitutions in the PToV and BToV hairpins compared to that of BEV; note that base pairing is maintained. (Right panel) Current working model for the discontinuous synthesis of BEV mRNA2 and for the nondiscontinuous transcription of mRNA3 to -5. Details are explained in the text (adapted from reference 73).

virus, driven merely by chance identity between ORF1b and 5′ UTR sequences. In the new situation, however, it would have given rise to a minor transcription-competent subgenomic minus-strand RNA species through which the new S protein could be expressed. With a strong selection advantage provided by this novel S protein, even inefficient expression at first may have created a window of opportunity for the recombinant virus to survive and further optimize mRNA2 synthesis (73).

## The Torovirus Replicase Polyproteins: Domain Organization and Processing

Computer-assisted analysis of torovirus replicase polyprotein sequences has revealed an array of characteristic domains, the presence and order of which are conserved among (most) nidoviruses (Fig. 4); conspicuous differences notwithstanding, the 1ab polyproteins of toro- and coronaviruses are essentially collinear, with all key domains located at cognate positions (15, 60, 62, 63; see also chapters 2, 3, 5, and 6). ADP-ribose 1″-phosphatase and papain-like proteinase (PLP), transmembrane, and chymotrypsin-like "main proteinase" ($M^{pro}$) domains are found at equivalent locations in pp1a (15, 60), but sequence identity is most prominent in the ORF1b-encoded part of pp1ab, which comprises the RNA-dependent RNA polymerase (RdRp), a zinc-binding domain, the helicase, the 3′-to-5′ exoribonuclease domain, the nidoviral uridylate-specific endoribonuclease, and a ribose-2′-O methyltransferase domain (62, 63).

The N terminus of pp1a/pp1ab is highly divergent and, except from the ADP-ribose 1″-phosphatase and PLP domains, there is no obvious sequence similarity between toroviruses and other members of the *Nidovirales* in this region. A comparison of the BEV and BRV-1 proteomes shows that this part of the polyprotein is in fact least conserved, with sequence identities plummeting to 40% and below, particularly in the regions formed by residues 650 through 800 and residues 2150 through 2300 (Fig. 4). The variation within these regions arises not only from numerous substitutions but also from large insertions (in BEV) and/or deletions (in BRV-1). What function the protein domains in question might have and the why and how of the extensive sequence heterogeneity in these regions are all questions begging answers.

Proteolytic processing of the N-terminal part of pp1a/pp1ab is presumably mediated by the PLP (15). However, most processing steps in *cis* and in *trans* are thought to be carried out by $M^{pro}$, a 33-kDa chymotrypsin-like serine proteinase with $S^{3416}$ and $H^{3304}$ as its main catalytic residues (60). Given the pivotal role

of $M^{pro}$ in the nidoviral life cycle, one would expect stringent sequence conservation, as even minor changes affecting cleavage efficiency or specificity should come at a heavy fitness penalty. Paradoxically, however, the $M^{pro}$s of arteri-, roni-, corona-, and toroviruses have diverged almost beyond recognition (60; see also chapters 2, 5, and 6).

As in all other nidoviruses studied so far, the torovirus $M^{pro}$ domain in pp1a/pp1ab is flanked by hydrophobic regions typical for multispanning membrane proteins. BEV $M^{pro}$ autocatalytically releases itself from these adjoining sequences by cutting at the locations $^{3244}$FSFQ↓$S^{3252}$ and $^{3540}$FKKQ↓$S^{3544}$ (↓ indicating the scissile bond). Surprisingly, in an *Escherichia coli* expression system, cleavage also occurred at a site internal to $M^{pro}$ ($^{3394}$FATQ↓$A^{3398}$). Although the resulting 16-kDa products have not been detected in BEV-infected cells so far, it is too early to decide whether cleavage at this site is an artifact resulting from bacterial overexpression and misfolding or yet a relevant phenomenon during the natural infection (60).

The BEV $M^{pro}$ cleavage sites identified by protein sequence analysis conform to the consensus FXXQ↓(S,A). However, from alignments of coronavirus and torovirus pp1ab sequences, it would seem that Y/M/L and G/K may also be tolerated at the P4 and P1′ positions, respectively. A tentative processing scheme of the torovirus replicase polyproteins, based upon predicted $M^{pro}$ cleavage sites conserved between BEV and BRV, is shown in Fig. 4. Several points are of note. (i) A putative $M^{pro}$ cleavage site is found halfway through pp1a at a position topologically similar to that of a PLP site within coronavirus pp1a. (ii) Of the predicted sites in the ORF1b-encoded part of pp1ab, only the one between RdRp and the zinc finger/helicase domains conforms to the proposed consensus sequence. Future studies should determine whether the predicted sites are actually cleaved by $M^{pro}$. (iii) A cleavage site that would separate the cyclic phosphodiesterase homolog and the RdRp is not immediately apparent, raising questions as to whether $M^{pro}$ utilizes a noncanonical site, whether another viral or host proteinase is involved, or whether processing of pp1ab yields an RdRp with the cyclic phosphodiesterase still attached (60).

## THE TOROVIRUS LIFE CYCLE

In cultured cells, single-cycle replication of BEV is completed within 10 to 12 h, with viral progeny first being detected in the tissue culture supernatant around 6 h postinfection (38, 74; van Vliet and de Groot, unpublished). Cytopathic effect becomes noticeable only late in infection (>18 h postinfection), with cells rounding off; syncytia, however, are never observed (for a schematic overview of the reproductive cycle of BEV, see Fig. 7a).

Under natural conditions, toroviruses might initially attach to their host cells via the HE spikes binding to sialic acid receptor determinants. Conceivably, this would increase the likelihood of S peplomers finding their own dedicated receptor, presumably a host-specific glycoprotein. It is not known whether entry occurs via fusion at the plasma membrane or via an endocytotic route. It seems unlikely that

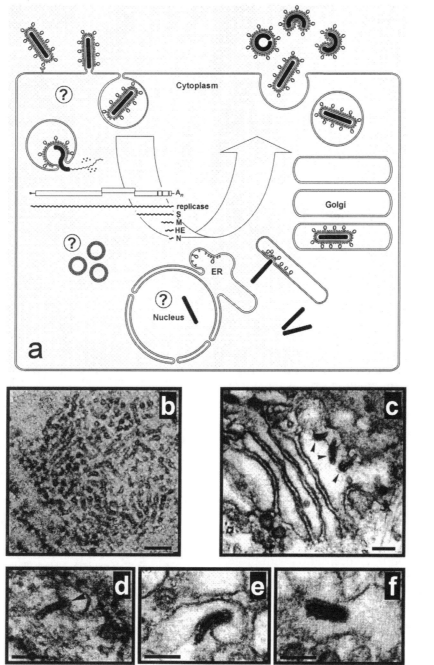

**Figure 7.** Single-cell replicative cycle of BEV. (a) Replicative cycle of BEV, with the open arrow indicating the chronological order of the various stages. It is not known whether entry occurs at the plasma membrane or via the endocytotic route. Similarly, it is not known whether torovirus replication occurs in association with double membrane vesicles. (b) Deposits of tubular structures in the cytoplasm of a BEV-infected cell. (c) Viruses budding through membranes of Golgi cisternae (arrowheads). (d to f) Various stages of viral budding into smooth membrane vesicles. Bar markers represent 100 nm (micrographs reprinted from the *Journal of General Virology* [74, 76] with permission of the publisher).

membrane fusion during entry of BEV (solely) involves a pH-induced conformational change in S protein: the virus is remarkably stable over a wide range of pH values and even retains full infectivity after incubation at pH 2.5 for 1 h at 37°C (75).

Fusion of the viral envelope and host membrane releases the nucleocapsid into the cytoplasm. Upon uncoating, the genome becomes available for replication, a process which most likely occurs in the cytoplasm. In analogy with corona- and arteriviruses, RNA synthesis may take place in association with double-membrane vesicles, although such structures were not specifically noted in torovirus-infected cells in ultrastructural studies published so far (22, 25, 74). Presumably, during the early hours of infection, the emphasis will be on synthesis of replicase proteins and genome amplification. Later in infection, a shift may occur towards production of sgRNAs and structural proteins. The N protein and the viral genomic RNA apparently autoassemble into tubular structures; whether the N protein can also form empty capsids is not known, nor is there information about the mechanism and specificity of the encapsidation process. In any case, agglomerates of nucleocapsid-like tubuli can be seen in the cytoplasm and consistently also in the nuclei of BEV- and BRV-infected cells (Fig. 7b) (22, 25, 74). The putative ARM in the N protein, proposed to mediate RNA binding, contains a conserved cluster of four or five arginine residues that might also function—fortuitously or by design—as a nuclear import signal (7); the imported N proteins might form tubuli in situ, as these structures were never seen entering or leaving the nucleus (74). Whether nuclear import of the N protein is relevant for viral replication or merely an epiphenomenon is not known.

The envelope (glyco)proteins are produced in the endoplasmic reticulum (ER) and largely retained in premedial Golgi compartments. The S protein acquires endoglycosidase H resistance only with a half-life of ~3.5 h (67), while the M protein accumulates in the ER Golgi-intermediate compartment (ERGIC) as indicated by colocalization with protein marker ERGIC-53 (25). Budding occurs intracellularly, predominantly at smooth membrane compartments consistent with the ERGIC and/or the Golgi system (Fig. 7c), although late in infection occasional budding through the rough ER and even the nuclear membrane was also observed (74). The first step of the budding process entails the attachment of a preassembled nucleocapsid with one pole to the cytoplasmic face of the membrane, after which the capsid is enwrapped sideways and the completed particle is released into the vesicular lumen (Fig. 7d to 7f) (74). It is assumed that the virions are subsequently transported along the exocytotic pathway and become secreted into the extracellular medium through fusion of secretory vesicles and the plasma membrane.

## CONCLUDING REMARKS

The existing body of literature on toroviruses may be modest in volume, but it offers decidedly more than a passing glimpse into the biology of these viruses. Even so, this chapter also shows how much remains to be discovered. We now have a decent road map of the viral life cycle, but the details are blurry. The mechanisms of entry, replication, transcription, and viral assembly (72) all make choice subjects for future study. We know even less about the behavior of toroviruses in the field, about their host range, their pathogenic potential, and their genetic diversity. For certain, surprising and exciting new findings that will significantly add to our understanding of nidoviruses and RNA viruses in general lie in store.

**Acknowledgments.** I am grateful to Peter J. M. Rottier, Marian C. Horzinek, and Jolanda D. F. de Groot-Mijnes for their careful and critical reading of the manuscript.

## REFERENCES

1. **Bayer, T. S., L. N. Booth, S. M. Knudsen, and A. D. Ellington.** 2005. Arginine-rich motifs present multiple interfaces for specific binding by RNA. *RNA* **11:**1848–1857.

2. **Beards, G. M., D. W. Brown, J. Green, and T. H. Flewett.** 1986. Preliminary characterisation of torovirus-like particles of humans: comparison with Berne virus of horses and Breda virus of calves. *J. Med. Virol.* **20:**67–78.

3. **Beards, G. M., C. Hall, J. Green, T. H. Flewett, F. Lamouliatte, and P. Du Pasquier.** 1984. An enveloped virus in stools of children and adults with gastroenteritis that resembles the Breda virus of calves. *Lancet* **i:**1050–1052.

4. **Blom, N., T. Sicheritz-Ponten, R. Gupta, S. Gammeltoft, and S. Brunak.** 2004. Prediction of post-translational glycosylation and phosphorylation of proteins from the amino acid sequence. *Proteomics* **4:**1633–1649.

5. **Bosch, B. J., B. E. Martina, R. Van Der Zee, J. Lepault, B. J. Haijema, C. Versluis, A. J. Heck, R. De Groot, A. D. Osterhaus, and P. J. Rottier.** 2004. Severe acute respiratory syndrome coronavirus (SARS-CoV) infection inhibition using spike protein heptad repeat-derived peptides. *Proc. Natl. Acad. Sci. USA* **101:**8455–8460.

6. **Bosch, B. J., R. van der Zee, C. A. de Haan, and P. J. Rottier.** 2003. The coronavirus spike protein is a class I virus fusion protein: structural and functional characterization of the fusion core complex. *J. Virol.* **77:**8801–8811.

7. **Boulikas, T.** 1993. Nuclear localization signals (NLS). *Crit. Rev. Eukaryot. Gene Expr.* **3:**193–227.

8. **Cavanagh, D., D. A. Brian, M. A. Brinton, L. Enjuanes, K. V. Holmes, M. C. Horzinek, M. M. Lai, H. Laude, P. G. Plagemann, S. G. Siddell, et al.** 1993. The Coronaviridae now comprises two genera, coronavirus and torovirus: report of

the Coronaviridae Study Group. *Adv. Exp. Med. Biol.* **342**:255–257.

9. Cavanagh, D., and M. C. Horzinek. 1993. Genus Torovirus assigned to the Coronaviridae. *Arch. Virol.* **128**:395–396.

10. Cornelissen, L. A., P. A. van Woensel, R. J. de Groot, M. C. Horzinek, N. Visser, and H. F. Egberink. 1998. Cell culture-grown putative bovine respiratory torovirus identified as a coronavirus. *Vet. Rec.* **142**:683–686.

11. Cornelissen, L. A., C. M. Wierda, F. J. van der Meer, A. A. Herrewegh, M. C. Horzinek, H. F. Egberink, and R. J. de Groot. 1997. Hemagglutinin-esterase, a novel structural protein of torovirus. *J. Virol.* **71**:5277–5286.

12. de Groot, R. J. 2006. Structure, function and evolution of the hemagglutinin-esterase proteins of corona- and toroviruses. *Glycoconj. J.* **23**:59–72.

13. de Groot, R. J., W. Luytjes, M. C. Horzinek, B. A. van der Zeijst, W. J. Spaan, and J. A. Lenstra. 1987. Evidence for a coiled-coil structure in the spike proteins of coronaviruses. *J. Mol. Biol.* **196**:963–966.

14. Den Boon, J. A., E. J. Snijder, J. K. Locker, M. C. Horzinek, and P. J. Rottier. 1991. Another triple-spanning envelope protein among intracellularly budding RNA viruses: the torovirus E protein. *Virology* **182**:655–663.

15. Draker, R., R. L. Roper, M. Petric, and R. Tellier. 2006. The complete sequence of the bovine torovirus genome. *Virus Res.* **115**:56–68.

16. Duckmanton, L., S. Carman, E. Nagy, and M. Petric. 1998. Detection of bovine torovirus in fecal specimens of calves with diarrhea from Ontario farms. *J. Clin. Microbiol.* **36**:1266–1270.

17. Duckmanton, L., B. Luan, J. Devenish, R. Tellier, and M. Petric. 1997. Characterization of torovirus from human fecal specimens. *Virology* **239**:158–168.

18. Duckmanton, L., R. Tellier, C. Richardson, and M. Petric. 1999. The novel hemagglutinin-esterase genes of human torovirus and Breda virus. *Virus Res.* **64**:137–149.

19. Duckmanton, L. M., R. Tellier, P. Liu, and M. Petric. 1998. Bovine torovirus: sequencing of the structural genes and expression of the nucleocapsid protein of Breda virus. *Virus Res.* **58**:83–96.

20. Durham, P. J., L. E. Hassard, G. R. Norman, and R. L. Yemen. 1989. Viruses and virus-like particles detected during examination of feces from calves and piglets with diarrhea. *Can. Vet. J.* **30**:876–881.

21. Dutch, R. E., T. S. Jardetzky, and R. A. Lamb. 2000. Virus membrane fusion proteins: biological machines that undergo a metamorphosis. *Biosci. Rep.* **20**:597–612.

22. Fagerland, J. A., J. F. Pohlenz, and G. N. Woode. 1986. A morphological study of the replication of Breda virus (proposed family Toroviridae) in bovine intestinal cells. *J. Gen. Virol.* **67**:1293–1304.

23. Falk, K., V. Aspehaug, R. Vlasak, and C. Endresen. 2004. Identification and characterization of viral structural proteins of infectious salmon anemia virus. *J. Virol.* **78**:3063–3071.

24. Finlaison, D. S. 1995. Faecal viruses of dogs—an electron microscope study. *Vet. Microbiol.* **46**:295–305.

25. Garzon, A., A. M. Maestre, J. Pignatelli, and M. T. Rejas, and D. Rodriguez. 2006. New insights on the structure and morphogenesis of Berne virus. *Adv. Exp. Med. Biol.* **581**:175–180.

26. Gonzalez, J. M., P. Gomez-Puertas, D. Cavanagh, A. E. Gorbalenya, and L. Enjuanes. 2003. A comparative sequence analysis to revise the current taxonomy of the family Coronaviridae. *Arch. Virol.* **148**:2207–2235.

27. Haschek, B., D. Klein, V. Benetka, C. Herrera, I. Sommerfeld-Stur, S. Vilcek, K. Moestl, and W. Baumgartner. 2006. Detection of bovine torovirus in neonatal calf diarrhoea in Lower Austria and Styria (Austria). *J. Vet. Med. Ser. B* **53**:160–165.

28. Hellebo, A., U. Vilas, K. Falk, and R. Vlasak. 2004. Infectious salmon anemia virus specifically binds to and hydrolyzes 4-O-acetylated sialic acids. *J. Virol.* **78**:3055–3062.

29. Hoet, A. E., K. O. Chang, and L. J. Saif. 2003. Comparison of ELISA and RT-PCR versus immune electron microscopy for detection of bovine torovirus (Breda virus) in calf fecal specimens. *J. Vet. Diagn. Investig.* **15**:100–106.

30. Hoet, A. E., K. O. Cho, K. O. Chang, S. C. Loerch, T. E. Wittum, and L. J. Saif. 2002. Enteric and nasal shedding of bovine torovirus (Breda virus) in feedlot cattle. *Am. J. Vet. Res.* **63**:342–348.

31. Hoet, A. E., P. R. Nielsen, M. Hasoksuz, C. Thomas, T. E. Wittum, and L. J. Saif. 2003. Detection of bovine torovirus and other enteric pathogens in feces from diarrhea cases in cattle. *J. Vet. Diagn. Investig.* **15**:205–212.

32. Hoet, A. E., and L. J. Saif. 2004. Bovine torovirus (Breda virus) revisited. *Anim. Health Res. Rev.* **5**:157–171.

33. Horzinek, M. C. 1984. Nonarbo animal togaviruses and control perspectives, p. 163–177. *In* E. Kurstak (ed.), *Control of Virus Diseases.* Academic Press, New York, NY.

34. Horzinek, M. C. 1993. Toroviruses—members of the coronavirus superfamily? *Arch. Virol. Suppl.* **7**:75–80.

35. Horzinek, M. C., J. Ederveen, B. Kaeffer, D. de Boer, and M. Weiss. 1986. The peplomers of Berne virus. *J. Gen. Virol.* **67**:2475–2483.

36. Horzinek, M. C., J. Ederveen, and M. Weiss. 1985. The nucleocapsid of Berne virus. *J. Gen. Virol.* **66**(Pt. 6):1287–1296.

37. Horzinek, M. C., T. H. Flewett, L. J. Saif, W. J. Spaan, M. Weiss, and G. N. Woode. 1987. A new family of vertebrate viruses: Toroviridae. *Intervirology* **27**:17–24.

38. Horzinek, M. C., and M. Weiss. 1984. Toroviridae: a taxonomic proposal. *Zbl. Veted. Reihe B* **31**:649–659.

39. Horzinek, M. C., M. Weiss, and J. Ederveen. 1984. Berne virus is not 'coronavirus-like'. *J. Gen. Virol.* **65**:645–649.

40. Kaeffer, B., P. van Kooten, J. Ederveen, W. van Eden, and M. C. Horzinek. 1989. Properties of monoclonal antibodies against Berne virus (Toroviridae). *Am. J. Vet. Res.* **50**:1131–1137.

41. Kielian, M., and F. A. Rey. 2006. Virus membrane-fusion proteins: more than one way to make a hairpin. *Nat. Rev. Microbiol.* **4**:67–76.

42. Koonin, E. V. 1991. The phylogeny of RNA-dependent RNA polymerases of positive-strand RNA viruses. *J. Gen. Virol.* **72**:2197–2206.

43. Koopmans, M., and M. C. Horzinek. 1994. Toroviruses of animals and humans: a review. *Adv. Virus Res.* **43**:233–273.

44. Koopmans, M., E. J. Snijder, and M. C. Horzinek. 1991. cDNA probes for the diagnosis of bovine torovirus (Breda virus) infection. *J. Clin. Microbiol.* **29**:493–497.

45. Koopmans, M., U. van den Boom, G. Woode, and M. C. Horzinek. 1989. Seroepidemiology of Breda virus in cattle using ELISA. *Vet. Microbiol.* **19**:233–243.

46. Krishnan, T., and T. N. Naik. 1997. Electronmicroscopic evidence of torovirus like particles in children with diarrhoea. *Indian J. Med. Res.* **105**:108–110.

47. Kroneman, A., L. A. Cornelissen, M. C. Horzinek, R. J. de Groot, and H. F. Egberink. 1998. Identification and characterization of a porcine torovirus. *J. Virol.* **72**:3507–3511.

48. Lissenberg, A., M. M. Vrolijk, A. L. van Vliet, M. A. Langereis, J. D. de Groot-Mijnes, P. J. Rottier, and R. J. de Groot. 2005. Luxury at a cost? Recombinant mouse hepatitis viruses expressing the accessory hemagglutinin esterase protein display reduced fitness in vitro. *J. Virol.* **79**:15054–15063.

49. Matiz, K., S. Kecskemeti, I. Kiss, Z. Adam, J. Tanyi, and B. Nagy. 2002. Torovirus detection in faecal specimens of calves and pigs in Hungary: short communication. *Acta Vet. Hung.* **50:**293–296.

50. Moussa, A., G. Dannacher, and M. Fedida. 1983. Nouveaux virus intervenant dans l'etiologie des enteritis neonatales des bovins. *Recl. Med. Vet.* **159:**185–190.

51. Muir, P., D. A. Harbour, T. J. Gruffydd-Jones, P. E. Howard, C. D. Hopper, E. A. Gruffydd-Jones, H. M. Broadhead, C. M. Clarke, and M. E. Jones. 1990. A clinical and microbiological study of cats with protruding nictitating membranes and diarrhoea: isolation of a novel virus. *Vet. Rec.* **127:**324–330.

52. Penrith, M. L., and G. H. Gerdes. 1992. Breda virus-like particles in pigs in South Africa. *J. S. Afr. Vet. Assoc.* **63:**102.

53. Rosenthal, P. B., X. Zhang, F. Formanowski, W. Fitz, C. H. Wong, H. Meier-Ewert, J. J. Skehel, and D. C. Wiley. 1998. Structure of the haemagglutinin-esterase-fusion glycoprotein of influenza C virus. *Nature* **396:**92–96.

54. Schibli, D. J., and W. Weissenhorn. 2004. Class I and class II viral fusion protein structures reveal similar principles in membrane fusion. *Mol. Membr. Biol.* **21:**361–371.

55. Schütze, H., R. Ulferts, B. Schelle, S. Bayer, H. Granzow, B. Hoffmann, T. C. Mettenleiter, and J. Ziebuhr. 2006. Characterization of *white bream virus* reveals a novel genetic cluster of nidoviruses. *J. Virol.* **80:**8493–8502.

56. Scott, A. C., M. J. Chaplin, M. J. Stack, and L. J. Lund. 1987. Porcine torovirus? *Vet. Rec.* **120:**583.

57. Scott, F. M., A. Holliman, G. W. Jones, E. W. Gray, and J. Fitton. 1996. Evidence of torovirus infection in diarrhoeic cattle. *Vet. Rec.* **138:**284–285.

58. Smits, S. L., G. J. Gerwig, A. L. van Vliet, A. Lissenberg, P. Briza, J. P. Kamerling, R. Vlasak, and R. J. de Groot. 2005. Nidovirus sialate-O-acetylesterases: evolution and substrate specificity of coronaviral and toroviral receptor-destroying enzymes. *J. Biol. Chem.* **280:**6933–6941.

59. Smits, S. L., A. Lavazza, K. Matiz, M. C. Horzinek, M. P. Koopmans, and R. J. de Groot. 2003. Phylogenetic and evolutionary relationships among torovirus field variants: evidence for multiple intertypic recombination events. *J. Virol.* **77:**9567–9577.

60. Smits, S. L., E. J. Snijder, and R. J. de Groot. 2006. Characterization of a torovirus main proteinase. *J. Virol.* **80:**4157–4167.

61. Smits, S. L., A. L. van Vliet, K. Segeren, H. el Azzouzi, M. van Essen, and R. J. de Groot. 2005. Torovirus non-discontinuous transcription: mutational analysis of a subgenomic mRNA promoter. *J. Virol.* **79:**8275–8281.

62. Snijder, E. J., P. J. Bredenbeek, J. C. Dobbe, V. Thiel, J. Ziebuhr, L. L. Poon, Y. Guan, M. Rozanov, W. J. Spaan, and A. E. Gorbalenya. 2003. Unique and conserved features of genome and proteome of SARS-coronavirus, an early split-off from the coronavirus group 2 lineage. *J. Mol. Biol.* **331:**991–1004.

63. Snijder, E. J., J. A. den Boon, P. J. Bredenbeek, M. C. Horzinek, R. Rijnbrand, and W. J. Spaan. 1990. The carboxyl-terminal part of the putative Berne virus polymerase is expressed by ribosomal frameshifting and contains sequence motifs which indicate that toro- and coronaviruses are evolutionarily related. *Nucleic Acids Res.* **18:**4535–4542.

64. Snijder, E. J., J. A. den Boon, M. C. Horzinek, and W. J. Spaan. 1991. Characterization of defective interfering RNAs of Berne virus. *J. Gen. Virol.* **72:**1635–1643.

65. Snijder, E. J., J. A. den Boon, M. C. Horzinek, and W. J. Spaan. 1991. Comparison of the genome organization of toro- and coronaviruses: evidence for two nonhomologous RNA recombination events during Berne virus evolution. *Virology* **180:**448–452.

66. Snijder, E. J., J. A. den Boon, W. J. Spaan, G. M. Verjans, and M. C. Horzinek. 1989. Identification and primary structure of the gene encoding the Berne virus nucleocapsid protein. *J. Gen. Virol.* **70**(Pt. 12):3363–3370.

67. Snijder, E. J., J. A. Den Boon, W. J. Spaan, M. Weiss, and M. C. Horzinek. 1990. Primary structure and post-translational processing of the Berne virus peplomer protein. *Virology* **178:**355–363.

68. Snijder, E. J., J. Ederveen, W. J. Spaan, M. Weiss, and M. C. Horzinek. 1988. Characterization of Berne virus genomic and messenger RNAs. *J. Gen. Virol.* **69:**2135–2144.

69. Snijder, E. J., and M. C. Horzinek. 1993. Toroviruses: replication, evolution and comparison with other members of the coronavirus-like superfamily. *J. Gen. Virol.* **74:**2305–2316.

70. Snijder, E. J., M. C. Horzinek, and W. J. Spaan. 1990. A 3'-coterminal nested set of independently transcribed mRNAs is generated during Berne virus replication. *J. Virol.* **64:**331–338.

71. Snijder, E. J., M. C. Horzinek, and W. J. Spaan. 1993. The coronaviruslike superfamily. *Adv. Exp. Med. Biol.* **342:**235–244.

72. Spann, K. M., and R. J. G. Lester. 1997. Special topic review: viral diseases of penaeid shrimp with particular reference to four viruses recently found in shrimp from Queensland. *World J. Microbiol. Biotechnol.* **13:**419–426.

73. van Vliet, A. L., S. L. Smits, P. J. Rottier, and R. J. de Groot. 2002. Discontinuous and non-discontinuous subgenomic RNA transcription in a nidovirus. *EMBO J.* **21:**6571–6580.

74. Weiss, M., and M. C. Horzinek. 1986. Morphogenesis of Berne virus (proposed family Toroviridae). *J. Gen. Virol.* **67:**1305–1314.

75. Weiss, M., and M. C. Horzinek. 1986. Resistance of Berne virus to physical and chemical treatment. *Vet. Microbiol.* **11:**41–49.

76. Weiss, M., F. Steck, and M. C. Horzinek. 1983. Purification and partial characterization of a new enveloped RNA virus (Berne virus). *J. Gen. Virol.* **64:**1849–1858.

77. Weiss, M., F. Steck, R. Kaderli, and M. C. Horzinek. 1984. Antibodies to Berne virus in horses and other animals. *Vet. Microbiol.* **9:**523–531.

78. Woode, G. N., D. E. Reed, P. L. Runnels, M. A. Herrig, and H. T. Hill. 1982. Studies with an unclassified virus isolated from diarrheic calves. *Vet. Microbiol.* **7:**221–240.

79. Woode, G. N., L. J. Saif, M. Quesada, N. J. Winand, J. F. Pohlenz, and N. K. Gourley. 1985. Comparative studies on three isolates of Breda virus of calves. *Am. J. Vet. Res.* **46:**1003–1010.

*Nidoviruses*
Edited by S. Perlman, T. Gallagher, and E. J. Snijder
© 2008 ASM Press, Washington, DC

Chapter 10

# Angiotensin-Converting Enzyme 2, the Cellular Receptor for Severe Acute Respiratory Syndrome Coronavirus and Human Coronavirus NL63

WENHUI LI, HYERYUN CHOE, AND MICHAEL FARZAN

Viruses use receptors for a variety of purposes (14). First, the receptor provides a specific, high-affinity docking site for the virion. Second, the receptor can, in the process of binding, induce conformational changes in the entry or spike protein that primes for or induces downstream steps in fusion. Third, the receptor can facilitate internalization of the virus, in many cases to a low-pH compartment where subsequent fusion events can occur. Fourth, the receptor can bring the virus to additional proteins, for example, a coreceptor (in the case of human immunodeficiency virus type 1) or a necessary protease (in the case of filoviruses and, as discussed below, severe acute respiratory syndrome coronavirus [SARS-CoV]). Fifth, the receptor can serve to identify cells that are advantageous for the virus to infect. For example, the SARS-CoV receptor marks pulmonary and gastrointestinal epithelial cells that are useful for a virus that transmits rapidly from animal to animal, before the emergence of adaptive immunity (29, 92).

The identification of a viral receptor can make a significant contribution to our understanding of viral pathogenesis and viral evolution, and to the development of vaccines and antiviral therapeutics. Knowing the receptor makes it possible to identify the target cells in the infected host, which is useful for understanding viral pathogenesis (92). In some cases, notably that of the SARS-CoV receptor angiotensin-converting enzyme 2 (ACE2), interference with natural receptor function many contribute to viral disease (40, 45). The receptor-entry protein interaction is frequently a major or sole restriction on the ability of viruses to infect new hosts (28, 91). Characterizing entry proteins of viruses from reservoir species and from humans, and their respective receptors, can tell us how a zoonotic transmission occurred and, therefore, how likely a zoonotic transmission may be from a related virus (57). In some cases—again, SARS-CoV is a good example—the efficiency with which a virus utilizes its receptor correlates with the severity of disease caused (57).

Here we describe the shared cellular receptor for SARS-CoV and human coronavirus NL63 (HCoV-NL63). Identification of this receptor contributed to our understanding of the zoonotic transmission of SARS-CoV and of the distinctive entry mechanisms of both SARS-CoV and HCoV-NL63. These are discussed below in the context of the structure of the SARS-CoV S protein receptor-binding domain (RBD) bound to this common receptor, ACE2.

## ZOONOTIC TRANSMISSION OF SARS-CoV TO HUMANS

SARS first emerged in November of 2002, when inhabitants of Guangdong Province, China, presented with an influenza-like illness that began with headache, myalgia, and fever, often followed by acute atypical pneumonia, respiratory failure, and death. In the winter and spring of 2002–2003, the outbreak spread over Asia and to Europe and North America. More than 8,000 people were infected, including nearly 2,000 health care workers. Nearly 10% of infected individuals died (10, 51, 71, 106, 108). The etiological agent of SARS was identified as a novel coronavirus, SARS-CoV (16, 20, 44, 47, 108). The 2002–2003 SARS-CoV epidemic was successfully contained by conventional public health measures by July 2003 (59, 107).

**Wenhui Li and Michael Farzan** • Department of Microbiology and Molecular Genetics, Harvard Medical School, Southborough, MA 01772.   **Hyeryun Choe** • Department of Pediatrics, Harvard Medical School, Boston, MA 02215.

SARS-CoV reemerged in Guangdong Province in the winter of 2003–2004, when it infected four individuals, all of whom recovered (19, 59, 83). No subsequent human-to-human transmission was observed in these cases. The infections in 2002–2003 and 2003–2004 were unlikely to be the first instances of SARS-CoV transmission to humans; almost 2% (17 of 938) of serum samples collected in 2001 from one Hong Kong cohort recognized and neutralized SARS-CoV (59). Additional SARS cases resulted from accidental laboratory infections in 2003 and 2004 (60, 69).

Exotic animals from the Guandong marketplace are likely to have been the immediate origin of SARS-CoV that infected humans in the winters of both 2002–2003 and 2003–2004. Marketplace Himalayan palm civets (*Paguma larvata*) and raccoon dogs (*Nyctereutes procyonoides*) harbored viruses highly similar to SARS-CoV (27). Palm civets are of special interest because virus could be isolated from most marketplace civets, and SARS-CoV can persist in palm civets for weeks (101). Moreover, the sporadic infections observed in 2003–2004 were associated with restaurants in which palm civet meat was prepared and consumed (59, 83). Additionally, culling of palm civets dramatically reduced the number of infected animals in the Guandong marketplace and may be responsible for the absence of virus in humans after the winter of 2003–2004 (96, 107). Finally, functional studies of the viral receptor, described below, also support a critical role for palm civets in transmitting virus to humans (58). Evidence of SARS-CoV infection has also been observed in many other marketplace species, including the domestic cat (*Felis catus*), the red fox (*Vulpes vulpes*), and the Chinese ferret-badger (*Melogale moschata*) (27, 96).

Although marketplace animals may be the immediate source of virus found in humans, evidence suggests that they may serve as a conduit for virus from another reservoir or precursor host. For example, although SARS antisera and virus were overwhelmingly present in marketplace palm civets in Guangdong, the vast majority of civets on farms and in the wild were found to be free of infection (43, 73, 92). Further, analysis of the rates of coding changes in the genomes of viruses isolated from palm civets suggests that the genome is not at equilibrium in the palm civet host (43, 83). Recently, SARS-CoV-like viruses have been isolated from several bat species, predominately horseshoe bats (genus *Rhinolophus*) (50, 56). The genetic diversity of this virus in bat hosts, and the absence of overt disease, is consistent with a role for bats as a reservoir for SARS-CoV. However, as described below, substantial genetic changes in the spike protein (S protein) of bat SARS-CoV are likely necessary for this virus to infect humans.

SARS-CoV isolated from humans can efficiently infect and be transmitted by domestic cats (*Felis catus*) and ferrets (*Mustela putorius furo*) (63). BALB/c mice (86, 98), Syrian hamsters (76), and cynomolgus and rhesus macaques (74, 78) are currently being used as animal models for SARS-CoV infection, although transmission has not been observed in these species. Most of these marketplace and laboratory animals, with the notable exception of palm civets, spontaneously clear the virus (63, 101). However, the number of species in which the virus can replicate indicates that SARS-CoV is capable of efficient zoonotic transmission. Nonetheless, as described below, interaction between the SARS-CoV S protein and its human cellular receptor initially limited efficient transmission to and among humans. The variant that emerged in 2002–2003 had distinctive properties that facilitated efficient replication in humans. These included changes in the SARS-CoV S protein, discussed below.

## CORONAVIRAL RECEPTORS

Three distinct genetic and serological groups of coronaviruses have been defined (23, 77). Coronaviruses from groups 1 and 2 are known to cause disease in humans (67). HCoV-229E, a group 1 virus, and HCoV-OC43, a group 2 virus, cause mild upper respiratory infections that result in self-resolving common colds in otherwise healthy individuals or severe pneumonia in immunocompromised people (67, 77). HCoV-NL63 (also referred to as HCoV-NH and HCoV-NL) has recently been identified as a group 1 virus causing conjunctivitis, croup, and sometimes serious respiratory infections in children (18, 70, 94). As described below, HCoV-NL63 is also notable for its use of the SARS-CoV cellular receptor ACE2 to infect cells (25). Another group 2 coronavirus (HCoV-HKU1) was recently isolated from a 71-year-old man with pneumonia (15). SARS-CoV and SARS-CoV-like viruses found in animals also cluster with group 2 viruses, although they are outliers of group 2 and have been also described as group 4 or, more recently, group 2b viruses (22, 24).

Like that of other RNA viruses, coronaviral diversity is generated by mutations due to polymerase infidelity. In addition, a key feature of coronavirus evolution is the propensity of the viral genomic RNA to recombine (37). Recombination permits the virus to acquire genes and gene regions from other transcripts, including those of other coronaviruses. Targeted recombination has been effectively used in the laboratory to manipulate and study coronaviral genomes (6, 28, 48, 52, 79). Natural recombination permits the rapid transformation of viral proteins such as the S protein. For example, acquisition of a small region of the S protein by a SARS-CoV precursor, perhaps originally more similar to the SARS-CoV found in bats, may have allowed it to utilize ACE2. In general, recombination can alter the tissue tropism of a virus and provide new avenues for further evolution and interspecies transmission.

The host spectrum of a specific coronavirus is largely determined by its S protein (48, 72, 79). In many cases, subtle alterations of the S protein are sufficient to alter tissue and species tropism and virulence of a coronavirus (6, 28, 48, 80). Coronaviral S proteins are type I transmembrane and class I fusion proteins that consist of distinct N-terminal (S1) and C-terminal (S2) domains, which mediate receptor binding and virus-cell fusion, respectively (4, 14, 21). Following association with the cell surface receptor, a conformational change of the S protein exposes a fusion peptide embedded in the S2 domain and induces reorganization of S2's large heptad repeats into coiled coils. This conformational change brings the virion membrane into close apposition to the cellular membrane for subsequent fusion (11, 14, 49).

Some coronavirus S proteins, for example, that of murine hepatitis virus, are cleaved between their S1 and S2 domains by a furin-like protease in the producer cell (41, 84, 85). Others, for example, HCoV-229E and SARS-CoV, do not retain furin recognition sites and are uncleaved on the virion (1, 68, 102). SARS-CoV is nonetheless dependent, following receptor association, on protease activity in the target cell (38, 39, 65, 82). This proteolysis can be mediated by cathepsin L in an endosomal or lysosomal compartment, or by exogenous proteases such as trypsin, thermolysin, and elastase. The role of proteolysis in the target cell remains to be determined, but it is likely that its function may be distinct from that of furin cleavage in the producer cell. For example, filovirus GP1,2 proteins, analogous to coronavirus S proteins, retain dependency on cathepsin B and L despite their cleavage into GP1 and GP2 in the producer cell (8). Not all coronaviruses are dependent on cathepsins or other lysosomal cysteine proteases; infection by HCoV-NL63 is not dependent on these enzymes despite its utilization of the same receptor as SARS-CoV (38, 39). Variation in cathepsin activity may, like receptor expression, govern the efficiency of infection in different tissues.

Several coronavirus cell surface receptors have been identified. Aminopeptidase N (CD13) was shown to be the receptor for canine coronavirus, feline infectious peritonitis virus, HCoV-229E, porcine epidemic diarrhea virus, and transmissible gastroenteritis virus, all of which are group 1 coronaviruses (13, 105). Members of the pleiotropic family of carcinoembryonic antigen adhesion molecules were identified as receptors for the group 2 pathogen murine hepatitis virus (17, 99), whereas bovine group 2 coronaviruses bind to 9-O-acetylated sialic acids (81). In 2003, ACE2 was identified as a functional cellular receptor for SARS-CoV (55). The role of ACE2 in HCoV-NL63 infection was demonstrated following isolation and characterization of this recently described group 1 coronavirus (25).

## ACE2, THE SARS-CoV AND HCoV-NL63 RECEPTOR

ACE2 was identified as a functional receptor for SARS-CoV using a direct biochemical approach (55). The S1 region of the SARS-CoV S protein was used to precipitate ACE2 from Vero E6 cells, an African green monkey kidney cell line previously shown to support efficient viral replication. Robust syncytia formed between HEK 293T cells expressing the S protein and those overexpressing ACE2. Transfection of cell lines with ACE2 rendered them permissive to infection with SARS-CoV and with retroviruses pseudotyped with S protein (55, 68). Anti-ACE2 antisera, but not identically prepared anti-ACE1 sera, blocked replication of SARS-CoV, as did a soluble form of ACE2. The surprising observation that the group 1 coronavirus also utilized ACE2, despite its far greater similarity with the group 1 virus HCoV-229E than with group 2 SARS-CoV, was made in 2005 (35, 36, 94).

Many lines of evidence further implicate ACE2 as the principal receptor utilized in vivo by SARS-CoV. ACE2 is expressed in the lung and in the gastrointestinal tract, the major sites of replication of the virus (7, 29, 30, 61). The efficiency of infection in humans, mice, rats, and palm civets correlates with the ability of the ACE2 of each species to support viral replication (54, 58, 86, 98, 101). ACE2 binds S protein specifically, with approximately 2 nM affinity (87). Although many cell lines do not express ACE2, all cell lines shown to support efficient SARS-CoV infection express this receptor (64). The ACE2-binding region of the S protein raises a protective neutralizing antibody response in mice, and anti-S-protein antibodies that block ACE2 association protect mice and hamsters against infection (26, 32, 34, 88). Also, little or no viral replication is observed in ACE2$^{-/-}$ mice (45), whereas mice transgenic for human ACE2 die of a SARS-like syndrome (66). Additional factors may also contribute to the efficiency of infection. DC-SIGNR (L-SIGN, CD209L), DC-SIGN (CD209), and L-SECTIN have been shown to enhance infection of ACE2-expressing cells (25, 42, 64, 103); these proteins do not appear to mediate efficient infection in the absence of ACE2 (42, 64). As described previously, cathepsin L or other alternative proteases are also necessary for efficient infection following ACE2 association (65, 82).

ACE2 is a type I transmembrane protein with a single metalloprotease active site with an HEXXH zinc-binding motif (15, 89). The physiological function of ACE2 remains unclear. The enzyme has been shown to cleave a variety of regulatory peptides in vitro, among them angiotensins I and II, des-Arg-bradykinin, kinetensin, and neurotensin (15, 95). Some cleavage products have been shown to be potent vasodilators with antidiuretic effects. This finding suggests that ACE2 counterbalances the actions of ACE1, which mediates vasoconstriction (12). Furthermore, targeted disruption of ACE2 in mice resulted in severe cardiac contractility defects (12). The enzymatic activity of ACE2 does not contribute to its ability to mediate fusion and viral entry, and small-molecule inhibitors that block catalysis do not inhibit SARS-CoV infection (58). However, ACE2 proteolysis has been implicated in SARS pathogenesis and in acute respiratory distress syndrome caused by other viruses (40, 45). These studies also demonstrated that SARS-CoV S protein can down-regulate pulmonary ACE2 and that soluble ACE2 can protect mice from lung injury in a model of acute respiratory distress syndrome.

## S-PROTEIN RBDs

Discrete, independently folded RBDs of the S proteins of several coronaviruses have been described (2, 3, 5, 46, 100, 102). The first 330 amino acids of the 769-residue S1 subunit of the murine hepatitis virus S protein are sufficient to bind its receptor, carcinoembryonic antigen adhesion molecule 1 (46). A very different region of the S1 domain of HCoV-229E, between residues 407 and 547, is sufficient to associate with CD13 (3, 5). A 192-amino-acid fragment of the SARS-CoV S1 domain, residues 319 to 510, binds human ACE2 with greater efficiency than does the full-length S1 domain (2, 100, 102). The RBDs of these coronaviruses are found in distinct regions of the primary structure of the S protein. This pattern may suggest that coronavirus S proteins are adapted for easy acquisition of novel binding domains or for rapid shifts in receptor usage. However, a larger, less discrete RBD has also been described for HCoV-NL63, perhaps reflecting its longer evolution and selection in the human host (36).

The crystal structure of the SARS-CoV RBD is consistent with this speculative possibility (53). The RBD contains two subdomains: a core and an extended loop. The core is a five-stranded, antiparallel β-sheet, with three short connecting α-helices. The loop, residues 424 to 494, termed the receptor-binding motif (RBM), is the only domain that contacts ACE2 directly. Although the RBD core is homologous with similar regions of other group 2 coronaviruses, the RBM is unique to SARS-CoV. The RBM may have been acquired from another coronavirus, perhaps a group 1 virus relative of HCoV-NL63. As indicated, HCoV-NL63 also enters cells through ACE2 (25), and its extended RBD region includes a stretch of residues with weak homology to the SARS-CoV RBM (36).

Moreover, the recently described SARS-CoV-like viruses isolated from bats lack this stretch of residues, including most residues directly contacting ACE2 (50, 53, 56). The absence of these RBM residues is consistent with the inability of these viruses to grow on tissue culture cells permissive for SARS-CoV (50, 56). If indeed bats are reservoir animals for a SARS-CoV predecessor, acquisition of this ACE2-binding region is likely to have been a critical event in the evolution of the virus. According to this scenario, the virus found in bats utilizes another receptor. A recombination event, perhaps with a group 1 virus similar to HCoV-NL63, occurring in bats, palm civets, or another host may have given rise to SARS-CoV.

Humoral responses are sufficient to protect animals from SARS-CoV infection. A number of independent studies have found the RBD to be the major immunodominant and a potent neutralizing epitope on the S protein (9, 32, 34, 59, 90, 93, 97). Inoculation of the RBD induces potent neutralizing antibody responses in rabbits and mice (33). Neutralizing antibodies are relatively easy to generate against the SARS-CoV RBD, consistent with exposure of this domain (59, 87). Monoclonal antibodies targeted to the SARS-CoV RBD are effective in protecting mice at doses usable in humans (26, 88, 90). Collectively, the data suggest that the SARS-CoV RBD readily elicits antibodies that block replication. The exposure of this domain may reflect its recent acquisition or a strategy in which rapid transmission is favored over immune escape.

## THE S-PROTEIN-BINDING REGIONS OF ACE2

The ability of the ACE2 proteins of mice, rats, and palm civets to support SARS-CoV infection has been compared with that of human ACE2 (54, 58). SARS-CoV infection was less efficient in cells expressing murine ACE2 than in cells expressing the human receptor. Infection was nearly absent in those expressing rat ACE2. Consistent with a role for palm civets in transmitting virus, palm civet ACE2 supported SARS-CoV infection as efficiently as human ACE2. These results correlated with the affinity of each of these receptors for the S protein and its RBD (54, 58). Chimeras between human and rat ACE2 receptors were used to identify the S-protein-binding site on ACE2 (58). Alteration of four rat ACE2 residues (82 to 84 and 353) to their human equivalents converted rat ACE2 to an efficient SARS-CoV receptor. Residues 82 to 84 comprise a glycosylation site on the rat receptor that is not present on the mouse, palm civet, or human receptor. Residue 353 is a histidine in the mouse and rat receptors and a lysine in palm civet and human ACE2. Strikingly, alteration of histidine 353 of mouse ACE2 to the human lysine results in a receptor that supports infection as efficiently as human ACE2 (W. Li, unpublished observation). Alterations of additional residues along the first helix of human ACE2 (lysine 31 and tyrosine 41) to alanine interfered with S-protein-mediated infection and RBD association. Collectively these data localize the S-protein-binding region to the membrane-distal lobe of the cleft that contains the catalytic site of ACE2 (53, 58). Recent data indicate that the HCoV-NL63 S-protein-binding region on ACE2 largely overlaps with that of SARS-CoV, consistent with a recombination event contributing to the latter's use of ACE2 (W. Li and M. Farzan, unpublished data). Of note, a palm civet ACE2 residue, aspartic acid 354, immediately adjacent to critical ACE2 lysine 353, precludes HCoV-NL63 use of this ACE2. Alterations of residues in helix 1 that interfere with SARS-CoV entry also interfere with use of ACE2 by HCoV-NL63 (unpublished data).

## S-PROTEIN VARIATION AMONG SARS-CoV ISOLATES

Three S proteins of distinct origins have been compared for the ability to use human and palm civet ACE2 (58, 75, 104). The first, TOR2, was isolated during the 2002–2003 epidemic (62). The second, designated GD03, was isolated from the sporadic infections in 2003–2004 (31). The third, SZ3, was obtained from palm civets (27). Both SZ3 and, less expectedly, GD03 bound and utilized palm civet ACE2 much more efficiently than human ACE2 (58). In contrast, TOR2 utilized both receptors efficiently. The efficiency with which virus from both human outbreaks utilized the palm civet receptor is consistent with recent transfer of SARS-CoV from palm civets to humans. The lower efficiency with which GD03 utilized human ACE2 compared with TOR2

may in part account for the mildness of symptoms and the absence of subsequent transmission observed during the 2003–2004 infections (59, 83).

The differences in these three S proteins were also reflected in the ability of their RBDs to bind human and palm civet ACE2. Two amino acids, residues 479 and 487, largely determined the much greater efficiency with which the TOR2 RBD bound human ACE2 (58, 75). Residue 479 is an asparagine or serine in all S proteins isolated from humans either during the 2002–2003 epidemic or during 2003–2004 infections. However, most sequences isolated from palm civets or raccoon dogs encode a lysine at this position. This lysine is incompatible with human ACE2, but palm civet ACE2 can efficiently bind S proteins expressing either lysine or asparagine, without an apparent preference for either (58). Palm civets may therefore be an important intermediate in the transfer of SARS-CoV to humans, permitting the emergence of viruses that express a small, uncharged amino acid at S protein residue 479.

Residue 487 is also of interest. Residue 487 is a threonine in all of the more than 100 S protein sequences obtained during the 2002–2003 outbreak (31). It is a serine in S proteins from viruses isolated during the mild 2003–2004 infections and in all but one of the approximately 20 S-protein sequences obtained from palm civets and raccoon dogs. The relatively modest change of threonine in the TOR2 RBD to serine resulted in an approximately 20-fold decrease in binding to human ACE2 (58). A corresponding increase was observed when a threonine was introduced into the SZ3 RBD. A threonine at position 487 also substantially increased association with palm civet ACE2. Notably, the single palm civet-derived S protein sequence that encoded a threonine at position 487 also encoded an asparagine at position 479 (Z. Hu, personal communication). The emergence of this rare combination of S protein residues in palm civet-derived virus may have been necessary to generate a SARS-CoV that could efficiently transmit between humans. The infrequency of threonine 487 in animal-derived viruses may suggest that the receptor of the ultimate reservoir of SARS-CoV better utilizes a serine at this position.

The recently published cocrystal of ACE2 with the SARS-CoV RBD clarifies these observations (53) (Color Plate 4 [see color insert]). TOR2 S-protein asparagine 479, most commonly a lysine in palm civet virus, interacts with a network of residues that include lysine 31 of human ACE2. Palm civet and murine ACE2 express small, uncharged residues at this position, presumably better accommodating an S-protein lysine. S-protein residue 487, a threonine in all epidemic SARS-CoV isolates, directly contacts critical ACE2 lysine 353. Interaction of the threonine methyl group with lysine 353 provides a clear explanation for the decrease in affinity for human and palm civet ACE2 when this threonine is altered to serine.

## REMAINING QUESTIONS

The ability of the group 2 coronavirus SARS-CoV and the group 1 coronavirus HCoV-NL63 to use the same ACE2 receptor raises a number of interesting questions. Did use of ACE2 arise through convergent evolution or, as argued here, through a recombination event and divergent evolution? Are bats indeed the reservoir species of SARS-CoV? What receptor does the SARS-CoV-like virus found in bats use? Did SARS-CoV acquire the ability to use ACE2 in bats or in a marketplace animal that served as a mixing vessel? How can two viruses use the same receptor but nonetheless only one, SARS-CoV, remain dependent on cathepsin L and low pH? Perhaps relatedly, if ACE2 contributes to SARS pathogenesis, why does HCoV-NL63 cause only mild symptoms in infected individuals? Can HCoV-NL63 alter to become more pathogenic through either polymerase errors or recombination? Answers to these questions will be important as we assess the future risk of SARS-CoV and other coronaviruses.

## REFERENCES

1. Arpin, N., and P. J. Talbot. 1990. Molecular characterization of the 229E strain of human coronavirus. *Adv. Exp. Med. Biol.* **276:**73–80.
2. Babcock, G. J., D. J. Esshaki, W. D. Thomas, Jr., and D. M. Ambrosino. 2004. Amino acids 270 to 510 of the severe acute respiratory syndrome coronavirus spike protein are required for interaction with receptor. *J. Virol.* **78:**4552–4560.
3. Bonavia, A., B. D. Zelus, D. E. Wentworth, P. J. Talbot, and K. V. Holmes. 2003. Identification of a receptor-binding domain of the spike glycoprotein of human coronavirus HCoV-229E. *J. Virol.* **77:**2530–2538.
4. Bosch, B. J., R. van der Zee, C. A. de Haan, and P. J. Rottier. 2003. The coronavirus spike protein is a class I virus fusion protein: structural and functional characterization of the fusion core complex. *J. Virol.* **77:**8801–8811.
5. Breslin, J. J., I. Mørk, M. K. Smith, L. K. Vogel, E. M. Hemmila, A. Bonavia, P. J. Talbot, H. Sjöström, O. Norén, and K. V. Holmes. 2003. Human coronavirus 229E: receptor binding domain and neutralization by soluble receptor at 37°C. *J. Virol.* **77:**4435–4438.
6. Casais, R., B. Dove, D. Cavanagh, and P. Britton. 2003. Recombinant avian infectious bronchitis virus expressing a heterologous spike gene demonstrates that the spike protein is a determinant of cell tropism. *J. Virol.* **77:**9084–9089.
7. Chan, P. K., K. F. To, A. W. Lo, J. L. Cheung, I. Chu, F. W. Au, J. H. Tong, J. S. Tam, J. J. Sung, and H. K. Ng. 2004. Persistent infection of SARS coronavirus in colonic cells in vitro. *J. Med. Virol.* **74:**1–7.

8. Chandran, K., N. J. Sullivan, U. Felbor, S. P. Whelan, and J. M. Cunningham. 2005. Endosomal proteolysis of the Ebola virus glycoprotein is necessary for infection. *Science* **308:**1643–1645. [Epub 14 April 2005.]
9. Chen, Z., L. Zhang, C. Qin, L. Ba, C. E. Yi, F. Zhang, Q. Wei, T. He, W. Yu, J. Yu, H. Gao, X. Tu, A. Gettie, M. Farzan, K. Y. Yuen, and D. D. Ho. 2005. Recombinant modified vaccinia virus Ankara expressing the spike glycoprotein of severe acute respiratory syndrome coronavirus induces protective neutralizing antibodies primarily targeting the receptor binding region. *J. Virol.* **79:**2678–2688.
10. Cherry, J. D. 2004. The chronology of the 2002-2003 SARS mini pandemic. *Paediatr. Respir. Rev.* **5:**262–269.
11. Colman, P. M., and M. C. Lawrence. 2003. The structural biology of type I viral membrane fusion. *Nat. Rev. Mol. Cell Biol.* **4:**309–319.
12. Crackower, M. A., R. Sarao, G. Y. Oudit, C. Yagil, I. Kozieradzki, S. E. Scanga, A. J. Oliveira-dos-Santos, J. da Costa, L. Zhang, Y. Pei, J. Scholey, C. M. Ferrario, A. S. Manoukian, M. C. Chappell, P. H. Backx, Y. Yagil, and J. M. Penninger. 2002. Angiotensin-converting enzyme 2 is an essential regulator of heart function. *Nature* **417:**822–828.
13. Delmas, B., J. Gelfi, R. L'Haridon, L. K. Vogel, H. Sjostrom, O. Noren, and H. Laude. 1992. Aminopeptidase N is a major receptor for the entero-pathogenic coronavirus TGEV. *Nature* **357:**417–420.
14. Dimitrov, D. S. 2004. Virus entry: molecular mechanisms and biomedical applications. *Nat. Rev. Microbiol.* **2:**109–122.
15. Donoghue, M., F. Hsieh, E. Baronas, K. Godbout, M. Gosselin, N. Stagliano, M. Donovan, B. Woolf, K. Robison, R. Jeyaseelan, R. E. Breitbart, and S. Acton. 2000. A novel angiotensin-converting enzyme-related carboxypeptidase (ACE2) converts angiotensin I to angiotensin 1–9. *Circ. Res.* **87:**E1–E9.
16. Drosten, C., S. Gunther, W. Preiser, S. van der Werf, H. R. Brodt, S. Becker, H. Rabenau, M. Panning, L. Kolesnikova, R. A. Fouchier, A. Berger, A. M. Burguiere, J. Cinatl, M. Eickmann, N. Escriou, K. Grywna, S. Kramme, J. C. Manuguerra, S. Muller, V. Rickerts, M. Sturmer, S. Vieth, H. D. Klenk, A. D. Osterhaus, H. Schmitz, and H. W. Doerr. 2003. Identification of a novel coronavirus in patients with severe acute respiratory syndrome. *N. Engl. J. Med.* **348:**1967–1976.
17. Dveksler, G. S., M. N. Pensiero, C. B. Cardellichio, R. K. Williams, G. S. Jiang, K. V. Holmes, and C. W. Dieffenbach. 1991. Cloning of the mouse hepatitis virus (MHV) receptor: expression in human and hamster cell lines confers susceptibility to MHV. *J. Virol.* **65:**6881–6891.
18. Esper, F., C. Weibel, D. Ferguson, M. L. Landry, and J. S. Kahn. 2005. Evidence of a novel human coronavirus that is associated with respiratory tract disease in infants and young children. *J. Infect. Dis.* **191:**492–498. [Epub 14 January 2005.]
19. Fleck, F. 2004. SARS virus returns to China as scientists race to find effective vaccine. *Bull. W. H. O.* **82:**152–153.
20. Fouchier, R. A., T. Kuiken, M. Schutten, G. van Amerongen, G. J. van Doornum, B. G. van den Hoogen, M. Peiris, W. Lim, K. Stohr, and A. D. Osterhaus. 2003. Aetiology: Koch's postulates fulfilled for SARS virus. *Nature* **423:**240.
21. Gallagher, T. M., and M. J. Buchmeier. 2001. Coronavirus spike proteins in viral entry and pathogenesis. *Virology* **279:**371–374.
22. Gibbs, A. J., M. J. Gibbs, and J. S. Armstrong. 2004. The phylogeny of SARS coronavirus. *Arch. Virol.* **149:**621–624. [Epub 5 January 2004.]

23. Gonzalez, J. M., P. Gomez-Puertas, D. Cavanagh, A. E. Gorbalenya, and L. Enjuanes. 2003. A comparative sequence analysis to revise the current taxonomy of the family Coronaviridae. *Arch. Virol.* **148:**2207–2235.

24. Gorbalenya, A. E., E. J. Snijder, and W. J. Spaan. 2004. Severe acute respiratory syndrome coronavirus phylogeny: toward consensus. *J. Virol.* **78:**7863–7866.

25. Gramberg, T., H. Hofmann, P. Moller, P. F. Lalor, A. Marzi, M. Geier, M. Krumbiegel, T. Winkler, F. Kirchhoff, D. H. Adams, S. Becker, J. Munch, and S. Pohlmann. 2005. LSECtin interacts with filovirus glycoproteins and the spike protein of SARS coronavirus. *Virology* **340:**224–236.

26. Greenough, T. C., G. J. Babcock, A. Roberts, H. J. Hernandez, W. D. Thomas, Jr., J. A. Coccia, R. F. Graziano, M. Srinivasan, I. Lowy, R. W. Finberg, K. Subbarao, L. Vogel, M. Somasundaran, K. Luzuriaga, J. L. Sullivan, and D. M. Ambrosino. 2005. Development and characterization of a severe acute respiratory syndrome-associated coronavirus-neutralizing human monoclonal antibody that provides effective immunoprophylaxis in mice. *J. Infect. Dis.* **191:**507–514. [Epub 14 January 2005.]

27. Guan, Y., B. J. Zheng, Y. Q. He, X. L. Liu, Z. X. Zhuang, C. L. Cheung, S. W. Luo, P. H. Li, L. J. Zhang, Y. J. Guan, K. M. Butt, K. L. Wong, K. W. Chan, W. Lim, K. F. Shortridge, K. Y. Yuen, J. S. Peiris, and L. L. Poon. 2003. Isolation and characterization of viruses related to the SARS coronavirus from animals in southern China. *Science* **302:**276–278.

28. Haijema, B. J., H. Volders, and P. J. M. Rottier. 2003. Switching species tropism: an effective way to manipulate the feline coronavirus genome. *J. Virol.* **77:**4528–4538.

29. Hamming, I., W. Timens, M. L. Bulthuis, A. T. Lely, G. J. Navis, and H. van Goor. 2004. Tissue distribution of ACE2 protein, the functional receptor for SARS coronavirus. A first step in understanding SARS pathogenesis. *J. Pathol.* **203:**631–637.

30. Harmer, D., M. Gilbert, R. Borman, and K. L. Clark. 2002. Quantitative mRNA expression profiling of ACE 2, a novel homologue of angiotensin converting enzyme. *FEBS Lett.* **532:**107–110.

31. He, J.-F., G.-W. Peng, J. Min, D.-W. Yu, W.-J. Liang, S.-Y. Zhang, R.-H. Xu, H.-Y. Zheng, X.-W. Wu, J. Xu, Z.-H. Wang, L. Fang, X. Zhang, H. Li, X.-G. Yan, J.-H. Lu, Z.-H. Hu, J.-C. Huang, X. W. Wan, et al. 2004. Molecular evolution of the SARS coronavirus during the course of the SARS epidemic in China. *Science* **303:**1666–1669. [Epub 29 January 2004.]

32. He, Y., H. Lu, P. Siddiqui, Y. Zhou, and S. Jiang. 2005. Receptor-binding domain of severe acute respiratory syndrome coronavirus spike protein contains multiple conformation-dependent epitopes that induce highly potent neutralizing antibodies. *J. Immunol.* **174:**4908–4915.

33. He, Y., Y. Zhou, S. Liu, Z. Kou, W. Li, M. Farzan, and S. Jiang. 2004. Receptor-binding domain of SARS-CoV spike protein induces highly potent neutralizing antibodies: implication for developing subunit vaccine. *Biochem. Biophys. Res. Commun.* **324:**773–781.

34. He, Y., Y. Zhou, H. Wu, B. Luo, J. Chen, W. Li, and S. Jiang. 2004. Identification of immunodominant sites on the spike protein of severe acute respiratory syndrome (SARS) coronavirus: implication for developing SARS diagnostics and vaccines. *J. Immunol.* **173:**4050–4057.

35. Hofmann, H., K. Pyrc, L. van der Hoek, M. Geier, B. Berkhout, and S. Pohlmann. 2005. Human coronavirus NL63 employs the severe acute respiratory syndrome coronavirus receptor for cellular entry. *Proc. Natl. Acad. Sci. USA* **102:**7988–7993.

36. Hofmann, H., G. Simmons, A. J. Rennekamp, C. Chaipan, T. Gramberg, E. Heck, M. Geier, A. Wegele, A. Marzi, P. Bates, and S. Pohlmann. 2006. Highly conserved regions within the spike proteins of human coronaviruses 229E and NL63 determine recognition of their respective cellular receptors. *J. Virol.* **80:**8639–8652.

37. Holmes, E. C., and A. Rambaut. 2004. Viral evolution and the emergence of SARS coronavirus. *Philos. Trans. R. Soc. Lond. B* **359:**1059–1065.

38. Huang, I. C., B. J. Bosch, F. Li, W. Li, K. H. Lee, S. Ghiran, N. Vasilieva, T. S. Dermody, S. C. Harrison, P. R. Dormitzer, M. Farzan, P. J. Rottier, and H. Choe. 2006. SARS coronavirus, but not human coronavirus NL63, utilizes cathepsin L to infect ACE2-expressing cells. *J. Biol. Chem.* **281:**3198–3203.

39. Huang, I. C., B. J. Bosch, W. Li, M. Farzan, P. M. Rottier, and H. Choe. 2006. SARS-CoV, but not HCoV-NL63, utilizes cathepsins to infect cells: viral entry. *Adv. Exp. Med. Biol.* **581:**335–338.

40. Imai, Y., K. Kuba, S. Rao, Y. Huan, F. Guo, B. Guan, P. Yang, R. Sarao, T. Wada, H. Leong-Poi, M. A. Crackower, A. Fukamizu, C. C. Hui, L. Hein, S. Uhlig, A. S. Slutsky, C. Jiang, and J. M. Penninger. 2005. Angiotensin-converting enzyme 2 protects from severe acute lung failure. *Nature* **436:**112–116.

41. Jackwood, M. W., D. A. Hilt, S. A. Callison, C. W. Lee, H. Plaza, and E. Wade. 2001. Spike glycoprotein cleavage recognition site analysis of infectious bronchitis virus. *Avian Dis.* **45:**366–372.

42. Jeffers, S. A., S. M. Tusell, L. Gillim-Ross, E. M. Hemmila, J. E. Achenbach, G. J. Babcock, W. D. Thomas, Jr., L. B. Thackray, M. D. Young, R. J. Mason, D. M. Ambrosino, D. E. Wentworth, J. C. Demartini, and K. V. Holmes. 2004. CD209L (L-SIGN) is a receptor for severe acute respiratory syndrome coronavirus. *Proc. Natl. Acad. Sci. USA* **101:**15748–15753.

43. Kan, B., M. Wang, H. Jing, H. Xu, X. Jiang, M. Yan, W. Liang, H. Zheng, K. Wan, Q. Liu, B. Cui, Y. Xu, E. Zhang, H. Wang, J. Ye, G. Li, M. Li, Z. Cui, X. Qi, K. Chen, L. Du, K. Gao, Y.-T. Zhao, X.-Z. Zou, Y.-J. Feng, Y.-F. Gao, R. Hai, D. Yu, Y. Guan, and J. Xu. 2005. Molecular evolution analysis and geographic investigation of severe acute respiratory syndrome coronavirus-like virus in palm civets at an animal market and on farms. *J. Virol.* **79:**11892–11900.

44. Ksiazek, T. G., D. Erdman, C. S. Goldsmith, S. R. Zaki, T. Peret, S. Emery, S. Tong, C. Urbani, J. A. Comer, W. Lim, P. E. Rollin, S. F. Dowell, A. E. Ling, C. D. Humphrey, W. J. Shieh, J. Guarner, C. D. Paddock, P. Rota, B. Fields, J. DeRisi, J. Y. Yang, N. Cox, J. M. Hughes, J. W. LeDuc, W. J. Bellini, and L. J. Anderson. 2003. A novel coronavirus associated with severe acute respiratory syndrome. *N. Engl. J. Med.* **348:**1953–1966.

45. Kuba, K., Y. Imai, S. Rao, H. Gao, F. Guo, B. Guan, Y. Huan, P. Yang, Y. Zhang, W. Deng, L. Bao, B. Zhang, G. Liu, Z. Wang, M. Chappell, Y. Liu, D. Zheng, A. Leibbrandt, T. Wada, A. S. Slutsky, D. Liu, C. Qin, C. Jiang, and J. M. Penninger. 2005. A crucial role of angiotensin converting enzyme 2 (ACE2) in SARS coronavirus-induced lung injury. *Nat. Med.* **11:**875–879.

46. Kubo, H., Y. K. Yamada, and F. Taguchi. 1994. Localization of neutralizing epitopes and the receptor-binding site within the amino-terminal 330 amino acids of the murine coronavirus spike protein. *J. Virol.* **68:**5403–5410.

47. Kuiken, T., R. A. Fouchier, M. Schutten, G. F. Rimmelzwaan, G. van Amerongen, D. van Riel, J. D. Laman, T. de Jong, G. van Doornum, W. Lim, A. E. Ling, P. K. Chan, J. S. Tam,

M. C. Zambon, R. Gopal, C. Drosten, S. van der Werf, N. Escriou, J. C. Manuguerra, K. Stohr, J. S. Peiris, and A. D. Osterhaus. 2003. Newly discovered coronavirus as the primary cause of severe acute respiratory syndrome. *Lancet* **362**:263–270.

48. Kuo, L., G. J. Godeke, M. J. Raamsman, P. S. Masters, and P. J. Rottier. 2000. Retargeting of coronavirus by substitution of the spike glycoprotein ectodomain: crossing the host cell species barrier. *J. Virol.* **74**:1393–1406.

49. Lai, M. M., and D. Cavanagh. 1997. The molecular biology of coronaviruses. *Adv. Virus Res.* **48**:1–100.

50. Lau, S. K., P. C. Woo, K. S. Li, Y. Huang, H. W. Tsoi, B. H. Wong, S. S. Wong, S. Y. Leung, K. H. Chan, and K. Y. Yuen. 2005. Severe acute respiratory syndrome coronavirus-like virus in Chinese horseshoe bats. *Proc. Natl. Acad. Sci. USA* **102**:14040–14045. [Epub 16 September 2005.]

51. Lee, N., D. Hui, A. Wu, P. Chan, P. Cameron, G. M. Joynt, A. Ahuja, M. Y. Yung, C. B. Leung, K. F. To, S. F. Lui, C. C. Szeto, S. Chung, and J. J. Sung. 2003. A major outbreak of severe acute respiratory syndrome in Hong Kong. *N. Engl. J. Med.* **348**:1986–1994.

52. Leparc-Goffart, I., S. T. Hingley, M. M. Chua, J. Phillips, E. Lavi, and S. R. Weiss. 1998. Targeted recombination within the spike gene of murine coronavirus mouse hepatitis virus-A59: Q159 is a determinant of hepatotropism. *J. Virol.* **72**:9628–9636.

53. Li, F., W. Li, M. Farzan, and S. C. Harrison. 2005. Structure of SARS coronavirus spike receptor-binding domain complexed with receptor. *Science* **309**:1864–1868.

54. Li, W., T. C. Greenough, M. J. Moore, N. Vasilieva, M. Somasundaran, J. L. Sullivan, M. Farzan, and H. Choe. 2004. Efficient replication of severe acute respiratory syndrome coronavirus in mouse cells is limited by murine angiotensin-converting enzyme 2. *J. Virol.* **78**:11429–11433.

55. Li, W., M. J. Moore, N. Vasilieva, J. Sui, S. K. Wong, M. A. Berne, M. Somasundaran, J. L. Sullivan, C. Luzeriaga, T. C. Greenough, H. Choe, and M. Farzan. 2003. Angiotensin-converting enzyme 2 is a functional receptor for the SARS coronavirus. *Nature* **426**:450–454.

56. Li, W., Z. Shi, M. Yu, W. Ren, C. Smith, J. H. Epstein, H. Wang, G. Crameri, Z. Hu, H. Zhang, J. Zhang, J. McEachern, H. Field, P. Daszak, B. T. Eaton, S. Zhang, and L. F. Wang. 2005. Bats are natural reservoirs of SARS-like coronaviruses. *Science* **310**:676–679.

57. Li, W., S.-K. Wong, F. Li, J. H. Kuhn, I.-C. Huang, H. Choe, and M. Farzan. 2006. Animal origins of the severe acute respiratory syndrome coronavirus: insight from ACE2-S-protein interactions. *J. Virol.* **80**:4211–4219.

58. Li, W., C. Zhang, J. Sui, J. H. Kuhn, M. J. Moore, S. Luo, S. K. Wong, I. C. Huang, K. Xu, N. Vasilieva, A. Murakami, Y. He, W. A. Marasco, Y. Guan, H. Choe, and M. Farzan. 2005. Receptor and viral determinants of SARS-coronavirus adaptation to human ACE2. *EMBO J.* **24**:1634–1643.

59. Liang, G., Q. Chen, J. Xu, Y. Liu, W. Lim, J. S. Peiris, L. J. Anderson, L. Ruan, H. Li, B. Kan, B. Di, P. Cheng, K. H. Chan, D. D. Erdman, S. Gu, X. Yan, W. Liang, D. Zhou, L. Haynes, S. Duan, X. Zhang, H. Zheng, Y. Gao, S. Tong, D. Li, L. Fang, P. Qin, and W. Xu. 2004. Laboratory diagnosis of four recent sporadic cases of community-acquired SARS, Guangdong Province, China. *Emerg. Infect. Dis.* **10**:1774–1781.

60. Lim, P. L., A. Kurup, G. Gopalakrishna, K. P. Chan, C. W. Wong, L. C. Ng, S. Y. Se-Thoe, L. Oon, X. Bai, L. W. Stanton, Y. Ruan, L. D. Miller, V. B. Vega, L. James, P. L. Ooi, C. S. Kai, S. J. Olsen, B. Ang, and Y. S. Leo. 2004. Laboratory-acquired severe acute respiratory syndrome. *N. Engl. J. Med.* **350**:1740–1745.

61. Liu, B. H., D. L. Wu, D. W. Zhan, E. D. Qin, Q. Y. Zhu, C. E. Wang, Q. W. Meng, W. M. Peng, X. N. Yin, Y. H. Yang, Y. T. Guan, W. G. Han, C. W. Li, Y. G. Liu, M. P. Wang, Q. G. Liu, H. Y. Shi, and Z. F. Ding. 2004. Study on the animal model for severe acute respiratory syndrome. *Wei Sheng Wu Xue Bao* **44**:711–716. (In Mandarin Chinese.)

62. Marra, M. A., S. J. M. Jones, C. R. Astell, R. A. Holt, A. Brooks-Wilson, Y. S. N. Butterfield, J. Khattra, J. K. Asano, S. A. Barber, S. Y. Chan, A. Cloutier, S. M. Coughlin, D. Freeman, N. Girn, O. L. Griffith, S. R. Leach, M. Mayo, H. McDonald, S. B. Montgomery, P. K. Pandoh, A. S. Petrescu, A. G. Robertson, J. E. Schein, A. Siddiqui, D. E. Smailus, J. M. Stott, G. S. Yang, F. Plummer, A. Andonov, H. Artsob, N. Bastien, K. Bernard, T. F. Booth, D. Bowness, M. Czub, M. Drebot, L. Fernando, R. Flick, M. Garbutt, M. Gray, A. Grolla, S. Jones, H. Feldmann, A. Meyers, A. Kabani, Y. Li, S. Normand, U. Stroher, G. A. Tipples, S. Tyler, R. Vogrig, D. Ward, B. Watson, R. C. Brunham, M. Krajden, M. Petric, D. M. Skowronski, C. Upton, and R. L. Roper. 2003. The genome sequence of the SARS-associated coronavirus. *Science* **300**:1399–1404.

63. Martina, B. E., B. L. Haagmans, T. Kuiken, R. A. Fouchier, G. F. Rimmelzwaan, G. Van Amerongen, J. S. Peiris, W. Lim, and A. D. Osterhaus. 2003. Virology: SARS virus infection of cats and ferrets. *Nature* **425**:915.

64. Marzi, A., T. Gramberg, G. Simmons, P. Moller, A. J. Rennekamp, M. Krumbiegel, M. Geier, J. Eisemann, N. Turza, B. Saunier, A. Steinkasserer, S. Becker, P. Bates, H. Hofmann, and S. Pohlmann. 2004. DC-SIGN and DC-SIGNR interact with the glycoprotein of Marburg virus and the S protein of severe acute respiratory syndrome coronavirus. *J .Virol.* **78**:12090–12095.

65. Matsuyama, S., M. Ujike, S. Morikawa, M. Tashiro, and F. Taguchi. 2005. Protease-mediated enhancement of severe acute respiratory syndrome coronavirus infection. *Proc. Natl. Acad. Sci. USA* **102**:12543–12547.

66. McCray, P. B., Jr., L. Pewe, C. Wohlford-Lenane, M. Hickey, L. Manzel, L. Shi, J. Netland, H. P. Jia, C. Halabi, C. D. Sigmund, D. K. Meyerholz, P. Kirby, D. C. Look, and S. Perlman. 2007. Lethal Infection of K18-*hACE2* mice infected with severe acute respiratory syndrome coronavirus. *J. Virol.* **81**:813–821.

67. McIntosh, K. 2005. Coronaviruses in the limelight. *J. Infect. Dis.* **191**:489–491. [Epub 14 January 2005.]

68. Moore, M. J., T. Dorfman, W. Li, S. K. Wong, Y. Li, J. H. Kuhn, J. Coderre, N. Vasilieva, Z. Han, T. C. Greenough, M. Farzan, and H. Choe. 2004. Retroviruses pseudotyped with the severe acute respiratory syndrome coronavirus spike protein efficiently infect cells expressing angiotensin-converting enzyme 2. *J. Virol.* **78**:10628–10635.

69. Normile, D. 2004. Infectious diseases. Mounting lab accidents raise SARS fears. *Science* **304**:659–661.

70. Osterhaus, A. D., R. A. Fouchier, and T. Kuiken. 2004. The aetiology of SARS: Koch's postulates fulfilled. *Philos. Trans. R. Soc. Lond. B* **359**:1081–1082.

71. Peiris, J. S., S. T. Lai, L. L. Poon, Y. Guan, L. Y. Yam, W. Lim, J. Nicholls, W. K. Yee, W. W. Yan, M. T. Cheung, V. C. Cheng, K. H. Chan, D. N. Tsang, R. W. Yung, T. K. Ng, and K. Y. Yuen. 2003. Coronavirus as a possible cause of severe acute respiratory syndrome. *Lancet* **361**:1319–1325.

72. Phillips, J. J., M. M. Chua, E. Lavi, and S. R. Weiss. 1999. Pathogenesis of chimeric MHV4/MHV-A59 recombinant viruses: the murine coronavirus spike protein is a major determinant of neurovirulence. *J. Virol.* **73**:7752–7760.

73. Poon, L. L., D. K. Chu, K. H. Chan, O. K. Wong, T. M. Ellis, Y. H. Leung, S. K. Lau, P. C. Woo, K. Y. Suen, K. Y. Yuen,

Y. Guan, and J. S. Peiris. 2005. Identification of a novel coronavirus in bats. *J. Virol.* **79:**2001–2009.

74. Qin, C., J. Wang, Q. Wei, M. She, W. A. Marasco, H. Jiang, X. Tu, H. Zhu, L. Ren, H. Gao, L. Guo, L. Huang, R. Yang, Z. Cong, Y. Wang, Y. Liu, Y. Sun, S. Duan, J. Qu, L. Chen, W. Tong, L. Ruan, P. Liu, H. Zhang, J. Zhang, D. Liu, Q. Liu, T. Hong, and W. He. 2005. An animal model of SARS produced by infection of Macaca mulatta with SARS coronavirus. *J. Pathol.* **206:**251–259.

75. Qu, X. X., P. Hao, X. J. Song, S. M. Jiang, Y. X. Liu, P. G. Wang, X. Rao, H. D. Song, S. Y. Wang, Y. Zuo, A. H. Zheng, M. Luo, H. L. Wang, F. Deng, H. Z. Wang, Z. H. Hu, M. X. Ding, G. P. Zhao, and H. K. Deng. 2005. Identification of two critical amino acid residues of the severe acute respiratory syndrome coronavirus spike protein for its variation in zoonotic tropism transition via a double substitution strategy. *J. Biol. Chem.* **280:**29588–29595.

76. Roberts, A., L. Vogel, J. Guarner, N. Hayes, B. Murphy, S. Zaki, and K. Subbarao. 2005. Severe acute respiratory syndrome coronavirus infection of golden Syrian hamsters. *J. Virol.* **79:**503–511.

77. Rota, P. A., M. S. Oberste, S. S. Monroe, W. A. Nix, R. Campagnoli, J. P. Icenogle, S. Penaranda, B. Bankamp, K. Maher, M.-H. Chen, S. Tong, A. Tamin, L. Lowe, M. Frace, J. L. DeRisi, Q. Chen, D. Wang, D. D. Erdman, T. C. T. Peret, C. Burns, T. G. Ksiazek, P. E. Rollin, A. Sanchez, S. Liffick, B. Holloway, J. Limor, K. McCaustland, M. Olsen-Rasmussen, R. Fouchier, S. Gunther, A. D. M. E. Osterhaus, C. Drosten, M. A. Pallansch, L. J. Anderson, and W. J. Bellini. 2003. Characterization of a novel coronavirus associated with severe acute respiratory syndrome. *Science* **300:**1394–1399.

78. Rowe, T., G. Gao, R. J. Hogan, R. G. Crystal, T. G. Voss, R. L. Grant, P. Bell, G. P. Kobinger, N. A. Wivel, and J. M. Wilson. 2004. Macaque model for severe acute respiratory syndrome. *J. Virol.* **78:**11401–11404.

79. Sanchez, C. M., A. Izeta, J. M. Sanchez-Morgado, S. Alonso, I. Sola, M. Balasch, J. Plana-Duran, and L. Enjuanes. 1999. Targeted recombination demonstrates that the spike gene of transmissible gastroenteritis coronavirus is a determinant of its enteric tropism and virulence. *J. Virol.* **73:**7607–7618.

80. Schickli, J. H., L. B. Thackray, S. G. Sawicki, and K. V. Holmes. 2004. The N-terminal region of the murine coronavirus spike glycoprotein is associated with the extended host range of viruses from persistently infected murine cells. *J. Virol.* **78:**9073–9083.

81. Schultze, B., and G. Herrler. 1992. Bovine coronavirus uses N-acetyl-9-O-acetylneuraminic acid as a receptor determinant to initiate the infection of cultured cells. *J. Gen. Virol.* **73** (Pt. 4):901–906.

82. Simmons, G., D. N. Gosalia, A. J. Rennekamp, J. D. Reeves, S. L. Diamond, and P. Bates. 2005. Inhibitors of cathepsin L prevent severe acute respiratory syndrome coronavirus entry. *Proc. Natl. Acad. Sci. USA* **102:**11876–11881.

83. Song, H. D., C. C. Tu, G. W. Zhang, S. Y. Wang, K. Zheng, L. C. Lei, Q. X. Chen, Y. W. Gao, H. Q. Zhou, H. Xiang, H. J. Zheng, S. W. Chern, F. Cheng, C. M. Pan, H. Xuan, S. J. Chen, H. M. Luo, D. H. Zhou, Y. F. Liu, J. F. He, P. Z. Qin, L. H. Li, Y. Q. Ren, W. J. Liang, Y. D. Yu, L. Anderson, M. Wang, R. H. Xu, X. W. Wu, H. Y. Zheng, J. D. Chen, G. Liang, Y. Gao, M. Liao, L. Fang, L. Y. Jiang, H. Li, F. Chen, B. Di, L. J. He, J. Y. Lin, S. Tong, X. Kong, L. Du, P. Hao, H. Tang, A. Bernini, X. J. Yu, O. Spiga, Z. M. Guo, H. Y. Pan, W. Z. He, J. C. Manuguerra, A. Fontanet, A. Danchin, N. Niccolai, Y. X. Li, C. I. Wu, and G. P. Zhao. 2005. Cross-host evolution of severe acute respiratory syndrome coronavirus in palm civet and

human. *Proc. Natl. Acad. Sci. USA* **102:**2430–2435. [Epub 4 February 2005.]

84. Sturman, L. S., and K. V. Holmes. 1984. Proteolytic cleavage of peplomeric glycoprotein E2 of MHV yields two 90K subunits and activates cell fusion. *Adv. Exp. Med. Biol.* **173:** 25–35.

85. Sturman, L. S., C. S. Ricard, and K. V. Holmes. 1985. Proteolytic cleavage of the E2 glycoprotein of murine coronavirus: activation of cell-fusing activity of virions by trypsin and separation of two different 90K cleavage fragments. *J. Virol.* **56:**904–911.

86. Subbarao, K., J. McAuliffe, L. Vogel, G. Fahle, S. Fischer, K. Tatti, M. Packard, W. J. Shieh, S. Zaki, and B. Murphy. 2004. Prior infection and passive transfer of neutralizing antibody prevent replication of severe acute respiratory syndrome coronavirus in the respiratory tract of mice. *J. Virol.* **78:**3572–3577.

87. Sui, J., W. Li, A. Murakami, A. Tamin, L. J. Matthews, S. K. Wong, M. J. Moore, A. St-Clair Tallarico, M. Olurinde, H. Choe, L. J. Anderson, W. J. Bellini, M. Farzan, and W. A. Marasco. 2004. Potent neutralization of severe acute respiratory syndrome (SARS) coronavirus by a human mAb to S1 protein that blocks receptor association. *Proc. Natl. Acad. Sci. USA* **101:**2536–2541.

88. Sui, J., W. Li, A. Roberts, L. J. Matthews, A. Murakami, L. Vogel, S. K. Wong, K. Subbarao, M. Farzan, and W. A. Marasco. 2005. Evaluation of human monoclonal antibody 80R for immunoprophylaxis of severe acute respiratory syndrome by an animal study, epitope mapping, and analysis of spike variants. *J. Virol.* **79:**5900–5906.

89. Tipnis, S. R., N. M. Hooper, R. Hyde, E. Karran, G. Christie, and A. J. Turner. 2000. A human homolog of angiotensin-converting enzyme. Cloning and functional expression as a captopril-insensitive carboxypeptidase. *J. Biol. Chem.* **275:** 33238–33243.

90. Traggiai, E., S. Becker, K. Subbarao, L. Kolesnikova, Y. Uematsu, M. R. Gismondo, B. R. Murphy, R. Rappuoli, and A. Lanzavecchia. 2004. An efficient method to make human monoclonal antibodies from memory B cells: potent neutralization of SARS coronavirus. *Nat. Med.* **10:**871–875.

91. Tsai, J. C., B. D. Zelus, K. V. Holmes, and S. R. Weiss. 2003. The N-terminal domain of the murine coronavirus spike glycoprotein determines the CEACAM1 receptor specificity of the virus strain. *J. Virol.* **77:**841–850.

92. Tu, C., G. Crameri, X. Kong, J. Chen, Y. Sun, M. Yu, H. Xiang, X. Xia, S. Liu, T. Ren, Y. Yu, B. T. Eaton, H. Xuan, and L. F. Wang. 2004. Antibodies to SARS coronavirus in civets. *Emerg. Infect. Dis.* **10:**2244–2248.

93. van den Brink, E. N., J. Ter Meulen, F. Cox, M. A. Jongeneelen, A. Thijsse, M. Throsby, W. E. Marissen, P. M. Rood, A. B. Bakker, H. R. Gelderblom, B. E. Martina, A. D. Osterhaus, W. Preiser, H. W. Doerr, J. de Kruif, and J. Goudsmit. 2005. Molecular and biological characterization of human monoclonal antibodies binding to the spike and nucleocapsid proteins of severe acute respiratory syndrome coronavirus. *J. Virol.* **79:**1635–1644.

94. van der Hoek, L., K. Pyrc, M. F. Jebbink, W. Vermeulen-Oost, R. J. Berkhout, K. C. Wolthers, P. M. Wertheim-van Dillen, J. Kaandorp, J. Spaargaren, and B. Berkhout. 2004. Identification of a new human coronavirus. *Nat. Med.* **10:**368–373.

95. Vickers, C., P. Hales, V. Kaushik, L. Dick, J. Gavin, J. Tang, K. Godbout, T. Parsons, E. Baronas, F. Hsieh, S. Acton, M. Patane, A. Nichols, and P. Tummino. 2002. Hydrolysis of biological peptides by human angiotensin-converting enzyme-related carboxypeptidase. *J. Biol. Chem.* **277:**14838–14843.

96. Wang, M., H. Q. Jing, H. F. Xu, X. G. Jiang, B. Kan, Q. Y. Liu, K. L. Wan, B. Y. Cui, H. Zheng, Z. G. Cui, M. Y. Yan, W. L. Liang, H. X. Wang, X. B. Qi, Z. J. Li, M. C. Li, K. Chen, E. M. Zhang, S. Y. Zhang, R. Hai, D. Z. Yu, and J. G. Xu. 2005. Surveillance on severe acute respiratory syndrome associated coronavirus in animals at a live animal market of Guangzhou in 2004. *Zhonghua Liu Xing Bing Xue Za Zhi* **26**:84–87. (In Mandarin Chinese.)

97. Wang, S., T. H. Chou, P. V. Sakhatskyy, S. Huang, J. M. Lawrence, H. Cao, X. Huang, and S. Lu. 2005. Identification of two neutralizing regions on the severe acute respiratory syndrome coronavirus spike glycoprotein produced from the mammalian expression system. *J. Virol.* **79**: 1906–1910.

98. Wentworth, D. E., L. Gillim-Ross, N. Espina, and K. A. Bernard. 2004. Mice susceptible to SARS coronavirus. *Emerg. Infect. Dis.* **10**:1293–1296.

99. Williams, R. K., G. S. Jiang, and K. V. Holmes. 1991. Receptor for mouse hepatitis virus is a member of the carcinoembryonic antigen family of glycoproteins. *Proc. Natl. Acad. Sci. USA* **88**:5533–5536.

100. Wong, S. K., W. Li, M. J. Moore, H. Choe, and M. Farzan. 2004. A 193-amino acid fragment of the SARS coronavirus S protein efficiently binds angiotensin-converting enzyme 2. *J. Biol. Chem.* **279**:3197–3201. [Epub 11 December 2003.]

101. Wu, D., C. Tu, C. Xin, H. Xuan, Q. Meng, Y. Liu, Y. Yu, Y. Guan, Y. Jiang, X. Yin, G. Crameri, M. Wang, C. Li, S. Liu, M. Liao, L. Feng, H. Xiang, J. Sun, J. Chen, Y. Sun, S. Gu, N. Liu, D. Fu, B. T. Eaton, L. F. Wang, and X. Kong. 2005. Civets are equally susceptible to experimental infection by two different severe acute respiratory syndrome coronavirus isolates. *J. Virol.* **79**:2620–2625.

102. Xiao, X., S. Chakraborti, A. S. Dimitrov, K. Gramatikoff, and D. S. Dimitrov. 2003. The SARS-CoV S glycoprotein: expression and functional characterization. *Biochem. Biophys. Res. Commun.* **312**:1159–1164.

103. Yang, Z. Y., Y. Huang, L. Ganesh, K. Leung, W. P. Kong, O. Schwartz, K. Subbarao, and G. J. Nabel. 2004. pH-dependent entry of severe acute respiratory syndrome coronavirus is mediated by the spike glycoprotein and enhanced by dendritic cell transfer through DC-SIGN. *J. Virol.* **78**:5642–5650.

104. Yang, Z. Y., H. C. Werner, W. P. Kong, K. Leung, E. Traggiai, A. Lanzavecchia, and G. J. Nabel. 2005. Evasion of antibody neutralization in emerging severe acute respiratory syndrome coronaviruses. *Proc. Natl. Acad. Sci. USA* **102**:797–801. [Epub 10 January 2005.]

105. Yeager, C. L., R. A. Ashmun, R. K. Williams, C. B. Cardellichio, L. H. Shapiro, A. T. Look, and K. V. Holmes. 1992. Human aminopeptidase N is a receptor for human coronavirus 229E. *Nature* **357**:420–422.

106. Yu, I. T., Y. Li, T. W. Wong, W. Tam, A. T. Chan, J. H. Lee, D. Y. Leung, and T. Ho. 2004. Evidence of airborne transmission of the severe acute respiratory syndrome virus. *N. Engl. J. Med.* **350**:1731–1739.

107. Zhong, N. 2004. Management and prevention of SARS in China. *Philos. Trans. R. Soc. Lond. B* **359**:1115–1116.

108. Zhong, N., Y. Ding, Y. Mao, Q. Wang, G. Wang, D. Wang, Y. Cong, Q. Li, Y. Liu, L. Ruan, B. Chen, X. Du, Y. Yang, Z. Zhang, X. Zhang, J. Lin, J. Zheng, Q. Zhu, D. Ni, X. Xi, G. Zeng, D. Ma, C. Wang, W. Wang, B. Wang, J. Wang, D. Liu, X. Li, X. Liu, J. Chen, R. Chen, F. Min, P. Yang, Y. Zhang, H. Luo, Z. Lang, Y. Hu, A. Ni, W. Cao, S. Lei, S. Wang, Y. Wang, X. Tong, W. Liu, M. Zhu, W. Chen, X. Xhen, L. Lin, Y. Luo, J. Zhong, W. Weng, S. Peng, Z. Pan, R. Wang, J. Zuo, B. Liu, N. Zhang, J. Zhang, B. Zhang, L. Chen, P. Zhou, L. Jiang, E. Chao, L. Guo, X. Tan, and J. Pan. 2003. Consensus for the management of severe acute respiratory syndrome. *Chin. Med. J. (Engl. Ed.)* **116**:1603–1635.

*Nidoviruses*
Edited by S. Perlman, T. Gallagher, and E. J. Snijder
© 2008 ASM Press, Washington, DC

# Chapter 11

# Nidovirus Entry into Cells

BEREND JAN BOSCH AND PETER J. M. ROTTIER

Enveloped viruses enter cells by fusion of their membrane with that of the host cell. To this end they are equipped with surface structures that mediate this two-step process of cell attachment and membrane fusion. The general principles of this fascinating process have been elucidated during the last decades and have recently been described in several authoritative reviews (41, 78, 97, 131). Here we present an overview of cell entry by nidoviruses. Actually, the description is limited mainly to the *Coronaviridae,* simply because of the almost complete lack of information for the *Arteri-* and *Roniviridae,* let alone for the recently identified new nidovirus, white bream virus (WBV). In addition, we restrict ourselves to the post-receptor-binding part of the entry process, as the cell attachment and receptor binding aspects are dealt with in chapters 12 and 13. This review focuses on the functioning of the coronavirus fusion protein, in particular, on its proteolytic cleavage activation and on its conformation rearrangements in the process of membrane fusion.

## THE CORONAVIRUS SPIKE: KEY TO ENTRY

Coronavirus entry is mediated by the viral spike protein. Trimers of this envelope glycoprotein form the coronavirion surface spikes, which, by their characteristic manifestation in the electron microscope, give the viruses their corona-like appearance. The shape and dimensions of the spikes seem to vary among different coronaviruses, appearing, for instance, teardrop shaped in the case of infectious bronchitis virus (IBV) or cone shaped for mouse hepatitis virus (MHV, strain 3) (29). While the spikes measure 11 to 20 nm in length and 5 to 11 nm in width in

these examples, size variations can be attributed at least in part to different negative-staining procedures (29). Technical differences probably also explain the diverse outcomes of the first electron cryomicroscopy analyses of coronaviruses. Whereas in one study the dimensions of the reconstructed single-particle images of three coronaviruses, including the severe acute respiratory syndrome coronavirus (SARS-CoV), were consistent with those obtained by classical electron microscopy (109), in another study the SARS-CoV "club-shaped" spike was found to project 16 nm from the viral envelope and to exhibit an unusually broad bulbous end measuring 18 nm in diameter (4). Both studies documented three-lobed spike densities consistent with the trimeric stoichiometry of the spikes, as demonstrated biochemically for transmissible gastroenteritis virus (TGEV) (36) and SARS-CoV (142). Based on their spatial distribution, an average-size coronavirion with a full complement of spikes was estimated to be covered by approximately 65 (4) or some 50 to 100 (109) spike protein trimers.

Like in many other enveloped viruses such as retro-, rhabdo-, and orthomyxoviruses, the spike protein of coronaviruses performs both the binding and the fusion functions. These two functions can be attributed to two functionally distinct parts of the molecule. As detailed in the previous chapters, the amino-terminal half (S1), which supposedly constitutes the main part of the globular head of the spike, contains the receptor-binding domain. The carboxy-terminal, membrane-anchored half (S2) is responsible for membrane fusion. In some coronaviruses these two domains are actually separated by furin cleavage (see below). The length of the spike protein varies considerably among coronaviruses; the shortest and longest proteins presently known count 1,162

Berend Jan Bosch and Peter J. M. Rottier • Virology Division, Faculty of Veterinary Medicine, Utrecht University, Yalelaan 1, 3584 CL Utrecht, The Netherlands.

(IBV) (GenBank accession no. CAC39114) and 1,481 residues (canine coronavirus [CCoV]) (121) (GenBank accession no. AAP72150), respectively. The spike protein is a highly N-glycosylated type I membrane protein 150 to 220 kDa in size. Due to the formation of numerous disulfide bonds in its luminal domain, it folds slowly in the endoplasmic reticulum (ER) and assembles into trimers before being transported to the virion assembly sites or to the plasma membrane (113).

Little is known about the secondary structure of the spike protein. Based on structure predictions (http://www.predictprotein.org/ [124]), the SARS-CoV S1 domain consists for the most part of β-sheets (6% α-helical, 44% β-sheet, and 50% loop), whereas the S2 domain (residues 668 to 1255) has a predominantly α-helical fold (49% α-helical, 17% β-sheet, and 35% loop). Contributing to this α-helicity are two heptad repeat regions, HR1 and HR2, which have a propensity to form coiled coils (30). The HR1 region is located near the middle of the S2 domain, while the HR2 region occurs close to the transmembrane region (Fig. 1). Unlike S1, the structure of the S2 domain is highly conserved (30), as is illustrated for instance by the strong conservation of its cysteines (Fig. 1).

Enveloped viruses appear to use primarily one of two distinct mechanisms to achieve their membrane fusion. Accordingly, two types of fusion proteins, designated class I and class II, can be distinguished (for two recent reviews, see references 78 and 131). The spike protein of coronaviruses belongs to class I, together with fusion proteins like the influenza virus hemagglutinin (HA) and the human immunodeficiency virus type 1 (HIV-1) *env* protein. Class I fusion proteins share several features. They are type I glycoproteins that occur in virions as homotrimers.

Their ectodomain has an elongated shape and is oriented perpendicular to the viral membrane. They require proteolytic activation to become fusion active. Cleavage generally occurs N terminally or N proximally to a hydrophobic region called the fusion peptide, thereby providing the ectodomain of the resulting membrane-anchored polypeptide with a lipophilic terminus. This ectodomain typically also contains two heptad repeat regions, the main hallmark of class I fusion proteins. The positions of these regions—designated here as HR1 and HR2, with HR2 being membrane proximal—relative to the fusion peptide and the transmembrane domain vary considerably among class I proteins (Fig. 2).

While the coronavirus spike protein conforms to all of these typical class I features, it seems to deviate in one important aspect, its proteolytic activation. Activation of class I fusion proteins, a prerequisite for virus infectivity, is effected by cellular proteases. The cleavage primes the viral protein for membrane fusion, probably by affecting its conformational stability and thereby enabling molecular rearrangements essential for fusion. As spike proteins of a number of coronaviruses lack a furin cleavage site and actually occur in the virion in an uncleaved form, proteolytic activation was long believed not to be required for their fusion activation. Recently, however, it appeared that this activation step does not necessarily have to occur in the secretory pathway, i.e., during biogenesis of the virion, but that it can also take place during virus entry in an endocytic compartment of the target cell. Cleavage activation of the spike protein in the exo- and endocytic pathways might thus be considered two sides of the same coin. Below we begin first with a thorough discussion of this cleavage issue,

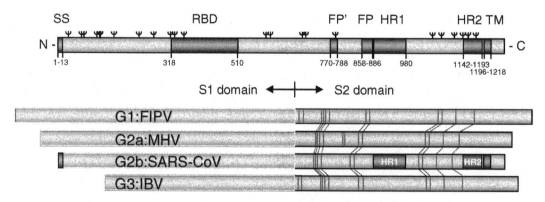

Figure 1. (Top) schematic diagram of the SARS-CoV spike protein (drawn to scale). The position of the signal sequence (SS), receptor-binding domain (RBD), putative fusion peptides (FP' and FP), heptad repeat domains (HR1 and HR2), and transmembrane domain (TM) are indicated, as well as the potential N glycosylation sites. (Lower part) Schematic diagram of the spike proteins of representatives of the three coronavirus groups 1, 2, and 3 (G1 to G3): FIPV (G1), MHV and SARS-CoV (G2a and G2b, respectively), and IBV (G3). Bars are drawn to scale and aligned at the S1-S2 domain junction. The cysteine residues in the S2 ectodomain are indicated by vertical gray lines. Most of these cysteines are strictly conserved among all coronavirus spike proteins, as indicated by the connecting dashed lines.

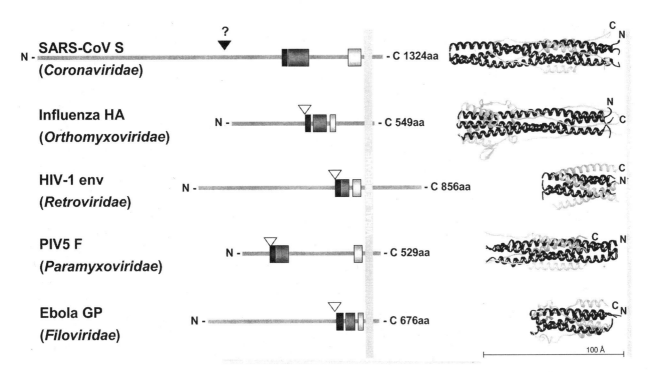

**Figure 2.** Schematic diagrams (left) and drawings of the postfusion core structures (right) of the fusion proteins of SARS-CoV, influenza virus, HIV-1, parainfluenza virus 5 (PIV5; formerly known as SV5), and Ebola virus. The fusion peptide is indicated by a black bar. The HR1 and HR2 regions are depicted by dark and light gray shaded bars, respectively. The positions of the furin cleavage sites are indicated by open arrowheads, and the position of the putative cathepsin L cleavage site is indicated by a filled arrowhead. The fusion proteins are C-terminally anchored in the viral membrane (gray bar). The ribbon diagrams of the postfusion core structures (PDB codes: 1WYV [40], 1QU1 [23], 1AIK [18], 1SVF [2], and 2EBO [96], respectively) were generated using RIBBONS (14). The interior HR1 coiled coil is depicted in black, and the HR2 polypeptide is indicated in gray. "N" and "C" indicate the N and C termini of one HR1 and HR2 peptide in each case, respectively. Their positions correspond to the approximate locations of the membrane-interacting segments of the protein, i.e., the N-terminal fusion peptide and the C-terminal transmembrane domain. aa, amino acids.

because of its importance, because of the new insights, and because of its significance for understanding the subsequent sections. Thereafter, we describe the routes of entry of coronaviruses, the conformational changes in the spike protein leading to fusion, and the domains actually functioning in the membrane fusion process.

## CLEAVAGE ACTIVATION

### Spike Protein Cleavage during Cell Exit: Furin(-Like) Proteases

In most of the group 2 and all of the group 3 coronaviruses, the spike protein is cleaved during its biogenesis into its subunits S1 and S2, which remain associated noncovalently. Sequencing analysis showed cleavage to take place after the last residue of a multibasic motif (often RRxRR) (16, 95) present in most group 2 and 3 coronaviruses but absent in almost all group 1 coronaviruses. This motif resembles the

RxxR sequence that is recognized by furin, a calcium-dependent serine proprotein endoprotease belonging to the family of proprotein convertases (104). Consistently, cleavage of the MHV strain A59 (MHV-A59) spike protein was shown to be dependent on furin or a furin-like host protease (34). Cleavage occurs at a late step of transport, on passage of the protein through the *trans*-Golgi network, where furin accumulates (151). The extent of cleavage is dependent on the particular cleavage sequence. Thus, cleavage of the MHV-A59 spike protein was abrogated by various mutations in the multibasic cleavage site, while, conversely, virtually complete cleavage was observed after changing the RRAHR sequence to RRARR, which comprises two overlapping furin cleavage sites (7, 55). Cleavage also depends on the type of cell or tissue in which the coronavirus replicates. Thus, spikes in MHV-A59 virions were fully cleaved when the virus was obtained from Sac⁻ cells but only about 50% cleaved when grown in 17Cl1 cells (47). The same spike proteins isolated from infected mouse brain or liver appeared not to be cleaved at all (61). The differences probably reflect variations in the expression levels of the cellular protease.

SARS-CoV is phylogenetically related to the group 2 coronaviruses, yet no substantial proteolytic cleavage of its spike protein in infected cells or on virions has been reported (5, 12, 53, 142, 175, 182). In this respect it resembles the coronaviruses of group 1, the spikes of which are known to remain uncleaved, as was demonstrated long ago for feline infectious peritonitis virus (FIPV; strain 79-1146), TGEV (strain FS772/70), and CCoV (strain K378) (31, 32, 43, 52, 162), which all lack a multibasic furin consensus motif (162). It now appears, however, that this is not a universal feature of group 1 coronaviruses. In the recently published sequence of the CCoV strain Elmö/02, a clear RRxRR motif occurs near the middle of the spike protein (121), as is also the case for the UCD strain of feline coronavirus, the spike protein of which was demonstrated to be actually cleaved (B. Haijema and P. Rottier, unpublished data).

By its fusion activity the spike protein often causes the formation of syncytia in cultures of coronavirus-infected cells and when being expressed independently. In the case of MHV, the most extensively studied virus, the efficiency of this process appeared to correlate with the extent of the protein's cleavage, as was demonstrated by using different strains (47, 129, 146, 149) or cleavage mutants (7, 8, 54), or by inhibiting cleavage by means of a furin protease inhibitor (34). An unexplained exception is an MHV-WB1 recombinant spike protein which, despite the lack of cleavage, caused extensive cell-cell fusion (144). Of all natural MHV isolates, MHV-2 is the only strain with an uncleaved spike protein (62, 74). Isolated mutants of MHV-2, which, in contrast to the parental virus, were capable of inducing syncytium formation, appeared to have acquired this ability through a single mutation restoring an apparently lost cleavage site (179). Fusion of MHV-2-infected cells can also be induced by exogenous cleavage of the spike protein, by addition of proteases like trypsin (123). Such treatment enhanced the fusion of cells infected by MHV-A59 (186) or bovine coronavirus (BCoV) (strain L9) (28, 117, 145), and partially restored syncytium formation by cleavage-defective MHV-A59 mutants (55). A trypsin-dependent effect was also observed for a process called "fusion from without," i.e., the rapid formation of syncytia induced by adding high concentrations of infectious virus to susceptible cells. Fusion occurred upon addition of 17Cl1 cell-derived MHV-A59, which carries partially cleaved spikes, onto L2 cells, but only after exogenous trypsin treatment of the virus (47, 146).

Consistent with the cleavage phenotype of its spike, SARS-CoV induces little or no syncytia in various types of cells. However, cell fusion could be elicited by treatment with exogenous proteases such as trypsin and thermolysin and resulted in two defined proteolytic products, suggesting an exposed cleavage site (53, 101, 139). The trypsin cleavage was recently mapped at a position that aligns precisely with the site that separates S1 and S2 in MHV (90). Introduction of a furin cleavage site at this position enabled efficient cleavage of the spike protein into S1 and S2 subunits and markedly increased syncytium formation upon its expression (46).

Despite the clear correlation between furin cleavage and cell-cell fusion, there is as yet no evidence that this cleavage also enhances coronavirus infectivity. Rather, in a direct comparison the specific infectivities of MHV-A59 with cleaved and uncleaved spikes appeared to be indistinguishable, as were the kinetics by which these viruses initiated infection (34). Consistently, though not specifically looked at, viruses with uncleaved spikes, such as most of the group 1 coronaviruses, MHV-2 (62, 74), and certain natural MHV-A59 isolates (54, 129), do not seem to exhibit conspicuously poor infectivity. Conversely, the introduction of the furin cleavage site at the S1-S2 junction of the SARS-CoV spike protein did not increase the infectivity of lentiviral particles pseudotyped with it (46). Collectively these data seem to indicate that the infectivity of coronaviruses does not depend on cleavage of the spike protein into the S1 and S2 subunits.

### Spike Protein Cleavage during Cell Entry: Endosomal Proteases

Exciting new light on the enigmatic cleavage issue was shed recently by observations that fusion activation can occur not only during virion biogenesis in the virus-producing cell but also during its entry into the target cell (Fig. 3). Evidence for this came from studies with protease inhibitors. Infection by SARS-CoV or by retroviruses pseudotyped with the SARS-CoV spike protein could be inhibited effectively by leupeptin, an inhibitor of serine and cysteine proteases, as well as—more specifically—by the cysteine protease inhibitors E64-c and E64-d (71, 138). The inhibitory effect of leupeptin could be overcome by trypsin treatment of cell surface-bound SARS-CoV, suggesting that the trypsin activity could compensate for the inhibition of cellular proteases (138). In addition, it was shown that specific inhibitors of the cathepsin L protease, a cysteine protease, potently inhibited infection by virus particles pseudotyped with the SARS-CoV spike protein (138) as well as by

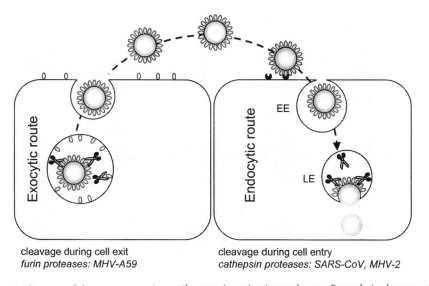

cleavage during cell exit
*furin proteases: MHV-A59*

cleavage during cell entry
*cathepsin proteases: SARS-CoV, MHV-2*

**Figure 3.** Schematic diagram of the two coronavirus spike protein activation pathways. Proteolytic cleavage of spikes occurs in the exocytic route by furin(-like) proteases or in the endocytic (entry) route by cathepsin proteases, as indicated by the scissors in the left and right panels, respectively.

SARS-CoV itself (71). Many cysteine proteases that occur in the endosomal/lysosomal compartment, such as cathepsin L, become activated and function optimally at acidic pH (68). This pH dependence correlates well with the observed entry inhibition of SARS-CoV virions and SARS-CoV spike protein-pseudotyped viruses by agents that prevent the acidification of endosomes (63, 76, 101, 138, 139, 157, 181). The effect of these lysosomotropic agents could again be overcome by trypsin treatment of cell surface-bound viral particles, further supporting a role for pH-dependent endosomal proteases in SARS-CoV entry (101, 138). Moreover, treatment of cell-bound viruses with other proteases such as elastase, which is produced in the lungs during inflammation, could also lift infection from its pH-dependence. This implies that proteases in the extracellular milieu can activate SARS-CoV, thereby allowing it to obviate the acid-dependent route and to enter through nonacidic pathways, including the plasma membrane. The presence of an appropriate protease in a given tissue, organ, or host might thus be an important determinant of tropism and hence of the pathogenesis of those coronaviruses that are dependent on activation by cellular proteases (101), as has also been observed for paramyxoviruses and influenza viruses (reviewed in reference 79).

Another coronavirus recently found to be sensitive to cathepsin B and L protease inhibitors is MHV-2 (123), the MHV with the uncleaved spikes that fails to induce syncytia. Interestingly, mutants of MHV-2 carrying a proper furin cleavage site appeared to have lost their sensitivity both to lysosomotropic agents

and to cathepsin inhibitors (123). The authors speculate that MHVs with spikes not cleaved by furin-like enzymes enter cells via receptor-mediated endocytosis and fusion through endosomal cathepsin-mediated proteolytic activation (Fig. 3) (123).

Although cleavage of the receptor or of other cellular factors cannot be fully ruled out, the cathepsin enzymes most likely act on the spike protein. However, no cathepsin L proteolytic target site has yet been identified in any coronavirus spike protein, and predictions are hampered by the enzyme's poorly defined sequence specificity. It has been hypothesized that cleavage of the spike protein is required to liberate the internally located fusion peptide (71, 138). Cleavage just upstream of this peptide would place it at the N terminus of the membrane-anchored S2 subunit, as it occurs in other class I fusion proteins. Alternatively, cathepsin L might cleave at the S1-S2 boundary, just like furin does (138). Exposure of the SARS-CoV spike protein expressed on infected cells to exogenous proteases such as trypsin, thermolysin, dispase, or elastase resulted in defined proteolytic products due to cleavage somewhere in the middle of the polypeptide (53, 101, 139). Similar products were observed after trypsin treatment of SARS-CoV spike protein expressed independently on cells or on pseudotyped viral particles (53, 139), suggesting the presence of an exposed cleavage site. The actual identification of the trypsin cleavage site (90) confirmed this suggestion. As this cleavage induces cell-cell fusion, it is conceivable that cathepsin L also targets the S1-S2 junction. This is consistent with the already-mentioned rescue of SARS-CoV entry inhibition by leupeptin and lysosomotropic agents by trypsin treatment of cell-bound virions (101, 138), as well as with the formation of syncytia in SARS-CoV spike protein-expressing cells (46, 123) and in MHV-2-infected cells (123) that is observed after introduction of a furin cleavage site at the S1-S2 junction of these viruses' spike proteins. Yet cleavage by cathepsin L protease might still occur at alternative positions but with similar activating effects. Treatment of SARS-CoV virions with trypsin before engagement with the receptor has been found to reduce infectivity (139). Perhaps the cathepsin L target site becomes exposed only upon receptor binding, or cleavage prior to receptor binding triggers a premature conformational change that results in inactivation of the spike protein.

The question arose whether cathepsin dependence is a general feature of coronavirus entry. This appeared not to be the case after several coronaviruses—including the group 1 human coronavirus NL63 (HCoV-NL63) (71), the group 2 viruses MHV-A59 and MHV-JHM (123, 190), and the group 3 virus IBV (24)—were found to be insensitive to the action of cathepsin protease inhibitors. It is of note that HCoV-NL63 uses the same receptor as SARS-CoV but has apparently different entry requirements. Early studies already showed HCoV-229E, a group 1 coronavirus, to be inhibited by leupeptin, but only when added within the first 2 h of infection (1). Both HCoV-229E and HCoV-OC43 (group 2) were found to be also sensitive to cystatins (25, 26), which are natural inhibitors of cysteine proteases (3). Accordingly, HCoV-229E infection appeared to be inhibited by E64-d and by lysosomotropic agents, while, just like for SARS-CoV, treatment of plasma membrane-bound HCoV-229E virions with exogenous trypsin could relieve the inhibitory effect of E64-d (B. J. Bosch and P. Rottier, unpublished data).

Considering the strict cleavage requirements of other class I fusion proteins, it can be speculated that proteolytic processing is also an obligatory requisite of the coronavirus fusion protein, but that coronaviruses have evolved different ways to accomplish it. One might argue that all spike proteins, including those of group 1 coronaviruses, originally contained a furin cleavage site. Spike protein cleavage during biogenesis might have been unfavorable for some coronaviruses, as it could lead to spike inactivation through S1-S2 dissociation (66). Viruses with uncleaved spikes might thus have benefited somehow from the loss of furin cleavage. This idea is supported by the presence of what has been suggested to be a vestigial furin cleavage site (DRTRG) approximately in the middle of the TGEV spike protein (87). Viruses like this might have become furin protease independent while becoming dependent on cleavage in the

extracellular environment or after endocytosis, an adjustment that might also have occurred to MHV-2 and SARS-CoV. Similarly, the spike protein of porcine epidemic diarrhea virus (PEDV; strain CV777), a group 1 coronavirus, lacks the minimal furin recognition sequence in its ectodomain, yet the protein was found in a cleaved form in the gut of infected pigs (43). Presumably, PEDV is proteolytically activated by enzymes occurring in the gut, consistent with its trypsin requirement for productive infection of Vero cells (65). Unlike the intracellular processing at a multibasic cleavage site mediated by furin, a number of viral fusion proteins, such as the Sendai virus F protein (67, 130) and several subtypes of the influenza virus HA protein (77), are cleaved at single basic residues by extracellular proteases restricted to tissues to which the infection is hence localized (79). Like PEDV, these viruses require trypsin to allow replication in vitro.

The available data point to proteolytic activation as a quite general requirement for coronaviruses. However, whether the requirement is absolute remains to be established. Activation cleavage can occur during any phase of the virus lifetime, i.e., during virion maturation and exit from the infected cell, in the extracellular environment, or during cell entry in an endosome. The situation partly resembles that of the paramyxoviruses and of Ebola virus. Interestingly, however, the cathepsin L-mediated activation of the Hendra and Nipah paramyxovirus fusion proteins appears to occur while the protein recycles between the endosome and the cell surface before being incorporated into virions (114, 115). For Ebola virus, furin cleavage of the fusion glycoprotein into GP1 and GP2 (158) is not required for infection (110, 172). Rather, the activity of cathepsin proteases B and L is required (20, 134) to proteolytically process the GP1 subunit (20, 134), presumably to trigger the fusion reaction mediated by GP2.

## ROUTES OF ENTRY

The cellular membranes with which enveloped viruses fuse to enter cells are the plasma membrane and the limiting membrane of an endocytic organelle. Class I fusion proteins are known to act in both of these pathways, the low pH in the latter being a distinguishing feature. Thus, the fusion and Env proteins of Sendai virus and HIV-1, respectively, mediate pH-independent fusion with the plasma membrane, while for the influenza virus HA protein acidic conditions are instrumental in catalyzing fusion with the endosomal membrane (for elegant reviews, see references 39 and 97). Coronaviruses do not uniformly exploit one single entry pathway. Rather, a picture is emerging in which infections by viruses carrying uncleaved spikes are mostly pH sensitive, in contrast to infections by viruses with cleaved spikes.

Acidic pH dependence of virus entry is often studied by establishing the sensitivity of infection to lysosomotropic agents such as the weak basic amines chloroquine and ammonium chloride, which prevent endosomal acidification, or to the drug bafilomycin A1, an inhibitor of the vacuolar $H^+$ V-ATPase. As already discussed, the cathepsin-dependent SARS-CoV, MHV-2, and HCoV-229E are all sensitive to such treatments. Also, TGEV was inhibited by ammonium chloride and bafilomycin A1 (6, 59, 112), consistent with electron microscopic observations that showed TGEV particles in endocytic pits shortly after inoculation of susceptible cells (59). HCoV-229E infection was additionally inhibited by nocodazole, a microtubule depolymerizing drug affecting the transport from early to late endosomes. Interestingly, infection with the cathepsin-insensitive HCoV-NL63 appeared to be sensitive to ammonium chloride (64, 71), though to a lesser extent than SARS-CoV, which also uses ACE2 as a receptor.

Coronaviruses carrying cleaved spikes are generally pH independent. Most strains of MHV, such as MHV-A59 and MHV-4, are relatively insensitive to lysosomotropic agents (51, 80, 107), although two studies reported a delay and a clear inhibition of infection by MHV-A59 (102) and MHV-3 (84), respectively. A slight sensitivity to ammonium chloride was also reported for another group 2 virus, BCoV strain L9. This virus was, however, shown by electron microscopy to fuse with the plasma membrane of HRT-18 cells, while no fusion with endosomal membranes was observed, leading the authors to conclude that BCoV enters directly through the cell membrane (118).

The picture is, however, not completely clear yet, as illustrated by the MHV-4 variant OBLV60 and the group 3 coronavirus IBV, both of which carry cleaved spikes. Infection by these viruses was found to be acid dependent (24, 51, 107), indicative of endocytic entry. Thus, infection of Vero cells with the Beaudette strain of IBV was sensitive to ammonium chloride during the first 2 h (89). Remarkably, however, in the same study infection of CK cells with the UK/123/82 strain of IBV appeared to be insensitive to this treatment. These MHV and IBV examples suggest that different virus strains may have different pH requirements. For MHV-OBLV60 and IBV-Beaudette, acidic pH treatment was shown to actively induce cell-cell and virus-cell fusion, respectively, suggesting that acid pH per se can directly trigger the spike protein for membrane fusion (24, 51, 107).

pH independence of infection does not necessarily imply entry by plasma membrane fusion. Both MHV-4 and its neuron-adapted variant OBLV60 were observed in endosomal vesicles of inoculated cells by electron microscopy. After protease-mediated removal of extracellular virus, the productive infection by OBLV60 but not that of the parental virus was significantly inhibited by lysosomotropic agents (107). Apparently, both viruses can utilize the endocytic pathway. Considering the role of cathepsins in cell entry, one might even speculate that for some pH-insensitive coronaviruses, internalization through the endocytic route could still be mandatory for establishing infection, as would for instance be the case when the spike protein would require fusion activation by acid-independent proteases present in endocytic organelles.

## MEMBRANE FUSION: TRIGGERS, ACTORS, AND STRUCTURAL REARRANGEMENTS

The molecular mechanisms by which class I fusion proteins mediate the merging of viral and cellular membranes are only beginning to be understood. Current insights are based for the major part on studies with the influenza virus HA and the paramyxovirus fusion proteins, the only fusion proteins for which both pre- and postfusion crystal structures are available (13, 168, 184, 185). The process—which appears to apply to the coronavirus spike protein as well (Fig. 2)—involves a homotrimeric complex that is synthesized as a fusion-inactive, metastable structure stabilized by noncovalent intermolecular contacts, notably by coiled-coil interactions between its carboxy-terminal subunits. As discussed above, furin cleavage often renders the complex fusion competent already before or immediately after assembly into virions; alternatively, this essential activation step occurs extracellularly or endosomally. The actual fusion reaction is primed by interaction with the target cell where any of a number of triggers—receptor binding, proteolytic cleavage, or acidic pH—can spark off a cascade of conformational changes by which the metastable trimer eventually ends up in a trimer-of-hairpins conformation that is characterized by two main features: a six-helix bundle structure formed by the antiparallel association of the HR1 and HR2 domains, and the juxtaposed fusion peptides and transmembrane domains anchored together in the fused lipid bilayer. The energy released during the conformational transitions to this highly stable postfusion form is used to draw viral and target membrane together and to force their coalescence. With regard to the intermediate conformational states, experimental support has only been obtained for the occurrence of a prehairpin intermediate in which the fusion peptides, originally hidden away in the native trimeric structure, have become exposed, pointing away from the viral membrane and into the target membrane (41, 42, 98). In the following section we describe how coronavirus membrane fusion fits in this picture by discussing the triggers, the key structural elements in the spike protein, its conformational states, and the actual fusion process.

## Fusion Triggers

The key event that initiates the membrane fusion reaction seems to vary quite remarkably among different coronaviruses. This is due mostly to variation in the cleavage state in which coronavirions present themselves to their target cells. Assuming that most, if not all, coronaviruses require proteolytic activation at one stage or another, it thus appears that, generally, both cleavage and receptor binding are essential to allow fusion, the actual fusion trigger being whichever event comes last. A third condition triggering fusion by some coronaviruses is acidic pH. As illustrated below, these triggers elicit changes in the spike protein that apparently assist in overcoming a critical energy barrier needed to set off the irreversible reaction leading to membrane fusion.

## Receptor binding

For many coronaviruses, particularly those that have furin-cleaved spikes and fuse at neutral pH, engagement with the cellular receptor initiates the fusion process. That this interaction affects the spike structure has been demonstrated most extensively with MHV upon binding to its CEACAM receptor (48, 88, 100, 189). Changes were, for instance, revealed using a soluble form of the receptor by showing the induction of alternative disulfide bonds in the S1 domain (88). Soluble receptor binding was also found to affect the integrity of the S1-S2 complex by causing the dissociation of the S1 subunit (88, 147, 189). Soluble CEACAM binding even appeared to transmit conformational changes to the S2 subunit, as observed by alterations in its protease sensitivity. Thus, a 58-kDa fragment comprising the HR1 and HR2 domains remained after proteinase K digestion of MHV-JHM virions bound to its soluble receptor, while no resistant material was found after digestion in the absence of the receptor (100). When MHV-A59 virions were preincubated with or without a soluble receptor and subsequently treated with trypsin, the S2 protein appeared to be degraded but only in the receptor-triggered virus, while the S1 protein

was unaffected in either case (189). Interestingly, conformational changes in response to receptor binding are apparently not dependent on preceding furin cleavage of the spike protein. When the trypsin assay was applied to virions of a cleavage-defective MHV-A59 spike protein mutant (H716D), a novel 120-kDa fragment remained in the presence of soluble CEACAM, while the spike protein was not degraded in its absence. Another elegant assay by which these authors detected conformational changes in the MHV spike in response to receptor binding was by showing that the virions became hydrophobic and bound to liposomes (189). These receptor-induced conformational changes play a functional role in MHV entry, as illustrated by the potential of soluble CEACAM receptor to mediate targeting of MHV to nonsusceptible cells (150, 159, 173). A particular case is presented by viruses for which interaction with the receptor seems less critical for the spike protein to be fusogenic. The best example is the neurovirulent MHV-JHM strain, which is able to spread from cell to cell in a receptor-independent manner by syncytium formation with CEACAM-negative BHK cells (50). This feature was found to correlate with spike stability, more specifically, with the strength of the interaction between the S1 and S2 subunits. Thus, sequence analysis of in vitro-passaged mutants that had lost the ability to induce CEACAM-independent fusion revealed these viruses to exhibit increased S1-S2 stability due to deletions in the S1 gene and substitutions (V870A and A1046V) in HR regions in S2 (83). The observations suggest the existence of fusion triggers other than receptor binding (reviewed in reference 49).

## Proteolytic cleavage

Cleavage is a fusion trigger for several coronaviruses that require an additional activating event subsequent to receptor binding. This holds for viruses such as SARS-CoV and HCoV-229E, which need proteolytic activation by acid-activated endosomal enzymes. Acidic conditions per se do not seem to be a direct trigger for entry of these viruses. Infection could also be established effectively at neutral pH by trypsin, thermolysin, or elastase treatment of cell surface-bound SARS-CoV (101, 138), SARS-CoV spike protein-pseudotyped retrovirions (101, 138), and HCoV-229E (Bosch and Rottier, unpublished); these treatments enabled the viruses to bypass the inhibition of infection caused by lysosomotropic agents. Consistently, trypsin treatment at neutral pH strongly induced formation of syncytia in cultures of cells expressing the SARS-CoV spike protein and triggered membrane fusion in a virion-virion fusion assay, while low-pH treatment did not have such effects (101, 138, 139).

The SARS-CoV spike protein needs to bind to the ACE2 receptor for trypsin to be able to activate fusion. The prior interaction with the receptor may be required to induce conformational changes within the spike protein, either to expose the cleavage site or for the protein to undergo some of the initial steps towards fusion. Though direct evidence is lacking, the temperature dependence of protease activation suggests such conformational changes do occur. In the intervirion fusion assay, trypsin treatment at 4°C did not give rise to membrane fusion if the interacting virions had been kept at this low temperature; fusion occurred after the mixture had been briefly incubated at 37°C before trypsin treatment in the cold (101, 138). When not associated with the receptor, virions appeared to be vulnerable to the action of trypsin, as judged by the significant drop in infectivity after cell-free virions had been incubated with the enzyme (101, 138). Apparently, the effect of proteolysis is dependent on the context in which it occurs.

## Acidic pH

For only a few coronaviruses, fusion appears to be triggered truly by low pH. Documented examples are the MHV-4 mutant OBLV60 and the Beaudette and M41 strains of IBV. Infection by these viruses is normally dependent on the acidic conditions in the endosome. The viruses were found, however, to be able to enter susceptible cells directly through the plasma membrane if the pH was made permissive for fusion. Thus, while endosomal entry was blocked using the ionophore monensin, the cell surface-bound viruses were triggered to fuse by exposure to acidified culture medium (24, 107). Consistently, a low-pH treatment induced spike-mediated syncytium formation by cells infected by OBLV60 or expressing its spike protein (51). How the three critical mutations in the HR1 domain of this spike protein (Q1067H, Q1094H, and L1114R) alter the fusion requirements so dramatically is unclear. In contrast to influenza virus, which is inactivated by low-pH exposure and subsequent neutralization of the pH, the infectivity of IBV (strain Beaudette) was almost completely resistant to this treatment (24). Under these conditions the spike protein appeared to undergo reversible conformational changes, as was indirectly shown by the reversible binding of a fluorophore, 4,4′-bis(1-anilinonaphthalene 8-sulfonate), to hydrophobic sites exposed only at acidic pH. Whether the same conformational changes occur when the virus is associated with its receptor is unknown yet. Cell entry by IBV and OBLV60 is reminiscent of infection by avian sarcoma and leukosis virus, a retrovirus also requiring both receptor binding and low-pH triggering (106).

## From Native to Prehairpin Conformation: Exposure of the Fusion Peptide

Once effectively triggered for fusion, the coronavirus spike opens up to liberate the previously hidden fusion peptides, to stretch them out towards the target cell and to insert them, presumably jointly, into its membrane. Though possibly not static at any time, the resulting prehairpin state represents at least a conceptual intermediate of the fusion process.

### Initial conformational changes induced by the fusion triggers

In the absence of ultrastructural information, little is known about the interactions that stabilize the spike proteins in the metastable prefusion trimer. The S1 and S2 subunits appear to occur as rather independently folded structures, as is suggested by the ready dissociation of S1 subunits from cleaved spikes (147). Hence, the intersubunit contacts are supposedly weak. The trimeric state seems to be stabilized primarily by interactions between the S2 subunits. As judged by the difficulty in obtaining trimeric spikes by expression of truncated ectodomain constructs (90, 142), interactions between the transmembrane and/or between the carboxy-terminal domains are likely to contribute to trimer stability. Additional contributions probably come from the HR2 domains. Peptides corresponding to the SARS-CoV spike protein HR2 region have a propensity to assemble into a parallel trimeric coiled-coil structure (30, 58, 153, 180). In the native spike this structure probably constitutes the stalk region (4, 58). Accordingly, the group 1 feline coronavirus spikes were found by cryo-electron microscopic reconstructions to have an elongated stalk compared to that of the group 2 SARS-CoV (109), which is consistent with the 14-residue (i.e., two-heptad-repeat) difference in the lengths of their HR domains (11). In further support of the occurrence of an HR2 trimer are the defects in the oligomerization of the spike protein observed after mutagenesis of the HR2 domain (94), which were presumably due to destabilization of the trimeric HR2 coiled coil.

The HR1 domains do not seem to occur in a trimeric configuration in the prefusion spike. Circular-dichroism data suggest that synthetic HR1-based peptides by themselves adopt a less helical conformation than after their assembly into the postfusion six-helix bundle structure (92, 153). The crystal structure of this complex, discussed below, reveals how a hydrophilic cavity in the otherwise hydrophobic interior of the HR1 coiled coil indeed destabilizes the HR1 trimer, and how this effect is compensated by interactions with the helical portion of HR2 (40). Accordingly, HR1 peptides in isolation were found by sedimentation analysis to be associated mainly as a tetramer (153). Like in the paramyxovirus SV5 fusion protein (185), the HR1 domain probably plays a role in stabilizing intersubunit S1-S2 interactions in the prefusion state, possibly through direct contacts with the S1 subunit, as is suggested by several observations (for examples, see references 35, 51, and 99).

The structural rearrangements occurring in response to fusion activation and leading to the prehairpin state are still completely obscure. Essential at this stage is the erection of a parallel triple-stranded coiled coil by the HR1 domains, which thereby projects the fusion peptides away from the virion surface, but direct evidence for this intermediate structure is lacking. However, significant work by the Holmes laboratory (154, 189) revealed that interaction of the (soluble) CEACAM1 receptor with spikes on MHV virions rendered these virions hydrophobic, as demonstrated by a liposome-binding assay. Apparently, receptor binding causes a destabilization of the spike structure that results in the release of the fusion peptide. The conformational change, which occurred irreversibly at pH 6.5 and 37°C, but not at 4°C, could also be induced in the absence of a receptor by incubation of the virions at pH 8 and 37°C (189). This condition had been shown earlier to irreversibly inactivate the virus, leading to conformational changes in (160) and dissociation of the S1 subunit and to aggregation of virions and of detergent-released S2 subunits (147). The changes induced at pH 8 supposedly mimic the receptor-induced rearrangements in the spike and give rise to structures that may either represent or approach the prefusion intermediate. The effect has not yet been reported for other coronaviruses.

### The fusion peptide

The fusion peptide has not been identified yet. Unlike the case with other class I viral fusion proteins, coronaviruses lack a hydrophobic sequence at or near the amino terminus of their S2 subunit (95, 132). Consequently, their fusion peptide is positioned internally, analogous to the class I proteins of Ebola virus, Rous sarcoma virus, and avian sarcoma and leukosis virus; to the class II viral fusion proteins; and to the unclassified vesicular stomatitis virus glycoprotein (44, 164). Sequence analyses predict the internal fusion peptide to be located immediately upstream of the HR1 region (SARS-CoV spike residues 858 to 886) (10, 17). As is typical for internal fusion peptides (163, 164), it contains bulky apolar residues, harbors a proline near its center, and is enriched in alanines and glycines (30.8%), all of these features that are well conserved among coronavirus spike proteins (Fig. 4). Its location

```
A)
                                                          a  d
HCoV-NL63    924 RMAMYTGSLIGGMVLGGLTSAAAIPFSLALQARLNYV  960
HCoV-229E    744 RMAMYTGSLIGGIALGGLTSAVSIPFSLAIQARLNYV  780
FIPV        1022 MTMYTASLAGGITLGALGGGAVAIPFAVAVQARLNYV 1053
HCoV-OC43    965 QISGYTLAATSASLFPPWTAAAGVPFYLNVQYRINGL 1001
MHV-A59      923 QISGYTTGATAAAMFPPWSAAAGVPFSLSVQYRINGL  959
SARS-CoV     855 YTAALVSGTATAGWTFGAGAALQIPFAMQMAYRFNGI  891
IBV          746 MQALYTSSLVASMAFGGITAAGAIPFATQLQARINHL  782
WBV          815 HDLEQPSWVYDLGGTAIVPWIGTAVAVGKLANRVASI  851
EToV        1100 KASTLSKIGSVLSSGLSIASLGLSIFSIVEDRRVTEL 1136
BToV        1101 KASTLSTIGSVLSSGLSIASLGLSIFSIIEDRRVIEL 1137
                                                 *
                                                  |-->
                                                   HR1
B)
HPIV-3         110 FFGGVIGTIALGVATSA-QITAAVALV 135
HCoV-229E      750   GSLIGGIALGGLTSAVSIPFSLAIQ 974
                     *.:** ****  *** .*. ::*:
```

**Figure 4.** (A) Sequence alignment of the putative fusion peptides of coronavirus, WBV, and torovirus spike proteins. The sequences encompassing the putative fusion peptides of the coronaviruses HCoV-NL63 (AAS89767), HCoV-229E (VGIHHC), FIPV (strain 79-1146; VGIH79), HCoV-OC43 (CAA83661), MHV-A59 (P11224), SARS-CoV (strain TOR2; P59594), and IBV (strain Beaudette; P11223), the unclassified WBV (strain DF24/00; YP_803215), equine torovirus (EToV; strain P138/72; P23052), and bovine torovirus (BToV; strain B145; CAE01339) were manually aligned at the first heptad repeat of the HR1 region, of which the hydrophobic "a" and "d" residues are boxed. The start of the HR1 domain is just after a conserved arginine marked by an asterisk. The predicted fusion peptide sequences are underlined. The helix-breaking glycines and prolines within the putative fusion peptides are indicated by dark gray shading. (B) Sequence alignment of the (putative) fusion peptides of the human parainfluenza virus type 3 (HPIV-3; genus *Respirovirus;* strain NIH 47885; P06828) with that of the HCoV-229E. Identical residues are indicated by asterisks. Similar and strongly similar residues are indicated by periods and colons, respectively.

upstream of the HR1 domain is consistent with that of fusion peptides in other class I fusion proteins (17). Mutagenesis of the predicted SARS-CoV fusion peptide severely compromised the cell fusion capacity of the spike protein (120). Also, biophysical experiments support the candidacy of this segment as a fusion peptide. By using a peptide library covering the entire SARS-CoV spike protein in a membrane leakage assay, this region was identified as having membrane interaction capabilities (57). Another fusion peptide was proposed to be located further upstream of the HR1 region (SARS-CoV spike protein residues 770 to 788; FP′ in Fig. 1) based on theoretical and lipid vesicle interaction studies (128). This less hydrophobic (net charge, +2) region also contains bulky residues but has a lower alanine/glycine content (10.5%); moreover, its sequence is poorly conserved among coronavirus spike proteins. While a synthetic peptide with this sequence was more membrane active than a peptide representing the other fusion peptide candidate (128), it was not recognized in the peptide library screen by the membrane leakage assay (57). Other membrane-active regions that were additionally identified by these methods include a hydrophobic segment between the two HR regions (SARS-CoV spike protein residues 1077 to 1092) and the extremely conserved tryptophan-rich pretransmembrane region (SARS-CoV spike protein residues 1094 to 1199) (57, 126, 127). As suggested by these authors, multiple membrane-active regions in S2 might work in conjunction during the fusion process, implying that more work is required to unambiguously annotate these segments for their role in membrane fusion.

### From Prehairpin to Trimer of Hairpins: Structure of the HR1-HR2 Fusion Core

Subsequent to insertion of the fusion peptides into the target cell membrane, the three proteins in the spike undergo a dramatic, concerted refolding process by which the S2 subunit polypeptides assemble into a trimer-of-hairpins structure. Instrumental in this process are the heptad repeat regions, domains characterized by the occurrence of hydrophobic residues at the "a" and "d" positions of seven-residue repeats that can form the interface of two or more interlocking helices. These domains, identified in coronavirus spike proteins long before their functional significance could be truly valued (30), coalesce into a rigid coiled coil. During prehairpin formation, the HR2 domains become separated due to destabilization of the trimeric structure. They subsequently reposition, approach the trimeric HR1 bundle formed also during the prehairpin stage, and nestle in an

antiparallel orientation in the interhelical HR1 grooves, giving rise to a six-helix bundle.

There is ample evidence for the key role of the HR regions in spike protein-mediated membrane fusion. Thus, peptides corresponding to its HR2 domain inhibit MHV-A59 entry and syncytium formation in the low micromolar range (11). Infections by SARS-CoV and HCoV-NL63 were similarly shown to be inhibited by their corresponding HR2-derived peptides (10, 92, 122, 188). Also, HR1-based peptides appeared to block entry in the case of SARS-CoV and FIPV (92, 174). In addition, mutations in the HR1 or HR2 domains of SARS-CoV (19, 45, 120) and MHV-A59 (94) severely compromised or completely inhibited spike fusion function. The functional involvement of the HR2 region in entry was further illustrated by the ability of monoclonal antibodies targeting the HR2 region or the region just upstream of HR2 to inhibit SARS-CoV infection (75, 85, 91). Also, a monoclonal antibody abrogating MHV (strain JHM)-induced cell fusion was shown to target an epitope in the HR2 region (125). At what stage and how these antibodies interfere with the fusion process are unknown.

The six-helix bundle structure has been studied biochemically and crystallographically. A hexameric complex consisting of HR1 and HR2 in an antiparallel orientation assembles spontaneously when combining peptides corresponding to the HR1 and HR2 regions, as was demonstrated for MHV-A59, SARS-CoV, and HCoV-NL63 (10, 11, 122, 153, 178). The complex is highly stable, resisting harsh chemical and proteolytic conditions as well as high temperatures (10, 11, 92). Crystal structures were obtained of the fusion cores of MHV (176) and SARS-CoV (40, 148, 176, 177). In the most complete HR1-HR2 complex structure of SARS-CoV, the HR1 peptide (residues 890 to 973) forms a 12-nm-long coiled coil consisting of three helices, each encompassing 22 helical turns. HR2 (residues 1148 to 1188) is folded in an extended-helical-extended conformation (with residues 1160 to 1178 folded as a helix), intimately folded into the groove of the HR1 coiled coil (residues 902 to 951) (40). The abundance of hydrophobic, electrostatic, and hydrogen bond interactions observed in the crystal structure explains the high (thermo)stability of the HR1-HR2 complex. The infection and cell-cell fusion-inhibitory capacity of the HR peptides, most likely through competitive binding, supports the notion that the HR1-HR2 complex is not present in the prefusion state.

The peculiar structure of the HR2 peptide in the core complex suggests that its secondary conformation underwent significant change during the fusion process, losing part of its α-helical organization. In their homotrimeric state in the prefusion native spike, the HR2 segments apparently have a high α-helicity. The nuclear magnetic resonance structure of the SARS-CoV HR2 peptide (residues 1141 to 1193), in the absence of HR1, shows an ~10-nm-long trimeric coiled coil, with the middle 31 residues (residues 1155 to 1185) being folded in a helical configuration comprising eight turns (58). However, in the complex the HR2 region makes only five helical turns (residues 1160 to 1178), the remainder being in an extended conformation (40, 148, 177). The unfolding of the helical part of HR2 into the extended HR2 domains is enforced by newly formed hydrogen bond interactions of the HR2 main chain with conserved asparagine/glutamine in the HR1 helices (40). Hence, except for its helical part, HR2 stretches out like a leash into the grooves of the HR1 coiled coil in a way similar to what has been described for the fusion core of the influenza virus HA protein (116).

Interestingly, the essence of the conformational process undergone by the spike has apparently been reproduced in vitro recently (90). Purified recombinant SARS-CoV spike ectodomain, produced in monomeric form by expression in insect cells, was shown to stably trimerize into clove-like structures just by lowering the pH. Trypsin was found to cleave the proteins precisely at the S1-S2 boundary. Subsequent dissociation of the S1 subunit, either spontaneously or assisted by urea, caused the S2 trimers to rearrange into 250-Å long rods that clustered at one end into rosettes. The rosettes probably represent clusters of elongated postfusion trimers of S2 associated through their fusion peptides (90).

## Membrane Fusion

The mechanism by which viral and cell membranes actually fuse is not well understood. Clearly, as a result of the formation of the six-helix structure, the fusion peptides and transmembrane domains of the spike, previously anchored in opposite membranes

during the prehairpin stage, have joined at one pole of the helix bundle to bring the membranes together and effect their fusion. Membrane fusion is currently viewed as a process with defined events: merging first of the apposing leaflets (lipid stalk formation or hemifusion) and then of the distal leaflets (fusion pore formation), followed by fusion pore enlargement (41, 60). Though more membrane-active domains might be involved, at this stage the most prominent roles are played by the fusion peptide, the transmembrane domain, and the cytoplasmic tail.

### The fusion peptide

Fusion peptides may act at different steps during the fusion reaction (41, 60). The internal fusion peptide of coronaviruses is likely to be involved at least in the early part, when it inserts into the cellular membrane presumably as a loop, penetrating only the outer leaflet. It is subsequently expected to meet with the pretransmembrane region, i.e., the amino-terminal part of the transmembrane domain. The interaction of these hydrophobic domains might promote the destabilization and merger of the two apposing outer membrane leaflets to effect hemifusion. Fusion peptides from the same spike and perhaps from different spikes might act together in this process. Whether these peptides have roles in the subsequent steps of fusion is unclear. Peptides corresponding to the two putative fusion peptides of SARS-CoV spike protein appeared to inhibit plaque formation (126), possibly by competitive binding to the endogenous fusion peptide segment in the target membrane.

### The transmembrane domain

Coronavirus fusion proteins have relatively large transmembrane domains. Though their boundaries have not been exactly defined, they may comprise as much as 33 (SARS-CoV) to 45 (FIPV) residues as judged by the charged residues flanking them (Fig. 5).

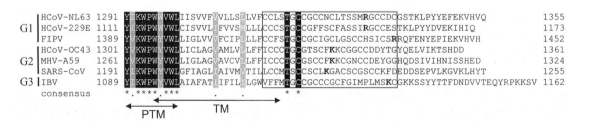

**Figure 5.** Alignment of the spike protein endodomains of the group 1 (G1) coronaviruses HCoV-NL63, HCoV-229E, and FIPV; of the group 2 (G2) coronaviruses HCoV-OC43, MHV-A59, and SARS-CoV; and of the group 3 (G3) coronavirus IBV-Beaudette. Indicated are the pretransmembrane region (PTM), the transmembrane region (TM; as predicted by the TMHMM program [143] for SARS-CoV spike protein), and the cysteine-rich region (boxed). The charged residues first encountered downstream of the predicted TM are in bold. Identical residues are indicated by asterisks, and strongly similar residues are indicated by periods. Residue numbers are indicated on either side of each sequence.

However, according to the TMHMM program (143), presently considered the best transmembrane prediction program (103), the SARS-CoV transmembrane domain consists of only a stretch of 23 residues (residues 1196 to 1218), which includes two cysteines of the cysteine-rich region discussed below.

At its amino-terminal boundary the transmembrane domain of coronavirus spike proteins contains a decameric segment (Y[V/I]KWPW[Y/W]VWL) that is extremely well conserved, suggesting a key role in the functioning of the protein (15). It has been argued that this region may in fact precede the actual transmembrane domain and interact with the membrane like the pretransmembrane region of HIV (57, 127). Peptides corresponding to this region were shown to be membrane active and to inhibit coronavirus infection (57, 126, 127). The region has a high content of aromatic residues, known for their high tendency to locate at membrane interfaces between fatty acids and head group layers (169). This suggests that the region partitions at the virion membrane outer interface rather than dwelling deep in the lipid bilayer. The tryptophan and tyrosine side chains were suggested to destabilize the viral membrane and, together with the fusion peptide, to provide a flow of lipids allowing fusion pore formation to occur (127). It has also been hypothesized that interaction of the transmembrane domains within and possibly between fusion protein trimers is essential for (complete) fusion (135).

### The cytoplasmic tail

The cytoplasmic tail of the coronavirus spike protein has multiple but distinct functions. It is involved in virion assembly, intracellular transport, cell surface expression, and cell-cell fusion. It mediates incorporation of spikes into viral particles through interaction with the viral membrane (M) protein, the key player in virion assembly (9, 183). Signals in the tail also regulate the spike protein's intracellular localization and its transport to the cell surface (93, 187). An important role in fusion has been shown as well (7, 9, 22, 120).

The carboxy-terminal tail of the spike protein counts 36 (MHV-A59, residues 1289 to 1324) to 46 residues (IBV, residues 1117 to 1162). Two domains can be distinguished: a membrane-proximal, conserved cysteine-rich region and a less well-conserved terminal domain (15). The cysteine-rich region (Fig. 5) encompasses some 18 to 24 residues, of which 7 to 10 are cysteines. Deletion of the region in the MHV-A59 and SARS-CoV spike protein abrogated cell-cell fusion (7, 9, 22, 120). Partial deletion (residues 1290 to 1302) removing 4 of the 9 cysteines yielded a viable virus displaying dramatically delayed syncytium formation (183). Deletion of the amino-terminal half (residues 1287 to 1297), taking out 6 cysteines, completely abolished cell-cell fusion by the expressed protein despite its ability to promote hemifusion, as shown in a lipid mixing assay, suggesting that this part of the cysteine-rich region is involved at a post-hemifusion stage of the membrane fusion process (Fig. 6) (22). Substitution of the cysteines in this region, including Cys-1292, which is part of a strictly conserved TxC motif, severely impaired cell-cell fusion (7, 22). Insertion of alanines before the TxC motif (Fig. 5) diminished fusion strongly, whereas alanine insertions downstream of this motif had no detrimental effect (21). The data demonstrate the importance of the identity and of the spacing of at least part of the cysteines in the cysteine-rich region for membrane fusion.

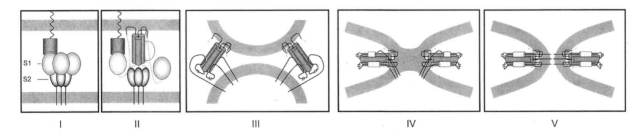

**Figure 6.** Model for coronavirus spike-mediated membrane fusion. (I) Spike in its native, prefusion state interacts with a receptor. Subsequently, dissociation of S1 and S2 is triggered by a cellular factor or condition (receptor binding, proteolytic cleavage, low pH) (II). This, in turn, primes the S2 protein to refold, to expose its fusion peptide, and to insert it into the target cell membrane, resulting in a state defined as the prefusion intermediate (II). Upon continued refolding, the HR2 region zippers alongside the HR1 trimeric coiled coil (III), thereby colocalizing the fusion peptide inserted in the target cell membrane and the transmembrane domain anchored in the viral membrane, and driving the juxtaposition of both membranes. This step can be blocked by heptad repeat corresponding peptides. Completion of the zippering process results in the formation of the HR1-HR2 six-helix bundle and leads to the creation of a hemifusion stalk and eventually to a fusion pore (IV and V), by processes that are presumably mediated by the membrane-interacting domains (e.g., fusion peptide, transmembrane domain, and cytoplasmic tail).

Its involvement in fusion suggests an association of the cysteine-rich region with the membrane. As mentioned above, theoretical predictions with the SARS-CoV spike protein place the amino-terminal two cysteines of the region within the membrane bilayer (Fig. 5). Alternatively, or additionally, the cysteines might also be associated with the membrane through acylation. The S2 domain is known to be palmitoylated (111, 133, 146, 155). At least two cysteine residues in the cysteine-rich region of the MHV-A59 spike protein appear to be palmitoylated, consistent with membrane association (7). Acylation often targets proteins to lipid raft domains. Besides having detrimental effects on complexing with the M proteins, inhibition of palmitoylation of the MHV-A59 spike protein caused them to partition out of detergent-resistant membranes and prevented syncytium formation (152).

Syncytium formation is strictly dependent on the spike protein's surface expression, which is, in turn, often regulated by the cytoplasmic tail. Partial truncation of the SARS-CoV and the MHV spike cytoplasmic tail by 17 residues substantially increased cell-cell fusion (21, 22, 120). This region of the tail might influence the fusion function by regulating cell surface expression through intracellular sorting signals such as ER retrieval signals or internalization signals. Group 1 and 3 coronaviruses, but not group 2 coronaviruses, except SARS-CoV, harbor a dibasic ER retrieval motif in the tail (93). Mutation of this dibasic motif in the otherwise ER-retained IBV spike protein resulted in surface expression, indicating that it is a bona fide ER retrieval signal (93). The cytoplasmic tails of group 1 and 3 coronavirus spike proteins contain an endocytosis signal (YxxΦ) (93, 137), mutation of which surprisingly produced a lethal phenotype for IBV (187). Coronaviruses are assembled at intracellular membranes, where incorporation of spikes is mediated by interactions with the M protein (for a review, see reference 33). How the various cytoplasmic tail transport signals affect this process remains to be established.

## FUSION MODEL

The available data lead us to the working model for coronavirus spike-mediated fusion that is depicted in Fig. 6. It is based in part on observations with other class I fusion proteins, particularly with the influenza virus HA protein, the HIV-1 Env protein, and the paramyxovirus fusion protein (41, 42, 86, 105, 185). Its features have been discussed in the previous sections.

The fusion process is triggered by an event that destabilizes the interaction between the spike subunits.

Interestingly, in the case of coronaviruses this priming event can be any of very different actions or conditions—receptor binding, proteolytic cleavage, or acidic pH—and can hence occur at different cellular locations, i.e., the plasma membrane or an endocytic organelle. The destabilization of the spike leads to a weakening of the interaction between the S1 and S2 subunits and even, in spikes that are cleaved, to the actual dissociation of S1. Apparently, the triggering event allows the metastable spike to overcome a certain low-energy threshold, which, once taken, sets off the irreversible reaction cascade. Accordingly, premature S1-S2 dissociation inactivates the virus.

Once released from the constraints apparently imposed by the chaperoning behavior of the S1 subunit, the S2 protein enters into a dramatic refolding process. During the first part of this process the trimeric S2 structure relaxes, the HR2 trimer opens up, and the previously hidden fusion peptide becomes exposed and is directed toward and inserted into the target membrane, while the HR1 domains associate into a parallel trimer. At this prehairpin stage the extended S2 trimer connects the two opposing membranes, which are subsequently brought closer together by the continued refolding, particularly of the more carboxy-terminal parts of the S2 ectodomains. These rearrangements direct the HR2 regions to the HR1 bundle, where they dock into the grooves exposed by the trimer, zipping up in the direction of the fusion peptides and eventually giving rise to the stable six-helix bundle. This process, and hence the actual fusion reaction, can be inhibited by peptides mimicking the HR domains.

In the last part of the process the fusion peptides and the (pre)transmembrane domains, each associated with its own membrane, come together. Somehow their interaction is supposed to locally destabilize the bilayers and to trigger the flow of lipids, resulting in the hemifusion state. Additional rearrangements, in which also carboxy-terminal tails of the spike protein may play a role, ultimately lead to the creation of a pore, which subsequently enlarges to complete the process.

It is clear that the entire course of actions is an energy-costly process. This energy is obtained from various events such as the spike-receptor interaction, the formation of the HR1 trimeric coiled coil, the insertion of the fusion peptides into the cell membrane, and, particularly, the formation of the trimer-of-hairpins structure.

The coronavirus entry process as we described it here follows in many respects the principles that govern entry by other viruses that use class I fusion proteins. It stands out, however, in a number of interesting aspects, notably with regard to the cleavage issue, the variation in fusion triggers, and the internal position of the fusion peptide. These aspects as well as many other questions concerning the conformational rearrangements, the fusion mechanism, the kinetics, and the possible cooperativity between spikes remain to be elucidated.

## CELL ENTRY BY NONCORONAVIRUS NIDOVIRUSES

Actually, as they have not been the subjects of much study, nothing is really known about the entry mechanisms of the noncoronavirus nidoviruses. Hence, what follows is just a brief summary of the present situation for each virus group.

### Torovirus

Toroviruses, which constitute the second genus—*Torovirus*—in the *Coronaviridae* family, resemble coronaviruses in the composition of their envelope components (for a review on these viruses, see chapter 9). Besides a triple-spanning M protein, the structural hallmark of all nidoviruses, and a hemagglutinin-esterase (HE) protein, a characteristic of group 2 coronaviruses, they exhibit a coronavirus-like spike protein. The spike protein of the prototype equine torovirus (previously known as the Berne virus) measures 1,581 amino acids (141). It is a type I membrane protein synthesized as a highly N-glycosylated 190-kDa precursor glycoprotein, which is processed into 75- and 100-kDa species, both of which are also present in the virion (69, 70). Cleavage most likely takes place at the multibasic arginine motif at position 1006/1007 (141), supposedly by furin or a furin-like enzyme. The spike protein forms peplomers of about 20 nm in length on the virion surface that consist of a globular structure on top of an elongated stem (161). Like in coronaviruses, the membrane-anchored subunit of the spike protein contains two heptad repeat regions, located also at similar positions (HR1, residues 1158 to 1230; HR2, residues 1504 to 1545) (141). When applying the TMAP program, designed to detect transmembrane regions in proteins (119), on a multiple alignment of the porcine and bovine torovirus spike proteins, a putative fusion peptide is predicted immediately amino terminal of HR1 (residues 1107 to 1128) (Bosch and Rottier, unpublished). Its sequence is indeed enriched in glycines but not in alanines, and it conspicuously lacks a proline (Fig. 4). It thus appears that torovirus spike proteins are class I fusion proteins that mediate cell entry similar to their coronavirus counterparts.

### Arteriviridae

As detailed in chapter 17, the envelope of arteriviruses contains six different envelope proteins. In addition to the M protein, it has a second triple-spanning membrane protein, the glycoprotein GP5. These are the major envelope components, occurring in virions in equimolar amounts, consistent with their disulfide linkage. The M-GP5 heterodimers supposedly constitute the tiny virion surface projections (72). The minor envelope constituents are the glycoproteins GP2b, GP3, and GP4 and the small, hydrophobic E protein. These proteins, of which the glycoproteins were shown in equine arteritis virus to occur as a disulfide-bonded heterotrimeric complex (166), are cooperatively incorporated into virions (165, 170). While the GP5 and M proteins are both essential for particle assembly, the minor proteins are not, yet particles lacking the minor protein complex are not infectious (167, 170), indicating that this complex is somehow critical for cell entry. It is, however, fully unclear what its contribution is. Heparan sulfate and sialoadhesin have been identified on porcine macrophages as receptors for porcine reproductive and respiratory syndrome virus (PRRSV) (38, 156), the former by attachment to the M protein and the latter probably by binding to sialic acids on viral glycoproteins (37). PRRSV infects cells by low-pH-dependent endocytic entry (82, 108), as seems also the case for lactate dehydrogenase-elevating virus (81), but it is unclear what confers the target specificity to the infection. It is also unclear which proteins effect the fusion of viral and endosomal membrane. Neither of the envelope proteins nor their complexes bears similarity to either class I or class II fusion proteins. It has been suggested that the minor protein complex, positioned in virions above the vertices of the putatively icosahedral nucleocapsid, may be involved in mediating membrane fusion (167). In any case, it seems like arteriviruses have an original entry mechanism to be discovered.

### Roniviridae

Only two viruses have presently been assigned to the *Roniviridae* family, yellow head virus and gill-associated virus, both members of *Okavirus*, the single genus in this family. Yellow head virus, the causative agent of yellow head disease in shrimp, is an enveloped, rod-shaped particle with prominent ~11-nm surface projections. These spikes are composed of either one or both of the glycoproteins gp116 and gp64, which arise by cleavage from a precursor, presumably cotranslationally by signal peptidases (73, 140). gp64 is predicted to be a type I membrane glycoprotein; gp116 is predicted to be a membrane protein of type III with two transmembrane regions in its carboxy-terminal region and having both the N and C termini oriented externally. gp116 and gp64 are not covalently associated. They do not show any sequence homology with spike proteins of other nidoviruses. Both proteins lack heptad repeat regions and significant amphipathic helices, suggesting the absence of coiled-coil structures (27, 73). As for the arteriviruses, the data indicate a different and so far unknown entry mechanism for these roniviruses.

## WBV

A novel enveloped virus named WBV was recently isolated from white bream fish (*Blicca bjoerkna* L.). It has a bacilliform shape and an array of 20- to 25-nm-long spikes on its envelope reminiscent of those of corona- and toroviruses (56). Analysis of its 26.6-kb genomic RNA revealed a nidovirus-like genome organization. The virus, which appears to represent a taxonomically separate cluster, encodes a 1,220-residue protein with homology to the torovirus and, to a lesser extent, the coronavirus spike protein, and it is hence predicted to represent the WBV spike protein (136). Accordingly, it has a type I membrane topology with features characteristic of class I fusion proteins. It contains a putative furin cleavage site (RRYR↓; residues 802 to 805). Three heptad repeat regions are predicted by the program Multicoil (171): the canonical regions HR1 (residues 840 to 972) and HR2 (residues 1113 to 1171), and an additional region, HR3 (residues 762 to 799), located just upstream of the putative furin cleavage site. In addition to the carboxy-terminal membrane anchor, a second hydrophobic membrane-interacting segment (residues 820 to 847) is detected in the spike protein by the program TMAP (119). This segment is enriched in alanines, glycines, and bulky apolar residues, which are characteristics of (internal) fusion peptides (163). Interestingly, in contrast to the corona- and torovirus spike proteins, the predicted fusion peptide of WBV is located only 14 residues away from the furin cleavage consensus sequence and partly overlaps with the HR1 region. The remote yet significant sequence conservation with the spike proteins of the *Coronaviridae* in combination with the preservation of structural features suggests mechanistic homology with respect to the entry, at least to the membrane fusion machinery.

## PERSPECTIVES

The increased scientific interest in coronaviruses as a result of the outbreak of SARS has given research on these viruses, particularly of their mechanism of cell entry, a strong boost. This has, for instance, led to the elucidation of the atomic structures of portions of the spike protein such as the receptor-binding domain and the pre- and postfusion structures of HR bundles, which gave rise to the classification of the coronavirus spike protein as a class I fusion protein. Though the general picture of the fusion process has become clear, our knowledge is still rudimentary. In fact, there are important fundamental questions to be answered on all the issues that we described in this review, whether related to cleavage activation, entry pathways, functioning of triggers, conformational changes, or mechanism of membrane bilayer fusion. What is urgently needed to enhance our insight is structural information about the spike. Crystal structures of native and postfusion forms will be extremely helpful for our understanding of the process, for the development of models and hypotheses, and for the proper design of experiments to test the ideas. Because coronavirions themselves have appeared inappropriate as sources of spikes, such studies will rely heavily on expressed forms of the spikes. Progress with these technologies, as demonstrated recently by the elucidation of the paramyxovirus fusion protein native structure (185), obviously trigger our expectations. As far as the noncoronavirus nidoviruses are concerned, there is still a very long way to go, but it is already clear that—also—these viruses have a lot of excitement for us in store.

**Acknowledgments.** We thank Stephane Duqueroy for his help in preparing figures and Raoul de Groot for critical reading of the manuscript.

## REFERENCES

1. Appleyard, G., and M. Tisdale. 1985. Inhibition of the growth of human coronavirus 229E by leupeptin. *J. Gen. Virol.* **66** (Pt. 2):363–366.
2. Baker, K. A., R. E. Dutch, R. A. Lamb, and T. S. Jardetzky. 1999. Structural basis for paramyxovirus-mediated membrane fusion. *Mol. Cell* **3**:309–319.
3. Barrett, A. J. 1986. The cystatins: a diverse superfamily of cysteine peptidase inhibitors. *Biomed. Biochim. Acta* **45**:1363–1374.
4. Beniac, D. R., A. Andonov, E. Grudeski, and T. F. Booth. 2006. Architecture of the SARS coronavirus prefusion spike. *Nat. Struct. Mol. Biol.* **13**:751–752.
5. Bisht, H., A. Roberts, L. Vogel, A. Bukreyev, P. L. Collins, B. R. Murphy, K. Subbarao, and B. Moss. 2004. Severe acute respiratory syndrome coronavirus spike protein expressed by attenuated vaccinia virus protectively immunizes mice. *Proc. Natl. Acad. Sci. USA* **101**:6641–6646.
6. Blau, D. M., and K. V. Holmes. 2001. Human coronavirus HCoV-229E enters susceptible cells via the endocytic pathway. *Adv. Exp. Med. Biol.* **494**:193–198.
7. Bos, E. C., L. Heijnen, W. Luytjes, and W. J. Spaan. 1995. Mutational analysis of the murine coronavirus spike protein: effect on cell-to-cell fusion. *Virology* **214**:453–463.
8. Bos, E. C., W. Luytjes, and W. J. Spaan. 1997. The function of the spike protein of mouse hepatitis virus strain A59 can be

studied on virus-like particles: cleavage is not required for infectivity. *J. Virol.* **71:**9427–9433.

9. Bosch, B. J., C. A. de Haan, S. L. Smits, and P. J. Rottier. 2005. Spike protein assembly into the coronavirion: exploring the limits of its sequence requirements. *Virology* **334:**306–318.

10. Bosch, B. J., B. E. Martina, R. Van Der Zee, J. Lepault, B. J. Haijema, C. Versluis, A. J. Heck, R. De Groot, A. D. Osterhaus, and P. J. Rottier. 2004. Severe acute respiratory syndrome coronavirus (SARS-CoV) infection inhibition using spike protein heptad repeat-derived peptides. *Proc. Natl. Acad. Sci. USA* **101:**8455–8460.

11. Bosch, B. J., R. van der Zee, C. A. de Haan, and P. J. Rottier. 2003. The coronavirus spike protein is a class I virus fusion protein: structural and functional characterization of the fusion core complex. *J. Virol.* **77:**8801–8811.

12. Bukreyev, A., E. W. Lamirande, U. J. Buchholz, L. N. Vogel, W. R. Elkins, M. St. Claire, B. R. Murphy, K. Subbarao, and P. L. Collins. 2004. Mucosal immunisation of African green monkeys (Cercopithecus aethiops) with an attenuated parainfluenza virus expressing the SARS coronavirus spike protein for the prevention of SARS. *Lancet* **363:**2122–2127.

13. Bullough, P. A., F. M. Hughson, J. J. Skehel, and D. C. Wiley. 1994. Structure of influenza haemagglutinin at the pH of membrane fusion. *Nature* **371:**37–43.

14. Carson, M. 1997. Ribbons. *Methods Enzymol.* **277:**493–505.

15. Cavanagh, D. 1995. *The Coronavirus Surface Glycoprotein.* Plenum Press, New York, NY.

16. Cavanagh, D., P. J. Davis, D. J. Pappin, M. M. Binns, M. E. Boursnell, and T. D. Brown. 1986. Coronavirus IBV: partial amino terminal sequencing of spike polypeptide S2 identifies the sequence Arg-Arg-Phe-Arg-Arg at the cleavage site of the spike precursor propolypeptide of IBV strains Beaudette and M41. *Virus Res.* **4:**133–143.

17. Chambers, P., C. R. Pringle, and A. J. Easton. 1990. Heptad repeat sequences are located adjacent to hydrophobic regions in several types of virus fusion glycoproteins. *J. Gen. Virol.* **71**(Pt. 12):3075–3080.

18. Chan, D. C., D. Fass, J. M. Berger, and P. S. Kim. 1997. Core structure of gp41 from the HIV envelope glycoprotein. *Cell* **89:**263–273.

19. Chan, W. E., C. K. Chuang, S. H. Yeh, M. S. Chang, and S. S. Chen. 2006. Functional characterization of heptad repeat 1 and 2 mutants of the spike protein of severe acute respiratory syndrome coronavirus. *J. Virol.* **80:**3225–3237.

20. Chandran, K., N. J. Sullivan, U. Felbor, S. P. Whelan, and J. M. Cunningham. 2005. Endosomal proteolysis of the Ebola virus glycoprotein is necessary for infection. *Science* **308:**1643–1645.

21. Chang, K. W., and J. L. Gombold. 2001. Effects of amino acid insertions in the cysteine-rich domain of the MHV-A59 spike protein on cell fusion. *Adv. Exp. Med. Biol.* **494:**205–211.

22. Chang, K. W., Y. Sheng, and J. L. Gombold. 2000. Coronavirus-induced membrane fusion requires the cysteine-rich domain in the spike protein. *Virology* **269:**212–224.

23. Chen, J., J. J. Skehel, and D. C. Wiley. 1999. N- and C-terminal residues combine in the fusion-pH influenza hemagglutinin HA(2) subunit to form an N cap that terminates the triple-stranded coiled coil. *Proc. Natl. Acad. Sci. USA* **96:**8967–8972.

24. Chu, V. C., L. J. McElroy, V. Chu, B. E. Bauman, and G. R. Whittaker. 2006. The avian coronavirus infectious bronchitis virus undergoes direct low-pH-dependent fusion activation during entry into host cells. *J. Virol.* **80:**3180–3188.

25. Collins, A. R., and A. Grubb. 1991. Inhibitory effects of recombinant human cystatin C on human coronaviruses. *Antimicrob. Agents Chemother.* **35:**2444–2446.

26. Collins, A. R., and A. Grubb. 1998. Cystatin D, a natural salivary cysteine protease inhibitor, inhibits coronavirus replication at its physiologic concentration. *Oral Microbiol. Immunol.* **13:**59–61.

27. Cowley, J. A., and P. J. Walker. 2002. The complete genome sequence of gill-associated virus of Penaeus monodon prawns indicates a gene organisation unique among nidoviruses. *Arch. Virol.* **147:**1977–1987.

28. Cyr-Coats, K. S., H. R. Payne, and J. Storz. 1988. The influence of the host cell and trypsin treatment on bovine coronavirus infectivity. *Zentbl. Vetmed. Reihe B* **35:**752–759.

29. Davies, H. A., and M. R. Macnaughton. 1979. Comparison of the morphology of three coronaviruses. *Arch. Virol.* **59:**25–33.

30. de Groot, R. J., W. Luytjes, M. C. Horzinek, B. A. van der Zeijst, W. J. Spaan, and J. A. Lenstra. 1987. Evidence for a coiled-coil structure in the spike proteins of coronaviruses. *J. Mol. Biol.* **196:**963–966.

31. de Groot, R. J., J. Maduro, J. A. Lenstra, M. C. Horzinek, B. A. van der Zeijst, and W. J. Spaan. 1987. cDNA cloning and sequence analysis of the gene encoding the peplomer protein of feline infectious peritonitis virus. *J. Gen. Virol.* **68** (Pt. 10):2639–2346.

32. de Groot, R. J., R. J. ter Haar, M. C. Horzinek, and B. A. van der Zeijst. 1987. Intracellular RNAs of the feline infectious peritonitis coronavirus strain 79-1146. *J. Gen. Virol.* **68** (Pt. 4):995–1002.

33. de Haan, C. A., and P. J. Rottier. 2005. Molecular interactions in the assembly of coronaviruses. *Adv. Virus. Res.* **64:**165–230.

34. de Haan, C. A., K. Stadler, G. J. Godeke, B. J. Bosch, and P. J. Rottier. 2004. Cleavage inhibition of the murine coronavirus spike protein by a furin-like enzyme affects cell-cell but not virus-cell fusion. *J. Virol.* **78:**6048–6054.

35. de Haan, C. A., E. Te Lintelo, Z. Li, M. Raaben, T. Wurdinger, B. J. Bosch, and P. J. Rottier. 2006. Cooperative involvement of the s1 and s2 subunits of the murine coronavirus spike protein in receptor binding and extended host range. *J. Virol.* **80:**10909–10918.

36. Delmas, B., and H. Laude. 1990. Assembly of coronavirus spike protein into trimers and its role in epitope expression. *J. Virol.* **64:**5367–5375.

37. Delputte, P. L., S. Costers, and H. J. Nauwynck. 2005. Analysis of porcine reproductive and respiratory syndrome virus attachment and internalization: distinctive roles for heparan sulphate and sialoadhesin. *J. Gen. Virol.* **86:**1441–1445.

38. Delputte, P. L., N. Vanderheijden, H. J. Nauwynck, and M. B. Pensaert. 2002. Involvement of the matrix protein in attachment of porcine reproductive and respiratory syndrome virus to a heparinlike receptor on porcine alveolar macrophages. *J. Virol.* **76:**4312–4320.

39. Dimitrov, D. S. 2004. Virus entry: molecular mechanisms and biomedical applications. *Nat. Rev. Microbiol.* **2:**109–122.

40. Duquerroy, S., A. Vigouroux, P. J. Rottier, F. A. Rey, and B. J. Bosch. 2005. Central ions and lateral asparagine/glutamine zippers stabilize the post-fusion hairpin conformation of the SARS coronavirus spike glycoprotein. *Virology* **335:**276–285.

41. Earp, L. J., S. E. Delos, H. E. Park, and J. M. White. 2005. The many mechanisms of viral membrane fusion proteins. *Curr. Top. Microbiol. Immunol.* **285:**25–66.

42. Eckert, D. M., and P. S. Kim. 2001. Mechanisms of viral membrane fusion and its inhibition. *Annu. Rev. Biochem.* **70:**777–810.

43. Egberink, H. F., J. Ederveen, P. Callebaut, and M. C. Horzinek. 1988. Characterization of the structural proteins of porcine epizootic diarrhea virus, strain CV777. *Am. J. Vet. Res.* **49:**1320–1324.

44. Epand, R. M. 2003. Fusion peptides and the mechanism of viral fusion. *Biochim. Biophys. Acta* **1614:**116–121.

45. Follis, K. E., J. York, and J. H. Nunberg. 2005. Serine-scanning mutagenesis studies of the C-terminal heptad repeats in the SARS coronavirus S glycoprotein highlight the important role of the short helical region. *Virology* **341:**122–129.

46. Follis, K. E., J. York, and J. H. Nunberg. 2006. Furin cleavage of the SARS coronavirus spike glycoprotein enhances cell-cell fusion but does not affect virion entry. *Virology* **350:**358–369.

47. Frana, M. F., J. N. Behnke, L. S. Sturman, and K. V. Holmes. 1985. Proteolytic cleavage of the E2 glycoprotein of murine coronavirus: host-dependent differences in proteolytic cleavage and cell fusion. *J. Virol.* **56:**912–920.

48. Gallagher, T. M. 1997. A role for naturally occurring variation of the murine coronavirus spike protein in stabilizing association with the cellular receptor. *J. Virol.* **71:**3129–3137.

49. Gallagher, T. M., and M. J. Buchmeier. 2001. Coronavirus spike proteins in viral entry and pathogenesis. *Virology* **279:**371–374.

50. Gallagher, T. M., M. J. Buchmeier, and S. Perlman. 1992. Cell receptor-independent infection by a neurotropic murine coronavirus. *Virology* **191:** 517–522.

51. Gallagher, T. M., C. Escarmis, and M. J. Buchmeier. 1991. Alteration of the pH dependence of coronavirus-induced cell fusion: effect of mutations in the spike glycoprotein. *J. Virol.* **65:**1916–1928.

52. Garwes, D. J., and D. H. Pocock. 1975. The polypeptide structure of transmissible gastroenteritis virus. *J. Gen. Virol.* **29:**25–34.

53. Giroglou, T., J. Cinatl, Jr., H. Rabenau, C. Drosten, H. Schwalbe, H. W. Doerr, and D. von Laer. 2004. Retroviral vectors pseudotyped with severe acute respiratory syndrome coronavirus S protein. *J. Virol.* **78:**9007–9015.

54. Gombold, J. L., S. T. Hingley, and S. R. Weiss. 1993. Fusion-defective mutants of mouse hepatitis virus A59 contain a mutation in the spike protein cleavage signal. *J. Virol.* **67:**4504–4512.

55. Gombold, J. L., S. T. Hingley, and S. R. Weiss. 1993. Identification of peplomer cleavage site mutations arising during persistence of MHV-A59. *Adv. Exp. Med. Biol.* **342:**157–163.

56. Granzow, H., F. Weiland, D. Fichtner, H. Schutze, A. Karger, E. Mundt, B. Dresenkamp, P. Martin, and T. C. Mettenleiter. 2001. Identification and ultrastructural characterization of a novel virus from fish. *J. Gen. Virol.* **82:**2849–2859.

57. Guillén, J., A. J. Pérez-Berná, M. R. Moreno, and J. Villalaín. 2005. Identification of the membrane-active regions of the severe acute respiratory syndrome coronavirus spike membrane glycoprotein using a 16/18-mer peptide scan: implications for the viral fusion mechanism. *J. Virol.* **79:**1743–1752.

58. Hakansson-McReynolds, S., S. Jiang, L. Rong, and M. Caffrey. 2006. Solution structure of the severe acute respiratory syndrome-coronavirus heptad repeat 2 domain in the prefusion state. *J. Biol. Chem.* **281:**11965–11971.

59. Hansen, G. H., B. Delmas, L. Besnardeau, L. K. Vogel, H. Laude, H. Sjostrom, and O. Noren. 1998. The coronavirus transmissible gastroenteritis virus causes infection after receptor-mediated endocytosis and acid-dependent fusion with an intracellular compartment. *J. Virol.* **72:**527–534.

60. Hernandez, L. D., L. R. Hoffman, T. G. Wolfsberg, and J. M. White. 1996. Virus-cell and cell-cell fusion. *Annu. Rev. Cell Dev. Biol.* **12:**627–661.

61. Hingley, S. T., I. Leparc-Goffart, and S. R. Weiss. 1998. The mouse hepatitis virus A59 spike protein is not cleaved in primary hepatocyte and glial cell cultures. *Adv. Exp. Med. Biol.* **440:**529–535.

62. Hirano, N., K. Fujiwara, S. Hino, and M. Matumoto. 1974. Replication and plaque formation of mouse hepatitis virus (MHV-2) in mouse cell line DBT culture. *Arch. Gesamte. Virusforsch.* **44:**298–302.

63. Hofmann, H., K. Hattermann, A. Marzi, T. Gramberg, M. Geier, M. Krumbiegel, S. Kuate, K. Uberla, M. Niedrig, and S. Pohlmann. 2004. S protein of severe acute respiratory syndrome-associated coronavirus mediates entry into hepatoma cell lines and is targeted by neutralizing antibodies in infected patients. *J. Virol.* **78:**6134–6142.

64. Hofmann, H., G. Simmons, A. J. Rennekamp, C. Chaipan, T. Gramberg, E. Heck, M. Geier, A. Wegele, A. Marzi, P. Bates, and S. Pohlmann. 2006. Highly conserved regions within the spike proteins of human coronaviruses 229E and NL63 determine recognition of their respective cellular receptors. *J. Virol.* **80:**8639–8652.

65. Hofmann, M., and R. Wyler. 1988. Propagation of the virus of porcine epidemic diarrhea in cell culture. *J. Clin. Microbiol.* **26:**2235–2239.

66. Holmes, K. V., and S. R. Compton. 1995. *Coronavirus Receptors.* Plenum Press, New York, NY.

67. Homma, M. 1971. Trypsin action on the growth of Sendai virus in tissue culture cells. I. Restoration of the infectivity for L cells by direct action of trypsin on L cell-borne Sendai virus. *J. Virol.* **8:**619–629.

68. Honey, K., and A. Y. Rudensky. 2003. Lysosomal cysteine proteases regulate antigen presentation. *Nat. Rev. Immunol.* **3:**472–482.

69. Horzinek, M. C., J. Ederveen, B. Kaeffer, D. de Boer, and M. Weiss. 1986. The peplomers of Berne virus. *J. Gen. Virol.* **67**(Pt. 11)**:**2475–2483.

70. Horzinek, M. C., M. Weiss, and J. Ederveen. 1984. Berne virus is not 'coronavirus-like.' *J. Gen. Virol.* **65**(Pt. 3)**:**645–649.

71. Huang, I. C., B. J. Bosch, F. Li, W. Li, K. H. Lee, S. Ghiran, N. Vasilieva, T. S. Dermody, S. C. Harrison, P. R. Dormitzer, M. Farzan, P. J. Rottier, and H. Choe. 2006. SARS coronavirus, but not human coronavirus NL63, utilizes cathepsin L to infect ACE2-expressing cells. *J. Biol. Chem.* **281:**3198–3203.

72. Hyllseth, B. 1973. Structural proteins of equine arteritis virus. *Arch. Gesamte Virusforsch.* **40:**177–188.

73. Jitrapakdee, S., S. Unajak, N. Sittidilokratna, R. A. Hodgson, J. A. Cowley, P. J. Walker, S. Panyim, and V. Boonsaeng. 2003. Identification and analysis of gp116 and gp64 structural glycoproteins of yellow head nidovirus of Penaeus monodon shrimp. *J. Gen. Virol.* **84:**863–873.

74. Keck, J. G., L. H. Soe, S. Makino, S. A. Stohlman, and M. M. Lai. 1988. RNA recombination of murine coronaviruses: recombination between fusion-positive mouse hepatitis virus A59 and fusion-negative mouse hepatitis virus 2. *J. Virol.* **62:**1989–1998.

75. Keng, C. T., A. Zhang, S. Shen, K. M. Lip, B. C. Fielding, T. H. Tan, C. F. Chou, C. B. Loh, S. Wang, J. Fu, X. Yang, S. G. Lim, W. Hong, and Y. J. Tan. 2005. Amino acids 1055 to 1192 in the S2 region of severe acute respiratory syndrome coronavirus S protein induce neutralizing antibodies: implications for the development of vaccines and antiviral agents. *J. Virol.* **79:**3289–3296.

76. Keyaerts, E., L. Vijgen, P. Maes, J. Neyts, and M. Van Ranst. 2004. In vitro inhibition of severe acute respiratory syndrome coronavirus by chloroquine. *Biochem. Biophys. Res. Commun.* **323:**264–268.

77. Kido, H., Y. Yokogoshi, K. Sakai, M. Tashiro, Y. Kishino, A. Fukutomi, and N. Katunuma. 1992. Isolation and characterization of a novel trypsin-like protease found in rat bronchiolar epithelial Clara cells. A possible activator of the viral fusion glycoprotein. *J. Biol. Chem.* **267:**13573–13579.

78. Kielian, M., and F. A. Rey. 2006. Virus membrane-fusion proteins: more than one way to make a hairpin. *Nat. Rev. Microbiol.* **4:**67–76.

79. Klenk, H. D., and W. Garten. 1994. Host cell proteases controlling virus pathogenicity. *Trends Microbiol.* **2:**39–43.

80. Kooi, C., M. Cervin, and R. Anderson. 1991. Differentiation of acid-pH-dependent and -nondependent entry pathways for mouse hepatitis virus. *Virology* **180:**108–119.

81. Kowalchyk, K., and P. G. Plagemann. 1985. Cell surface receptors for lactate dehydrogenase-elevating virus on subpopulation of macrophages. *Virus Res.* **2:**211–229.

82. Kreutz, L. C., and M. R. Ackermann. 1996. Porcine reproductive and respiratory syndrome virus enters cells through a low pH-dependent endocytic pathway. *Virus Res.* **42:**137–147.

83. Krueger, D. K., S. M. Kelly, D. N. Lewicki, R. Ruffolo, and T. M. Gallagher. 2001. Variations in disparate regions of the murine coronavirus spike protein impact the initiation of membrane fusion. *J. Virol.* **75:**2792–2802.

84. Krzystyniak, K., and J. M. Dupuy. 1984. Entry of mouse hepatitis virus 3 into cells. *J. Gen. Virol.* **65**(Pt. 1):227–231.

85. Lai, S. C., P. C. Chong, C. T. Yeh, L. S. Liu, J. T. Jan, H. Y. Chi, H. W. Liu, A. Chen, and Y. C. Wang. 2005. Characterization of neutralizing monoclonal antibodies recognizing a 15-residues epitope on the spike protein HR2 region of severe acute respiratory syndrome coronavirus (SARS-CoV). *J. Biomed. Sci.* **12:**711–727.

86. Lamb, R. A., R. G. Paterson, and T. S. Jardetzky. 2006. Paramyxovirus membrane fusion: lessons from the F and HN atomic structures. *Virology* **344:**30–37.

87. Laude, H., D. Rasschaert, B. Delmas, M. Godet, J. Gelfi, and B. Charley. 1990. Molecular biology of transmissible gastroenteritis virus. *Vet. Microbiol.* **23:**147–154.

88. Lewicki, D. N., and T. M. Gallagher. 2002. Quaternary structure of coronavirus spikes in complex with carcinoembryonic antigen-related cell adhesion molecule cellular receptors. *J. Biol. Chem.* **277:**19727–19734.

89. Li, D., and D. Cavanagh. 1992. Coronavirus IBV-induced membrane fusion occurs at near-neutral pH. *Arch. Virol.* **122:**307–316.

90. Li, F., M. Berardi, W. Li, M. Farzan, P. R. Dormitzer, and S. C. Harrison. 2006. Conformational states of the severe acute respiratory syndrome coronavirus spike protein ectodomain. *J. Virol.* **80:**6794–6800.

91. Lip, K. M., S. Shen, X. Yang, C. T. Keng, A. Zhang, H. L. Oh, Z. H. Li, L. A. Hwang, C. F. Chou, B. C. Fielding, T. H. Tan, J. Mayrhofer, F. G. Falkner, J. Fu, S. G. Lim, W. Hong, and Y. J. Tan. 2006. Monoclonal antibodies targeting the HR2 domain and the region immediately upstream of the HR2 of the S protein neutralize in vitro infection of severe acute respiratory syndrome coronavirus. *J. Virol.* **80:**941–950.

92. Liu, S., G. Xiao, Y. Chen, Y. He, J. Niu, C. R. Escalante, H. Xiong, J. Farmar, A. K. Debnath, P. Tien, and S. Jiang. 2004. Interaction between heptad repeat 1 and 2 regions in spike protein of SARS-associated coronavirus: implications for virus fusogenic mechanism and identification of fusion inhibitors. *Lancet* **363:**938–947.

93. Lontok, E., E. Corse, and C. E. Machamer. 2004. Intracellular targeting signals contribute to localization of coronavirus spike proteins near the virus assembly site. *J. Virol.* **78:**5913–5922.

94. Luo, Z., A. M. Matthews, and S. R. Weiss. 1999. Amino acid substitutions within the leucine zipper domain of the murine coronavirus spike protein cause defects in oligomerization and the ability to induce cell-to-cell fusion. *J. Virol.* **73:**8152–8159.

95. Luytjes, W., L. S. Sturman, P. J. Bredenbeek, J. Charite, B. A. van der Zeijst, M. C. Horzinek, and W. J. Spaan. 1987.

Primary structure of the glycoprotein E2 of coronavirus MHV-A59 and identification of the trypsin cleavage site. *Virology* **161:**479–487.

96. Malashkevich, V. N., B. J. Schneider, M. L. McNally, M. A. Milhollen, J. X. Pang, and P. S. Kim. 1999. Core structure of the envelope glycoprotein GP2 from Ebola virus at 1.9-A resolution. *Proc. Natl. Acad. Sci. USA* **96:**2662–2667.

97. Marsh, M., and A. Helenius. 2006. Virus entry: open sesame. *Cell* **124:**729–740.

98. Matsuyama, S., S. E. Delos, and J. M. White. 2004. Sequential roles of receptor binding and low pH in forming prehairpin and hairpin conformations of a retroviral envelope glycoprotein. *J. Virol.* **78:**8201–8209.

99. Matsuyama, S., and F. Taguchi. 2002. Communication between S1N330 and a region in S2 of murine coronavirus spike protein is important for virus entry into cells expressing CEACAM1b receptor. *Virology* **295:**160–171.

100. Matsuyama, S., and F. Taguchi. 2002. Receptor-induced conformational changes of murine coronavirus spike protein. *J. Virol.* **76:**11819–11826.

101. Matsuyama, S., M. Ujike, S. Morikawa, M. Tashiro, and F. Taguchi. 2005. Protease-mediated enhancement of severe acute respiratory syndrome coronavirus infection. *Proc. Natl. Acad. Sci. USA* **102:**12543–12547.

102. Mizzen, L., A. Hilton, S. Cheley, and R. Anderson. 1985. Attenuation of murine coronavirus infection by ammonium chloride. *Virology* **142:**378–388.

103. Moller, S., M. D. Croning, and R. Apweiler. 2001. Evaluation of methods for the prediction of membrane spanning regions. *Bioinformatics* **17:**646–653.

104. Molloy, S. S., P. A. Bresnahan, S. H. Leppla, K. R. Klimpel, and G. Thomas. 1992. Human furin is a calcium-dependent serine endoprotease that recognizes the sequence Arg-X-X-Arg and efficiently cleaves anthrax toxin protective antigen. *J. Biol. Chem.* **267:**16396–16402.

105. Morrison, T. G. 2003. Structure and function of a paramyxovirus fusion protein. *Biochim. Biophys. Acta.* **1614:**73–84.

106. Mothes, W., A. L. Boerger, S. Narayan, J. M. Cunningham, and J. A. Young. 2000. Retroviral entry mediated by receptor priming and low pH triggering of an envelope glycoprotein. *Cell* **103:**679–689.

107. Nash, T. C., and M. J. Buchmeier. 1997. Entry of mouse hepatitis virus into cells by endosomal and nonendosomal pathways. *Virology* **233:**1–8.

108. Nauwynck, H. J., X. Duan, H. W. Favoreel, P. Van Oostveldt, and M. B. Pensaert. 1999. Entry of porcine reproductive and respiratory syndrome virus into porcine alveolar macrophages via receptor-mediated endocytosis. *J. Gen. Virol.* **80**(Pt. 2):297–305.

109. Neuman, B. W., B. D. Adair, C. Yoshioka, J. D. Quispe, G. Orca, P. Kuhn, R. A. Milligan, M. Yeager, and M. J. Buchmeier. 2006. Supramolecular architecture of severe acute respiratory syndrome coronavirus revealed by electron cryomicroscopy. *J. Virol.* **80:**7918–7928.

110. Neumann, G., H. Feldmann, S. Watanabe, I. Lukashevich, and Y. Kawaoka. 2002. Reverse genetics demonstrates that proteolytic processing of the Ebola virus glycoprotein is not essential for replication in cell culture. *J. Virol.* **76:**406–410.

111. Niemann, H., and H. D. Klenk. 1981. Coronavirus glycoprotein E1, a new type of viral glycoprotein. *J. Mol. Biol.* **153:**993–1010.

112. Nomura, R., A. Kiyota, E. Suzaki, K. Kataoka, Y. Ohe, K. Miyamoto, T. Senda, and T. Fujimoto. 2004. Human coronavirus 229E binds to CD13 in rafts and enters the cell through caveolae. *J. Virol.* **78:**8701–8708.

113. Opstelten, D. J., P. de Groote, M. C. Horzinek, H. Vennema, and P. J. Rottier. 1993. Disulfide bonds in folding and transport of mouse hepatitis coronavirus glycoproteins. *J. Virol.* 67:7394–7401.

114. Pager, C. T., W. W. Craft, Jr., J. Patch, and R. E. Dutch. 2006. A mature and fusogenic form of the Nipah virus fusion protein requires proteolytic processing by cathepsin L. *Virology* 346:251–257.

115. Pager, C. T., and R. E. Dutch. 2005. Cathepsin L is involved in proteolytic processing of the Hendra virus fusion protein. *J. Virol.* 79:12714–12720.

116. Park, H. E., J. A. Gruenke, and J. M. White. 2003. Leash in the groove mechanism of membrane fusion. *Nat. Struct. Biol.* 10:1048–1053.

117. Payne, H. R., and J. Storz. 1988. Analysis of cell fusion induced by bovine coronavirus infection. *Arch. Virol.* 103:27–33.

118. Payne, H. R., J. Storz, and W. G. Henk. 1990. Initial events in bovine coronavirus infection: analysis through immunogold probes and lysosomotropic inhibitors. *Arch. Virol.* 114:175–189.

119. Persson, B., and P. Argos. 1997. Prediction of membrane protein topology utilizing multiple sequence alignments. *J. Protein Chem.* 16:453–457.

120. Petit, C. M., J. M. Melancon, V. N. Chouljenko, R. Colgrove, M. Farzan, D. M. Knipe, and K. G. Kousoulas. 2005. Genetic analysis of the SARS-coronavirus spike glycoprotein functional domains involved in cell-surface expression and cell-to-cell fusion. *Virology* 341:215–230.

121. Pratelli, A., V. Martella, N. Decaro, A. Tinelli, M. Camero, F. Cirone, G. Elia, A. Cavalli, M. Corrente, G. Greco, D. Buonavoglia, M. Gentile, M. Tempesta, and C. Buonavoglia. 2003. Genetic diversity of a canine coronavirus detected in pups with diarrhoea in Italy. *J. Virol. Methods* 110:9–17.

122. Pyrc, K., B. J. Bosch, B. Berkhout, M. F. Jebbink, R. Dijkman, P. Rottier, and L. van der Hoek. 2006. Inhibition of human coronavirus NL63 infection at early stages of the replication cycle. *Antimicrob. Agents Chemother.* 50:2000–2008.

123. Qiu, Z., S. T. Hingley, G. Simmons, C. Yu, J. Das Sarma, P. Bates, and S. R. Weiss. 2006. Endosomal proteolysis by cathepsins is necessary for murine coronavirus mouse hepatitis virus type 2 spike-mediated entry. *J. Virol.* 80:5768–5776.

124. Rost, B., G. Yachdav, and J. Liu. 2004. The Predict Protein server. *Nucleic Acids Res.* 32:W321–W326.

125. Routledge, E., R. Stauber, M. Pfleiderer, and S. G. Siddell. 1991. Analysis of murine coronavirus surface glycoprotein functions by using monoclonal antibodies. *J. Virol.* 65:254–262.

126. Sainz, B., Jr., E. C. Mossel, W. R. Gallaher, W. C. Wimley, C. J. Peters, R. B. Wilson, and R. F. Garry. 2006. Inhibition of severe acute respiratory syndrome-associated coronavirus (SARS-CoV) infectivity by peptides analogous to the viral spike protein. *Virus Res.* 120:146–155.

127. Sainz, B., Jr., J. M. Rausch, W. R. Gallaher, R. F. Garry, and W. C. Wimley. 2005. The aromatic domain of the coronavirus class I viral fusion protein induces membrane permeabilization: putative role during viral entry. *Biochemistry* 44:947–958.

128. Sainz, B., Jr., J. M. Rausch, W. R. Gallaher, R. F. Garry, and W. C. Wimley. 2005. Identification and characterization of the putative fusion peptide of the severe acute respiratory syndrome-associated coronavirus spike protein. *J. Virol.* 79:7195–7206.

129. Sawicki, S. G. 1987. Characterization of a small plaque mutant of the A59 strain of mouse hepatitis virus defective in cell fusion. *Adv. Exp. Med. Biol.* 218:169–174.

130. Scheid, A., and P. W. Choppin. 1974. Identification of biological activities of paramyxovirus glycoproteins. Activation of cell fusion, hemolysis, and infectivity of proteolytic cleavage of an inactive precursor protein of Sendai virus. *Virology* 57:475–490.

131. Schibli, D. J., and W. Weissenhorn. 2004. Class I and class II viral fusion protein structures reveal similar principles in membrane fusion. *Mol. Membr. Biol.* 21:361–371.

132. Schmidt, I., M. Skinner, and S. Siddell. 1987. Nucleotide sequence of the gene encoding the surface projection glycoprotein of coronavirus MHV-JHM. *J. Gen. Virol.* 68(Pt. 1):47–56.

133. Schmidt, M. F. 1982. Acylation of viral spike glycoproteins: a feature of enveloped RNA viruses. *Virology* 116:327–338.

134. Schornberg, K., S. Matsuyama, K. Kabsch, S. Delos, A. Bouton, and J. White. 2006. Role of endosomal cathepsins in entry mediated by the Ebola virus glycoprotein. *J. Virol.* 80:4174–4178.

135. Schroth-Diez, B., K. Ludwig, B. Baljinnyam, C. Kozerski, Q. Huang, and A. Herrmann. 2000. The role of the transmembrane and of the intraviral domain of glycoproteins in membrane fusion of enveloped viruses. *Biosci. Rep.* 20:571–595.

136. Schütze, H., R. Ulferts, B. Schelle, S. Bayer, H. Granzow, B. Hoffmann, T. C. Mettenleiter, and J. Ziebuhr. 2006. Characterization of *White bream virus* reveals a novel genetic cluster of nidoviruses. *J. Virol.* 80:11598–11609.

137. Schwegmann-Wessels, C., M. Al-Falah, D. Escors, Z. Wang, G. Zimmer, H. Deng, L. Enjuanes, H. Y. Naim, and G. Herrler. 2004. A novel sorting signal for intracellular localization is present in the S protein of a porcine coronavirus but absent from severe acute respiratory syndrome-associated coronavirus. *J. Biol. Chem.* 279:43661–43666.

138. Simmons, G., D. N. Gosalia, A. J. Rennekamp, J. D. Reeves, S. L. Diamond, and P. Bates. 2005. Inhibitors of cathepsin L prevent severe acute respiratory syndrome coronavirus entry. *Proc. Natl. Acad. Sci. USA* 102:11876–11881.

139. Simmons, G., J. D. Reeves, A. J. Rennekamp, S. M. Amberg, A. J. Piefer, and P. Bates. 2004. Characterization of severe acute respiratory syndrome-associated coronavirus (SARS-CoV) spike glycoprotein-mediated viral entry. *Proc. Natl. Acad. Sci. USA* 101:4240–4245.

140. Sittidilokratna, N., N. Phetchampai, V. Boonsaeng, and P. J. Walker. 2006. Structural and antigenic analysis of the yellow head virus nucleocapsid protein p20. *Virus Res.* 116:21–29.

141. Snijder, E. J., J. A. Den Boon, W. J. Spaan, M. Weiss, and M. C. Horzinek. 1990. Primary structure and post-translational processing of the Berne virus peplomer protein. *Virology* 178:355–363.

142. Song, H. C., M. Y. Seo, K. Stadler, B. J. Yoo, Q. L. Choo, S. R. Coates, Y. Uematsu, T. Harada, C. E. Greer, J. M. Polo, P. Pileri, M. Eickmann, R. Rappuoli, S. Abrignani, M. Houghton, and J. H. Han. 2004. Synthesis and characterization of a native, oligomeric form of recombinant severe acute respiratory syndrome coronavirus spike glycoprotein. *J. Virol.* 78:10328–10335.

143. Sonnhammer, E. L., G. von Heijne, and A. Krogh. 1998. A hidden Markov model for predicting transmembrane helices in protein sequences. *Proc. Int. Conf. Intell. Syst. Mol. Biol.* 6:175–182.

144. Stauber, R., M. Pfleiderera, and S. Siddell. 1993. Proteolytic cleavage of the murine coronavirus surface glycoprotein is not required for fusion activity. *J. Gen. Virol.* 74(Pt. 2):183–191.

145. Storz, J., R. Rott, and G. Kaluza. 1981. Enhancement of plaque formation and cell fusion of an enteropathogenic coronavirus by trypsin treatment. *Infect. Immun.* 31:1214–1222.

146. Sturman, L. S., C. S. Ricard, and K. V. Holmes. 1985. Proteolytic cleavage of the E2 glycoprotein of murine coronavirus: activation of cell-fusing activity of virions by trypsin and separation of two different 90K cleavage fragments. *J. Virol.* **56:**904–911.

147. Sturman, L. S., C. S. Ricard, and K. V. Holmes. 1990. Conformational change of the coronavirus peplomer glycoprotein at pH 8.0 and 37°C correlates with virus aggregation and virus-induced cell fusion. *J. Virol.* **64:**3042–3050.

148. Supekar, V. M., C. Bruckmann, P. Ingallinella, E. Bianchi, A. Pessi, and A. Carfi. 2004. Structure of a proteolytically resistant core from the severe acute respiratory syndrome coronavirus S2 fusion protein. *Proc. Natl. Acad. Sci. USA* **101:**17958–17963.

149. Taguchi, F. 1993. Fusion formation by the uncleaved spike protein of murine coronavirus JHMV variant cl-2. *J. Virol.* **67:**1195–1202.

150. Taguchi, F., and S. Matsuyama. 2002. Soluble receptor potentiates receptor-independent infection by murine coronavirus. *J. Virol.* **76:**950–958.

151. Thomas, G. 2002. Furin at the cutting edge: from protein traffic to embryogenesis and disease. *Nat. Rev. Mol. Cell. Biol.* **3:**753–766.

152. Thorp, E. B., J. A. Boscarino, H. L. Logan, J. T. Goletz, and T. M. Gallagher. 2006. Palmitoylations on murine coronavirus spike proteins are essential for virion assembly and infectivity. *J. Virol.* **80:**1280–1289.

153. Tripet, B., M. W. Howard, M. Jobling, R. K. Holmes, K. V. Holmes, and R. S. Hodges. 2004. Structural characterization of the SARS-coronavirus spike S fusion protein core. *J. Biol. Chem.* **279:**20836–20849.

154. Tsai, J. C., B. D. Zelus, K. V. Holmes, and S. R. Weiss. 2003. The N-terminal domain of the murine coronavirus spike glycoprotein determines the CEACAM1 receptor specificity of the virus strain. *J. Virol.* **77:**841–850.

155. van Berlo, M. F., W. J. van den Brink, M. C. Horzinek, and B. A. van der Zeijst. 1987. Fatty acid acylation of viral proteins in murine hepatitis virus-infected cells. Brief report. *Arch. Virol.* **95:**123–128.

156. Vanderheijden, N., P. L. Delputte, H. W. Favoreel, J. Vandekerckhove, J. Van Damme, P. A. van Woensel, and H. J. Nauwynck. 2003. Involvement of sialoadhesin in entry of porcine reproductive and respiratory syndrome virus into porcine alveolar macrophages. *J. Virol.* **77:**8207–8215.

157. Vincent, M. J., E. Bergeron, S. Benjannet, B. R. Erickson, P. E. Rollin, T. G. Ksiazek, N. G. Seidah, and S. T. Nichol. 2005. Chloroquine is a potent inhibitor of SARS coronavirus infection and spread. *Virol. J.* **2:**69.

158. Volchkov, V. E., H. Feldmann, V. A. Volchkova, and H. D. Klenk. 1998. Processing of the Ebola virus glycoprotein by the proprotein convertase furin. *Proc. Natl. Acad. Sci. USA* **95:**5762–5767.

159. Watanabe, R., S. Matsuyama, and F. Taguchi. 2006. Receptor-independent infection of murine coronavirus: analysis by spinoculation. *J. Virol.* **80:**4901–4908.

160. Weismiller, D. G., L. S. Sturman, M. J. Buchmeier, J. O. Fleming, and K. V. Holmes. 1990. Monoclonal antibodies to the peplomer glycoprotein of coronavirus mouse hepatitis virus identify two subunits and detect a conformational change in the subunit released under mild alkaline conditions. *J. Virol.* **64:**3051–3055.

161. Weiss, M., F. Steck, and M. C. Horzinek. 1983. Purification and partial characterization of a new enveloped RNA virus (Berne virus). *J. Gen. Virol.* **64**(Pt. 9):1849–1858.

162. Wesseling, J. G., H. Vennema, G. J. Godeke, M. C. Horzinek, and P. J. Rottier. 1994. Nucleotide sequence and expression of the spike (S) gene of canine coronavirus and comparison with the S proteins of feline and porcine coronaviruses. *J. Gen. Virol.* **75**(Pt. 7):1789–1794.

163. White, J. M. 1990. Viral and cellular membrane fusion proteins. *Annu. Rev. Physiol.* **52:**675–697.

164. White, J. M. 1992. Membrane fusion. *Science* **258:**917–924.

165. Wieringa, R., A. A. De Vries, S. M. Post, and P. J. Rottier. 2003. Intra- and intermolecular disulfide bonds of the GP2b glycoprotein of equine arteritis virus: relevance for virus assembly and infectivity. *J. Virol.* **77:**12996–13004.

166. Wieringa, R., A. A. de Vries, and P. J. Rottier. 2003. Formation of disulfide-linked complexes between the three minor envelope glycoproteins (GP2b, GP3, and GP4) of equine arteritis virus. *J. Virol.* **77:**6216–6226.

167. Wieringa, R., A. A. de Vries, J. van der Meulen, G. J. Godeke, J. J. Onderwater, H. van Tol, H. K. Koerten, A. M. Mommaas, E. J. Snijder, and P. J. Rottier. 2004. Structural protein requirements in equine arteritis virus assembly. *J. Virol.* **78:** 13019–13027.

168. Wilson, I. A., J. J. Skehel, and D. C. Wiley. 1981. Structure of the haemagglutinin membrane glycoprotein of influenza virus at 3 A resolution. *Nature* **289:**366–373.

169. Wimley, W. C., and S. H. White. 1993. Membrane partitioning: distinguishing bilayer effects from the hydrophobic effect. *Biochemistry* **32:**6307–6312.

170. Wissink, E. H., M. V. Kroese, H. A. van Wijk, F. A. Rijsewijk, J. J. Meulenberg, and P. J. Rottier. 2005. Envelope protein requirements for the assembly of infectious virions of porcine reproductive and respiratory syndrome virus. *J. Virol.* **79:** 12495–12506.

171. Wolf, E., P. S. Kim, and B. Berger. 1997. MultiCoil: a program for predicting two- and three-stranded coiled coils. *Protein Sci.* **6:**1179–1189.

172. Wool-Lewis, R. J., and P. Bates. 1999. Endoproteolytic processing of the Ebola virus envelope glycoprotein: cleavage is not required for function. *J. Virol.* **73:**1419–1426.

173. Wurdinger, T., M. H. Verheije, K. Broen, B. J. Bosch, B. J. Haijema, C. A. de Haan, V. W. van Beusechem, W. R. Gerritsen, and P. J. Rottier. 2005. Soluble receptor-mediated targeting of mouse hepatitis coronavirus to the human epidermal growth factor receptor. *J. Virol.* **79:**15314–15322.

174. Wurdinger, T., M. H. Verheije, M. Raaben, B. J. Bosch, C. A. de Haan, V. W. van Beusechem, P. J. Rottier, and W. R. Gerritsen. 2005. Targeting non-human coronaviruses to human cancer cells using a bispecific single-chain antibody. *Gene Ther.* **12:**1394–1404.

175. Xiao, X., S. Chakraborti, A. S. Dimitrov, K. Gramatikoff, and D. S. Dimitrov. 2003. The SARS-CoV S glycoprotein: expression and functional characterization. *Biochem. Biophys. Res. Commun.* **312:**1159–1164.

176. Xu, Y., Y. Liu, Z. Lou, L. Qin, X. Li, Z. Bai, H. Pang, P. Tien, G. F. Gao, and Z. Rao. 2004. Structural basis for coronavirus-mediated membrane fusion. Crystal structure of mouse hepatitis virus spike protein fusion core. *J. Biol. Chem.* **279:**30514–30522.

177. Xu, Y., Z. Lou, Y. Liu, H. Pang, P. Tien, G. F. Gao, and Z. Rao. 2004. Crystal structure of severe acute respiratory syndrome coronavirus spike protein fusion core. *J. Biol. Chem.* **279:**49414–49419.

178. Xu, Y., J. Zhu, Y. Liu, Z. Lou, F. Yuan, D. K. Cole, L. Ni, N. Su, L. Qin, X. Li, Z. Bai, J. I. Bell, H. Pang, P. Tien, G. F. Gao, and Z. Rao. 2004. Characterization of the heptad repeat regions, HR1 and HR2, and design of a fusion core structure model of the spike protein from severe acute respiratory syndrome (SARS) coronavirus. *Biochemistry* **43:** 14064–14071.

179. Yamada, Y. K., K. Takimoto, M. Yabe, and F. Taguchi. 1998. Requirement of proteolytic cleavage of the murine coronavirus MHV-2 spike protein for fusion activity. *Adv. Exp. Med. Biol.* **440:**89–93.

180. Yan, Z., B. Tripet, and R. S. Hodges. 2006. Biophysical characterization of HRC peptide analogs interaction with heptad repeat regions of the SARS-coronavirus Spike fusion protein core. *J. Struct. Biol.* **155:**162–175.

181. Yang, Z. Y., Y. Huang, L. Ganesh, K. Leung, W. P. Kong, O. Schwartz, K. Subbarao, and G. J. Nabel. 2004. pH-dependent entry of severe acute respiratory syndrome coronavirus is mediated by the spike glycoprotein and enhanced by dendritic cell transfer through DC-SIGN. *J. Virol.* **78:**5642–5650.

182. Yao, Y. X., J. Ren, P. Heinen, M. Zambon, and I. M. Jones. 2004. Cleavage and serum reactivity of the severe acute respiratory syndrome coronavirus spike protein. *J. Infect. Dis.* **190:**91–98.

183. Ye, R., C. Montalto-Morrison, and P. S. Masters. 2004. Genetic analysis of determinants for spike glycoprotein assembly into murine coronavirus virions: distinct roles for charge-rich and cysteine-rich regions of the endodomain. *J. Virol.* **78:**9904–9917.

184. Yin, H. S., R. G. Paterson, X. Wen, R. A. Lamb, and T. S. Jardetzky. 2005. Structure of the uncleaved ectodomain of the paramyxovirus (hPIV3) fusion protein. *Proc. Natl. Acad. Sci. USA* **102:**9288–9293.

185. Yin, H. S., X. Wen, R. G. Paterson, R. A. Lamb, and T. S. Jardetzky. 2006. Structure of the parainfluenza virus 5 F protein in its metastable, prefusion conformation. *Nature* **439:**38–44.

186. Yoshikura, H., and S. Tejima. 1981. Role of protease in mouse hepatitis virus-induced cell fusion. Studies with a cold-sensitive mutant isolated from a persistent infection. *Virology* **113:**503–511.

187. Youn, S., E. W. Collisson, and C. E. Machamer. 2005. Contribution of trafficking signals in the cytoplasmic tail of the infectious bronchitis virus spike protein to virus infection. *J. Virol.* **79:**13209–13217.

188. Yuan, K., L. Yi, J. Chen, X. Qu, T. Qing, X. Rao, P. Jiang, J. Hu, Z. Xiong, Y. Nie, X. Shi, W. Wang, C. Ling, X. Yin, K. Fan, L. Lai, M. Ding, and H. Deng. 2004. Suppression of SARS-CoV entry by peptides corresponding to heptad regions on spike glycoprotein. *Biochem. Biophys. Res. Commun.* **319:**746–752.

189. Zelus, B. D., J. H. Schickli, D. M. Blau, S. R. Weiss, and K. V. Holmes. 2003. Conformational changes in the spike glycoprotein of murine coronavirus are induced at 37°C either by soluble murine CEACAM1 receptors or by pH 8. *J. Virol.* **77:**830–840.

190. Zhou, H., and S. Perlman. 2006. Preferential infection of mature dendritic cells by mouse hepatitis virus strain JHM. *J. Virol.* **80:**2506–2514.

*Nidoviruses*
Edited by S. Perlman, T. Gallagher, and E. J. Snijder
© 2008 ASM Press, Washington, DC

Chapter 12

# Coronavirus Structural Proteins and Virus Assembly

BRENDA G. HOGUE AND CAROLYN E. MACHAMER

Coronaviruses are ubiquitous pathogens in vertebrates and cause a variety of diseases, including respiratory infections, gastroenteritis, encephalitis, and hepatitis (194). They are enveloped viruses that contain a positive-strand RNA genome of approximately 30 kb. Their name comes from the typical crown or corona surrounding virions observed by electron microscopy (Fig. 1A). All coronaviruses encode at least three envelope proteins: membrane (M), spike (S), and envelope (E), which use the host cell secretory system for biosynthesis. Some coronaviruses have additional envelope proteins, including the hemagglutinin-esterase (HE) protein found in some group 2 coronaviruses. The other structural protein is the nucleocapsid (N) protein, which encapsidates the RNA genome. Unlike many well-studied enveloped viruses that assemble at the plasma membrane, coronaviruses assemble by budding into the lumen of the endoplasmic reticulum-Golgi intermediate compartment (ERGIC) (82), a dynamic compartment between the endoplasmic reticulum (ER) and Golgi complex (2). The Golgi complex plays an essential role in processing and sorting of secretory and membrane cargo in all eukaryotic cells, with cargo from the ER entering on the *cis* face and exiting on the *trans* face. The ERGIC (also called the *cis* Golgi network) is at the *cis* face of the Golgi complex and is an active site of protein and lipid sorting. The viral envelope proteins are integral M proteins that are targeted to the ERGIC by independent targeting signals and by interactions with each other. M protein also interacts with the viral nucleocapsid, resulting in virion formation by budding into the lumen of the ERGIC (Fig. 1B). After budding, virions are released from infected cells by exocytosis. The advantage of intracellular assembly is unknown. Here, we review the processing, targeting, and assembly of the coronavirus structural proteins,

and the release of assembled virions from infected cells. Several other excellent reviews have also recently covered this topic (39, 118).

## STRUCTURAL PROTEINS OF CORONAVIRUS VIRIONS

### N Protein

Coronavirus N protein is a multifunctional phosphoprotein that encapsidates the genomic RNA into a helical nucleocapsid within the mature virion (35, 112). The helical nature of the nucleocapsid, which is a common characteristic of negative-stranded animal RNA viruses, is unique for a positive-stranded RNA virus. Through its interactions with the viral RNA, the M protein, and itself, N protein plays important roles in virus assembly (50, 74, 125, 127, 190). The protein is also involved in viral RNA transcription and/or replication (6, 21, 28, 44, 186). Recent studies with coronavirus infectious clones provided direct evidence for N protein in these roles (1, 15, 157, 206). Transmissible gastroenteritis virus (TGEV) and severe acute respiratory syndrome coronavirus (SARS-CoV) N proteins both exhibit RNA chaperone activity in vitro (215). It was suggested that this activity may play a role in template switching during transcription of viral subgenomic transcription, but it remains to be demonstrated that the activity exists in virus-infected cells. The protein may also play a role in viral mRNA translation (171). Additionally, it was recently shown that the N proteins of both mouse hepatitis virus (MHV)-A59 and SARS-CoV are type I interferon antagonists (84, 202).

A three-domain model for the N protein was proposed a number of years ago based on sequence comparison of many MHV strains (Fig. 2) (137).

**Brenda G. Hogue** • Biodesign Institute, School of Life Sciences, Arizona State University, Tempe, AZ 85257-5401. **Carolyn E. Machamer** • Department of Cell Biology, Johns Hopkins University School of Medicine, Baltimore, MD 21205-2196.

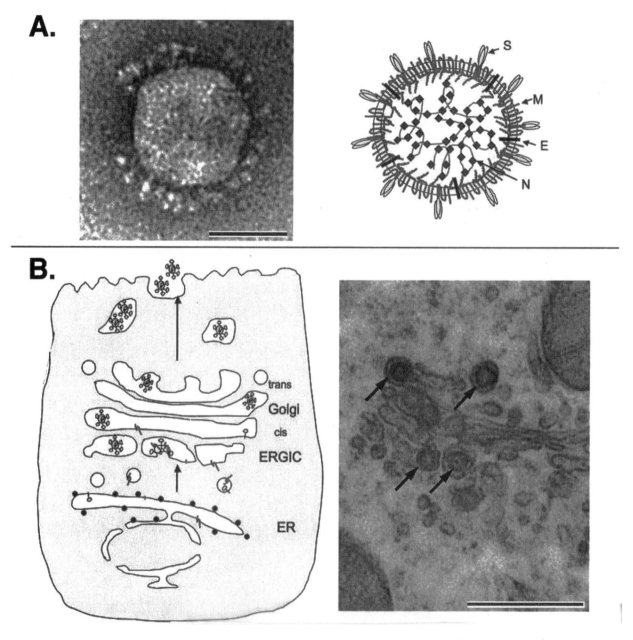

**Figure 1.** Coronavirus structure and intracellular assembly site. (A) Electron micrograph of purified IBV particle after negative staining (left). Bar, 50 nm. Virion schematic showing the major structural proteins (right). Note that some coronaviruses contain additional E proteins (e.g., HE in some group 2 viruses and several accessory proteins in SARS-CoV). (B) Schematic of virus assembly in cells (left). The E proteins are synthesized in the ER and transported to the ERGIC/Golgi complex. Independent targeting signals and interactions with the other E proteins allow accumulation in the ERGIC, and after interaction with the nucleocapsid, virions bud into the lumen of the ERGIC. They are released from infected cells by exocytosis. The right panel is an electron micrograph of Vero cells infected with IBV, showing a Golgi region with budded virions inside (arrows). Bar, 500 nm.

A serine- and arginine-rich (SR) region in domain II is conserved in different coronavirus N proteins, which is likely involved in some function of the protein. Recently, a modular organization for SARS-CoV N protein was proposed based on results from a number of analytical approaches, including nuclear magnetic resonance (NMR) spectroscopy (19). The new model suggests that the protein consists of two noninteracting domains, the RNA-binding and dimerization domains, with the remainder of the protein being disordered. Bioinformatic analyses suggest that other coronavirus N proteins may have a similar modular organization.

Sequence-specific and nonspecific binding of N protein to RNA has been reported (27, 117, 121, 129, 144, 166, 214). RNA-binding domains have

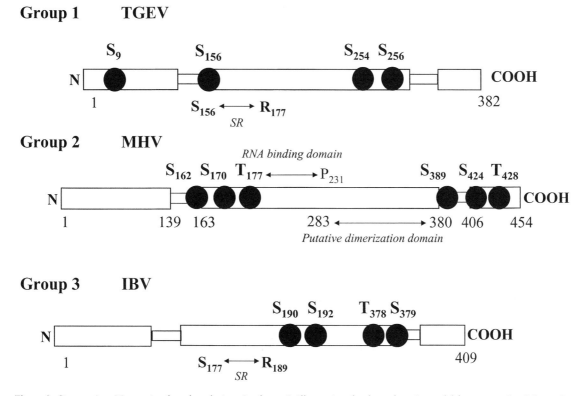

**Figure 2.** Coronavirus N-protein phosphorylation. A schematic illustrating the three-domain model for coronavirus N proteins with A and B spacer domains (137) is shown at the top. The relative positions of the phosphorylated sites identified on intracellular N protein from TGEV-infected cells (14) and MHV-infected cells (196) and IBV N protein expressed alone (22) are shown below. The positions of the RNA-binding domain that includes the SR region (129) and putative dimerization domain (208) are indicated for MHV. The positions of the SR regions are indicated for TGEV and IBV.

been mapped for MHV, SARS-CoV, and infectious bronchitis virus (IBV) N proteins (51, 72, 129, 214). The domain maps to domain II in MHV N protein, which includes the SR region, whereas the domain is N terminal of the SR region in SARS-CoV and IBV N proteins. The SARS-CoV SR region was reported, based on mammalian two-hybrid screens, to be important for N protein oligomerization and also interaction with M protein, which could be important for assembly of nucleocapsids (62, 63).

All coronavirus N proteins are highly basic, with isoelectric points of 10.3 to 10.7 (90). In addition, all coronavirus N proteins are phosphorylated. The role of phosphorylation is not known, and only very recently were phosphorylated sites identified for IBV, TGEV, and MHV N proteins. There are a large number of potential phosphorylation sites in all coronavirus N proteins, but few of these are actually modified (Fig. 2). Phosphoserines at positions 9, 156, 254, and 256 were identified for the TGEV N protein in virus-infected cells, whereas sites S156 and S256 were identified on N protein in purified virions (14). The sites that are phosphorylated on the IBV N protein expressed with baculovirus in insect Sf9 cells were

found to be identical to those present on the N protein expressed alone in Vero cells (22). Data from this study suggest that S190, S192, T378, and S379 are phosphorylated on intracellular IBV N protein. Six residues that cluster on the amino and carboxy ends of the RNA-binding and putative dimerization domains, respectively, are phosphorylated on both intracellular and extracellular virion MHV N proteins (196).

Phosphorylation can regulate protein function, so deciphering the role(s) of phosphorylation of coronavirus N proteins is important. N protein is multifunctional, and phosphorylation could be involved in modulating any of its functions during the virus life cycle, including virus assembly. The RNA-binding affinities of phosphorylated and nonphosphorylated IBV N protein were recently shown to be equivalent when measured by surface plasmon resonance (22). Interestingly, however, the phosphorylated form of the protein bound viral RNA with a higher binding affinity than nonviral RNA. It is possible that the modification alters the structure of the protein and, in turn, presentation of the RNA binding domain(s) that is important for recognition of the packaging signal, transcription regulatory sequences, or other signature sequences in the viral RNA(s).

Another modification reported for SARS-CoV N protein is sumoylation at lysine 62 (96). Ubc9, a ubiquitin-conjugating enzyme that participates in sumoylation, may be involved in modifying SARS-CoV N protein, as it was shown to interact with N protein in a yeast two-hybrid screen (52). This modification has not been reported for N proteins from other coronaviruses.

Very recently, structural information has become available for IBV and SARS-CoV N proteins (51, 72, 77, 208). The three-dimensional structures are based on NMR analysis of amino acids 45 to 181 from SARS-CoV N protein and X-ray crystal structures of residues 19 to 162, 219 to 349, and 29 to 160 from IBV-CoV N protein and 270 to 370 from SARS-CoV N protein. The structures of the N-terminal domains of IBV and SARS-CoV N proteins are similar, adopting the same general polypeptide fold consisting of a four- or five-stranded antiparallel β-sheet with a positively charged β-hairpin or loop extension and a hydrophobic core or platform structure (51, 72, 77). High-resolution structures for the C termini of SARS-CoV and IBV N proteins indicate that subunits interact extensively through hydrogen-bonding and hydrophobic interactions to form dimers, strongly suggesting that the oligomer is the major functional unit for the protein (77, 208). NMR structures of the N- and C-terminal domains agree with the crystal structures (18, 19).

## M Protein

The M protein is the most abundant protein in the viral envelope, with a short amino terminus exposed on the outside of the virion, three hydrophobic transmembrane domains, and a long carboxy-terminal tail located inside the virion that consists of an amphiphilic region followed by a hydrophilic domain (153) (Fig. 3). The amphiphilic region of the carboxy tail appears to be tightly associated with the membrane (153), which may result in formation of a matrix-like structure that lines the inner virion envelope. All known coronavirus M proteins assume this topology with the exception of that of the group 1 coronavirus TGEV. The TGEV M protein exhibits two topologies in the viral envelope: one population with the amino$_{exo}$-carboxy$_{endo}$ orientation and another population with an amino$_{exo}$-carboxy$_{exo}$ orientation (50, 143) (Fig. 3). Most M proteins do not have N-terminal cleaved signal sequences. The group 1 viruses TGEV, feline infectious peritonitis virus, and canine coronavirus do have potentially cleavable signal sequences located at their N termini, but these sequences do not appear to be required for membrane insertion (79, 91, 189). However, the topology of the M proteins lacking the putative signal sequences was not determined, so the signal may be required for proper translocation of the N terminus and the correct orientation of the transmembrane domains.

Coronavirus M proteins are composed of 220 to 262 amino acids, and all are glycosylated on the N-terminal domain. M proteins from group 1 and 3 coronaviruses and SARS-CoV are glycosylated with N-linked oligosaccharides, whereas the M proteins of group 2 viruses exhibit O-linked glycosylation (17, 68, 76, 124, 132, 133, 151, 165). The M protein of MHV strain 2 is modified with both N- and O-linked oligosaccharides (200). The role of glycosylation is unclear, since elimination of the sites for carbohydrate addition in MHV M protein, or swapping the sites from O to N linked, has no effect on targeting or virus production (38). However, the glycosylation

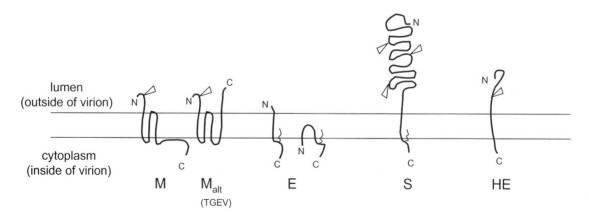

**Figure 3.** Topology of coronavirus E proteins. Two topologies are shown for M and E proteins, as supported by evidence discussed in the text. Small triangles represent glycosylation but are not meant to indicate the number or type of oligosaccharides, which differ in the proteins from different coronaviruses. S proteins and some E proteins are palmitoylated on their cytoplasmic tails (indicated by the squiggly line).

status of MHV M protein may contribute to induction of interferon by the virus. Cells infected with MHV containing N-glycosylated M protein induce interferon better than those infected with MHV containing the normal O-glycosylated M protein, and cells infected with MHV containing nonglycosylated M protein are very poor interferon inducers (37). Interestingly, growth of these MHV variants in the liver corresponded to their ability to induce interferon (37). However, an earlier study showed that swapping the N-terminal domain of TGEV (N glycosylated) with that of bovine coronavirus (BCoV) (O glycosylated) had no effect on interferon induction by virus-like particles (VLPs) produced by coexpression of TGEV M and E proteins (7).

## E Protein

Coronavirus E proteins are small (76- to 109-amino-acid) integral membrane proteins that lack a cleaved N-terminal signal sequence and have fairly long membrane anchor domains. The protein is a minor structural component of virions but plays an important, not yet fully defined, role in virus production (33, 55, 88, 101, 136, 209). Two topologies for E protein have been proposed, with either one or two transmembrane domains (Fig. 3). Studies on different E proteins agree that the C terminus is cytoplasmic. If the protein spans the membrane once, this would indicate a type III membrane protein with the N terminus translocated across the membrane in the absence of a cleaved signal sequence. IBV E protein appears to adopt this orientation, since the N terminus was accessible to antibody only after permeabilization of Golgi membranes (29). In addition, IBV E protein's hydrophobic region can replace the membrane-spanning domain of a type I membrane protein, showing that it can adopt a transmembrane configuration with an $N_{exo}$-to-$C_{endo}$ orientation (31). However, several studies have shown that the epitope-tagged N termini of MHV and SARS-CoV E proteins are in the cytoplasm (115, 210). This would result in a protein with two transmembrane domains, or a "hairpin" conformation, with a loop inserted into the cytoplasmic face of the bilayer. Caution must be used in interpreting these results, since extending the N terminus with an epitope tag could block its translocation, altering the topology of the protein. However, synthetic peptides corresponding to the SARS-CoV E protein's hydrophobic region inserted into model membranes adopt the hairpin conformation (3, 81). An epitope tag inserted at the N terminus of IBV E protein allows translocation of the N terminus, whereas the same N-terminal tag on SARS-CoV E protein does not (210), which supports the idea that

IBV and SARS-CoV E proteins may adopt different topologies. Perhaps coronavirus E protein can adopt two membrane conformations, each with a specific function. Antibodies that recognize the N termini of MHV and SARS-CoV E proteins will be required to confirm the topology of the native proteins.

Coronavirus E proteins are not glycosylated. The only modification that has been documented is palmitoylation for some coronavirus E proteins. IBV and SARS-CoV E proteins are palmitoylated on cytoplasmic cysteine residues near the hydrophobic segment (31, 98). Palmitoylation of MHV E protein in infected L2 cells was inferred from a mobility shift that is sensitive to alkaline hydroxylamine cleavage (209), but it has not been directly demonstrated. However, another group did not observe the hydroxylamine sensitivity of MHV E protein when expressed by transfection in OST-7 cells (141). The function of palmitoylation is unknown.

Coronavirus E proteins share characteristics with small hydrophobic membrane viroporin proteins of other viruses (60). Viroporins are defined as proteins that alter cellular permeability, and some viroporins are ion channels. Viroporins contain at least one highly hydrophobic domain that forms an amphipathic (-helix in the membrane. The proteins are generally oligomeric, with hydrophobic residues facing the phospholipid bilayer and hydrophilic residues lining the pore (60). Recently, the SARS-CoV and MHV E proteins were shown to exhibit viroporin activity (97, 98, 113). In addition, peptides corresponding to the E proteins from SARS-CoV, MHV, IBV, and human coronavirus strain 229E form cation-specific ion channels in planar bilayer systems (197, 198). Ion channel activity of E proteins would require formation of homo-oligomers. Multimers that are resistant to sodium dodecyl sulfate during electrophoresis have been observed for some coronavirus E proteins, although it is not clear if oligomers form in cells. However, molecular dynamic simulations predict that homo-oligomers are possible for these proteins (182). These predictions are based on E proteins with an $N_{exo}$ and $C_{endo}$ orientation and a single transmembrane domain.

## S Protein

S protein extends from the envelope to give coronaviruses their characteristic "crowned" appearance. S protein binds the host cell receptor and mediates virus-to-cell and cell-to-cell fusion (57). S proteins are large, between 1,160 and 1,450 amino acids in length, and are heavily glycosylated to yield 150- to 200-kDa monomers. They are type I membrane proteins, with a cleaved signal sequence, a single transmembrane domain, and a short C-terminal tail inside the virion (Fig. 3).

MHV-A59 S protein contains 22 sites for N-linked glycosylation, many of which are used. In addition, there are many intrachain disulfide bonds that are essential for proper folding (134). Homo-oligomerization of coronavirus S proteins has also been reported. Such oligomerization is expected to occur in the ER after folding but prior to export to the Golgi complex, like many other viral envelope proteins that have been examined (45). IBV S protein was reported to form a homodimer or homotrimer (16). The shed S1 subunit of MHV S protein behaves as a homodimer (94), although the S2 subunit appeared to run as a trimer on immunoblots (58). Homotrimers of TGEV S protein were shown to form early after synthesis, prior to Golgi-specific carbohydrate processing (43). Trimers of SARS S proteins have also been reported (95, 124). MHV S protein is slow to fold, and "older" S molecules interact with "newer" M molecules, suggesting that S protein folding rates influence its ER export and assembly (135). However, this does not seem to be the case for BCoV, where newly synthesized S protein interacted immediately with newly synthesized M protein (and HE; see below) (131). In addition to glycosylation, S proteins are palmitoylated on one or more cysteine residues in the cytoplasmic domain near the transmembrane domain (9, 168, 185). These cysteine residues have been implicated in cell-to-cell fusion by MHV S (9, 20). A recent study showed that palmitoylation of MHV S protein is important for interaction of S protein with M protein, and assembly of infectious virus (176).

Some coronavirus S proteins are cleaved into S1 and S2 subunits by furin or a related enzyme in the Golgi complex (39). S proteins of group 1 coronaviruses and SARS-CoV lack a furin cleavage site. Although SARS-CoV S protein is not cleaved during biogenesis, cleavage upon entry by endosomal proteases is required for efficient infection (71, 162). Cleavage of MHV S protein is not essential for infectivity but may enhance cell-to-cell fusion (41).

## HE Protein

Some group 2 coronaviruses express another structural protein, HE, that is anchored in the envelope as a second spike. HE protein is synthesized as a 42.5-kDa protein that is subsequently glycosylated to 65-kDa disulfide-linked dimers (67). It is a type I membrane protein with a cleaved signal sequence, a single transmembrane domain, and a short cytoplasmic tail (Fig. 3). HE dimers associate with M and S proteins in virus-infected cells (131). Proper oligomerization appears to be necessary for incorporation of HE into these complexes.

HE hydrolyzes O-acetylated sialic acid on oligosaccharides to which S protein binds, presumably allowing reversible attachment. Interestingly, the specificity of HE differs in different coronaviruses, likely due to host species variability in sialic acid modifications (164). In MHV, strains expressing functional HE are more neuropathic than those that do not express HE (80). However, the functional gene is rapidly lost with passage in cell culture (100).

## TARGETING OF VIRAL STRUCTURAL PROTEINS

### Targeting of N Protein

N protein is synthesized in the cytoplasm, where it interacts with newly synthesized viral genomes to form nucleocapsids. MHV N protein can also be detected at RNA replication sites at membranes early in infection (12, 186). IBV N protein was reported to localize to nucleoli as well as the cytoplasm, both in infected and in transfected cells (65). Hiscox and colleagues have shown that IBV N protein interacts with cellular nucleolar proteins, and IBV infection induces morphological changes in nucleoli (23, 46). The same group showed that N proteins of TGEV and MHV could also be found in nucleoli of transfected cells (199). The localization of N protein to nucleoli could influence host ribosome biogenesis and cell growth and division. However, most investigators have not detected nuclear or nucleolar localization of the N protein in cells infected with TGEV or MHV (14, 163). In addition, several groups have reported that SARS-CoV N protein is cytoplasmic, even when nuclear export is blocked with leptomycin B (154, 169, 204). Thus, the localization of coronavirus N proteins to nuclear subdomains does not appear to be a universal property. A recent report showing that individually expressed fragments of SARS-CoV N protein did localize to the nucleus or nucleolus (177) raises the possibility that at least some of the discrepancies reported for targeting of coronavirus N proteins could be due to proteolytic processing in some situations.

### Targeting of M Protein

MHV, IBV, TGEV, feline infectious peritonitis virus, BCoV, and SARS-CoV M proteins are all targeted to the Golgi region when expressed individually from cDNA (82, 110, 124, 131, 152). Given the abundance of M protein in viral envelopes and its targeting to the Golgi region, it was surprising when localization at the electron microscopic level showed that M protein does not, on its own, determine the site of virus assembly. In transfected cells, IBV M protein is localized to the *cis* side of the Golgi stack (109), whereas MHV M protein reaches the *trans* side of the organelle (82). Thus, neither IBV nor MHV M protein is retained in the ERGIC, the site of assembly. Association with other viral proteins is believed to restrict trafficking of the M protein, to collect it in the ERGIC for assembly.

Golgi region targeting of coronavirus M proteins has been most extensively studied for MHV and IBV. For IBV M protein, a signal for Golgi localization was identified in the first of the three transmembrane domains (110). Deletion of the second and third transmembrane domains has no effect on Golgi localization, but deletion of the first and second membrane spans results in transport to the plasma membrane. Deletion of most of the cytoplasmic tail also has no effect on Golgi localization. The first transmembrane domain of IBV M protein retains a plasma membrane reporter protein, vesicular stomatitis virus G protein (VSV-G), in the *cis* Golgi region when it is inserted in place of the normal VSV-G transmembrane domain (170). The sequence appears to function as a true retention signal, since VSV-G containing the IBV M protein first transmembrane domain (Gm1) forms large, detergent-insoluble oligomers upon arrival at the Golgi complex (195). The critical sequence in the transmembrane domain was mapped to polar uncharged residues that line one face of a predicted $\propto$-helix. Mutation of any one of these four polar residues results in transport of the Gm1 chimera to the cell surface (108). Although quite surprising at the time, Golgi resident proteins were subsequently shown to use targeting information within their transmembrane domains as well (25). However, there is no sequence conservation or motifs that are shared within these proteins. A popular model for the mechanism of Golgi protein localization originated from the observation that some Golgi membrane proteins had shorter predicted transmembrane domains than did plasma membrane proteins (123). Membrane thickness, commonly believed to increase from the ER to the plasma membrane due to a cholesterol gradient, could thus mediate localization of Golgi membrane proteins due to a membrane partitioning effect (13). However, it was subsequently shown that transmembrane domains themselves determine the membrane thickness, rather than the other way around (120). Other factors must therefore contribute to efficient localization of Golgi membrane proteins, although the lipid composition of Golgi membranes is likely to play a role.

MHV M protein requires sequences in both its cytoplasmic tail and its transmembrane domains for Golgi localization. When the first and second transmembrane domains of MHV M protein are deleted, the protein is transported past the Golgi complex to endosomes and lysosomes, suggesting that this region of the protein contributes to Golgi localization (5, 102). The cytoplasmic tail of MHV M is essential but not sufficient for Golgi targeting, with C-terminal residues playing a key role (5, 102). In addition, other regions of MHV M protein contribute to targeting as well (4). The first transmembrane domain of MHV M protein is unable to retain VSV-G in the Golgi complex, confirming that IBV and MHV M proteins use different mechanisms for steady-state localization (108). Perhaps the differences in the Golgi targeting domains for IBV and MHV M proteins are not so surprising, considering that the two M proteins are targeted to opposite faces of the Golgi complex.

### Targeting of E Protein

Different investigators reported that IBV E protein is targeted to the Golgi region (29) or to the ER (99) when expressed from cDNA. The latter study implicated a dibasic ER retrieval signal in targeting of IBV E protein containing a C-terminal epitope tag (99). By immunoelectron microscopy, untagged IBV E protein is localized to *cis* and *medial* Golgi membranes when expressed in BHK-21 cells (30). It is also localized to the Golgi region in many other cell types at the light microscopic level. One possible explanation for the different results for IBV E protein targeting is the use of epitope tags or different expression systems. The Golgi targeting reported by Corse and Machamer depends on a central region of the cytoplasmic tail (31). This region shares some homology with the cytoplasmic tail of the G1 protein from Uukuniemi virus (a bunyavirus), which is also targeted to Golgi membranes (145). The targeting signal in the cytoplasmic tail of IBV E protein is likely to interact with cellular Golgi proteins, but these have not yet been identified.

MHV E protein is localized to the ERGIC when expressed independently (141). The same study showed that overexpression of MHV E induces smooth, convoluted membrane accumulations, presumably derived from the ER. Targeting signals have not been reported.

The localization of SARS-CoV E protein when expressed from cDNA may vary with the cell type and expression system. Using a vaccinia virus T7 expression system, epitope-tagged SARS-CoV E protein is localized in the ER in HeLa cells, but in BHK-21 cells, both tagged and untagged SARS-CoV E proteins are localized to the Golgi region (98). Using a Semliki Forest virus expression system, tagged

SARS-CoV E protein was reported to partially overlap with ER markers in BHK-21 cells (124). However, using a plasmid expression system, tagged SARS-CoV E protein is localized to the Golgi region in BHK-21 cells (105). Mutations in the hydrophobic region of SARS-CoV E protein disrupt membrane localization (98), but specific targeting signals for ER or Golgi localization have not yet been reported. These collected findings warrant caution in determining intracellular localization of coronavirus E proteins when expressed from cDNA, as well as ER and Golgi targeting signals.

## Targeting of S Protein

Some coronavirus S proteins contain information in their cytoplasmic tails that contributes to targeting. IBV and other group 3 coronaviruses possess canonical dilysine ER retrieval signals (104). This type of signal requires a lysine residue in the $-3$ and the $-4$ or $-5$ position from the C terminus. The dilysine signal binds a coat complex known as COPI, which coats vesicles that form on Golgi membranes that are subsequently targeted to the ER (175). The signal is found on ER and ERGIC resident membrane proteins and is required for retrieval if they escape these compartments. The dilysine signal on IBV S protein ($KKSV_{COOH}$) contributes to its localization near the virus assembly site, although at high expression levels the machinery is saturated and IBV S protein reaches the plasma membrane. When a mutation in the dilysine signal was introduced into an infectious clone of IBV, the resulting virus had a growth defect, including premature formation of syncytia (205). Interestingly, the S proteins of group 1 coronaviruses and SARS-CoV contain a related dibasic signal, $KXHXX_{COOH}$. In SARS-CoV S protein, this dibasic signal functions similarly to the dilysine signal in IBV S protein, although less efficiently (119). Mutation of the dibasic signal results in faster trafficking of SARS-CoV S protein through the secretory pathway, which, in turn, prevents efficient interaction with SARS-CoV M protein when these proteins are coexpressed (119). Thus, cycling between the Golgi region and ER induced by the dibasic signal may be critical for allowing sufficient opportunity for SARS-CoV S and M proteins to interact. Group 2 coronavirus S proteins, including MHV S protein, lack a dibasic signal in their cytoplasmic tails. Slower folding and assembly of S protein, or more robust interaction with M protein, might preclude the necessity for ER retrieval in S proteins from group 2 coronaviruses. It is currently unknown whether the presence or absence of an ER retrieval signal on S proteins influences virus pathogenesis.

TGEV S protein contains the $KXHXX_{COOH}$ dibasic signal found on the SARS-CoV S protein mentioned above. However, Schwegmann-Wessels et al. reported that TGEV S protein was localized to the ER by a tyrosine-based motif found upstream of the dibasic signal (158). In a different study, the last 11 amino acids of the TGEV S tail (containing both the dibasic signal and the tyrosine motif) were able to retain a reporter construct in the ERGIC, and this localization was dependent only on the dibasic motif (104). The different results from the two groups could reflect different cell types, expression systems, or the fact that the chimeric reporter construct does not accurately reflect the behavior of the full-length protein. Alternatively, the tyrosine-based motif could contribute to rapid endocytosis of TGEV S protein from the plasma membrane, which would have been missed in the steady-state experiments that were used to analyze the localization of full-length TGEV S protein (158).

IBV S protein contains a second targeting signal in its cytoplasmic tail: a canonical endocytosis signal (YTTF) upstream of its dilysine signal. This type of sequence binds the AP2 adaptor complex that, in turn, binds clathrin to induce endocytosis (8). IBV S protein is endocytosed from the plasma membrane in both infected and transfected cells (205). Mutation of the tyrosine residue blocks endocytosis, and mutation of both ER retrieval and endocytosis signals allows accumulation of IBV S protein at the surface of transfected cells, with a concomitant increase in syncytium formation. Interestingly, recombinant virus could not be recovered when the tyrosine in the endocytosis signal was mutated (205), suggesting that too much IBV S protein at the surface of infected cells is incompatible with virus replication, or that the tyrosine residue plays another important role in the virus life cycle.

## SARS-CoV Accessory Proteins Present in Virions

Several proteins encoded by the "group-specific" open reading frames in SARS-CoV are incorporated into virions. In other coronaviruses, these accessory proteins are expressed in infected cells, but none have been reported to be structural proteins. SARS-CoV 3a protein has a topology similar to M protein, with three membrane-spanning domains and an O-glycosylated N terminus (133). It is the largest of the SARS-CoV accessory proteins, with 274 amino acids. Several reports have shown that SARS-CoV 3a protein is present in purified virions (75, 161). One group reported that when it is expressed from cDNA, SARS-CoV 3a protein is transported to the plasma membrane and is endocytosed (173). However, deletion of several motifs that are often involved in endocytosis actually blocked surface delivery. Other investigators have reported that SARS-CoV 3a protein is localized to the Golgi region (211) or plasma membrane (106) in infected cells, and to the Golgi region (133) or the ER (93) in transfected cells.

SARS-CoV 7a protein is a type I membrane protein of 122 amino acids, with a cleaved signal sequence and a single transmembrane domain (54). Like the 3a protein, SARS-CoV 7a protein is incorporated into virions (70). The structure of the 7a ectodomain shares features with the immunoglobulin superfamily (128). The protein contains a canonical ER retrieval signal at its C terminus ($KRKTE_{COOH}$) and when expressed from cDNA is localized in the ER and ERGIC region. However, both the transmembrane and cytoplasmic domains are required to retain a reporter protein in the ER-Golgi region (128).

SARS-CoV 7b protein is a small hydrophobic integral membrane protein of 44 amino acids that is produced from subgenomic RNA7 by leaky ribosome scanning (156). The C terminus of SARS-CoV 7b protein is in the cytoplasm, but it is not clear whether the protein spans the bilayer or is inserted as a hairpin. The protein is targeted to the Golgi region in both transfected and infected cells and is incorporated into virions (156).

It will be important to determine the level of these accessory proteins incorporated into SARS-CoV virions. Are only a few molecules present, or are they present at substantial levels? Deletion of all of the accessory proteins from the SARS-CoV genome has no effect on virus production from cultured cells (207), so none of the three proteins discussed above are essential for virus production. Like accessory proteins from other coronaviruses, SARS-CoV accessory proteins are believed to impact the host antiviral response. SARS-CoV 3a protein induces apoptosis when expressed in Vero E6 cells (93) and up-regulates fibrinogen expression in lung epithelium (174). SARS-CoV 7a protein has been reported to induce apoptosis (172), to block cell cycle progression (212), and to inhibit host protein synthesis and activate p38 mitogen-activated protein kinase (85). It will be important to determine if these any of these reported activities depend on incorporation of the accessory proteins into virions.

## VIRUS ASSEMBLY

Coronaviruses assemble at internal membranes of the ERGIC (82, 179). Exactly what determines the site of assembly is still not fully understood, although the localization of E proteins near this compartment certainly contributes to the process. S, M, E, and N proteins all form complexes that through multiple interactions presumably drive assembly. Interestingly, only M and E proteins are required for assembly of the viral envelope. Coexpression of M and E proteins in the absence of the other viral components is sufficient for assembly of MHV, IBV, BCoV, and SARS-CoV VLPs (7, 10, 29, 69, 122, 188). S protein is incorporated into VLPs when coexpressed with M and E proteins (10, 188). One exception is a report indicating that SARS-CoV M and N proteins are sufficient and required for VLP assembly (73), although this study did not analyze the release of VLPs. Thus, in contrast to most enveloped viruses, coronavirus envelope proteins are able to assemble and form particles independent of nucleocapsids. The unusual structure of M protein (membrane spanning with a cytoplasmic tail that is also tightly associated with the bilayer), coupled with its ability to oligomerize, may promote nucleocapsid-independent budding in the presence of E protein, which might increase membrane curvature. The unique lipid composition of the ERGIC (24) may also contribute to this unusual property of nucleocapsid-independent budding.

### Role of M Protein in Assembly

M protein is a major player in assembly of the viral envelope through interactions with itself, the other E proteins, and the nucleocapsid (40, 42, 47, 87, 131, 135). M protein is the most abundant protein in the mature virion, and VLPs consist primarily of M protein with only a few molecules of E protein. Thus, M-M protein interactions are thought to provide the overall scaffold for assembly of the envelope. M protein forms large multimeric complexes, and M-M lateral interactions in the membrane are thought to be primarily responsible for assembly of the viral envelope, even though the protein is not capable of driving the process when expressed alone (103).

Interactions between M protein molecules appear to be mediated by multiple domains. MHV M proteins with deletions in the luminal domain, transmembrane domains, the amphipathic domain, or the hydrophilic C-terminal tail are unable to assemble into VLPs (38). However, when the mutants were analyzed for the ability to associate with assembly-competent M proteins, only mutant proteins with replacement of the three transmembrane domains were not incorporated into VLPs, suggesting that M-M interactions are mediated through their transmembrane domains (42). Targeted RNA recombination demonstrated that complete virions are more tolerant of changes in the C terminus of the M protein tail than VLPs, since some mutants could be assembled into virions. Both VLP and virus assembly are sensitive to deletion and changes of the two C-terminal residues (38, 87, 191).

## E-M Protein Interactions

The role of E protein in virus assembly is far from understood, but it is clear that the protein is important for virus assembly. As mentioned above, VLP assembly is dependent on coexpression of E and M proteins, which are sufficient for their production and release (7, 10, 29, 122, 188). This strongly implies that the two proteins must interact at some level. Interaction between IBV E and M proteins was demonstrated in IBV-infected cells and in transfected cells by cross-linking and coimmunoprecipitation (32). The IBV E protein cytoplasmic tail mediates its interaction with the cytoplasmic tail of M protein (32, 99). M protein is far more abundant in virions and VLPs than E protein, but expression of M protein alone does not produce VLPs. As originally proposed by Vennema and colleagues (188), E protein could induce curvature at precise sites in a lattice composed of M protein or could promote particle scission. However, E protein is not a universal requirement for coronavirus particle formation (see below). Another observation is that E protein-containing vesicles are released from cells when E protein is expressed alone (29, 114). The significance of this is not known, but it suggests that the activity provided by the protein can function in the absence of M protein or the other viral proteins.

Deletion of the E protein gene from MHV results in severely crippled virus (88), whereas removal of the protein from TGEV-CoV blocks virus production (33, 136). SARS-CoV E protein is important for virus production, but not absolutely essential, since a mutant virus lacking the gene yielded titers ranging from 20- to 200-fold less than the wild-type virus (depending on the cell type used to grow the virus) (36). The specificity of E protein interaction with the M protein was recently investigated by replacing MHV E protein with the heterologous counterpart from other coronaviruses (86). MHV E protein could be replaced by E protein from the related group 2 viruses BCoV and SARS-CoV and, surprisingly, by E protein from group 3 IBV. However, E protein from group 1 TGEV could not substitute for MHV E protein. Even though there is little sequence homology between MHV and IBV E proteins, IBV E protein was incorporated into the complemented MHV virions, suggesting a specific interaction with M protein, or at least a precise role in particle formation (86).

The importance of the MHV E protein transmembrane domain in assembly has recently been illustrated. Alanine scanning insertion mutagenesis was used to examine the effect of disruption of the domain and gain insight into its possible function beyond serving to anchor the protein in the membrane (203). MHV mutants with insertions in the transmembrane domain exhibited a small-plaque phenotype and were significantly crippled in their growth. The most striking difference between the crippled viruses and recovered viruses that grew similarly to the wild-type virus was the positions of four hydrophilic polar residues along one face of the predicted α-helix. The positions of these residues on one face of the predicted α-helix are conserved in essentially all E proteins, suggesting that this is a functionally important feature of the proteins. These residues and their positioning along one face of the transmembrane α-helix may be essential for the overall structure of the transmembrane domain or of the entire protein. The transmembrane domain could play a role in protein-protein interactions or some other function that impacts the protein's ion channel activity, which, in turn, plays a role in assembly of the viral envelope and/or release of assembled virions as they mature through the exocytic pathway via transport vesicles. A second study clearly demonstrated that the transmembrane domain of E protein is required for efficient release of IBV (111) (see "Release of Virus from Infected Cells" below).

## S-M Protein Interactions

Most coronavirus S proteins are transported past the virus assembly site, and interaction with M protein is required for incorporation into virions. Recently, the requirement for incorporation of S protein into MHV virions was mapped to the juxtamembrane cysteine-rich and central regions of the cytoplasmic tail (11, 201). Palmitoylation of multiple cysteine residues of the MHV S tail is required for efficient interaction with the M protein (176). Dissection of the domain(s) of M protein that interacts with S protein is incomplete and has been studied only by coimmunoprecipitation (40). Deletion of the amphipathic domain has a severe affect on M-S interaction, whereas deletion of the amino and extreme carboxy domains does not.

## N-M Protein Interactions

Interactions between M and N proteins have been analyzed both in vitro and by reverse genetics. For TGEV, an in vitro binding assay using a panel of M protein substitution and deletion mutants and purified nucleocapsids mapped a 16-amino-acid domain located 10 residues from the C terminus of the protein that is responsible for M-nucleocapsid interaction (49). Two different amino acid stretches in the central region (residues 211 to 254 and 168 to 208) of SARS-CoV N protein were reported to be required for interaction with M protein (53, 63). These results are based primarily on in vitro pull-down assays and mammalian two-hybrid analysis; thus, further studies are required to validate the significance of these interactions in SARS-CoV-infected cells.

More recently, genetic analysis has provided evidence for MHV N-M protein interactions and new insight about the interactions. Initial attempts to isolate by recombination a virus lacking the two C-terminal amino acids in M protein suggested that the mutation was lethal; however, virus lacking these residues was subsequently isolated using more stringent host range selection (38, 87). The recovered MΔ2 viruses had an extremely defective phenotype, with very small plaques and low titers, but viruses were recovered after several passages with second-site changes in the M or N proteins, some of which were shown to compensate for deletion of the terminal two amino acids (87). The second-site changes mapped to regions in the C terminus of the M or N proteins.

Two additional studies showed that negatively charged amino acids in the C terminus of MHV-A59 N protein are important for virus assembly. Two aspartic acid residues (D440 and D441) in N protein were independently identified by two groups as residues necessary for virus assembly (74, 191). One of the studies identified second-site suppressor changes that compensated for mutations in the D440 and D441 residues, which provides strong evidence for genetic cross talk between the two proteins (74), whereas the other study identified compensatory changes only in the C terminus of N protein (191). Replacement of the penultimate positively charged R227 in MHV M protein with negative charges resulted in very crippled virus. Adaptive second-site changes restoring growth to the R227A mutant were identified in M protein, changes that were identical to those M protein alterations restoring growth to the D440A-D441A mutant virus (191). It is interesting that when key charged residues (D440 and D441 in N protein or R227 in M protein) are modified, these independently give rise to overlapping second-site suppressor or adaptive changes in the same region of M protein. Results from these studies strongly argue that M-N interactions are complex, indicating that more than just the single R227 and D440-D441 charges are important. This idea is supported further by the fact that reciprocal exchange of the charges between the two proteins was unsuccessful (74, 191).

## M-Nucleocapsid and M-RNA Interactions

A number of early studies demonstrated that M proteins from different coronaviruses copurified with nucleocapsids when purified virions were disrupted with nonionic detergents in low-salt buffers (59, 89, 193). More detailed analysis of MHV showed that M protein interacts with nucleocapsids in a temperature-dependent manner when virions were solubilized with nonionic detergent, which appeared to be mediated by M-RNA binding (167). More recent studies demonstrated that TGEV M protein is part of an internal virion core surrounding the helical ribonucleoprotein complex (47, 142).

Interaction between M protein and nucleocapsids containing genome-length RNA has been demonstrated for MHV (126). N protein was associated with all viral RNAs, whereas antibodies specific for M protein only coimmunoprecipitated N protein complexed with genomic RNA. The interaction between M and the N-genomic RNA complexes is dependent on the presence of the packaging signal (see below) that is located in gene 1b of the genome (127). Significantly, the packaging signal was shown to mediate selective interaction between M protein and viral RNA. Coexpression of M and E proteins with a reporter RNA containing the packaging signal was sufficient for selective packaging of the RNA into VLPs without expression of N protein (125). It is interesting that a number of studies over the years have noted potential M-RNA interactions. The suggestion from the latest studies that a viral envelope protein contributes to the selective packaging of genomic RNA is novel. Future studies that focus on further characterization of the M-RNA interaction and mechanistically how it contributes to selectivity of packaging are warranted.

## Packaging Signals

Packaging signals specify selective encapsidation of viral genomic RNA into virions. Coronaviruses synthesize a nested set of 3' coterminal subgenomic RNAs that share a common 5' leader sequence, but most package only the full-length genomic RNA in the mature virion. Subgenomic RNAs have been detected in purified BCoV, TGEV, and IBV (66, 116, 159, 160, 213). However, recent analysis demonstrated that subgenomic mRNAs are not present in extensively purified TGEV virions (48). Packaging signals have been identified for a number of coronaviruses. The MHV signal was the first to be identified and requires a 61-nucleotide stem-loop structure that is present approximately 21 kb from the 5' end of the genome in gene 1b for RNA packaging (56). A similar sequence in BCoV is a functional packaging signal

(26). The packaging signal for TGEV is located within the first 649 nucleotides at the 5′ end of the genome (48). Sequences within the 5′ and/or 3′ untranslated region of IBV are thought to be required for packaging, but signals necessary for RNA replication are also located in these regions, making it difficult to completely distinguish between these functions (34).

## RELEASE OF VIRUS FROM INFECTED CELLS

### Post-Golgi Transport of Constitutive Cargo

Coronaviruses are believed to follow the constitutive secretory pathway for exocytosis. Originally, it was thought that coronavirus release might be an unusual type of exocytosis, since virions are larger (~100 nm) than typical secretory vesicles (80 nm). Large vacuoles containing virions are usually greater than 500 nm in diameter. However, recent characterization of post-Golgi carriers used by cellular cargo (described below) suggests that virus release could follow a normal cellular route.

Until recently, constitutive transport of cargo from the Golgi complex to the plasma membrane was believed to follow a conventional vesicle-mediated pathway similar to that of cargo leaving the Golgi complex that is diverted to other destinations, like lysosomes. The cargo that is sorted at the *trans* Golgi network for other destinations is concentrated and requires the coat protein clathrin and associated adaptor proteins (183). However, constitutive cargo leaving the Golgi complex en route to the plasma membrane has been shown to exit in large, pleomorphic carriers lacking a coat (107). Experiments following fluorescent protein-tagged cargo in live cells identified transport carriers leaving the Golgi complex that are tubular with saccular regions and quite long, averaging between 1 and 2 μm in length (64, 139, 178). The molecular requirements for formation and fusion of these post-Golgi carriers are currently under active study. It was reported that small and large cargo (VSV-G and procollagen) can exit the Golgi complex in the same transport carriers (138). However, it is not known if large spherical cargo like coronaviruses can be packaged into the same type of transport carriers as other cargo, and whether these large cargoes require additional cellular machinery.

### Coronavirus Exocytosis

Few studies have directly examined coronavirus release. Drugs that perturb the late secretory pathway (e.g., monensin and weak bases) also block release of TGEV (155). A characteristic maturation of TGEV virions that occurs during transport was also reported in this study. Mature particles (which are not present in monensin-treated cells) are smaller and more condensed than immature particles. The only other study to examine exocytosis of coronavirions was one that analyzed MHV in cells that perform regulated secretion (AtT20 cells). It was demonstrated that virions are sorted away from regulated secretory products at the Golgi complex (181), suggesting that MHV release follows a constitutive pathway. A characteristic morphological change was also noted for virions in this study; empty-looking particles are present in the Golgi region, whereas those present in post-Golgi vacuoles are more electron dense.

Another factor in virus release may be the significant cellular alterations that occur in infected cells. Late in infection, the Golgi complex is disrupted, with fragmentation of the Golgi ribbon and dispersion of stacks (92, 180). This may hinder transport of virions through the Golgi complex or their incorporation into secretory vesicles. This idea is supported by the observation that late in infection, MHV budding was shown to occur in ER membranes, where large numbers of virions accumulated (179). In coronaviruses that induce syncytia, cellular alternations may also significantly impact virus release. After cell fusion, the microtubule network is rearranged and Golgi complexes from individual cells move together to form one organelle near the center of the syncytium (92). Given these alterations, post-Golgi transport intermediates containing virions may have a greater distance to travel to reach the plasma membrane, and they might not have the appropriate microtubule tracks for efficient delivery.

### Polarized Release of Coronaviruses from Epithelial Cells

Polarized epithelial cells are the first cells infected during coronavirus infection. These cells line all internal and external surfaces of the body and are characterized by two distinct plasma membrane domains (apical and basolateral) separated by tight junctions. The apical or basolateral localization of the virus receptor determines the site of coronavirus entry in polarized epithelial cells. In respiratory epithelial cells, SARS-CoV and human coronavirus strain 229E preferentially enter and are exocytosed from the apical surface (78, 184, 192). In a similar way, TGEV preferentially enters and exits from the apical surface of a polarized porcine kidney line (147). However, although MHV also preferentially infects cells from the apical surface, the polarity of release varies depending on the cell line. In a mouse kidney line and a porcine kidney line (expressing the MHV receptor), release occurs preferentially from the basolateral side, whereas in a canine kidney line (also expressing the receptor), release is apical (146, 149, 150).

The polarity of release of infectious virus will impact the ability to generate a localized versus systemic infection. How is sorting of virus-containing exocytic vesicles achieved? Sorting into vesicles destined for the apical or basolateral surface requires signals in the cargo itself and occurs in the last Golgi compartment (the *trans* Golgi network) in simple epithelia (130). Since coronaviruses assemble by budding into the ERGIC, these signals would have to be present in intact virions as they move into the *trans* Golgi network. S protein projects from the surface of virions and could be recognized by cellular sorting machinery. However, one study showed that MHV S protein was not involved in determining the polarized release of virus (148). Thus, the mechanism for polarized sorting of virions into transport carriers destined for different plasma membrane domains is still not understood.

## Role for Coronavirus E Protein in Virion Exocytosis?

Recent evidence suggests that coronavirus E proteins form cation-specific ion channels when reconstituted into planar lipid bilayers (197, 198). This activity may be important during infection, since drugs that block the in vitro channel activity reduced infectivity in an E protein-dependent manner (197). The E protein is absolutely required for replication of TGEV (136) but is not essential for MHV or SARS-CoV (36, 88). There may be more than one function for E protein, and these functions may be virus and cell type specific. Although a specific effect on release of virions was not reported, cells infected with a recombinant SARS-CoV lacking E protein have reduced numbers of intracellular mature virions relative to those infected with wild-type virus, and intracellular vacuoles contain potentially aborted assembly intermediates or degraded material (36).

A recent study on IBV supports the idea that the transmembrane domain of E protein is critical for exocytosis of infectious virions. IBV E protein with a complete replacement of its transmembrane domain (called EG3) is targeted to the Golgi region, is palmitoylated, and assembles with M protein to form particles normally (31, 32). However, cells infected with a recombinant virus encoding EG3 instead of E protein are significantly deficient in release of infectious particles (111). Examination of infected cells by electron microscopy showed the accumulation of large, virion-containing vacuoles, many of which contained degraded structures (Fig. 4A). Most S protein in

purified particles released from cells infeated with IBV encoding EG-3 is cleaved near the surface of the virion envelope, resulting in noninfectious particles. These data suggest that the transmembrane domain of IBV E protein is required for exocytosis of intact virions. Replacing the transmembrane domain of an ion channel should inactivate it, so channel activity may be required to promote fusion of transport carriers containing virions with the plasma membrane, or to prevent their fusion with lysosomes. Alternatively, the transmembrane domain of E protein could also promote interactions with cellular trafficking machinery. These potential functions for E protein would be required postassembly, and they suggest an additional nonstructural role for the protein (Fig. 4B). E protein is expressed in excess in infected cells relative to what is incorporated into virions, so an additional role(s) as a nonstructural protein is possible.

Why would coronaviruses need a protein that alters intracellular ion concentrations (or interacts with trafficking machinery) to promote release of virions if exocytosis follows normal cellular pathways? Perhaps the sheer number of particles per transport carrier or their spherical structure prevents the carriers from moving normally along microtubules. Another possibility is that the cell recognizes the carriers containing virions as abnormal and targets them for fusion with lysosomes. Rapid progress in this area of coronavirus research is expected.

## UNANSWERED QUESTIONS

One of the biggest remaining questions for coronavirus assembly is why these viruses assemble at intracellular membranes. Although most well-studied enveloped viruses bud from the plasma membrane, there are a number of enveloped viruses that assemble by budding into intracellular compartments (61). What are the advantages that compensate for the complication of virion exocytosis after budding? One possibility is that complete assembly inside the cell helps the virus "hide" from the immune system. However, since cytotoxic T cells (the predominant antiviral defense arm of the immune system) recognize viral peptides generated intracellularly (83), it is unlikely that the virus could hide for long. Another interesting possibility is that the lipid composition of viral envelopes provides an advantage. The lipid composition of the ERGIC is distinct from that of the plasma membrane (24), and this difference is reflected in the lipid composition of coronavirus envelopes (24, 187). This distinct lipid composition could promote budding, virus-cell fusion, and/or stability of virions in different environments in the host.

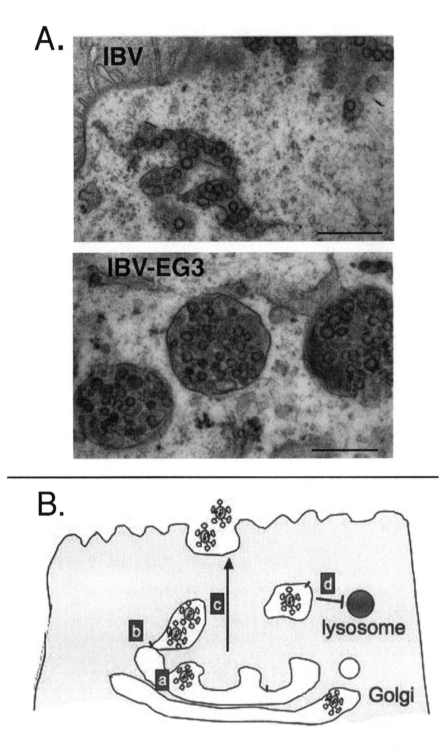

**Figure 4.** Potential roles for the E protein transmembrane domain in release of infectious virus. (A) Electron micrographs of Vero cells infected for 14 h with IBV or IBV containing an E protein with a heterologous transmembrane domain (IBV-EG3). Typical pleomorphic transport intermediates are present in cells infected with wild-type IBV, but large spherical vacuoles containing virions and degraded material are prominent in cells infected with IBV-EG3. Bars, 500 nm. (B) Results from mutations in the E protein transmembrane domain suggest that this domain could promote maturation of virions in late Golgi or post-Golgi compartments (a), promote formation of virus containing transport intermediates (b), promote fusion of transport intermediates with the plasma membrane (c), or prevent fusion of transport intermediates with lysosomes (d). The three last roles could be as a nonstructural protein. Ion channel activity or other interactions of the E protein transmembrane domain could be involved.

Coronaviruses or VLPs with altered lipid compositions will be required to test these ideas.

It remains to be determined what components actually initiate coronavirus budding. It was initially assumed that M-nucleocapsid interactions drive the budding process, with the long cytoplasmic tail of M functioning like a "receptor" for the nucleocapsid. M-nucleocapsid interactions do occur, and it is likely these interactions drive budding of nucleocapsids into the virion envelope. Do the M protein tails form a matrix-like structure along the membrane that ultimately lines the inner virion envelope (like matrix proteins of negative-strand viruses) to facilitate budding? The structure of coronaviruses should be more extensively investigated to determine if association of M protein with the nucleocapsid to form a core is a common characteristic of these viruses. This will require careful state-of-the-art microscopy studies of morphogenesis and of virions. Does the M protein play a role in encapsidation? Studies that address whether coronavirus RNA encapsidation is mediated by interactions between N and M proteins or directly between the M protein and RNA genomic packaging signals should answer this question.

At a fundamental level it is clear that the envelope can assemble in the absence of nucleocapsids, since coexpression of M and E proteins is sufficient for formation of VLPs, which resemble "spikeless" virions lacking a genome. The function(s) of the coronavirus E protein in assembly is still a mystery. Does it induce curvature of membranes containing a scaffold of the M protein, or promote the scission step at the conclusion of budding? Is the proposed hairpin topology conformation of E protein the form that promotes virus assembly? One important issue is how much E protein is actually incorporated into virions. Is there a fixed ratio of M to E protein in virions? This would be expected if E protein is required to perturb an M scaffold at precise places to induce curvature. If E protein does promote assembly, how do MHV and SARS-CoV replicate in its absence?

It will also be important to examine the role of the putative ion channel activity in assembly and release of infectious virions. Further experiments to define the sequence requirements of the transmembrane domain are essential. Is the ion channel required in assembled virions, or as a nonstructural protein in Golgi or post-Golgi membranes? If this activity is required in virions, does it promote "maturation" observed for some coronaviruses (which could be required for subsequent stability of virions)? One important piece of the puzzle that is missing is the localization of E protein at the electron microscopic level in infected cells. Knowing if E protein moves past the Golgi complex late in infection should help

define the compartment in which a potential nonstructural role may be required. If E protein promotes efficient release of infectious virus, why is TGEV absolutely dependent on its expression, whereas MHV and SARS-CoV are not?

Finally, nothing is known about the role of host proteins in coronavirus assembly. Human immunodeficiency virus and other enveloped viruses co-opt cellular machinery for budding (140). It is likely that cellular factors are recruited to assist with coronavirus envelope biogenesis and budding, but these have not been identified and the processes in which they may be involved are unknown at this time. This is an area that requires significant investigation.

The emergence of SARS-CoV sparked tremendous interest in and recognition of coronaviruses as intriguing for their molecular and cellular biology and as significant pathogens. As a result, the number of investigators involved in research on coronaviruses has significantly increased, which has brought new ideas and experience to the field. The availability of new tools such as infectious clones provides the opportunity to use reverse genetics to address many important questions. Answers to many of the remaining issues regarding coronavirus assembly should be forthcoming, which will no doubt raise new interesting questions to ponder and investigate.

**Acknowledgments.** We thank the members of our labs for helpful discussions and comments on the manuscript.

The work in our labs is supported by grants from the NIH (AI54704 and GM64647).

## REFERENCES

1. **Almazan, F., C. Galan, and L. Enjuanes.** 2004. The nucleoprotein is required for efficient coronavirus genome replication. *J. Virol.* **78:**12683–12688.
2. **Appenzeller-Herzog, C., and H. P. Hauri.** 2006. The ER-Golgi intermediate compartment (ERGIC): in search of its identity and function. *J. Cell Sci.* **119:**2173–2183.
3. **Arbely, E., Z. Khattari, G. Brotons, M. Akkawi, T. Salditt, and I. T. Arkin.** 2004. A highly unusual palindromic transmembrane helical hairpin formed by SARS coronavirus E protein. *J. Mol. Biol.* **341:**769–779.
4. **Armstrong, J., and S. Patel.** 1991. The Golgi sorting domain of coronavirus E1 protein. *J. Cell Sci.* **98**( Pt. 4):567–575.
5. **Armstrong, J., S. Patel, and P. Riddle.** 1990. Lysosomal sorting mutants of coronavirus E1 protein, a Golgi membrane protein. *J. Cell Sci.* **95**(Pt. 2) :191–197.
6. **Baric, R. S., G. W. Nelson, J. O. Fleming, R. J. Deans, J. G. Keck, N. Casteel, and S. A. Stohlman.** 1988. Interactions between coronavirus nucleocapsid protein and viral RNAs: implications for viral transcription. *J. Virol.* **62:**4280–4287.
7. **Baudoux, P., C. Carrat, L. Besnardeau, B. Charley, and H. Laude.** 1998. Coronavirus pseudoparticles formed with recombinant M and E proteins induce alpha interferon synthesis by leukocytes. *J. Virol.* **72:**8636–8643.
8. **Bonifacino, J. S., and L. M. Traub.** 2003. Signals for sorting of transmembrane proteins to endosomes and lysosomes. *Annu. Rev. Biochem.* **72:**395–447.

9. Bos, E. C., L. Heijnen, W. Luytjes, and W. J. Spaan. 1995. Mutational analysis of the murine coronavirus spike protein: effect on cell-to-cell fusion. *Virology* **214**:453–463.

10. Bos, E. C., W. Luytjes, H. V. van der Meulen, H. K. Koerten, and W. J. Spaan. 1996. The production of recombinant infectious DI-particles of a murine coronavirus in the absence of helper virus. *Virology* **218**:52–60.

11. Bosch, B. J., C. A. de Haan, S. L. Smits, and P. J. Rottier. 2005. Spike protein assembly into the coronavirion: exploring the limits of its sequence requirements. *Virology* **334**:306–318.

12. Bost, A. G., E. Prentice, and M. R. Denison. 2001. Mouse hepatitis virus replicase protein complexes are translocated to sites of M protein accumulation in the ERGIC at late times of infection. *Virology* **285**:21–29.

13. Bretscher, M. S., and S. Munro. 1993. Cholesterol and the Golgi apparatus. *Science* **261**:1280–1281.

14. Calvo, E., D. Escors, J. A. Lopez, J. M. Gonzalez, A. Alvarez, E. Arza, and L. Enjuanes. 2005. Phosphorylation and subcellular localization of transmissible gastroenteritis virus nucleocapsid protein in infected cells. *J. Gen. Virol.* **86:** 2255–2267.

15. Casais, R., V. Thiel, S. G. Siddell, D. Cavanagh, and P. Britton. 2001. Reverse genetics system for the avian coronavirus infectious bronchitis virus. *J. Virol.* **75**:12359–12369.

16. Cavanagh, D. 1983. Coronavirus IBV: structural characterization of the spike protein. *J. Gen. Virol.* **64**(Pt. 12):2577–2583.

17. Cavanagh, D., and P. J. Davis. 1988. Evolution of avian coronavirus IBV: sequence of the matrix glycoprotein gene and intergenic region of several serotypes. *J. Gen. Virol.* **69**(Pt. 3):621–629.

18. Chang, C. K., S. C. Sue, T. H. Yu, C. M. Hsieh, C. K. Tsai, Y. C. Chiang, S. J. Lee, H. H. Hsiao, W. J. Wu, C. F. Chang, and T. H. Huang. 2005. The dimer interface of the SARS coronavirus nucleocapsid protein adapts a porcine respiratory and reproductive syndrome virus-like structure. *FEBS Lett.* **579**:5663–5668.

19. Chang, C. K., S. C. Sue, T. H. Yu, C. M. Hsieh, C. K. Tsai, Y. C. Chiang, S. J. Lee, H. H. Hsiao, W. J. Wu, W. L. Chang, C. H. Lin, and T. H. Huang. 2006. Modular organization of SARS coronavirus nucleocapsid protein. *J. Biomed. Sci.* **13**:59–72.

20. Chang, K. W., Y. Sheng, and J. L. Gombold. 2000. Coronavirus-induced membrane fusion requires the cysteine-rich domain in the spike protein. *Virology* **269**:212–224.

21. Chang, R. Y., and D. A. Brian. 1996. *cis* requirement for N-specific protein sequence in bovine coronavirus defective interfering RNA replication. *J. Virol.* **70**:2201–2207.

22. Chen, H., A. Gill, B. K. Dove, S. R. Emmett, C. F. Kemp, M. A. Ritchie, M. Dee, and J. A. Hiscox. 2005. Mass spectroscopic characterization of the coronavirus infectious bronchitis virus nucleoprotein and elucidation of the role of phosphorylation in RNA binding by using surface plasmon resonance. *J. Virol.* **79**:1164–1179.

23. Chen, H., T. Wurm, P. Britton, G. Brooks, and J. A. Hiscox. 2002. Interaction of the coronavirus nucleoprotein with nucleolar antigens and the host cell. *J. Virol.* **76**:5233–5250.

24. Cluett, E. B., E. Kuismanen, and C. E. Machamer. 1997. Heterogeneous distribution of the unusual phospholipid semilysobisphosphatidic acid through the Golgi complex. *Mol. Biol. Cell.* **8**:2233–2240.

25. Colley, K. J. 1997. Golgi localization of glycosyltransferases: more questions than answers. *Glycobiology* **7**:1–13.

26. Cologna, R., and B. G. Hogue. 2000. Identification of a bovine coronavirus packaging signal. *J. Virol.* **74**:580–583.

27. Cologna, R., J. F. Spagnolo, and B. G. Hogue. 2000. Identification of nucleocapsid binding sites within coronavirus-defective genomes. *Virology* **277**:235–249.

28. Compton, S. R., D. B. Rogers, K. V. Holmes, D. Fertsch, J. Remenick, and J. J. McGowan. 1987. In vitro replication of mouse hepatitis virus strain A59. *J. Virol.* **61**:1814–1820.

29. Corse, E., and C. E. Machamer. 2000. Infectious bronchitis virus E protein is targeted to the Golgi complex and directs release of virus-like particles. *J. Virol.* **74**:4319–4326.

30. Corse, E., and C. E. Machamer. 2001. Infectious bronchitis virus envelope protein targeting: implications for virus assembly. *Adv. Exp. Med. Biol.* **494**:571–576.

31. Corse, E., and C. E. Machamer. 2002. The cytoplasmic tail of infectious bronchitis virus E protein directs Golgi targeting. *J. Virol.* **76**:1273–1284.

32. Corse, E., and C. E. Machamer. 2003. The cytoplasmic tails of infectious bronchitis virus E and M proteins mediate their interaction. *Virology* **312**:25–34.

33. Curtis, K. M., B. Yount, and R. S. Baric. 2002. Heterologous gene expression from transmissible gastroenteritis virus replicon particles. *J. Virol.* **76**:1422–1434.

34. Dalton, K., R. Casais, K. Shaw, K. Stirrups, S. Evans, P. Britton, T. D. K. Brown, and D. Cavanagh. 2001. *cis*-Acting sequences required for coronavirus infectious bronchitis virus defective-RNA replication and packaging. *J. Virol.* **75**:125–133.

35. Davies, H. A., R. R. Dourmashkin, and M. R. Macnaughton. 1981. Ribonucleoprotein of avian infectious bronchitis virus. *J. Gen. Virol.* **53**:67–74.

36. DeDiego, M. L., E. Álvarez, F. Almazán, M. T. Rejas, E. Lamirande, A. Roberts, W. J. Shieh, S. R. Zaki, K. Subbarao, and L. Enjuanes. 2007. A severe acute respiratory syndrome coronavirus that lacks the E gene is attenuated in vitro and in vivo. *J. Virol.* **81**:1701–1713.

37. de Haan, C. A., M. de Wit, L. Kuo, C. Montalto-Morrison, B. L. Haagmans, S. R. Weiss, P. S. Masters, and P. J. Rottier. 2003. The glycosylation status of the murine hepatitis coronavirus M protein affects the interferogenic capacity of the virus in vitro and its ability to replicate in the liver but not the brain. *Virology* **312**:395–406.

38. de Haan, C. A., L. Kuo, P. S. Masters, H. Vennema, and P. J. Rottier. 1998. Coronavirus particle assembly: primary structure requirements of the membrane protein. *J. Virol.* **72:** 6838–6850.

39. de Haan, C. A., and P. J. Rottier. 2005. Molecular interactions in the assembly of coronaviruses. *Adv. Virus Res.* **64**:165–230.

40. de Haan, C. A., M. Smeets, F. Vernooij, H. Vennema, and P. J. Rottier. 1999. Mapping of the coronavirus membrane protein domains involved in interaction with the spike protein. *J. Virol.* **73**:7441–7452.

41. de Haan, C. A., K. Stadler, G. J. Godeke, B. J. Bosch, and P. J. Rottier. 2004. Cleavage inhibition of the murine coronavirus spike protein by a furin-like enzyme affects cell-cell but not virus-cell fusion. *J. Virol.* **78**:6048–6054.

42. de Haan, C. A., H. Vennema, and P. J. Rottier. 2000. Assembly of the coronavirus envelope: homotypic interactions between the M proteins. *J. Virol.* **74**:4967–4978.

43. Delmas, B., and H. Laude. 1990. Assembly of coronavirus spike protein into trimers and its role in epitope expression. *J. Virol.* **64**:5367–5375.

44. Denison, M. R., W. J. Spaan, Y. van der Meer, C. A. Gibson, A. C. Sims, E. Prentice, and X. T. Lu. 1999. The putative helicase of the coronavirus mouse hepatitis virus is processed from the replicase gene polyprotein and localizes in complexes that are active in viral RNA synthesis. *J. Virol.* **73**:6862–6871.

45. Doms, R. W., R. A. Lamb, J. K. Rose, and A. Helenius. 1993. Folding and assembly of viral membrane proteins. *Virology* 193:545–562.

46. Dove, B. K., J. H. You, M. L. Reed, S. R. Emmett, G. Brooks, and J. A. Hiscox. 2006. Changes in nucleolar morphology and proteins during infection with the coronavirus infectious bronchitis virus. *Cell. Microbiol.* 8:1147–1157.

47. Escors, D., E. Camafeita, J. Ortego, H. Laude, and L. Enjuanes. 2001. Organization of two transmissible gastroenteritis coronavirus membrane protein topologies within the virion and core. *J. Virol.* 75:12228–12240.

48. Escors, D., A. Izeta, C. Capiscol, and L. Enjuanes. 2003. Transmissible gastroenteritis coronavirus packaging signal is located at the 5′ end of the virus genome. *J. Virol.* 77:7890–7902.

49. Escors, D., J. Ortego, and L. Enjuanes. 2001. The membrane M protein of the transmissible gastroenteritis coronavirus binds to the internal core through the carboxy-terminus. *Adv. Exp. Med. Biol.* 494:589–593.

50. Escors, D., J. Ortego, H. Laude, and L. Enjuanes. 2001. The membrane M protein carboxy terminus binds to transmissible gastroenteritis coronavirus core and contributes to core stability. *J. Virol.* 75:1312–1324.

51. Fan, H., A. Ooi, Y. W. Tan, S. Wang, S. Fang, D. X. Liu, and J. Lescar. 2005. The nucleocapsid protein of coronavirus infectious bronchitis virus: crystal structure of its N-terminal domain and multimerization properties. *Structure* 13:1859–1868.

52. Fan, Z., Y. Zhuo, X. Tan, Z. Zhou, J. Yuan, B. Qiang, J. Yan, X. Peng, and G. F. Gao. 2006. SARS-CoV nucleocapsid protein binds to hUbc9, a ubiquitin conjugating enzyme of the sumoylation system. *J. Med. Virol.* 78:1365–1373.

53. Fang, X., L. B. Ye, Y. Zhang, B. Li, S. Li, L. Kong, Y. Wang, H. Zheng, W. Wang, and Z. Wu. 2006. Nucleocapsid amino acids 211 to 254, in particular, tetrad glutamines, are essential for the interaction between the nucleocapsid and membrane proteins of SARS-associated coronavirus. *J. Microbiol.* 44:577–580.

54. Fielding, B. C., Y. J. Tan, S. Shuo, T. H. Tan, E. E. Ooi, S. G. Lim, W. Hong, and P. Y. Goh. 2004. Characterization of a unique group-specific protein (U122) of the severe acute respiratory syndrome coronavirus. *J. Virol.* 78:7311–7318.

55. Fischer, F., C. F. Stegen, P. S. Masters, and W. A. Samsonoff. 1998. Analysis of constructed E gene mutants of mouse hepatitis virus confirms a pivotal role for E protein in coronavirus assembly. *J. Virol.* 72:7885–7894.

56. Fosmire, J. A., K. Hwang, and S. Makino. 1992. Identification and characterization of a coronavirus packaging signal. *J. Virol.* 66:3522–3530.

57. Gallagher, T. M., and M. J. Buchmeier. 2001. Coronavirus spike proteins in viral entry and pathogenesis. *Virology* 279:371–374.

58. Gallagher, T. M., S. E. Parker, and M. J. Buchmeier. 1990. Neutralization-resistant variants of a neurotropic coronavirus are generated by deletions within the amino-terminal half of the spike glycoprotein. *J. Virol.* 64:731–741.

59. Garwes, D. J., D. H. Pocock, and B. V. Pike. 1976. Isolation of subviral components from transmissible gastroenteritis virus. *J. Gen. Virol.* 32:283–294.

60. Gonzalez, M. E., and L. Carrasco. 2003. Viroporins. *FEBS Lett.* 552:28–34.

61. Griffiths, G., and P. Rottier. 1992. Cell biology of viruses that assemble along the biosynthetic pathway. *Semin. Cell Biol.* 3:367–381.

62. He, R., F. Dobie, M. Ballantine, A. Leeson, Y. Li, N. Bastien, T. Cutts, A. Andonov, J. Cao, T. F. Booth, F. A. Plummer, S. Tyler, L. Baker, and X. Li. 2004. Analysis of multimerization

63. He, R., A. Leeson, M. Ballantine, A. Andonov, L. Baker, F. Dobie, Y. Li, N. Bastien, H. Feldmann, U. Strocher, S. Theriault, T. Cutts, J. Cao, T. F. Booth, F. A. Plummer, S. Tyler, and X. Li. 2004. Characterization of protein-protein interactions between the nucleocapsid protein and membrane protein of the SARS coronavirus. *Virus Res.* 105:121–125.

64. Hirschberg, K., C. M. Miller, J. Ellenberg, J. F. Presley, E. D. Siggia, R. D. Phair, and J. Lippincott-Schwartz. 1998. Kinetic analysis of secretory protein traffic and characterization of Golgi to plasma membrane transport intermediates in living cells. *J. Cell Biol.* 143:1485–1503.

65. Hiscox, J. A., T. Wurm, L. Wilson, P. Britton, D. Cavanagh, and G. Brooks. 2001. The coronavirus infectious bronchitis virus nucleoprotein localizes to the nucleolus. *J. Virol.* 75:506–512.

66. Hofmann, M. A., P. B. Sethna, and D. A. Brian. 1990. Bovine coronavirus mRNA replication continues throughout persistent infection in cell culture. *J. Virol.* 64:4108–4114.

67. Hogue, B. G., T. E. Kienzle, and D. A. Brian. 1989. Synthesis and processing of the bovine enteric coronavirus haemagglutinin protein. *J. Gen. Virol.* 70(Pt. 2):345–352.

68. Holmes, K. V., E. W. Doller, and L. S. Sturman. 1981. Tunicamycin resistant glycosylation of coronavirus glycoprotein: demonstration of a novel type of viral glycoprotein. *Virology* 115:334–344.

69. Hsieh, P. K., S. C. Chang, C. C. Huang, T. T. Lee, C. W. Hsiao, Y. H. Kou, I. Y. Chen, C. K. Chang, T. H. Huang, and M. F. Chang. 2005. Assembly of severe acute respiratory syndrome coronavirus RNA packaging signal into virus-like particles is nucleocapsid dependent. *J. Virol.* 79:13848–13855.

70. Huang, C., N. Ito, C. T. Tseng, and S. Makino. 2006. Severe acute respiratory syndrome coronavirus 7a accessory protein is a viral structural protein. *J. Virol.* 80:7287–7294.

71. Huang, I. C., B. J. Bosch, F. Li, W. Li, K. H. Lee, S. Ghiran, N. Vasilieva, T. S. Dermody, S. C. Harrison, P. R. Dormitzer, M. Farzan, P. J. Rottier, and H. Choe. 2006. SARS coronavirus, but not human coronavirus NL63, utilizes cathepsin L to infect ACE2-expressing cells. *J. Biol. Chem.* 281:3198–3203.

72. Huang, Q., L. Yu, A. M. Petros, A. Gunasekera, Z. Liu, N. Xu, P. Hajduk, J. Mack, S. W. Fesik, and E. T. Olejniczak. 2004. Structure of the N-terminal RNA-binding domain of the SARS CoV nucleocapsid protein. *Biochemistry* 43:6059–6063.

73. Huang, Y., Z. Y. Yang, W. P. Kong, and G. J. Nabel. 2004. Generation of synthetic severe acute respiratory syndrome coronavirus pseudoparticles: implications for assembly and vaccine production. *J. Virol.* 78:12557–12565.

74. Hurst, K. R., L. Kuo, C. A. Koetzner, R. Ye, B. Hsue, and P. S. Masters. 2005. A major determinant for membrane protein interaction localizes to the carboxy-terminal domain of the mouse coronavirus nucleocapsid protein. *J. Virol.* 79:13285–13297.

75. Ito, N., E. C. Mossel, K. Narayanan, V. L. Popov, C. Huang, T. Inoue, C. J. Peters, and S. Makino. 2005. Severe acute respiratory syndrome coronavirus 3a protein is a viral structural protein. *J. Virol.* 79:3182–3186.

76. Jacobs, L., B. A. van der Zeijst, and M. C. Horzinek. 1986. Characterization and translation of transmissible gastroenteritis virus mRNAs. *J. Virol.* 57:1010–1015.

77. Jayaram, H., H. Fan, B. R. Bowman, A. Ooi, J. Jayaram, E. W. Collisson, J. Lescar, and B. V. Prasad. 2006. X-ray structures of the N- and C-terminal domains of a coronavirus

nucleocapsid protein: implications for nucleocapsid formation. *J. Virol.* **80**:6612–6620.

78. Jia, H. P., D. C. Look, L. Shi, M. Hickey, L. Pewe, J. Netland, M. Farzan, C. Wohlford-Lenane, S. Perlman, and P. B. McCray, Jr. 2005. ACE2 receptor expression and severe acute respiratory syndrome coronavirus infection depend on differentiation of human airway epithelia. *J. Virol.* **79**:14614–14621.

79. Kapke, P. A., F. Y. Tung, B. G. Hogue, D. A. Brian, R. D. Woods, and R. Wesley. 1988. The amino-terminal signal peptide on the porcine transmissible gastroenteritis coronavirus matrix protein is not an absolute requirement for membrane translocation and glycosylation. *Virology* **165**:367–376.

80. Kazi, L., A. Lissenberg, R. Watson, R. J. de Groot, and S. R. Weiss. 2005. Expression of hemagglutinin esterase protein from recombinant mouse hepatitis virus enhances neurovirulence. *J. Virol.* **79**:15064–15073.

81. Khattari, Z., G. Brotons, M. Akkawi, E. Arbely, I. T. Arkin, and T. Salditt. 2006. SARS coronavirus E protein in phospholipid bilayers: an x-ray study. *Biophys J.* **90**:2038–2050.

82. Klumperman, J., J. K. Locker, A. Meijer, M. C. Horzinek, H. J. Geuze, and P. J. Rottier. 1994. Coronavirus M proteins accumulate in the Golgi complex beyond the site of virion budding. *J. Virol.* **68**:6523–6534.

83. Koch, J., and R. Tampe. 2006. The macromolecular peptide-loading complex in MHC class I-dependent antigen presentation. *Cell. Mol. Life. Sci.* **63**:653–662.

84. Kopecky-Bromberg, S. A., L. Martinez-Sobrido, M. Frieman, R. A. Baric, and P. Palese. 2007. Severe acute respiratory syndrome coronavirus 3b, open reading frame (ORF) 3b, ORF6, and nucleocapsid proteins function as interferon antagonists. *J. Virol.* **81**:548–557.

85. Kopecky-Bromberg, S. A., L. Martinez-Sobrido, and P. Palese. 2006. 7a protein of severe acute respiratory syndrome coronavirus inhibits cellular protein synthesis and activates p38 mitogen-activated protein kinase. *J. Virol.* **80**:785–793.

86. Kuo, L., K. R. Hurst, and P. S. Masters. 2007. Exceptional flexibility in the sequence requirements for coronavirus small envelope protein function. *J. Virol.* **81**:2249–2262.

87. Kuo, L., and P. S. Masters. 2002. Genetic evidence for a structural interaction between the carboxy termini of the membrane and nucleocapsid proteins of mouse hepatitis virus. *J. Virol.* **76**:4987–4999.

88. Kuo, L., and P. S. Masters. 2003. The small envelope protein E is not essential for murine coronavirus replication. *J. Virol.* **77**:4597–4608.

89. Lancer, J. A., and C. R. Howard. 1980. The disruption of infectious bronchitis virus (IBV-41 strain) with Triton X-100 detergent. *J. Virol. Methods* **1**:121–131.

90. Laude, H., and P. S. Masters. 1995. The coronavirus nucleocapsid protein, p. 141–163. *In* S. G. Siddell (ed.), *The Coronaviridae*. Plenum, New York, NY.

91. Laude, H., D. Rasschaert, and J. C. Huet. 1987. Sequence and N-terminal processing of the transmembrane protein E1 of the coronavirus transmissible gastroenteritis virus. *J. Gen. Virol.* **68**(Pt. 6):1687–1693.

92. Lavi, E., Q. Wang, S. R. Weiss, and N. K. Gonatas. 1996. Syncytia formation induced by coronavirus infection is associated with fragmentation and rearrangement of the Golgi apparatus. *Virology* **221**:325–334.

93. Law, P. T., C. H. Wong, T. C. Au, C. P. Chuck, S. K. Kong, P. K. Chan, K. F. To, A. W. Lo, J. Y. Chan, Y. K. Suen, H. Y. Chan, K. P. Fung, M. M. Waye, J. J. Sung, Y. M. Lo, and S. K. Tsui. 2005. The 3a protein of severe acute respiratory syndrome-associated coronavirus induces apoptosis in Vero E6 cells. *J. Gen. Virol.* **86**:1921–1930.

94. Lewicki, D. N., and T. M. Gallagher. 2002. Quaternary structure of coronavirus spikes in complex with carcinoembryonic antigen-related cell adhesion molecule cellular receptors. *J. Biol. Chem.* **277**:19727–19734.

95. Li, F., M. Berardi, W. Li, M. Farzan, P. R. Dormitzer, and S. C. Harrison. 2006. Conformational states of the severe acute respiratory syndrome coronavirus spike protein ectodomain. *J. Virol.* **80**:6794–6800.

96. Li, F. Q., H. Xiao, J. P. Tam, and D. X. Liu. 2005. Sumoylation of the nucleocapsid protein of severe acute respiratory syndrome coronavirus. *FEBS Lett.* **579**:2387–2396.

97. Liao, Y., J. Lescar, J. P. Tam, and D. X. Liu. 2004. Expression of SARS-coronavirus envelope protein in Escherichia coli cells alters membrane permeability. *Biochem. Biophys. Res. Commun.* **325**:374–380.

98. Liao, Y., Q. Yuan, J. Torres, J. P. Tam, and D. X. Liu. 2006. Biochemical and functional characterization of the membrane association and membrane permeabilizing activity of the severe acute respiratory syndrome coronavirus envelope protein. *Virology* **349**:264–275.

99. Lim, K. P., and D. X. Liu. 2001. The missing link in coronavirus assembly. Retention of the avian coronavirus infectious bronchitis virus envelope protein in the pre-Golgi compartments and physical interaction between the envelope and membrane proteins. *J. Biol. Chem.* **276**:17515–17523.

100. Lissenberg, A., M. M. Vrolijk, A. L. van Vliet, M. A. Langereis, J. D. de Groot-Mijnes, P. J. Rottier, and R. J. de Groot. 2005. Luxury at a cost? Recombinant mouse hepatitis viruses expressing the accessory hemagglutinin esterase protein display reduced fitness in vitro. *J. Virol.* **79**:15054–15063.

101. Liu, D. X., and S. C. Inglis. 1991. Association of the infectious bronchitis virus 3c protein with the virion envelope. *Virology* **185**:911–917.

102. Locker, J. K., J. Klumperman, V. Oorschot, M. C. Horzinek, H. J. Geuze, and P. J. Rottier. 1994. The cytoplasmic tail of mouse hepatitis virus M protein is essential but not sufficient for its retention in the Golgi complex. *J. Biol. Chem.* **269**:28263–28269.

103. Locker, J. K., D. J. Opstelten, M. Ericsson, M. C. Horzinek, and P. J. Rottier. 1995. Oligomerization of a trans-Golgi/trans-Golgi network retained protein occurs in the Golgi complex and may be part of its retention. *J. Biol. Chem.* **270**:8815–8821.

104. Lontok, E., E. Corse, and C. E. Machamer. 2004. Intracellular targeting signals contribute to localization of coronavirus spike proteins near the virus assembly site. *J. Virol.* **78**:5913–5922.

105. Lopez, L. A., A. Jones, W. D. Arndt, and B. G. Hogue. 2006. Subcellular localization of SARS-CoV structural proteins. *Adv. Exp. Med. Biol.* **581**:297–300.

106. Lu, W., B. J. Zheng, K. Xu, W. Schwarz, L. Du, C. K. Wong, J. Chen, S. Duan, V. Deubel, and B. Sun. 2006. Severe acute respiratory syndrome-associated coronavirus 3a protein forms an ion channel and modulates virus release. *Proc. Natl. Acad. Sci. USA* **103**:12540–12545.

107. Luini, A., A. Ragnini-Wilson, R. S. Polishchuck, and M. A. De Matteis. 2005. Large pleiomorphic traffic intermediates in the secretory pathway. *Curr. Opin. Cell. Biol.* **17**:353–361.

108. Machamer, C. E., M. G. Grim, A. Esquela, S. W. Chung, M. Rolls, K. Ryan, and A. M. Swift. 1993. Retention of a cis Golgi protein requires polar residues on one face of a predicted alpha-helix in the transmembrane domain. *Mol. Biol. Cell* **4**:695–704.

109. Machamer, C. E., S. A. Mentone, J. K. Rose, and M. G. Farquhar. 1990. The E1 glycoprotein of an avian coronavirus

is targeted to the cis Golgi complex. *Proc. Natl. Acad. Sci. USA* **87:**6944–6948.

110. **Machamer, C. E., and J. K. Rose.** 1987. A specific transmembrane domain of a coronavirus E1 glycoprotein is required for its retention in the Golgi region. *J. Cell Biol.* **105:**1205–1214.

111. **Machamer, C. E., and S. Youn.** 2006. The transmembrane domain of the infectious bronchitis virus E protein is required for efficient virus release. *Adv. Exp. Med. Bio.l* **581:**193–198.

112. **Macneughton, M. R., and H. A. Davies.** 1978. Ribonucleoprotein-like structures from coronavirus particles. *J. Gen. Virol.* **39:**545–549.

113. **Madan, V., J. Garcia Mde, M. A. Sanz, and L. Carrasco.** 2005. Viroporin activity of murine hepatitis virus E protein. *FEBS Lett.* **579:**3607–3612.

114. **Maeda, J., A. Maeda, and S. Makino.** 1999. Release of coronavirus E protein in membrane vesicles from virus-infected cells and E protein-expressing cells. *Virology* **263:**265–272.

115. **Maeda, J., J. F. Repass, A. Maeda, and S. Makino.** 2001. Membrane topology of coronavirus E protein. *Virology* **281:**163–169.

116. **Makino, S., K. Yokomori, and M. M. Lai.** 1990. Analysis of efficiently packaged defective interfering RNAs of murine coronavirus: localization of a possible RNA-packaging signal. *J. Virol.* **64:**6045–6053.

117. **Masters, P. S.** 1992. Localization of an RNA-binding domain in the nucleocapsid protein of the coronavirus mouse hepatitis virus. *Arch. Virol.* **125:**141–160.

118. **Masters, P. S.** 2006. The molecular biology of coronaviruses. *Adv. Virus Res.* **66:**193–292.

119. **McBride, C. E., J. Li, and C. E. Machamer.** 2007. The cytoplasmic tail of the severe acute respiratory syndrome coronavirus spike protein contains a novel endoplasmic reticulum retrieval signal that binds COPI and promotes interaction with membrane protein. *J. Virol.* **81:**2418–2428.

120. **Mitra, K., I. Ubarretxena-Belandia, T. Taguchi, G. Warren, and D. M. Engelman.** 2004. Modulation of the bilayer thickness of exocytic pathway membranes by membrane proteins rather than cholesterol. *Proc. Natl. Acad. Sci. USA* **101:**4083–4088.

121. **Molenkamp, R., and W. J. Spaan.** 1997. Identification of a specific interaction between the coronavirus mouse hepatitis virus A59 nucleocapsid protein and packaging signal. *Virology* **239:**78–86.

122. **Mortola, E., and P. Roy.** 2004. Efficient assembly and release of SARS coronavirus-like particles by a heterologous expression system. *FEBS Lett.* **576:**174–178.

123. **Munro, S.** 1995. An investigation of the role of transmembrane domains in Golgi protein retention. *EMBO J.* **14:**4695–4704.

124. **Nal, B., C. Chan, F. Kien, L. Siu, J. Tse, K. Chu, J. Kam, I. Staropoli, B. Crescenzo-Chaigne, N. Escriou, S. van der Werf, K. Y. Yuen, and R. Altmeyer.** 2005. Differential maturation and subcellular localization of severe acute respiratory syndrome coronavirus surface proteins S, M and E. *J. Gen. Virol.* **86:**1423–1434.

125. **Narayanan, K., K. H. Kim, and S. Makino.** 2003. Characterization of N protein self-association in coronavirus ribonucleoprotein complexes. *Virus Res.* **98:**131–140.

126. **Narayanan, K., A. Maeda, J. Maeda, and S. Makino.** 2000. Characterization of the coronavirus M protein and nucleocapsid interaction in infected cells. *J. Virol.* **74:**8127–8134.

127. **Narayanan, K., and S. Makino.** 2001. Cooperation of an RNA packaging signal and a viral envelope protein in coronavirus RNA packaging. *J. Virol.* **75:**9059–9067.

128. **Nelson, C. A., A. Pekosz, C. A. Lee, M. S. Diamond, and D. H. Fremont.** 2005. Structure and intracellular targeting of the SARS-coronavirus Orf7a accessory protein. *Structure* **13:**75–85.

129. **Nelson, G. W., S. A. Stohlman, and S. M. Tahara.** 2000. High affinity interaction between nucleocapsid protein and leader/intergenic sequence of mouse hepatitis virus RNA. *J. Gen. Virol.* **81:**181–188.

130. **Nelson, W. J., and C. Yeaman.** 2001. Protein trafficking in the exocytic pathway of polarized epithelial cells. *Trends Cell Biol.* **11:**483–486.

131. **Nguyen, V. P., and B. G. Hogue.** 1997. Protein interactions during coronavirus assembly. *J. Virol.* **71:**9278–9284.

132. **Niemann, H., G. Heisterberg-Moutsis, R. Geyer, H. D. Klenk, and M. Wirth.** 1984. Glycoprotein E1 of MHV-A59: structure of the O-linked carbohydrates and construction of full length recombinant cDNA clones. *Adv. Exp. Med. Biol.* **173:**201–213.

133. **Oostra, M., C. A. M. de Haan, R. J. de Groot, and P. J. M. Rottier.** 2006. Glycosylation of the severe acute respiratory syndrome coronavirus triple-spanning membrane proteins 3a and M. *J. Virol.* **80:**2326–2336.

134. **Opstelten, D. J., P. de Groote, M. C. Horzinek, H. Vennema, and P. J. Rottier.** 1993. Disulfide bonds in folding and transport of mouse hepatitis coronavirus glycoproteins. *J. Virol.* **67:**7394–7401.

135. **Opstelten, D. J., M. J. Raamsman, K. Wolfs, M. C. Horzinek, and P. J. Rottier.** 1995. Envelope glycoprotein interactions in coronavirus assembly. *J. Cell Biol.* **131:**339–349.

136. **Ortego, J., D. Escors, H. Laude, and L. Enjuanes.** 2002. Generation of a replication-competent, propagation-deficient virus vector based on the transmissible gastroenteritis coronavirus genome. *J. Virol.* **76:**11518–11529.

137. **Parker, M. M., and P. S. Masters.** 1990. Sequence comparison of the N genes of five strains of the coronavirus mouse hepatitis virus suggests a three domain structure for the nucleocapsid protein. *Virology* **179:**463–468.

138. **Polishchuk, E. V., A. Di Pentima, A. Luini, and R. S. Polishchuk.** 2003. Mechanism of constitutive export from the Golgi: bulk flow via the formation, protrusion, and en bloc cleavage of large trans-Golgi network tubular domains. *Mol. Biol. Cell* **14:**4470–4485.

139. **Polishchuk, R. S., E. V. Polishchuk, P. Marra, S. Alberti, R. Buccione, A. Luini, and A. A. Mironov.** 2000. Correlative light-electron microscopy reveals the tubular-saccular ultrastructure of carriers operating between Golgi apparatus and plasma membrane. *J. Cell Biol.* **148:**45–58.

140. **Pornillos, O., J. E. Garrus, and W. I. Sundquist.** 2002. Mechanisms of enveloped RNA virus budding. *Trends Cell Biol.* **12:**569–579.

141. **Raamsman, M. J., J. K. Locker, A. de Hooge, A. A. de Vries, G. Griffiths, H. Vennema, and P. J. Rottier.** 2000. Characterization of the coronavirus mouse hepatitis virus strain A59 small membrane protein E. *J. Virol.* **74:**2333–2342.

142. **Risco, C., I. M. Anton, L. Enjuanes, and J. L. Carrascosa.** 1996. The transmissible gastroenteritis coronavirus contains a spherical core shell consisting of M and N proteins. *J. Virol.* **70:**4773–4777.

143. **Risco, C., I. M. Anton, C. Sune, A. M. Pedregosa, J. M. Martin-Alonso, F. Parra, J. L. Carrascosa, and L. Enjuanes.** 1995. Membrane protein molecules of transmissible gastroenteritis coronavirus also expose the carboxy-terminal region on the external surface of the virion. *J. Virol.* **69:**5269–5277.

144. **Robbins, S. G., M. F. Frana, J. J. McGowan, J. F. Boyle, and K. V. Holmes.** 1986. RNA-binding proteins of coronavirus

MHV: detection of monomeric and multimeric N protein with an RNA overlay-protein blot assay. *Virology* **150**:402–410.

145. **Rönnholm, R.** 1992. Localization to the Golgi complex of Uukuniemi virus glycoproteins G1 and G2 expressed from cloned cDNAs. *J. Virol.* **66**:4525–4531.

146. **Rossen, J. W., C. P. Bekker, G. J. Strous, M. C. Horzinek, G. S. Dveksler, K. V. Holmes, and P. J. Rottier.** 1996. A murine and a porcine coronavirus are released from opposite surfaces of the same epithelial cells. *Virology* **224**:345–351.

147. **Rossen, J. W., C. P. Bekker, W. F. Voorhout, G. J. Strous, A. van der Ende, and P. J. Rottier.** 1994. Entry and release of transmissible gastroenteritis coronavirus are restricted to apical surfaces of polarized epithelial cells. *J. Virol.* **68**:7966–7973.

148. **Rossen, J. W., R. de Beer, G. J. Godeke, M. J. Raamsman, M. C. Horzinek, H. Vennema, and P. J. Rottier.** 1998. The viral spike protein is not involved in the polarized sorting of coronaviruses in epithelial cells. *J. Virol.* **72**:497–503.

149. **Rossen, J. W., G. J. Strous, M. C. Horzinek, and P. J. Rottier.** 1997. Mouse hepatitis virus strain A59 is released from opposite sides of different epithelial cell types. *J. Gen. Virol.* **78**(Pt. 1):61–69.

150. **Rossen, J. W., W. F. Voorhout, M. C. Horzinek, A. van der Ende, G. J. Strous, and P. J. Rottier.** 1995. MHV-A59 enters polarized murine epithelial cells through the apical surface but is released basolaterally. *Virology* **210**:54–66.

151. **Rottier, P. J., M. C. Horzinek, and B. A. van der Zeijst.** 1981. Viral protein synthesis in mouse hepatitis virus strain A59-infected cells: effect of tunicamycin. *J. Virol.* **40**:350–357.

152. **Rottier, P. J., and J. K. Rose.** 1987. Coronavirus E1 glycoprotein expressed from cloned cDNA localizes in the Golgi region. *J. Virol.* **61**:2042–2045.

153. **Rottier, P. J., G. W. Welling, S. Welling-Wester, H. G. Niesters, J. A. Lenstra, and B. A. Van der Zeijst.** 1986. Predicted membrane topology of the coronavirus protein E1. Biochemistry **25**:1335–1339.

154. **Rowland, R. R., V. Chauhan, Y. Fang, A. Pekosz, M. Kerrigan, and M. D. Burton.** 2005. Intracellular localization of the severe acute respiratory syndrome coronavirus nucleocapsid protein: absence of nucleolar accumulation during infection and after expression as a recombinant protein in Vero cells. *J. Virol.* **79**:11507–11512.

155. **Salanueva, I. J., J. L. Carrascosa, and C. Risco.** 1999. Structural maturation of the transmissible gastroenteritis coronavirus. *J. Virol.* **73**:7952–7964.

156. **Schaecher, S. R., J. M. Mackenzie, and A. Pekosz.** 2006. The ORF7b protein of severe acute respiratory syndrome coronavirus (SARS-CoV) is expressed in virus-infected cells and incorporated into SARS-CoV particles. *J. Virol.* **81**:718–731.

157. **Schelle, B., N. Karl, B. Ludewig, S. G. Siddell, and V. Thiel.** 2005. Selective replication of coronavirus genomes that express nucleocapsid protein. *J. Virol.* **79**:6620–6630.

158. **Schwegmann-Wessels, C., M. Al-Falah, D. Escors, Z. Wang, G. Zimmer, H. Deng, L. Enjuanes, H. Y. Naim, and G. Herrler.** 2004. A novel sorting signal for intracellular localization is present in the S protein of a porcine coronavirus but absent from severe acute respiratory syndrome-associated coronavirus. *J. Biol. Chem.* **279**:43661–43666.

159. **Sethna, P. B., M. A. Hofmann, and D. A. Brian.** 1991. Minus-strand copies of replicating coronavirus mRNAs contain antileaders. *J. Virol.* **65**:320–325.

160. **Sethna, P. B., S. L. Hung, and D. A. Brian.** 1989. Coronavirus subgenomic minus-strand RNAs and the potential for mRNA replicons. *Proc. Natl. Acad. Sci. USA* **86**:5626–5630.

161. **Shen, S., P. S. Lin, Y. C. Chao, A. Zhang, X. Yang, S. G. Lim, W. Hong, and Y. J. Tan.** 2005. The severe acute respiratory syndrome coronavirus 3a is a novel structural protein. *Biochem. Biophys. Res. Commun.* **330**:286–292.

162. **Simmons, G., D. N. Gosalia, A. J. Rennekamp, J. D. Reeves, S. L. Diamond, and P. Bates.** 2005. Inhibitors of cathepsin L prevent severe acute respiratory syndrome coronavirus entry. *Proc. Natl. Acad. Sci. USA* **102**:11876–11881.

163. **Sims, A. C., J. Ostermann, and M. R. Denison.** 2000. Mouse hepatitis virus replicase proteins associate with two distinct populations of intracellular membranes. *J. Virol.* **74**:5647–5654.

164. **Smits, S. L., G. J. Gerwig, A. L. van Vliet, A. Lissenberg, P. Briza, J. P. Kamerling, R. Vlasak, and R. J. de Groot.** 2005. Nidovirus sialate-O-acetylesterases: evolution and substrate specificity of coronaviral and toroviral receptor-destroying enzymes. *J. Biol. Chem.* **280**:6933–6941.

165. **Stern, D. F., and B. M. Sefton.** 1982. Coronavirus proteins: structure and function of the oligosaccharides of the avian infectious bronchitis virus glycoproteins. *J. Virol.* **44**:804–812.

166. **Stohlman, S. A., R. S. Baric, G. N. Nelson, L. H. Soe, L. M. Welter, and R. J. Deans.** 1988. Specific interaction between coronavirus leader RNA and nucleocapsid protein. *J. Virol.* **62**:4288–4295.

167. **Sturman, L. S., K. V. Holmes, and J. Behnke.** 1980. Isolation of coronavirus envelope glycoproteins and interaction with the viral nucleocapsid. *J. Virol.* **33**:449–462.

168. **Sturman, L. S., C. S. Ricard, and K. V. Holmes.** 1985. Proteolytic cleavage of the E2 glycoprotein of murine coronavirus: activation of cell-fusing activity of virions by trypsin and separation of two different 90K cleavage fragments. *J. Virol.* **56**:904–911.

169. **Surjit, M., R. Kumar, R. N. Mishra, M. K. Reddy, V. T. Chow, and S. K. Lal.** 2005. The severe acute respiratory syndrome coronavirus nucleocapsid protein is phosphorylated and localizes in the cytoplasm by 14-3-3-mediated translocation. *J. Virol.* **79**:11476–11486.

170. **Swift, A. M., and C. E. Machamer.** 1991. A Golgi retention signal in a membrane-spanning domain of coronavirus E1 protein. *J. Cell Biol.* **115**:19–30.

171. **Tahara, S. M., T. A. Dietlin, C. C. Bergmann, G. W. Nelson, S. Kyuwa, R. P. Anthony, and S. A. Stohlman.** 1994. Coronavirus translational regulation: leader affects mRNA efficiency. *Virology* **202**:621–630.

172. **Tan, Y. J., B. C. Fielding, P. Y. Goh, S. Shen, T. H. Tan, S. G. Lim, and W. Hong.** 2004. Overexpression of 7a, a protein specifically encoded by the severe acute respiratory syndrome coronavirus, induces apoptosis via a caspase-dependent pathway. *J. Virol.* **78**:14043–14047.

173. **Tan, Y. J., E. Teng, S. Shen, T. H. Tan, P. Y. Goh, B. C. Fielding, E. E. Ooi, H. C. Tan, S. G. Lim, and W. Hong.** 2004. A novel severe acute respiratory syndrome coronavirus protein, U274, is transported to the cell surface and undergoes endocytosis. *J. Virol.* **78**:6723–6734.

174. **Tan, Y. J., P. Y. Tham, D. Z. Chan, C. F. Chou, S. Shen, B. C. Fielding, T. H. Tan, S. G. Lim, and W. Hong.** 2005. The severe acute respiratory syndrome coronavirus 3a protein up-regulates expression of fibrinogen in lung epithelial cells. *J. Virol.* **79**:10083–10087.

175. **Teasdale, R. D., and M. R. Jackson.** 1996. Signal-mediated sorting of membrane proteins between the endoplasmic reticulum and the Golgi apparatus. *Annu. Rev. Cell Dev. Biol.* **12**:27–54.

176. **Thorp, E. B., J. A. Boscarino, H. L. Logan, J. T. Goletz, and T. M. Gallagher.** 2006. Palmitoylations on murine

coronavirus spike proteins are essential for virion assembly and infectivity. *J. Virol.* **80:**1280–1289.

177. **Timani, K. A., Q. Liao, L. Ye, Y. Zeng, J. Liu, Y. Zheng, X. Yang, K. Lingbao, J. Gao, and Y. Zhu.** 2005. Nuclear/nucleolar localization properties of C-terminal nucleocapsid protein of SARS coronavirus. *Virus Res.* **114:**23–34.

178. **Toomre, D., P. Keller, J. White, J. C. Olivo, and K. Simons.** 1999. Dual-color visualization of trans-Golgi network to plasma membrane traffic along microtubules in living cells. *J. Cell Sci.* **112**(Pt. 1):21–33.

179. **Tooze, J., S. Tooze, and G. Warren.** 1984. Replication of coronavirus MHV-A59 in sac− cells: determination of the first site of budding of progeny virions. *Eur. J. Cell Biol.* **33:**281–293.

180. **Tooze, J., and S. A. Tooze.** 1985. Infection of AtT20 murine pituitary tumour cells by mouse hepatitis virus strain A59: virus budding is restricted to the Golgi region. *Eur. J. Cell Biol.* **37:**203–212.

181. **Tooze, J., S. A. Tooze, and S. D. Fuller.** 1987. Sorting of progeny coronavirus from condensed secretory proteins at the exit from the trans-Golgi network of AtT20 cells. *J. Cell Biol.* **105:**1215–1226.

182. **Torres, J., J. Wang, K. Parthasarathy, and D. X. Liu.** 2005. The transmembrane oligomers of coronavirus protein E. *Biophys. J.* **88:**1283–1290.

183. **Traub, L. M.** 2005. Common principles in clathrin-mediated sorting at the Golgi and the plasma membrane. *Biochim. Biophys. Acta* **1744:**415–437.

184. **Tseng, C. T., J. Tseng, L. Perrone, M. Worthy, V. Popov, and C. J. Peters.** 2005. Apical entry and release of severe acute respiratory syndrome-associated coronavirus in polarized Calu-3 lung epithelial cells. *J. Virol.* **79:**9470–9479.

185. **van Berlo, M. F., W. J. van den Brink, M. C. Horzinek, and B. A. van der Zeijst.** 1987. Fatty acid acylation of viral proteins in murine hepatitis virus-infected cells. Brief report. *Arch. Virol.* **95:**123–128.

186. **van der Meer, Y., E. J. Snijder, J. C. Dobbe, S. Schleich, M. R. Denison, W. J. Spaan, and J. K. Locker.** 1999. Localization of mouse hepatitis virus nonstructural proteins and RNA synthesis indicates a role for late endosomes in viral replication. *J. Virol.* **73:**7641–7657.

187. **van Genderen, I. L., G. J. Godeke, P. J. Rottier, and G. van Meer.** 1995. The phospholipid composition of enveloped viruses depends on the intracellular membrane through which they bud. *Biochem. Soc. Trans.* **23:**523–526.

188. **Vennema, H., G. J. Godeke, J. W. Rossen, W. F. Voorhout, M. C. Horzinek, D. J. Opstelten, and P. J. Rottier.** 1996. Nucleocapsid-independent assembly of coronavirus-like particles by co-expression of viral envelope protein genes. *EMBO J.* **15:**2020–2028.

189. **Vennema, H., R. Rijnbrand, L. Heijnen, M. C. Horzinek, and W. J. Spaan.** 1991. Enhancement of the vaccinia virus/phage T7 RNA polymerase expression system using encephalomyocarditis virus 5′-untranslated region sequences. *Gene* **108:**201–209.

190. **Verma, S., V. Bednar, A. Blount, and B. G. Hogue.** 2006. Identification of functionally important negatively charged residues in the carboxy end of mouse hepatitis coronavirus A59 nucleocapsid protein. *J. Virol.* **80:**4344–4355.

191. **Verma, S., L. A. Lopez, V. Bednar, and B. G. Hogue.** 2007. Importance of the penultimate positive charge in mouse hepatitis coronavirus A59 membrane protein. *J. Virol.* **81:**5339–5348.

192. **Wang, G., C. Deering, M. Macke, J. Shao, R. Burns, D. M. Blau, K. V. Holmes, B. L. Davidson, S. Perlman, and P. B. McCray, Jr.** 2000. Human coronavirus 229E infects polarized airway epithelia from the apical surface. *J. Virol.* **74:**9234–9239.

193. **Wege, H., K. Nagashima, and V. ter Meulen.** 1979. Structural polypeptides of the murine coronavirus JHM. *J. Gen. Virol.* **42:**37–47.

194. **Weiss, S. R., and S. Navas-Martin.** 2005. Coronavirus pathogenesis and the emerging pathogen severe acute respiratory syndrome coronavirus. *Microbiol. Mol. Biol. Rev.* **69:**635–664.

195. **Weisz, O. A., A. M. Swift, and C. E. Machamer.** 1993. Oligomerization of a membrane protein correlates with its retention in the Golgi complex. *J. Cell Biol.* **122:**1185–1196.

196. **White, T. C., Z. Yi, and B. G. Hogue.** 2007. Identification of mouse hepatitis coronavirus A59 nucleocapsid protein phosphorylation sites. *Virus Res.* **126:**139–148.

197. **Wilson, L., P. Gage, and G. Ewart.** 2006. Hexamethylene amiloride blocks E protein ion channels and inhibits coronavirus replication. *Virology* **353:**294–306.

198. **Wilson, L., C. McKinlay, P. Gage, and G. Ewart.** 2004. SARS coronavirus E protein forms cation-selective ion channels. *Virology* **330:**322–331.

199. **Wurm, T., H. Chen, T. Hodgson, P. Britton, G. Brooks, and J. A. Hiscox.** 2001. Localization to the nucleolus is a common feature of coronavirus nucleoproteins, and the protein may disrupt host cell division. *J. Virol.* **75:**9345–9356.

200. **Yamada, Y. K., M. Yabe, T. Ohtsuki, and F. Taguchi.** 2000. Unique N-linked glycosylation of murine coronavirus MHV-2 membrane protein at the conserved O-linked glycosylation site. *Virus Res.* **66:**149–154.

201. **Ye, R., C. Montalto-Morrison, and P. S. Masters.** 2004. Genetic analysis of determinants for spike glycoprotein assembly into murine coronavirus virions: distinct roles for charge-rich and cysteine-rich regions of the endodomain. *J. Virol.* **78:**9904–9917.

202. **Ye, Y., K. Hauns, J. O. Langland, B. L. Jacobs, and B. G. Hogue.** 2006. Mouse hepatitis coronavirus A59 nucleocapsid protein is a type I interferon antagonist. *J. Virol.* **81:**2554–2563.

203. **Ye, Y., and B. G. Hogue.** 2007. Role of the coronavirus E viroporin protein transmembrane domain in virus assembly. *J. Virol.* **81:**3597–3607.

204. **You, J., B. K. Dove, L. Enjuanes, M. L. DeDiego, E. Alvarez, G. Howell, P. Heinen, M. Zambon, and J. A. Hiscox.** 2005. Subcellular localization of the severe acute respiratory syndrome coronavirus nucleocapsid protein. *J. Gen. Virol.* **86:**3303–3310.

205. **Youn, S., E. W. Collisson, and C. E. Machamer.** 2005. Contribution of trafficking signals in the cytoplasmic tail of the infectious bronchitis virus spike protein to virus infection. *J. Virol.* **79:**13209–13217.

206. **Yount, B., K. M. Curtis, and R. S. Baric.** 2000. Strategy for systematic assembly of large RNA and DNA genomes: transmissible gastroenteritis virus model. *J. Virol.* **74:**10600–10611.

207. **Yount, B., R. S. Roberts, A. C. Sims, D. Deming, M. B. Frieman, J. Sparks, M. R. Denison, N. Davis, and R. S. Baric.** 2005. Severe acute respiratory syndrome coronavirus group-specific open reading frames encode nonessential functions for replication in cell cultures and mice. *J. Virol.* **79:**14909–14922.

208. **Yu, I. M., M. L. Oldham, J. Zhang, and J. Chen.** 2006. Crystal structure of the severe acute respiratory syndrome (SARS) coronavirus nucleocapsid protein dimerization domain reveals evolutionary linkage between corona- and arteriviridae. *J. Biol. Chem.* **281:**17134–17139.

209. Yu, X., W. Bi, S. R. Weiss, and J. L. Leibowitz. 1994. Mouse hepatitis virus gene 5b protein is a new virion envelope protein. *Virology* **202:**1018–1023.

210. Yuan, Q., Y. Liao, J. Torres, J. P. Tam, and D. X. Liu. 2006. Biochemical evidence for the presence of mixed membrane topologies of the severe acute respiratory syndrome coronavirus envelope protein expressed in mammalian cells. *FEBS Lett.* **580:**3192–3200.

211. Yuan, X., J. Li, Y. Shan, Z. Yang, Z. Zhao, B. Chen, Z. Yao, B. Dong, S. Wang, J. Chen, and Y. Cong. 2005. Subcellular localization and membrane association of SARS-CoV 3a protein. *Virus Res.* **109:**191–202.

212. Yuan, X., J. Wu, Y. Shan, Z. Yao, B. Dong, B. Chen, Z. Zhao, S. Wang, J. Chen, and Y. Cong. 2006. SARS coronavirus 7a protein blocks cell cycle progression at G0/G1 phase via the cyclin D3/pRb pathway. *Virology* **346:**74–85.

213. Zhao, X., K. Shaw, and D. Cavanagh. 1993. Presence of subgenomic mRNAs in virions of coronavirus IBV. *Virology* **196:**172–178.

214. Zhou, M., and E. W. Collisson. 2000. The amino and carboxyl domains of the infectious bronchitis virus nucleocapsid protein interact with 3′ genomic RNA. *Virus Res.* **67:**31–39.

215. Zúñiga, S., I. Sola, J. L. Moreno, P. Sabella, J. Plana-Durán, and L. Enjuanes. 2007. Coronavirus nucleocapsid protein is an RNA chaperone. *Virology* **357:**215–227.

*Nidoviruses*
Edited by S. Perlman, T. Gallagher, and E. J. Snijder
© 2008 ASM Press, Washington, DC

Chapter 13

# Supramolecular Architecture of the Coronavirus Particle

BENJAMIN W. NEUMAN

The significance of virion architecture to the study of viral pathogenesis is twofold. As a vehicle for nucleic acid transport, the virus particle shepherds its genome through intercellular space, ultimately depositing its cargo in the particular subcellular environment suited to its mode of replication. Scientific inquiry has focused with somewhat less intensity on the virion as the culmination of the multifaceted process of virogenesis. A central theme of the work presented here is that investigation of the supramolecular design of the virion, in the context of a molecular understanding of its component parts, can illuminate the machinations of viral assembly. In the coronaviruses, both criteria are met: recent advances in image analysis technology have brought ultrastructural analysis to bear on a growing molecular biology database. The analysis presented here hints at the exquisite interplay of interactions that contribute both form and transience to the coronavirus particle.

A closer focus on coronavirus structure brings out a central conundrum in the order *Nidovirales*. Despite considerable similarity at the level of genomic organization, virion morphology is quite divergent across the family. For example, spherical arterivirus particles may house an icosahedral nucleocapsid (37), ronivirus particles are typically rod-like or pleomorphic (6), torovirus particles are toroidal or pleomorphic (2, 22), and coronaviruses display a variety of pleomorphic forms (3, 9). Coronaviruses can be recognized by their eponymous coronal fringe of protruding spike glycoproteins (S proteins). The viral ribonucleoprotein (RNP) core is populated by the single-stranded RNA genome and molecules of nucleocapsid protein (N protein). The major protein species present in the viral membrane is the triple-pass membrane glycoprotein (M protein), which is central to the virus assembly process. A suite of minor membrane-localized components in each species of coronavirus typically includes the minor envelope protein (E protein) and a selection of the group-specific accessory proteins encoded in the 3′-terminal region of the genome.

## ANALYSIS TECHNIQUES

Previous investigations of virion organization have harnessed X-ray crystallography and electron microscopy (EM) to analyze homogeneous virion populations. Features of this class of viral particles, including consistent long-range order and helical or icosahedral exterior symmetry, have come to symbolize virion structure in general despite the increasing profile of pathogenic viruses that do not adhere to this structural type. Coronaviruses have proven more challenging to study in detail, because as electron micrographs show, coronavirus particles are neither homogeneous nor symmetric (9, 24, 30, 31). Examination of coronaviruses by atomic-force microscopy (24) and scanning EM (25) has produced little insight into particle architecture, to date. Cryo-EM and single-particle image analysis techniques do not require homogeneity or symmetry and can be adapted to study pleomorphic specimens (28, 29). In this methodology, statistical algorithms are used to group and average similar images. Images selected at the virion edge, designated "edge views," provide data on the radial stacking of features. Complementary information on the lateral distribution of features can be extracted from "axial views" selected near the virion center. A relatively complete picture of virion supramolecular architecture can be compiled by integrating structural data from axial and edge views.

**Benjamin W. Neuman** • Department of Molecular and Integrative Neurosciences, The Scripps Research Institute, 10550 N. Torrey Pines Rd., La Jolla, CA 92037.

## CRYO-EM OF CORONAVIRUS PARTICLES

In preparation for cryo-EM, viral particles were fixed with buffered formalin and applied to a porous carbon support film. Samples were flash-frozen by immersion in liquid ethane slush. Images were recorded over holes in the support film, and they show particles suspended in a thin layer of vitreous ice (Fig. 1). Three coronaviruses deriving from two of the three coronavirus phylogenetic divisions were analyzed in detail using cryo-EM and single-particle image analysis techniques: severe acute respiratory syndrome coronavirus (SARS-CoV), feline coronavirus (FCoV), and murine hepatitis virus (MHV). Particles of all three coronaviruses appear largely similar in size, shape, and organization. Regions of electron density include viral proteins, nucleic acid, and the lipid bilayer that forms a double halo around each particle core. Finer details such as the internal RNP-related densities are visible in images recorded nearer true focus, while more strongly defocused images highlight larger and more widely spaced features such as the surface spikes (Fig. 1). To assist in the analysis of particle structure, spike-depleted MHV grown in the presence of tunicamycin (TUN) was imaged and analyzed alongside native virus particles. TUN treatment sharply reduces the spike protein content of the virion by inhibiting glycosylation of newly synthesized S protein (32, 33). Conventional electron micrographs illustrate the difference in surface appearance between native and spike-depleted TUN-treated MHV particles but confirm the similarity of particle size and morphology (Fig. 2).

## VIRION CHARACTERISTICS

Coronavirus particle diameter ranges from approximately 50 to 150 nm in these cryo-EM images. Particle diameters were clustered about means of 82 to 94 nm, with typical standard deviations of 10 to 20 nm. The mean diameters of TUN-grown and native MHV particles did not differ significantly, an indication that the level of S protein incorporation is not an important factor in particle morphogenesis, as previously reported (5, 18, 21, 36). The particle diameter distribution (Fig. 3) appears not to follow a Gaussian "bell curve" distribution, an

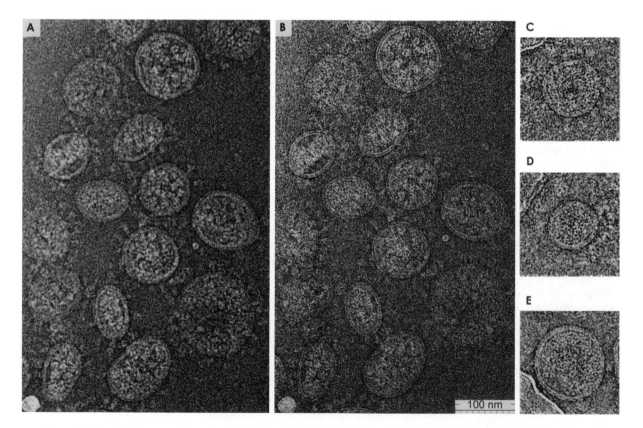

**Figure 1.** Cryo-EM of coronaviruses in vitreous ice. SARS-CoV-Tor2 (A and B), FCoV-Black (C), MHV-OBLV60 (D), and TUN-grown MHV-OBLV60 (E) are shown in "reversed" contrast with density in white. Images were recorded at either ~2.5 μm below true focus (B to E) or ~4.0 μm under focus (A).

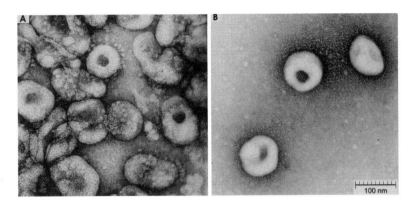

**Figure 2.** Transmission EM comparison of native and spike-depleted coronavirus. Purified MHV-OBLV60 (A) and TUN-grown MHV-OBLV60 (B) were stained with uranyl acetate prior to imaging in order to enhance contrast.

observation that is confirmed by the Kolmogorov-Smirnov test of normality. The teardrop-shaped distribution suggests instead that minimum particle size is constrained, perhaps by the volume of the packaged genome, while maximum particle size shows a greater degree of flexibility.

A radial-density plot reveals stratification within the particle and is often taken as a useful starting point for image analysis. The analysis of coronavirus particles is aided by their relative structural simplicity: only three conserved high-copy-number structural proteins have been described, and each has distinct

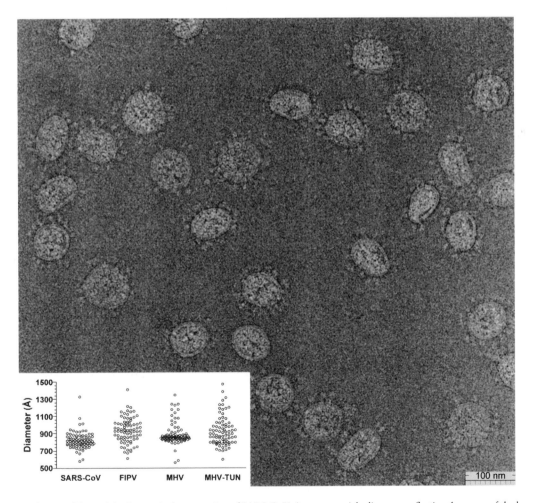

**Figure 3.** Pleomorphic particles in a typical preparation of SARS-CoV. Average particle diameter, reflecting the mean of the longest and shortest particle diameters (inset), was calculated from cryo-EM images. The cryo-EM image shown here depicts SARS-CoV.

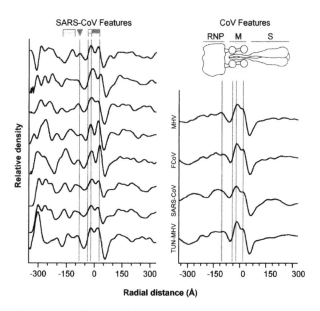

**Figure 4.** Stratification of density near the viral membrane. Rotationally averaged radial-density profiles were generated for ~30° wedges taken from intact coronavirus particles. Wedges from SARS-CoV ($n = 80$), FCoV ($n = 41$), MHV ($n = 53$), and TUN-MHV ($n = 82$) particles were aligned on the minimum density node between the headgroup densities of the lipid bilayer. Radial-density plots demonstrate typical interparticle variability in SARS-CoV (left) and an averaged density from different coronaviruses (right). The schematic at the top interprets densities in the spike, membrane-proximal and M protein, and RNP regions.

biophysical properties that can be used to further assist in identification. The analysis of several related viruses at once is another important factor in attribution of observed cryo-EM features to specific viral proteins; a guiding principle applied throughout the analysis is that common features are most likely achieved through common means. Analysis of the radial distribution of density in coronavirus particles revealed a characteristic signature, with external spikes increasingly visible at higher defocus (as in SARS-CoV images), a thin M protein-related density directly apposed to the lipid bilayer, and a somewhat heterogeneous RNP-related feature distributed in the core region (Fig. 4).

## THE SPIKE IN PROFILE

Crystal structures of peptides from two small regions of the spike, comprising receptor-binding (23) and fusion-motor (11, 13, 19, 34, 35, 38, 39) domains, have been reported. For the time being, EM techniques offer the clearest insight into the structure of the intact spike. Negatively stained EM (Fig. 1) and unstained cryo-EM (Fig. 2 and 3) images show that spike ectodomains extend up to 17 nm (SARS-CoV and MHV) and 19 nm (FCoV) from the outer edge of

the viral membrane. The globular head region of the spike is approximately 10 nm long by 10 nm wide. The distinction between the head and stalk densities is somewhat arbitrary, but careful observation reveals that the difference in spike length appears to reside mainly in the stalk region. If so, this may be explained by the observation that the FCoV S protein fusion motor domain contains two additional heptad repeat units in each predicted amphipathic helix compared to MHV and SARS-CoV S protein, as pointed out by Bosch et al. (4).

Single-particle cryo-EM image analysis techniques provide a more detailed picture of the two-dimensional structure of the spike. In analyzing spike structure, the boundaries of the region being analyzed (also called the "boxed" region) are critical to the quality of the final model. A general tenet of single-particle analysis is that resolution improves as variable regions are removed from the analysis. In the case of coronavirus side views, the positions of adjacent spikes and the curvature of the membrane are variable. As would be expected, images of the coronavirus spike improve as contributions from the variably curved lipid bilayer are minimized. In principle, the results of a boxing analysis can be used to draw conclusions about the degree of connectedness between observed features; regions of the image that can be refined simultaneously can be described as being consistently aligned or "in register." Class averages of the spike are crispest and most consistent when membrane-proximal subjacent RNP densities are included in the alignment (Fig. 5). Edge view class averages from similarly boxed and masked images of particles of TUN-treated MHV show multiple RNP densities with no external spikes. These analyses and results presented elsewhere (29) indicate that the inter-RNP density distribution is relatively consistent, but spikes are in register with the only outermost layer of RNP densities. The existence of a membrane-proximal structural protein complex, likely mediated through S-M, and M-RNP, interactions, is also implicit.

## OLIGOMERIZATION OF S PROTEIN

Coronavirus spikes have been described in the literature as homodimeric or homotrimeric. Some of the discrepancy likely derives from differences in technique and the boundaries of protein constructs used. An estimation of the volume of one spike, based on measurements from side views, can serve as a check on this calculation by relating the observed volume to the average partial specific volume of folded protein (20). Estimates of spike ectodomain volume from cryo-EM images ranged between $4.9 \times 10^2$ and

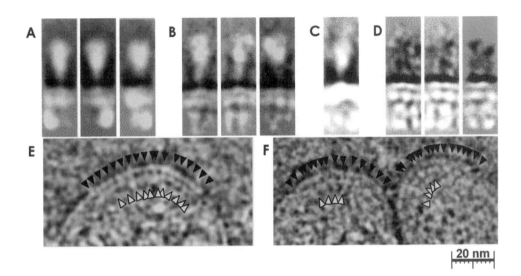

**Figure 5.** Analysis of the structural proteins as seen in edge views. Boxed images centered on the viral membrane below one spike were subjected to iterative reference-free alignment and averaging to produce class average images representative of hundreds to thousands of individual images. Edge view class averages show the ultrastructure of the membrane-associated structural protein complex from SARS-CoV (A), FCoV (B), MHV (C), and spike-depleted TUN-treated MHV (D). Intramembrane densities ascribed to SARS-CoV (E) and TUN-treated MHV (F) M protein are indicated with black arrowheads positioned outside each particle. Connecting densities located between the RNP and membrane regions are indicated with white arrowheads.

$5.9 \times 10^2$ nm$^3$ for SARS-CoV, FCoV, and MHV. Each copy of the SARS-CoV (130 kDa), FCoV (151 kDa), or MHV (137 kDa) S ectodomain is predicted to occupy a partial specific volume of $1.8 \times 10^2$ to $2.1 \times 10^2$ nm$^3$, for a hypothetical volume of $5.4 \times 10^2$ to $6.3 \times 10^2$ nm$^3$ per trimer. The estimated volume of each S ectodomain is therefore most consistent with a homotrimer. For the sake of comparison, the volumes of SARS-CoV, FCoV, MHV, and TUN-treated MHV RNP densities were also estimated. Volumes based on refined cryo-EM images ranged between 53 and 73 nm$^3$ per RNP density. The expected partial specific volume of a single SARS-CoV, FCoV, or MHV N protein is between 51 and 60 nm$^3$. Each RNP density is therefore most likely an RNA protein complex containing one molecule of N protein.

Image analysis techniques provide a second check on the stoichiometry calculation. Principal-component analysis (PCA) provides a method to analyze the distribution of densities represented in several thousand axial images. In PCA, a reference-free alignment is performed, and the "principal components" held in common throughout the data set, termed eigenvectors, are extracted from the set of aligned images (15). Prominent eigenvectors extracted from reference-free alignments of SARS-CoV, FCoV, and MHV axial views feature round $\sim$10-nm spikes, situated $\sim$15 nm apart. Less prominent eigenvectors from these data sets feature closely packed arrays of oblong $\sim$6-nm densities, related to

the RNP. Confirmation of this assignment comes from PCA of axial images of TUN-treated MHV. Axial eigenimages and reconstructed images of TUN-treated MHV show only the RNP lattice (Fig. 6).

PCA also offers an avenue to further refinement. Reconstructing individual axial views using the weighted-contributions spike-related eigenvectors produces relatively clear images showing three-lobed spike densities for SARS-CoV (Fig. 6), and also for FCoV and MHV (data not shown). In contrast, PCA-based reconstruction of images of TUN-treated MHV clarifies only the RNP lattice (Fig. 6). PCA results therefore support a trimeric interpretation of spike stoichiometry. It should be noted that while PCA is a powerful tool, results are dependent on the quality and accuracy of the initial alignment and thus should not be taken as definitive in the absence of strong corroborating evidence. However, the accumulation of molecular and crystallographic data, together with the observations of spike size, volume, and shape provided by conventional EM and cryo-EM, indicates that the metastable, prefusion conformation of the spike is trimeric.

## ARRANGEMENT OF STRUCTURAL PROTEINS

Direct observation, density distribution profiles, image analysis of edge views, and PCA all suggest the presence of some form of a multicomponent structural

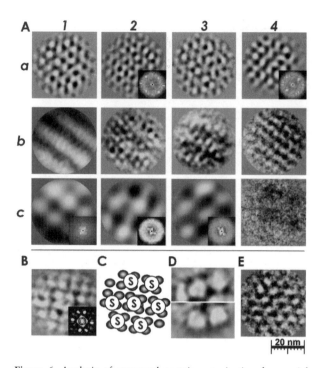

**Figure 6.** Analysis of structural protein organization from axial views. Axial spike images were selected from the central region of each virion. (A) Axial images of SARS-CoV (column *1*), FCoV (column *2*), MHV (column *3*), and TUN-treated MHV (column *4*), were aligned and averaged iteratively until a stable averaged image emerged (row *b*). Axial images were filtered in Fourier space to remove image data greater than (row *a*) or smaller than (row *c*) 9 nm. Filtered axial images were averaged; the averaged image was refined by 10 rounds of iterative alignment and averaging, and then unfiltered images were aligned to the averaged filtered image for a further two cycles to produce the images shown (rows *a* and *c*). Insets show FTs of the corresponding averaged images. The SARS-CoV RNP lattice was used as a reference for iterative alignment and averaging (B). Reflections were selected from the FT of this image (inset) and back-transformed to reveal the overlapping RNP and spike lattices, which are illustrated schematically in panel C. PCA reconstruction was used to clarify spike images from axial views (D). An example eigenimage from PCA of TUN-treated MHV, showing only RNP densities, is presented for comparison (E).

network at the virion surface. A network of M proteins was invoked by de Haan and colleagues to explain how protein-protein interactions might lead to the exclusion of certain host proteins from the viral membrane (10). Cryo-EM image analysis makes it possible to examine the structure of the membrane region directly, using reciprocal space analysis. Fourier transformation (FT) is a mathematical operation that resolves a signal into amplitude and phase components as a function of frequency, interconverting image data between real space and reciprocal space (for a review of single-particle EM techniques including FT, see reference 15). FT is particularly useful in analyzing the degree of periodicity in EM images. For example, intraimage periodicity deriving from the

characteristic minimum spacing between phospholipid headgroup densities in a lipid bilayer becomes readily apparent and quantifiable after FT (Fig. 7).

Consider FTs of images showing only membranes, released viral RNP, intact virions, and background ice, as shown in Fig. 7. Fluctuations in the FT of background ice approximate the shape of the contrast transfer function, which describes the effects of focal distance, particle size, and the optics of the electron microscope on the resulting EM image. The intensity of the signal generated by background ice can be interpreted as an approximation of the distribution of image "noise" in reciprocal space. It is apparent from Fig. 7, for instance, that image data (here, recorded at ~2 μm under focus) converges rapidly below ~30 Å, making interpretation beyond this resolution problematic. It is also apparent that FT amplitude in RNP and virions rises above background at frequencies of 5 to 8 nm$^{-1}$, with a more precipitous feature found only in the virions at a frequency of 15 nm$^{-1}$. FT analysis, and further analysis presented elsewhere (29), suggests that the prominent reciprocal space features arise from intermolecular spacing between adjacent spikes (separated by ~15 nm) and adjacent RNP densities (separated by ~5 to 8 nm).

The characteristic spacing of densities revealed by PCA and corroborated by FT analysis provides a means of discriminating spike and RNP densities in axial views. Reciprocal space filtration with a filtration cutoff falling between the 5- to 8-nm inter-RNP spacing and 15-nm interspike spacing provides a means of examining spike and RNP organization separately. Iterative refinement of filtered images serves to clarify images of the spike and RNP lattices that were revealed previously by PCA. SARS-CoV, FCoV, and MHV spike-related features are refined as round densities, 10 nm in diameter, arranged in an oblique planar lattice with a unit cell of ~14 by 15 nm and an angle of ~100° (Fig. 6). Analysis of an equivalent number of axial images of spike-depleted TUN-treated MHV reveals no such lattice, confirming the assignment to the glycoprotein spikes (Fig. 6). RNP-related features from SARS-CoV, FCoV, MHV, and TUN-treated MHV axial images are refined as arrays of oval, 5- by 6-nm RNP densities arranged in an ~100° oblique lattice with unit cell edges of 6 and 7.5 nm (Fig. 6). Further FT analysis reveals discrete first-order reflections from RNP and spike lattices (Fig. 6, insets). The presence of a signal consisting solely of first-order reflections is consistent with a level of organization in which interparticle spacing is relatively consistent and alignment of fine features is inconsistent. A reconstruction based only on FT reflections shows that each spike density appears to be aligned with four RNP densities in the membrane-proximal lattice,

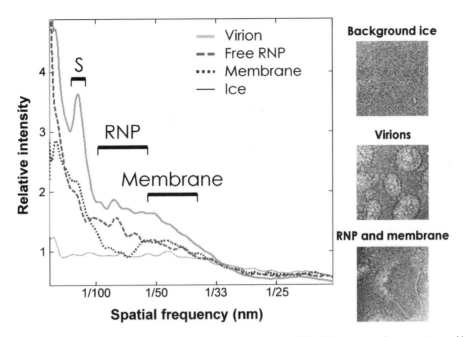

**Figure 7.** FT analysis of SARS-CoV virion components. One hundred entire SARS-CoV virions, adjacent regions of background vitrified ice, phospholipid membranes, and images of released RNP from spontaneously disrupted particles were selected for analysis. Results are presented as reciprocal space power spectra, showing the intensity of the FT as a function of spatial frequency. Prominent features are noted in the $\sim$15-nm$^{-1}$ (spike), $\sim$5- to 8-nm$^{-1}$ (RNP), and $\sim$4- to 6-nm$^{-1}$ (membrane) frequency ranges.

giving a proposed structural module with a stoichiometry of $4N:1S_3$ (Fig. 6).

The analysis of M protein organization has been problematic because of the small size of each M molecule and overlapping signal from the phospholipid headgroups in edge views; however, estimation of M spacing from the virion edge (Fig. 5) indicates that four or five M molecules could fit along an edge of the $4N:1S_3$ module (Fig. 8). Assuming that each intramembrane density represents one M protein, at best estimate the coronavirus surface structural module

would contain 16 to 25 M protein molecules. Closely packed $\sim$1-nm transmembrane M protein densities are readily visible in the membrane region (Fig. 5) but are not clearly resolved in class averages showing spike and RNP densities. Since the location of M relative to the viral envelope is presumably fixed by the presence of three transmembrane segments, it follows that the M-N interaction should constrain some N molecules in the envelope region, as is apparent from radial-density and edge view image analyses. Connecting densities are spaced 5 to 8 nm apart

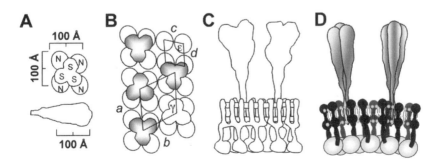

**Figure 8.** Description of the structural module present at the coronavirus membrane. Conserved structural proteins are drawn as they appear in axial views (A and B) and edge views (C and D). Images were either compiled from traced densities in class averages (A and C) or composed according to experimentally determined specifications (B and D). Trimeric spikes (shaded midtones) can be seen projecting outward from the membrane, M proteins (solid black) appear as membrane striations, and oval RNP densities are shown in the form of an interior scaffold (lightly shaded). The dimensions of lattices of S trimers ($a = 14.0$ nm, $b = 15.0$ nm, and $\gamma = 100°$) and RNP molecules ($c = 6.0$ nm, $d = 7.5$ nm, and $\varepsilon = 100°$) were determined from the reflections shown in Fig. 6B and were consistent with real-space measurements of the same parameters. All components are drawn to the scale shown in panel A.

(Fig. 5) and may represent interacting M protein and RNP. While the observation of spike and N protein lattices, connected by mutual interaction with M, supports the hypothesis that M protein is organized to a similar extent, investigation of the precise arrangement of M protein in the virion remains a subject for future work.

## OVERALL VIRION ARCHITECTURE

The preceding analyses describe the organization within and among the structural modules that populate the virion surface. However, they do not directly address the nature of the "global" virion structure. One analysis that is particularly informative in this respect is a scatterplot relating virion diameter and ellipticity, which is defined for these purposes as the percent difference between the longest and shortest axes in a virion image. Keeping in mind that an ellipsoid can appear circular when viewed end-on, but a spherical particle appears circular from all angles, it can be presumed that observed ellipticity in a two-dimensional cryo-EM image underestimates the actual ellipticity of the imaged particles. As shown in Fig. 9, a plot of diameter versus ellipticity for 500 coronavirus particles yields a scattered cloud of data points. This distribution confirms that frozen hydrated coronaviruses are pleomorphic.

Occasionally, membrane-enclosed vesicles lacking any visible spikes or RNP content are found alongside coronaviruses in cryo-EM images, likely through incidental copurification. It is thus possible to analyze the distribution of size and ellipticity across non-RNP-containing particles, spikeless (TUN-treated MHV) particles, and normal CoV particles and form conclusions as to the role of a particular feature in particle morphology. Morphologically typical coronaviruses have an average ellipticity approaching 20% and a range of 0% to more than 70% ellipticity. TUN-treated MHV particles are similar, with 25% ellipticity on average. The structure of empty vesicles should be shaped primarily by fluid forces and should reflect the natural state of a phospholipid bilayer of a particular size in solution. Empty vesicles that fall within the size range observed for coronavirus particles, between 50 and 150 nm in diameter, appear no more than 6% elliptical on average, ranging from 0 to 15% ellipticity. Therefore, while a lack of spikes correlates with a slight increase in ellipticity, a lack of RNP renders a particle almost completely spherical. Another piece of data that should be considered is the structure of the RNP itself. RNP has been reported to form a sphere (14, 31) that can dissociate to more chaotic states that may include a roughly helical form (8, 14, 26). Cryo-EM images of spontaneously released RNP also show mostly chaotic forms, as exemplified in Fig. 7. In the absence of other viral proteins, RNP appears to lack a characteristic global form, as reported by Escors et al. (14). These observations do not indicate an apparent mechanism by which the RNP would, on its own, elliptically distort coronavirus particles. Global virion structure is primarily imparted through the interaction of membrane-embedded structural M protein with RNP, the same set of interactions that produces the structural module extending from the spike, through the viral membrane, to the outermost RNP shell. Observed macromolecular structures for bona fide two-dimensional protein lattices, as formed by retroviral matrix proteins, for example, include planar sheets and tubes of variable dimensions (reference 17 and references therein). Coronaviruses morphology is consistent with that of a nonrigid two-dimensional lattice incorporating distortions particularly at the tips of the ellipsoidal virion. Further research may provide structural and compositional explanations for curvature at the tips. Particularly, the distribution of minor structural proteins, such as the budding factor E, may be quite interesting with respect to the global architecture of the virion.

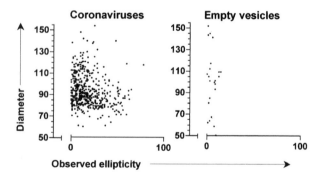

**Figure 9.** Scatterplot relating diameter and size for coronavirus particles and empty vesicles. Shown are results for combined SARS-CoV, FCoV, and MHV particles (left; $n = 500$ total) and, for comparison, vesicles of similar size that were present in coronavirus cryo-EM images but that lacked any visible RNP or spike content (right; $n = 23$). Diameter refers to the mean diameter for oblong particles, and ellipticity refers to the difference between maximum and minimum observed diameters, expressed as a percentage of the maximum diameter.

## MODULAR ARCHITECTURE IN THE VIRAL WORLD

In light of the present description of coronavirus ultrastructure, a modified scheme can be proposed for classification of viral architecture. Some viruses exhibit an integrated design in which precise positioning of a defined number of components is essential to the functionality and structural integrity of the particle. Examples of integrated architecture include tailed bacteriophages and both encapsidated and enveloped icosahedral particles. Viruses in the second structural class are organized along modular principles, in which the assembly nucleation event is followed by serial addition of a potentially variable number of structurally equivalent units. In addition to filamentous viruses, exemplars of modular architecture would also include viruses previously classified as pleomorphic that appear to be composed of structural modules. Emerging data indicate that coronaviruses may share a modular architectural design with members of the *Poxviridae* (7, 12), *Paramyxoviridae* (1), *Arenaviridae* (28), and, possibly, *Retroviridae* (16, 27, 40). The significance of the proposed new high-level structural classification is that the terms "integrated" and "modular" are related to similarities of construction, as opposed to differences in ultimate form. As in the world of architecture, modular virion architecture implies a degree of interchangeability at the point of construction that will require further experimental validation. The observation that overlapping lattices of RNP and S protein complexes are present at the viral membrane strongly suggests that two-dimensional structural protein lattices are present at the site of budding, either as an intermediate step or perhaps as a necessary by-product of the coronavirus assembly process. Investigation of the pathways leading to membrane-proximal protein organization may be essential in understanding not only coronavirus assembly but also the assembly processes of modular viruses in general.

**Acknowledgments.** I thank Michael Buchmeier for essential guidance and support in this endeavor and Mark Yeager and Brian Adair for computational and technical assistance.

Funding for this work was provided by the NIH/NIAID contract "Functional and Structural Proteomics of SARS Coronavirus" (HHSN266200400058C) and by the Pacific-Southwest Regional Center of Excellence (AI-065359). Some of the work presented here was conducted at the National Resource for Automated Molecular Microscopy, which is supported by the National Institutes of Health though the National Center for Research Resources' P41 program (RR17573).

## REFERENCES

1. Bächi, T. 1980. Intramembrane structural differentiation in Sendai virus maturation. *Virology* **106**:41–49.
2. Beards, G. M., D. W. Brown, J. Green, and T. H. Flewett. 1986. Preliminary characterisation of torovirus-like particles of humans: comparison with Berne virus of horses and Breda virus of calves. *J. Med. Virol.* **20**:67–78.
3. Beniac, D. R., A. Andonov, E. Grudeski, and T. F. Booth. 2006. Architecture of the SARS coronavirus prefusion spike. *Nat. Struct. Mol. Biol.* **13**:751–752.
4. Bosch, B. J., R. van der Zee, C. A. de Haan, and P. J. Rottier. 2003. The coronavirus spike protein is a class I virus fusion protein: structural and functional characterization of the fusion core complex. *J. Virol.* **77**:8801–8811.
5. Corse, E., and C. E. Machamer. 2003. The cytoplasmic tails of infectious bronchitis virus E and M proteins mediate their interaction. *Virology* **312**:25–34.
6. Cowley, J. A., C. M. Dimmock, K. M. Spann, and P. J. Walker. 2000. Gill-associated virus of Penaeus monodon prawns: an invertebrate virus with ORF1a and ORF1b genes related to arteri- and coronaviruses. *J. Gen. Virol.* **81**:1473–1484.
7. Cyrklaff, M., C. Risco, J. J. Fernández, M. V. Jiménez, M. Estéban, W. Baumeister, and J. L. Carrascosa. 2005. Cryo-electron tomography of vaccinia virus. *Proc. Natl. Acad. Sci. USA* **102**:2772–2777.
8. Davies, H. A., R. R. Dourmashkin, and M. R. Macnaughton. 1981. Ribonucleoprotein of avian infectious bronchitis virus. *J. Gen. Virol.* **53**:67–74.
9. Davies, H. A., and M. R. Macnaughton. 1979. Comparison of the morphology of three coronaviruses. *Arch. Virol.* **59**:25–33.
10. de Haan, C. A., H. Vennema, and P. J. Rottier. 2000. Assembly of the coronavirus envelope: homotypic interactions between the M proteins. *J. Virol.* **74**:4967–4978.
11. Deng, Y., J. Liu, Q. Zheng, W. Yong, and M. Lu. 2006. Structures and polymorphic interactions of two heptad-repeat regions of the SARS virus S2 protein. *Structure* **14**:889–899.
12. Dubochet, J., M. Adrian, K. Richter, J. Garces, and R. Wittek. 1994. Structure of intracellular mature vaccinia virus observed by cryoelectron microscopy. *J. Virol.* **68**:1935–1941.
13. Duquerroy, S., A. Vigouroux, P. J. Rottier, F. A. Rey, and B. J. Bosch. 2005. Central ions and lateral asparagine/glutamine zippers stabilize the post-fusion hairpin conformation of the SARS coronavirus spike glycoprotein. *Virology* **335**:276–285.
14. Escors, D., J. Ortego, H. Laude, and L. Enjuanes. 2001. The membrane M protein carboxy terminus binds to transmissible gastroenteritis coronavirus core and contributes to core stability. *J. Virol.* **75**:1312–1324.
15. Frank, J. 1990. Classification of macromolecular assemblies studied as 'single particles.' *Q. Rev. Biophys.* **23**:281–329.
16. Fuller, S. D., T. Wilk, B. E. Gowen, H. G. Krausslich, and V. M. Vogt. 1997. Cryo-electron microscopy reveals ordered domains in the immature HIV-1 particle. *Curr. Biol.* **7**:729–738.
17. Ganser, B. K., A. Cheng, W. I. Sundquist, and M. Yeager. 2003. Three-dimensional structure of the M-MuLV CA protein on a lipid monolayer: a general model for retroviral capsid assembly. *EMBO J.* **22**:2886–2892.
18. Godeke, G. J., C. A. de Haan, J. W. Rossen, H. Vennema, and P. J. Rottier. 2000. Assembly of spikes into coronavirus particles is mediated by the carboxy-terminal domain of the spike protein. *J. Virol.* **74**:1566–1571.
19. Hakansson-McReynolds, S., S. Jiang, L. Rong, and M. Caffrey. 2006. Solution structure of the severe acute respiratory syndrome-coronavirus heptad repeat 2 domain in the prefusion state. *J. Biol. Chem.* **281**:11965–11971.
20. Harpaz, Y., M. Gerstein, and C. Chothia. 1994. Volume changes on protein folding. *Structure* **2**:641–649.
21. Ho, Y., P. H. Lin, C. Y. Liu, S. P. Lee, and Y. C. Chao. 2004. Assembly of human severe acute respiratory syndrome coronavirus-like particles. *Biochem. Biophys. Res. Commun.* **318**:833–838.
22. Hoet, A. E., and L. J. Saif. 2004. Bovine torovirus (Breda virus) revisited. *Anim. Health Res. Rev.* **5**:157–171.
23. Li, F., W. Li, M. Farzan, and S. C. Harrison. 2005. Structure of SARS coronavirus spike receptor-binding domain complexed with receptor. *Science* **309**:1864–1868.

24. Lin, S., C. K. Lee, S. Y. Lee, C. L. Kao, C. W. Lin, A. B. Wang, S. M. Hsu, and L. S. Huang. 2005. Surface ultrastructure of SARS coronavirus revealed by atomic force microscopy. *Cell. Microbiol.* **7:**1763–1770.

25. Lin, Y., X. Yan, W. Cao, C. Wang, J. Feng, J. Duan, and S. Xie. 2004. Probing the structure of the SARS coronavirus using scanning electron microscopy. *Antivir. Ther.* **9:**287–289.

26. Macnaughton, M. R., H. A. Davies, and M. V. Nermut. 1978. Ribonucleoprotein-like structures from coronavirus particles. *J. Gen. Virol.* **39:**545–549.

27. Nermut, M. V., C. Grief, S. Hashmi, and D. J. Hockley. 1993. Further evidence of icosahedral symmetry in human and simian immunodeficiency virus. *AIDS Res. Hum. Retrovir.* **9:**929–938.

28. Neuman, B. W., B. D. Adair, J. W. Burns, R. A. Milligan, M. J. Buchmeier, and M. Yeager. 2005. Complementarity in the supramolecular design of arenaviruses and retroviruses revealed by electron cryomicroscopy and image analysis. *J. Virol.* **79:**3822–3830.

29. Neuman, B. W., B. D. Adair, C. Yoshioka, J. D. Quispe, G. Orca, P. Kuhn, R. A. Milligan, M. Yeager, and M. J. Buchmeier. 2006. Supramolecular architecture of severe acute respiratory syndrome coronavirus revealed by electron cryomicroscopy. *J. Virol.* **80:**7918–7928.

30. Ng, M. L., J. W. Lee, M. L. Leong, A. E. Ling, H. C. Tan, and E. E. Ooi. 2004. Topographic changes in SARS coronavirus-infected cells at late stages of infection. *Emerg. Infect. Dis.* **10:**1907–1914.

31. Risco, C., I. M. Anton, L. Enjuanes, and J. L. Carrascosa. 1996. The transmissible gastroenteritis coronavirus contains a spherical core shell consisting of M and N proteins. *J. Virol.* **70:**4773–4777.

32. Rossen, J. W., R. de Beer, G. J. Godeke, M. J. Raamsman, M. C. Horzinek, H. Vennema, and P. J. Rottier. 1998. The viral spike protein is not involved in the polarized sorting of coronaviruses in epithelial cells. *J. Virol.* **72:**497–503.

33. Rottier, P. J., M. C. Horzinek, and B. A. van der Zeijst. 1981. Viral protein synthesis in mouse hepatitis virus strain A59-infected cells: effect of tunicamycin. *J. Virol.* **40:**350–357.

34. Supekar, V. M., C. Bruckmann, P. Ingallinella, E. Bianchi, A. Pessi, and A. Carfi. 2004. Structure of a proteolytically resistant core from the severe acute respiratory syndrome coronavirus S2 fusion protein. *Proc. Natl. Acad. Sci. USA* **101:**17958–17963.

35. Tripet, B., M. W. Howard, M. Jobling, R. K. Holmes, K. V. Holmes, and R. S. Hodges. 2004. Structural characterization of the SARS-coronavirus spike S fusion protein core. *J. Biol. Chem.* **279:**20836–20849.

36. Vennema, H., G. J. Godeke, J. W. Rossen, W. F. Voorhout, M. C. Horzinek, D. J. Opstelten, and P. J. Rottier. 1996. Nucleocapsid-independent assembly of coronavirus-like particles by co-expression of viral envelope protein genes. *EMBO J.* **15:**2020–2028.

37. Wieringa, R., A. A. de Vries, J. van der Meulen, G. J. Godeke, J. J. Onderwater, H. van Tol, H. K. Koerten, A. M. Mommaas, E. J. Snijder, and P. J. Rottier. 2004. Structural protein requirements in equine arteritis virus assembly. *J. Virol.* **78:**13019–13027.

38. Xu, Y., Y. Liu, Z. Lou, L. Qin, X. Li, Z. Bai, H. Pang, P. Tien, G. F. Gao, and Z. Rao. 2004. Structural basis for coronavirus-mediated membrane fusion. Crystal structure of mouse hepatitis virus spike protein fusion core. *J. Biol. Chem.* **279:**30514–30522.

39. Xu, Y., Z. Lou, Y. Liu, H. Pang, P. Tien, G. F. Gao, and Z. Rao. 2004. Crystal structure of severe acute respiratory syndrome coronavirus spike protein fusion core. *J. Biol. Chem.* **279:**49414–49419.

40. Yeager, M., E. M. Wilson-Kubalek, S. G. Weiner, P. O. Brown, and A. Rein. 1998. Supramolecular organization of immature and mature murine leukemia virus revealed by electron cryomicroscopy: implications for retroviral assembly mechanisms. *Proc. Natl. Acad. Sci. USA* **95:**7299–7304.

*Nidoviruses*
Edited by S. Perlman, T. Gallagher, and E. J. Snijder
© 2008 ASM Press, Washington, DC

Chapter 14

# Arterivirus Structural Proteins and Assembly

### Kay S. Faaberg

This chapter reviews the structural characteristics of the *Arteriviridae,* including the basic molecular details of all of the proteins involved, the interactions of these proteins and where they occur, and further functional characterization. Most recent available literature has been focused on equine arteritis virus (EAV) and porcine reproductive and respiratory syndrome virus (PRRSV), and thus this review concentrates primarily on these viruses. However, early studies on murine lactate dehydrogenase-elevating virus (LDV) and simian hemorrhagic fever virus (SHFV) were often critical to understanding the later work, particularly in the subject of viral attachment, and thus are prominently mentioned when appropriate. Space limitations prevented any discussion of the clinical diseases caused by arteriviruses, the immense evolutionary variation that exists, and, except, briefly, the immune response to these proteins. Lastly, a current model of virus propagation is displayed.

## BIOSYNTHESIS OF ARTERIVIRUS STRUCTURAL PROTEINS

The structural proteins of arteriviruses are expressed through a nested set of subgenomic mRNAs (sg mRNAs) that each include the genome 5′ leader sequence, a portion of untranslated nucleotides followed by one or more open reading frames (ORFs), the 3′ noncoding sequence, and a poly(A) tail. The virus-specific sg mRNAs are listed in Table 1 along with their respective length, the body transcription-regulating sequence (TRS) utilized in their biosynthesis, and the nucleotide distance between the TRS and the first AUG of the mRNA (17, 32, 54, 93, 107, 169). Each arteriviral sg mRNA has its own

individual length, TRS, and distance to the first AUG, suggesting an extensive time frame of evolution from a putative common ancestor. Meaningful nucleotide alignment of the structural region of all arteriviruses is not easily produced, as SHFV is proposed to contain a duplication of its ORF2a to ORF3 acquired by recombination during arteriviral evolution (54). The structural region architecture reveals how similar the various arteriviruses are to each other (Fig. 1). Discounting SHFV, each arterivirus contains the same number of structural proteins. In addition, the ORFs are also in the same relative position, with the exception of the ORF for the envelope protein (E protein), which appears first in sg mRNA2 for EAV, LDV (ORF2a/E), and SHFV (ORF4a/E) and second in sg mRNA2 for PRRSV-EU (genotype 1) and PRRSV-NA (genotype 2). However, the individual ORF lengths vary among viruses. Nearly all ORFs overlap with another, and there is no consistency as to which reading frame a particular ORF occupies with respect to the initial gene of the structural region (Fig. 1).

This relatively simplistic view does not include the sg mRNAs produced from atypical TRSs, which are present in most arteriviruses. In EAV, investigators found four different species of sg mRNA3 and two species for sg mRNA4 and -5 (32, 112). An alternate species for sg mRNA3 was also detected in infected cells of a PRRSV-NA (type 2) strain, ISU79 (90). For type 2 strain VR-2332 sg mRNA4 and -7, two genomic TRSs were identified. In addition, another sg mRNA (5-1) utilized a site downstream of the starting AUG for ORF5, and it appears to encode a truncated protein utilizing the second ORF5 methionine (107). One additional PRRSV sg mRNA7 was found in cells infected with a Taiwanese type 2 strain (82). With cells infected with PRRSV type 2 strains VR-2332, Ingelvac PRRS

Kay S. Faaberg • Department of Veterinary and Biomedical Sciences, College of Veterinary Medicine, University of Minnesota, St. Paul, MN 55108.

Table 1. sg mRNAs utilized to produce structural proteins[a]

| mRNA | Virus | Length (bases) | Body TRS | Distance to first AUG (nt[b]) |
|------|-------|----------------|----------|-------------------------------|
| 2/2a | EAV | 3,200 | UCAACU | 34 |
|      | LDV | 3,335 | UAUACC | 80 |
|      | PRRSV-EU | 3,562 | UAAACC | 38 |
|      | PRRSV-NA | 3,548 | UGAACC | 20 |
|      | SHFV | 5,049 | UUAACU | 87 |
| 3/2b | EAV | 2,716 | UCAAUA | 105 |
|      | LDV | 2,718 | GUAACC | 74 |
|      | PRRSV-EU | 2,927 | UUGACC | 11 |
|      | PRRSV-NA | 2,988 | GUAACC | 83 |
|      | SHFV | 5,049 | UUAACU | 620 |
| 4/3  | EAV | 2,251 | UCAACU | 34 |
|      | LDV | 2,232 | GUAACC | 35 |
|      | PRRSV-EU | 2,457 | UCAACC | 83 |
|      | PRRSV-NA | 2,364 | UUCACC | 4 |
|      | SHFV | 4,032 | UUCACC | 55 |
| 5/7  | EAV | 1,883 | UCAACU | 112 |
|      | LDV | 1,699 | AUAACC | 26 |
|      | PRRSV-EU | 1,858 | ACAACC | 32 |
|      | PRRSV-NA | 1,853 | UUAGCC | 40 |
|      | SHFV | 1,921 | UUAACU | 8 |
| 6/8  | EAV | 1,041 | UCAACC | 25 |
|      | LDV | 1,100 | AAAACC | 14 |
|      | PRRSV-EU | 1,257 | UCAACC | 24 |
|      | PRRSV-NA | 1,243 | AUAACC | 17 |
|      | SHFV | 1,210 | UCAACC | 127 |
| 7/9  | EAV | 659 | UCAACU | 55 |
|      | LDV | 719 | UAACCA | 135 |
|      | PRRSV-EU | 731 | UUAACC | 9 |
|      | PRRSV-NA | 835 | UUAACC | 123 |
|      | SHFV | 629 | UUAACC | 9 |

[a]Only major and SHFV-specific mRNAs are listed. Body TRSs were based upon the primary data but sometimes were modified to account for nucleotide sequences not available when originally published. sg mRNA base lengths do not include a poly(A) tail. Full-length sequences used in the analyses include EAV (NC_002532), LDV (U15146), PRRSV-EU (M96262), PRRSV-NA (U87392) and SHFV (NC_003092).
[b]nt, nucleotides.

MLV, and PrimePac MLV as well as packaged virus, researchers also identified constitutive expression of atypical sg mRNAs (heteroclites) with aberrant TRSs that could code for proteins expressing fusions of part of ORF1 linked to parts of different structural proteins (166, 167). These data provide evidence that the TRSs utilized by arteriviruses are more heterogeneous than is commonly described, adding questions about the preciseness of the mechanism by which the abundant structural proteins are expressed. TRS mutation studies with EAV suggest that the degree of nucleotide sequence homology between the leader and body TRSs does not completely correlate with the abundance of the individual sg mRNAs. The RNA secondary structures of the different body TRSs and/or flanking sequences also determine the translational activity of the sg mRNAs (112). However, manipulation of the leader-body junction sites in EAV also correlated with the amount of expression of the structural proteins needed for producing competent nascent virus (112).

Only the 3′-terminal sg mRNA, encoding the nucleocapsid protein (N protein), is structurally monocistronic. It has been suggested that most other sg mRNAs are essentially monocistronic, expressing only the first encoded ORF, but the fact that sg mRNA2 encodes at least two important viral proteins implies that this concept has not been fully investigated.

In in vitro translation studies with PRRSV-NA strain VR-2332, abundant protein expression of ORF2, ORF5, and ORF7 was dependent on the respective entire sg mRNA. Deletion of the poly(A) tract or the 5′ or 3′ untranslated region reduced the amount of protein produced as much as 50-fold. It thus appears as if the sg mRNAs have inherent secondary or tertiary structures that also determine the quantity of the protein produced, not just the amount of mRNA produced for the individual ORFs. Whether other viral or cellular components are also necessary for translation has not yet been evaluated (46, 99; unpublished results).

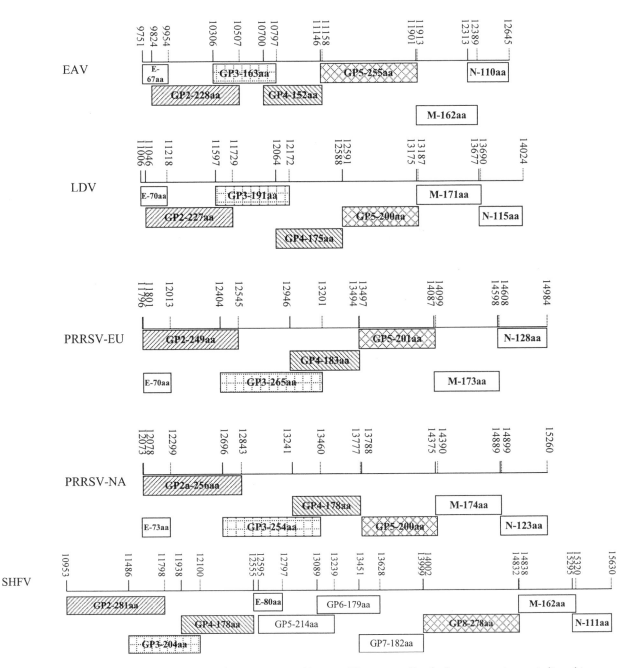

**Figure 1.** Schematic of arterivirus structural protein gene architecture. The genes coding for known proteins are indicated in the respective reading frame, with the nucleotide start site indicated by a vertical solid line and the stop codon indicated by a dotted line. Identified components of mature viruses are identified by boldface type, and main structural glycoproteins are further indicated by hatched boxes. Publications used for analysis were as follows: for EAV, reference 32; for SHFV, references 54 and 169; for LDV, reference 17; for PRRSV-EU, reference 93; and for PRRSV-NA, reference 107. aa, amino acids.

## ARTERIVIRUS STRUCTURAL PROTEINS

### E Protein

All arteriviruses have a small ORF protein encoded in sg mRNA2 (130). In EAV as well as in LDV, this small ORF protein is encoded upstream of glycoprotein 2 (GP2) and is not N glycosylated. The SHFV homolog of this protein is found in potentially bicistronic sg mRNA4, thought to arise from gene duplication (54, 130). However, in both PRRSV type 1 and type 2, the starting AUG placement for the ORF is 6 nucleotides downstream of the GP2 initiation codon. In all arteriviruses, this small E protein (67 to 80 amino acids, 7.3 to 8.7 kDa, pI of 7.0 to 9.7) is predicted by structural-algorithm programs to encode an N-myristoylation site followed by a casein kinase II phosphorylation site, a central hydrophobic domain, and a region of basic amino acid residues in its hydrophilic C-terminal domain (130). In addition, the cysteine residues seen in all arterivirus E proteins appear not to be covalently linked in any intra- or intermolecular disulfide bonds (79, 130), but studies with PRRSV-NA strain SDSU-23983 suggest a noncovalent association with the N protein (161). Although the protein is quite conserved between the two genotypes of PRRSV, little sequence identity exists among the other arteriviruses. However, an amino acid alignment reveals that many residues represent conserved or semiconserved mutations, illustrating the importance of retention of protein structure. The E protein is situated in the cellular and viral membranes of EAV (130) and type 1 and type 2 PRRSV (154, 160, 161). Fluorescence assays with PRRSV 2b/E fused to an enhanced green fluorescent protein (EGFP) tag revealed that the protein was localized to the perinuclear region in transfected cells (160). Further work using reverse genetics has shown that E protein is essential for EAV and PRRSV-EU infectivity (130, 152, 154). A study of LDV ORF2S (E protein), however, did not reveal a significant quantity of the molecule in virions, but it also did not rule out a role for the protein in virion morphogenesis (116). An essential membrane protein, also named E, exists in the *Coronaviridae*, yet the coronavirus envelope structure differs greatly from that in the *Arteriviridae* (28, 116, 127).

The E protein most likely presents with an uncleaved signal anchor sequence in the central part of the molecule. Two predictions of E protein conformation in the membrane have been proposed. If the small acidic N terminus is translocated to the cytosol and the C-terminal basic residues remain on the cytoplasmic side of the membrane (144), a type III orientation is predicted (131). However, if the E protein spans the membrane twice, both termini would be located at the cytoplasmic face (Fig. 2) (130). Snijder and coinvestigators could not

rule out multiple transmembrane configurations for the E protein of EAV.

## Glycoprotein 2

The identification of GP2 (25.5 to 31.8 kDa and pI of 8.7 to 10.2 [unprocessed]) as a structural protein of an arterivirus was first demonstrated in EAV studies (35). These early studies involved expression of ORFs identified within nucleotide sequences, and by immunoidentification these investigators identified an N-glycosylated Gs (now GP2) that was abundant in infected cells but only a very minor component of virions. They also revealed by endoglycosidase digestion that the single N-linked glycan of GP2 becomes sialylated during transport of the virus particles through the secretory pathway. Shortly afterwards, the generation of LDV and PRRSV-EU nucleotide sequences led to the suggestion that these arteriviruses also contained similar N-glycosylated proteins (24, 53). However, work describing the placement of VP-3M of LDV (now GP2) as a structural component of virions was not completed for 2 more years (48). The investigators also showed, using in vitro transcription and translation experiments with and without canine pancreatic microsomal membranes followed by enzyme digestions, that VP-3M is predicted to be a standard class I glycoprotein with a single C-terminal membrane anchor segment and that its signal peptide is removed during membrane-associated synthesis (Fig. 2). Later studies on PRRSV type 1 strain LV (94) and PRRSV type 2 strain SDSU-23983 (160) established that GP2 is a minor component of virions. Although SHFV was predicted to encode an N-glycosylated protein in sg mRNA2, no biochemical work has been documented (53). Aligned by the Lipman-Pearson method (83) (default parameters), the EU and NA genotypes of PRRSV share 62.1% amino acid similarity and LDV shares approximately 33 to 39% amino acid identity with the two PRRSV types. EAV and SHFV share very little homology with the other three arteriviruses or with each other.

All three N-glycosylation sites of LDV GP2 are modified by oligosaccharides to an approximate molecular mass of 35 to 40 kDa (48), as well as both sites of PRRSV type 1 strain LV, which has a molecular mass of 29 to 30 kDa (94). In PRRSV-EU, GP2 was recognized by ORF2-specific antipeptide serum from infected CL2621 cell lysates and extracellular virus. A fraction of the GP2 protein contains an intrachain disulfide bond in infected-cell lysates, but no disulfide-linked oligomers of GP2 are easily detected in purified virus. Furthermore, the endoglycosidase H-sensitive N-glycans of PRRSV-EU GP2 become

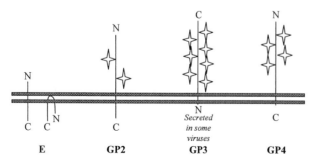

**Figure 2.** Predicted conformations of the E protein and GP2, GP3, and GP4 in eukaryotic membranes.

endoglycosidase H resistant during passage through the Golgi compartment, indicating that GP2 acquired complex N-glycans (94). But N-linked glycans normally present on GP2 are apparently not essential for particle formation or for viral infectivity (153). The original study also found that GP2 expressed individually in a recombinant Semliki Forest virus is trapped in the endoplasmic reticulum (ER), indicating that other viral factors are needed to derive mature GP2 (94). Later studies, using a series of mutant infectious clones of PRRSV-EU strain LV that individually knocked out expression of individual structural proteins, confirmed that the PRRSV-EU minor glycoproteins GP2, GP3, and GP4, and probably the E protein, interact with each other in order to be transported through the Golgi compartment (154).

In work with EAV, researchers first used traditional methods of biochemistry to establish the interactions of GP2, GP3, and GP4 (151). When purified virions were isolated and subjected to immunoprecipitation in the presence of specific antisera and then analyzed by sodium dodecyl sulfate-polyacrylamide gel electrophoresis (SDS-PAGE) under reducing or nonreducing conditions, it became clear that GP2 (25 kDa) was present as a disulfide-bonded heterotrimer (not the homodimer originally proposed [35]) with GP3 and GP4 in a 1:1:1 ratio, as well as in another disulfide-bonded complex of equimolar ratios of GP2 and GP4. They went on to establish that this heterodimer was loosely associated with GP3. The GP2 cysteine residues involved in these interactions were also localized (149). In addition, the investigators showed through pulse-chase experiments that only the heterodimeric complex of GP2 and GP4 was seen in EAV-infected cells. Following the gradual diminishment of the heterodimeric complex and concomitant increase of the heterotrimeric complex over time as virions were produced, they were able to establish that shortly after EAV particles are released from infected cells, they contain mainly disulfide-bonded GP2/GP4 heterodimers that are then converted into cysteine-linked GP2b/GP3/GP4 heterotrimers (149).

Even though it has been firmly established that GP2 is an essential component of infectious arterivirions, antibodies to GP2 appear to be nonneutralizing, no function has been described for this protein, and it has no apparent homology with any other viral or cellular component. Since it is conserved throughout the *Arteriviridae* and has been documented biochemically to be an essential minor glycoprotein for productive infection of different cultured cells as well as host-derived macrophages, the function may be involved with proper transport of the viral membrane components through infected cells, primary or

secondary identification of proper hosts, as a decoy antigen to target the immune response away from the primary viral attachment protein, or some other undescribed function. In PRRSV particularly, investigators have shown that GP2 is subject to evolutionary pressure and most probably immune selection based on the number of unique GP2 nucleotide sequences (60 to 100% amino acid similarity to GP2 of VR-2332) derived from all over the world (first noted in references 71 and 91).

## Glycoprotein 3

GP3 (18.0 to 30.5 kDa and pI of 5.0 to 9.2 [unprocessed]), originally identified by nucleotide sequence homologies as mentioned for GP2, varies greatly in arteriviruses, even between the two genotypes of PRRSV. However, an amino acid alignment reveals that there are several conserved cysteines and putative N-glycan addition sites among the five representative strains. The first demonstration that GP3 was expressed in PRRSV-EU strain LV used antipeptide sera to first identify in vitro translation products of the same LV ORF, followed by a positive immunoperoxidase monolayer assay of LV-infected alveolar lung macrophages (95). Confirmation of the structural nature of GP3 was completed through the use of monoclonal antibodies (MAbs). Western blot analyses using two MAbs, purified virions, and glycosidase digestion clearly established the structural nature of GP3 in PRRSV-EU strain LV and identified the processed protein as a molecule that migrated in an SDS-PAGE gel as a diffuse band of 45 to 50 kDa that was modified by complex N-glycans, indicating that GP3 had been processed through the Golgi compartment (140). Two other investigators also found evidence of GP3 in purified PRRSV-EU of a different strain by biochemical means (41, 146). As mentioned above, later studies concluded that the heterotrimeric nature of PRRSV-EU GP2, GP3, and GP4 was necessary for fully glycosylating all of the molecules (154). The next arterivirus to be analyzed for its GP3 characteristics was LDV-P (49). An established host cell line is not available for this virus, so the investigators utilized in vitro translation in the presence and absence of canine microsomal membranes, incubation in different buffer systems, and further centrifugation to establish the fact that ORF3 encodes a highly glycosylated (∼31 kDa; core glycosylated at all six N-glycan sites) and soluble protein when expressed individually. Furthermore, the size of GP3 after removal of the sugar residues suggested that the putative signal sequence was not cleaved after transport through the artificial membranes, most likely because of rapid core N glycosylation close to the site of cleavage. This proposed N glycosylation of the signal peptide may also have prevented its reinsertion into the membrane to form a class II integral membrane protein (Fig. 2) (142, 143). LDV-specific antisera recognized the product of ORF3 in in vitro translation, signifying its presence in infected mouse macrophages, but an anti-ORF3 MAb could not identify a ≥31-kDa protein in purified virions (49). Studies with PRRSV-NA strain IAF-KLOP suggested that GP3 appeared not to be a structural glycoprotein, but a portion of it was soluble and could be found in the supernatant of infected cells (58, 87). Initial studies expressed ORF3 as a fusion protein in replication-defective recombinant adenovirus to raise monospecific antiserum, which identified a highly N-glycosylated 42-kDa GP3 in infected-cell extracts in amounts equivalent to those of GP5, N protein, and M protein but not in purified virions (58). Further pulse-chase experiments, either in the context of PRRSV infection or upon individual GP3 expression, showed that the protein remained completely sensitive to endo-β-$N$-acetylglucosaminidase H (endo-H) and was thus restricted to the premedial Golgi compartment, in contrast to PRRSV-EU (87). Surprisingly, they also discovered a minor fraction (∼10%) in the culture medium, membrane free, both from individually expressed GP3 in the context of adenovirus and from authentic PRRSV-NA IAF-KLOP infection, which they named sGP3. sGP3 acquired Golgi-specific complex carbohydrate side chains and was found as a disulfide-linked homodimer of 97 kDa. Brefeldin A treatment, which collapses the Golgi compartment into the ER, completely abolished cellular secretion of sGP3 (87). Thus, GP3 appears to be differentially expressed between the two genotypes of PRRSV. EAV studies, similar to the in vitro translation studies on LDV ORF3, showed that in the presence of canine pancreatic microsomal membranes, a 36- to 42-kDa protein was produced, again purporting that all six available N-glycan sites (in the ATCC strain of EAV) were modified by sugar residues (62). In addition, the EAV GP3 proposed signal peptide was not cleaved, as the protein produced in the presence of membranes, once deglycosylated, was the same size as the protein produced in the absence of membranes and remained membrane bound after incubation in vesicle disruption buffer. Further studies revealed that there was little available EAV GP3 for protease digestion in closed vesicles, suggesting that the N-terminal hydrophobic sequence did not act as a signal sequence but remained as part of the protein serving to anchor the protein to the membrane. These data concluded unequivocally that the EAV protein is not a soluble protein, as was the case for LDV and PRRSV-NA (62). EAV studies by another

group confirmed these conclusions by the same means but also used prepared ORF3-specific antisera to localize the 37- to 42-kDa protein to the ER when expressed individually or in EAV-infected cells. No GP3 with mature N-linked glycans, indicating movement through the Golgi apparatus, was detected (150). However, EAV GP3 was detected in purified virions as a protein with a mixture of mature and immature N-linked oligosaccharides, signifying that at least some of the protein was processed through the Golgi compartment and did not remain in the ER (150). Finally, as detailed above, EAV GP3 was resolved to be a structural component of mature virions and is part of a heterotrimer with GP2 and GP4 that gradually forms after release from infected cells (149). The ORF3 protein of SHFV has not been investigated.

Completed studies with both PRRSV-EU and EAV do not discount the fact that the GP3s of LDV and PRRSV-NA may somehow be loosely linked to other viral structural components such as GP2 and GP4 at some point in the maturation of the virus (149, 154) and then sloughed off, possibly as a homodimer (87). All work to date suggests that all structural genes, including the GP3 gene, are essential in arteriviruses, but no work has been done to further investigate the structural nature of GP3 for LDV or PRRSV-NA using reverse genetics (109, 137, 147). It is difficult to pinpoint amino acid differences between the two genotypes of PRRSV that could account for the different sequelae, yet IAF-KLOP is remarkably different from strain LV (54.9% protein similarity). The GP3 action in different arteriviruses may instead reflect individual protein use and cellular localization, corresponding to their radically diverse sizes, the placement of the N-glycan residues in the context of the putative signal sequence, and total amino acid composition and placement.

All arterivirus GP3s appear to be highly antigenic and under selective pressure (3, 50, 62, 87, 111, 171). Since GP3 was found to be nonstructural in the case of PRRSV-NA strain IAF-KLOP and LDV, secretion of a minor fraction of GP3 might be an explanation for its high degree of immunogenicity in infected pigs, acting to provide a nonneutralizing decoy for the virus or another host disruption function (72, 87).

## Glycoprotein 4

The minor glycoprotein GP4 (17 to 23 kDa and pI of 6.0 to 8.3 [unprocessed]) is more conserved than GP3 among all arteriviruses except EAV. This interesting protein, identified in the sequence analyses of all arteriviruses (35, 53, 89, 93, 128), was first analyzed for its biochemical properties in the initial in vitro translation studies on PRRSV-EU strain LV alongside GP3 (95). Again, the investigators found that GP4 was present in PRRSV-EU-infected alveolar macrophages using immunoperoxidase monolayer assays, but they could not locate the protein in purified virions. They produced MAbs against purified strain LV, tested the antibodies for reactivity with baculovirus-expressed GP4, and performed Western blot analysis using the GP4 MAbs and purified virus to demonstrate that it was a structural protein. GP4 was identified as a 31- to 35-kDa protein without glycosidase treatment and was measured at 16 kDa after digestion with N-glycosidase F, which removes all oligosaccharides from N-linked glycoproteins; the latter finding signifies that the original high-mannose residues had been processed to complex N-glycans upon transport through the Golgi compartment (140). Another group confirmed their findings at a later date (146). Again, detailed studies reveal that PRRSV-EU GP2/GP3/GP4 heterotrimer formation was necessary for full complex N-glycan modification of the proteins (154). In LDV, in vitro transcription and translation of the ORF4 protein (predicted at 19 kDa) in the presence of canine pancreatic microsomal membranes produced a GP4 protein that was core N glycosylated at all of its putative sites (31 kDa) (49). GP4 remained in the membrane fraction after incubation with buffer that lyses membranes, showing it is a class I integral membrane protein with a signal sequence removed and a hydrophobic C-terminal tail (Fig. 2). The first evidence that GP4 was produced in PRRSV-NA-infected cells came when MAb to a baculovirus recombinant expressing the ORF4 protein produced strong perinuclear fluorescence in PRRSV-NA strain VR2385-infected cells (170). No reactivity was seen upon Western blot analysis with infected-cell lysate as well as purified virus, suggesting that the MAb was to a conformational epitope, and no PRRSV neutralization activity was detected with any of four MAbs against GP4 on CRL11171 cell monolayers (170). Further work was done using an infectious clone of PRRSV-NA isolate P129, partially deleting ORF4 and rescuing the replication-impaired deletion mutant virus with an established MARC-145 cell line expressing the full ORF4 by complementation. The mutant virus, without complementation, did not replicate in porcine alveolar macrophages. Thus, the investigators concluded that the PRRSV-NA GP4 gene was an essential gene. GP4 of EAV was studied biochemically alongside GP3, as detailed above (150). The investigators concluded that the GP4 gene produced a 28-kDa class I integral membrane protein with little if any carboxyl terminus exposed, as suggested by the C-terminal transmembrane region predicted by modeling (76) (Fig. 2).

Furthermore, EAV GP4 was modified by three N-glycans out of four predicted glycosylation sites, and in EAV-infected cells, most of the GP4 protein is retained in the ER with immature oligosaccharide side chains. However, in purified virions, GP4 is found with both mature and immature N-glycans. It was concluded also that only a small fraction of GP4 ends up in virions, establishing structural status for the protein (150). Later studies showed conclusively that EAV GP4 exists in infected cells first as a cysteine-linked heterodimer with GP2, and after viral budding, it becomes part of a disulfide-lined heterotrimer of GP2/GP3/GP4 (151).

GP4 was shown to harbor neutralization sites on PRRSV type 1 strain LV (140). A PRRSV-EU strain LV plaque reduction assay on CL2621 cells in the presence of any of four GP4 MAbs diminished the number of viral plaques seen by more than 50%. The analysis was repeated on other PRRSV-EU isolates adapted to replicate efficiently on CL2621 cells. One isolate was effectively neutralized, while the other was not. Further work by the laboratory went on to show that the neutralization domain could be localized to amino acids 40 to 79, found to be the most variable region in PRRSV GP4, with the part of the region shown to partially overlap the core domain (SAAQEKISF) not present in North American isolates (97). In contrast, investigators working with PRRSV-NA strain VR2385 and four conformationally dependent MAbs that reacted with 22 out of 23 different PRRSV-NA isolates could not detect neutralizing activity in GP4 (170). However, another study suggested that DNA vaccines incorporating either ORF4 or ORF5 nucleotides were able to elicit neutralizing antibodies (78). Weiland and coinvestigators examined the neutralization properties of MAbs against GP4 and GP5 more closely (146). Using the Dutch isolate Intervet-10, they developed immunoglobulin G MAbs to both GP4 and GP5 of this PRRSV-EU strain. They first tested the reactivity of the MAb preparations with different PRRSV isolates from Europe and North America. They found that the anti-GP4 MAbs could also react in immunoperoxidase monolayer assays with isolates from the United Kingdom (L1), The Netherlands (LV), and West Germany (2.25/2.35) but not isolates from East Germany (L01; Cobbelsdorf), Spain (2.93/2.96), or the United States (12 isolates). They also demonstrated (data not shown) that the four isolates recognized by these anti-GP4 MAbs were also neutralized by the same antibody preparations. Only plaque-purified isolate Intervet-10 was recognized and neutralized by three anti-GP5 MAbs, showing that the neutralization site was strain specific. Using plaque-purified Intervet-10, an extensive panel of MAbs

(11 GP4 and 13 GP5 MAbs) was tested for neutralization index (antibody mixed with graded doses of virus) as well as the neutralizing titer (100 50% tissue culture infective doses [TCID$_{50}$] of virus mixed with graded antibody dilutions). The results of the two assays on either MARC-145 cells or porcine alveolar macrophages clearly showed that anti-GP5 MAbs were more effective at viral neutralization of isolate Intervet-10 than anti-GP4 MAbs (146). While past viral neutralization studies of LDV (15, 25) and EAV (6–8, 21, 34, 52) have suggested that only the protein encoded by arteriviral ORF5 contains the major neutralizing site for macrophage infection, the analyses discussed here suggest that viral neutralization may be more complex than previously thought and may signal that separate neutralization mechanisms (blocking entry, fusion, and uncoating) play a role in different host cells or that different cell receptor specificities exist for the various arteriviruses.

## Glycoprotein 5

GP5 (22.4 to 31.2 kDa and pI of 4.9 to 9.2 [unprocessed]) is the most studied of the arteriviral proteins. In the early 1970s, investigators described the morphology of the LDV virion and determined through classical virological methods that the virus consisted of three proteins, one of which was an envelope glycoprotein named VP-3 (24 to 44 kDa; now GP5) (13, 98). EAV VP3 was first described in 1976 (168). Both groups placed the respective viruses in the *Togaviridae* family, where they were classified until 1989 (LDV) and 1991 (EAV) (13, 33, 56, 168). Genotypic

variation of both viruses was noted early in their study (12, 23, 104). Work further describing the virion proteins did not progress until the 1990s, when the nucleotide sequences of the complete or 3′ termini of genomes of all of the arteriviruses were derived, including the new members of this viral family, SHFV and PRRSV (newly emerged) (24, 33, 53, 57, 92, 105). The structural proteins of EAV were further described in 1992, when researchers assigned the 3′ ORFs detected in the EAV genome with the use of sequence analysis, vaccinia virus recombinant protein expression in BHK-21 cells, radiolabeled virions, and virus-specific antisera. Two glycoproteins were noted at that time and named Gl (now GP5) and Gs (now GP2). EAV GP5 migrated in SDS-PAGE analysis as a smear of 30 to 42 kDa with one N-linked oligosaccharide (35). PRRSV-NA and PRRSV-EU GP5s were established as having similar sizes (11, 86, 90, 95). The membrane topology was analyzed biochemically only for LDV, but since all arteriviral GP5s display similar hydrophobicity profiles, they were predicted to have the same membrane orientation (48). Using in vitro transcription and translation of individual ORFs in the presence or absence of artificial membranes, enzyme digests, and antiserum and based on the derived hydrophobicity plots (44), researchers were able to establish the membrane topology of the proteins encoded by ORF2, ORF5, and ORF6, deriving three membrane-spanning regions in the glycoprotein encoded by ORF5, classifying it as a polytopic class I glycoprotein (VP-3, now GP5 [Fig. 3]). EAV, LDV, and PRRSV-NA GP5s were found to be linked to the membrane protein (M protein) by

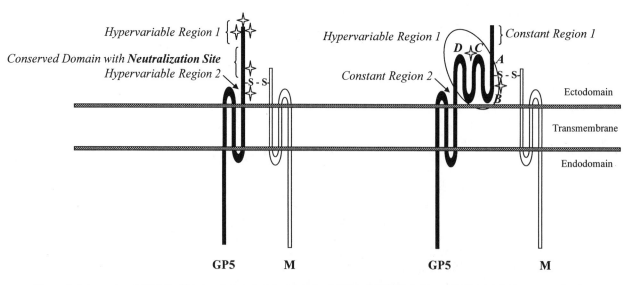

**Figure 3.** Schematics of GP5 disulfide bonded to the M protein for LDV and PRRSV (left) and EAV (right). One neutralization domain has been identified on LDV and PRRSV, and four (*A-D*) have been identified on EAV. N-glycan addition (✧) varies for all arteriviruses, but the N-glycans closest to the disulfide bond between GP5 and M (S-S) are mostly conserved.

disulfide bonds through analysis of reducing and nonreducing SDS-PAGE and coimmunoprecipitation experiments (36, 45, 88). Investigators showed in pulse-chase experiments that the covalent interaction between the cysteine residues of the heterodimer of EAV and PRRSV-NA was found to take place in the ER (36, 88). The covalent interaction through disulfide bonds between the conserved cysteine of GP5 (amino acid 48 in strain VR-2332 and amino acid 34 in EAV) and the only cysteine predicted to be located on the ectodomain of M protein was shown to be critical for LDV and EAV infectivity (45, 129). EAV has additional cysteine residues that cannot be altered, suggesting that there may be additional intramolecular covalent interactions (129). Lastly, the N-linked oligosaccharides were shown to be of a complex nature, since the GP5s of EAV and PRRSV were both sensitive to endoglycosidase F/N-glycosidase F and somewhat cleaved by endo-H (11, 36, 88). Researchers working with EAV clearly showed that the single N-linked sugar was modified with N-acetyllactosamine since GP5 was susceptible to endo-β-galactosidase (endo-β), an enzyme that cleaves the internal galactoside linkage of such polylactosaminoglycans (36). PRRSV-NA GP5 was not sensitive to endo-β and thus is thought to be modified by complex sugars other than polylactosaminoglycans (88). LDV GP5 has never been examined with endo-β, primarily due to the difficulties associated with the lack of an established cell line for viral growth. The other interesting point is that both EAV and SHFV have approximately 90 amino acids on their GP5 ectodomains and LDV and both genotypes of PRRSV possess a GP5 ectodomain of only around 32 amino acids. This may have a marked effect on the properties of the respective viral subgroups, particularly on host cell tropism.

The GP5s of LDV, EAV, and both PRRSV genotypes have been long recognized as the major structural proteins to which neutralizing antibodies are synthesized. Investigators working with several isolates of PRRSV-EU found that GP5 was quantitatively more effective in neutralization than GP4, but that neutralization escape mutants were fairly easily derived (146). The same conclusion was reached by researchers working with PRRSV-NA (59). In 1982, researchers noted that one-hit kinetics (one antibody molecule to one virion) would neutralize LDV, and although the viral component could not be pinpointed at that time, this observation suggests that there is only one LDV protein involved (16). This group of researchers established the viral protein that induced neutralizing antibodies as VP-3 (GP5) (15). All later studies on LDV confirmed that GP5 possessed the neutralizing epitope (25, 119). In addition, it was noted that when MAbs were prepared using formalin-inactivated LDV, all neutralizing MAbs recognized a single contiguous epitope, nonneutralizing antibodies reacted with two other distinct epitopes on the virion, and infection of mice or immunization of rabbits with nondenatured LDV did not elicit neutralizing antibodies (61). However, the mechanism of neutralization was not defined until Plagemann and coworkers established through sedimentation studies that LDV neutralization results from the binding of antibodies to specific epitopes on GP5 that lead to destruction of virions, suggesting that the protein could be considered the viral attachment protein (119). Later work showed that the neutralizing MAbs that were developed against a mixture of formalin-inactivated LDV strains reacted strongly in an indirect enzyme-linked immunosorbent assay (ELISA) with synthetic peptides consisting of the strain-specific 30-amino-acid ectodomains of several LDV variants, while nonneutralizing antibodies did not, confirming the protein as the target of viral neutralization (80). Since LDV infectivity was correlated with the disulfide bond between GP5 and M protein (48), and considering the membrane topology and conformation, the fact that the neutralization site was situated on the short ectodomain of GP5 (80), and the addition of N-glycans to all GP5 ectodomain asparagine residues (48) (all derived through biochemical evidence), investigators reasoned that the viral attachment site on GP5 was masked by the N-linked oligosaccharides and covalent linkage between GP5 and M protein (117). Lastly, the neutralization site on LDV GP5 was pinpointed through an indirect ELISA study (117). This series of work built upon previous work (80) and sought to determine the exact location on GP5 that induced neutralizing antibodies. Using the neutralizing MAb binding to the 30-amino-acid peptide mimicking the GP5 epitope and N- and C-terminal truncations of the peptide, and then using peptide inhibition in solution, these seminal ELISA studies revealed that the neutralizing epitope could be shortened to an 8-amino-acid segment (SSTKNLIY).

For PRRSV, findings similar to those for LDV were obtained. Pirzadeh and Dea developed MAbs that recognized the PRRSV type 2 ORF5 product expressed in *Escherichia coli* and found that they exclusively recognized a 25-kDa product of expressed nonglycosylated GP5 and, when PRRSV virions were immunoprecipitated or analyzed by Western blotting under reducing conditions, recognized the 42-kDa GP5 (113). To determine the capacity of these MAbs to neutralize the virus, microneutralization assays were done in which dilutions of the antibodies were incubated with 100 TCID$_{50}$ of PRRSV-NA and then the monolayers were examined for inhibition of infection or inhibition of N protein expression visualized by immunofluorescence. They found that although all five MAbs neutralized the homologous PRRSV-NA strain IAF-KLOP, only two were capable of neutralizing another NA strain, VR-2332. Because all MAbs bound to GP5 of IAF-KLOP in a Western blot and could recognize the protein in both its nonglycosylated and its N-glycosylated forms, they concluded that the MAb recognized a linear epitope on the protein. Furthermore, the researchers suggested that PRRSV GP5 might play a role in virus infectivity and that it may function in attachment to cell receptors and/or in virus penetration (113). GP5 of IAF-KLOP (Canadian strain) was compared to predicted ORF proteins of eight other Canadian viruses as well as three other type 2 strains derived from the United States (115). Amino acids 26 to 39 (AALVI-NASSSSSSQL) represented a region on GP5 that was hypervariable between the aligned strains (hypervariable region 1 [Fig. 3]). In addition, the predicted number of N-glycans added to this segment of the protein differed from zero to three, whereas two other putative N-glycosylation sites downstream (N44 and N51) were conserved. By expressing five of these GP5 regions (LV, IAF-KLOP, Ingelvac MLV, IAF-93-653, and ONT-TS, representing phylogenetically distinct viruses) in *E. coli* glutathione *S*-transferase (GST)-ORF5 protein recombinant fusion constructs, preparing hyperimmune antisera against each protein, and subsequently performing indirect immunofluorescence assays, it was determined that the specific antisera recognized the parental GP5 but had less ability to recognize the other expressed proteins. The investigators concluded that the occurrence of antigenic variability among the different strains might involve specific neutralizing epitopes that, again because the antisera detected virus-specific GP5 in a Western blot, were most likely linear in nature. Research by another group revealed the apparent identity of three distinct antigenic groups of PRRSV, based on profiles of reactivity of MAbs to N and M proteins, GP5, and GP3 with a panel of 69 PRRSV-NA isolates and PRRSV-EU strain LV, again suggesting viral variability (163). The neutralizing domain previously mapped by the original MAb studies was not located in this hypervariable region (113, 115). The same laboratory went on to reveal that GP5 was the protein recognized by porcine anti-PRRSV neutralizing sera and, due to the failure of porcine antisera to recognize bacterially expressed ORF5 protein, suggested that GP5 is modified by proper folding, oligosaccharide addition, and/or disulfide binding to obtain its final antigenic conformation on the virion (114). Earlier work had already shown that PRRSV GP5 and M protein were disulfide linked as well as modified by endo-β-resistant N-glycans (45, 88). In

order to more closely pinpoint the neutralization epitope of PRRSV-NA GP5, the strategy employed in derivation of the epitope for LDV (SSTKNLIY) was used (121). In such synthetic-peptide studies, it was revealed that pigs mount a response to the GP5 ectodomain, that the ectodomain residues that were most correlative with neutralization activity encompassed amino acids 36 to 52 of PRRSV-NA strain VR-2332, and that flanking N-glycans probably interfere with immunorecognition by the swine host (121). The ectodomain sequence of strain VR-2332 was further analyzed in this manner, deriving the minimal epitope recognized by neutralizing sera to be amino acids 37 to 45 (SHLQLIYNL) (118). Further exploration of this epitope showed that peptides that were mutated at 42IT and 38HLTY blocked antibody recognition. The same GP5 neutralization epitope (amino acids 37 to 45) was recognized by a neutralizing anti-PRRSV MAb and hyperimmune sera to two other North American PRRSV isolates, PRRSV IA 97-7895 and PRRSV KY-35 (110). These investigators identified the region by analyzing synthetic peptides that were generated on the basis of mimotope antibodies selected from phage display library. The latter study suggested that H38, I42, and Y43 in the GP5 ectodomain are essential residues for interaction with the neutralizing antibodies. They also surmised that a nonneutralizing epitope corresponded to amino acids 27 to 30 of PRRSV-NA strain KY-35. In addition, *Mycobacterium bovis* strain bacillus Calmette-Guérin (BCG) expressing 30 amino acids of the GP5 ectodomain of PRRSV-NA strain 16244B along with the M protein was found to induce neutralizing antibody responses in mice and pigs (9, 10). Less work has been done on PRRSV-EU strains. Plagemann used indirect and competition ELISA with 8- to 10-amino-acid peptides to demonstrate that that sera from swine infected with strain LV recognized an ectodomain segment composed of 38SSTYQYIYN-LTICELNG, analogous to the region identified for LDV and PRRSV-NA. However, other investigators used Pepscan analysis to produce 12-mer peptides of strain Intervet-10 and found that all three neutralizing MAbs tested specifically reacted with peptides containing the sequence 29WSFADGN. The fact that this region partially lies in the predicted signal sequence, upstream from the homologous region of PRRSV-NA, suggests that the actual cleavage occurs at an unexpected site or not at all, at least in this EU virus. It also suggests that viral neutralization may occur by more than one molecular mechanism.

A bioinformatic approach, based on 916 PRRSV-NA and -EU unique isolates (>2% amino acid difference), was useful in investigating how much variability could be seen among the viruses in the entire predicted ectodomain region. Two hypervariable regions spanning a region containing the proposed neutralization epitope were discerned by this method (Fig. 3). Furthermore, the analysis revealed that the amino acids at positions 36 to 39 of the core neutralizing epitope were quite variable but that the rest of the region was very conserved (Fig. 4) (my unpublished data). In particular, I42, C48 (predicted to be covalently linked to M protein through a disulfide bond), and L50 were found to be invariant, and most of the other amino acid positions had very few variants. The range of deviations seen in the proposed neutralizing site located at amino acids 37 to 45 among 3,188 field viruses (18 EU isolates) collected at the University of Minnesota Veterinary Diagnostic Laboratory was evaluated to more closely analyze the viral neutralization site encoded by ORF5 (SHLQLIYNL) (118). The results of the query determined that there are more than 100 amino acid variations within this 9-amino-acid stretch (data not shown). Several conserved amino acids are located in the identified neutralizing epitope, with very few substitutions occurring in nature (S37, Q40, I42, Y43, L45). A few amino acids show moderate variation (H38, L39, L41, N44), with N44 usually displaying the N-glycosylation motif NXS/T (Fig. 4) (my unpublished results). The other amino acids in the core epitope may be important to development of effective PRRSV vaccines and to understanding the serospecificity of different PRRSV isolates. Perhaps the variability in

some of these areas may be partially responsible for the observed lack of cross protection between PRRSV strains. The remaining conserved amino acids (amino acids 46 to 53) may be necessary for appropriate interaction with the M protein, attachment to the host cell, and/or some other uncharacterized GP5 function.

In 1993, the fact that a 29-kDa protein of EAV expressed a neutralization determinant was demonstrated by production of MAbs and further characterization of their binding properties by Western immunoblotting and competitive ELISA (8). All MAbs were found to recognize a single neutralization site on this glycosylated protein. Furthermore, equine anti-EAV serum bound the same protein and blocked the binding of selected MAbs. This finding was further supported by five other MAbs that recognized vaccinia virus-expressed GP5 of EAV (34). The MAbs were found to bind in a reciprocal manner in a competitive binding assay, but only one effectively neutralized EAV infectivity. The work suggested that these MAbs recognized an antigenic domain on GP5 that was composed of overlapping or closely adjacent epitopes. The location of this domain was further mapped to amino acids 55 to 98 through the use of GST fusion proteins expressing full-length GP5 and truncated mutants and subsequent screening with an ELISA for immunoreactive regions (21). A fusion peptide expressing amino acids 55 to 98 was found to induce EAV-neutralizing antibody in horses. The

| 36 | 37 | 38 | 39 | 40 | 41 | 42 | 43 | 44 | 45 | 46 | 47 | 48 | 49 | 50 | 51 | 52 | 53 |
|---|---|---|---|---|---|---|---|---|---|---|---|---|---|---|---|---|---|
| **S** | **S** | **H** | **L** | **Q** | **L** | **I** | **Y** | **N** | **L** | **T** | **L** | **C** | **E** | **L** | **N** | **G** | **T** |
| N | F | Y | F | H(1) | S | | N(2) | S(<10) | M(<10) | K(<5) | I | | K(2) | | S(2) | S(1) | P(2) |
| A | C | P | S | | | | | D(<10) | | P(<5) | V(<10) | | S(1) | | | | |
| G | P | Q | T | | | | | K(<10) | | | | | | | | | |
| | | N | Y | | | | | T(<10) | | | | | | | | | |
| - | | | | | | | | | | | | | | | | | |

↓ N⁴⁴ - conserved N-glycosylation            ↓ C⁴⁸ - Invariant cysteine; disulfide linked to M    ↓ N⁵¹ - conserved N-glycosylation

**Figure 4.** Variation among 916 unique isolates of PRRSV-NA and -EU in amino acids 36 to 53 of GP5. The sequence in boldface is the sequence of PRRSV-NA strain VR-2332. The smaller letters below indicate other amino acids seen at the same relative positions, and if these are also in boldface, they represent an approximately equal number of PRRSV isolates as for strain VR-2332. Numbers in parentheses point out how few isolates were seen with the indicated residue for amino acids 40 to 53. I42, C48 (predicted to covalently link to M protein through a disulfide bond), and L50 were found to be invariant, and most of the other amino acid positions from 40 to 53 had very few variants.

29-kDa protein identified in 1993 was then shown to be equivalent to GP5 of EAV, and the amino acids contributing to a neutralization domain were determined to be amino acids 98 to 104 (6). Another group identified a similar neutralization determinant (52). Eleven additional MAbs were prepared and used with previously studied MAbs to examine the neutralization of EAV in more depth (7). The 11 additional MAbs again neutralized EAV, and they recognized GP5 by Western immunoassay (4 MAbs) or by competitive ELISA (7 MAbs). The 7 MAbs detected through ELISA were determined to recognize conformation-dependent GP5 epitopes. Work with the EAV neutralization escape mutants and microneutralization assays with polyclonal anti-EAV serum suggested that there were both linear and conformational epitopes on GP5. Nucleotide sequence analysis of many field strains showed that these epitopes could differ, suggesting that the regions selected by the MAbs correlate with immune targets in the host. Lastly, four immunogenic epitopes (A to D) were derived from this work, one before the conserved N-glycosylation site and conserved cysteine and the other three downstream. The research, combined with work by others, also showed the immense variety of sequences that exist in field isolates of EAV (7, 52, 63, 145). Further studies preparing additional MAbs to GP5 using the Venezuelan equine encephalitis virus replicon vector system led to the discovery that neutralizing antibodies to GP5 were only produced in mice when GP5 was disulfide linked to the M protein (4). However, the fact that neutralizing MAbs could be prepared in mice using just the expressed EAV ORF5 argues against that observation (6, 135, 145). This may suggest that neutralization can be derived by different mechanisms. Recently, an infectious clone of EAV was used to reexamine the GP5 interaction with the neutralizing MAbs. Constructed chimeras of the ORF5 sequences of multiple isolates and strains and traditional neutralization techniques were used. The data clearly confirmed that the four neutralization domains are on the N-terminal ectodomain of GP5 and that the amino acids within those domains contribute to both linear and conformational epitopes (2). As the putative viral receptor protein and perhaps also the EAV protein that mediates fusion with the host macrophage, GP5 may have alternative domains that perform discrete functions. Regardless of the number of potential neutralization mechanisms—such as direct hindrance of critical sites by early components of complement, viral lysis by late complement components or other immune cells, or inhibition of interactions between the virus and the cell that prevents release of the viral genome (37)—research on EAV has only shown GP5 to be recognized

by over 25 neutralizing MAbs (5). In an effort to examine the viral determinant of cell tropism for EAV (viral attachment protein), researchers took advantage of engineered chimeric recombinant viruses displaying the GP5s of LDV, PRRSV-NA, and SHFV and/or the M epitope of LDV or PRRSV-NA fused to the transmembrane and C-terminal region of the respective proteins of EAV (40). Remarkably, although the viruses are slow growing, the GP5s of LDV/EAV and PRRSV-NA/EAV retained their infectivity for BHK-21 cells and were processed to the Golgi apparatus just as wild-type EAV. This was unexpected, as LDV and PRRSV cannot normally infect BHK-21 cells. The investigators concluded that the GP5 domain is not the main determinant of tropism in cell culture. The suggestion was made that the results implied that the major glycoprotein is not required for cell receptor binding or virus entry, or the ectodomain is involved in cell binding but an alternative EAV protein determines host specificity. However, the fact that BHK-21 cells are not the EAV host cell in vivo and are extraordinarily unrestrictive to many viruses also suggests that the system used in this study may not be reflective of the tropism for the natural equine host cell, the macrophage.

The variability of N-glycan addition to LDV, PRRSV, and EAV GP5 is one other component to be considered when examining structure-function determinants. Neuropathogenic isolates of LDV are approximately 100 times more susceptible to antibody neutralization than nonneuropathogenic strains, and neutralizing antibodies are generated more rapidly and to a higher level in the same mice, leading to low-level viremia (19). These phenotypic properties of the neuropathic strains of LDV were genetically linked to the loss of two out of three N-glycosylation sites on the short ectodomain of LDV GP5 (47). In addition, neutralization escape mutants were isolated that regained the ability to cause high-level viremia concomitant with the loss in neuropathogenicity and the regaining of full N glycosylation. It was concluded that the resistance of the nonneuropathogenic LDVs to the humoral immune response is due to masking of the single neutralization epitope by the GP5 N-glycans. Instead, the loss of the N-glycans allowed GP5 of the neuropathic LDVs to attach to alternate host cell receptors on motor neurons of C58/AKR mice (18). Polyclonal activation of B cells, recognized as a $\geq$10-fold increase in plasma immunoglobulin G levels, was also correlated with LDV GP5 N glycosylation (81). Field isolates of EAV contain a GP5 that is also differentially glycosylated (2, 52). Decreased N glycosylation of PRRSV type 1 and 2 GP5 has also been seen to negatively influence viral replication (153) as well as increase sensitivity to neutralization in infectious clone models (1). Although not yet investigated fully for PRRSV, the addition or loss of N-glycosylation sites has also been studied by examining the amount of natural variation that can occur in the N-terminal region of GP5, after cleavage of the signal sequence (Fig. 3). A selection of 916 PRRSV-NA and -EU unique field isolates revealed 219 different patterns for an 8-amino-acid stretch in hypervariable region 1. In addition, hypervariable region 1 was also seen to have additions (up to 6 amino acids) or deletions (1 amino acid). PRRSV strains have been noted to have up to five predicted N-glycosylation sites within the entire ∽30-amino-acid GP5 ectodomain (my unpublished results). Thus, the suggested masking of the PRRSV GP5 neutralization epitope by N-glycans (18) but also potential immune evasion through amino acid variability make the study of this PRRSV protein extremely interesting.

## M Protein

Although the existence of the nonglycosylated M protein (formerly VP2; 17.7 to 19.0 kDa; pI of 9.6 to 10.5) has been known for more than 30 years, relatively little has been clarified about its structure and role in virion morphogenesis (13, 168). The M protein sequence is the most conserved of all the structural proteins, perhaps due to the critical nature of this protein in the virion. The M protein was assigned to ORF6 for EAV, LDV, and PRRSV and ORF8 for SHFV based on the predicted protein size and the fact that it is not glycosylated (24, 35, 53, 77, 93). ORF6 was predicted to have two or three transmembrane helices (35, 77), confirmed as three by topology studies for LDV (48). As a polytopic class III membrane protein, there is no cleaved signal sequence, and it consists of a very short N-terminal ectodomain (∽9 to 11 amino acids), three membrane-spanning regions, and a longer endodomain (∽77 to 85 amino acids) (Fig. 3). Although arterivirus ORF6 (outside of SHFV) encodes a potentially myristoylated protein with a glycine residue next to the initiating AUG, amino acids directly downstream suggest that this is not likely, and experiments with EAV concur (36). The major emphasis has been on its disulfide heterodimerization with GP5, shown to be critical in EAV and LDV infectivity (36, 45, 129). As such, it is an essential protein for the virus. Several anti-M-protein antibody preparations against predominately the putative intravirion region of M protein have been obtained by predicted antigenic peptide synthesis (95), by prokaryotic or eukaryotic expression of ORF6 (4, 26, 68, 73, 122, 132), or with MAbs prepared against purified virions (26, 85, 140), but most are virus strain specific. One MAb shown to

cross-react with many PRRSV-NA isolates was described (85). By far, antibody preparations that have been described appear to recognize the C terminus of the protein (68) over the N-terminal ectodomain region (141). In one study, the M ectodomain of PRRSV-EU strain LV was replaced by those of LDV, EAV, and PRRSV-NA strain VR-2332 (141). One chimeric virus, LDV-M, was able to replicate on porcine alveolar macrophages, suggesting that M protein did not play a role in cell targeting. Other chimeric viruses were unable to replicate in the macrophages until the infectious construct was altered to express the GP5 and M protein genes separately instead of as overlapping proteins in the genome (Fig. 1). However, all chimeric viruses were defective in viral growth, as detected in growth curves obtained by using infected porcine alveolar macrophages and measuring TCID$_{50}$ per milliliter. The results led the authors to conclude that the ectodomain of M protein is not involved in host cell tropism in vitro. They also speculated that the binding of the GP5/M heterodimer recruits the virus to the cell surface through a heparin-like cell receptor, when other minor viral envelope proteins act to determine cell specificity (141). Alternatively, perhaps the GP5/M heterodimer does determine cell specificity, but the chimeric viruses have a reduced capacity to recognize specific host macrophages, leading to lower replication rates. The conserved M ectodomain may serve instead to provide a mostly stabilizing influence on GP5 through the cysteine interaction, contributing little else to the virus neutralization domain. However, another interesting finding was that the M proteins of both genotypes of PRRSV, mainly as a disulfide-linked complex with GP5, were involved in attachment of the virus to a heparin-like receptor on porcine alveolar macrophages in a dose-dependent manner (31). Clearly, the exact molecular mechanism(s) that the arteriviruses utilize to infect cells demands further research.

## N Protein

The most abundant viral protein in arterivirus-infected cells is the N protein, which forms a spherical, potentially icosahedral core 20 to 30 nm in diameter (27). N protein with bound RNA can be isolated from the envelope proteins by disruption with nonionic detergent (98). The N protein of arteriviruses has long been known to associate with the viral RNA in a spherical or cubic morphology (13, 66, 98, 136, 138, 168). In all arteriviruses, N protein is a very basic protein and the second shortest structural protein. Also, comparison of the N proteins of EAV, LDV, PRRSV, and SHFV shows that they are not as conserved as the M and E proteins, even though the

N protein is essential for infectivity and performs the same function in each virus. The first evidence that the protein (then VP-1; 12.4 kDa and pI of 10.6) was encoded just upstream of the 3′ untranslated region came from initial sequence analysis of LDV compared to direct VP-1 protein sequencing, which also revealed that the structure of the genome was not togavirus-like, as thought previously (55). Shortly thereafter, the complete nucleotide sequence of EAV was determined, with the most 3′ ORF (ORF7) putatively encoding the N protein (12.3 kDa and pI of 11.9), suggesting that the virus was evolutionarily related to LDV and the coronavirus-like superfamily (35). Investigators first realized that PRRSV isolates from Europe were antigenically distinct from U.S. isolates based on differential activity of MAbs prepared against the putative N protein (108). The last gene (ORF7) of PRRSV-EU (13.8 kDa and pI of 10.5 for its product) (24, 92) and PRRSV-NA (13.6 kDa and pI of 10.1 for its product) (90) was determined to code for the N protein and was established decisively by in vitro translation of ORF7 followed by antibody recognition of both the ORF7 translation product and the N protein of PRRSV-EU (95) and PRRSV-NA (11, 89) virions. SHFV was shown to be of a similar genomic structure, with the last ORF in the genome putatively representing the capsid (12.3 kDa and pI of 11.1) protein. Amino-terminal sequencing of gel-purified nucleocapsid-associated protein established conclusively that this peptide was encoded by the ultimate 3′ ORF (57). Several antibody studies with EU and NA isolates of PRRSV have been developed and used to define common and genotype-specific immunogenic epitopes on the N protein (20, 26, 41, 51, 84, 96, 108, 123, 148, 156, 157, 164). Less research has been documented for the N protein of EAV (22, 145), and the antigenic structures of the N proteins of LDV and SHFV have not been studied. However, antibodies to the N protein are predominately made in all the arteriviruses and do not neutralize virions. In a study designed to lend understanding of the action of the N protein in viral assembly, PRRSV type 2 strain PA8 N protein oligomerization properties were studied (159). Under nonreducing conditions, immunoprecipitation of N protein from PRRSV-infected cells showed that the protein forms disulfide-linked homodimers, but this could be prevented by addition of the alkylating agent N-ethylmaleimide (NEM), perhaps suggesting that the intermolecular disulfide bonds were merely oxidized during infected-cell lysis prior to immunoprecipitation. The study also found that homodimers of N protein were isolated from extracellular virus and that these disulfide linkages were NEM resistant. When infected cells were subjected to pulse-chase

analysis, N protein disulfide-linked homodimers as well as monomers were found. Because there are three cysteine residues in PRRSV-NA N protein, the investigators reasoned that both inter- and intramolecular disulfide bonds could form, giving rise to both N homodimers and monomers. They next investigated when the disulfide interaction took place during the virus replication cycle. Pulse-chase labeling of infected cells, followed by cell lysis and immunoprecipitation under nonreducing conditions at various times postinfection, showed that the homodimers were evident as a minor component of N protein at 2 h and became more abundant over time. However, the majority of N protein in infected cells was present in noncovalently linked forms or as monomers. In contrast, virus particles released from these PRRSV-infected cells showed that homodimers of N protein were more numerous, and evidence of higher-ordered structures of N protein was also seen. The researchers concluded that in the virus-infected cell, N homodimers are formed as the virus particle buds into the oxidizing environment of the ER, when cysteine-cysteine bonds could form, but that a substantial amount of N protein remained noncovalently associated. Next, it was determined through mutational analysis that only the cysteine at PRRSV-NA N protein position 23 seemed to be involved in the disulfide linkage between homodimers. However, evidence that the N protein dimer seemed to be stable in both the absence and presence of intermolecular disulfide bonds was obtained by analysis of sucrose-purified virion N protein formed in the presence and absence of NEM, immunoprecipitation, and PAGE analysis under nonreducing and reducing conditions. The results suggested that N dimers were present in purified virions as homodimers, some covalently linked through disulfide bridges and some noncovalently linked. The authors concluded that perhaps N dimers first form as noncovalently linked proteins and acquire disulfide linkages when removed from the reducing environment of the infected-cell cytoplasm. Amino acids 30 to 37 seem to be essential for this noncovalent interaction between N molecules. RNA may be involved in bridging the N protein monomers because RNase A treatment dramatically reduced N-N interactions. Lastly, cross-linking experiments suggested that the N protein assembles into higher-ordered structures of dimers, trimers, tetramers, and pentamers. The overall finding of the complex series of studies was that N protein possesses properties that lend themselves to self-association, likely providing the basis for nucleocapsid assembly.

Investigators have found that N proteins of PRRSV-NA (124) and EAV (101, 134), as well as coronaviruses (65, 162), can be found in both the

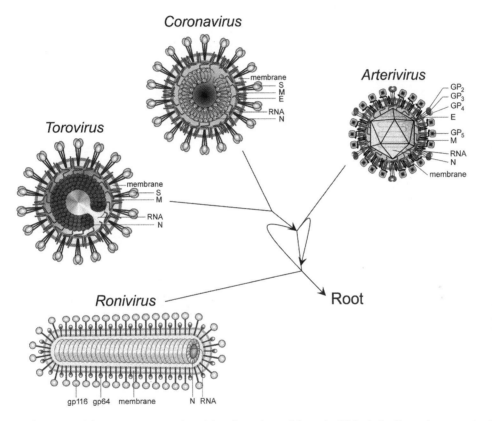

**Color Plate 1 (chapter 1).** Schematic structure of particles of members of the order *Nidovirales*. E, envelope protein; GP and gp, glycoprotein; M, membrane protein; N, nucleoprotein; S, spike glycoprotein. The HEs of some group 2 coronaviruses and some toroviruses are not illustrated. The stoichiometry of the virion components is shown arbitrarily. Adapted from reference 44a.

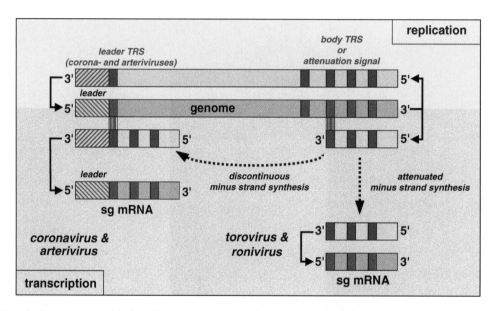

**Color Plate 2 (chapter 1).** Models for nidovirus replication and transcription using hypothetical viruses that produce four subgenomic mRNAs. Plus-strand RNA is depicted in red, and minus-strand RNA is depicted in blue. In the case of coronaviruses and arteriviruses, discontinuous extension during minus-strand RNA synthesis is proposed as the mechanism to produce subgenome-length minus-strand templates. The RTC is proposed to be attenuated at one of the body TRSs in the 3′-proximal part of the genome, after which the nascent minus strand would be extended with the antileader sequence by a process of discontinuous extension. The completed subgenome-length minus strands would serve as templates for mRNA synthesis. In the case of roniviruses and all but the largest subgenome-length mRNA of toroviruses, conserved attenuation sequences, found upstream of each of the genes in the 3′-proximal part of the genome, direct the termination of nascent minus-strand synthesis. The attenuated subgenome-length minus-strand RNAs would serve directly as templates for transcription of mRNA. Adapted from reference 37.

| anti-replicase | RNA detection | overlay |
| --- | --- | --- |

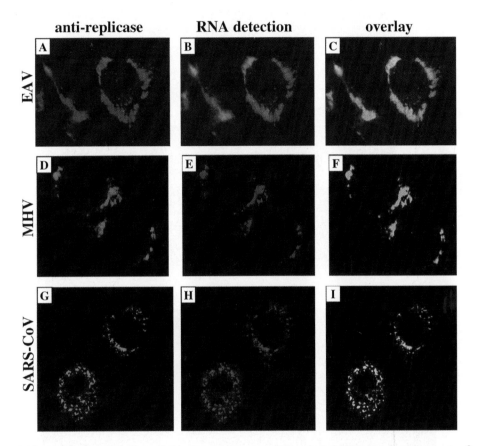

**Color Plate 3 (chapter 7).** Colocalization of nidovirus replicase proteins and viral RNA visualized by immunofluorescence assays. EAV, EAV-infected BHK-21 cells at 10 h postinfection. (A) Detection of EAV nsp3, one of the viral replicase TM proteins, using specific antiserum. (B) In situ hybridization using a fluorescently labeled RNA probe complementary to a part of the EAV replicase gene, and thus recognizing genome-length plus-strand RNA. (C) Overlay showing colocalization of nsp3 and plus-strand RNA. (Courtesy of Yvonne van der Meer, Jessika Zevenhoven-Dobbe, and Eric Snijder, Leiden University Medical Center, Leiden, The Netherlands). MHV, MHV-A59-infected 17cl-1 cells at 8.5 h postinfection. (D) Detection of MHV nsp5 (3CL$^{\text{pro}}$) using specific antiserum. (E) Detection of newly synthesized viral RNA labeled with BrUTP in the presence of actinomycin D, using antiserum directed against BrdU. (F) Overlay showing colocalization of nsp5 and newly synthesized viral RNA (reproduced with permission from Shi et al., 1999). SARS-CoV, SARS-CoV-infected Vero-E6 cells. (G) Detection of nsp3 using specific antiserum. (H) Detection of newly synthesized viral RNA labeled with BrUTP in the presence of actinomycin D, using antiserum directed against BrdU. (I) Overlay showing colocalization of nsp3 and newly synthesized viral RNA (reproduced with permission from reference 25.)

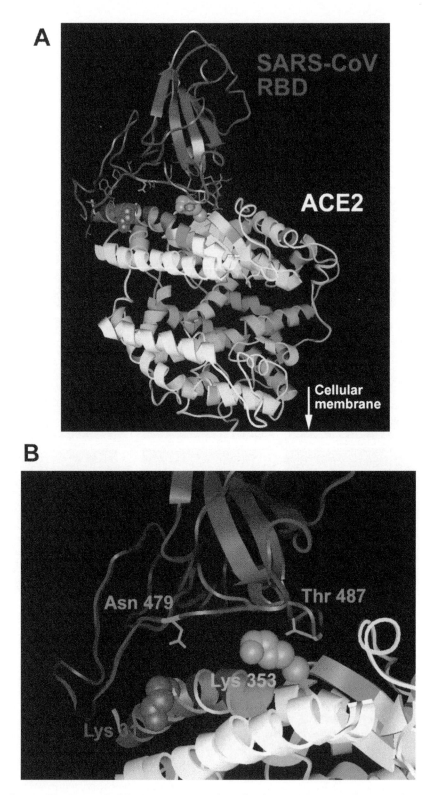

**Color Plate 4 (chapter 10).** Cocrystal of the SARS-CoV RBD bound to human ACE2. (A) The RBD of SARS CoV, residues 319 to 511, is shown in red, bound to the ectodomain of human ACE2, shown in white. ACE2 regions that contact the SARS-CoV RBD are indicated in orange ribbon. Residues within these same regions also contribute to HCoV-NL63 entry, indicating substantial overlap between HCoV-NL63 and SARS-CoV binding regions on ACE2. SARS-CoV RBD residues 479 and 487, whose alteration from lysine to asparagine and serine to threonine, respectively, permits efficient use of human ACE2, are shown in green. ACE2 lysine 31, which precludes association with S proteins bearing lysine 479, found in most palm civet viruses, is shown in magenta. ACE2 threonine 487, critical for efficient use of human and palm civet ACE2, and found only in SARS-CoV isolated from humans during the 2002–2003 epidemic, is shown in green. Lysine 353 is shown in cyan. (B) Closeup view of the ACE2-RBD contact region, in which RBD residues other than 479 and 487 are hidden. Note the close contact between the methyl group of threonine 487 of the RBD and the stalk of ACE2 lysine 353, critical to SARS-CoV entry.

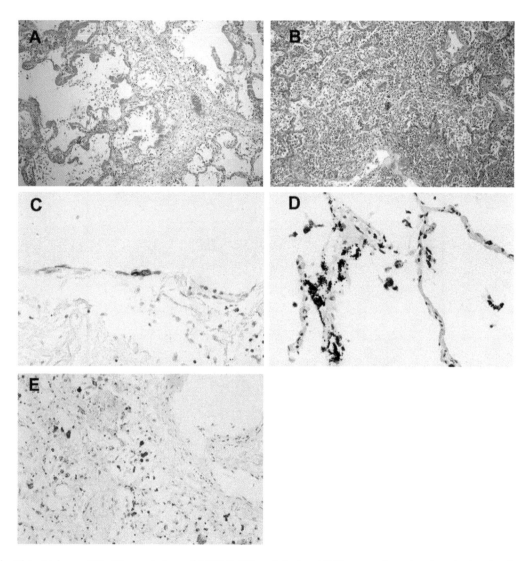

**Color Plate 5 (chapter 19).** Histopathology of SARS-CoV lung infection. (A) Hematoxylin and eosin stain showing the early phase of SARS pneumonia; pink hyaline membranes within the alveoli and increased inflammatory cells in the interstitium can be seen. (B) Hematoxylin and eosin stain showing the organizing phase of SARS. There is obliteration of the alveoli by fibrous tissue and reactive pneumocytes. A giant cell is identified in the center of the field. (C) AEC (3-amino-9-ethylcarbazole) with hematoxylin counterstain immunochemistry for SARS-CoV nucleoprotein in early-stage SARS pneumonia; positive staining for nucleoprotein in flattened pneumocytes can be seen. (D) AEC with hematoxylin counterstain immunochemistry for SARS-CoV nucleoprotein in early-stage SARS pneumonia with evidence that the carbon-containing macrophages are also positive for SARS nucleoprotein. (E) AEC with hematoxylin counterstain showing early SARS pneumonia; shown are results of in situ hybridization with pooled SARS-CoV genes, with red positive staining of the bronchial epithelium, flattened pneumocytes, and macrophages. Magnification for all panels, ×200.

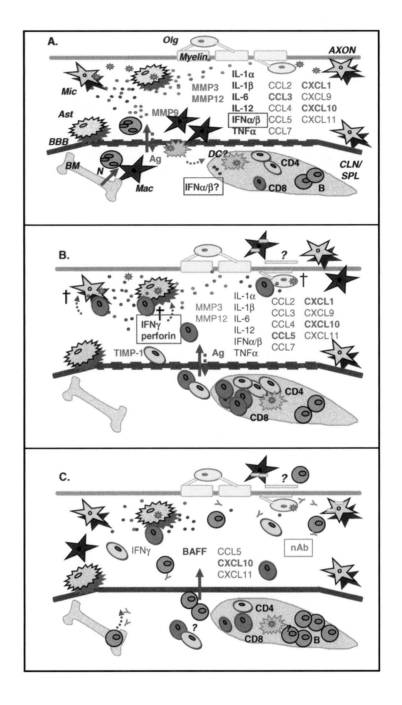

**Color Plate 6 (chapter 22).** Critical immune parameters controlling MHV infection within the CNS during the innate (A), acute (B), and persistent (C) stages of infection. Crucial effector molecules are boxed for each phase. (A) Infection by the MHV-JHM variant V2.2-1 is initiated in ependymal cells and spreads to glial cells, but only rarely to neurons. Microglia (Mic), macrophages (Mac), and astrocytes (Ast) are infected prior to oligodendrocytes (Olg), the cell type maintaining myelin and thus axonal function. Early viral replication induces expression of MMP-3 and MMP-12, as well as numerous chemokines (green) and cytokines (purple). The earliest chemokines detected are CCL3, CXCL1, and CXCL10. Neutrophils (N) and monocytes/macrophages (Mac) are recruited from the bone marrow (BM) as an integral part of the acute-phase response. By releasing MMP-9, N enhance breakdown of the extracellular matrix and facilitate subsequent entry of lymphocytes. Induction of type I IFN (boxed) is critical to stem initial viral spread, prior to expansion and recruitment of antiviral T cells. The extent to which DC subsets contribute to IFN-α/β secretion in lymphoid tissue is being investigated rigorously. Similarly, the migration pattern of DC detected in the CNS and CLN, as well as their acquisition of viral antigen, remains to be elucidated. (B) Viral antigen presentation in lymphoid tissue results in activation, expansion, and extravasation of virus-specific CD8 and CD4 T cells. Proinflammatory cytokines and chemokines act as guiding signals for recruitment to the site of infection. While CD8 T cells localize to parenchymal CNS sites, CD4 T cells initially remain perivascular, correlated with TIMP-1 production. CD8 T cells exert antiviral function via IFN-γ and perforin-mediated cytolytic pathways. IFN-γ is critical in control of viral replication and host survival, presumably by enhancing MHC molecule antigen presentation. The apparent resistance of oligodendrocytes to both perforin-mediated viral clearance and infection-induced apoptosis, contrasting with disintegration of myelin sheaths, remains an enigma. Nevertheless, T-cell effector function is tightly associated with macrophage/microglial activation and uptake of myelin debris. As T cells are recruited, viral replication diminishes and levels of MMPs, chemokines, and innate cytokines decline. CCL5 and CXCL10 expression remains prominent. (C) Despite control of infectious virus, virus persists in astrocytes and oligodendrocytes. There is little evidence of an antiviral role for T cells retained or still recruited during persistence, as cytolytic activity is lost and IFN-γ secretion is significantly reduced. Local Ab prevents viral recrudescence, which is achieved by accumulation and retention of virus-specific ASC (vASC). Accumulation of vASC in BM is modest, suggesting preferential recruitment to the CNS. Continued CXCL10 and up-regulation of the B-cell survival factor BAFF might underlie ongoing B-cell/ASC recruitment, differentiation, and survival. The vital humoral component keeping persistent virus in check is neutralizing Ab (nAb).

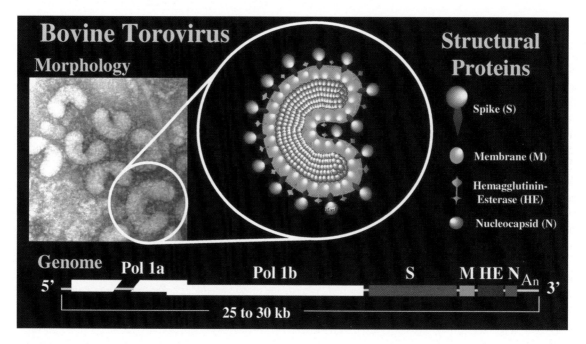

**Color Plate 7 (chapter 23).** Schematic representation of the typical extracellular morphology of torovirus (as visualized by EM) and its structural proteins and genome (single-stranded RNA of positive polarity, polyadenylated tail, and six open reading frames).

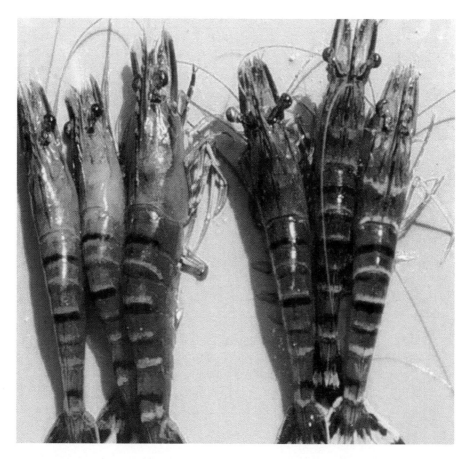

**Color Plate 8 (chapter 24).** Gross signs of YHD in the giant tiger shrimp (*Penaeus monodon*). The three diseased shrimp to the left display bleached yellowish discoloration of the cephalothorax caused by paleness of the underlying hepatopancreas and brownish discoloration of the gills. Photograph kindly supplied by T. W. Flegel, CENTEX Shrimp, Mahidol University, Bangkok, Thailand.

cytoplasm and the nucleus of infected cells. Moreover, only small quantities of the N proteins of these viruses home to the nucleolus, leading to a possible posttranslational modification of some molecules of N protein, such as phosphorylation, or modulation of host cell function (134), possibly common to all nidoviruses. Phosphorylation of the N protein of EAV (168) has long been known. As an initial step in determining a possible link between these observations, investigators first established through [$^{32}$P$_i$]orthophosphate labeling of virus-infected cells and subsequent immunoprecipitation that N protein phosphorylation also occurred in both genotypes of PRRSV (158). After determining that N protein phosphorylation occurred in the absence of other viral components, it was revealed that a cellular kinase was responsible and that the N protein of PRRSV type 2 strain PA8 was a serine phosphoprotein. Further cell fractionation studies established that equivalent amounts of N protein, labeled with [$^{35}$S]methionine or [$^{32}$P$_i$]orthophosphate and then immunoprecipitated, were found in the cytoplasm and nucleus of PRRSV-NA-infected MARC-145 cells as well as cells transfected with vaccinia virus expressing the PRRSV-NA N protein gene. A pulse-chase experiment designed to assess the kinetics of phosphorylation determined that N protein is rapidly phosphorylated after translation and was stable for at least 12 h after infection. Another series of studies examined whether multiple isoforms of the N protein existed. Following two types of two-dimensional isoelectric focusing and/or electrophoresis, the investigators were able to conclude that the N protein existed as only one isoform and was therefore not differentially phosphorylated despite containing multiple serine residues. The PRRSV-NA serine residue that participates in phosphorylation has not been identified. A final experiment revealed that the N protein is also phosphorylated in mature virions. The researchers concluded that the mechanism determining subcellular distribution was apparently not phosphorylation, since only one isoform of N protein existed in both the cytoplasm and nucleus of PRRSV-NA-infected cells. They also suggested that the biological function of N protein phosphorylation might be similar to what was found for mouse hepatitis virus, where upon virus entry into neutral endosomes, dephosphorylation of the N protein occurs, which is essential for uncoating and release of the viral RNA (70). However, since phosphorylation may also regulate dimer formation/oligomerization and PRRSV-NA N protein exists as a dimer in the mature virion (159), phosphorylation may be involved in dimerization and subsequent oligomerization of the N protein for capsid assembly.

Using various full-length, deletion, and mutated constructs of PRRSV type 2 strain SDSU-23983 N protein fused to EGFP and expressed in MARC-145 cells as well as alveolar macrophages, it was determined that both nuclear localization signals contained in N protein could serve to mediate transport to the nucleus and nucleolus but that residues 43-KKNKK formed the actual core localization domain, as determined by examination of full-length N protein (125). In addition, residues outside this core domain could also modulate nuclear localization. Through additional mutation and nuclear localization studies, it was also revealed that the first nuclear localization signal (10-KRKK) was prevented from its nuclear targeting action by the conformation of full-length N protein alone. Deletion of the C-terminal amino acids (and mutation of the second nuclear localization signal) uncovered this domain. In the same study, the researchers investigated whether the N protein interacted with importin-α and -β, cellular proteins shown to be critical for nuclear localization signal-dependent transport to the nucleus (60, 64, 103). Using GST pull-down assays, both importin shuttle proteins were shown to interact specifically with the N protein. There are two identified mechanisms for further transport to the nucleolus. One identified way is that after N protein obtains entrance into the nucleoplasm, a nucleolar targeting signal functioning through a specific interaction with another nucleolar component may mediate N protein transport to the nucleolus. Alternatively, translocation to the nucleolus is direct from the cytoplasm, occurring through cotransport with a nucleolar shuttle protein, such as fibrillarin. Further study showed that in PRRSV-NA, nucleolar localization was mediated by an unconventional nucleolar targeting sequence contained in amino acids 41 to 72 of the N protein. Subsequent to this, another research aim was to examine the ability of viral N protein to colocalize with the nucleolar molecule fibrillarin, which associates with RNA in uninfected cells (165). The study revealed that the N protein did not stain throughout the nucleolus but was instead found in clusters in the dense fibrillar component region. There was a direct colocalization of N protein with fibrillarin molecules in this area, but not in Cajal bodies, with which fibrillarin is also associated. In a yeast two-hybrid system, evidence that N protein may actually interact with fibrillarin was also obtained. The region on N protein and the region on fibrillarin were investigated through the use of protein deletion mutants. The results of GST fusion protein pull-down assays suggested that the region included in amino acids 30 to 37 of N protein was responsible for the interaction with fibrillarin, and the glycine-arginine rich domain in the N-terminal region of fibrillarin was associated with its interaction with the N protein. The N protein was also found to interact with PRRSV genomic RNA, and using deletions constructs, the investigators located the RNA-binding domain between residues 37 and 57 of the N protein, which overlaps one nucleolar localization signal. The N protein was also found to bind to both the 28S and 18S subunits of rRNA. Finally, the investigators provided evidence that RNA is required for the interaction of the N protein with fibrillarin, and both the phosphorylated and unphosphorylated forms of N protein can bind to RNA and fibrillarin. The authors concluded that N protein and fibrillarin may compete for the same rRNA substrate, potentially modifying fibrillarin function, or that N protein binding of nucleolar RNAs may lead to a conformational change in N protein facilitating a stable interaction with other nucleolar proteins. One such protein may be fibrillarin, and the binding of N protein would then serve to down-regulate a fibrillarin function such as RNA methylation.

The EAV N protein contains a potential nuclear export signal (NES) sequence starting at residue 54 (125), which may participate in the translocation of N protein from the nucleus into the cytoplasm through a cellular transporter protein (134). When investigating the mechanism for transport to and from the nucleus of EAV nonstructural protein 1, researchers discovered that the CRM1 transporter, inactivated by the drug leptomycin B, which blocks its interaction with NES-containing proteins, had an effect on N protein localization. EAV-infected BHK-21 cells were treated with 10 ng of leptomycin B per ml at various times both pre- and postinfection, and N protein was found to now accumulate only in the nucleus, which usually has only minor amounts of N protein during EAV infection. The authors suggested that perhaps all N protein is immediately targeted to the nucleus after translation and reasoned that it must be shuttled back to the cytoplasm to complete cytoplasmic virion assembly. Similar findings were recently reported for PRRSV (126). The PRRSV-NA N protein contains two regions that could be NES sequences, the region between amino acids 19 and 30 and the peptide starting at amino acid 106 (LPTHHTVRLIRV). PRRSV-EU has a very similar sequence (125, 126). Some evidence of the involvement of the C-terminal region of PRRSV-NA N protein in nuclear export was provided through MARC-145 cell transfection of an EGFP fusion protein expressing amino acids 90 to 123, which showed that localization could be modified to be mostly cytoplasmic (126).

Although several theories have been put forward, the biological function of N protein in the nucleus or nucleolus is presently unknown. Such theories include a viral strategy to divert biosynthetic resources, a novel innate protection strategy whereby the host cell would deplete viruses of an essential protein, and down-regulation of cellular functions such as RNA methylation (126, 134, 165). Alternatively, the N protein, because of its basic charge and function in the virus, is transported to the nucleus as a side effect of viral infection.

N is the only arteriviral structural protein that has been examined for its three-dimensional makeup (38, 39). The C-terminal half, representing the putative capsid-forming domain of residues 58 to 123, was expressed abundantly in *E. coli* by N-terminal fusion to a histidine tag and rigorously purified. The polypeptide was then crystallized, and the structure was subsequently analyzed by single-wavelength anomalous diffraction using the two sulfur groups located in the N protein segment and resolved to 2.6 Å. The capsid-forming region existed as a dimer in the crystal. Perhaps this structure represents a conformation similar to the authentic protein as detected in PRRSV-NA-infected cells (159). Monomeric N protein was found to contain two antiparallel β strands flanked by α helices (39). As a dimer, the four strands together form a continuous, flat antiparallel β-sheet floor, superposed by the two long α helices and flanked by two N- and two C-terminal α helices. The investigators suggested that the arteriviral N protein structure might present a novel class of viral capsid-forming domains that is so far unseen in other enveloped viruses.

## STRUCTURAL PROTEINS AND ARTERIVIRUS ENTRY

Arteriviruses have been suggested to enter cells through a receptor-mediated pathway. For LDV, Ia antigens were originally proposed to mediate attachment (67), but later studies suggested that the major receptor was not Ia (14). No viral receptor has been found for EAV on equine macrophages or for SHFV on simian macrophages. Attachment of the arteriviruses has been best described for PRRSV. Early studies suggested that PRRSV-EU has a restricted tropism for a subpopulation of porcine macrophages (43), just as was proposed for LDV (75), and the protein nature of the macrophage receptor was established by blocking binding of PRRSV with proteases (133). PRRSV-EU was also determined to enter cells by receptor-mediated endocytosis, and because the addition of cytochalasin D and because PRRSV and clathrin were determined to colocalize, virus uptake into vesicles was deemed a clathrin-dependent process (106). A 210-kDa membrane protein was first identified as a putative receptor for PRRSV (42). Heparin was shown to block PRRSV-EU and -NA replication, and treatment of MARC-145 cells as well as porcine alveolar macrophages with heparanase prevented PRRSV infection (31, 69). Investigators then established that a heparinlike receptor on macrophages (heparan sulfate) was a PRRSV ligand, and the viral proteins that bound to heparin-Sepharose included M protein and M protein disulfide bound to GP5 (31). It was noted, however, that another cellular molecule might be involved, as viral infection could not be totally blocked, and suggested that the 210-kDa protein noted previously may also be involved. Purification of the 210-kDa protein using a MAb that blocked binding of PRRSV, followed by tryptic digestion and mass spectrometry, established that the molecule was the porcine homolog of mouse sialoadhesin (139). Sialoadhesin was found to mediate PRRSV entry into nonpermissive cells and to participate in clathrin-mediated endocytosis. In later studies, it was found that sialoadhesin bound to sialic acid and that treatment of PRRSV with neuraminidase (to remove all sialic acid) or with N-glycosidase F (to remove all N-linked glycans) reduced PRRSV infection (30). Linkage-specific neuraminidase treatment established that 2-3- and 2-6-linked sialic acids on the virion are important for infection of porcine alveolar macrophages with PRRSV. Recent work by the same laboratory established that heparan sulfate and sialoadhesin have distinctive roles in attachment and internalization (29). When porcine alveolar macrophages were treated with both heparin and anti-sialoadhesin MAb at 4°C, 99% reduction in PRRSV attachment was seen. Based on the finding that either heparin or MAb alone could not completely abolish infection, the investigators surmised that heparan sulfate and sialoadhesin acted in attachment via different mechanisms. The researchers also concluded that because the added effect of the inhibitors completely abolished PRRSV infection, most likely heparan sulfate glycoaminoglycans and sialoadhesin were the only two cellular receptors on porcine alveolar macrophages. Heparan sulfate glycoaminoglycans was shown merely to attach and concentrate the virus onto the cell surface, but only sialoadhesin could serve for entry into permissive cells. Another group developed MAbs that also blocked PRRSV infection, finding that a 150-kDa polypeptide doublet and a 220-kDa protein were recognized by separate antibodies (155). Evidence was obtained that these two proteins were N glycosylated, and it thus appeared that perhaps multiple glycoproteins might be involved in PRRSV infection of porcine alveloar macrophages. Lastly, another group also reported that simian vimentin, a molecule expressed on the surface of MARC-145 cells, could render the nonsusceptible cell lines BHK-21 and CRFK susceptible to PRRSV

infection (74). Thus, PRRSV may utilize different cell surface molecules to establish infection of different cells, a notion that clearly must be evaluated further. The fact that arteriviruses have four glycoproteins available for attachment, entry, and uncoating suggests that the viruses use multiple ways, via perhaps different cell components, to infect permissive cells via receptor-mediated endocytosis.

## STRUCTURAL PROTEINS AND ARTERIVIRUS ASSEMBLY

A diagram of arterivirus replication, based mostly on the data obtained for PRRSV, is shown in Fig. 5. Predominant findings by several groups suggest that GP5, complexed in a disulfide interaction with M protein, is the major viral attachment protein. PRRSV GP5 has been the most well studied, and while the regions surrounding the core attachment domain (SHLQLIYNL) are hypervariable, only a limited number of residue alterations with the core domain are accepted. Alternatively, epitopes on other arterivirus glycoproteins such as GP4 may contribute to the initial binding by GP5, perhaps mediating another stage in virus entry. After attachment to heparan sulfate moieties, entry by noncovalent association with cellular sialoadhesin, uncoating (perhaps through a potential pore-forming protein such as E protein), subgenomic transcription ensues, followed by translation on ribosomes of the rough ER (RER). Following translation, N protein is phosphorylated on serine residues and begins to form homodimers and eventually multimers that encase the newly replicated full-length as well as defective interfering particles, presumably through a packaging signal. This packaging signal has been located near the N terminus of PRRSV ORF1a (166, 167) or near the 5' terminus and/or within ORF1b of EAV (100). N protein is also translocated to the nucleus and nucleolus of infected cells. Perhaps the ribonucleocapsid complex then migrates to places within the RER to associate noncovalently with the M and/or E protein cytoplasmic tail. In the RER, core N-glycan addition ensues for the major glycoprotein, GP5, as well as the minor glycoproteins, GP2 to GP4. At the same time, heterodimers of unglycosylated M protein disulfide bound to N-glycan-modified GP5 as well as heterodimers of GP2 and GP4 are formed, with an apparently noncovalent association of GP3 in a 1:1:1 ratio (151, 154). Since additional molecules of M are synthesized, it may be that these serve to shuttle associated N protein to sites of virion assembly. The role of E protein at this stage is unknown, but as it is an essential protein for EAV and PRRSV-EU infectivity, it must somehow

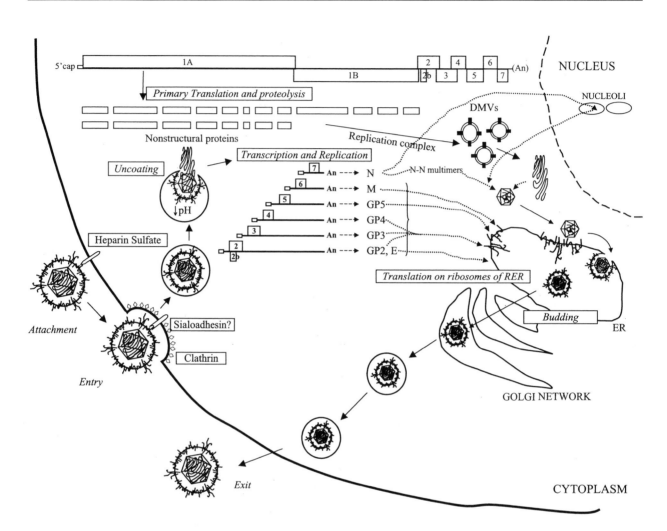

**Figure 5.** Model of arteriviral replication based primarily on PRRSV (see text for details).

interchelate with the other known components of the virus. Only when all structural components are localized to the same site is the ribonucleocapsid thought to begin transversing the membrane, eventually budding into the cisternae of the RER. It is thought that noncovalently associated molecules of N protein may become linked through cysteine residues (amino acid 23) as a consequence of attaining the oxidizing environment of the ER cisternae (159). This may mean that the nucleocapsid forms a tighter complex at this stage, perhaps attaining the conformational structure needed to fully protect the viral RNA and to stably interact with other proteins of the virion, such as E protein. As the newly formed immature virion now proceeds through the Golgi network, core high-mannose N-glycan residues on the glycoproteins are trimmed and replaced with complex sugars, such that EAV GP5 is modified by polylactosaminoglycans (36) while GP5 of PRRSV is terminally modified by complex sugars other than polylactosaminoglycans (88). In the Golgi network, the GP2/GP4 heterodimer may

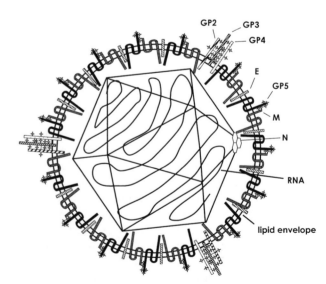

**Figure 6.** Schematic of the PRRSV virion. N-glycan addition for the glycoproteins (✧) varies for all arteriviruses.

also become covalently attached to GP3 via disulfide linkages, as shown for EAV and PRRSV-EU. However, the protein has not been detected in LDV mature virions, and only minimal amounts of PRRSV-NA GP3 have been found in extracellular virus. It is assumed that the virus is released to the extracellular space, as cytopathic effect does not appear until after a substantial quantity of nascent virus is released. PRRSV virions are released as 52- to 70-nm spherical particles (30), LDV as 62- to 80-nm particles (68), SHFV as 45- to 50-nm particles (138), and EAV as 50- to 70-nm particles (37). A diagram of a PRRSV virion is shown in Fig. 6. One replication cycle takes 4 to 6 h for the arteriviruses studied, with maximum virus yield at 16 hours postinfection (hpi) for LDV (120), 60 hpi for PRRSV-NA strain VR-2332 and PRRSV-EU strain LV viruses grown on MA-104 cells, and 36 hpi for virulent strains of EAV on primary equine cells (102). No information was found for SHFV. Arteriviruses, as far as is known, have no visible effect on translation of cellular proteins.

## REFERENCES

1. Ansari, I. H., B. Kwon, F. A. Osorio, and A. K. Pattnaik. 2006. Influence of N-linked glycosylation of porcine reproductive and respiratory syndrome virus GP5 on virus infectivity, antigenicity, and ability to induce neutralizing antibodies. *J. Virol.* 80:3994–4004.

2. Balasuriya, U. B., J. C. Dobbe, H. W. Heidner, V. L. Smalley, A. Navarrette, E. J. Snijder, and N. J. MacLachlan. 2004. Characterization of the neutralization determinants of equine arteritis virus using recombinant chimeric viruses and site-specific mutagenesis of an infectious cDNA clone. *Virology* 321:235–246.

3. Balasuriya, U. B., J. F. Hedges, V. L. Smalley, A. Navarrette, W. H. McCollum, P. J. Timoney, E. J. Snijder, and N. J. MacLachlan. 2004. Genetic characterization of equine arteritis virus during persistent infection of stallions. *J. Gen. Virol.* 85:379–390.

4. Balasuriya, U. B., H. W. Heidner, J. F. Hedges, J. C. Williams, N. L. Davis, R. E. Johnston, and N. J. MacLachlan. 2000. Expression of the two major envelope proteins of equine arteritis virus as a heterodimer is necessary for induction of neutralizing antibodies in mice immunized with recombinant Venezuelan equine encephalitis virus replicon particles. *J. Virol.* 74:10623–10630.

5. Balasuriya, U. B., and N. J. MacLachlan. 2004. The immune response to equine arteritis virus: potential lessons for other arteriviruses. *Vet. Immunol. Immunopathol.* 102:107–129.

6. Balasuriya, U. B., N. J. Maclachlan, A. A. De Vries, P. V. Rossitto, and P. J. Rottier. 1995. Identification of a neutralization site in the major envelope glycoprotein (GL) of equine arteritis virus. *Virology* 207:518–527.

7. Balasuriya, U. B., J. F. Patton, P. V. Rossitto, P. J. Timoney, W. H. McCollum, and N. J. MacLachlan. 1997. Neutralization determinants of laboratory strains and field isolates of equine arteritis virus: identification of four neutralization sites in the amino-terminal ectodomain of the G(L) envelope glycoprotein. *Virology* 232:114–128.

8. Balasuriya, U. B., P. V. Rossitto, C. D. DeMaula, and N. J. MacLachlan. 1993. A 29K envelope glycoprotein of equine

arteritis virus expresses neutralization determinants recognized by murine monoclonal antibodies. *J. Gen. Virol.* 74:2525–2529.

9. Bastos, R. G., O. A. Dellagostin, R. G. Barletta, A. R. Doster, E. Nelson, and F. A. Osorio. 2002. Construction and immunogenicity of recombinant Mycobacterium bovis BCG expressing GP5 and M protein of porcine reproductive respiratory syndrome virus. *Vaccine* 21:21–29.

10. Bastos, R. G., O. A. Dellagostin, R. G. Barletta, A. R. Doster, E. Nelson, F. Zuckermann, and F. A. Osorio. 2004. Immune response of pigs inoculated with Mycobacterium bovis BCG expressing a truncated form of GP5 and M protein of porcine reproductive and respiratory syndrome virus. *Vaccine* 22:467–474.

11. Bautista, E. M., J. J. Meulenberg, C. S. Choi, and T. W. Molitor.. 1996. Structural polypeptides of the American (VR-2332) strain of porcine reproductive and respiratory syndrome virus. *Arch. Virol.* 141:1357–1365.

12. Brinton, M. A., E. I. Gavin, and A. V. Fernandez. 1986. Genotypic variation among six isolates of lactate dehydrogenase-elevating virus. *J. Gen. Virol.* 67:2673–2684.

13. Brinton-Darnell, M., and P. G. Plagemann. 1975. Structure and chemical-physical characteristics of lactate dehydrogenase-elevating virus and its RNA. *J. Virol.* 16:420–433.

14. Buxton, I. K., S. P. Chan, and P. G. Plagemann. 1988. The IA antigen is not the major receptor for lactate dehydrogenase-elevating virus on macrophages from CBA and BALB/c mice. *Virus Res.* 9:205–219.

15. Cafruny, W. A., S. P. Chan, J. T. Harty, S. Yousefi, K. Kowalchyk, D. McDonald, B. Foreman, G. Budweg, and P. G. Plagemann. 1986. Antibody response of mice to lactate dehydrogenase-elevating virus during infection and immunization with inactivated virus. *Virus Res.* 5:357–375.

16. Cafruny, W. A., and P. G. Plagemann. 1982. Immune response to lactate dehydrogenase-elevating virus: serologically specific rabbit neutralizing antibody to the virus. *Infect. Immun.* 37:1007–1012.

17. Chen, Z., L. Kuo, R. R. Rowland, C. Even, K. S. Faaberg, and P. G. Plagemann. 1993. Sequences of 3′ end of genome and of 5′ end of open reading frame 1a of lactate dehydrogenase-elevating virus and common junction motifs between 5′ leader and bodies of seven subgenomic mRNAs. *J. Gen. Virol.* 74:643–659.

18. Chen, Z., K. Li, and P. G. Plagemann. 2000. Neuropathogenicity and sensitivity to antibody neutralization of lactate dehydrogenase-elevating virus are determined by polylactosaminoglycan chains on the primary envelope glycoprotein. *Virology* 266:88–98.

19. Chen, Z., K. Li, R. R. Rowland, and P. G. Plagemann. 1999. Selective antibody neutralization prevents neuropathogenic lactate dehydrogenase-elevating virus from causing paralytic disease in immunocompetent mice. *J. Neurovirol.* 5:200–208.

20. Cheon, D. S., and C. Chae. 2000. Antigenic variation and genotype of isolates of porcine reproductive and respiratory syndrome virus in Korea. *Vet. Rec.* 147:215–218.

21. Chirnside, E. D., A. A. de Vries, J. A. Mumford, and P. J. Rottier. 1995. Equine arteritis virus-neutralizing antibody in the horse is induced by a determinant on the large envelope glycoprotein GL. *J. Gen. Virol.* 76:1989–1998.

22. Chirnside, E. D., P. M. Francis, and J. A. Mumford. 1995. Expression cloning and antigenic analysis of the nucleocapsid protein of equine arteritis virus. *Virus Res.* 39:277–288.

23. Contag, C. H., E. F. Retzel, and P. G. Plagemann. 1986. Genomic differences between strains of lactate dehydrogenase-elevating virus. *Intervirology* 26:228–233.

24. Conzelmann, K. K., N. Visser, P. Van Woensel, and H. J. Thiel. 1993. Molecular characterization of porcine reproductive and

respiratory syndrome virus, a member of the arterivirus group. *Virology* **193:**329–339.

25. Coutelier, J. P., and J. Van Snick. 1988. Neutralization and sensitization of lactate dehydrogenase-elevating virus with monoclonal antibodies. *J. Gen. Virol.* **69:**2097–2100.

26. Dea, S., C. A. Gagnon, H. Mardassi, and G. Milane. 1996. Antigenic variability among North American and European strains of porcine reproductive and respiratory syndrome virus as defined by monoclonal antibodies to the matrix protein. *J. Clin. Microbiol.* **34:**1488–1493.

27. Dea, S., C. A. Gagnon, H. Mardassi, B. Pirzadeh, and D. Rogan. 2000. Current knowledge on the structural proteins of porcine reproductive and respiratory syndrome (PRRS) virus: comparison of the North American and European isolates. *Arch. Virol.* **145:**659–688.

28. de Haan, C. A., H. Vennema, and P. J. Rottier. 2000. Assembly of the coronavirus envelope: homotypic interactions between the M proteins. *J. Virol.* **74:**4967–4978.

29. Delputte, P. L., S. Costers, and H. J. Nauwynck. 2005. Analysis of porcine reproductive and respiratory syndrome virus attachment and internalization: distinctive roles for heparan sulphate and sialoadhesin. *J. Gen. Virol.* **86:**1441–1445.

30. Delputte, P. L., and H. J. Nauwynck. 2004. Porcine arterivirus infection of alveolar macrophages is mediated by sialic acid on the virus. *J. Virol.* **78:**8094–8101.

31. Delputte, P. L., N. Vanderheijden, H. J. Nauwynck, and M. B. Pensaert. 2002. Involvement of the matrix protein in attachment of porcine reproductive and respiratory syndrome virus to a heparinlike receptor on porcine alveolar macrophages. *J. Virol.* **76:**4312–4320.

32. den Boon, J. A., M. F. Kleijnen, W. J. Spaan, and E. J. Snijder. 1996. Equine arteritis virus subgenomic mRNA synthesis: analysis of leader-body junctions and replicative-form RNAs. *J. Virol.* **70:**4291–4298.

33. den Boon, J. A., E. J. Snijder, E. D. Chirnside, A. A. de Vries, M. C. Horzinek, and W. J. Spaan. 1991. Equine arteritis virus is not a togavirus but belongs to the coronaviruslike superfamily. *J. Virol.* **65:**2910–2920.

34. Deregt, D., A. A. de Vries, M. J. Raamsman, L. D. Elmgren, and P. J. Rottier. 1994. Monoclonal antibodies to equine arteritis virus proteins identify the GL protein as a target for virus neutralization. *J. Gen. Virol.* **75:**2439–2444.

35. de Vries, A. A., E. D. Chirnside, M. C. Horzinek, and P. J. Rottier. 1992. Structural proteins of equine arteritis virus. *J. Virol.* **66:**6294–6303.

36. de Vries, A. A., S. M. Post, M. J. Raamsman, M. C. Horzinek, and P. J. Rottier. 1995. The two major envelope proteins of equine arteritis virus associate into disulfide-linked heterodimers. *J. Virol.* **69:**4668–4674.

37. Dimmock, N. J. 1993. Neutralization of animal viruses. *Curr. Top. Microbiol. Immunol.* **183:**1–149.

38. Doan, D. N., and T. Dokland. 2003. Cloning, expression, purification, crystallization and preliminary X-ray diffraction analysis of the structural domain of the nucleocapsid N protein from porcine reproductive and respiratory syndrome virus (PRRSV). *Acta Crystallogr. Sect. D* **59:**1504–1506.

39. Doan, D. N., and T. Dokland. 2003. Structure of the nucleocapsid protein of porcine reproductive and respiratory syndrome virus. *Structure* **11:**1445–1451.

40. Dobbe, J. C., Y. van der Meer, W. J. Spaan, and E. J. Snijder. 2001. Construction of chimeric arteriviruses reveals that the ectodomain of the major glycoprotein is not the main determinant of equine arteritis virus tropism in cell culture. *Virology* **288:**283–294.

41. Drew, T. W., J. J. Meulenberg, J. J. Sands, and D. J. Paton. 1995. Production, characterization and reactivity of monoclonal antibodies to porcine reproductive and respiratory syndrome virus. *J. Gen. Virol.* **76:**1361–1369.

42. Duan, X., H. J. Nauwynck, H. W. Favoreel, and M. B. Pensaert. 1998. Identification of a putative receptor for porcine reproductive and respiratory syndrome virus on porcine alveolar macrophages. *J. Virol.* **72:**4520–4523.

43. Duan, X., H. J. Nauwynck, and M. B. Pensaert. 1997. Effects of origin and state of differentiation and activation of monocytes/macrophages on their susceptibility to porcine reproductive and respiratory syndrome virus (PRRSV). *Arch. Virol.* **142:**2483–2497.

44. Eisenberg, D., E. Schwarz, M. Komaromy, and R. Wall. 1984. Analysis of membrane and surface protein sequences with the hydrophobic moment plot. *J. Mol. Biol.* **179:**125–142.

45. Faaberg, K. S., C. Even, G. A. Palmer, and P. G. Plagemann. 1995. Disulfide bonds between two envelope proteins of lactate dehydrogenase-elevating virus are essential for viral infectivity. *J. Virol.* **69:**613–617.

46. Faaberg, K. S., C. J. Nelsen, and T. M. Truong. 1998. Effects of 5′ and 3′ untranslated regions on *in vitro* expression of porcine reproductive and respiratory syndrome virus (PRRSV) mRNA7, abstr. W33-6. *Abstr. 17th Annu. Meet. Am. Soc. Virol.*

47. Faaberg, K. S., G. A. Palmer, C. Even, G. W. Anderson, and P. G. Plagemann. 1995. Differential glycosylation of the ectodomain of the primary envelope glycoprotein of two strains of lactate dehydrogenase-elevating virus that differ in neuropathogenicity. *Virus Res.* **39:**331–340.

48. Faaberg, K. S., and P. G. Plagemann. 1995. The envelope proteins of lactate dehydrogenase-elevating virus and their membrane topography. *Virology* **212:**512–525.

49. Faaberg, K. S., and P. G. Plagemann. 1997. ORF 3 of lactate dehydrogenase-elevating virus encodes a soluble, nonstructural, highly glycosylated, and antigenic protein. *Virology* **227:**245–251.

50. Forsberg, R., M. B. Oleksiewicz, A. M. Petersen, J. Hein, A. Botner, and T. Storgaard. 2001. A molecular clock dates the common ancestor of European-type porcine reproductive and respiratory syndrome virus at more than 10 years before the emergence of disease. *Virology* **289:**174–179.

51. Gagnon, C. A., and S. Dea. 1998. Differentiation between porcine reproductive and respiratory syndrome virus isolates by restriction fragment length polymorphism of their ORFs 6 and 7 genes. *Can. J. Vet. Res.* **62:**110–116.

52. Glaser, A. L., A. A. de Vries, and E. J. Dubovi. 1995. Comparison of equine arteritis virus isolates using neutralizing monoclonal antibodies and identification of sequence changes in GL associated with neutralization resistance. *J. Gen. Virol.* **76:**2223–2233.

53. Godeny, E. K., L. Chen, S. N. Kumar, S. L. Methven, E. V. Koonin, and M. A. Brinton. 1993. Complete genomic sequence and phylogenetic analysis of the lactate dehydrogenase-elevating virus (LDV). *Virology* **194:**585–596.

54. Godeny, E. K., A. A. de Vries, X. C. Wang, S. L. Smith, and R. J. de Groot. 1998. Identification of the leader-body junctions for the viral subgenomic mRNAs and organization of the simian hemorrhagic fever virus genome: evidence for gene duplication during arterivirus evolution. *J. Virol.* **72:**862–867.

55. Godeny, E. K., D. W. Speicher, and M. A. Brinton. 1990. Map location of lactate dehydrogenase-elevating virus (LDV) capsid protein (Vp1) gene. *Virology* **177:**768–771.

56. Godeny, E. K., M. R. Werner, and M. A. Brinton. 1989. The 3′ terminus of lactate dehydrogenase-elevating virus genome RNA does not contain togavirus or flavivirus conserved sequences. *Virology* **172:**647–650.

57. Godeny, E. K., L. Zeng, S. L. Smith, and M. A. Brinton. 1995. Molecular characterization of the 3′ terminus of the

simian hemorrhagic fever virus genome. *J. Virol.* **69:**2679–2683.

58. Gonin, P., H. Mardassi, C. A. Gagnon, B. Massie, and S. Dea. 1998. A nonstructural and antigenic glycoprotein is encoded by ORF3 of the IAF-Klop strain of porcine reproductive and respiratory syndrome virus. *Arch. Virol.* **143:**1927–1940.

59. Gonin, P., B. Pirzadeh, C. A. Gagnon, and S. Dea. 1999. Seroneutralization of porcine reproductive and respiratory syndrome virus correlates with antibody response to the GP5 major envelope glycoprotein. *J. Vet. Diagn. Investig.* **11:**20–26.

60. Gorlich, D., and I. W. Mattaj. 1996. Nucleocytoplasmic transport. *Science* **271:**1513–1518.

61. Harty, J. T., and P. G. Plagemann. 1988. Formalin inactivation of the lactate dehydrogenase-elevating virus reveals a major neutralizing epitope not recognized during natural infection. *J. Virol.* **62:**3210–3216.

62. Hedges, J. F., U. B. Balasuriya, and N. J. MacLachlan. 1999. The open reading frame 3 of equine arteritis virus encodes an immunogenic glycosylated, integral membrane protein. *Virology* **264:**92–98.

63. Hedges, J. F., U. B. Balasuriya, P. J. Timoney, W. H. McCollum, and N. J. MacLachlan. 1999. Genetic divergence with emergence of novel phenotypic variants of equine arteritis virus during persistent infection of stallions. *J. Virol.* **73:**3672–3681.

64. Henderson, B. R., and P. Percipalle. 1997. Interactions between HIV Rev and nuclear import and export factors: the Rev nuclear localisation signal mediates specific binding to human importin-beta. *J. Mol. Biol.* **274:**693–707.

65. Hiscox, J. A., T. Wurm, L. Wilson, P. Britton, D. Cavanagh, and G. Brooks. 2001. The coronavirus infectious bronchitis virus nucleoprotein localizes to the nucleolus. *J. Virol.* **75:**506–512.

66. Horzinek, M. C., and P. S. Wielink. 1975. Purification and electron microscopy of lactic dehydrogenase virus of mice. *J. Gen. Virol.* **26:**217–226.

67. Inada, T., and C. A. Mims. 1984. Mouse Ia antigens are receptors for lactate dehydrogenase virus. *Nature* **309:**59–61.

68. Jeronimo, C., and D. Archambault. 2002. Importance of M-protein C terminus as substrate antigen for serodetection of equine arteritis virus infection. *Clin. Diagn. Lab. Immunol.* **9:**698–703.

69. Jusa, E. R., Y. Inaba, M. Kouno, and O. Hirose. 1997. Effect of heparin on infection of cells by porcine reproductive and respiratory syndrome virus. *Am J. Vet. Res.* **58:**488–491.

70. Kalicharran, K., D. Mohandas, G. Wilson, and S. Dales. 1996. Regulation of the initiation of coronavirus JHM infection in primary oligodendrocytes and L-2 fibroblasts. *Virology* **225:**33–43.

71. Kapur, V., M. R. Elam, T. M. Pawlovich, and M. P. Murtaugh. 1996. Genetic variation in porcine reproductive and respiratory syndrome virus isolates in the midwestern United States. *J. Gen. Virol.* **77:**1271–1276.

72. Katz, J. B., A. L. Shafer, K. A. Eernisse, J. G. Landgraf, and E. A. Nelson. 1995. Antigenic differences between European and American isolates of porcine reproductive and respiratory syndrome virus (PRRSV) are encoded by the carboxyterminal portion of viral open reading frame 3. *Vet. Microbiol.* **44:**65–76.

73. Kheyar, A., S. Martin, G. St-Laurent, P. J. Timoney, W. H. McCollum, and D. Archambault. 1997. Expression cloning and humoral immune response to the nucleocapsid and membrane proteins of equine arteritis virus. *Clin. Diagn. Lab. Immunol.* **4:**648–652.

74. Kim, J. K., A. M. Fahad, K. Shanmukhappa, and S. Kapil. 2006. Defining the cellular target(s) of porcine reproductive

75. Kowalchyk, K., and P. G. Plagemann. 1985. Cell surface receptors for lactate dehydrogenase-elevating virus on subpopulation of macrophages. *Virus Res.* **2:**211–229.

76. Krogh, A., B. Larsson, G. von Heijne, and E. L. Sonnhammer. 2001. Predicting transmembrane protein topology with a hidden Markov model: application to complete genomes. *J. Mol. Biol.* **305:**567–580.

77. Kuo, L., Z. Chen, R. R. Rowland, K. S. Faaberg, and P. G. Plagemann. 1992. Lactate dehydrogenase-elevating virus (LDV): subgenomic mRNAs, mRNA leader and comparison of 3′-terminal sequences of two LDV isolates. *Virus Res.* **23:**55–72.

78. Kwang, J., F. Zuckermann, G. Ross, S. Yang, F. Osorio, W. Liu, and S. Low. 1999. Antibody and cellular immune responses of swine following immunisation with plasmid DNA encoding the PRRS virus ORF9s 4, 5, 6 and 7. *Res. Vet. Sci.* **67:**199–201.

79. Lee, C., and D. Yoo. 2005. Cysteine residues of the porcine reproductive and respiratory syndrome virus small envelope protein are non-essential for virus infectivity. *J. Gen. Virol.* **86:**3091–3096.

80. Li, K., Z. Chen, and P. Plagemann. 1998. The neutralization epitope of lactate dehydrogenase-elevating virus is located on the short ectodomain of the primary envelope glycoprotein. *Virology* **242:**239–245.

81. Li, X., B. Hu, J. Harty, C. Even, and P. G. Plagemann. 1990. Polyclonal B cell activation of IgG2a and IgG2b production by infection of mice with lactate dehydrogenase-elevating virus is partly dependent on CD4+ lymphocytes. *Viral Immunol.* **3:**273–288.

82. Lin, Y. C., R. Y. Chang, and L. L. Chueh. 2002. Leader-body junction sequence of the viral subgenomic mRNAs of porcine reproductive and respiratory syndrome virus isolated in Taiwan. *J. Vet. Med. Sci.* **64:**961–965.

83. Lipman, D. J., and W. R. Pearson. 1985. Rapid and sensitive protein similarity searches. *Science* **227:**1435–1441.

84. Magar, R., R. Larochelle, S. Dea, C. A. Gagnon, E. A. Nelson, J. Christopher-Hennings, and D. A. Benfield. 1995. Antigenic comparison of Canadian and US isolates of porcine reproductive and respiratory syndrome virus using monoclonal antibodies to the nucleocapsid protein. *Can. J. Vet. Res.* **59:**232–234.

85. Magar, R., R. Larochelle, E. A. Nelson, and C. Charreyre. 1997. Differential reactivity of a monoclonal antibody directed to the membrane protein of porcine reproductive and respiratory syndrome virus. *Can. J. Vet. Res.* **61:**69–71.

86. Mardassi, H., R. Athanassious, S. Mounir, and S. Dea. 1994. Porcine reproductive and respiratory syndrome virus: morphological, biochemical and serological characteristics of Quebec isolates associated with acute and chronic outbreaks of porcine reproductive and respiratory syndrome. *Can. J. Vet. Res.* **58:**55–64.

87. Mardassi, H., P. Gonin, C. A. Gagnon, B. Massie, and S. Dea. 1998. A subset of porcine reproductive and respiratory syndrome virus GP3 glycoprotein is released into the culture medium of cells as a non-virion-associated and membrane-free (soluble) form. *J. Virol.* **72:**6298–6306.

88. Mardassi, H., B. Massie, and S. Dea. 1996. Intracellular synthesis, processing, and transport of proteins encoded by ORFs 5 to 7 of porcine reproductive and respiratory syndrome virus. *Virology* **221:**98–112.

89. Mardassi, H., S. Mounir, and S. Dea. 1995. Molecular analysis of the ORFs 3 to 7 of porcine reproductive and respiratory

syndrome virus, Quebec reference strain. *Arch. Virol.* **140:**1405–1418.

90. **Meng, X. J., P. S. Paul, and P. G. Halbur.** 1994. Molecular cloning and nucleotide sequencing of the 3'-terminal genomic RNA of the porcine reproductive and respiratory syndrome virus. *J. Gen. Virol.* **75:**1795–1801.

91. **Meng, X. J., P. S. Paul, P. G. Halbur, and I. Morozov.** 1995. Sequence comparison of open reading frames 2 to 5 of low and high virulence United States isolates of porcine reproductive and respiratory syndrome virus. *J. Gen. Virol.* **76:**3181–3188.

92. **Meulenberg, J. J., M. M. Hulst, E. J. de Meijer, P. L. Moonen, A. den Besten, E. P. de Kluyver, G. Wensvoort, and R. J. Moormann.** 1993. Lelystad virus, the causative agent of porcine epidemic abortion and respiratory syndrome (PEARS), is related to LDV and EAV. *Virology* **192:**62–72.

93. **Meulenberg, J. J., M. M. Hulst, E. J. de Meijer, P. L. Moonen, A. den Besten, E. P. de Kluyver, G. Wensvoort, and R. J. Moormann.** 1994. Lelystad virus belongs to a new virus family, comprising lactate dehydrogenase-elevating virus, equine arteritis virus, and simian hemorrhagic fever virus. *Arch. Virol. Suppl.* **9:**441–448.

94. **Meulenberg, J. J., and A. Petersen-den Besten.** 1996. Identification and characterization of a sixth structural protein of Lelystad virus: the glycoprotein GP2 encoded by ORF2 is incorporated in virus particles. *Virology* **225:**44–51.

95. **Meulenberg, J. J., A. Petersen-den Besten, E. P. De Kluyver, R. J. Moormann, W. M. Schaaper, and G. Wensvoort.** 1995. Characterization of proteins encoded by ORFs 2 to 7 of Lelystad virus. *Virology* **206:**155–163.

96. **Meulenberg, J. J., A. P. van Nieuwstadt, A. van Essen-Zandbergen, J. N. Bos-de Ruijter, J. P. Langeveld, and R. H. Meloen.** 1998. Localization and fine mapping of antigenic sites on the nucleocapsid protein N of porcine reproductive and respiratory syndrome virus with monoclonal antibodies. *Virology* **252:**106–114.

97. **Meulenberg, J. J., A. P. van Nieuwstadt, A. van Essen-Zandbergen, and J. P. M. Langeveld.** 1997. Posttranslational processing and identification of a neutralization domain of the GP$_4$ protein encoded by ORF4 of Lelystad virus. *J. Virol.* **71:**6061–6067.

98. **Michaelides, M. C., and S. Schlesinger.** 1973. Structural proteins of lactic dehydrogenase virus. *Virology* **55:**211–217.

99. **Mickelson, D. J., and K. S. Faaberg.** 1999. Effects of 5' and 3' untranslated regions on *in vitro* expression of porcine reproductive and respiratory syndrome virus (PRRSV) mRNA2, abstr. W13-1. *Abstr. 18th Annu. Meet. Am. Soc. Virol.*

100. **Molenkamp, R., B. C. Rozier, S. Greve, W. J. Spaan, and E. J. Snijder.** 2000. Isolation and characterization of an arterivirus defective interfering RNA genome. *J. Virol.* **74:**3156–3165.

101. **Molenkamp, R., H. van Tol, B. C. Rozier, Y. van der Meer, W. J. Spaan, and E. J. Snijder.** 2000. The arterivirus replicase is the only viral protein required for genome replication and subgenomic mRNA transcription. *J. Gen. Virol.* **81:**2491–2496.

102. **Moore, B. D., U. B. Balasuriya, J. F. Hedges, and N. J. MacLachlan.** 2002. Growth characteristics of a highly virulent, a moderately virulent, and an avirulent strain of equine arteritis virus in primary equine endothelial cells are predictive of their virulence to horses. *Virology* **298:**39–44.

103. **Moroianu, J., G. Blobel, and A. Radu.** 1996. The binding site of karyopherin alpha for karyopherin beta overlaps with a nuclear localization sequence. *Proc. Natl. Acad. Sci. USA* **93:**6572–6576.

104. **Murphy, T. W., W. H. McCollum, P. J. Timoney, B. W. Klingeborn, B. Hyllseth, W. Golnik, and B. Erasmus.** 1992. Genomic variability among globally distributed isolates of equine arteritis virus. *Vet. Microbiol.* **32:**101–115.

105. **Murtaugh, M. P., M. R. Elam, and L. T. Kakach.** 1995. Comparison of the structural protein coding sequences of the VR-2332 and Lelystad virus strains of the PRRS virus. *Arch. Virol.* **140:**1451–1460.

106. **Nauwynck, H. J., X. Duan, H. W. Favoreel, P. Van Oostveldt, and M. B. Pensaert.** 1999. Entry of porcine reproductive and respiratory syndrome virus into porcine alveolar macrophages via receptor-mediated endocytosis. *J. Gen. Virol.* **80:**297–305.

107. **Nelsen, C. J., M. P. Murtaugh, and K. S. Faaberg.** 1999. Porcine reproductive and respiratory syndrome virus comparison: divergent evolution on two continents. *J. Virol.* **73:**270–280.

108. **Nelson, E. A., J. Christopher-Hennings, T. Drew, G. Wensvoort, J. E. Collins, and D. A. Benfield.** 1993. Differentiation of U.S. and European isolates of porcine reproductive and respiratory syndrome virus by monoclonal antibodies. *J. Clin. Microbiol.* **31:**3184–3189.

109. **Nielsen, H. S., G. Liu, J. Nielsen, M. B. Oleksiewicz, A. Botner, T. Storgaard, and K. S. Faaberg.** 2003. Generation of an infectious clone of VR-2332, a highly virulent North American-type isolate of porcine reproductive and respiratory syndrome virus. *J. Virol.* **77:**3702–3711.

110. **Ostrowski, M., J. A. Galeota, A. M. Jar, K. B. Platt, F. A. Osorio, and O. J. Lopez.** 2002. Identification of neutralizing and nonneutralizing epitopes in the porcine reproductive and respiratory syndrome virus GP5 ectodomain. *J. Virol.* **76:**4241–4250.

111. **Palmer, G. A., L. Kuo, Z. Chen, K. S. Faaberg, and P. G. Plagemann.** 1995. Sequence of the genome of lactate dehydrogenase-elevating virus: heterogenicity between strains P and C. *Virology* **209:**637–642.

112. **Pasternak, A. O., A. P. Gultyaev, W. J. Spaan, and E. J. Snijder.** 2000. Genetic manipulation of arterivirus alternative mRNA leader-body junction sites reveals tight regulation of structural protein expression. *J. Virol.* **74:**11642–11653.

113. **Pirzadeh, B., and S. Dea.** 1997. Monoclonal antibodies to the ORF5 product of porcine reproductive and respiratory syndrome virus define linear neutralizing determinants. *J. Gen. Virol.* **78:**1867–1873.

114. **Pirzadeh, B., and S. Dea.** 1998. Immune response in pigs vaccinated with plasmid DNA encoding ORF5 of porcine reproductive and respiratory syndrome virus. *J. Gen. Virol.* **79:**989–999.

115. **Pirzadeh, B., C. A. Gagnon, and S. Dea.** 1998. Genomic and antigenic variations of porcine reproductive and respiratory syndrome virus major envelope GP5 glycoprotein. *Can. J. Vet. Res.* **62:**170–177.

116. **Plagemann, P. G.** 2001. An ORF-2a protein is not present at a significant level in virions of the arterivirus lactate dehydrogenase-elevating virus. *Virus Res.* **74:**47–52.

117. **Plagemann, P. G.** 2001. Complexity of the single linear neutralization epitope of the mouse arterivirus lactate dehydrogenase-elevating virus. *Virology* **290:**11–20.

118. **Plagemann, P. G.** 2004. The primary GP5 neutralization epitope of North American isolates of porcine reproductive and respiratory syndrome virus. *Vet. Immunol. Immunopathol.* **102:**263–275.

119. **Plagemann, P. G., J. T. Harty, and C. Even.** 1992. Mode of neutralization of lactate dehydrogenase-elevating virus by polyclonal and monoclonal antibodies. *Arch. Virol.* **123:**89–100.

120. Plagemann, P. G., R. R. Rowland, C. Even, and K. S. Faaberg. 1995. Lactate dehydrogenase-elevating virus: an ideal persistent virus? *Springer Semin. Immunopathol.* **17**:167–186.

121. Plagemann, P. G., R. R. Rowland, and K. S. Faaberg. 2002. The primary neutralization epitope of porcine respiratory and reproductive syndrome virus strain VR-2332 is located in the middle of the GP5 ectodomain. *Arch. Virol.* **147**:2327–2347.

122. Qian, P., X. Li, G. Tong, and H. Chen. 2003. High-level expression of the ORF6 gene of porcine reproductive and respiratory syndrome virus (PRRSV) in Pichia pastoris. *Virus Genes* **27**:189–196.

123. Rodriguez, M. J., J. Sarraseca, J. Garcia, A. Sanz, J. Plana-Duran, and J. Ignacio Casal. 1997. Epitope mapping of the nucleocapsid protein of European and North American isolates of porcine reproductive and respiratory syndrome virus. *J. Gen. Virol.* **78**:2269–2278.

124. Rowland, R. R., R. Kervin, C. Kuckleburg, A. Sperlich, and D. A. Benfield. 1999. The localization of porcine reproductive and respiratory syndrome virus nucleocapsid protein to the nucleolus of infected cells and identification of a potential nucleolar localization signal sequence. *Virus Res.* **64**:1–12.

125. Rowland, R. R., P. Schneider, Y. Fang, S. Wootton, D. Yoo, and D. A. Benfield. 2003. Peptide domains involved in the localization of the porcine reproductive and respiratory syndrome virus nucleocapsid protein to the nucleolus. *Virology* **316**:135–145.

126. Rowland, R. R., and D. Yoo. 2003. Nucleolar-cytoplasmic shuttling of PRRSV nucleocapsid protein: a simple case of molecular mimicry or the complex regulation by nuclear import, nucleolar localization and nuclear export signal sequences. *Virus Res.* **95**:23–33.

127. Siddell, S. G. 1995. *The Coronaviridae.* Plenum Press, New York, NY.

128. Smith, S. L., X. Wang, and E. K. Godeny. 1997. Sequence of the 3' end of the simian hemorrhagic fever virus genome. *Gene* **191**:205–210.

129. Snijder, E. J., J. C. Dobbe, and W. J. Spaan. 2003. Heterodimerization of the two major envelope proteins is essential for arterivirus infectivity. *J. Virol.* **77**:97–104.

130. Snijder, E. J., H. van Tol, K. W. Pedersen, M. J. Raamsman, and A. A. de Vries. 1999. Identification of a novel structural protein of arteriviruses. *J. Virol.* **73**:6335–6345.

131. Spiess, M. 1995. Heads or tails—what determines the orientation of proteins in the membrane. *FEBS Lett.* **369**:76–79.

132. Takahashi-Omoe, H., K. Omoe, M. Sakaguchi, Y. Kameoka, S. Matsushita, and T. Inada. 2004. Production of virus-specific antiserum corresponding to sequences in the lactate dehydrogenase-elevating virus (LDV) ORF6 protein. *Comp. Immunol. Microbiol. Infect. Dis.* **27**:47–55.

133. Therrien, D., Y. St-Pierre, and S. Dea. 2000. Preliminary characterization of protein binding factor for porcine reproductive and respiratory syndrome virus on the surface of permissive and non-permissive cells. *Arch. Virol.* **145**:1099–1116.

134. Tijms, M. A., Y. van der Meer, and E. J. Snijder. 2002. Nuclear localization of non-structural protein 1 and nucleocapsid protein of equine arteritis virus. *J. Gen. Virol.* **83**:795–800.

135. Tobiasch, E., R. Kehm, U. Bahr, C. A. Tidona, N. J. Jakob, M. Handermann, G. Darai, and M. Giese. 2001. Large envelope glycoprotein and nucleocapsid protein of equine arteritis virus (EAV) induce an immune response in Balb/c mice by DNA vaccination; strategy for developing a DNA-vaccine against EAV-infection. *Virus Genes* **22**:187–199.

136. Trousdale, M. D., D. W. Trent, and A. Shelokov. 1975. Simian hemorrhagic fever virus: a new togavirus. *Proc. Soc. Exp. Biol. Med.* **150**:707–711.

137. Truong, H. M., Z. Lu, G. F. Kutish, J. Galeota, F. A. Osorio, and A. K. Pattnaik. 2004. A highly pathogenic porcine reproductive and respiratory syndrome virus generated from an infectious cDNA clone retains the in vivo virulence and transmissibility properties of the parental virus. *Virology* **325**:308-319.

138. van Berlo, M. F., P. J. Rottier, W. J. Spaan, and M. C. Horzinek. 1986. Equine arteritis virus-induced polypeptide synthesis. *J. Gen. Virol.* **67**:1543–1549.

139. Vanderheijden, N., P. L. Delputte, H. W. Favoreel, J. Vandekerckhove, J. Van Damme, P. A. van Woensel, and H. J. Nauwynck. 2003. Involvement of sialoadhesin in entry of porcine reproductive and respiratory syndrome virus into porcine alveolar macrophages. *J. Virol.* **77**:8207–8215.

140. van Nieuwstadt, A. P., J. J. Meulenberg, A. van Essen-Zanbergen, A. Petersen-den Besten, R. J. Bende, R. J. Moormann, and G. Wensvoort. 1996. Proteins encoded by open reading frames 3 and 4 of the genome of Lelystad virus (Arteriviridae) are structural proteins of the virion. *J. Virol.* **70**:4767–4772.

141. Verheije, M. H., T. J. Welting, H. T. Jansen, P. J. Rottier, and J. J. Meulenberg. 2002. Chimeric arteriviruses generated by swapping of the M protein ectodomain rule out a role of this domain in viral targeting. *Virology* **303**:364–373.

142. von Heijne, G. 1988. Transcending the impenetrable: how proteins come to terms with membranes. *Biochim. Biophys. Acta* **947**:307–333.

143. von Heijne, G. 1990. The signal peptide. *J. Membr. Biol.* **115**:195–201.

144. Wahlberg, J. M., and M. Spiess. 1997. Multiple determinants direct the orientation of signal-anchor proteins: the topogenic role of the hydrophobic signal domain. *J. Cell Biol.* **137**:555–562.

145. Weiland, E., S. Bolz, F. Weiland, W. Herbst, M. J. Raamsman, P. J. Rottier, and A. A. De Vries. 2000. Monoclonal antibodies directed against conserved epitopes on the nucleocapsid protein and the major envelope glycoprotein of equine arteritis virus. *J. Clin. Microbiol.* **38**:2065–2075.

146. Weiland, E., M. Wieczorek-Krohmer, D. Kohl, K. K. Conzelmann, and F. Weiland. 1999. Monoclonal antibodies to the GP5 of porcine reproductive and respiratory syndrome virus are more effective in virus neutralization than monoclonal antibodies to the GP4. *Vet. Microbiol.* **66**:171–186.

147. Welch, S. K., R. Jolie, D. S. Pearce, W. D. Koertje, E. Fuog, S. L. Shields, D. Yoo, and J. G. Calvert. 2004. Construction and evaluation of genetically engineered replication-defective porcine reproductive and respiratory syndrome virus vaccine candidates. *Vet. Immunol. Immunopathol.* **102**:277–290

148. Wieczorek-Krohmer, M., F. Weiland, K. Conzelmann, D. Kohl, N. Visser, P. van Woensel, H. J. Thiel, and E. Weiland. 1996. Porcine reproductive and respiratory syndrome virus (PRRSV): monoclonal antibodies detect common epitopes on two viral proteins of European and U.S. isolates. *Vet Microbiol.* **51**:257–266.

149. Wieringa, R., A. A. F. de Vries, S. M. Post, and P. J. M. Rottier. 2003. Intra- and intermolecular disulfide bonds of the GP$_{2b}$ glycoprotein of equine arteritis virus: relevance for virus assembly and infectivity. *J. Virol.* **77**:12996–13004.

150. Wieringa, R., A. A. F. de Vries, M. J. B. Raamsman, and P. J. M. Rottier. 2002. Characterization of two new structural glycoproteins, GP$_3$ and GP$_4$, of equine arteritis virus. *J. Virol.* **76**:10829–10840.

151. Wieringa, R., A. A. F. de Vries, and P. J. M. Rottier. 2003. Formation of disulfide-linked complexes between the three minor envelope glycoproteins (GP$_{2b}$, GP$_3$, and GP$_4$) of equine arteritis virus. *J. Virol.* 77:6216–6226.

152. Wieringa, R., A. A. F. de Vries, J. van der Meulen, G.-J. Godeke, J. J. M. Onderwater, H. van Tol, H. K. Koerten, A. M. Mommaas, E. J. Snijder, and P. J. M. Rottier. 2004. Structural protein requirements in equine arteritis virus assembly. *J. Virol.* 78:13019–13027.

153. Wissink, E. H., M. V. Kroese, J. G. Maneschijn-Bonsing, J. J. Meulenberg, P. A. van Rijn, F. A. Rijsewijk, and P. J. Rottier. 2004. Significance of the oligosaccharides of the porcine reproductive and respiratory syndrome virus glycoproteins GP2a and GP5 for infectious virus production. *J. Gen. Virol.* 85:3715–3723.

154. Wissink, E. H., M. V. Kroese, H. A. van Wijk, F. A. Rijsewijk, J. J. Meulenberg, and P. J. Rottier. 2005. Envelope protein requirements for the assembly of infectious virions of porcine reproductive and respiratory syndrome virus. *J. Virol.* 79:12495–12506.

155. Wissink, E. H., H. A. van Wijk, J. M. Pol, G. J. Godeke, P. A. van Rijn, P. J. Rottier, and J. J. Meulenberg. 2003. Identification of porcine alveolar macrophage glycoproteins involved in infection of porcine respiratory and reproductive syndrome virus. *Arch. Virol.* 148:177–187.

156. Wootton, S., G. Koljesar, L. Yang, K. J. Yoon, and D. Yoo. 2001. Antigenic importance of the carboxy-terminal beta-strand of the porcine reproductive and respiratory syndrome virus nucleocapsid protein. *Clin. Diagn. Lab. Immunol.* 8:598–603.

157. Wootton, S. K., E. A. Nelson, and D. Yoo. 1998. Antigenic structure of the nucleocapsid protein of porcine reproductive and respiratory syndrome virus. *Clin. Diagn. Lab. Immunol.* 5:773–779.

158. Wootton, S. K., R. R. Rowland, and D. Yoo. 2002. Phosphorylation of the porcine reproductive and respiratory syndrome virus nucleocapsid protein. *J. Virol.* 76:10569–10576.

159. Wootton, S. K., and D. Yoo. 2003. Homo-oligomerization of the porcine reproductive and respiratory syndrome virus nucleocapsid protein and the role of disulfide linkages. *J. Virol.* 77:4546–4557.

160. Wu, W. H., Y. Fang, R. Farwell, M. Steffen-Bien, R. R. Rowland, J. Christopher-Hennings, and E. A. Nelson. 2001. A 10-kDa structural protein of porcine reproductive and respiratory syndrome virus encoded by ORF2b. *Virology* 287:183–191.

161. Wu, W. H., Y. Fang, R. R. Rowland, S. R. Lawson, J. Christopher-Hennings, K. J. Yoon, and E. A. Nelson. 2005. The 2b protein as a minor structural component of PRRSV. *Virus Res.* 114:177–181.

162. Wurm, T., H. Chen, T. Hodgson, P. Britton, G. Brooks, and J. A. Hiscox. 2001. Localization to the nucleolus is a common feature of coronavirus nucleoproteins, and the protein may disrupt host cell division. *J. Virol.* 75:9345–9356.

163. Yang, L., M. L. Frey, K. J. Yoon, J. J. Zimmerman, and K. B. Platt. 2000. Categorization of North American porcine reproductive and respiratory syndrome viruses: epitopic profiles of the N, M, GP5 and GP3 proteins and susceptibility to neutralization. *Arch. Virol.* 145:1599–1619.

164. Yang, L., K. J. Yoon, Y. Li, J. H. Lee, J. J. Zimmerman, M. L. Frey, K. M. Harmon, and K. B. Platt. 1999. Antigenic and genetic variations of the 15 kD nucleocapsid protein of porcine reproductive and respiratory syndrome virus isolates. *Arch. Virol.* 144:525–546.

165. Yoo, D., S. K. Wootton, G. Li, C. Song, and R. R. Rowland. 2003. Colocalization and interaction of the porcine arterivirus nucleocapsid protein with the small nucleolar RNA-associated protein fibrillarin. *J. Virol.* 77:12173–12183.

166. Yuan, S., M. P. Murtaugh, and K. S. Faaberg. 2000. Heteroclite subgenomic RNAs are produced in porcine reproductive and respiratory syndrome virus infection. *Virology* 275:158–169.

167. Yuan, S., M. P. Murtaugh, F. A. Schumann, D. Mickelson, and K. S. Faaberg. 2004. Characterization of heteroclite subgenomic RNAs associated with PRRSV infection. *Virus Res.* 105:75–87.

168. Zeegers, J. J., B. A. Van der Zeijst, and M. C. Horzinek. 1976. The structural proteins of equine arteritis virus. *Virology* 73:200–205.

169. Zeng, L., E. K. Godeny, S. L. Methven, and M. A. Brinton. 1995. Analysis of simian hemorrhagic fever virus (SHFV) subgenomic RNAs, junction sequences, and 5′ leader. *Virology* 207:543–548.

170. Zhang, Y., R. D. Sharma, and P. S. Paul. 1998. Monoclonal antibodies against conformationally dependent epitopes on porcine reproductive and respiratory syndrome virus. *Vet. Microbiol.* 63:125–136.

171. Zhou, Y. J., T. Q. An, Y. X. He, J. X. Liu, H. J. Qiu, Y. F. Wang, and G. Tong. 2006. Antigenic structure analysis of glycosylated protein 3 of porcine reproductive and respiratory syndrome virus. *Virus Res.* 118:98–104.

*Nidoviruses*
Edited by S. Perlman, T. Gallagher, and E. J. Snijder
© 2008 ASM Press, Washington, DC

# Chapter 15

# Coronavirus Accessory Proteins

KRISHNA NARAYANAN, CHENG HUANG, AND SHINJI MAKINO

Coronaviruses are classified, based on comparative sequence analyses and other studies, into three major groups: 1, 2, and 3. The basic steps in the coronavirus replication cycle are conserved among several groups and are regulated by viral proteins encoded by a set of genes essential for viral replication and assembly. The essential genes include open reading frame 1ab (ORF 1ab), which occupies about two-thirds of the genome towards the 5′ end and encodes two large polyprotein precursors whose cleavage products are responsible for RNA replication and transcription. The other essential genes encode the common structural proteins, the spike protein (S protein), membrane protein (M protein), envelope protein (E protein), and nucleocapsid protein (N protein); these genes occupy the remaining one-third of the genome proximal to the 3′ end and are involved in infectious-virus assembly. In addition to these genes, the coronavirus genome also contains several other genes that have homologous versions in viruses within each group but have no similarity with genes in different groups (47). The locations and numbers of these genes, initially called group-specific genes, vary among viruses (Fig. 1), and their functions in the viral life cycle have not been fully established as yet. These group-specific genes are now called nonessential or accessory genes, and the gene products are termed accessory proteins because they are not expressed by all coronaviruses and are not required for virus growth in vitro. Several studies using reverse genetics and targeted mutagenesis analysis have shown that many of these genes are indeed dispensable for growth of virus in cell culture. Nevertheless, many of the accessory proteins encoded by these genes could be important for virus replication and virulence in the natural host. In this review, we have compiled the current knowledge about the coronavirus accessory proteins to provide insight into the possible role of these proteins in the propagation of coronavirus under natural conditions.

## GROUP 1 CORONAVIRUS ACCESSORY PROTEINS

Group 1 coronaviruses have two or three accessory ORFs in the region between the S and E protein genes and two other ORFs 3′ to the N protein gene. The accessory gene cluster located between the S and E protein genes contains ORF3a and -3b in transmissible gastroenteritis virus (TGEV) and the ORF3a, -3b, and -3c in feline infectious peritonitis virus (FIPV) (Fig. 1). Amino acid sequence analysis suggests that TGEV ORF3a and -3b are highly homologous to FIPV ORF3a and -3c, respectively. Protein sequence similarity searches using BLAST (Basic Local Alignment Search Tool) shows that other group 1 coronaviruses, like human coronavirus 229E (HCoV-229E), porcine respiratory coronavirus, and porcine enteric diarrhea virus, also have an accessory ORF homologous to TGEV ORF3b (9, 40, 69, 70, 91).

In the Purdue strain of TGEV, gene 3b was shown to produce a 31-kDa glycosylated, integral membrane protein in vitro (62). The following studies have established that the accessory genes 3a and 3b are dispensable for TGEV replication in cell culture: a truncated form of gene 3b was observed after passage of TGEV twice in cell culture (91); a naturally occurring TGEV variant had a large deletion in the 3a gene (58); a genetically manipulated TGEV mutant lacking gene 3a, which was generated using a reverse-genetics system, is viable (14, 96); and deletion of TGEV genes 3a and 3b and replacement with the heterologous gene encoding the green fluorescent

**Krishna Narayanan, Cheng Huang, and Shinji Makino** • Department of Microbiology and Immunology, The University of Texas Medical Branch at Galveston, Galveston, TX 77555-1019.

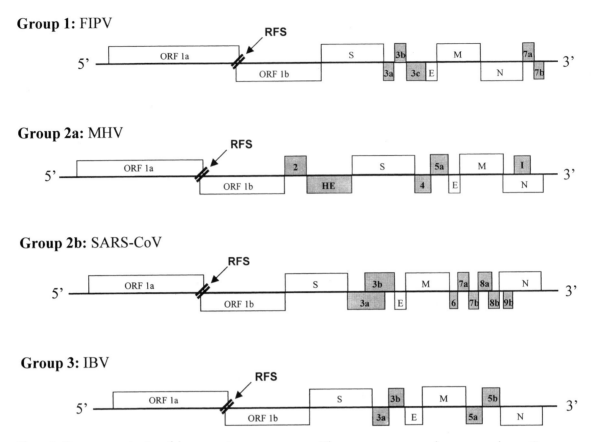

**Figure 1.** Genome organization of the coronavirus accessory genes. The accessory genes are shown as gray boxes. One member of each group is shown as a representative example. The figure is not drawn to scale. RFS, ribosomal frameshift.

protein (GFP) had very little effect on virus growth in cell culture (81). Similarly, FIPV accessory genes 3a, 3b, and 3c are also not required for virus replication in cell culture; naturally occurring mutations have been observed in FIPV gene 3c (92), and deletion of FIPV ORF3abc did not affect the growth of the mutant virus in cell culture (27).

TGEV has a mortality rate of nearly 100% in infected newborn piglets, its natural host (65). Infection of newborn piglets with a TGEV mutant lacking both the 3a and 3b genes showed only a marginal reduction in virulence, compared to the lethal wild-type virus, and did not severely affect viral replication efficiency or tissue tropism in infected animals (81). In contrast, an FIPV 3abc deletion mutant showed severely attenuated virulence in cats with no typical clinical signs of the disease relative to the lethal phenotype of the wild-type virus, suggesting the important role for this gene cluster in FIPV pathogenesis (27).

Accessory gene 7, located at the 3' end of the genome, is a group 1-specific gene that is present in TGEV, FIPV, and canine enteric coronavirus (47) with no homologous counterparts in group 2 and 3 coronaviruses. In TGEV, gene 7 encodes a 78-amino-acid,

9-kDa hydrophobic protein (22, 90). Immunofluorescence studies suggested that this protein is associated not only with the nucleus (22) but also with endoplasmic reticulum and cell surface membranes in infected cells (90); the latter observation suggested a role for this protein in virus replication or assembly (90). Analysis of a TGEV mutant lacking gene 7, generated by using a TGEV reverse-genetics system, shows that deletion of gene 7 has very little effect on virus replication in cell culture, whereas the in vivo growth of the deletion mutant is more than 100-fold less efficient in the lung and gut, its target organs, and its virulence is attenuated in infected newborn piglets (65). Similarly, analysis of FIPV carrying naturally occurring deletion mutants of ORF7a, which is homologous to TGEV gene 7, suggests a possible role for the 7a gene in viral virulence in cats (42). In feline coronavirus, a virus closely related to FIPV, deletions of ORF7b readily occur in cultured cells, and a correlation between ORF7b deletion and loss of virulence is observed (28, 92). Deletion of the FIPV accessory gene cluster 7ab using the reverse-genetics system results in a mutant that replicates well in cell culture but is phenotypically attenuated in cats (27); infection with the FIPV 7ab deletion mutant, using doses that are considered to be fatal in the case of wild-type virus, does not cause any clinical signs of illness in cats (27).

## GROUP 2 CORONAVIRUS ACCESSORY PROTEINS

Group 2 coronaviruses form a diverse phylogenetic cluster. The recent emergence of severe acute respiratory syndrome coronavirus (SARS-CoV) has led to further classification of group 2 into groups 2a and 2b. Members of group 2a include mouse hepatitis virus (MHV), bovine coronavirus (BCoV), HCoV-OC43, and others, while SARS-CoV belongs to the more distant group 2b.

### Group 2a Coronavirus Accessory Proteins

#### General properties

Coronaviruses belonging to group 2a have two accessory ORFs, the 2a and 2b genes, encoding hemagglutinin-esterase (HE), located between ORF1b and the S protein gene, and two additional group-specific accessory ORFs, the 4 and 5a genes, located between the S and E protein genes (Fig. 1). Also, an internal (I) accessory gene is located in the +1 reading frame within the N protein gene in BCoV, several strains of MHV, and the rat coronavirus (Fig. 1) (15, 32, 45, 48, 66, 78); MHV I protein is a hydrophobic 23-kDa protein that is incorporated into the virus particles (21).

The 30-kDa protein 2a is expressed in the cytoplasm of MHV-, BCoV-, and HCoV-OC43-infected cells (8, 13, 46, 73, 105). BCoV 2a protein was shown to be a phosphoprotein (13). The 2a protein of the group 2a coronaviruses is predicted to have a cyclic phosphodiesterase function; cyclic phosphodiesterase is an enzyme involved in tRNA maturation pathways (80).

ORF2b encodes HE, a group 2-specific, 65-kDa accessory structural protein found in MHV, BCoV, and HCoV-OC43 particles (41, 76); HE is a viral structural protein. It is an N-glycosylated, type I transmembrane envelope protein that forms disulfide-linked homodimers and has hemagglutinating and sialate O-acetylesterase enzymatic activities (31, 43, 76, 77). This gene is expressed only in some strains of MHV. While the MHV-JHM and MHV-S strains express HE, the gene is inactivated in strain MHV-A59 due to a mutation in the transcription-regulating sequence and a nonsense mutation in the ORF (56, 76).

The gene 4 region is variable among different members of group 2a coronaviruses. In strains MHV-JHM and MHV-S, the gene 4 region consists of a single ORF, but in BCoV and strain MHV-A59, it consists of two ORFs, 4a and ORF4b (60, 79, 93, 94). The ORF4 gene product is predicted to be an integral membrane protein, and the gene expresses a 15-kDa protein in MHV-JHM-infected cells (17, 79, 93).

MHV has an accessory ORF5a downstream of the ORF4 gene. Expression of the putative ORF5a protein product has not yet been demonstrated in MHV-infected cells.

#### Known functions and roles in virulence

Evidence for the nonessential role of MHV ORF2a for virus replication in cell culture comes from a study that describes an MHV-JHM isolate lacking ORF2a expression as having no effect on growth in transformed murine cells (73). Analysis of an MHV mutant generated using a reverse-genetics system shows that although a single amino acid mutation in the ORF2a product has no measurable effect on virus replication in cell culture, this mutation does have a partially attenuating effect on the virulence of the virus in mice, implying a role for MHV 2a protein in virus pathogenesis (83).

Genetic inactivation of MHV-JHM gene 4, using targeted recombination, results in a mutant virus that exhibits replication kinetics similar to those of the parental virus in cell culture, and the mutant and parental viruses have similar degrees of virulence in a murine model of encephalitis (63); the biological function of MHV accessory protein 4 remains unclear.

Analysis of MHV mutants with deletions of the gene clusters 2a/HE and 4/5a revealed that these accessory genes are nonessential for virus growth in cell culture (16); no significant effect on growth of the 2a/HE deletion mutant is observed, while the 4/5a deletion mutant replicates to a 10-fold-lower level (16). Whether the reduction in growth of the 4/5a deletion mutant is due to lack of expression of these proteins or to the deletions per se is unknown. Infection of both deletion mutants in their natural host, the mouse, shows an attenuated phenotype (16); infection with the wild-type virus is lethal, while mice infected with the deletion mutants exhibit mild signs of clinical illness and no mortality (16). Further studies will determine whether the deletion of both the 4 and 5a genes or the deletion of the 5a gene alone is responsible for the altered virulence.

Among the group 2a-specific accessory proteins, HE is one of the most well-characterized accessory gene products. The nonessential nature of the gene for virus replication in cell culture is suggested by the inactivation of this gene in several tissue culture-adapted MHV strains (56, 76). Also, MHV strains lacking the HE gene can establish a productive infection in mice leading to hepatitis and diseases of the central nervous system (5, 49, 72). Nevertheless, a study using recombinant MHVs generated by a targeted recombination method shows that HE, which is expressed on the surface of virus particles, might enhance viral infectivity by binding sialic acid residues on the cell surface (41). MHV HE also enhances the neurovirulence in mice by promoting the dissemination and entry of virus in the brain, possibly by acting as a coreceptor-binding protein mediating attachment to sialic acid residues (52), while the enzymatic activity of HE is not required for this function (52). Furthermore, HE reduces the in vitro propagation efficiency of the virus, suggesting that MHV maintains the expression of luxury proteins, i.e., HE, at the cost of viral fitness (52).

An MHV mutant lacking I protein expression, created by site-directed mutagenesis using a targeted recombination method, is viable in cell culture, and its replication is not affected in mice (21). The titers of the mutant virus are comparable to those of the wild-type virus in the brains and livers of mice (21). The biological function of MHV I protein is currently unclear.

## SARS-CoV Accessory Proteins

The SARS-CoV genome contains eight accessory genes, 3a, 3b, 6, 7a, 7b, 8a, 8b, and 9b (57, 71); the 3a and 3b genes are located between the S and E protein genes (ORF4 gene); genes 6, 7a, 7b, 8a, and 8b are located between the M protein gene (ORF5 gene) and the N protein gene (ORF9); and gene 9b is found within the N protein gene (Fig. 1). Analysis of SARS-CoV deletion mutants generated using a reverse-genetics system confirmed that genes 3a, 3b, 6, 7a, and 7b are dispensable for SARS-CoV replication in cell culture, establishing that these genes are indeed SARS-CoV accessory genes (97). No significant amino acid sequence similarity exists between the accessory proteins encoded by these SARS-CoV accessory genes and any known viral or cellular proteins. Several reports have demonstrated expression of SARS-CoV accessory proteins 3a, 3b, 6, 7a, and 9b in infected cells as well as in SARS patients (12, 20, 23, 38, 82, 88, 103). Evidence suggests that proteins 7b and 8a are also produced during infection, as antibodies against these proteins are detected in sera from SARS patients (26). As described below, the biological functions of these SARS-CoV accessory proteins have been investigated primarily by expressing

each protein in cultured cells. Whether each SARS-CoV accessory protein exerts the same biological functions in infected cells and/or infected animals as is observed in expression studies is largely unknown.

## SARS-CoV 3a protein

The 274-amino-acid-long SARS-CoV 3a protein, also known as X1 protein or U274 protein, is an O-glycosylated triple-membrane-spanning protein carrying an N-terminal ectodomain and a C-terminal endodomain; 3a protein is localized in both intracellular and plasma membranes in infected cells (38, 64, 82, 88, 98). Within the C terminus of 3a protein are two intracellular protein sorting and trafficking signals, the YxxΦ and diacidic motifs (88). One expression study describes these motifs as being important for the transportation of 3a protein to the cell surface, where it rapidly undergoes endocytosis (88). Another expression study further indicates that 3a protein can form a homotetramer complex through interprotein disulfide bridges and that this 3a protein homotetramer complex functions as a potassium channel (55).

Zeng et al. propose that 3a protein might be incorporated into virus particles by direct association with S protein in infected cells (103). Expression studies revealed that 3a protein interacts with S and M proteins in the Golgi apparatus close to where virus assembly and budding occur (88, 98). 3a protein also interacts with E and 7a proteins (88). The idea that 3a protein is a novel viral structural protein was therefore expected because of its multiple interactions with other viral proteins, including structural proteins (38, 74). Several studies report production of virus-like particles (VLPs) of SARS-CoV after expressing viral structural proteins in the absence of 3a protein expression (29, 33, 34, 36, 59), which demonstrates that 3a protein is not necessary for VLP production. And in cells coexpressing 3a, S, E, M, and N proteins, 3a protein is incorporated into VLPs (34, 74), probably through interaction between 3a protein and other SARS-CoV envelope proteins, e.g., S, M, or E protein (74). That the SARS-CoV mutant virus lacking gene 3a is viable and replicates efficiently in cell culture (97) verifies that 3a protein is not essential for SARS-CoV assembly in cell culture. How virion-associated 3a protein functions biologically is unknown.

In addition to being a SARS-CoV structural protein, 3a protein is released from SARS-CoV-infected and 3a protein-expressing cells; the released 3a protein is probably associated with detergent-resistant membrane structures (35). The presence of the YxxΦ and diacidic motifs, located within the cytoplasmic tail of 3a protein, is not required for its efficient release (35). The release of 3a protein from SARS-CoV-infected cells hints that SARS-CoV, by secreting 3a protein, might affect neighboring cells or more remote cells, although ascribing any such biological significance to released 3a protein requires experimental proof.

Several lines of data suggest that 3a protein is a highly antigenic protein that may affect SARS pathogenesis. Antibodies against 3a protein are readily detected in convalescent SARS patients (87). The amino terminus of 3a protein appears to elicit a strong and potentially protective humoral response in SARS patients (104). Furthermore, injection of amino acids 15 to 28 from the amino-terminal region of 3a protein into rabbits results in generation of neutralizing antibodies against SARS-CoV (1). In lung epithelial cells, 3a protein up-regulates expression of fibrinogen (89), which might contribute to SARS pathogenesis.

Although SARS-CoV 3a protein is one of the better-characterized coronavirus accessory proteins, its biological functions in infected cells and its role in viral pathogenesis remain unclear.

### SARS-CoV 7a protein

The 122-amino-acid-long SARS-CoV 7a protein, also known as X4 protein or U122 protein, is a type I transmembrane protein, consisting of a 15-amino-acid-long signal peptide sequence, an 81-amino-acid luminal domain, a 21-amino-acid transmembrane domain, and a short C-terminal tail (61). Analysis of the crystal structure of the luminal domain of 7a protein reveals a compact seven-stranded beta sandwich, which is similar in folding and topology to members of the immunoglobulin superfamily (61). SARS-CoV 7a protein is detected at the perinuclear region in SARS-CoV-infected cells (20, 61). In 7a protein-expressing cells, one study reports colocalization of most of 7a protein with the endoplasmic reticulum marker GRP94 or the intermediate compartment marker Sec-31 (20). Of two studies with 7a-GFP fusion protein, the first shows that 7a-GFP fusion protein mainly colocalizes with a trans-Golgi marker, Golgin 97 (61); in the second study, independently expressed 7a-GFP fusion protein, untagged 7a protein- and 7a-hemagglutinin fusion protein were all shown to move to the Golgi compartment but not the endoplasmic reticulum, mitochondria, or nucleus (44).

Like protein 3a, the accessory protein 7a is also a viral structural protein (34). Expression studies suggest that 7a protein incorporates into VLPs by interacting with other viral structural proteins, M protein and E protein (19, 34). 7a protein also binds to 3a protein (88) and S protein (34), but these interactions appear to be nonessential for the assembly of 7a into VLPs (34). Unlike 3a protein, 7a protein is not released from 7a-expressing cells (34).

Expression studies show that 7a protein functions in a variety of ways. These activities include induction of apoptosis in various cell lines through a caspase-dependent pathway (86), inhibition of cellular protein synthesis, activation of p38 mitogen-activated protein kinase (44), and suppression of the cell cycle progression at the $G_0/G_1$ phase (101). Expressed 7a protein also interacts with a small glutamine-rich tetratricopeptide repeat-containing protein (19). An existing SARS-CoV mutant lacking the 7a and 7b genes is known to be viable and replicates efficiently in cell culture (97); this mutant could be used to determine whether 7a protein exerts these functions in SARS-CoV-infected cells as well.

### Other SARS-CoV accessory proteins

Although expression of the 63-amino-acid-long 6 protein, also known as the X3 protein, is not required for SARS-CoV replication in cell culture (97), it accumulates in SARS-CoV-infected Vero-E6 cells and in the lung and intestine tissues of the SARS patients (23). Expression studies locate the 6 protein mainly in the endoplasmic reticulum and Golgi compartments (23, 68). Interestingly, an attenuated MHV carrying SARS-CoV accessory gene 6 replicates to a higher titer than the parental MHV in cell culture and exhibits increased virulence to mice (68). In contrast, MHV carrying each of other SARS-CoV accessory genes, 3a, 3b, 7a, 7b, and 8, shows no changes in viral virulence (68), suggesting that SARS-CoV 6 protein may play a role in SARS-CoV pathogenesis.

The 154-amino-acid-long SARS-CoV 3b protein is detected in infected cells (12) and is dispensable for SARS-CoV replication in cell culture (99, 102). In 3b protein-expressing cells, 3b protein shows nucleolar and mitochondrial localization (98, 99) and induces cell growth arrest in $G_0/G_1$ phase as well as apoptosis (100).

Early human and animal SARS-CoV isolates have one intact ORF8, while most human isolates of SARS-CoV from the outbreak of SARS in 2003 have a naturally occurring 29-nucleotide (nt) deletion in ORF8, resulting in ORF8a and -8b, in this gene (25). These observations may indicate that the deletion of those 29 nt may represent an adaptation of SARS-CoV to humans. Insertion of this 29-nt sequence into later-date human isolates, which effectively merges ORF8a and -8b into a continuous ORF8 using reverse genetics, has little impact on virus growth and RNA replication in cell culture (97). Although these results clearly indicate that ORF8 is not required for virus infection in cell culture (97), the biological significance of the 29-nt deletion in pathogenesis of SARS-CoV is unclear.

### Role of SARS-CoV accessory proteins in viral pathogenesis

Studies of SARS-CoV accessory proteins are still in their infancy, and understanding the roles of the SARS-CoV accessory proteins in virus replication and pathogenesis requires further study. One major obstacle to determining the roles of SARS-CoV accessory proteins in viral pathogenesis is that there is no single ideal animal model for SARS (85). Intranasal inoculation of SARS-CoV into mice results in SARS-CoV replication in the lung, yet infected mice do not show any clinical signs (84). Nevertheless, Yount et al. have examined the role of SARS-CoV accessory proteins in virus replication in mice (97). They found that intranasal inoculation of 6-week-old female BALB/c mice with the Urbani strain-derived SARS-CoV or its mutants, each of which lacks SARS-CoV accessory genes individually or in combinations, results in similar virus titers in the lung at 2 days postinfection (97). Exploring the roles of SARS-CoV accessory protein in viral pathogenesis awaits a relevant animal disease model that reproduces the severe symptoms observed in SARS patients.

## GROUP 3 CORONAVIRUS ACCESSORY PROTEINS

The prototypic group 3 avian coronavirus, infectious bronchitis virus (IBV) contains two group-specific genes, genes 3 and 5 (7) (Fig. 1), which are functionally tricistronic (53) and bicistronic (54), respectively. Gene 3 encodes three small proteins, the 58-amino-acid-long 3a protein, the 65-amino-acid-long 3b protein, and the 94-amino-acid-long E protein. E protein, originally named 3c protein, is a minor viral structural protein. These proteins are translated from the same subgenomic RNA3 in three ways: directly from the first translational initiation codon (for 3a protein), from leaky ribosomal scanning (for 3b protein) (53), or from an internal ribosome entry site (for E protein) (50, 54). IBV 3a protein is expressed in infected cells but is not detected in virions. In both infected and transfected cells, IBV 3a protein localizes to the cytoplasm in a diffuse pattern as well as in sharp puncta. These puncta do not overlap cellular organelles or other punctate structures. IBV 3a puncta line up along smooth endoplasmic reticulum tubules and often are partially surrounded by these tubules. These observations suggest that IBV 3a protein is partially

targeted to a novel domain of the smooth endoplasmic reticulum (67). IBV 3b protein is detected in the nucleus of infected cells (75).

Gene 5 encodes two accessory proteins, the 66-amino-acid-long 5a protein and the 83-amino-acid-long 5b protein, both of which are expressed in IBV-infected cells (54). Like 3b protein, 5b protein is probably produced by leaky ribosome scanning.

Sequence homology analysis of different IBV strains indicates that genes 3 and 5 are highly conserved. Overall nucleotide sequence homologies for genes 3 and 5 are 84.1 to 90.8% and 90.4 to 96.4%, respectively. Comparison of predicted amino acid sequence homologies further reveals that genes 3b and 5b are more conserved than genes 3a, 3c, and 5a (39). Indeed, the 3a and 3b ORFs are remarkably conserved in other group 3 coronaviruses from turkeys and pheasants (11).

Evidence is accumulating that the IBV accessory proteins 3a, 3b, 5a, and 5b are not essential for virus replication in cultured cells. Serial passage of the Beaudette strain of IBV in Vero cells results in accumulation of viruses carrying an insertion of a single adenine in a six-adenine stretch of the 3b gene. This nucleotide insertion causes a frameshift event, resulting in generation of a C-terminally truncated protein. The mutant viruses carrying the truncated 3b gene replicate equally as well in Vero cells and chicken embryos as the wild-type virus, indicating that the entire length of gene 3b is not essential for virus replication (75). Analysis of recombinant IBV demonstrates that 3a and 3b proteins are not essential for virus replication in primary chick kidney cells and in chicken embryos, although in chicken tracheal organ cultures, the titer of viruses lacking the 3a gene declines earlier than that of the parental virus carrying gene 3a (30). Similarly, gene 5 of IBV is not required for virus replication in chick kidney cell culture, embryonated eggs, or chicken tracheal organ cultures (10, 95). These studies have firmly established that IBV 3a, 3b, 5a, and 5b proteins are indeed viral accessory proteins. Biological functions of IBV accessory proteins and their roles in viral pathogenesis remain to be elucidated.

## CONCLUDING REMARKS

A precise role for the coronavirus accessory proteins in the viral replication cycle, as evidenced from this overview, is still an enigma. Despite their accessory role in cell culture, the corresponding genes are maintained within the genome, suggesting that they provide a selective advantage that adapts the virus to its natural host. These genes might manipulate and regulate the fundamental host cell pathways and responses to achieve optimal efficiency of replication for the virus in infected hosts.

In other virus families, there are several examples of accessory proteins performing regulatory roles in modulating virus replication and pathogenesis. In human immunodeficiency virus, the four accessory genes, *nef, vif, vpr,* and *vpu,* perform several critical functions at different stages in the virus life cycle. The corresponding specialized viral accessory proteins are multifunctional proteins involved in regulation of host cell functions and viral immune evasion to achieve enhanced virus infectivity in the host (18). Several viruses use their accessory proteins to circumvent the interferon (IFN) response by targeting the transcription factors involved in IFN induction, by suppressing the functions of IFN-induced antiviral proteins, or by interfering with IFN signal transduction. Many such examples are found in negative-strand RNA viruses, including the influenza virus NS1 protein, Ebola virus VP35 protein, respiratory syncytial virus NS1 and NS2 proteins, and paramyxovirus V and C proteins (2, 3, 24). Note that Rift Valley fever virus accessory protein NSs (37) is a major viral virulence factor (6); efficient replication of Rift Valley fever virus in host animals requires expression of NSs protein, which blocks the production of IFN by suppressing host gene transcription (4, 37, 51).

A detailed analysis of the mode of action of the accessory proteins in coronaviruses is warranted, which will not only provide insights into the molecular interactions of the virus with the host cell but also give clues to help elucidate the mechanism of viral pathogenesis. Uncovering the unique role played by these proteins, along with their cellular cofactors, will provide attractive targets for designing novel antiviral drugs as well as recombinant live vaccines.

### REFERENCES

1. **Akerstrom, S., Y. J. Tan, and A. Mirazimi.** 2006. Amino acids 15–28 in the ectodomain of SARS coronavirus 3a protein induces neutralizing antibodies. *FEBS Lett.* **580:**3799–3803.
2. **Basler, C. F., and A. Garcia-Sastre.** 2002. Viruses and the type I interferon antiviral system: induction and evasion. *Int. Rev. Immunol.* **21:**305–337.
3. **Basler, C. F., X. Wang, E. Muhlberger, V. Volchkov, J. Paragas, H. D. Klenk, A. Garcia-Sastre, and P. Palese.** 2000. The Ebola virus VP35 protein functions as a type I IFN antagonist. *Proc. Natl. Acad. Sci. USA* **97:**12289–12294.
4. **Billecocq, A., M. Spiegel, P. Vialat, A. Kohl, F. Weber, M. Bouloy, and O. Haller.** 2004. NSs protein of Rift Valley fever virus blocks interferon production by inhibiting host gene transcription. *J. Virol.* **78:**9798–9806.
5. **Blau, D. M., C. Turbide, M. Tremblay, M. Olson, S. Létourneau, E. Michaliszyn, S. Jothy, K. V. Holmes, and N. Beauchemin.** 2001. Targeted disruption of the *Ceacam1*

6. **Bouloy, M., C. Janzen, P. Vialat, H. Khun, J. Pavlovic, M. Huerre, and O. Haller.** 2001. Genetic evidence for an interferon-antagonistic function of rift valley fever virus nonstructural protein NSs. *J. Virol.* **75:**1371–1377.
7. **Boursnell, M. E., T. D. Brown, I. J. Foulds, P. F. Green, F. M. Tomley, and M. M. Binns.** 1987. Completion of the sequence of the genome of the coronavirus avian infectious bronchitis virus. *J. Gen. Virol.* **68**(Pt. 1)**:**57–77.
8. **Bredenbeek, P. J., A. F. Noten, M. C. Horzinek, and W. J. Spaan.** 1990. Identification and stability of a 30-kDa nonstructural protein encoded by mRNA 2 of mouse hepatitis virus in infected cells. *Virology* **175:**303–306.
9. **Britton, P., K. L. Mawditt, and K. W. Page.** 1991. The cloning and sequencing of the virion protein genes from a British isolate of porcine respiratory coronavirus: comparison with transmissible gastroenteritis virus genes. *Virus Res.* **21:**181–198.
10. **Casais, R., M. Davies, D. Cavanagh, and P. Britton.** 2005. Gene 5 of the avian coronavirus infectious bronchitis virus is not essential for replication. *J. Virol.* **79:**8065–8078.
11. **Cavanagh, D., K. Mawditt, B. Welchman Dde, P. Britton, and R. E. Gough.** 2002. Coronaviruses from pheasants (Phasianus colchicus) are genetically closely related to coronaviruses of domestic fowl (infectious bronchitis virus) and turkeys. *Avian Pathol.* **31:**81–93.
12. **Chan, W. S., C. Wu, S. C. Chow, T. Cheung, K. F. To, W. K. Leung, P. K. Chan, K. C. Lee, H. K. Ng, D. M. Au, and A. W. Lo.** 2005. Coronaviral hypothetical and structural proteins were found in the intestinal surface enterocytes and pneumocytes of severe acute respiratory syndrome (SARS). *Mod. Pathol.* **18:**1432–1439.
13. **Cox, G. J., M. D. Parker, and L. A. Babiuk.** 1991. Bovine coronavirus nonstructural protein ns2 is a phosphoprotein. *Virology* **185:**509–512.
14. **Curtis, K. M., B. Yount, and R. S. Baric.** 2002. Heterologous gene expression from transmissible gastroenteritis virus replicon particles. *J. Virol.* **76:**1422–1434.
15. **Decimo, D., H. Philippe, M. Hadchouel, M. Tardieu, and M. Meunier-Rotival.** 1993. The gene encoding the nucleocapsid protein: sequence analysis in murine hepatitis virus type 3 and evolution in Coronaviridae. *Arch. Virol.* **130:**279–288.
16. **de Haan, C. A., P. S. Masters, X. Shen, S. Weiss, and P. J. Rottier.** 2002. The group-specific murine coronavirus genes are not essential, but their deletion, by reverse genetics, is attenuating in the natural host. *Virology* **296:**177–189.
17. **Ebner, D., T. Raabe, and S. G. Siddell.** 1988. Identification of the coronavirus MHV-JHM mRNA 4 product. *J. Gen. Virol.* **69**(Pt. 5)**:**1041–1050.
18. **Emerman, M., and M. H. Malim.** 1998. HIV-1 regulatory/accessory genes: keys to unraveling viral and host cell biology. *Science* **280:**1880–1884.
19. **Fielding, B. C., V. Gunalan, T. H. Tan, C. F. Chou, S. Shen, S. Khan, S. G. Lim, W. Hong, and Y. J. Tan.** 2006. Severe acute respiratory syndrome coronavirus protein 7a interacts with hSGT. *Biochem. Biophys. Res. Commun.* **343:**1201–1208.
20. **Fielding, B. C., Y. J. Tan, S. Shuo, T. H. Tan, E. E. Ooi, S. G. Lim, W. Hong, and P. Y. Goh.** 2004. Characterization of a unique group-specific protein (U122) of the severe acute respiratory syndrome coronavirus. *J. Virol.* **78:**7311–7318.
21. **Fischer, F., D. Peng, S. T. Hingley, S. R. Weiss, and P. S. Masters.** 1997. The internal open reading frame within the nucleocapsid gene of mouse hepatitis virus encodes a structural protein that is not essential for viral replication. *J. Virol.* **71:**996–1003.

The (MHVR) gene leads to reduced susceptibility of mice to mouse hepatitis virus infection. *J. Virol.* **75:**8173–8186.

22. **Garwes, D. J., F. Stewart, and P. Britton.** 1989. The polypeptide of Mr 14,000 of porcine transmissible gastroenteritis virus: gene assignment and intracellular location. *J. Gen. Virol.* 70 (Pt. 9):2495–2499.

23. **Geng, H., Y. M. Liu, W. S. Chan, A. W. Lo, D. M. Au, M. M. Waye, and Y. Y. Ho.** 2005. The putative protein 6 of the severe acute respiratory syndrome-associated coronavirus: expression and functional characterization. *FEBS Lett.* 579:6763–6768.

24. **Gotoh, B., T. Komatsu, K. Takeuchi, and J. Yokoo.** 2001. Paramyxovirus accessory proteins as interferon antagonists. *Microbiol. Immunol.* 45:787–800.

25. **Guan, Y., B. J. Zheng, Y. Q. He, X. L. Liu, Z. X. Zhuang, C. L. Cheung, S. W. Luo, P. H. Li, L. J. Zhang, Y. J. Guan, K. M. Butt, K. L. Wong, K. W. Chan, W. Lim, K. F. Shortridge, K. Y. Yuen, J. S. Peiris, and L. L. Poon.** 2003. Isolation and characterization of viruses related to the SARS coronavirus from animals in southern China. *Science* 302:276–278.

26. **Guo, J. P., M. Petric, W. Campbell, and P. L. McGeer.** 2004. SARS corona virus peptides recognized by antibodies in the sera of convalescent cases. *Virology* 324:251–256.

27. **Haijema, B. J., H. Volders, and P. J. Rottier.** 2004. Live, attenuated coronavirus vaccines through the directed deletion of group-specific genes provide protection against feline infectious peritonitis. *J. Virol.* 78:3863–3871.

28. **Herrewegh, A. A., H. Vennema, M. C. Horzinek, P. J. Rottier, and R. J. de Groot.** 1995. The molecular genetics of feline coronaviruses: comparative sequence analysis of the ORF7a/7b transcription unit of different biotypes. *Virology* 212:622–631.

29. **Ho, Y., P. H. Lin, C. Y. Liu, S. P. Lee, and Y. C. Chao.** 2004. Assembly of human severe acute respiratory syndrome coronavirus-like particles. *Biochem. Biophys. Res. Commun.* 318: 833–838.

30. **Hodgson, T., P. Britton, and D. Cavanagh.** 2006. Neither the RNA nor the proteins of open reading frames 3a and 3b of the coronavirus infectious bronchitis virus are essential for replication. *J. Virol.* 80:296–305.

31. **Hogue, B. G., T. E. Kienzle, and D. A. Brian.** 1989. Synthesis and processing of the bovine enteric coronavirus haemagglutinin protein. *J. Gen. Virol.* 70(Pt. 2):345–352.

32. **Homberger, F. R.** 1995. Sequence analysis of the nucleoprotein genes of three enterotropic strains of murine coronavirus. *Arch. Virol.* 140:571–579.

33. **Hsieh, P. K., S. C. Chang, C. C. Huang, T. T. Lee, C. W. Hsiao, Y. H. Kou, I. Y. Chen, C. K. Chang, T. H. Huang, and M. F. Chang.** 2005. Assembly of severe acute respiratory syndrome coronavirus RNA packaging signal into virus-like particles is nucleocapsid dependent. *J. Virol.* 79:13848–13855.

34. **Huang, C., N. Ito, C. T. Tseng, and S. Makino.** 2006. Severe acute respiratory syndrome coronavirus 7a accessory protein is a viral structural protein. *J. Virol.* 80:7287–7294.

35. **Huang, C., K. Narayanan, N. Ito, C. J. Peters, and S. Makino.** 2006. Severe acute respiratory syndrome coronavirus 3a protein is released in membranous structures from 3a protein-expressing cells and infected cells. *J. Virol.* 80:210–217.

36. **Huang, Y., Z. Y. Yang, W. P. Kong, and G. J. Nabel.** 2004. Generation of synthetic severe acute respiratory syndrome coronavirus pseudoparticles: implications for assembly and vaccine production. *J. Virol.* 78:12557–12565.

37. **Ikegami, T., S. Won, C. J. Peters, and S. Makino.** 2006. Rescue of infectious Rift Valley fever virus entirely from cDNA, analysis of virus lacking the NSs gene, and expression of a foreign gene. *J. Virol.* 80:2933–2940.

38. **Ito, N., E. C. Mossel, K. Narayanan, V. L. Popov, C. Huang, T. Inoue, C. J. Peters, and S. Makino.** 2005. Severe respiratory syndrome coronavirus 3a protein is a viral structural protein. *J. Virol.* 79:3182–3186.

39. **Jia, W., and S. A. Naqi.** 1997. Sequence analysis of gene 3, gene 4 and gene 5 of avian infectious bronchitis virus strain CU-T2. *Gene* 189:189–193.

40. **Jouvenne, P., S. Mounir, J. N. Stewart, C. D. Richardson, and P. J. Talbot.** 1992. Sequence analysis of human coronavirus 229E mRNAs 4 and 5: evidence for polymorphism and homology with myelin basic protein. *Virus Res.* 22:125–141.

41. **Kazi, L., A. Lissenberg, R. Watson, R. J. de Groot, and S. R. Weiss.** 2005. Expression of hemagglutinin esterase protein from recombinant mouse hepatitis virus enhances neurovirulence. *J. Virol.* 79:15064–15073.

42. **Kennedy, M., N. Boedeker, P. Gibbs, and S. Kania.** 2001. Deletions in the 7a ORF of feline coronavirus associated with an epidemic of feline infectious peritonitis. *Vet. Microbiol.* 81:227–334.

43. **King, B., B. J. Potts, and D. A. Brian.** 1985. Bovine coronavirus hemagglutinin protein. *Virus Res.* 2:53–59.

44. **Kopecky-Bromberg, S. A., L. Martinez-Sobrido, and P. Palese.** 2006. 7a protein of severe acute respiratory syndrome coronavirus inhibits cellular protein synthesis and activates p38 mitogen-activated protein kinase. *J. Virol.* 80:785–793.

45. **Kunita, S., M. Mori, and E. Terada.** 1993. Sequence analysis of the nucleocapsid protein gene of rat coronavirus SDAV-681. *Virology* 193:520–523.

46. **Labonte, P., S. Mounir, and P. J. Talbot.** 1995. Sequence and expression of the ns2 protein gene of human coronavirus OC43. *J. Gen. Virol.* 76(Pt. 2):431–435.

47. **Lai, M. M., and D. Cavanagh.** 1997. The molecular biology of coronaviruses. *Adv. Virus Res.* 48:1–100.

48. **Lapps, W., B. G. Hogue, and D. A. Brian.** 1987. Sequence analysis of the bovine coronavirus nucleocapsid and matrix protein genes. *Virology* 157:47–57.

49. **Lavi, E., D. H. Gilden, M. K. Highkin, and S. R. Weiss.** 1986. The organ tropism of mouse hepatitis virus A59 in mice is dependent on dose and route of inoculation. *Lab. Anim. Sci.* 36:130–135.

50. **Le, S. Y., N. Sonenberg, and J. V. Maizel, Jr.** 1994. Distinct structural elements and internal entry of ribosomes in mRNA3 encoded by infectious bronchitis virus. *Virology* 198:405–411.

51. **Le May, N., S. Dubaele, L. Proietti De Santis, A. Billecocq, M. Bouloy, and J. M. Egly.** 2004. TFIIH transcription factor, a target for the Rift Valley hemorrhagic fever virus. *Cell* 116: 541–550.

52. **Lissenberg, A., M. M. Vrolijk, A. L. van Vliet, M. A. Langereis, J. D. de Groot-Mijnes, P. J. Rottier, and R. J. de Groot.** 2005. Luxury at a cost? Recombinant mouse hepatitis viruses expressing the accessory hemagglutinin esterase protein display reduced fitness in vitro. *J. Virol.* 79:15054–15063.

53. **Liu, D. X., D. Cavanagh, P. Green, and S. C. Inglis.** 1991. A polycistronic mRNA specified by the coronavirus infectious bronchitis virus. *Virology* 184:531–544.

54. **Liu, D. X., and S. C. Inglis.** 1992. Identification of two new polypeptides encoded by mRNA5 of the coronavirus infectious bronchitis virus. *Virology* 186:342–347.

55. **Lu, W., B. J. Zheng, K. Xu, W. Schwarz, L. Du, C. K. Wong, J. Chen, S. Duan, V. Deubel, and B. Sun.** 2006. Severe acute respiratory syndrome-associated coronavirus 3a protein forms an ion channel and modulates virus release. *Proc. Natl. Acad. Sci. USA* 103:12540–12545.

56. **Luytjes, W., P. J. Bredenbeek, A. F. Noten, M. C. Horzinek, and W. J. Spaan.** 1988. Sequence of mouse hepatitis virus A59 mRNA 2: indications for RNA recombination between coronaviruses and influenza C virus. *Virology* 166:415–422.

57. **Marra, M. A., S. J. Jones, C. R. Astell, R. A. Holt, A. Brooks-Wilson, Y. S. Butterfield, J. Khattra, J. K. Asano, S. A. Barber, S. Y. Chan, A. Cloutier, S. M. Coughlin, D. Freeman, N. Girn,**

O. L. Griffith, S. R. Leach, M. Mayo, H. McDonald, S. B. Montgomery, P. K. Pandoh, A. S. Petrescu, A. G. Robertson, J. E. Schein, A. Siddiqui, D. E. Smailus, J. M. Stott, G. S. Yang, F. Plummer, A. Andonov, H. Artsob, N. Bastien, K. Bernard, T. F. Booth, D. Bowness, M. Czub, M. Drebot, L. Fernando, R. Flick, M. Garbutt, M. Gray, A. Grolla, S. Jones, H. Feldmann, A. Meyers, A. Kabani, Y. Li, S. Normand, U. Stroher, G. A. Tipples, S. Tyler, R. Vogrig, D. Ward, B. Watson, R. C. Brunham, M. Krajden, M. Petric, D. M. Skowronski, C. Upton, and R. L. Roper. 2003. The genome sequence of the SARS-associated coronavirus. *Science* **300:**1399–1404.

58. **McGoldrick, A., J. P. Lowings, and D. J. Paton.** 1999. Characterisation of a recent virulent transmissible gastroenteritis virus from Britain with a deleted ORF 3a. *Arch. Virol.* **144:**763–770.

59. **Mortola, E., and P. Roy.** 2004. Efficient assembly and release of SARS coronavirus-like particles by a heterologous expression system. *FEBS Lett.* **576:**174–178.

60. **Mounir, S., and P. J. Talbot.** 1993. Human coronavirus OC43 RNA 4 lacks two open reading frames located downstream of the S gene of bovine coronavirus. *Virology* **192:**355–360.

61. **Nelson, C. A., A. Pekosz, C. A. Lee, M. S. Diamond, and D. H. Fremont.** 2005. Structure and intracellular targeting of the SARS-coronavirus Orf7a accessory protein. *Structure* (Cambridge) **13:**75–85.

62. **O'Connor, J. B., and D. A. Brian.** 1999. The major product of porcine transmissible gastroenteritis coronavirus gene 3b is an integral membrane glycoprotein of 31 kDa. *Virology* **256:**152–161.

63. **Ontiveros, E., L. Kuo, P. S. Masters, and S. Perlman.** 2001. Inactivation of expression of gene 4 of mouse hepatitis virus strain JHM does not affect virulence in the murine CNS. *Virology* **289:**230–238.

64. **Oostra, M., C. A. de Haan, R. J. de Groot, and P. J. Rottier.** 2006. Glycosylation of the severe acute respiratory syndrome coronavirus triple–spanning membrane proteins 3a and M. *J. Virol.* **80:**2326–2336.

65. **Ortego, J., I. Sola, F. Almazan, J. E. Ceriani, C. Riquelme, M. Balasch, J. Plana, and L. Enjuanes.** 2003. Transmissible gastroenteritis coronavirus gene 7 is not essential but influences in vivo virus replication and virulence. *Virology* **308:**13–22.

66. **Parker, M. M., and P. S. Masters.** 1990. Sequence comparison of the N genes of five strains of the coronavirus mouse hepatitis virus suggests a three domain structure for the nucleocapsid protein. *Virology* **179:**463–468.

67. **Pendleton, A. R., and C. E. Machamer.** 2005. Infectious bronchitis virus 3a protein localizes to a novel domain of the smooth endoplasmic reticulum. *J. Virol.* **79:**6142–6151.

68. **Pewe, L., H. Zhou, J. Netland, C. Tangudu, H. Olivares, L. Shi, D. Look, T. Gallagher, and S. Perlman.** 2005. A severe acute respiratory syndrome-associated coronavirus-specific protein enhances virulence of an attenuated murine coronavirus. *J. Virol.* **79:**11335–11342.

69. **Raabe, T., and S. Siddell.** 1989. Nucleotide sequence of the human coronavirus HCV 229E mRNA 4 and mRNA 5 unique regions. *Nucleic Acids Res.* **17:**6387.

70. **Rasschaert, D., M. Duarte, and H. Laude.** 1990. Porcine respiratory coronavirus differs from transmissible gastroenteritis virus by a few genomic deletions. *J. Gen. Virol.* **71**(Pt. 11):2599–2607.

71. **Rota, P. A., M. S. Oberste, S. S. Monroe, W. A. Nix, R. Campagnoli, J. P. Icenogle, S. Penaranda, B. Bankamp, K. Maher, M. H. Chen, S. Tong, A. Tamin, L. Lowe, M. Frace, J. L. DeRisi, Q. Chen, D. Wang, D. D. Erdman, T. C. Peret, C. Burns, T. G. Ksiazek, P. E. Rollin, A. Sanchez, S. Liffick, B. Holloway, J. Limor, K. McCaustland, M. Olsen-Rasmussen,

R. Fouchier, S. Gunther, A. D. Osterhaus, C. Drosten, M. A. Pallansch, L. J. Anderson, and W. J. Bellini. 2003. Characterization of a novel coronavirus associated with severe acute respiratory syndrome. *Science* **300:**1394–1399.

72. **Sarma, J. D., L. Fu, S. T. Hingley, and E. Lavi.** 2001. Mouse hepatitis virus type-2 infection in mice: an experimental model system of acute meningitis and hepatitis. *Exp. Mol. Pathol.* **71:**1–12.

73. **Schwarz, B., E. Routledge, and S. G. Siddell.** 1990. Murine coronavirus nonstructural protein ns2 is not essential for virus replication in transformed cells. *J. Virol.* **64:**4784–4791.

74. **Shen, S., P. S. Lin, Y. C. Chao, A. Zhang, X. Yang, S. G. Lim, W. Hong, and Y. J. Tan.** 2005. The severe acute respiratory syndrome coronavirus 3a is a novel structural protein. *Biochem. Biophys. Res. Commun.* **330:**286–292.

75. **Shen, S., Z. L. Wen, and D. X. Liu.** 2003. Emergence of a coronavirus infectious bronchitis virus mutant with a truncated 3b gene: functional characterization of the 3b protein in pathogenesis and replication. *Virology* **311:**16–27.

76. **Shieh, C. K., H. J. Lee, K. Yokomori, N. La Monica, S. Makino, and M. M. Lai.** 1989. Identification of a new transcriptional initiation site and the corresponding functional gene 2b in the murine coronavirus RNA genome. *J. Virol.* **63:**3729–3736.

77. **Siddell, S. G.** 1982. Coronavirus JHM: tryptic peptide fingerprinting of virion proteins and intracellular polypeptides. *J. Gen. Virol.* **62**(Pt. 2):259–269.

78. **Skinner, M. A., and S. G. Siddell.** 1983. Coronavirus JHM: nucleotide sequence of the mRNA that encodes nucleocapsid protein. *Nucleic Acids Res.* **11:**5045–5054.

79. **Skinner, M. A., and S. G. Siddell.** 1985. Coding sequence of coronavirus MHV-JHM mRNA 4. *J. Gen. Virol.* **66**(Pt. 3):593–596.

80. **Snijder, E. J., P. J. Bredenbeek, J. C. Dobbe, V. Thiel, J. Ziebuhr, L. L. Poon, Y. Guan, M. Rozanov, W. J. Spaan, and A. E. Gorbalenya.** 2003. Unique and conserved features of genome and proteome of SARS-coronavirus, an early split-off from the coronavirus group 2 lineage. *J. Mol. Biol.* **331:**991–1004.

81. **Sola, I., S. Alonso, S. Zuniga, M. Balasch, J. Plana-Duran, and L. Enjuanes.** 2003. Engineering the transmissible gastroenteritis virus genome as an expression vector inducing lactogenic immunity. *J. Virol.* **77:**4357–4369.

82. **Song, H. D., C. C. Tu, G. W. Zhang, S. Y. Wang, K. Zheng, L. C. Lei, Q. X. Chen, Y. W. Gao, H. Q. Zhou, H. Xiang, H. J. Zheng, S. W. Chern, F. Cheng, C. M. Pan, H. Xuan, S. J. Chen, H. M. Luo, D. H. Zhou, Y. F. Liu, J. F. He, P. Z. Qin, L. H. Li, Y. Q. Ren, W. J. Liang, Y. D. Yu, L. Anderson, M. Wang, R. H. Xu, X. W. Wu, H. Y. Zheng, J. D. Chen, G. Liang, Y. Gao, M. Liao, L. Fang, L. Y. Jiang, H. Li, F. Chen, B. Di, L. J. He, J. Y. Lin, S. Tong, X. Kong, L. Du, P. Hao, H. Tang, A. Bernini, X. J. Yu, O. Spiga, Z. M. Guo, H. Y. Pan, W. Z. He, J. C. Manuguerra, A. Fontanet, A. Danchin, N. Niccolai, Y. X. Li, C. I. Wu, and G. P. Zhao.** 2005. Cross-host evolution of severe acute respiratory syndrome coronavirus in palm civet and human. *Proc. Natl. Acad. Sci. USA* **102:**2430–2435.

83. **Sperry, S. M., L. Kazi, R. L. Graham, R. S. Baric, S. R. Weiss, and M. R. Denison.** 2005. Single-amino-acid substitutions in open reading frame (ORF) 1b-nsp14 and ORF 2a proteins of the coronavirus mouse hepatitis virus are attenuating in mice. *J. Virol.* **79:**3391–3400.

84. **Subbarao, K., J. McAuliffe, L. Vogel, G. Fahle, S. Fischer, K. Tatti, M. Packard, W. J. Shieh, S. Zaki, and B. Murphy.** 2004. Prior infection and passive transfer of neutralizing antibody prevent replication of severe acute respiratory syndrome coronavirus in the respiratory tract of mice. *J. Virol.* **78:**3572–3577.

85. Subbarao, K., and A. Roberts. 2006. Is there an ideal animal model for SARS? *Trends Microbiol.* **14:**299–303.

86. Tan, Y. J., B. C. Fielding, P. Y. Goh, S. Shen, T. H. Tan, S. G. Lim, and W. Hong. 2004. Overexpression of 7a, a protein specifically encoded by the severe acute respiratory syndrome coronavirus, induces apoptosis via a caspase-dependent pathway. *J. Virol.* **78:**14043–14047.

87. Tan, Y. J., P. Y. Goh, B. C. Fielding, S. Shen, C. F. Chou, J. L. Fu, H. N. Leong, Y. S. Leo, E. E. Ooi, A. E. Ling, S. G. Lim, and W. Hong. 2004. Profiles of antibody responses against severe acute respiratory syndrome coronavirus recombinant proteins and their potential use as diagnostic markers. *Clin. Diagn. Lab. Immunol.* **11:**362–371.

88. Tan, Y. J., E. Teng, S. Shen, T. H. Tan, P. Y. Goh, B. C. Fielding, E. E. Ooi, H. C. Tan, S. G. Lim, and W. Hong. 2004. A novel severe acute respiratory syndrome coronavirus protein, u274, is transported to the cell surface and undergoes endocytosis. *J. Virol.* **78:**6723–6734.

89. Tan, Y. J., P. Y. Tham, D. Z. Chan, C. F. Chou, S. Shen, B. C. Fielding, T. H. Tan, S. G. Lim, and W. Hong. 2005. The severe acute respiratory syndrome coronavirus 3a protein up-regulates expression of fibrinogen in lung epithelial cells. *J. Virol.* **79:**10083–10087.

90. Tung, F. Y., S. Abraham, M. Sethna, S. L. Hung, P. Sethna, B. G. Hogue, and D. A. Brian. 1992. The 9-kDa hydrophobic protein encoded at the 3' end of the porcine transmissible gastroenteritis coronavirus genome is membrane-associated. *Virology* **186:**676–683.

91. Vaughn, E. M., P. G. Halbur, and P. S. Paul. 1995. Sequence comparison of porcine respiratory coronavirus isolates reveals heterogeneity in the S, 3, and 3-1 genes. *J. Virol.* **69:**3176–3184.

92. Vennema, H., A. Poland, J. Foley, and N. C. Pedersen. 1998. Feline infectious peritonitis viruses arise by mutation from endemic feline enteric coronaviruses. *Virology* **243:**150–157.

93. Weiss, S. R., P. W. Zoltick, and J. L. Leibowitz. 1993. The ns 4 gene of mouse hepatitis virus (MHV), strain A 59 contains two ORFs and thus differs from ns 4 of the JHM and S strains. *Arch. Virol.* **129:**301–309.

94. Yokomori, K., and M. M. Lai. 1991. Mouse hepatitis virus S RNA sequence reveals that nonstructural proteins ns4 and ns5a are not essential for murine coronavirus replication. *J. Virol.* **65:**5605–5608.

95. Youn, S., J. L. Leibowitz, and E. W. Collisson. 2005. In vitro assembled, recombinant infectious bronchitis viruses demonstrate that the 5a open reading frame is not essential for replication. *Virology* **332:**206–215.

96. Yount, B., K. M. Curtis, and R. S. Baric. 2000. Strategy for systematic assembly of large RNA and DNA genomes: transmissible gastroenteritis virus model. *J. Virol.* **74:**10600–10611.

97. Yount, B., R. S. Roberts, A. C. Sims, D. Deming, M. B. Frieman, J. Sparks, M. R. Denison, N. Davis, and R. S. Baric. 2005. Severe acute respiratory syndrome coronavirus group-specific open reading frames encode nonessential functions for replication in cell cultures and mice. *J. Virol.* **79:**14909–14922.

98. Yuan, X., J. Li, Y. Shan, Z. Yang, Z. Zhao, B. Chen, Z. Yao, B. Dong, S. Wang, J. Chen, and Y. Cong. 2005. Subcellular localization and membrane association of SARS-CoV 3a protein. *Virus Res.* **109:**191–202.

99. Yuan, X., Y. Shan, Z. Yao, J. Li, Z. Zhao, J. Chen, and Y. Cong. 2006. Mitochondrial location of severe acute respiratory syndrome coronavirus 3b protein. *Mol. Cells* **21:**186–191.

100. Yuan, X., Y. Shan, Z. Zhao, J. Chen, and Y. Cong. 2005. G0/G1 arrest and apoptosis induced by SARS-CoV 3b protein in transfected cells. *Virol. J.* **2:**66.

101. Yuan, X., J. Wu, Y. Shan, Z. Yao, B. Dong, B. Chen, Z. Zhao, S. Wang, J. Chen, and Y. Cong. 2006. SARS coronavirus 7a protein blocks cell cycle progression at G0/G1 phase via the cyclin D3/pRb pathway. *Virology* **346:**74–85.

102. Yuan, X., Z. Yao, Y. Shan, B. Chen, Z. Yang, J. Wu, Z. Zhao, J. Chen, and Y. Cong. 2005. Nucleolar localization of nonstructural protein 3b, a protein specifically encoded by the severe acute respiratory syndrome coronavirus. *Virus Res.* **114:**70–79.

103. Zeng, R., R. F. Yang, M. D. Shi, M. R. Jiang, Y. H. Xie, H. Q. Ruan, X. S. Jiang, L. Shi, H. Zhou, L. Zhang, X. D. Wu, Y. Lin, Y. Y. Ji, L. Xiong, Y. Jin, E. H. Dai, X. Y. Wang, B. Y. Si, J. Wang, H. X. Wang, C. E. Wang, Y. H. Gan, Y. C. Li, J. T. Cao, J. P. Zuo, S. F. Shan, E. Xie, S. H. Chen, Z. Q. Jiang, X. Zhang, Y. Wang, G. Pei, B. Sun, and J. R. Wu. 2004. Characterization of the 3a protein of SARS-associated coronavirus in infected vero E6 cells and SARS patients. *J. Mol. Biol.* **341:**271–279.

104. Zhong, X., Z. Guo, H. Yang, L. Peng, Y. Xie, T. Y. Wong, S. T. Lai, and Z. Guo. 2006. Amino terminus of the SARS coronavirus protein 3a elicits strong, potentially protective humoral responses in infected patients. *J. Gen. Virol.* **87:**369–373.

105. Zoltick, P. W., J. L. Leibowitz, E. L. Oleszak, and S. R. Weiss. 1990. Mouse hepatitis virus ORF 2a is expressed in the cytosol of infected mouse fibroblasts. *Virology* **174:**605–607.

*Nidoviruses*
Edited by S. Perlman, T. Gallagher, and E. J. Snijder
© 2008 ASM Press, Washington, DC

Chapter 16

# Host Cell Responses to Coronavirus Infections

GIJS A. VERSTEEG AND WILLY J. M. SPAAN

RNA viruses have developed a high level of pleiotropy as a result of their limited genomic coding capacity. Although a substantial part of viral protein functions in the life cycle of coronaviruses (CoVs) has been determined, the role of the majority of the viral proteins in their interaction with the host cell has not yet been fully characterized. Microarray technology provides an efficient method to investigate the entire cellular transcriptome and has emerged as the preferred method for large-scale gene expression studies. Several microarray studies have been performed to further elucidate host responses to CoV infection in vitro. We have compared differentially expressed genes from these studies and categorized them based on their presence in only a single study (unique) or during the majority of other CoV infections in vitro as well (common). In this chapter, common as well as unique alterations in host gene expression during CoV infection in vitro are discussed and compared to those in other RNA virus infections. Transcriptional profiling and studies using other approaches have led to a more comprehensive understanding of CoV-induced (immune) responses. Several common responses on the topics of apoptosis, cell cycle regulation, unfolded-protein response, ubiquitin-proteasome-mediated degradation, autophagy, heterogeneous nuclear ribonucleoprotein (hnRNP)-involved viral transcription, and modulation of cellular translation are addressed in more detail.

To distinguish reference to genes and associated mRNA from reference to proteins, mouse gene and protein nomenclature has been used in this chapter (http://www.informatics.jax.org/mgihome/nomen/gene.shtml). Gene and mRNA symbols begin with a capital letter, followed by lowercase letters. Protein abbreviations are all capital letters.

## GLOBAL TRANSCRIPTIONAL PROFILING OF CoV INFECTIONS IN VITRO

The type, kinetics, and extent of cellular responses during infection are related to cell type as well as infection outcome. All nucleated cells are believed to have several types of intracellular sensor molecules with CARD, PYRIN, or TIR domains, such as the retinoic acid inducible gene I (RIG-I) and melanoma differentiation-associated gene 5 (MDA-5) proteins, which can recognize viral RNA and protein (105). Some specialized cells possess Toll-like receptors (TLRs), allowing fast mounting of antiviral tactics even in the absence of viral replication (61). Cellular responses during CoV infection in vitro have been studied in various different cell types on a genome-wide scale by microarray analysis. Virus-induced changes in host cell morphology are often accompanied by marked changes in gene expression. Although these studies can be organized in various ways, a logical arrangement is to compare cellular responses in lytic and nonlytic infections. Comparison of the microarray data sets revealed common as well as CoV-specific host gene expression patterns that provide further insights into the host (transcriptional) response (Fig. 1). Common differentially regulated genes during nonlytic CoV infections in vitro mainly encompass chemokine genes (47%) and interferon (IFN)-stimulated genes (ISGs) (43%). The remaining 10% consists of nuclear factor κb (NF-κB)-related and other genes. In contrast, lytically infected cells differentially express a much more diverse set of genes. The expression of substantially fewer genes of the chemokine family is commonly changed than in the previous group, while anti-inflammatory, apoptosis-, Fos/Jun-, and NF-κB-related genes show common changes during infection. Yet, the majority of the

**Gijs A. Versteeg and Willy J. M. Spaan** • Molecular Virology Laboratory, Department of Medical Microbiology, Leiden University Medical Center, P.O. Box 9600, 2300 RC Leiden, The Netherlands.

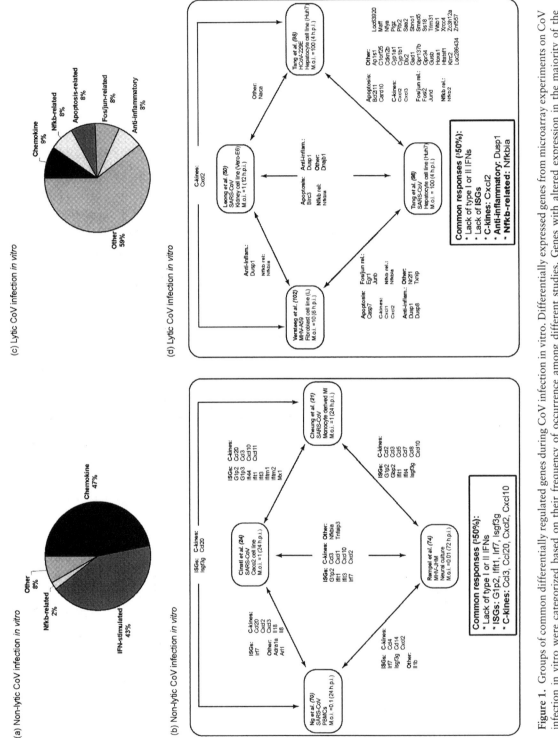

**Figure 1.** Groups of common differentially regulated genes during CoV infection in vitro. Differentially expressed genes from microarray experiments on CoV infection in vitro were categorized based on their frequency of occurrence among different studies. Genes with altered expression in the majority of the analyzed CoV infections were identified as "common regulated genes." Since virus-induced changes in host cell morphology often result in changes in gene expression, these studies were organized in lytically and nonlytically infected cells. (a and c) Common regulated genes during nonlytic CoV infections mainly encompass chemokines and IFN-stimulated genes. (b and d) Lytic CoV infection in vitro shows a much more diverse set of common differentially expressed genes. The number of differentially regulated chemokine genes is substantially lower than for nonlytic infections. Induction of IFN and IFN-stimulated genes is completely absent. M.o.i., multiplicity if infection.

common differentially expressed genes (59%) falls in none of the above categories, underlining the broader diversity in this type of in vitro infection (Fig. 1). Common responses that are also induced during replication of a wide variety of other pathogens mainly encompass induction of mRNA coding inflammatory and anti-inflammatory mediators, cytokines and chemokines (40). Both common and unique responses during CoV infection have been described in several publications. The expression of genes involved in apoptosis, cell cycle regulation, coagulation, endoplasmic reticulum (ER) stress, and transcription/translation was only changed in a subset of these studies (23, 49, 68, 97, 100) and is most likely specific for certain CoV infections.

## CYTOKINE AND CHEMOKINE INDUCTION

Cytokines and chemokines are secreted messenger proteins whose major function is to mediate inflammatory responses and attract immune cells to sites of infection (29). Various microarray (Fig. 1) and non-microarray (Fig. 2) studies have shown extensive cytokine and chemokine up-regulation during CoV infection in vitro (12, 20, 23, 47, 49, 53, 68, 69, 74, 89, 90, 97, 98, 100, 113, 120), consistent with in vivo infection (73). Nonlytic CoV infections in primary cells of lymphoid origin resulted in induction of a wide range of CC as well as CXC chemokines (Fig. 1b and 2a). These lymphoid primary cells are likely to express TLRs and induce innate immune responses by virus replication-independent routes. Transcriptional up-regulation of IFN regulatory factor (IRF-7) in these cells, which is the key transcription factor involved in TLR-mediated IFN induction, supports this view (32). Mouse hepatitis virus (MHV) infection in peritoneal macrophages (Fig. 2a) is marked by induction of tumor necrosis factor alpha, interleukin 4 (IL-4), leutotriene B$_4$, and transcription growth factor β. Moreover, procoagulant activity (PCA) is induced in macrophages during infection and is involved in the marked liver fibrosis observed in MHV-infected mice (7). Similarly, MHV-3 induced PCA (50) and severe acute respiratory syndrome CoV (SARS-CoV) up-regulated several coagulation genes (68) in peripheral blood mononuclear cells (PBMCs). Lymphocyte-macrophage collaboration is necessary for the full induction of PCA (50).

Lytic infections in nonlymphoid cell lines result in less prominent induction of chemokine genes (Fig. 1d and 2b). Only certain CXC-type chemokines are differentially expressed. More selective induction of a particular subset of chemokine genes is likely to be cell type dependent. Most of the nonlymphoid cell lines lack TLRs and means to express "specialized" cytokines. Up-regulation of chemokine transcription in these cells is most likely the result of other intracellular interactions between viral components and the host cell. For example, SARS-CoV and MHV spike expression induces the cytokine IL-8 and its murine functional counterpart Cxcl2, respectively. Intracellular interactions between the spike protein (S protein) and still-unidentified host cell components are thought to be responsible for enhanced IL-8/Cxcl2 expression (G. A. Versteeg, P. S. van de Nes, P. J. Bredenbeek, and W. J. M. Spaan, unpublished data). NF-κB inhibitor expression is up-regulated in most CoV-infected cells (Fig. 1b and 1d). The NF-κB inhibitor gene encodes an NF-κB inhibitor that is up-regulated in various other viral infections (40). It may play a role in limiting inflammatory responses or in regulation of apoptosis-related genes, such as Casp7, Bcl2l11, Card10, and Birc3. In addition, CoV infection stimulates genes coding for transcription factors Fos and Jun, which have been known for their role in regulation of inflammatory responses. Moreover, some dual-specificity phosphatases involved in limiting inflammatory responses are up-regulated (Dusp1/8 [Fig. 1d]).

In summary, CoV infections in vitro activate expression of numerous cytokines. The set of differentially expressed cytokines depends on the infected cell type and outcome of infection. Cytokine expression in primary cultures of lymphoid cells most likely results from virus-TLR interactions. Yet other intracellular interactions between viral components and the host cell may be responsible for cytokine induction during lytic infection in nonlymphoid cells.

## EVASION OF IFN INDUCTION

IFNs are secreted messenger proteins that induce an antiviral state upon infection. Viruses interfere at essentially all possible steps of the IFN induction cascades as well as with the activation of effector molecules (32). IFN genes are not induced during lytic CoV infection in vitro (Fig. 1d), suggesting that induction through intracellular detection by RNA helicases such as RIG-I and MDA-5 does not occur in cells that lack TLR expression. In contrast, TLR-mediated IFN induction does occur during CoV infection. In nonlytically CoV-infected lymphoid cells, IFN can be induced (Fig. 2), and ISGs are up-regulated in the absence of detectable IFN mRNA induction (Fig. 1b). Up-regulated ISGs include Irf7, Mx1, Isgf3g, Ifit1/3/4, Ifitm1/2, Ifi44, G1p2/3, and Gbp2. These genes are possibly stimulated directly by the infection

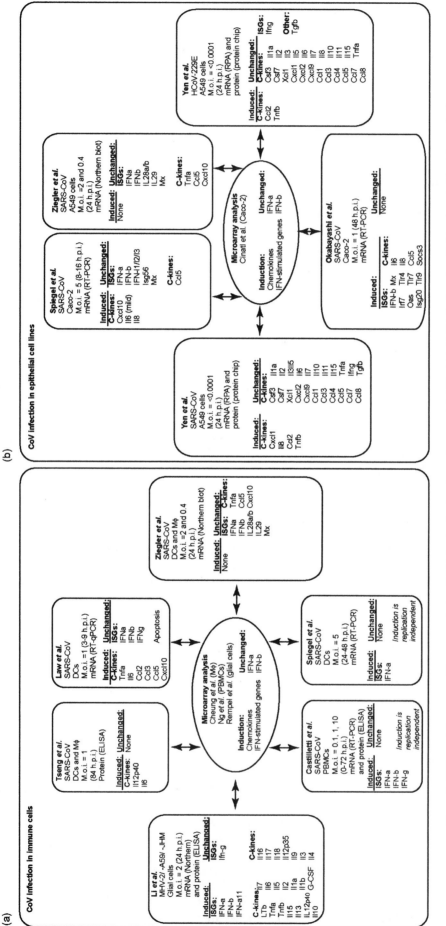

**Figure 2.** Differentially expressed host genes during CoV infection in vitro (nonmicroarray). (a) Nonlytic CoV infections in cells from lymphoid origin resulted in induction of a wide range of CC as well as CXC chemokines partially induced by activation of TLRs. (b) Lytic infections in nonlymphoid cell lines result in less prominent induction of chemokine genes. The more selective induction of a particular subset of chemokine genes is likely cell type dependent. Most of the nonlymphoid cell lines lack TLRs and means to express "specialized" cytokines. Up-regulation of chemokine transcription in these cells is most likely the result of other intracellular interactions between viral components and the host cell. M.o.i., multiplicity of infection; ELISA, enzyme-linked immunosorbent assay.

or by low concentrations of IFN. In support of the latter possibility, up-regulation of the ISGs occurs relatively late after the onset of infection, suggestive of paracrine signaling. IFN induction has been reported in four studies (Fig. 2). Two reports have shown that induction is independent of virus replication, suggesting that IFN is most likely induced by recognition of components of virus particles by TLRs. The membrane and envelope proteins (M and E proteins) can trigger viral replication-independent IFN induction during CoV infection (6, 25). MHV infection in primary astrocyte/microglial culture also stimulated IFN expression (53). Astrocytes and microglia express TLRs and are considered the "immune cells" of the brain (39). It is therefore feasible that IFN induction in glial cell culture was mediated through TLR activation, consistent with other CoV infections (Fig. 1 and 2). SARS-CoV infection in Caco-2 cells did not induce IFNs up to 24 h postinfection (h p.i.) by microarray analysis as well as reverse transcription-PCR (RT-PCR) (23, 90). In contrast, in another report it was described that infection in the same cells under similar conditions induced a wide range of IFNs and ISGs at 48 h p.i. (69). Although the underlying reason for this apparent discrepancy remains elusive, the longer infection period could be involved. It remains unclear whether mounting of antiviral responses during these infections determines the low productivity and limited development of cytopathic effect (CPE) (76) or whether other cellular factors underlie restricted viral production.

The absence of IFN-β induction in CoV-infected nonlymphoid cells might indicate that CoVs interfere with the induction of IFN-β or hide from recognition by RNA helicases. Various viruses block early IFN production (32) by preventing (i) recognition by RNA helicases via double-stranded RNA (dsRNA) sequestering (influenza A virus), (ii) RNA helicase function by direct binding (paramyxoviruses), and (iii) IFN-β promoter stimulator (1) or TANK-binding kinase 1 function (hepatitis C virus and Borna disease virus). Finally, some lytic viruses (e.g., poliovirus and vesicular stomatitis virus) cause a general inhibition of host gene transcription, thereby preventing IFN mRNA synthesis. In contrast to the case with poliovirus and vesicular stomatitis virus, no general transcriptional shutoff is induced by CoVs (85). Nevertheless, the accumulation of several mRNAs is down-regulated in MHV- and SARS-CoV-infected cells (43, 45, 100), suggesting that CoVs may have devised means to specifically lower the concentration of IFN transcripts. SARS-CoV infection and ectopic nonstructural protein 1 (nsp 1) expression resulted in degradation of cellular mRNAs, while rRNA was not affected (43). Although nsp1 expression resulted in degradation

of Sendai virus-induced IFN-β transcription, the biological relevance of these findings remains to be established since some CoVs seem to interfere with earlier steps of the IFN induction pathway as well. IFN-3 is a key transcription factor involved in the induction of IFN-β. Upon activation it translocates from the cytoplasm to the nucleus, where it initiates IFN-β mRNA transcription. No nuclear IRF-3 localization occurs during MHV infection (G. A. Versteeg, P. J. Bredenbeek, and W. J. M. Spaan, unpublished data). In contrast, IRF-3 localizes to the nucleus of SARS-CoV-infected 293 cells late in infection (16 h p.i.) (88). This suggests that SARS-CoV interferes with the steps following IRF-3 translocation or that interference with preceding steps is not complete. Up to now, no viral product responsible for blocking of IRF-3 activation during CoV infection has been identified. Therefore, it is possible that CoVs possess sophisticated mechanisms to hide their dsRNA replication intermediates and other molecules that could trigger an IFN response. Double-membrane vesicles (DMVs) are believed to represent the sites of virus replication (30) and form tightly controlled viral structures that could fulfill such a role.

In conclusion, CoV structural proteins can trigger TLR-mediated IFN production; however, IFN induction by viral RNA via RNA helicases is absent. This suggests possible viral interference with RIG-I or MDA-5 pathways or prevention of dsRNA detection by cellular sensory molecules. Furthermore, degradation of IFN transcripts by SARS-CoV nsp1 has been shown.

## APOPTOSIS

Apoptosis can be triggered in response to viral infection to limit viral spread and to promote clearance of infected cells without inflammation. Numerous viruses induce apoptosis in infected cells. A broad range of viruses has developed strategies to inhibit or delay apoptosis in order to promote cell survival and hence viral production (33). In contrast, other viruses benefit from apoptosis, as it is involved in viral spread or subversion of the host's immune response (10). Some CoVs induce apoptosis in vivo (4, 46, 78, 108) as well as in various different cell lines (Table 1). Several viral proteins involved in this process have been identified. The mechanisms of apoptosis induction seem to vary significantly among different CoVs, and the use of various infection models in different cell types makes it challenging to draw general conclusions about routes of apoptosis induction by CoVs. Moreover, a significant number of studies has been based on the effect of (over)expression of single viral

**Table 1.** Apoptosis induction during CoV infection[a]

| Reference(s) | Virus | Cells | Apoptosis | Protein | Infection and expression |
|---|---|---|---|---|---|
| Liu et al. (54) | IBV | Vero-E6 | Yes | p58 | Both |
| Eléouët et al. (28) | TGEV | HRT18 | Yes | | Infection |
| Collins (24) | HCoV-229E | Macrophages | Yes | | Infection |
| Collins (24) | HCoV-OC43 | Macrophages | No | | Infection |
| Belyavski et al. (7, 8) | MHV | Macrophages | Yes | | Infection |
| An et al. (1), Chen and Makino (14) | | 17Cl1 | Yes | E | Both |
| An et al. (1), Cai et al. (11), Chen and Makino (14) | | DBT | No | | Infection |
| Chen and Makino (14) | | J774.1 | No | | Infection |
| Chen and Makino (14) | | L2 | No | | Infection |
| Liu et al. (56–58) | | Oligodendrocytes | Yes | | Infection |
| Surjit et al. (93) | SARS-CoV | COS-1 | Yes | N | Both |
| Wong et al. (107) | | *Drosophila* | Yes | 3a | Expression |
| Surjit et al. (93) | | Huh-7 | No | | Infection |
| Yang et al. (112) | | T cells | Yes | E | Expression |
| Law et al. (48) | | Vero-E6 | Yes | 3a | Expression |
| Chow et al. (22) | | Vero-E6 | Yes | S | Expression |
| Mizutani et al. (62) | | Vero-E6 | Yes | | Infection |
| Yan et al. (111) | | Vero-E6 | Yes | | Infection |
| Tan et al. (96) | | Vero-E6 and other | Yes | 7a | Expression |
| Tan et al. (96) | | Vero-E6 and other | No | 3a | Expression |

[a]CoVs induce apoptosis in various cell lines. Several viral proteins involved in this process have been identified. The mechanisms of apoptosis induction vary to a large extent among different CoVs.

genes on apoptosis. Importantly, the effects of single-gene (over)expression are unpredictable, and verification with infection experiments will be required to pinpoint their role in apoptosis induction.

Activation of the apoptosis program can lead to degradation of viral proteins. Transmissible gastroenteritis virus (TGEV) activates a broad range of apoptosis markers in HRT18 cells, such as caspases and cytochrome *c* release into the cytoplasm (28). Moreover, the nucleocapsid protein (N protein) of TGEV is cleaved by caspase 3 or downstream effector molecules at Asp-359. Other CoVs have potential caspase cleavage sites in their N proteins as well, indicating that many viruses might be targeted by host caspases (119). Cleavage of the N protein has also been described for other viruses, such as influenza A virus (28). MHV triggers apoptosis in macrophages (8). Induction occurs only in cells that have not been fused into syncytia. Strikingly, macrophages from MHV-resistant mice show five times more apoptosis than similar cells from susceptible mice. Additionally, the extent of apoptosis is inversely correlated with the up-regulation of coagulant gene Fgl2 and the onset of CPE. This illustrates the protective potential of apoptosis in preventing viral pathogenesis. Infection of macrophages with human coronavirus 229E (HCoV-229E) induces apoptosis as well, while infection with HCoV-OC43 does not (24). The cellular stress caused by the more efficiently replicating HCoV-229E probably determines this difference with HCoV-OC43. Oligodendrocytes are involved in myelination of neural cells

and can be infected with neurotropic strains of MHV. UV-inactivated MHV induces programmed death in these cells (57, 58) and uncoating during MHV entry is sufficient to induce caspase-dependent apoptosis and cytochrome *c* release into the cytoplasm, a hallmark of apoptosis (56). Several other viruses induce apoptosis via replication-independent routes as well, such as avian leukosis virus, bovine herpesvirus, vaccinia virus, reovirus, and Sindbis virus (56).

MHV infection of murine fibroblast-like cell line 17Cl1 induces the mitochondrial apoptosis pathway and caspase activation (1, 14). The apoptotic process is characterized by the absence of cytochrome *c* release into the cytoplasm and the formation of an unusual apoptome near mitochondria. It remains unclear if incomplete activation of apoptosis is restricted to 17Cl1 cells or if MHV interferes with the induction of certain apoptosis pathways. Expression of the small E protein is sufficient to trigger apoptosis in 17Cl1 cells. Strikingly, MHV did not induce programmed cell death in other cell lines such as DBT, L2, or J774.1, indicating that apoptosis induction is not a universal effect of MHV infection (14). Also, the SARS-CoV E protein induces apoptosis in T lymphocytes, possibly by interacting with antiapoptotic protein Bcl-xL and preventing its action (112). Potentially lower MHV E protein concentrations in DBT, L2, and J774.1 cells compared to 17Cl1 cells could explain the absence of programmed death in these cells. However, an alternative possibility could be down-regulation of proapoptotic genes in certain cell types. For instance, transcription of proapoptotic gene Bnip3 is down-regulated in MHV-JHM-infected DBT cells in a replication-independent manner (11). This effect might be specific for MHV in DBT cells, as Ng and coworkers demonstrated a 56-fold up-regulation of the related Bnip2 gene by SARS-CoV in PBMCs instead of down-regulation (68). In addition, no other microarray study (Fig. 1b and 1d) reported differential Bnip3 expression. SARS-CoV infection has been studied extensively in the green monkey kidney cell line Vero-E6. In these cells, the antiapoptotic molecule Akt was not sufficiently activated during infection to prevent SARS-CoV-induced programmed cell death (62, 111). The SARS-CoV-unique accessory proteins 3b and 7a can induce apoptosis in Vero-E6 cells (96, 116), whereas conflicting reports about the potential of the 3a protein to induce programmed cell death have been published (48, 96, 107). Also, adenovirus-mediated expression of the SARS-CoV S protein, in particular the S2 part, has been demonstrated to induce DNA fragmentation at 36 to 84 h p.i. (22). These results should be verified during SARS-CoV infection, especially since MHV and infectious bronchitis virus (IBV) S proteins do not play a role in apoptosis induction (1, 54). The IBV nonstructural protein p58 (110) and structural protein E can trigger cell death accompanied by nuclear fragmentation and condensation, yet only p58 induced caspase-dependent apoptosis (54). SARS-CoV N protein expression in COS-1, cells, but not in Huh-7 cells, down-regulates several molecules from the integrin pathway, which leads to apoptosis only in the absence of serum (93). Serum deprivation is considered to be a method to enhance apoptosis, by lowering the concentration of antiapoptotic mediators. Akt was only weakly activated in COS-1 cells, similar to the case in Vero-E6 cells (62).

In summary, many CoVs induce caspase-dependent programmed cell death in vitro. Several studies with MHV suggest that induction of apoptosis can depend on uncoating of the virus or expression of the E protein. Also, SARS-CoV N protein, S protein, and 3a and 7a protein expression might play a role. Apoptosis induction by CoVs seems to be cell line dependent, which suggests that a variety of host-specific interactions are involved in the induction of programmed cell death.

## CELL CYCLE REGULATION

Many viruses interfere with cell cycle progression (70, 77). Genome replication of DNA viruses benefits from arrest in the S phase of the cell cycle, in which nuclear DNA replication is maximal. The role of cell cycle perturbations by RNA viruses is less well understood. Nonetheless, cell cycle deregulation by several RNA viruses has been reported. The $\sigma 1s$ protein of reoviruses inhibits DNA synthesis and cellular proliferation by arresting the cell cycle in the $G_2/M$ phase (71). Also, members of the *Paramyxoviridae,* simian virus 5 and measles virus, slow the progression of the cell cycle by blocking the cell cycle at $G_0$ or $G_1$ (65). Infection with the CoV IBV results in accumulation of infected cells in $G_2/M$ phase (26). Several cell cycle-regulatory proteins were down-regulated, and cytokinesis was disturbed. Furthermore, $G_2/M$-synchronized cells exhibited increased viral protein production, suggesting that IBV induces $G_2/M$ arrest to promote viral replication and translation.

Ectopically expressed N proteins of several group 1, 2, and 3 CoVs have been reported to localize to the nucleolus in a subset of transfected cells (109). Nucleolar localization has been shown during IBV infection in vitro as well, although the efficiency and frequency of nucleolar localization remain debated (36). SARS-CoV and MHV nucleoproteins exclusively localize in the cytoplasm during infection in vitro (99, 114). Overexpression of a single viral gene may have unpredictable effects on subcellular localization, and nucleic acid-binding proteins can localize to nuclei as fixation artifacts (59), indicating that these data should be validated in infected cells. Nonetheless, nucleolar localization of CoV nucleocapsids, altered nucleolar morphology, and redistribution of nucleolar proteins were observed in IBV-infected Vero cells (27). The main function of the nucleolus is rRNA biogenesis. Nucleolar sequestration of proteins appears to be a common way to regulate the eukaryote cell cycle (101). The N phosphoprotein interacts with two nucleolar antigens, nucleolin and fibrillarin (18, 109), thereby potentially disturbing correct cellular functioning of these proteins in rRNA metabolism and cell proliferation. In agreement with these observations, CoV N protein expression could interfere with cell cycle regulation. CoVs might delay the cell cycle in order to promote virus assembly or to sequester ribosomes for translation of viral proteins and keep the cell in the interphase that is most favorable for translation of cap-containing viral RNAs (18). Expressed SARS-CoV N protein is phosphorylated in the nucleus and subsequently transported to the perinuclear region in the cytoplasm by interaction with 14-3-3 proteins (91). These 14-3-3 proteins modulate interactions between components of various cell cycle-regulatory pathways through phosphorylation-dependent protein-protein interactions. This indicates that while transport to the nucleus of the N protein could be a property of all CoVs, nuclear localization is not (75).

Cell cycle regulation is mediated by cyclin-dependent kinases (CDKs) that in association with cyclins trigger entry into the cell cycle S and M phases. SARS-CoV N protein is phosphorylated by the cyclin-CDK complex (91) and prevents S phase progression in infected cells by directly inhibiting the activity of the cyclin-CDK complex (92). This results in hypophosphorylation of retinoblastoma protein (pRb) and subsequent down-regulation of E2F transcription factor 1-mediated transactivation. In line with these observations, cytoplasmic MHV nsp1 (p28) expression mediates hypophosphorylation of pRb and induces cell cycle arrest in the $G_0/G_1$ phase (16). In MHV-infected DBT and 17Cl1 cells, cyclins D1, D2, D3, and E as well as CDK2 are clearly reduced. This suggests that MHV reduces cyclin-CDK complexes, leading to pRb hypophosphorylation and subsequent prevention of $G_0/G_1$-to-S cell cycle transition (15, 16). Also, ectopic expression of SARS-CoV 3b and 7a proteins arrests the cell cycle in $G_0/G_1$ phase (116, 117). Expression of the SARS-CoV 7a protein reduced cyclin D3 expression, which may cause subsequent $G_0/G_1$ arrest. However, it remains questionable whether the results of single-gene (over)-expression can be extrapolated to the complex events during virus infection. Virus-induced cell cycle perturbation by deregulation of pRb has been described before for several large-DNA viruses, as well as for RNA viruses such as measles virus. Measles virus infection of T lymphocytes is accompanied by down-regulation of several cyclins as well as a lack of pRb up-regulation, effectively resulting in $G_0$ cell cycle arrest (65).

In summary, several CoVs interfere with cell cycle progression. For some CoVs, nucleolar localization of the N protein has been implicated in this process. In SARS-CoV- and MHV-infected cells cyclin-CDK complexes are reduced, resulting in pRb hypophosphorylation and possibly arresting the cell cycle in $G_0/G_1$ phase. It remains elusive whether these interactions yield any benefit to the virus. Notwithstanding, $G_2/M$ arrest by IBV enhances viral replication and translation, suggesting that CoVs could benefit from cell cycle alterations (26).

## UNFOLDED-PROTEIN RESPONSE, UBIQUITIN SYSTEM, AND AUTOPHAGY

Ubiquitin additions target a substrate to the proteasome, where it is unfolded and degraded to amino acids. Deubiquitinating enzymes can reverse substrate fate, preventing degradation in proteasomes or autophagosomes (84). The ubiquitin-proteasome system and autophagy play roles in the life cycle of

CoVs. Entry of most MHV strains appears to occur through a pH-independent pathway (66). However, some strains utilize the endosomal route, which involves proteasome-dependent processes. Treatment with proteasome inhibitors during early infection with an MHV strain that enters the cell through the endosomal route reduces virus production and prevents release of virus from endosomes and lysosomes into the cytoplasm (72). However, MHV-A59, which presumably enters via plasma-membrane fusion, was less sensitive to treatment with proteasome inhibtors. These data suggest that the ubiquitin-proteasome system is involved in release of virus from endosomes to the cytoplasm during entry. In addition, CoVs could interfere with the ubiquitin-proteasome system at later stages during infection. SARS-CoV papain-like protease ($PL^{pro}$) has been shown to possess deubiquitinating activity in *trans*-cleavage assays (5). Furthermore, $PL^{pro}$ can deconjugate ISG-15 in vitro, suggesting that it could have a role in circumventing IFN-mediated innate immunity, as was shown for the adenovirus protease and influenza virus NS1 (5). Lastly, it has been speculated that deubiquitination by $PL^{pro}$ might prevent maturation of replication complex-bearing DMVs into degradative organelles (72). Strikingly, no ubiquitinated viral (interacting) proteins have been found during SARS-CoV infection (72). Although many scenarios can explain these data, SARS-CoV $PL^{pro}$ could actively deubiquitinate viral and cellular factors to prevent degradation by the proteasome system and proper functioning of (antiviral) cellular responses.

Autophagy is a cellular quality control system that removes damaged organelles and long-lived proteins from the cytoplasm. It can function as an innate cellular defense against pathogens by directing them to lysosomes. Autophagosomes are formed by sequestration of an area of cytoplasm into double-membraned structures that eventually fuse with endosomes and lysosomes (106). CoVs and enteroviruses assemble their replication complexes on DMVs in the cytoplasm of infected cells (99). One of the proposed mechanisms by which these structures form is as part of the autophagy system (106). Although no differentially expressed host genes controlling authophagy were measured by transcriptional profiling (Fig. 1), several observations suggest the importance of autophagy during MHV infection (72). Firstly, infection up-regulates autophagy, and markers for the replication complex and autophagy colocalize in cells. Secondly, virus production is impaired more than 1,000-fold in cells lacking functional autophagy. Finally, infection of autophagy-negative cells results in hyperswollen ER membranes and the absence of DMV formation. This study suggested the rough ER as the possible source of membranes for MHV replication complexes (72). Recently, immunofluorescence and electron microscopy indicated that the ER is the most likely donor of SARS-CoV DMVs as well (86). However, other immunofluorescence studies suggested that MHV may generate DMVs from the Golgi complex or endosomal membranes (82). The use of different cell lines, compartment marker proteins, and antisera against different nonstructural proteins may underlie this ambiguity.

## CELLULAR FACTORS IN VIRAL REPLICATION

CoVs redirect and utilize host cell components to participate in subgenomic RNA (sgRNA) synthesis and replication. Replication involves recognition of the genomic RNA by the replicase as well as other viral and cellular proteins mainly at the 3′ end (55, 115). Also, sgRNA synthesis is dependent on host proteins. Members of the hnRNP family shuttle between the nucleus and cytoplasm and play a role in regulation of alternative RNA splicing. They participate in sgRNA synthesis and replication of MHV. hnRNPs bind to the MHV leader and body transcription-regulating sequences (TRSs) in both the plus and minus strands (51, 52). They play a role in altering RNA conformation in the 3′ untranslated region (3′ UTR) of the complementary strand. hnRNP A1, for example, interacts with the 5′ region of the MHV genome, and hnRNP I binds to the complementary strand. Association of these two proteins together with the nucleocapsid might play a role in RNA replication and transcription by mediating 5′→3′ interactions within the genomic RNA (37, 38, 80, 81, 104). Genomic circularization might be of importance in replication, as has been shown for poliovirus (34). hnRNP A1 can be functionally replaced by related type A/B hnRNPs in hnRNP A1-deficient cells (80, 83). In addition, several other proteins, including poly(A) binding protein, mitochondrial aconitase, and another hnRNP, synaptotagmin-binding cytoplasmic RNA-interacting protein, function as *trans*-regulatory factors for MHV replication (21, 64, 87). Supporting findings have been reported for SARS-CoV infection (60). Moreover, quantitative proteome analysis of a SARS-CoV-infected kidney cell line identified significant up-regulation of eight kinds of hnRNP factors. CoVs might enhance their expression in infected cells to stimulate viral replication (41). Among the hnRNPs, hnRNP A1, hnRNP I, hnRNP K, and hnRNP E2 have been previously shown to participate in plus-strand RNA virus replication (83, 103). Taken together, experimental findings support the view that several different hnRNP factors in infected cells may form a functional hnRNP complex participating in viral RNA metabolism in which one hnRNP factor can be replaced by another without disruption of the function of the hnRNP complex.

## CoV-INDUCED MODULATION OF TRANSLATION

Many lytic RNA viruses preferentially express their viral proteins at the expense of host proteins. Viruses interfere with host functions at the level of transcription, RNA export from the nucleus to the cytoplasm, and translation. Poliovirus, for example, shuts off cap-dependent protein synthesis by cleavage of eukaryotic transcription factor 4G (118). Since cap-dependent translation is used to produce 96% of all cellular proteins, poliovirus very effectively alters the cellular translation machinery to the benefit of its internal ribosome entry site (IRES)-containing genomic RNA. Translational attenuation occurs in CoV-infected cells as well. However, in the case of CoV infection, the translation machinery is not irreversibly altered and translational shutoff is not as complete as for poliovirus (35).

During acute MHV infection in vitro, total protein synthesis steeply drops to 7% of the original synthesis between 3 and 6 h p.i. (35). Viral protein synthesis increases from 3 h p.i. onwards and almost completely accounts for the translation in infected cells at 6 h p.i. This is likely to result from the exponential increase of viral RNA and competition with cellular mRNA for components of the host translation machinery. Polysome analysis has revealed a shift to lighter polysomes during MHV infection and an increase in number of free 80S ribosomes, suggesting a potential block at the translation initiation phase (35). Increased membrane permeability and $Na^+$ influx during cell-cell fusion has no influence on protein synthesis (63). Interestingly, a limited set of cellular mRNAs, such as the one encoding IL-6, is still efficiently translated in MHV-infected cells (3). This suggests that certain cellular messengers contain elements that allow competition for translation and can still be expressed in infected cells. Such an element could be an IRES, as is found in the 5′ UTR of some stress-induced mRNAs (9). Although several cytokine mRNAs are induced, the concentrations of several other cellular mRNAs, such as actin, tubulin, and major histocompatibility complex class I, decrease during MHV infection (35, 45, 100). It is yet undetermined whether this decrease follows from specific transcriptional repression or increased mRNA degradations, which was shown to be a function of nsp1 of SARS-CoV (43).

CoVs produce a nested set of sgRNAs that share a common 5′ leader sequence. Secondary structures in this virus-unique sequence could be involved in enhanced translation of viral RNAs. A first indication for this hypothesis came from the observation that accumulation of leader sequence mutations during persistent MHV infection affects translation rates (19). Furthermore, the 5′ UTRs of bovine coronavirus (BCoV) RNA1 and RNA7 enhance cap-dependent reporter RNA translation without affecting RNA stability (79). Comparable to what is observed during BCoV infection, the 5′ UTR of IBV RNA7 results in more efficient translation of reporter RNA than the 5′ UTR of RNA1. In support of this finding, translation of chimeric RNAs containing the MHV leader sequence fused to the alpha-globulin gene was enhanced in cell extract without a major effect on mRNA stability (94). Translation was most enhanced in extracts from MHV-infected cells, suggesting that a virus-induced viral or cellular factor is involved in leader-mediated preferential translation. The N protein has been proposed to be such a factor (94). Coexpression of N protein and reporter RNA containing the MHV leader provided the only evidence so far that N protein can enhance translation of such RNA twofold compared to RNA with a mutated leader sequence (95). Some studies suggest that binding of N protein to leader RNA may stimulate translation. However, direct mechanistic findings have been limited, and it remains to be investigated whether binding of N protein enhances RNA stability or affects other aspects of translation. Analysis of the IBV and MHV N proteins by surface plasmon resonance and solution-phase assays revealed that phosphorylation of N protein decreased binding to nonviral RNA, while it has no effect on binding to viral leader-containing RNA (17, 67). Stem-loops surrounding the TRS conferred high affinity of N protein binding to RNA (17, 67). Surprisingly, high-affinity binding to the antileader sequence was also described. Although translation of CoV RNAs has been extensively studied in MHV-infected cells, relatively little is known about this process during SARS-CoV infection. Although it is tempting to speculate that a similar mechanism of preferential translation could exist, since SARS-CoV RNAs possess unique leader sequences as well, this remains to be experimentally established. Recently though, a potential effect of the SARS-CoV unique 7a protein on cellular translation has been reported (44). Expression of the 7a protein induced p38 activation and apoptosis at 24 to 48 h p.i. (96) and diminished cellular translation at 8 to 12 h p.i. and translation of reporter RNAs. Furthermore, expression of SARS-CoV nsp1 degrades cellular mRNA and eventually

inhibits host protein synthesis, as was demonstrated by reduced incorporation of radioactively labeled amino acids (43). Additional experiments will have to determine whether these proteins have the same features in the context of a complete set of viral proteins during infection. Besides favored translation of viral RNAs, MHV mediates cleavage of 28S rRNA in multiple cell lines, which could influence translation in the later stages of cytopathic infection (2). Mature cytoplasmic 28S rRNA is cleaved into five major products from 4 h p.i. onwards, while 18S rRNA remains intact. Degradation of 28S rRNA is dependent on virus replication but is independent of apoptosis and RNase L activity, since it still occurred in the presence of apoptosis inhibitors and in RNase L$^{-/-}$ cells. The potential involvement of p38 or Fos/Jun in 28S rRNA degradation has been suggested (2).

In conclusion, MHV diminishes cellular protein synthesis during infection, without altering the translation machinery of the cell. Viral RNA competes with cellular mRNA for ribosomes. In addition, interaction of the N protein with the unique 5′ UTR in the MHV RNAs could mediate preferential translation of viral RNA. Furthermore, specific 28S rRNA cleavage in the later stages of infection could affect translation. It is currently unknown if other CoVs modulate translation efficiency in a similar way.

## PERSPECTIVES FOR THE USE OF "-OMICS" IN CoV HOST RESEARCH

Over the last years, transcriptomics and, more recently, proteomics have taken a prominent place in studies of virus-host interactions. One of the main advantages of microarray analysis is that a large set of differentially expressed genes and pathways can be studied within the same experiment. However, there can be a significant discrepancy between changes in cellular mRNA and its corresponding protein concentrations (31). Although differential expression of mRNA and proteins within similar cellular pathways yields a more pronounced correlation (102), profiling data should be treated with caution. Microarray analysis of polysome-associated mRNAs can be performed to assess changes in mRNAs that are still being translated in infected cells, as has been shown for poliovirus (42). Since changes in ribosome-bound mRNAs still do not fully reflect changes in effector molecules, virus infections will require analysis at the level of protein concentration, modification, or interaction as well.

Cellular responses during SARS-CoV infection in Vero-E6 cells have been addressed by transcriptomic as well as proteomic approaches (41, 49).

Although the times p.i. at which analysis was performed differed, overlapping groups of genes were found. They included heat shock proteins and ribosomal proteins. Yet a substantial part of the differentially expressed mRNAs and proteins did not match. It is unclear if the bias resulted from the methods used or whether attenuation of translation in SARS-CoV-infected cells underlies this observation. Despite the fact that poor correlation may exist between differential expression at the levels of mRNA and functional protein, transcriptional profiling will remain a valuable tool in the future when incorporated in parallel analyses using transcriptomics as well as proteomic and interactomic approaches. Also, changes in small-RNA species that have been implemented in multiple cellular regulatory processes which may play a role in viral replication or transcription could be studied in more detail using microarrays. Combinational analysis will increasingly depend on the development and accessibility of sophisticated analysis software.

## REFERENCES

1. **An, S., C. J. Chen, X. Yu, J. L. Leibowitz, and S. Makino.** 1999. Induction of apoptosis in murine coronavirus-infected cultured cells and demonstration of E protein as an apoptosis inducer. *J. Virol.* **73:**7853–7859.

2. **Banerjee, S., S. An, A. Zhou, R. H. Silverman, and S. Makino.** 2000. RNase L-independent specific 28S rRNA cleavage in murine coronavirus-infected cells. *J. Virol.* **74:**8793–8802.

3. **Banerjee, S., K. Narayanan, T. Mizutani, and S. Makino.** 2002. Murine coronavirus replication-induced p38 mitogen-activated protein kinase activation promotes interleukin-6 production and virus replication in cultured cells. *J. Virol.* **76:**5937–5948.

4. **Barac-Latas, V., G. Suchanek, H. Breitschopf, A. Stuehler, H. Wege, and H. Lassmann.** 1997. Patterns of oligodendrocyte pathology in coronavirus-induced subacute demyelinating encephalomyelitis in the Lewis rat. *Glia* **19:**1–12.

5. **Barretto, N., D. Jukneliene, K. Ratia, Z. Chen, A. D. Mesecar, and S. C. Baker.** 2005. The papain-like protease of severe acute respiratory syndrome coronavirus has deubiquitinating activity. *J. Virol.* **79:**15189–15198.

6. **Baudoux, P., C. Carrat, L. Besnardeau, B. Charley, and H. Laude.** 1998. Coronavirus pseudoparticles formed with recombinant M and E proteins induce alpha interferon synthesis by leukocytes. *J. Virol.* **72:**8636–8643.

7. **Belyavskyi, M., G. A. Levy, and J. L. Leibowitz.** 1998. The pattern of induction of apoptosis during infection with MHV-3 correlates with strain variation in resistance and susceptibility to lethal hepatitis. *Adv. Exp. Med. Biol.* **440:**619–625.

8. **Belyavsky, M., E. Belyavskaya, G. A. Levy, and J. L. Leibowitz.** 1998. Coronavirus MHV-3-induced apoptosis in macrophages. *Virology* **250:**41–49.

9. **Bert, A. G., R. Grepin, M. A. Vadas, and G. J. Goodall.** 2006. Assessing IRES activity in the HIF-1alpha and other cellular 5' UTRs. *RNA* **12:**1074–1083.

10. **Boya, P., A. L. Pauleau, D. Poncet, R. A. Gonzalez-Polo, N. Zamzami, and G. Kroemer.** 2004. Viral proteins targeting mitochondria: controlling cell death. *Biochim. Biophys. Acta* **1659:**178–189.

11. **Cai, Y., Y. Liu, D. Yu, and X. Zhang.** 2003. Down-regulation of transcription of the proapoptotic gene BNip3 in cultured astrocytes by murine coronavirus infection. *Virology* **316:**104–115.

12. **Castilletti, C., L. Bordi, E. Lalle, G. Rozera, F. Poccia, C. Agrati, I. Abbate, and M. R. Capobianchi.** 2005. Coordinate induction of IFN-alpha and -gamma by SARS-CoV also in the absence of virus replication. *Virology* **341:**163–169.

13. **Chang, Y. J., C. Y. Liu, B. L. Chiang, Y. C. Chao, and C. C. Chen.** 2004. Induction of IL-8 release in lung cells via activator protein-1 by recombinant baculovirus displaying severe acute respiratory syndrome-coronavirus spike proteins: identification of two functional regions. *J. Immunol.* **173:**7602–7614.

14. **Chen, C. J., and S. Makino.** 2002. Murine coronavirus-induced apoptosis in 17Cl-1 cells involves a mitochondria-mediated pathway and its downstream caspase-8 activation and bid cleavage. *Virology* **302:**321–332.

15. **Chen, C.-J., and S. Makino.** 2004. Murine coronavirus replication induces cell cycle arrest in $G_0/G_1$ phase. *J. Virol.* **78:**5658–5669.

16. **Chen, C.-J., K. Sugiyama, H. Kubo, C. Huang, and S. Makino.** 2004. Murine coronavirus nonstructural protein p28 arrests cell cycle in $G_0/G_1$ phase. *J. Virol.* **78:**10410–10419.

17. **Chen, H., A. Gill, B. K. Dove, S. R. Emmett, C. F. Kemp, M. A. Ritchie, M. Dee, and J. A. Hiscox.** 2005. Mass spectroscopic characterization of the coronavirus infectious bronchitis virus nucleoprotein and elucidation of the role of phosphorylation in RNA binding by using surface plasmon resonance. *J. Virol.* **79:**1164–1179.

18. **Chen, H., T. Wurm, P. Britton, G. Brooks, and J. A. Hiscox.** 2002. Interaction of the coronavirus nucleoprotein with nucleolar antigens and the host cell. *J. Virol.* **76:**5233–5250.

19. **Chen, W., and R. S. Baric.** 1995. Function of a 5'-end genomic RNA mutation that evolves during persistent mouse hepatitis virus infection in vitro. *J. Virol.* **69:**7529–7540.

20. **Cheung, C. Y., L. L. Poon, I. H. Ng, W. Luk, S. F. Sia, M. H. Wu, K. H. Chan, K. Y. Yuen, S. Gordon, Y. Guan, and J. S. Peiris.** 2005. Cytokine responses in severe acute respiratory syndrome coronavirus-infected macrophages in vitro: possible relevance to pathogenesis. *J. Virol.* **79:**7819–7826.

21. **Choi, K. S., A. Mizutani, and M. M. Lai.** 2004. SYNCRIP, a member of the heterogeneous nuclear ribonucleoprotein family, is involved in mouse hepatitis virus RNA synthesis. *J. Virol.* **78:**13153–13162.

22. **Chow, K. Y., Y. S. Yeung, C. C. Hon, F. Zeng, K. M. Law, and F. C. Leung.** 2005. Adenovirus-mediated expression of the C-terminal domain of SARS-CoV spike protein is sufficient to induce apoptosis in Vero E6 cells. *FEBS Lett.* **579:**6699–6704.

23. **Cinatl, J., Jr., G. Hoever, B. Morgenstern, W. Preiser, J. U. Vogel, W. K. Hofmann, G. Bauer, M. Michaelis, H. F. Rabenau, and H. W. Doerr.** 2004. Infection of cultured intestinal epithelial cells with severe acute respiratory syndrome coronavirus. *Cell. Mol. Life Sci.* **61:**2100–2112.

24. **Collins, A. R.** 2002. In vitro detection of apoptosis in monocytes/macrophages infected with human coronavirus. *Clin. Diagn. Lab. Immunol.* **9:**1392–1395.

25. **de Haan, C. A., M. de Wit, L. Kuo, C. Montalto-Morrison, B. L. Haagmans, S. R. Weiss, P. S. Masters, and P. J. M. Rottier.** 2003. The glycosylation status of the murine hepatitis coronavirus M protein affects the interferogenic capacity of the virus in vitro and its ability to replicate in the liver but not the brain. *Virology* **312:**395–406.

26. **Dove, B., G. Brooks, K. Bicknell, T. Wurm, and J. A. Hiscox.** 2006. Cell cycle perturbations induced by infection with the coronavirus infectious bronchitis virus and their effect on virus replication. *J. Virol.* **80:**4147–4156.

27. Dove, B. K., J. H. You, M. L. Reed, S. R. Emmett, G. Brooks, and J. A. Hiscox. 2006. Changes in nucleolar morphology and proteins during infection with the coronavirus infectious bronchitis virus. *Cell. Microbiol.* **8**:1147–1157.

28. Eléouët, J.-F., E. A. Slee, F. Saurini, N. Castagné, D. Poncet, C. Garrido, E. Solary, and S. J. Martin. 2000. The viral nucleocapsid protein of transmissible gastroenteritis coronavirus (TGEV) is cleaved by caspase-6 and -7 during TGEV-induced apoptosis. *J. Virol.* **74**:3975–3983.

29. Esche, C., C. Stellato, and L. A. Beck. 2005. Chemokines: key players in innate and adaptive immunity. *J. Investig. Dermatol.* **125**:615–628.

30. Gosert, R., A. Kanjanahaluethai, D. Egger, K. Bienz, and S. C. Baker. 2002. RNA replication of mouse hepatitis virus takes place at double-membrane vesicles. *J. Virol.* **76**:3697–3708.

31. Griffin, T. J., S. P. Gygi, T. Ideker, B. Rist, J. Eng, L. Hood, and R. Aebersold. 2002. Complementary profiling of gene expression at the transcriptome and proteome levels in Saccharomyces cerevisiae. *Mol. Cell. Proteomics* **1**:323–333.

32. Haller, O., G. Kochs, and F. Weber. 2006. The interferon response circuit: induction and suppression by pathogenic viruses. *Virology* **344**:119–130.

33. Hay, S., and G. Kannourakis. 2002. A time to kill: viral manipulation of the cell death program. *J. Gen. Virol.* **83**:1547–1564.

34. Herold, J., and R. Andino. 2001. Poliovirus RNA replication requires genome circularization through a protein-protein bridge. *Mol. Cell* **7**:581–591.

35. Hilton, A., L. Mizzen, G. MacIntyre, S. Cheley, and R. Anderson. 1986. Translational control in murine hepatitis virus infection. *J. Gen. Virol.* **67**(Pt. 5):923–932.

36. Hiscox, J. A., T. Wurm, L. Wilson, P. Britton, D. Cavanagh, and G. Brooks. 2001. The coronavirus infectious bronchitis virus nucleoprotein localizes to the nucleolus. *J. Virol.* **75**:506–512.

37. Huang, P., and M. M. Lai. 1999. Polypyrimidine tract-binding protein binds to the complementary strand of the mouse hepatitis virus 3′ untranslated region, thereby altering RNA conformation. *J. Virol.* **73**:9110–9116.

38. Huang, P., and M. M. C. Lai. 2001. Heterogeneous nuclear ribonucleoprotein A1 binds to the 3′-untranslated region and mediates potential 5′-3′-end cross talks of mouse hepatitis virus RNA. *J. Virol.* **75**:5009–5017.

39. Jack, C. S., N. Arbour, J. Manusow, V. Montgrain, M. Blain, E. McCrea, A. Shapiro, and J. P. Antel. 2005. TLR signaling tailors innate immune responses in human microglia and astrocytes. *J. Immunol.* **175**:4320–4330.

40. Jenner, R. G., and R. A. Young. 2005. Insights into host responses against pathogens from transcriptional profiling. *Nat. Rev. Microbiol.* **3**:281–294.

41. Jiang, X. S., L. Y. Tang, J. Dai, H. Zhou, S. J. Li, Q. C. Xia, J. R. Wu, and R. Zeng. 2005. Quantitative analysis of severe acute respiratory syndrome (SARS)-associated coronavirus-infected cells using proteomic approaches: implications for cellular responses to virus infection. *Mol. Cell. Proteomics* **4**:902–913.

42. Johannes, G., M. S. Carter, M. B. Eisen, P. O. Brown, and P. Sarnow. 1999. Identification of eukaryotic mRNAs that are translated at reduced cap binding complex eIF4F concentrations using a cDNA microarray. *Proc. Natl. Acad. Sci. USA* **96**:13118–13123.

43. Kamitani, W., K. Narayanan, C. Huang, K. Lokugamage, T. Ikegami, N. Ito, H. Kubo, and S. Makino. 2006. Severe acute respiratory syndrome coronavirus nsp1 protein suppresses host gene expression by promoting host mRNA degradation. *Proc. Natl. Acad. Sci. USA* **103**:12885–12890.

44. Kopecky-Bromberg, S. A., L. Martinez-Sobrido, and P. Palese. 2006. 7a protein of severe acute respiratory syndrome coronavirus inhibits cellular protein synthesis and activates p38 mitogen-activated protein kinase. *J. Virol.* **80**:785–793.

45. Kyuwa, S., M. Cohen, G. Nelson, S. M. Tahara, and S. A. Stohlman. 1994. Modulation of cellular macromolecular synthesis by coronavirus: implication for pathogenesis. *J. Virol.* **68**:6815–6819.

46. Lampert, P. W., J. K. Sims, and A. J. Kniazeff. 1973. Mechanism of demyelination in JHM virus encephalomyelitis. Electron microscopic studies. *Acta Neuropathol.* **24**:76–85.

47. Law, H. K., C. Y. Cheung, H. Y. Ng, S. F. Sia, Y. O. Chan, W. Luk, J. M. Nicholls, J. S. Peiris, and Y. L. Lau. 2005. Chemokine up-regulation in SARS-coronavirus-infected, monocyte-derived human dendritic cells. *Blood* **106**:2366–2374.

48. Law, P. T., C. H. Wong, T. C. Au, C. P. Chuck, S. K. Kong, P. K. Chan, K. F. To, A. W. Lo, J. Y. Chan, Y. K. Suen, H. Y. Chan, K. P. Fung, M. M. Waye, J. J. Sung, Y. M. Lo, and S. K. Tsui. 2005. The 3a protein of severe acute respiratory syndrome-associated coronavirus induces apoptosis in Vero E6 cells. *J. Gen. Virol.* **86**:1921–1930.

49. Leong, W. F., H. C. Tan, E. E. Ooi, D. R. Koh, and V. T. Chow. 2005. Microarray and real-time RT-PCR analyses of differential human gene expression patterns induced by severe acute respiratory syndrome (SARS) coronavirus infection of Vero cells. *Microbes Infect.* **7**:248–259.

50. Levy, G. A., J. L. Leibowitz, and T. S. Edgington. 1981. Induction of monocyte procoagulant activity by murine hepatitis virus type 3 parallels disease susceptibility in mice. *J. Exp. Med.* **154**:1150–1163.

51. Li, H. P., P. Huang, S. Park, and M. M. Lai. 1999. Polypyrimidine tract-binding protein binds to the leader RNA of mouse hepatitis virus and serves as a regulator of viral transcription. *J. Virol.* **73**:772–777.

52. Li, H. P., X. Zhang, R. Duncan, L. Comai, and M. M. Lai. 1997. Heterogeneous nuclear ribonucleoprotein A1 binds to the transcription-regulatory region of mouse hepatitis virus RNA. *Proc. Natl. Acad. Sci. USA* **94**:9544–9549.

53. Li, Y., L. Fu, D. M. Gonzales, and E. Lavi. 2004. Coronavirus neurovirulence correlates with the ability of the virus to induce proinflammatory cytokine signals from astrocytes and microglia. *J. Virol.* **78**:3398–3406.

54. Liu, C., H. Y. Xu, and D. X. Liu. 2001. Induction of caspase-dependent apoptosis in cultured cells by the avian coronavirus infectious bronchitis virus. *J. Virol.* **75**:6402–6409.

55. Liu, Q., W. Yu, and J. L. Leibowitz. 1997. A specific host cellular protein binding element near the 3′ end of mouse hepatitis virus genomic RNA. *Virology* **232**:74–85.

56. Liu, Y., Y. Cai, and X. Zhang. 2003. Induction of caspase-dependent apoptosis in cultured rat oligodendrocytes by murine coronavirus is mediated during cell entry and does not require virus replication. *J. Virol.* **77**:11952–11963.

57. Liu, Y., Y. Pu, and X. Zhang. 2006. Role of the mitochondrial signaling pathway in murine coronavirus-induced oligodendrocyte apoptosis. *J. Virol.* **80**:395–403.

58. Liu, Y., and X. Zhang. 2005. Expression of cellular oncogene Bcl-xL prevents coronavirus-induced cell death and converts acute infection to persistent infection in progenitor rat oligodendrocytes. *J. Virol.* **79**:47–56.

59. Lundberg, M., and M. Johansson. 2001. Is VP22 nuclear homing an artifact? *Nat. Biotechnol.* **19**:713–714.

60. Luo, H., Q. Chen, J. Chen, K. Chen, X. Shen, and H. Jiang. 2005. The nucleocapsid protein of SARS coronavirus has a high binding affinity to the human cellular heterogeneous nuclear ribonucleoprotein A1. *FEBS Lett.* **579**:2623–2628.

61. Meylan, E., and J. Tschopp. 2006. Toll-like receptors and RNA helicases: two parallel ways to trigger antiviral responses. *Mol. Cell* 22:561–569.

62. Mizutani, T., S. Fukushi, M. Saijo, I. Kurane, and S. Morikawa. 2004. Importance of Akt signaling pathway for apoptosis in SARS-CoV-infected Vero E6 cells. *Virology* 327:169–174.

63. Mizzen, L., G. MacIntyre, F. Wong, and R. Anderson. 1987. Translational regulation in mouse hepatitis virus infection is not mediated by altered intracellular ion concentrations. *J. Gen. Virol.* 68(Pt. 8):2143–2151.

64. Nanda, S. K., and J. L. Leibowitz. 2001. Mitochondrial aconitase binds to the 3' untranslated region of the mouse hepatitis virus genome. *J. Virol.* 75:3352–3362.

65. Naniche, D., S. I. Reed, and M. B. A. Oldstone. 1999. Cell cycle arrest during measles virus infection: a $G_0$-like block leads to suppression of retinoblastoma protein expression. *J. Virol.* 73:1894–1901.

66. Nash, T. C., and M. J. Buchmeier. 1997. Entry of mouse hepatitis virus into cells by endosomal and nonendosomal pathways. *Virology* 233:1–8.

67. Nelson, G. W., S. A. Stohlman, and S. M. Tahara. 2000. High affinity interaction between nucleocapsid protein and leader/intergenic sequence of mouse hepatitis virus RNA. *J. Gen. Virol.* 81:181–188.

68. Ng, L. F., M. L. Hibberd, E. E. Ooi, K. F. Tang, S. Y. Neo, J. Tan, K. R. Murthy, V. B. Vega, J. M. Chia, E. T. Liu, and E. C. Ren. 2004. A human in vitro model system for investigating genome-wide host responses to SARS coronavirus infection. *BMC Infect. Dis.* 4:34.

69. Okabayashi, T., H. Kariwa, S. Yokota, S. Iki, T. Indoh, N. Yokosawa, I. Takashima, H. Tsutsumi, and N. Fujii. 2006. Cytokine regulation in SARS coronavirus infection compared to other respiratory virus infections. *J. Med. Virol.* 78:417–424.

70. Op De Beeck, A., and P. Caillet-Fauquet. 1997. Viruses and the cell cycle. *Prog. Cell Cycle Res.* 3:1–19.

71. Poggioli, G. J., T. S. Dermody, and K. L. Tyler. 2001. Reovirus-induced σ1s-dependent $G_2$/M phase cell cycle arrest is associated with inhibition of p34$^{cdc2}$. *J. Virol.* 75:7429–7434.

72. Prentice, E., W. G. Jerome, T. Yoshimori, N. Mizushima, and M. R. Denison. 2004. Coronavirus replication complex formation utilizes components of cellular autophagy. *J. Biol. Chem.* 279:10136–10141.

73. Rempel, J. D., S. J. Murray, J. Meisner, and M. J. Buchmeier. 2004. Differential regulation of innate and adaptive immune responses in viral encephalitis. *Virology* 318:381–392.

74. Rempel, J. D., L. A. Quina, P. K. Blakely-Gonzales, M. J. Buchmeier, and D. L. Gruol. 2005. Viral induction of central nervous system innate immune responses. *J. Virol.* 79:4369–4381.

75. Rowland, R. R., V. Chauhan, Y. Fang, A. Pekosz, M. Kerrigan, and M. D. Burton. 2005. Intracellular localization of the severe acute respiratory syndrome coronavirus nucleocapsid protein: absence of nucleolar accumulation during infection and after expression as a recombinant protein in Vero cells. *J. Virol.* 79:11507–11512.

76. Samuel, M. A., and M. S. Diamond. 2005. Alpha/beta interferon protects against lethal West Nile virus infection by restricting cellular tropism and enhancing neuronal survival. *J. Virol.* 79:13350–13361.

77. Schafer, K. A. 1998. The cell cycle: a review. *Vet. Pathol.* 35:461–478.

78. Schwartz, T., L. Fu, and E. Lavi. 2002. Differential induction of apoptosis in demyelinating and nondemyelinating infection by mouse hepatitis virus. *J. Neurovirol.* 8:392–399.

79. Senanayake, S. D., and D. A. Brian. 1999. Translation from the 5' untranslated region (UTR) of mRNA 1 is repressed, but that from the 5' UTR of mRNA 7 is stimulated in coronavirus-infected cells. *J. Virol.* 73:8003–8009.

80. Shen, X., and P. S. Masters. 2001. Evaluation of the role of heterogeneous nuclear ribonucleoprotein A1 as a host factor in murine coronavirus discontinuous transcription and genome replication. *Proc. Natl. Acad. Sci. USA* 98:2717–2722.

81. Shi, S. T., P. Huang, H. P. Li, and M. M. Lai. 2000. Heterogeneous nuclear ribonucleoprotein A1 regulates RNA synthesis of a cytoplasmic virus. *EMBO J.* 19:4701–4711.

82. Shi, S. T., J. J. Schiller, A. Kanjanahaluethai, S. C. Baker, J. W. Oh, and M. M. Lai. 1999. Colocalization and membrane association of murine hepatitis virus gene 1 products and de novo-synthesized viral RNA in infected cells. *J. Virol.* 73:5957–5969.

83. Shi, S. T., G. Y. Yu, and M. M. Lai. 2003. Multiple type A/B heterogeneous nuclear ribonucleoproteins (hnRNPs) can replace hnRNP A1 in mouse hepatitis virus RNA synthesis. *J. Virol.* 77:10584–10593.

84. Shintani, T., and D. J. Klionsky. 2004. Autophagy in health and disease: a double-edged sword. *Science* 306:990–995.

85. Siddell, S., H. Wege, A. Barthel, and V. ter Meulen. 1981. Intracellular protein synthesis and the in vitro translation of coronavirus JHM mRNA. *Adv. Exp. Med. Biol.* 142:193–207.

86. Snijder, E. J., Y. van der Meer, J. Zevenhoven-Dobbe, J. J. Onderwater, J. van der Meulen, H. K. Koerten, and A. M. Mommaas. 2006. Ultrastructure and origin of membrane vesicles associated with the severe acute respiratory syndrome coronavirus replication complex. *J. Virol.* 80:5927–5940.

87. Spagnolo, J. F., and B. G. Hogue. 2000. Host protein interactions with the 3' end of bovine coronavirus RNA and the requirement of the poly(A) tail for coronavirus defective genome replication. *J. Virol.* 74:5053–5065.

88. Spiegel, M., A. Pichlmair, L. Martinez-Sobrido, J. Cros, A. Garcia-Sastre, O. Haller, and F. Weber. 2005. Inhibition of beta interferon induction by severe acute respiratory syndrome coronavirus suggests a two-step model for activation of interferon regulatory factor 3. *J. Virol.* 79:2079–2086.

89. Spiegel, M., K. Schneider, F. Weber, M. Weidmann, and F. T. Hufert. 2006. Interaction of severe acute respiratory syndrome-associated coronavirus with dendritic cells. *J. Gen. Virol.* 87:1953–1960.

90. Spiegel, M., and F. Weber. 2006. Inhibition of cytokine gene expression and induction of chemokine genes in non-lymphatic cells infected with SARS coronavirus. *Virol. J.* 3:17.

91. Surjit, M., R. Kumar, R. N. Mishra, M. K. Reddy, V. T. Chow, and S. K. Lal. 2005. The severe acute respiratory syndrome coronavirus nucleocapsid protein is phosphorylated and localizes in the cytoplasm by 14-3-3-mediated translocation. *J. Virol.* 79:11476–11486.

92. Surjit, M., B. Liu, V. T. K. Chow, and S. K. Lal. 2006. The nucleocapsid protein of severe acute respiratory syndrome-coronavirus inhibits the activity of cyclin-cyclin-dependent kinase complex and blocks S phase progression in mammalian cells. *J. Biol. Chem.* 281:10669–10681.

93. Surjit, M., B. Liu, S. Jameel, V. T. Chow, and S. K. Lal. 2004. The SARS coronavirus nucleocapsid protein induces actin reorganization and apoptosis in COS-1 cells in the absence of growth factors. *Biochem. J.* 383:13–18.

94. Tahara, S. M., T. A. Dietlin, C. C. Bergmann, G. W. Nelson, S. Kyuwa, R. P. Anthony, and S. A. Stohlman. 1994. Coronavirus translational regulation: leader affects mRNA efficiency. *Virology* 202:621–630.

95. Tahara, S. M., T. A. Dietlin, G. W. Nelson, S. A. Stohlman, and D. J. Manno. 1998. Mouse hepatitis virus nucleocapsid protein as a translational effector of viral mRNAs. *Adv. Exp. Med. Biol.* **440:**313–318.

96. Tan, Y. J., B. C. Fielding, P. Y. Goh, S. Shen, T. H. Tan, S. G. Lim, and W. Hong. 2004. Overexpression of 7a, a protein specifically encoded by the severe acute respiratory syndrome coronavirus, induces apoptosis via a caspase-dependent pathway. *J. Virol.* **78:**14043–14047.

97. Tang, B. S., K. H. Chan, V. C. Cheng, P. C. Woo, S. K. Lau, C. C. Lam, T. L. Chan, A. K. Wu, I. F. Hung, S. Y. Leung, and K. Y. Yuen. 2005. Comparative host gene transcription by microarray analysis early after infection of the Huh7 cell line by severe acute respiratory syndrome coronavirus and human coronavirus 229E. *J. Virol.* **79:**6180–6193.

98. Tseng, C. T., L. A. Perrone, H. Zhu, S. Makino, and C. J. Peters. 2005. Severe acute respiratory syndrome and the innate immune responses: modulation of effector cell function without productive infection. *J. Immunol.* **174:**7977–7985.

99. van der Meer, Y., E. J. Snijder, J. C. Dobbe, S. Schleich, M. R. Denison, W. J. M. Spaan, and J. K. Locker. 1999. Localization of mouse hepatitis virus nonstructural proteins and RNA synthesis indicates a role for late endosomes in viral replication. *J. Virol.* **73:**7641–7657.

100. Versteeg, G. A., O. Slobodskaya, and W. J. Spaan. 2006. Transcriptional profiling of acute cytopathic murine hepatitis virus infection in fibroblast-like cells. *J. Gen. Virol.* **87:**1961–1975.

101. Visintin, R., and A. Amon. 2000. The nucleolus: the magician's hat for cell cycle tricks. *Curr. Opin. Cell Biol.* **12:**372–377.

102. Walhout, A. J., J. Reboul, O. Shtanko, N. Bertin, P. Vaglio, H. Ge, H. Lee, L. Doucette-Stamm, K. C. Gunsalus, A. J. Schetter, D. G. Morton, K. J. Kemphues, V. Reinke, S. K. Kim, F. Piano, and M. Vidal. 2002. Integrating interactome, phenome, and transcriptome mapping data for the C. elegans germline. *Curr. Biol.* **12:**1952–1958.

103. Walter, B. L., T. B. Parsley, E. Ehrenfeld, and B. L. Semler. 2002. Distinct poly(rC) binding protein KH domain determinants for poliovirus translation initiation and viral RNA replication. *J. Virol.* **76:**12008–12022.

104. Wang, Y., and X. Zhang. 1999. The nucleocapsid protein of coronavirus mouse hepatitis virus interacts with the cellular heterogeneous nuclear ribonucleoprotein A1 in vitro and in vivo. *Virology* **265:**96–109.

105. Werts, C., S. E. Girardin, and D. J. Philpott. 2006. TIR, CARD and PYRIN: three domains for an antimicrobial triad. *Cell Death Differ.* **13:**798–815.

106. Wileman, T. 2006. Aggresomes and autophagy generate sites for virus replication. *Science* **312:**875–878.

107. Wong, S. L., Y. Chen, C. M. Chan, C. S. Chan, P. K. Chan, Y. L. Chui, K. P. Fung, M. M. Waye, S. K. Tsui, and H. Y. Chan. 2005. In vivo functional characterization of the SARS-coronavirus 3a protein in Drosophila. *Biochem. Biophys. Res. Commun.* **337:**720–729.

108. Wu, G. F., and S. Perlman. 1999. Macrophage infiltration, but not apoptosis, is correlated with immune-mediated demyelination following murine infection with a neurotropic coronavirus. *J. Virol.* **73:**8771–8780.

109. Wurm, T., H. Chen, T. Hodgson, P. Britton, G. Brooks, and J. A. Hiscox. 2001. Localization to the nucleolus is a common feature of coronavirus nucleoproteins, and the protein may disrupt host cell division. *J. Virol.* **75:**9345–9356.

110. Xu, H. Y., K. P. Lim, S. Shen, and D. X. Liu. 2001. Further identification and characterization of novel intermediate and mature cleavage products released from the ORF 1b region of the avian coronavirus infectious bronchitis virus 1a/1b polyprotein. *Virology* **288:**212–222.

111. Yan, H., G. Xiao, J. Zhang, Y. Hu, F. Yuan, D. K. Cole, C. Zheng, and G. F. Gao. 2004. SARS coronavirus induces apoptosis in Vero E6 cells. *J. Med. Virol.* **73:**323–331.

112. Yang, Y., Z. Xiong, S. Zhang, Y. Yan, J. Nguyen, B. Ng, H. Lu, J. Brendese, F. Yang, H. Wang, and X. F. Yang. 2005. Bcl-xL inhibits T-cell apoptosis induced by expression of SARS coronavirus E protein in the absence of growth factors. *Biochem. J.* **392:**135–143.

113. Yen, Y. T., F. Liao, C. H. Hsiao, C. L. Kao, Y. C. Chen, and B. A. Wu-Hsieh. 2006. Modeling the early events of severe acute respiratory syndrome coronavirus infection in vitro. *J. Virol.* **80:**2684–2693.

114. You, J., B. K. Dove, L. Enjuanes, M. L. DeDiego, E. Alvarez, G. Howell, P. Heinen, M. Zambon, and J. A. Hiscox. 2005. Subcellular localization of the severe acute respiratory syndrome coronavirus nucleocapsid protein. *J. Gen. Virol.* **86:**3303–3310.

115. Yu, W., and J. L. Leibowitz. 1995. Specific binding of host cellular proteins to multiple sites within the 3′ end of mouse hepatitis virus genomic RNA. *J. Virol.* **69:**2016–2023.

116. Yuan, X., Y. Shan, Z. Zhao, J. Chen, and Y. Cong. 2005. G0/G1 arrest and apoptosis induced by SARS-CoV 3b protein in transfected cells. *Virol. J.* **2:**66.

117. Yuan, X., J. Wu, Y. Shan, Z. Yao, B. Dong, B. Chen, Z. Zhao, S. Wang, J. Chen, and Y. Cong. 2006. SARS coronavirus 7a protein blocks cell cycle progression at G0/G1 phase via the cyclin D3/pRb pathway. *Virology* **346:**74–85.

118. Zamora, M., W. E. Marissen, and R. E. Lloyd. 2002. Multiple eIF4GI-specific protease activities present in uninfected and poliovirus-infected cells. *J. Virol.* **76:**165–177.

119. Zhirnov, O. P., T. E. Konakova, W. Garten, and H. Klenk. 1999. Caspase-dependent N-terminal cleavage of influenza virus nucleocapsid protein in infected cells. *J. Virol.* **73:**10158–10163.

120. Ziegler, T., S. Matikainen, E. Ronkko, P. Osterlund, M. Sillanpaa, J. Siren, R. Fagerlund, M. Immonen, K. Melen, and I. Julkunen. 2005. Severe acute respiratory syndrome coronavirus fails to activate cytokine-mediated innate immune responses in cultured human monocyte-derived dendritic cells. *J. Virol.* **79:**13800–13805.

*Nidoviruses*
Edited by S. Perlman, T. Gallagher, and E. J. Snijder
© 2008 ASM Press, Washington, DC

Chapter 17

# Pathogenesis of Murine Coronavirus Infection

Susan R. Weiss and Julian L. Leibowitz

The murine coronavirus, mouse hepatitis virus (MHV), is actually a group of strains with various organ tropisms as well as pathogenic potentials. MHV strains may be divided into two groups according to general patterns of tropism. One group of strains is enterotropic; this includes MHV-D, -Y, -RI, -S/CDC, -LIVIM, and -DVIM. These are the viruses associated with infections of mouse colonies that generally produce infections confined to the gastrointestinal tract (53). The other major group contains polytropic strains, including MHV-1, -2, -3, -4 (or JHM), and -A59; experimental infections of rodents with these strains provide animal models for human diseases such as hepatitis and encephalitis, demyelinating diseases such as multiple sclerosis, and, most recently, respiratory disease such as severe acute respiratory syndrome (SARS). In this review we discuss primarily infections of the central nervous system (CNS) and the liver.

## MHV INFECTION OF THE CNS BY STRAINS JHM AND A59

MHV strains JHM and A59 cause acute encephalitis, which is sometimes followed by the development of chronic demyelination in surviving animals. There are many laboratory variants of MHV strain JHM with variable degrees of pathogenesis, making it difficult to compare results obtained using different isolates. In this chapter, we compare the various isolates of JHM in terms of CNS disease and, when possible, their origins (Table 1).

JHM was initially isolated by Cheever, Bailey, and colleagues in 1949 from a paralyzed mouse and demonstrated to induce encephalomyelitis with extensive destruction of myelin (4, 17). Hartley and Rowe

at NIH (49a) obtained JHM from Joan Daniels, a coworker of Cheever and Bailey, and deposited the virus with Microbiological Associates, which passed the virus to the American Type Culture Collection (ATCC). Leslie Weiner obtained the virus from Microbiological Associates and passaged it multiple times through mouse brains (174, 175). Many of the JHM isolates used since were derived from the virus passaged by Weiner. Two JHM isolates used for pathogenesis studies, those used by Lampert et al. (69) and Lucas et al. (88), were not directly derived from Weiner's virus but were obtained directly from Hartley and Rowe (NIH) and from the ATCC, respectively.

An obstacle to the study of demyelinating disease was that early isolates of JHM were highly encephalitic and lethal, leaving few survivors. This issue prompted the isolation of temperature-sensitive mutants, plaque size variants, and monoclonal antibody escape variants, all neuroattenuated, for studies of demyelination. The development of a mouse model using the neuroattenuated strain of MHV-A59 has also been useful in studies of chronic demyelinating diseases.

The JHM stock obtained by Weiner induced lethal encephalitis and thus was not useful for studies of demyelination. However, multiple mouse brain passages led to the selection of variants that were less lethal and, as a consequence, more demyelinating (174). Stohlman and colleagues isolated viruses from plaques of different sizes after eight passages through mouse brains. These viruses include DL (large-plaque virus that is highly neuron tropic and lethal, leaving few survivors for the study of demyelination), DM (medium-plaque virus that causes both encephalitis and demyelination), and DS (small-plaque virus that is weakly neurovirulent but does induce demyelination) (150). Viruses that are attenuated for acute

Susan R. Weiss • Department of Microbiology, University of Pennsylvania School of Medicine, Philadelphia, PA 19104-6076. Julian L. Leibowitz • Department of Microbial and Molecular Pathogenesis, Texas A&M University System College of Medicine, College Station, TX 77843-1114.

**Table 1.** Neurotropic MHV strains and variants of MHV[a]

| Strain(s) | Pathogenesis | Spike | Reference(s) |
|---|---|---|---|
| JHM$_{SD}$ (MHV-4) | Highly lethal; receptor-independent spread; no demyelination | Long HVR spike | 23, 118 |
| JHM$_{IA}$ | Highly lethal but less than JHM$_{SD}$; receptor-dependent spread | Long HVR, S310G substitution | 116, 118 |
| JHM-cl2 | Highly lethal; receptor-independent spread | Long HVR | 158 |
| JHM-X | Avirulent | HVR deletion | 101a |
| JHM-DL (large plaque) | Kills neurons, little demyelination | | 150 |
| JHM-DM (medium plaque) | Encephalitis and demyelination | | 150 |
| JHM-DS (small plaque) | Nonneuronal; demyelination | | 150 |
| 2.2-V-1 (from DL) MAb escape mutant | Subacute paralytic disease; reduced neurovirulence | | 39, 170 |
| 2.2/7.2-V-2 (from DL) MAb escape mutant | Attenuation of virulence and demyelination | | 39, 170 |
| V5A13.1(86), V4B11.3(86); derived from MHV-4 as MAb escape mutants | Subacute paralytic disease; reduced neurovirulence | HVR deletion | 23, 118 |
| JHM (Wurzburg) | Isolated from rats; attenuated | HVR deletion | 173 |
| A59 | Mild to moderate encephalitis, demyelination (hepatitis) | 52-amino-acid deletion in HVR | 74 |

[a]Neurotropic strains and variants are listed, along with their general pathogenic phenotype, status of HVR in the spike protein (where known), and reference. MAb, monoclonal antibody.

infection but that are still demyelinating were also obtained by the selection of monoclonal antibody escape mutants of DL. Variant 2.2-V-1, resistant to monoclonal antibody J.2.2 (specific for the spike protein), infects mainly glial cells and causes little encephalitis; despite its neuroattenuation, 2.2-V-1 induces extensive demyelination. Variant 2.2/7.2-V-2, which is resistant to both monoclonal antibodies J.2.2 and J.7.2 (also directed against spike protein), causes little encephalitis or demyelination (39, 170). Attenuation of 2.2/7.2-V-2 was associated with point mutations and/or deletions within the spike protein, as discussed below. These viruses have been used by Stohlman and Bergmann and colleagues in studies of pathogenesis and immune response. Some of the conclusions drawn from these studies are as follows. (i) JHM infects several cell types in the brain, including neurons, astrocytes, microglia, and oligodendrocytes, and the more neuroattenuated variants infect glial cells rather than neurons (100). (ii) Viral clearance requires T cells and B cells. During acute infections CD8[+] T cells are crucial for clearance of virus, and they are aided by CD4[+] T cells (154). Clearance is mediated by perforin in the case of astrocytes and microglia and by gamma interferon (IFN-γ) in oligodendrocytes (9, 121). Antibodies are needed to prevent virus recrudescence (10, 104). (iii) Demyelination requires a threshold level of replication during acute infection to promote spread of virus to the spinal cord (99). Viral RNA persists in the CNS probably accompanied by low levels of antigen but in the absence of detectable infectious virus. Persistence in accompanied by the presence of viral-epitope-specific CD8[+] T cells (101).

The MHV-4 isolate of JHM (12, 23), recently referred to as JHM$_{SD}$ (116), is highly neurovirulent and is used primarily by Buchmeier and Weiss and colleagues. Following intracranial inoculation of doses as low as 2 PFU into 4-week-old mice C57BL/6 mice, JHM$_{SD}$ spreads rapidly throughout the brain and spinal cord, infecting mostly neurons, and is nearly uniformly fatal. This high virulence is associated with a long hypervariable domain within the JHM$_{SD}$ spike protein, as discussed below. High neurovirulence is at least partly due to the ability of the JHM$_{SD}$ spike protein to carry out carcinoembryonic antigen adhesion molecule 1 (CEACAM1) receptor-independent spread (43) and to confer the ability to rapidly infect large numbers of neurons both in vivo and in neuronal cultures (unpublished data). JHM$_{SD}$ induces a strong innate immune response, including high and prolonged levels of type I IFN, neutrophils, and macrophage-attracting chemokines (54, 137). Unlike the JHM isolates utilized by Bergmann et al. (8), it fails to induce more than a minimal CD8[+] T-cell response, resulting in the inability to clear virus effectively from the CNS (54, 96, 137). The inability of JHM$_{SD}$ to induce an effective CD8[+] T-cell response is not due to general immunosuppression. While this model is not useful for the study of MHV-induced demyelination, it is used to dissect molecular determinants of high neurovirulence. Results show that multiple viral genes as well as the host genetic background contribute to the highly neuropathogenic phenotype of JHM$_{SD}$ (54, 95, 110, 137, 138), which is discussed further below.

Pathogenesis studies of mutants and variants of JHM$_{SD}$ have contributed to the understanding of

MHV-induced CNS disease. A set of temperature-sensitive mutants of MHV-4 (JHM$_{SD}$) was selected. Several of these mutants, most notably ts8, were less lethal and thus provided more surviving animals with which to study demyelination (50). Neutralization-resistant monoclonal antibody escape mutants containing mutations and/or deletions within two independent epitopes of the spike protein have been selected from wild-type JHM$_{SD}$ (23). These viruses, like the ones described above, are attenuated for encephalitis but induce significant demyelination, again demonstrating that encephalitis is not a prerequisite for the development of late demyelinating disease. The OBLV60 variant of JHM$_{SD}$ selected by infection of olfactory bulb-derived OBLV21 cells has a highly attenuated phenotype different from that of the escape mutants. After intranasal inoculation, OBLV60 infects primarily neurons in the olfactory bulb (123). This altered pathogenesis is associated with limited numbers of mutations in the spike protein and an altered pathway of cell entry (44, 108), which is discussed below.

The JHM$_{IA}$ isolate, (116) is also highly neurovirulent, although somewhat less so than JHM$_{SD}$ when inoculated into weanling C57Bl/6 mice (95). This virus was derived from the JHM obtained by Lampert, multiply passaged in mouse brains, and plaque purified. The spike protein of JHM$_{IA}$ differs from that of JHM$_{SD}$ by four amino acids; it is amino acid 310 in the spike that determines the difference in virulence (116). JHM$_{IA}$ is not capable of receptor-independent spread, and it induces a protective CD8$^+$ T-cell response (95, 116), both of which likely contribute to its less virulent phenotype.

A model has been developed in which JHM$_{IA}$ is used to infect suckling mice that are passively immunized by nursing on JHM-immune dams. These mice are protected from acute encephalitis, but 40 to 90% of the animals develop hind-limb paralysis and demyelination, and infectious virus can be isolated from symptomatic mice (127). This model is fundamentally different from those used by other investigators in that virus persists during the chronic demyelinating stage. Much of the virus isolated contains inactivating mutations within the immunodominant H-2D$^b$-restricted CD8$^+$ T-cell epitope, S510–518 (S510), encoded in the spike gene. It is inferred that persistence of virus and hence the demyelinating disease depend on the selection of epitope escape mutants. It is difficult to generalize about the role of epitope escape mutation in demyelinating disease because the selection of these "epitope escape" mutants depends on the lack of detectable neutralizing antibody present in the CNS of these infected mice (24). Epitope escape does not occur in similarly

aged BALB/c mice of the H-2$^b$ haplotype, which have higher levels of neutralizing antibodies, nor does it occur in adult mice. This is discussed further below.

JHM induces acute encephalitis followed by demyelinating disease in the rat (147, 173). Viruses with different pathogenic potential may be recovered from the brains of infected rats. The cl-2 isolate of JHM was isolated from the brain of an infected rat and is almost identical to JHM$_{SD}$ (158). Another study reported isolation of viruses from the rat spinal cord that were either primarily encephalitic or primarily demyelinating (107).

The dual tropic A59 strain of MHV induces mild to moderate encephalitis as well as moderate to severe hepatitis, in a dose-dependent fashion. A59 was originally isolated from a mouse with leukemia in 1961 (97). A59 is considerably less neurovirulent than wild-type JHM isolates, requiring about 1,000 times more virus to kill mice than JHM$_{SD}$. Thus, following intracranial inoculation of C57Bl/6 mice with a moderate dose of A59, there are many survivors with which to study demyelination (74). A59 infects both neurons and glial cells and induces a robust CD8$^+$ T-cell response that is essential for viral clearance (48, 130). A59 does not express the immunodominant S510 epitope encoded within the JHM spike; thus, the response against the subdominant S598–605 epitope (S598), common to both the A59 and JHM spike proteins, is sufficient to mediate viral clearance. Interestingly, while T cells are sufficient for clearance of virus from the CNS (84), antibodies are needed to prevent reemergence of infectious virus in the CNS as in JHM (2.2-V-1)-infected mice. In contrast, T cells are sufficient for complete virus clearance from the liver, even in the absence of antibodies (104).

The importance of the epitope-specific CD8$^+$ T-cell response in virus clearance is supported by adoptive-transfer experiments using a recombinant A59 expressing a foreign CD8$^+$ T-cell epitope, GP33–41 (GP33), derived from lymphocytic choriomeningitis virus glycoprotein. Adoptive transfer of splenocytes from the P14 mouse, transgenic for a T-cell receptor for GP33, resulted in decreased viral spread in the CNS and significantly reduced levels of demyelination (94). Thus, consistent with the findings using attenuated JHM strains (101), it is the balance between replication and spread during acute infection and clearance by T cells that determines whether virus spreads adequately into the spinal cord to cause demyelination.

Adoptive transfer of GP33-specific CD8$^+$ T cells or immunization against the GP33 epitope results in the selection of epitope escape variants (18, 94). Thus, selection of GP33 epitope escape mutants occurs in adult animals, unlike S510 escape; it is likely that GP33 escape occurs more readily than S510 escape because the former is in a nonessential protein, while S510 is expressed within the spike protein. Indeed, S510 mutant viruses express a slightly less functional spike and are slightly attenuated in adult animals (95). Thus, epitope escape depends on host genetics, viral genes, and the level of viral replication (18, 95) as well as antibody status. Importantly, viral clearance occurs in adult mice, showing that selection of epitope escape mutants is not sufficient to promote viral persistence.

Animals surviving acute infection with A59 or the less virulent JHM isolate develop demyelination (25, 74, 94). Clinical signs may range from mild paresis with awkward gait to total paralysis. Lesions show predominantly primary demyelination with axons intact (74). Demyelination is accompanied by inflammatory infiltrates containing lymphocytes and macrophages containing lipid (72, 73, 151, 179). With the exception of the suckling mouse and rat models described above (125), MHV-induced demyelination occurs in the absence of detectable infectious virus.

While the mechanism of MHV-induced demyelination is not well understood, it is clear that both immune-mediated damage and virus cytotoxicity contribute to the process. Early studies by Weiner (174) and Lampert et al. (69) suggested that demyelination was mediated directly by infection and due to cytopathic effects of virus on oligodendrocytes, the myelin-producing cells (69). It later became clear that the immune response plays a major role in the development of demyelination, in terms of modulating the amount of virus that spreads into the spinal cord and by participating more directly in the demyelinating process through cytokine production and macrophage infiltration. Firstly, as mentioned above, the amount of spread of virus during acute infection is an important predictor of the likelihood of the development of demyelination in the later stages of disease (94, 99). This is dictated by the inherent ability of the virus strain to spread, balanced by the ability of the host to clear virus, which is largely determined by the $CD8^+$ T-cell response. The contributions of the immune response to the pathology of demyelination are not well understood. Viral RNA and likely low levels of viral antigen persist within the CNS, and it is possible that this antigen is responsible for the maintenance of T cells in the CNS during the chronic disease stage (134, 136). During the later stages of MHV-induced disease, levels of CXCL10 (IP-10) and CCL5 (RANTES) remain elevated. These two chemokines are believed to be responsible for recruitment of macrophages and T cells, respectively, and depletion of either one reduces the level of demyelination (47). Macrophages are associated with the chronic CNS

pathology observed in mice infected with MHV. While JHM-infected $RAG^{-/-}$ mice do not develop demyelination, adoptive transfers of splenocytes from infected immunocompetent mice into $RAG^{-/-}$ mice results in demyelination, which is associated with extensive recruitment of activated macrophages and microglia to the sites of spinal cord demyelination (40, 179). The development of demyelination in $RAG^{-/-}$ mice is restored by the transfer of either $CD4^+$ or $CD8^+$ T cells, indicating that either cell type is sufficient but not necessary to promote demyelination (178). In addition to secreting macrophage-attracting chemokines during acute infection, it is likely that the secretion of tumor necrosis factor alpha (TNF-$\alpha$), interleukin 1$\beta$ (IL-1$\beta$), IL-6, and type 2 nitric oxide synthase by chronically activated astrocytes during the persistent infection more directly contributes to the dysregulation of oligodendrocytes, resulting in myelin loss (49, 153).

Watanabe et al. (172) showed that lymphocytes harvested from the CNS of JHM-infected Lewis rats, when stimulated with myelin basic protein and adoptively transferred into naïve animals, induced lesions similar to experimental allergic encephalomyelitis, suggesting that JHM infection could initiate an autoimmune disease. There has been little further study of autoimmunity following MHV infection.

## MHV-INDUCED HEPATITIS

The MHV-3 strain has been used most commonly to study MHV-induced hepatitis. MHV-3 was first isolated from a strain VS weanling mouse that developed acute hepatitis after inoculation with serum from a patient with acute hepatitis (29). A liver homogenate from this initial isolate produced no clinical signs when inoculated into weanling mice, although about half of the mice had pathological evidence of acute hepatitis. Intraperitoneal inoculation into 2- to 4-day-old suckling mice, however, produced lethal hepatitis with massive hepatic necrosis. After serial passage in suckling or weanling mice, a virus that was lethal for weanling VS mice emerged. This virus was primarily hepatotropic and produced massive hepatic necrosis when inoculated, independent of the route of inoculation (29). While MHV-2 causes severe hepatitis and A59 causes moderate hepatitis, we primarily review MHV-3-induced disease.

The pattern of disease obtained after MHV-3 infection is dependent on the age and strain of mouse (78). Most mouse strains are susceptible or semisusceptible (require much larger inocula to produce lethality). DBA/2, BALB/c, and C57BL/6 strains are highly sensitive to lethal disease, with a 50% lethal dose for 4- to 8-week-old mice of 1 to 10 PFU. A/J mice are highly resistant and C3H mice are semisusceptible (78). As early as 12 h after intraperitoneal infection of susceptible mice, small discrete foci of necrotic hepatocytes can be seen, accompanied by a focal inflammatory infiltrate of neutrophils and mononuclear cells (29). Over the next 3 days these lesions progressively increase in size and number and become confluent (Fig. 1). Virus replication in the liver generally parallels the development of histologic lesions, reaching peak titers between 3 and 4 days postinfection, and remains at high levels until death 4 to 7 days after infection. Bloch et al. (11) and Levy et al. (80) demonstrated abnormalities in liver blood flow, including sinusoidal microthrombi, as early as 6 h after infection of susceptible BALB/c mice, preceding the development of hepatic lesions. Liver cell edema and small focal necrotic lesions developed over the next 36 h, and by 48 h thrombi and hepatocellular necrosis were widespread and blood was shunted from damaged areas into patent sinusoids.

Extrahepatic viral replication in the spleen and other lymphoid tissues, brain, heart, and muscle generally parallels that observed in the liver. In the spleen there is intense congestion and follicular necrosis (52). In the brain signs of viral replication are observed in meninges, ependymal cells, and neurons accompanied by focal necrosis (29).

Strain A mice (A/J) more than 4 weeks of age are highly resistant to disease and do not succumb to challenges even with $10^7$ PFU (78, 79). Resistance to MHV-3 infection in A/J mice is not present at birth, and mice younger than 14 days uniformly develop fatal hepatitis (78). In resistant A/J mice a wide range of peak titers have been reported, ranging from titers almost equivalent to those seen in susceptible animals (80) to approximately 100-fold less (78).

Immunofluorescent labeling for viral antigens reveals a large number of infected hepatocytes (80). Remarkably, virtually no hepatic pathology is observed even in the presence of substantial virus replication. At approximately day 6 to 7 postinfection, virus titers in the liver and other organs abruptly drop, coincident with development of adaptive T- and B-cell immune responses. The changes observed in the microcirculation of the liver after infection of susceptible mice are not present in MHV-3-infected A/J mice (80).

Twelve-week-old C3H mice and $F_1$ offspring of crosses of C57BL/6 or DBA/2 mice with resistant A/J mice have intermediate susceptibility, with 50% mortality in the first 14 days after infection. Surviving mice develop a persistent infection with low levels of infectious virus in the liver, brain, spleen, and lymph nodes (78). Persistently infected semisusceptible mice appear normal until 2 to 12 weeks after infection, but they eventually develop a progressive illness with ruffled fur, failure to gain weight, and decreased activity. This is followed by the development of neurological signs progressing to hind-limb paralysis and death. Pathological changes in the CNS include meningitis, ependymitis, and inflammatory cuffs around small vessels, particularly in the choroid plexus, and hydrocephalus. In C3H mice a widespread vasculitis with thrombosis and necrosis of vessel walls develops as the disease progresses (167). Viral antigens and bound immunoglobulins are found in vessel walls, suggesting an immunopathological basis for the lesions (167). Immunosuppression with cyclophosphamide or cyclosporine ameliorated the CNS disease when given from 2 weeks postinfection, consistent with an inflammatory basis for the pathology observed in the CNS (159). Persistently infected mice also have foci of necrosis in their livers, with an accompanying inflammatory reaction (167).

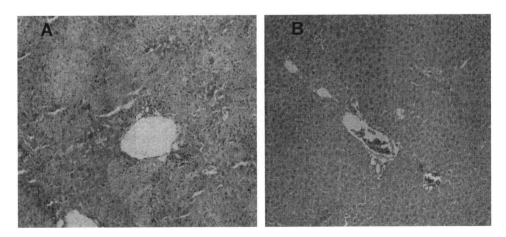

**Figure 1.** Histopathology of livers of MHV-3-infected mice. BALB/c (A) or A/J (B) mice were inoculated intraperitoneally with 1,000 PFU of MHV-3 and sacrificed at 5 days postinfection. Liver sections were stained with hematoxylin and eosin.

Studies examining the intrinsic resistance/susceptibility of macrophages to MHV-3 were spurred by the observation that the resistance of mouse strains to MHV-2-induced lethal hepatitis reflected viral replication in liver-derived macrophages (5). Unlike MHV-2, splenic and peritoneal macrophages from resistant A/J mice support viral replication when infected with MHV-3, although the characteristic syncytial cytopathic effect observed in susceptible macrophages is not observed (33, 34). The kinetics of viral replication in macrophages and hepatocytes derived from A/J mice are slower than that observed in C57BL/6-derived macrophages, and much lower titers are achieved (3, 33, 34). Extension of these studies to mouse embryonic fibroblasts (MEFs) showed that MHV-3 replicated to similar titers in A/J MEFs and C57BL/6 MEFs, but did so more slowly and without evidence of cytopathogenic effect (syncytium formation) in A/J MEFs (66). Studies of viral replication in Kupffer and endothelial cells from BALB/c (susceptible) and A/J mice produced similar results (124). Thus, most of these studies determined that MHV-3 replicated in cells derived from resistant A/J mice, often, but not uniformly, reaching the same final titer, albeit more slowly, as that achieved in cells derived from susceptible mice. This shows that infection of A/J-derived cells is not blocked at the level of virus attachment or penetration (60, 164).

A series of genetic studies by Levy-Leblond et al. demonstrated that at least two genes were implicated in resistance to lethal MHV-3 infection (82). One gene was not linked to H-2 and is inherited in a recessive manner. Another gene was H-2$^f$ linked and provided resistance to chronic disease. Dindzans et al. (31) further examined resistance and susceptibility in A/J and C57BL/6 mice and showed that resistance to lethal infection was regulated by two genes. The pattern of inheritance of resistance for both loci was recessive, and in this study neither gene was linked to H-2. The induction of macrophage procoagulant activity (PCA) by MHV-3 (see below) segregated among the recombinant inbred strains in a strain distribution pattern identical to that of susceptibility and resistance.

## Role of the fgl2 Prothrombinase in Pathogenesis of Hepatitis

Levy et al. (79) made the seminal observation that MHV-3 infection of peripheral blood mononuclear cells from susceptible, but not resistant (A/J), mice induces a PCA that accelerates the formation of a fibrin clot in recalcified plasma as early as 1 h postinfection. Monocytes from C3H mice of intermediate susceptibility produced levels of PCA

between those produced by monocytes from fully susceptible strains and resistant strains of mice. Thus, the elaboration of PCA in monocytes in response to MHV-3 infection paralleled susceptibility to disease. At least 50% of the PCA was present on the plasma membrane of infected monocytes, with the remainder located intracellularly (30, 79). Infection of macrophages by MHV-3 also induced PCA, with a strain distribution pattern identical to that observed in monocytes (21). The induction of PCA by MHV-3 infection was augmented by the presence of lymphocytes during the infection (21). This augmentation was primarily due to CD4$^+$ T cells and was also strain restricted in that lymphocytes from susceptible strains augmented PCA more efficiently than those from semisusceptible strains or resistant strains. Elaboration of PCA required both RNA and protein synthesis, showing that induction by MHV-3 infection was at the transcriptional level (21). PCA directly cleaved prothrombin to thrombin (prothrombinase) in assays with factor-deficient plasmas and in radiolabeled-prothrombinase cleavage assays (41). Studies with purified recombinant protein provided further evidence that fgl2 had serine protease activity, which required calcium and association with a phospholipid membrane for full enzymatic activity (15). Using site-directed mutagenesis, the active-site serine was identified at position 89 in the N-terminal domain.

The rapid formation of sinusoidal microthrombi prior to the development of histologic lesions in the liver (80), in combination with the correlation of PCA with susceptibility and resistance to lethal hepatitis (79), suggested that PCA played a role in the pathogenesis of MHV-3-induced hepatitis. This hypothesis was further supported by experiments demonstrating that PCA was induced in vivo (30). Pharmacological studies demonstrated that pretreatment with 16, 16-dimethyl prostaglandin E$_2$ (dmPGE$_2$) greatly decreased the severity of hepatitis in BALB/c mice, a strain which is otherwise fully susceptible to lethal MHV-3 hepatitis (1). Concordant with this decrease in hepatic damage, dmPGE$_2$ blocked the in vivo induction of PCA in macrophages recovered from infected animals, inhibited the induction of PCA in macrophages infected in vitro, and prevented the disturbances of the hepatic microcirculation that occur during infection of BALB/c mice (144). Viral titers present in the liver of dmPGE$_2$-treated mice were at least as high as those observed in untreated susceptible mice (144). Treatment of mice with an anti-PCA neutralizing monoclonal antibody also protected BALB/c mice from otherwise-lethal MHV-3-induced hepatitis (41, 83). Taken together, these data strongly supported a role for PCA in the pathogenesis of massive hepatic necrosis during MHV-3 infection of susceptible strains of mice.

The development of an anti-macrophage PCA monoclonal antibody enabled the molecular cloning of cDNAs encoding this enzyme (120). A BLAST search of the public databases revealed that the cDNA sequence of the murine MHV-3-induced PCA was almost identical to that of a gene cloned from T cells that had been designated musfiblp (later renamed fgl2), based on the presence of a fibrinogen-like domain at the C terminus of the encoded protein (58). This gene encodes a 432-amino-acid protein containing a fibrinogen-like domain at its C terminus and a N-terminal hydrophobic sequence that is predicted to be a secretory signal or a transmembrane domain for a type II membrane protein (58, 191). It is constitutively expressed at low levels in T cells, intestinal cells, trophoblasts, ovaries, and endothelial cells (58, 86) but not in macrophages. When a full-length cDNA was expressed in a macrophage-like cell line, transfected cells had prothombinase activity consistent with that of the MHV-3-induced PCA described previously (119). fgl2 RNA was not present in uninfected BALB/c macrophages, but transcription was rapidly and strongly induced by MHV-3 infection. Further studies demonstrated that MHV-3 infection of susceptible mice induced the expression of fgl2 mRNA and protein in hepatic reticuloendothelial cells, coincident with deposition of fibrin thrombi in the hepatic sinusoids, frequently outlining areas of hepatic necrosis (32). fgl2 mRNA was also induced in spleen and lungs, but not brain or kidneys, after infection of fully susceptible mice. The major cell types expressing fgl2 in these organs were macrophages (including Kupffer cells) and endothelial cells. Mice with disruption of the fgl2 gene had a survival rate of 40% after MHV-3 infection, in contrast to the 100% mortality in their fgl2$^{+/+}$ littermates (98). fgl2$^{+/-}$ heterozygote mice all succumbed but survived for longer periods. MHV-3 infection failed to induce the expression of PCA in macrophages from fgl2-null mice in vitro and in vivo. This loss of PCA was reflected by an almost complete absence of fibrin deposition in the liver and by an almost complete absence of hepatocellular necrosis at 3 days postinfection, although there was evidence of moderate hepatic necrosis at later times postinfection in surviving mice. Collectively, the data point out an important role for fgl2 prothrombinase in the pathogenesis of MHV-3-induced hepatitis.

In addition to its function as a prothrombinase, fgl2 has immunoregulatory activity; IFN-γ induces T cells to produce a soluble fgl2 that lacks prothrombinase activity (15). In susceptible BALB/cJ and C57BL/6J mice, soluble fgl2 binds to the FcγRIIB receptor, leading to inhibition of immune activation, suppression of T-cell proliferation, and inhibition of dendritic cell maturation (86, 87). These inhibitory activities can be blocked by a monoclonal antibody directed against the C-terminal fibrinogen-like domain, whereas an antibody directed against the N-terminal domain containing the prothrombinase activity did not block the activity (16).

Several studies investigated the transcriptional regulation of the fgl2 gene. Although MHV-3 and MHV-A59 induce fgl2 prothrombinase in BALB/c macrophages, several other viral strains do not (113). A series of recombinant viruses was utilized to implicate the MHV nucleocapsid protein (N protein) gene as the inducer of fgl2 in macrophages. A series of promoter truncations identified an N protein-responsive region 306 nucleotides upstream of the fgl2 translational start site containing several potential transcription factor binding sites. Electrophoretic gel mobility shift assays with infected and uninfected macrophage nuclear extracts implicated the transcription factor HNF4α in the induction of fgl2 by MHV-3 infection (114). This was supported by cotransfection experiments in which the activating effect of N protein on fgl2 promoter activity was abolished by mutation of the HNF4α binding site. The transcriptional activating and DNA binding activities of HNF4α are regulated by phosphorylation, an interesting finding considering that p38 and ERK mitogen-activated protein kinase (105) and tyrosine kinase (22) signaling pathways are implicated in macrophage fgl2 induction by MHV-3. Analysis of constitutive fgl2 transcription in endothelial cells (86) identified a positive regulatory domain binding the Oct-1, Ets-1, and Sp1 and Sp3 transcription factors required for constitutive expression of fgl2. This region was also required for induction of fgl2 by MHV infection of macrophages. Other molecules implicated in the regulation of fgl2 include the cytokines IFN-γ and TNF-α, which induce fgl2 expression in macrophages and hepatic sinusoidal lining cells (63, 87).

The basis for the failure of MHV-3 to induce fgl2 prothrombinase activity in A/J macrophages remains unknown. As noted above, fgl2 mRNA expression was rapidly induced during MHV-3-infection of BALB/c macrophages. Surprisingly, fgl2 mRNA was also induced in MHV-3-infected A/J macrophages, although at lower levels and with slower kinetics (119), even though fgl2 prothrombinase activity is not detected in these cells. Sequencing studies of the fgl2 gene demonstrated that the coding regions of the A/J and BALB/c genes only contained a single, synonymous nucleotide difference and that the promoters were identical. Together, these findings suggest that the differences in PCA and fgl2 gene induction after MHV-3 infection in these two strains may be due to differences in signaling pathways and posttranscriptional events rather than due to intrinsic differences in their fgl2 gene structures.

## Interaction of MHV-3 with the Immune System

In susceptible strains of mice, MHV-3 infection results in necrosis and destruction of splenic and lymphoid follicles of susceptible but not resistant mice (52, 65, 167, 181). Experiments by Lamontagne and colleagues demonstrated that T and B cells from susceptible, but not resistant, mice infected with MHV-3 in vitro were permissive for viral replication and underwent cell lysis (65). Concordant with the above work, antibody responses to MHV-3 were undetectable in BALB/c mice at any time postinfection up to death at 5 days postinfection, in contrast to A/J mice, which began to mount a robust antibody response by that time (81). Persistent infection of semisusceptible mice with MHV-3 depressed recall and primary antibody responses, decreased circulating total immunoglobulin G (IgG, and decreased spleen cell number (169). Lymphoid depletion can be reversed by adoptive transfer at 15 days postinfection (68). Transfer of CD4$^+$ and CD8$^+$ T cells was required to reverse IgG depletion; B-cell transfer alone was not effective. Thus, the ability of MHV-3 to grow in and destroy lymphocytes may be a key mechanism in the pathogenesis of this virus.

Host immune responses are critical for resistance of A/J mice to lethal infection with MHV-3. Immunosuppression induced by various methods converts an otherwise clinically and pathologically inapparent infection in this strain into lethal fulminant hepatitis (35). Methylprednisolone treatment abrogates viral clearance, which normally occurs on day 5 or 6 in untreated MHV-3-infected A/J mice, although the peak viral titers were not significantly different from those observed in untreated animals (37). Interestingly, treatment with methylprednisolone prior to infection with MHV-3 resulted in PCA expression in vivo; in vitro treatment of A/J macrophages with the drug resulted in the expression of fgl2 prothrombinase activity after MHV-3 infection (37). Passive transfer of antibody from mice that had recovered from MHV-3 infection did not fully protect susceptible mice, although it prolonged survival and protected a variable proportion of mice (78, 131). Studies with highly susceptible BALB/c mice that had recovered from infection with an attenuated mutant of MHV-3 (67) demonstrated that spleen cells from these mice failed to protect naïve BALB/c mice (131). CD4$^+$ T-cell lines derived from immunized BALB/c and A/J mice differed in that lines derived from A/J mice were

predominately Th1 cells (based on cytokine profiles), whereas lines derived from BALB/c mice had a Th2 phenotype (131). Additionally, the T-cell lines derived from BALB/c mice stimulated the production of PCA by macrophages from susceptible strains after MHV-3 infection (20, 131). Characterization of five A/J T-cell lines indicated that one line responsive to the spike protein was able to suppress the expression of MHV-3 PCA in macrophages, and when adoptively transferred into a susceptible major histocompatibility complex-compatible mouse, this line was able to completely protect it from MHV-3 hepatitis while only moderately decreasing virus yield (20). Surprisingly, this cell line secreted IFN-γ in response to MHV-3 antigen, a cytokine known to stimulate fgl2 expression.

Studies by Lucchiari et al. (89) demonstrated that antibody-mediated depletion of CD4$^+$ or CD8$^+$ T cells converted the benign course of MHV-3 infection in A/J mice to a lethal disease. Accompanying the depletion of CD4$^+$ or CD8$^+$ T cells was a marked decrease in levels of IFN-γ in serum. Treatment of CD4$^+$ cell-depleted mice with IFN-γ protected them from lethal disease (163), whereas treatment of A/J mice with anti-IFN-γ resulted in death upon MHV-3 challenge (89). Virelizier et al. showed that anti-IFN antibodies accelerated disease in C57BL/6 mice and rendered resistant A/J mice susceptible to lethal hepatitis, implicating IFN as an important factor for resistance to disease (166, 168). This work was extended by Lucchiari and Pereira, who demonstrated that A/J macrophages, unlike BALB/c macrophages, restrict MHV-3 replication in the presence of IFN-α/β and -γ (91). The mechanism by which IFN-γ restricts MHV-3 replication in macrophages may be related to downregulation of the MHV receptor, CEACAM1a, in A/J-derived macrophages, a response that is not observed in BALB/c-derived cells (164). Further, the age-dependent ability of macrophages and lymphocytes to synthesize IFN-α/β and -γ correlated with the development of resistance to MHV-3 in A/J mice (92). On balance, the data strongly support a role for IFNs in resistance to MHV-3 infection.

Another difference in the responses of A/J and BALB/c mice to MHV-3 infection is that macrophages from the former strain secrete less TNF-α and IL-1 than those from the latter (90, 132). Recently the simultaneous infusion of TNF-α and IFN-γ in C57BL/6 mice was reported to induce hepatocyte apoptosis and necrosis accompanied by fgl2 expression by endothelial cells and macrophages and fibrin deposition (87). Thus, the induction of these two cytokines during MHV-3 infection may up-regulate the expression of fgl2 and potentially plays a role in the evolution of MHV-3-induced hepatic lesions. Whether INF-γ has beneficial or adverse effects may depend on the genetics of the host, the amount of IFN-γ produced, or downstream signaling events.

Although it has been shown that A/J CD4[+] T cells recognize at least the MHV-3 N and spike proteins (20), T-cell epitopes recognized during infection of resistant or semisusceptible mice have not been identified, nor has their contribution to resistance been determined. However, H-2[d]-restricted CD8 and CD4 T-cell epitopes present in the MHV-JHM N protein (7, 162) are conserved in MHV-3. Further identification of viral determinants of virulence and of antigenic determinants recognized by the host merit further investigation.

## MHV MODELS OF PULMONARY INFECTION

With the increased interest in human coronavirus respiratory infections engendered by the 2002–2003 SARS outbreak and the isolation of several other new human coronavirus respiratory pathogens, there is renewed interest in a rodent coronavirus model of severe respiratory disease. Although the most extensively studied MHV strains, A59, JHM, and MHV-3, are primarily neurotropic or hepatotropic, these viruses typically enter the host by infection of the respiratory tract (13, 14). For these strains, either infection of the respiratory tract is confined to the nasal mucosa prior to spread to other sites or infection produces a mild interstitial pneumonitis. However, infection of CBA mice with MHV-1 produced a more severe interstitial pneumonia than obtained with the other viruses examined (14). Recent work by De Albuquerque et al. reexamined the ability of various strains MHV to produce pulmonary disease (26). Intranasal challenge of BALB/c mice with MHV-3, A59, JHM, or MHV-S produced much less severe respiratory disease than infection with MHV-1, confirming that MHV-1 is the most pneumotropic of the MHV strains. Intranasal infection of several different mouse strains revealed that A/J mice infected with MHV-1 developed a uniformly lethal pulmonary disease with a striking similarity to SARS. The pulmonary lesions largely recapitulated the pulmonary pathological changes observed in human SARS, including hyaline membrane formation, dense macrophage infiltrates, and occasional giant cells. Although focal hepatitis was also present, severe pulmonary disease was the predominant effect of MHV-1 infection. Intranasal inoculation of BALB/c and C57BL/6 mice with MHV-1 produced less severe disease with no mortality. C3H mice had a level of susceptibility that was intermediate to that in BALB/c and A/J mice, with 50% mortality. Although the basis for the more severe disease in A/J mice is not yet clear, several differences

were noted relative to the resistant C57BL/6 strain. A/J mice developed a much less robust type I IFN response to MHV-1 infection than resistant C57BL/6J mice. A/J infected mice had significantly higher levels of cytokines, particularly macrophage chemoattractant protein 1 (MCP-1/CCL-2), IFN-γ, and TNF-α. The expression of fgl2 and fibrin deposition in the lung were markedly increased. This is reminiscent of the situation during MHV-3 infection, where infection of susceptible strains such as C57BL/6 is associated with higher levels of these cytokines and infection of the resistant strain (A/J for MHV-3 infection) is associated with lower cytokine levels. Thus, although the strain susceptibility/resistance patterns for MHV-1 and MHV-3 are inverted in the respective models of pulmonary and hepatic disease, there appear to be common features to the host responses during lethal infection with these two viral pathogens.

## ROLE OF RECEPTOR IN MHV PATHOGENESIS

The receptor for murine coronavirus strains is CEACAM1a. In general, expression of CEACAM1a on cells nonpermissive for MHV replication renders them susceptible to infection; thus, the block to replication is at the entry level (36). While CEACAM1a expression is easily detected in the liver of susceptible mice, CEACAM1a is expressed at a very low level in the brain, and the only neural cell type demonstrated to express CEACAM1a is microglia (135). The very low level of expression in the brain might suggest that there is an additional receptor for MHV. However, transgenic mice with ablation of the expression of CEACAM1a are resistant to infection by the A59 strain of MHV following inoculation by either the intracranial or intranasal route (51), demonstrating that CEACAM1a is likely the only receptor at least for this strain. Spread of JHM may be enhanced by the ability to spread cell to cell in the absence of CEACAM1a receptor and also through expression of hemagglutinin-esterase (HE), which may interact with neural cell types (see below). Thus, it remains to be seen whether some strains of MHV use alternative receptors in the brain or other tissues. It is also striking that strains of MHV, such as A59 and JHM, show very high sequence homology and utilize the same receptor, yet have different organ tropisms.

## ROLES OF INDIVIDUAL MHV GENES IN PATHOGENESIS

A large body of literature supports the idea that the viral spike protein, which mediates entry, is a major determinant of pathogenesis. More recent studies with chimeric A59/JHM recombinant viruses demonstrated that while spike protein is a major determinant of the pathogenic properties of MHV, genes other than the spike gene play a major role in determining tropism and virulence. Furthermore, these genes are located in the 3′ end of the genome (46, 75, 110, 111) and include the remaining viral structural genes (membrane protein [M protein] gene, N protein gene, and the gene for the internal protein [I protein ] within the N protein) and small envelope protein gene, as well as the nonstructural proteins encoded in open reading frame 4 (ORF4) and ORF5a. The nonessential HE has been shown under some circumstances to enhance neurovirulence (55). We summarize below the roles of each protein in pathogenesis.

## Spike Protein

The coronavirus spike protein is a type I glycoprotein that forms the peplomers on coronavirus particles (Fig. 2). During synthesis and processing, the spike proteins of most MHV strains are cleaved into two noncovalently associated subunits of about 90 kDa by a furin-like enzymatic activity in the Golgi complex (152). The amino-terminal S1 subunit, which forms the globular head of the mature protein, contains a receptor-binding domain (RBD) within the first 330 amino acids (61) and, downstream of the RBD, a "hypervariable domain" (HVR) that varies in length among spikes of different strains (118). The carboxy-terminal S2 subunit, conserved among all coronavirus spikes and believed to form a stalk-like structure anchored in the membrane, contains two heptad repeat (HR) domains as well as the putative fusion peptide (44, 64, 93, 118, 155).

The development of reverse-genetics systems, facilitating selection of isogenic recombinant MHVs differing only in spike protein, has definitively demonstrated the important role of the spike protein during infection in the animal (54, 110, 129, 130). The replacement of the A59 spike gene with the spike gene of JHM$_{SD}$ confers high neurovirulence on the resulting virus (SJHM-RA59) (110, 129). As described above for wild-type JHM$_{SD}$, the high neurovirulence of the chimeric virus is due to rapid spread through the neurons of the CNS, which may partly occur in a CEACAM receptor-independent way (130). Figure 3 shows the spread of viral antigen in the brain following infection with wild types RA59 and RJHM as well as chimeric viruses with spike genes exchanged. The chimeric virus (SJHM-RA59) is, however, not as virulent as parental JHM$_{SD}$, at least partially because, in striking contrast to JHM$_{SD}$, it induces a robust CD8$^+$ T-cell response. Thus, the difference in T-cell response between JHM$_{SD}$ and A59 does not map to the spike gene, but rather is also influenced by viral background genes (54, 95, 138). The chimera with the A59 spike expressed from a JHM background (SA59-RJHM) has an intermediate level of virulence and spreads more like A59 (Fig. 3).

Spike protein also plays an important role in the induction of hepatitis. SJHM-RA59, expressing the spike protein of the nonhepatotropic JHM$_{SD}$ strain in the A59 background, induces only minimal hepatitis. Similarly, a chimeric virus with the spike protein of the highly hepatotropic MHV-2 strain, in the A59 background, is highly hepatotropic (109). However, SA59-RJHM causes minimal infection of the liver and induces hepatitis very poorly. Thus, in the presence of JHM background genes, the spike protein of the A59 strain is unable to mediate efficient infection

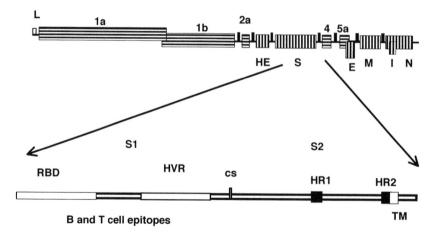

**Figure 2.** The MHV genome. Shown are structural genes (vertical stripes) and nonstructural genes (horizontal stripes). L denotes the 5′ leader sequence, and the hatches between genes denote the transcription-regulating sequences. In the A59 genome, the HE gene is a pseudogene and ORF4 is divided into ORF4a and ORF4b. Gene 1 is not to scale. Shown below is the spike gene, divided into subunits S1 and S2 with the major functional domains. CS, cleavage site; TM, transmembrane domain.

**RJHM** **RA59**

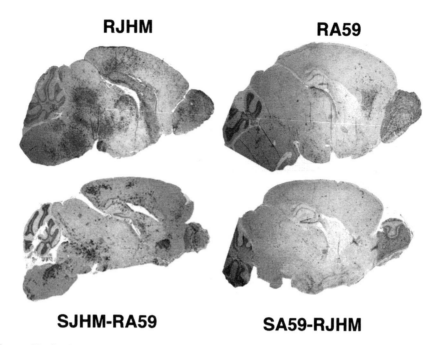

**SJHM-RA59** **SA59-RJHM**

**Figure 3.** Viral spread in the CNS. C57BL/6 mice were infected intracranially with 10 PFU of virus as follows: top left, RJHM; top right, RA59; bottom left, SJHM-RA59, expressing the A59 spike protein from a JHM background; bottom right, SA59-RJHM, expressing the A59 spike protein from a JHM background. Mice were sacrificed 5 days postinfection. Sagittal brain sections were prepared and stained by immunohistochemistry using a monoclonal antibody directed against viral nucleocapsid (×1 magnification). (This figure was modified from Figure 3 of reference 54 with permission from the ASM Journals Department.)

of the liver (110). The induction of hepatitis requires other A59 background genes and/or is suppressed by the presence of one or more JHM background genes. The mechanism by which this occurs is not understood and must involve steps in infection other than entry.

Among the JHM isolates, virulence is correlated with the presence of a long HVR within S1. $MHV_{SD}$ (MHV-4) (23, 116) has the longest MHV HVR among JHM spike proteins and is able to induce cell-to-cell fusion and viral spread in the absence of the CEACAM receptor (42, 43). The JHM-cl2 and DL variants express spike proteins with sequences nearly identical to that of $JHM_{SD}$ and carry out receptor-independent fusion, consistent with their high neurovirulence (150, 158). The neuroattenuated phenotypes of the monoclonal antibody escape variants of both JHM-DL and $JHM_{SD}$ described above are associated with single-site mutations and/or deletions within the HVR (23, 45, 95, 128). Spike proteins with full-length HVRs exhibit less stable association of S1 and S2 such that the conformational changes in spike protein that lead to fusion are more easily triggered. This, in turn, is at least partially responsible for very high neurovirulence (42, 59).

Mutations within the RBD have an influence on tropism and virulence. The enhanced neurovirulence of $JHM_{SD}$ compared with that of $JHM_{IA}$ maps to a

single amino acid substitution within the RBD, S310G, which confers the ability to spread in a CEACAM1-independent process (116). Furthermore, a single Q159L amino acid substitution in this region eliminates the ability of MHV-A59 to infect the liver while having no measurable effect on neurovirulence (76, 77).

Mutations within the HR domains can influence pathogenesis as well. Amino acid substitutions at L1114 within HR1 of the JHM spike protein (L1114R, F) are particularly intriguing in that they have been reported in multiple studies, in association with several mutant phenotypes. An L1114R substitution contributes to the neuroattenuation and restriction to olfactory bulbs of the OBLV60 mutant (44, 160). Substitutions at L1114 have also been identified in the spike protein of the 2.2-V-1 variant of JHM (170) and a soluble receptor-resistant mutant of JHM-cl2 (139, 140). These substitutions are associated with an inability to induce CEACAM-independent cell-to-cell fusion and neuroattenuation (102, 103, 157). Thus, small changes within the HR domains may result in major alterations in spike/receptor interaction, virus entry, and, finally, pathogenesis.

The spike proteins contain the only two H-2[b]-restricted CD8[+] T-cell epitopes thus far identified for MHV. The immunodominant CD8[+] T-cell epitope

S510 is located within the HVR (and therefore absent from the spikes of the neuroattenuated JHM variants with deletions in the HVR, as well as from the A59 strain). The subdominant CD8[+] T-cell epitope S598 is contained in a region adjacent to the carboxyl end of the HVR and is thus expressed by all MHVs. Variants with mutated JHM$_{IA}$ S510 epitope in the suckling mouse model discussed above have been reported and postulated as a mechanism to achieve viral persistence. Such epitope escape mutants were more virulent than wild-type virus (126). However, when the same inactivating mutation was introduced into a recombinant virus expressing the spike protein of JHM$_{SD}$, the resulting virus ranged from slightly to significantly attenuated in weanling mice, depending on the genetic background of the virus and the strain of the mouse infected (94). This suggests that mutations within the S510 epitope had negative effects on spike function. In contrast, escape mutants with inactivation of the foreign CD8[+] epitope, GP33, expressed within a nonessential gene from the A59 genome were rapidly selected in weanling mice immunized against this epitope (18). Thus, epitope escape depends on multiple factors such as the location of the epitope within an essential versus nonessential protein and its effect on function of the protein, the background genes of the virus, and the age and strain of mouse (19, 57, 95).

## Hemagglutinin-Esterase Protein

HE is a glycoprotein that forms a second, smaller spike on the envelope of some coronaviruses (56, 186) and has been recently studied in detail (145). For MHV, HE is expressed by a minority of strains, including some isolates of JHM (184). HE, expressed as a homodimer of a 65-kDa disulfide-bonded subunit, has both sialic acid binding and acetyl esterase (or receptor-destroying) activities and thus could potentially contribute to viral entry and/or release from the cell surface via interaction with sialic acid-containing moieties. While the highly tissue culture-adapted A59 genome contains an HE gene (143), HE is not expressed due to multiple mutations and its gene is considered a pseudogene. Expression of the viral HE glycoprotein is not necessary for virulence in the animal, as evidenced by the fact that A59 causes encephalitis and hepatitis, as well as demyelination, while it does not express HE.

HE expression is nonessential to the viral life cycle. Furthermore, during serial passage in cultures of recombinant A59 engineered to express HE, there is a selection for variants bearing mutations in the HE gene that preclude insertion into the viral membrane (85), suggesting that HE may play a role during infection of the animal (145). It has been speculated that HE may play a role in acute and/or chronic disease induced by MHV, possibly as a determinant of cellular tropism (182, 183, 187), or to aid spread of the virus by augmenting attachment and/or exit from the cell (56). There were early studies both supporting and arguing against this hypothesis (64, 156, 182, 183, 187). These studies, however, were not able to distinguish between effects of HE and the influence of other genes in the comparison of various MHV isolates. A recent study was carried out comparing the pathogenesis of isogenic recombinant viruses expressing wild-type HE, viruses expressing HE in which the acetylesterase activity was eliminated by mutation, and viruses in which HE polypeptide was not expressed. Surprisingly, viruses that expressed HE polypeptides (with or without a functional esterase activity) spread more extensively through the brain and were more virulent when inoculated intracranially into mice than were viruses not expressing an HE polypeptide (55). This demonstrates that enhanced virulence does not require an intact esterase activity and suggests that HE may enhance virus attachment and spread by binding to sialic acid-containing receptors. A role for HE in enhancement of infection in the brain is particularly intriguing, as this is a site of very poor expression of the CEACAM1 receptor.

## Membrane Protein

The M protein is the most abundant virion membrane protein. M proteins of coronaviruses may be N or O glycosylated. The M protein of MHV is O glycosylated, and while glycosylation is not essential for viral assembly or infectivity (27) and the glycosylation state of MHV M protein (N, O, or no glycosylation) does not alter the ability to replicate in vitro, it may affect the ability to induce IFN-α in vitro and also to replicate in the liver in the mouse (27). Indeed, in the case of the porcine coronavirus transmissible gastroenteritis virus, the M protein has been shown to have interferogenic activity, and mutations in the ectodomain of the M protein that reduce glycosylation decrease this activity (71).

## Nucleocapsid Protein

In addition to its role as a structural protein, N protein plays roles in transcription and in pathogenesis. Expression of N protein is necessary for efficient recovery of virus from infectious cDNA clones (188, 189). Some N protein of MHV enters the nucleus. While the role of N protein in the nucleus is not at all understood, N protein has been shown to interact with heterogeneous nuclear ribonucleoprotein A1, a protein involved in host cell mRNA genesis that is primarily nuclear (171, 180). Intracellular movement is especially important during neuronal spread because of the distances the virus must transverse and is accomplished through association with microtubules. Electron microscopy shows that JHM N protein is often found associated with microtubules and that virions assemble at sites near microtubules. If microtubules are disrupted, spread is also disrupted (122). Interestingly, N protein was found to share 44% similarity with the protein tau, a protein that cross-links microtubules, which may imply microtubule binding activity for N protein (122). Analysis of recombinant viruses in which the N protein of JHM is expressed within the background of A59 has shown that the JHM N protein confers increased neurovirulence and spread within the CNS (unpublished data).

In contrast to studies of CNS disease, little is known about viral determinants of pathogenesis in MHV-3-induced fulminant hepatitis. The lack of a convenient reverse-genetics system for MHV-3 has clearly limited work in this area. However, the N protein is involved in the induction of fgl2 by MHV-3 as documented above (113, 115, 119) and thus is an important determinant of pathogenesis in the liver. In a recent study by Hogue and colleagues, the N protein of A59 was shown to contribute to resistance to type I IFN during infection in vitro by interfering with the 2′-5′ oligoadenylate synthetase pathway (B. Hogue, personal communication). Expression of the N protein gene in a recombinant vaccinia virus in place of its IFN antagonist E3L gene rescued the VVΔ3L virus from IFN sensitivity. The N protein gene prevents cellular RNA degradation and partially rescues translation shutoff, both of which are characteristic of VVΔE3L.

## Small Envelope Protein

E protein is an integral membrane protein (190) that plays an important role in viral assembly (165). E protein, coexpressed with M protein, forms virus-like particles. Surprisingly, E protein is not an essential protein, as evidenced by the selection of a recombinant MHV lacking E protein expression. This virus, however replicates very inefficiently, consistent with an important role for E protein in production of infectious virus (62). The E proteins of several coronaviruses, including MHV, have ion channel activity (177); the function of the channel activity is unknown, but this activity may function at the site of budding to enhance assembly and morphogenesis. E protein also induces apoptosis in vitro in MHV-A59-infected 17Cl-1 cells via a caspase-dependent mechanism. Inhibition of MHV-induced apoptosis promotes virus production late in infection, suggesting that apoptosis

may be a host response that limits the level of virus production (2).

## Internal Protein

The genomes of several group II coronaviruses, including MHV, contain an I ORF within the N protein gene (38, 70). This ORF, translated in the +1 reading frame with respect to the N protein, encodes a 23-kDa polypeptide. The I ORF product is expressed in infected cells and is also found within virions. Selection and characterization of a recombinant virus in which the I protein gene is disrupted demonstrated that I protein is not essential for the replication of MHV; furthermore, this recombinant was indistinguishable from wild-type virus in terms of replication kinetics in tissue culture and pathogenesis in the mouse (38). However, expression of the I protein gene does confer a small-plaque morphology (38) and may have an as-yet-unknown role in pathogenesis.

## Replicase Proteins

The MHV replicase gene encompasses the 5′ two-thirds of the genome (approximately 21 kb) and encodes 16 proteins, including several enzymatic activities. One or more of these activities could affect tropism and pathogenesis by determining the rate of viral replication, perhaps via interactions with noncoding sequences in the viral genome, with cell-type-specific factors, or with elements of the immune response. In one example, a single amino acid substitution (Tyr6398His) in the MHV-A59 replicase ORF1b p59-nsp14 protein, an exoribonuclease (106, 146), does not effect replication in vitro, but it does result in attenuation of virulence for a recombinant A59 following intracranial infection of C57BL/6 mice (149). There are potentially as-yet-undiscovered roles in pathogenesis for other components of the replicase. Interestingly, studies of chimeric viruses in which the A59 replicase gene is expressed with the JHM structural genes and vice versa demonstrated that the replicase is not an important determinant of the ability to induce acute hepatitis or severe encephalitis, at least in the context of these chimeric viruses (112).

## Group-Specific Proteins

All coronaviruses encode, in addition to structural proteins and replicase proteins, small nonessential so-called "group-specific" or "accessory" proteins. While the functions of such proteins are not known, it has been speculated that in analogy with nonstructural proteins encoded by other RNA viruses, they may be involved in anti-host defense by interacting or subverting the host innate immune response (6, 142,

148, 161). The MHV genome contains ORF2a, ORF4, and ORF5a, all of which encode proteins that are nonessential for replication (141, 176, 185). The question of whether one or more of these ORFs encodes a protein with a role in pathogenesis remains unresolved, and the use of recombinant viruses makes it possible to address this question by the selection of isogenic viruses differing only in expression of a particular ORF. A recombinant MHV (JHM strain) lacking gene 4 has been shown to be as neurovirulent as the wild type in mice (117). In contrast, a recombinant MHV lacking ORF2a, ORF4, and ORF5a is avirulent in mice; however, because replication of this virus is inefficient in vitro, it is not possible to determine if the attenuation in mice is due to a specific function of a viral gene product or a more general inability of the virus to replicate efficiently (28). More recently it was shown that a recombinant virus with a deletion of ORF2a (as well as the HE pseudogene) was attenuated despite its ability to replicate to titers similar to those of wild-type virus in vitro; this suggests that ORF2a may play a role in virulence. In support of this, a recombinant MHV with a mutation in ORF2a is attenuated in animals (149).

## CONCLUSION

The group of viruses referred to collectively as murine coronavirus has for several decades provided animal models both for CNS disease, including encephalitis and demyelination, and hepatitis. It has become clear that MHV-1 infection may provide a model for severe respiratory diseases such as SARS. The facts that these viruses may be manipulated genetically and may induce variable host responses depending on the genetics of the host mouse strains makes them important and useful model pathogens with which to study human disease.

**Acknowledgments.** We thank Michael Buchmeier, Sam Dales, Janet Hartley, Stephen Stohlman, and Leslie Weiner for historical information and Gary Levy for reading the manuscript.

We acknowledge NIH grants AI17418, AI60021 (formerly NS21954), AI47800, and NS 54695 to S.R.W. and AI51493 to J.L.L.

## REFERENCES

1. **Abecassis, M., J. Falk, V. Dindzans, W. Lopatin, L. Makowka, G. Levy, and R. Falk.** 1987. Prostaglandin E2 (PGE2) alters the pathogenesis of MHV-3 infection in susceptible BALB/cJ mice. *Adv. Exp. Med. Biol.* **218:**465–466.
2. **An, S., C. J. Chen, X. Yu, J. L. Leibowitz, and S. Makino.** 1999. Induction of apoptosis in murine coronavirus-infected cultured cells and demonstration of E protein as an apoptosis inducer. *J. Virol.* **73:**7853–7859.
3. **Arnheiter, H., T. Baechi, and O. Haller.** 1982. Adult mouse hepatocytes in primary monolayer culture express genetic resistance to mouse hepatitis virus type 3. *J. Immunol.* **129:**1275–1281.
4. **Bailey, O. T., A. M. Pappenheimer, F. Sargent, M. D. Cheever, and J. B. Daniels.** 1949. A murine virus (JHM) causing disseminated encephalomyelitis with extensive destruction of myelin. II. Pathology. *J. Exp. Med.* **90:**195–212.
5. **Bang, F. B., and A. Warwick.** 1960. Mouse macrophages as host cells for the mouse hepatitis virus and the genetic basis of their susceptibility. *Proc. Natl. Acad. Sci. USA* **46:**1065–1075.
6. **Basler, C. F., X. Wang, E. Muhlberger, V. Volchkov, J. Paragas, H. D. Klenk, A. Garcia-Sastre, and P. Palese.** 2000. The Ebola virus vp35 protein functions as a type I IFN antagonist. *Proc. Natl. Acad. Sci. USA* **97:**12289–12294.
7. **Bergmann, C., M. McMillan, and S. Stohlman.** 1993. Characterization of the Ld-restricted cytotoxic T-lymphocyte epitope in the mouse hepatitis virus nucleocapsid protein. *J. Virol.* **67:**7041–7049.
8. **Bergmann, C. C., N. W. Marten, D. R. Hinton, B. Parra, and S. A. Stohlman.** 2001. CD8 T cell mediated immunity to neurotropic MHV infection. *Adv. Exp. Med. Biol.* **494:**299–308.
9. **Bergmann, C. C., B. Parra, D. R. Hinton, C. Ramakrishna, K. C. Dowdell, and S. A. Stohlman.** 2004. Perforin and gamma interferon-mediated control of coronavirus central nervous system infection by CD8 T cells in the absence of CD4 T cells. *J. Virol.* **78:**1739–1750.
10. **Bergmann, C. C., C. Ramakrishna, M. Kornacki, and S. A. Stohlman.** 2001. Impaired T cell immunity in B cell-deficient mice following viral central nervous system infection. *J. Immunol.* **167:**1575–1583.
11. **Bloch, E. H., K. S. Warren, and M. S. Rosenthal.** 1975. In vivo microscopic observations of the pathogenesis of acute mouse viral hepatitis. *Br. J. Exp. Pathol.* **56:**256–264.
12. **Buchmeier, M. J., R. G. Dalziel, M. J. Koolen, and P. W. Lampert.** 1987. Molecular determinants of CNS virulence of MHV-4. *Adv. Exp. Med. Biol.* **218:**287–295.
13. **Carrano, V. A., S. W. Barthold, D. S. Beck, and A. L. Smith.** 1984. Alteration of viral respiratory infections of mice by prior infection with mouse hepatitis virus. *Lab. Anim. Sci.* **34:**573–576.
14. **Carthrew, P., and S. Sparrow.** 1981. Murine coronaviruses: the histopathology of disease induced by intranasal inoculation. *Res. Vet. Sci.* **30:**270–273.
15. **Chan, C. W., M. W. Chan, M. Liu, L. Fung, E. H. Cole, J. L. Leibowitz, P. A. Marsden, D. A. Clark, and G. A. Levy.** 2002. Kinetic analysis of a unique direct prothrombinase, fgl2, and identification of a serine residue critical for the prothrombinase activity. *J. Immunol.* **168:**5170–5177.
16. **Chan, C. W., L. S. Kay, R. G. Khadaroo, M. W. Chan, S. Lakatoo, K. J. Young, L. Zhang, R. M. Gorczynski, M. Cattral, O. Rotstein, and G. A. Levy.** 2003. Soluble fibrinogen-like protein 2/fibroleukin exhibits immunosuppressive properties: suppressing T cell proliferation and inhibiting maturation of bone marrow-derived dendritic cells. *J. Immunol.* **170:**4036–4044.
17. **Cheever, F. S., J. B. Daniels, A. M. Pappenheimer, and O. T. Baily.** 1949. A murine virus (JHM) causing disseminated encephalomyelitis with extensive destruction of myelin. I. Isolation and biological properties of the virus. *J. Exp. Med.* **90:**181–194.
18. **Chua, M. M., K. C. MacNamara, L. San Mateo, H. Shen, and S. R. Weiss.** 2004. Effects of an epitope-specific CD8⁺ T-cell response on murine coronavirus central nervous system disease: protection from virus replication and antigen spread and selection of epitope escape mutants. *J. Virol.* **78:**1150–1159.

19. Chua, M. M., J. J. Phillips, S. H. Seo, E. Lavi, and S. R. Weiss. 2001. Mutation of the immunodominant CD8+ epitope in the MHV-4 spike protein. *Adv. Exp. Med. Biol.* **494:**121–125.

20. Chung, S., R. Gorczynski, B. Cruz, R. Fingerote, E. Skamene, S. Perlman, J. Leibowitz, L. Fung, M. Flowers, and G. Levy. 1994. A Th1 cell line (3E9.1) from resistant A/J mice inhibits induction of macrophage procoagulant activity in vitro and protects against MHV-3 mortality in vivo. *Immunology* **83:**353–361.

21. Chung, S., S. Sinclair, J. Leibowitz, E. Skamene, L. S. Fung, and G. Levy. 1991. Cellular and metabolic requirements for induction of macrophage procoagulant activity by murine hepatitis virus strain 3 in vitro. *J. Immunol.* **146:**271–278.

22. Dackiw, A. P., K. Zakrzewski, A. B. Nathens, P. Y. Cheung, R. Fingerote, G. A. Levy, and O. D. Rotstein. 1995. Induction of macrophage procoagulant activity by murine hepatitis virus strain 3: role of tyrosine phosphorylation. *J. Virol.* **69:**5824–5828.

23. Dalziel, R. G., P. W. Lampert, P. J. Talbot, and M. J. Buchmeier. 1986. Site-specific alteration of murine hepatitis virus type 4 peplomer glycoprotein E2 results in reduced neurovirulence. *J. Virol.* **59:**463–471.

24. Dandekar, A. A., G. Jacobsen, T. J. Waldschmidt, and S. Perlman. 2003. Antibody-mediated protection against cytotoxic T-cell escape in coronavirus-induced demyelination. *J. Virol.* **77:**11867–11874.

25. Das Sarma, J., L. Fu, J. C. Tsai, S. R. Weiss, and E. Lavi. 2000. Demyelination determinants map to the spike glycoprotein gene of coronavirus mouse hepatitis virus. *J. Virol.* **74:**9206–9213.

26. De Albuquerqur, N., E. Baig, M. Xuezhong, J. Zhang, W. He, A. Rowe, M. Habal, M. Liu, I. Shalev, G. P. Downey, R. Gorczynski, J. Butany, J. Leibowitz, S. R. Weiss, I. D. McGilvray, M. J. Phillips, E. N. Fish, and G. A. Levy. 2006. Murine hepatitis virus strain 1 produces a clinically relevant model of severe acute respiratory syndrome in A/J mice. *J. Virol.* **80:**10382–10394.

27. de Haan, C. A., M. de Wit, L. Kuo, C. Montalto-Morrison, B. L. Haagmans,, S. R. Weiss, P. S. Masters, and P. J. Rottier. 2003. The glycosylation status of the murine hepatitis coronavirus M protein affects the interferogenic capacity of the virus in vitro and its ability to replicate in the liver but not the brain. *Virology* **312:**395–406.

28. de Haan, C. A., P. S. Masters, X. Shen, S. Weiss, and P. J. Rottier. 2002. The group-specific murine coronavirus genes are not essential, but their deletion, by reverse genetics, is attenuating in the natural host. *Virology* **296:**177–189.

29. Dick, G. W., J. S. Niven, and A. W. Gledhill. 1956. A virus related to that causing hepatitis in mice (MHV). *Br. J. Exp. Pathol.* **37:**90–98.

30. Dindzans, V. J., P. J. MacPhee, L. S. Fung, J. L. Leibowitz, and G. A. Levy. 1985. The immune response to mouse hepatitis virus: expression of monocyte procoagulant activity and plasminogen activator during infection in vivo. *J. Immunol.* **135:**4189–4197.

31. Dindzans, V. J., E. Skamene, and G. A. Levy. 1986. Susceptibility/resistance to mouse hepatitis virus strain 3 and macrophage procoagulant activity are genetically linked and controlled by two non-H-2-linked genes. *J. Immunol.* **137:**2355–2360.

32. Ding, J. W., Q. Ning, M. F. Liu, A. Lai, J. Leibowitz, K. M. Peltekian, E. H. Cole, L. S. Fung, C. Holloway, P. A. Marsden, H. Yeger, M. J. Phillips, and G. A. Levy. 1997. Fulminant hepatic failure in murine hepatitis virus strain 3 infection: tissue-specific expression of a novel *fgl2* prothrombinase. *J. Virol.* **71:**9223–9230.

33. Dupuy, C., D. Lafforet-Cresteil, and J. M. Dupuy. 1980. Genetic study of MHV-3 infection in mice: in vitro replication of virus in macrophages, p. 241–246. *In* E. Skamene, P. A. L. Kongshavn, and M. Landy (ed.), *Genetic Control of Natural Resistance to Infection and Malignancy.* Academic Press, New York, NY.

34. Dupuy, J. M., and L. Lamontagne. 1987. Genetically-determined sensitivity to MHV3 infections is expressed in vitro in lymphoid cells and macrophages. *Adv. Exp. Med. Biol.* **218:**455–463.

35. Dupuy, J. M., E. Levey-Leblond, and C. Le Prevost. 1975. Immunopathology of mouse hepatitis virus type 3. II. Effect of immunosuppression in resistant mice. *J. Immunol.* **114:**226–230.

36. Dveksler, G. S., M. N. Pensiero, C. B. Cardellichio, R. K. Williams, G. S. Jiang, K. V. Holmes, and C. W. Dieffenbach. 1991. Cloning of the mouse hepatitis virus (MHV) receptor: expression in human and hamster cell lines confers susceptibility to MHV. *J. Virol.* **65:**6881–6891.

37. Fingerote, R. J., M. Abecassis, M. J. Phillips, Y. S. Rao, E. H. Cole, J. Leibowitz, and G. A. Levy. 1996. Loss of resistance to murine hepatitis virus strain 3 infection after treatment with corticosteroids is associated with induction of macrophage procoagulant activity. *J. Virol.* **70:**4275–4282.

38. Fischer, F., D. Peng, S. T. Hingley, S. R. Weiss, and P. S. Masters. 1997. The internal open reading frame within the nucleocapsid gene of mouse hepatitis virus encodes a structural protein that is not essential for viral replication. *J. Virol.* **71:**996–1003.

39. Fleming, J. O., M. D. Trousdale, F. A. K. El-Zaatari, S. A. Stohlman, and L. P. Weiner. 1986. Pathogenicity of antigenic variants of murine coronavirus JHM selected with monoclonal antibodies. *J. Virol.* **58:**869–875.

40. Fleming, J. O., F. I. Wang, M. D. Trousdale, D. R. Hinton, and S. A. Stohlman. 1990. Immunopathogenesis of demyelination induced by MHV-4. *Adv. Exp. Med. Biol.* **276:**565–572.

41. Fung, L. S., G. Neil, J. Leibowitz, E. H. Cole, S. Chung, A. Crow, and G. A. Levy. 1991. Monoclonal antibody analysis of a unique macrophage procoagulant activity induced by murine hepatitis virus strain 3 infection. *J. Biol. Chem.* **266:**1789–1795.

42. Gallagher, T. M., and M. J. Buchmeier. 2001. Coronavirus spike proteins in viral entry and pathogenesis. *Virology* **279:**371–374.

43. Gallagher, T. M., M. J. Buchmeier, and S. Perlman. 1992. Cell receptor-independent infection by a neurotropic murine coronavirus. *Virology* **191:**517–522.

44. Gallagher, T. M., C. Escarmis, and M. J. Buchmeier. 1991. Alteration of the pH dependence of coronavirus-induced cell fusion: effect of mutations in the spike glycoprotein. *J. Virol.* **65:**1916–1928.

45. Gallagher, T. M., S. E. Parker, and M. J. Buchmeier. 1990. Neutralization-resistant variants of a neurotropic coronavirus are generated by deletions within the amino-terminal half of the spike glycoprotein. *J. Virol.* **64:**731–741.

46. Gilmore, W., J. Correale, and L. P. Weiner. 1994. Coronavirus induction of class I major histocompatibility complex expression in murine astrocytes is virus strain specific. *J. Exp. Med.* **180:**1013–1023.

47. Glass, W. G., B. P. Chen, M. T. Liu, and T. E. Lane. 2002. Mouse hepatitis virus infection of the central nervous system: chemokine-mediated regulation of host defense and disease. *Viral Immunol.* **15:**261–272.

48. Gombold, J. L., R. M. Sutherland, E. Lavi, Y. Paterson, and S. R. Weiss. 1995. Mouse hepatitis virus A59-induced demyelination can occur in the absence of CD8+ T cells. *Microb. Pathog.* **18:**211–221.

49. Grzybicki, D. M., K. B. Kwack, S. Perlman, and S. P. Murphy. 1997. Nitric oxide synthase type II expression by different cell

types in MHV-JHM encephalitis suggests distinct roles for nitric oxide in acute versus persistent virus infection. *J. Neuroimmunol.* **73:**15–27.

49a.Hartley, J. W. 1963. Tissue culture cytopathic and plaque assays for mouse hepatitis viruses. *Proc. Soc. Exp. Biol. Med.* **113:**403–406.

50. Haspel, M. V., P. W. Lampert, and M. B. Oldstone. 1978. Temperature-sensitive mutants of mouse hepatitis virus produce a high incidence of demyelination. *Proc. Natl. Acad. Sci. USA* **75:**4033–4036.

51. Hemmila, E., C. Turbide, M. Olson, S. Jothy, K. V. Holmes, and N. Beauchemin. 2004. *Ceacam1a*$^{-/-}$ mice are completely resistant to infection by murine coronavirus mouse hepatitis virus A59. *J. Virol.* **78:**10156–10165.

52. Hirano, T., and B. H. Ruebner. 1965. The effect of murine hepatitis virus infection on lymphatic organs. *Lab. Investig.* **14:**488–500.

53. Homberger, F. R., L. Zhang, and S. W. Barthold. 1998. Prevalence of enterotropic and polytropic mouse hepatitis virus in enzootically infected mouse colonies. *Lab. Anim. Sci.* **48:**50–54.

54. Iacono, K. T., L. Kazi, and S. R. Weiss. 2006. Both spike and background genes contribute to murine coronavirus neurovirulence. *J. Virol.* **80:**6834–6843.

55. Kazi, L., A. Lissenberg, R. Watson, R. J. de Groot, and S. R. Weiss. 2005. Expression of hemagglutinin esterase protein from recombinant mouse hepatitis virus enhances neurovirulence. *J. Virol.* **79:**15064–15073.

56. Kienzle, T. E., S. Abraham, B. G. Hogue, and D. A. Brian. 1990. Structure and orientation of expressed bovine coronavirus hemagglutinin-esterase protein. *J. Virol.* **64:**1834–1838.

57. Kim, T. S., and S. Perlman. 2003. Protection against CTL escape and clinical disease in a murine model of virus persistence. *J. Immunol.* **171:**2006–2013.

58. Koyama, T., L. R. Hall, W. G. Haser, S. Tonegawa, and H. Saito. 1987. Structure of a cytotoxic T-lymphocyte-specific gene shows a strong homology to fibrinogen beta and gamma chains. *Proc. Natl. Acad. Sci. USA* **84:**1609–1613.

59. Krueger, D. K., S. M. Kelly, D. N. Lewicki, R. Ruffolo, and T. M. Gallagher. 2001. Variations in disparate regions of the murine coronavirus spike protein impact the initiation of membrane fusion. *J. Virol.* **75:**2792–2802.

60. Krzystyniak, K., and J. M. Dupuy. 1981. Early interaction between mouse hepatitis virus 3 and cells. *J. Gen. Virol.* **57:** 53–61.

61. Kubo, H., Y. K. Yamada, and F. Taguchi. 1994. Localization of neutralizing epitopes and the receptor-binding site within the amino-terminal 330 amino acids of the murine coronavirus spike protein. *J. Virol.* **68:**5403–5410.

62. Kuo, L., and P. S. Masters. 2003. The small envelope protein E is not essential for murine coronavirus replication. *J. Virol.* **77:**4597–4608.

63. Lafuse, W. P., L. Castle, D. Brown, and B. S. Zwilling. 1995. The cytotoxic T lymphocyte gene fiblp with homology to fibrinogen-beta and gamma subunits is also induced in mouse macrophages by IFN-gamma. *Cell. Immunol.* **163:**187–190.

64. LaMonica, N., L. R. Banner, V. L. Morris, and M. M. C. Lai. 1991. Localization of extensive deletions in the structural genes of two neurotropic variants of murine coronavirus JHM. *Virology* **182:**883–888.

65. Lamontagne, L., J. P. Descoteaux, and P. Jolicoeur. 1989. Mouse hepatitis virus 3 replication in T and B lymphocytes correlate with viral pathogenicity. *J. Immunol.* **142:**4458–4465.

66. Lamontagne, L., and J. M. Dupuy. 1984. Natural resistance of mice to mouse hepatitis virus type 3 infection is expressed in embryonic fibroblast cells. *J. Gen. Virol.* **65:**1165–1171.

67. Lamontagne, L., and P. Jolicoeur. 1991. Mouse hepatitis virus 3-thymic cell interactions correlating with viral pathogenicity. *J. Immunol.* **146:**3152–3159.

68. Lamontagne, L., P. Jolicoeur, D. Decarie, and J. Menezes. 1996. Effect of adoptive transfer of CD4, CD8 and B cells on recovery from MHV3-induced immunodeficiencies. *Immunology* **88:**220–229.

69. Lampert, P. W., J. K. Sims, and A. J. Kniazeff. 1973. Mechanism of demyelination in JHM virus encephalomyelitis. *Acta Neuropathol.* **24:**76–85.

70. Lapps, W., B. G. Hogue, and D. A. Brian. 1987. Sequence analysis of the bovine coronavirus nucleocapsid and matrix protein genes. *Virology* **157:**47–57.

71. Laude, H., J. Gelfi, I. Lavenant, and B. Charley. 1992. Single amino acid changes in the viral glycoprotein M affect 1induction of alpha interferon by the coronavirus transmissible gastroenteritis virus. *J. Virol.* **66:**743–749.

72. Lavi, E., P. S. Fishman, M. K. Highkin, and S. R. Weiss. 1988. Limbic encephalitis following inhalation of murine coronavirus MHV-A59. *Lab. Investig.* **58:**31–36.

73. Lavi, E., D. H. Gilden, M. K. Highkin,, and S. R. Weiss. 1986. The organ tropism of mouse hepatitis virus A59 in mice is dependent on dose and route of inoculation. *Lab. Anim. Sci.* **36:**130–135.

74. Lavi, E., D. H. Gilden, Z. Wroblewska, L. B. Rorke, and S. R. Weiss. 1984. Experimental demyelination produced by the A59 strain of mouse hepatitis virus. *Neurology* **34:**597–603.

75. Lavi, E., E. M. Murray, S. Makino, S. A. Stohlman, M. M. Lai, and S. R. Weiss. 1990. Determinants of coronavirus MHV pathogenesis are localized to 3′ portions of the genome as determined by ribonucleic acid-ribonucleic acid recombination. *Lab Investig.* **62:**570–578.

76. Leparc-Goffart, I., S. T. Hingley, M. M. Chua, X. Jiang, E. Lavi, and S. R. Weiss. 1997. Altered pathogenesis of a mutant of the murine coronavirus MHV-A59 is associated with a q159l amino acid substitution in the spike protein. *Virology* **239:**1–10.

77. Leparc-Goffart, I., S. T. Hingley, M. M. Chua, J. Phillips, E. Lavi, and S. R. Weiss. 1998. Targeted recombination within the spike gene of murine coronavirus mouse hepatitis virus-A59: Q159 is a determinant of hepatotropism. *J. Virol.* **72:**9628–9636.

78. Le Prevost, C., E. Levy-Leblond, J. L. Virelizier, and J. M. Dupuy. 1975. Immunopathology of mouse hepatitis virus type 3 infection. Role of humoral and cell-mediated immunity in resistance mechanisms. *J. Immunol.* **114:**221–225.

79. Levy, G. A., J. L. Leibowitz, and T. S. Edgington. 1981. Induction of monocyte procoagulant activity by murine hepatitis virus type 3 parallels disease susceptibility in mice. *J. Exp. Med.* **154:**1150–1163.

80. Levy, G. A., P. J. MacPhee, L. S. Fung, M. M. Fisher, and A. M. Rappaport. 1983. The effect of mouse hepatitis virus infection on the microcirculation of the liver. *Hepatology* **3:**964–973.

81. Levy, G. A., R. Shaw, J. L. Leibowitz, and E. Cole. 1984. The immune response to mouse hepatitis virus: genetic variation in antibody response and disease. *Adv. Exp. Med. Biol.* **173:**345–364.

82. Levy-Leblond, E., D. Oth, and J. M. Dupuy. 1979. Genetic study of mouse sensitivity to MHV3 infection: influence of the H-2 complex. *J. Immunol.* **122:**1359–1362.

83. Li, C., L. S. Fung, S. Chung, A. Crow, N. Myers-Mason, M. J. Phillips, J. L. Leibowitz, E. Cole, C. A. Ottaway, and G. Levy. 1992. Monoclonal antiprothrombinase (3d4.3) prevents mortality from murine hepatitis virus (MHV-3) infection. *J. Exp. Med.* **176:**689–697.

84. Lin, M. T., D. R. Hinton, N. W. Marten, C. C. Bergmann, and S. A. Stohlman. 1999. Antibody prevents virus reactivation within the central nervous system. *J. Immunol.* **162:**7358–7368.

85. Lissenberg, A., M. M. Vrolijk, A. L. vanVliet, M. A. Langereis, J. D. de Groot-Mijnes, P. J. Rottier, and R. J. de Groot. 2005. Luxury at a cost? Recombinant mouse hepatitis viruses expressing the accessory hemagglutinin esterase protein display reduced fitness in vitro. *J. Virol.* **79:**15054–15063.

86. Liu, M., J. L. Leibowitz, D. A. Clark, M. Mendicino, Q. Ning, J. W. Ding, C. D'Abreo, L. Fung, P. A. Marsden, and G. A. Levy. 2003. Gene transcription of fgl2 in endothelial cells is controlled by Ets-1 and Oct-1 and requires the presence of both Sp1 and Sp3. *Eur. J. Biochem.* **270:**2274–2286.

87. Liu, M., M. Mendicino, Q. Ning, A. Ghanekar, W. He, I. McGilvray, I. Shalev, D. Pivato, D. A. Clark, M. J. Phillips, and G. A. Levy. 2006. Cytokine-induced hepatic apoptosis is dependent on FGL2/fibroleukin: the role of Sp1/Sp3 and STAT1/PU.1 composite cis elements. *J. Immunol.* **176:**7028–7038.

88. Lucas, A., W. Flintoff, R. Anderson, D. Percy, M. Coulter, and S. Dales. 1977. *In vivo* and *in vitro* models of demyelinating diseases: tropism of the JHM strain of murine hepatitis virus for cells of glial origin. *Cell* **12:**553–560.

89. Lucchiari, M. A., M. Modolell, K. Eichmann, and C. A. Pereira. 1992. In vivo depletion of interferon-gamma leads to susceptibility of A/J mice to mouse hepatitis virus 3 infection. *Immunobiology* **185:**475–482.

90. Lucchiari, M. A., M. Modolell, R. C. Vassao, and C. A. Pereira. 1993. TNF alpha, IL-1 and O2 release by macrophages do not correlate with the anti-mouse hepatitis virus 3 effect induced by interferon gamma. *Microb. Pathog.* **15:**447–454.

91. Lucchiari, M. A., and C. A. Pereira. 1989. A major role of macrophage activation by interferon-gamma during mouse hepatitis virus type 3 infection. I. Genetically dependent resistance. *Immunobiology* **180:**12–22.

92. Lucchiari, M. A., and C. A. Pereira. 1990. A major role of macrophage activation by interferon-gamma during mouse hepatitis virus type 3 infection. II. Age-dependent resistance. *Immunobiology* **181:**31–39.

93. Luo, Z., and S. R. Weiss. 1998. Roles in cell-to-cell fusion of two conserved hydrophobic regions in the murine coronavirus spike protein. *Virology* **244:**483–494.

94. MacNamara, K. C., M. M. Chua, P. T. Nelson, H. Shen, and S. R. Weiss. 2005. Increased epitope-specific CD8$^+$ T cells prevent murine coronavirus spread to the spinal cord and subsequent demyelination. *J. Virol.* **79:**3370–3381.

95. MacNamara, K. C., M. M. Chua, J. J. Phillips, and S. R. Weiss. 2005. Contributions of the viral genetic background and a single amino acid substitution in an immunodominant CD8$^+$ T-cell epitope to murine coronavirus neurovirulence. *J. Virol.* **79:**9108–9118.

96. MacNamara, K. C., M. M. Chua, R. Watson, T. Cowley, and S. R. Weiss. Priming of CD8+ T cells during central nervous system infection with a murine coronavirus is strain-dependent and influences virulence. Submitted for publication.

97. Manaker, R. A., C. V. Piczak, A. A. Miller, and M. F. Stanton. 1961. A hepatitis virus complicating studies with mouse leukemia. *J. Natl. Cancer Inst.* **27:**29–51.

98. Marsden, P. A., Q. Ning, L. S. Fung, X. Luo, Y. Chen, M. Mendicino, A. Ghanekar, J. A. Scott, T. Miller, C. W. Chan, M. W. Chan, W. He, R. M. Gorczynski, D. R. Grant, D. A. Clark, M. J. Phillips, and G. A. Levy. 2003. The fgl2/fibroleukin prothrombinase contributes to immunologically mediated thrombosis in experimental and human viral hepatitis. *J. Clin. Investig.* **112:**58–66.

99. Marten, N. W., S. A. Stohlman, R. D. Atkinson, D. R. Hinton, J. O. Fleming, and C. C. Bergmann. 2000. Contributions of CD8+ T cells and viral spread to demyelinating disease. *J. Immunol.* **164:**4080–4088.

100. Marten, N. W., S. A. Stohlman, and C. C. Bergmann. 2001. MHV infection of the CNS: mechanisms of immune-mediated control. *Viral Immunol.* **14:**1–18.

101. Marten, N. W., S. A. Stohlman, and C. C. Bergmann. 2000. Role of viral persistence in retaining CD8$^+$ T cells within the central nervous system. *J. Virol.* **74:**7903–7910.

101a. Matsubara, Y., R. Watanabe, and F. Taguchi. 1991. Neurovirulence of six different murine coronavirus JHM variants for rats. *Virus Res.* **20:**45–58.

102. Matsuyama, S., and F. Taguchi. 2002. Communication between SlN330 and a region in S2 of murine coronavirus spike protein is important for virus entry into cells expressing CEACAM1b receptor. *Virology* **295:**160–171.

103. Matsuyama, S., and F. Taguchi. 2002. Receptor-induced conformational changes of murine coronavirus spike protein. *J. Virol.* **76:**11819–11826.

104. Matthews, A. E., S. R. Weiss, M. J. Shlomchik, L. G. Hannum, J. L. Gombold, and Y. Paterson. 2001. Antibody is required for clearance of infectious murine hepatitis virus A59 from the central nervous system, but not the liver. *J. Immunol.* **167:**5254–5263.

105. McGilvray, I. D., Z. Lu, A. C. Wei, A. P. Dackiw, J. C. Marshall, A. Kapus, G. Levy, and O. D. Rotstein. 1998. Murine hepatitis virus strain 3 induces the macrophage prothrombinase fgl-2 through p38 mitogen-activated protein kinase activation. *J. Biol. Chem.* **273:**32222–32229.

106. Minskaia, E., T. Hertzig, A. E. Gorbalenya, V. Campanacci, C. Cambillau, B. Canard, and J. Ziebuhr. 2006. Discovery of an RNA virus 3′→5′ exoribonuclease that is critically involved in coronavirus RNA synthesis. *Proc. Natl. Acad. Sci. USA* **103:**5108–5113.

107. Morris, V. L., C. Tieszer, J. Mackinnon, and D. Percy. 1989. Characterization of coronavirus JHM variants isolated from Wistar Furth rats with a viral-induced demyelinating disease. *Virology* **169:**127–136.

108. Nash, T. C., T. M. Gallagher, and M. J. Buchmeier. 1995. MHVR-independent cell-cell spread of mouse hepatitis virus infection requires neutral pH fusion. *Adv. Exp. Med. Biol.* **380:**351–357.

109. Navas, S., S. H. Seo, M. M. Chua, J. D. Sarma, E. Lavi, S. T. Hingley, and S. R. Weiss. 2001. Murine coronavirus spike protein determines the ability of the virus to replicate in the liver and cause hepatitis. *J. Virol.* **75:**2452–2457.

110. Navas, S., and S. R. Weiss. 2003. Murine coronavirus-induced hepatitis: JHM genetic background eliminates A59 spike-determined hepatotropism. *J. Virol.* **77:**4972–4978.

111. Navas-Martin, S., M. Brom, M.-M. Chua, R. Watson, Z. Qiu, and S. R. Weiss. 2007. Replicase genes of murine coronavirus strains A59 and JHM are interchangeable: differences in pathogenesis map to the 3′ one-third of the genome. *J. Virol.* **81:**1022–1026.

112. Navas-Martin, S., M. Brom, and S. R. Weiss. 2006. Role of the replicase gene of murine coronavirus JHM strain in hepatitis. *Adv. Exp. Med. Biol.* **581:**415–420.

113. Ning, Q., M. Liu, P. Kongkham, M. M. Lai, P. A. Marsden, J. Tseng, B. Pereira, M. Belyavskyi, J. Leibowitz, M. J. Phillips, and G. Levy. 1999. The nucleocapsid protein of murine hepatitis virus type 3 induces transcription of the novel fgl2 prothrombinase gene. *J. Biol. Chem.* **274:**9930–9936.

114. Ning, Q., X. P. Luo, Z. M. Wang, M. F. Han, W. M. Yan, M. F. Liu, and G. Levy. 2003. The study of cis-element hnf4

in the regulation of mfg12 prothrombinase/fibroleukin gene expression in response to nucleocapsid protein of MHV-3. *Zhonghua Yixue Zazhi* **83**:678–683. (In Chinese.)

115. Ning, Q., Y. Sun, M. Han, L. Zhang, C. Zhu, W. Zhang, H. Guo, J. Li, W. Yan, F. Gong, Z. Chen, W. He, C. Koscik, R. Smith, R. Gorczynski, G. Levy, and X. Luo. 2005. Role of fibrinogen-like protein 2 prothrombinase/fibroleukin in experimental and human allograft rejection. *J. Immunol.* **174**:7403–7411.

116. Ontiveros, E., T. S. Kim, T. M. Gallagher, and S. Perlman. 2003. Enhanced virulence mediated by the murine coronavirus, mouse hepatitis virus strain JHM, is associated with a glycine at residue 310 of the spike glycoprotein. *J. Virol.* **77**:10260–10269.

117. Ontiveros, E., L. Kuo, P. S. Masters, and S. Perlman. 2001. Inactivation of expression of gene 4 of mouse hepatitis virus strain JHM does not affect virulence in the murine CNS. *Virology* **289**:230–238.

118. Parker, S. E., T. M. Gallagher, and M. J. Buchmeier. 1989. Sequence analysis reveals extensive polymorphism and evidence of deletions within the E2 glycoprotein gene of several strains of murine hepatitis virus. *Virology* **173**:664–673.

119. Parr, R. L., L. Fung, J. Reneker, N. Myers-Mason, J. L. Leibowitz, and G. Levy. 1995. Association of mouse fibrinogen-like protein with murine hepatitis virus-induced prothrombinase activity. *J. Virol.* **69**:5033–5038.

120. Parr, R. L., L. Fung, J. Reneker, N. Myers-Mason, J. L. Leibowitz, and G. Levy. 1995. MHV-3 induced prothrombinase is encoded by musfiblp. *Adv. Exp. Med. Biol.* **380**:151–157.

121. Parra, B., D. R. Hinton, N. W. Marten, C. C. Bergmann, M. T. Lin, C. S. Yang, and S. A. Stohlman. 1999. IFN-gamma is required for viral clearance from central nervous system oligodendroglia. *J. Immunol.* **162**:1641–1647.

122. Pasick, J. M., K. Kalicharran, and S. Dales. 1994. Distribution and trafficking of JHM coronavirus structural proteins and virions in primary neurons and the OBL-21 neuronal cell line. *J. Virol.* **68**:2915–2928.

123. Pearce, B. D., M. V. Hobbs, T. S. McGraw, and M. J. Buchmeier. 1994. Cytokine induction during T-cell-mediated clearance of mouse hepatitis virus from neurons in vivo. *J. Virol.* **68**:5483–5495.

124. Pereira, C. A., A.-M. Steffan, and A. Kirn. 1984. Interaction between mouse hepatitis viruses and primary cultures of Kupffer and endothelial liver cells from resistant and susceptible inbred mouse strains. *J. Gen. Virol.* **65**:1617–1620.

125. Pewe, L., S. B. Heard, C. Bergmann, M. O. Dailey, and S. Perlman. 1999. Selection of CTL escape mutants in mice infected with a neurotropic coronavirus: quantitative estimate of TCR diversity in the infected central nervous system. *J. Immunol.* **163**:6106–6113.

126. Pewe, L., G. F. Wu, E. M. Barnett, R. F. Castro, and S. Perlman. 1996. Cytotoxic T cell-resistant variants are selected in a virus-induced demyelinating disease. *Immunity* **5**:253–262.

127. Pewe, L., S. Xue, and S. Perlman. 1997. Cytotoxic T-cell-resistant variants arise at early times after infection in C57BL/6 but not in SCID mice infected with a neurotropic coronavirus. *J. Virol.* **71**:7640–7647.

128. Phillips, J. J., M. Chua, S. H. Seo, and S. R. Weiss. 2001. Multiple regions of the murine coronavirus spike glycoprotein influence neurovirulence. *J. Neurovirol.* **7**:421–431.

129. Phillips, J. J., M. M. Chua, E. Lavi, and S. R. Weiss. 1999. Pathogenesis of chimeric MHV4/MHV-A59 recombinant viruses: the murine coronavirus spike protein is a major determinant of neurovirulence. *J. Virol.* **73**:7752–7760.

130. Phillips, J. J., M. M. Chua, G. F. Rall, and S. R. Weiss. 2002. Murine coronavirus spike glycoprotein mediates degree of viral spread, inflammation, and virus-induced immunopathology in the central nervous system. *Virology* **301**:109–120.

131. Pope, M., S. W. Chung, T. Mosmann, J. L. Leibowitz, R. M. Gorczynski, and G. A. Levy. 1996. Resistance of naive mice to murine hepatitis virus strain 3 requires development of a Th1, but not a Th2, response, whereas pre-existing antibody partially protects against primary infection. *J. Immunol.* **156**:3342–3349.

132. Pope, M., O. Rotstein, E. Cole, S. Sinclair, R. Parr, B. Cruz, R. Fingerote, S. Chung, R. Gorczynski, and L. Fung. 1995. Pattern of disease after murine hepatitis virus strain 3 infection correlates with macrophage activation and not viral replication. *J. Virol.* **69**:5252–5260.

133. Puntel, M., J. F. Curtin, J. M. Zirger, A. K. Muhammad, W. Xiong, C. Liu, J. Hu, K. M. Kroeger, P. Czer, S. Sciascia, S. Mondkar, P. R. Lowenstein, and M. G. Castro. 2006. Quantification of high-capacity helper-dependent adenoviral vector genomes in vitro and in vivo, using quantitative TaqMan real-time polymerase chain reaction. *Hum. Gene Ther.* **17**:531–544.

134. Ramakrishna, C., R. A. Atkinson, S. A. Stohlman, and C. C. Bergmann. 2006. Vaccine-induced memory CD8+ T cells cannot prevent central nervous system virus reactivation. *J. Immunol.* **176**:3062–3069.

135. Ramakrishna, C., C. C. Bergmann, K. V. Holmes, and S. A. Stohlman. 2004. Expression of the mouse hepatitis virus receptor by central nervous system microglia. *J. Virol.* **78**:7828–7832.

136. Ramakrishna, C., S. A. Stohlman, R. A. Atkinson, D. R. Hinton, and C. C. Bergmann. 2004. Differential regulation of primary and secondary CD8+ T cells in the central nervous system. *J. Immunol.* **173**:6265–6273.

137. Rempel, J. D., S. J. Murray, J. Meisner, and M. J. Buchmeier. 2004. Differential regulation of innate and adaptive immune responses in viral encephalitis. *Virology* **318**:381–392.

138. Rempel, J. D., S. J. Murray, J. Meisner, and M. J. Buchmeier. 2004. Mouse hepatitis virus neurovirulence: evidence of a linkage between S glycoprotein expression and immunopathology. *Virology* **318**:45–54.

139. Saeki, K., N. Ohtsuka, and F. Taguchi. 1997. Identification of spike protein residues of murine coronavirus responsible for receptor-binding activity by use of soluble receptor-resistant mutants. *J. Virol.* **71**:9024–9031.

140. Saeki, K., N. Ohtsuka, and F. Taguchi. 1998. Isolation and characterization of murine coronavirus mutants resistant to neutralization by soluble receptors. *Adv. Exp. Med. Biol.* **440**:11–16.

141. Schwarz, B., E. Routledge, and S. G. Siddell. 1990. Murine coronavirus nonstructural protein ns2 is not essential for virus replication in transformed cells. *J. Virol.* **64**:4784–4791.

142. Seo, S. H., E. Hoffmann, and R. G. Webster. 2002. Lethal H5N1 influenza viruses escape host anti-viral cytokine responses. *Nat. Med.* **8**:950–954.

143. Shieh, C. K., H. J. Lee, K. Yokomori, N. La Monica, S. Makino, and M. M. Lai. 1989. Identification of a new transcriptional initiation site and the corresponding functional gene 2b in the murine coronavirus RNA genome. *J. Virol.* **63**:3729–3736.

144. Sinclair, S., M. Abecassis, P. Y. Wong, A. Romaschin, L. S. Fung, and G. Levy. 1990. Mechanism of protective effect of prostaglandin E in murine hepatitis virus strain 3 infection: effects on macrophage production of tumour necrosis factor,

procoagulant activity and leukotriene B4. *Adv. Exp. Med. Biol.* **276:**533–542.

145. Smits, S. L., G. J. Gerwig, A. L. van Vliet, A. Lissenberg, P. Briza, J. P. Kamerling, R. Vlasak, and R. J. de Groot. 2005. Nidovirus sialate-O-acetylesterases: evolution and substrate specificity of coronaviral and toroviral receptor-destroying enzymes. *J. Biol. Chem.* **280:**6933–6941.

146. Snijder, E. J., P. J. Bredenbeek, J. C. Dobbe, V. Thiel, J. Ziebuhr, L. L. Poon, Y. Guan, M. Rozanov, W. J. Spaan, and A. E. Gorbalenya. 2003. Unique and conserved features of genome and proteome of SARS-coronavirus, an early split-off from the coronavirus group 2 lineage. *J. Mol. Biol.* **331:**991–1004.

147. Sorensen, O., and S. Dales. 1985. In vivo and in vitro models of demyelinating disease: JHM virus in the rat central nervous system localized by in situ cDNA hybridization and immunofluorescent microscopy. *J. Virol.* **56:**434–438.

148. Spann, K. M., K. C. Tran, B. Chi, R. L. Rabin, and P. L. Collins. 2004. Suppression of the induction of alpha, beta, and gamma interferons by the ns1 and ns2 proteins of human respiratory syncytial virus in human epithelial cells and macrophages. *J. Virol.* **78:**4363–4369.

149. Sperry, S. M., L. Kazi, R. L. Graham, R. S. Baric, S. R. Weiss, and M. R. Denison. 2005. Single-amino-acid substitutions in open reading frame (ORF) 1b-nsp14 and ORF 2a proteins of the coronavirus mouse hepatitis virus are attenuating in mice. *J. Virol.* **79:**3391–3400.

150. Stohlman, S. A., P. R. Brayton, J. O. Fleming, L. P. Weiner, and M. M. Lai. 1982. Murine coronaviruses: isolation and characterization of two plaque morphology variants of the JHM neurotropic strain. *J. Gen. Virol.* **63:**265–275.

151. Stohlman, S. A., and L. P. Weiner. 1981. Chronic central nervous system demyelination in mice after JHM virus infection. *Neurology* **31:**38–44.

152. Sturman, L. S., and K. V. Holmes. 1977. Characterization of coronavirus. II. Glycoproteins of the viral envelope: tryptic peptide analysis. *Virology* **77:**650–660.

153. Sun, N., D. Grzybicki, R. F. Castro, S. Murphy, and S. Perlman. 1995. Activation of astrocytes in the spinal cord of mice chronically infected with a neurotropic coronavirus. *Virology* **213:**482–493.

154. Sussman, M. A., R. A. Shubin, S. Kyuwa, and S. A. Stohlman. 1989. T-cell-mediated clearance of mouse hepatitis virus strain JHM from the central nervous system. *J. Virol.* **63:**3051–3061.

155. Taguchi, F. 1995. The S2 subunit of the murine coronavirus spike protein is not involved in receptor binding. *J. Virol.* **69:**7260–7263.

156. Taguchi, F., P. T. Massa, and V. ter Meulen. 1986. Characterization of a variant virus isolated from neural cell culture after infection of mouse coronavirus JHMV. *Virology* **155:**267–270.

157. Taguchi, F., and S. Matsuyama. 2002. Soluble receptor potentiates receptor-independent infection by murine coronavirus. *J. Virol.* **76:**950–958.

158. Taguchi, F., S. G. Siddell, H. Wege, and V. ter Meulen. 1985. Characterization of a variant virus selected in rat brains after infection by coronavirus mouse hepatitis virus JHM. *J. Virol.* **54:**429–435.

159. Tardieu, M., A. Goffinet, G. Harmant-van Rijckevorsel, and G. Lyon. 1982. Ependymitis, leukoencephalitis, hydrocephalus, and thrombotic vasculitis following chronic infection by mouse hepatitis virus 3 (MHV 3). *Acta Neuropathol.* **58:**168–176.

160. Tsai, J. C., L. de Groot, J. D. Pinon, K. T. Iacono, J. J. Phillips, S. H. Seo, E. Lavi, and S. R. Weiss. 2003. Amino acid

substitutions within the heptad repeat domain 1 of murine coronavirus spike protein restrict viral antigen spread in the central nervous system. *Virology* **312:**369–380.

161. Valarcher, J.-F., J. Furze, S. Wyld, R. Cook, K.-K. Conzelmann, and G. Taylor. 2004. Role of alpha/beta interferons in the attenuation and immunogenicity of recombinant bovine respiratory syncytial viruses lacking NS proteins. *J. Virol.* **77:**8426–8439.

162. van der Veen, R. C. 1996. Immunogenicity of JHM virus proteins: characterization of a CD4+ T cell epitope on nucleocapsid protein which induces different T-helper cell subsets. *Virology* **225:**339–346.

163. Vassão, R., and C. A. Pereira. 1994. Antiviral activity of interferon gamma in vivo during mouse hepatitis virus infection. *Braz. J. Med. Biol. Res.* **27:**2407–2411.

164. Vassao, R. C., M. T. de Franco, D. Hartz, M. Modolell, A. E. Sippel, and C. A. Pereira. 2000. Down-regulation of bgp1a viral receptor by interferon-gamma is related to the antiviral state and resistance to mouse hepatitis virus 3 infection. *Virology* **274:**278–283.

165. Vennema, H., G. J. Godeke, J. W. Rossen, W. F. Voorhout, M. C. Horzinek, D. J. Opstelten, and P. J. Rottier. 1996. Nucleocapsid-independent assembly of coronavirus-like particles by co-expression of viral envelope protein genes. *EMBO J.* **15:**2020–2028.

166. Virelizier, J. L., A. C. Allison, and E. de Maeyer. 1977. Production by mixed lymphocyte cultures of a type II interferon able to protect macrophages against virus infection. *Infect. Immun.* **17:**282–285.

167. Virelizier, J. L., A. D. Dayan, and A. C. Allison. 1975. Neuropathological effects of persistent infection of mice by mouse hepatitis virus. *Infect. Immun.* **12:**1127–1140.

168. Virelizier, J. L., and I. Gresser. 1978. Role of interferon in the pathogenesis of viral diseases of mice as demonstrated by the use of anti-interferon serum. V. Protective role in mouse hepatitis virus type 3 infection of susceptible and resistant strains of mice. *J. Immunol.* **120:**1616–1619.

169. Virelizier, J. L., A. M. Virelizier, and A. C. Allison. 1976. The role of circulating interferon in the modifications of immune responsiveness by mouse hepatitis virus (MHV-3). *J. Immunol.* **117:**748–753.

170. Wang, F. I., J. O. Fleming, and M. M. Lai. 1992. Sequence analysis of the spike protein gene of murine coronavirus variants: study of genetic sites affecting neuropathogenicity. *Virology* **186:**742–749.

171. Wang, Y., and X. Zhang. 1999. The nucleocapsid protein of coronavirus mouse hepatitis virus interacts with the cellular heterogeneous nuclear ribonucleoprotein A1 in vitro and in vivo. *Virology* **265:**96–109.

172. Watanabe, R., H. Wege, and V. ter Meulen. 1983. Adoptive transfer of EAE-like lesions from rats with coronavirus-induced demyelinating encephalomyelitis. *Nature* **305:**150–153.

173. Wege, H., H. Schluesener, R. Meyermann, V. Barac-Latas, G. Suchanek, and H. Lassmann. 1998. Coronavirus infection and demyelination. Development of inflammatory lesions in Lewis rats. *Adv. Exp. Med. Biol.* **440:**437–444.

174. Weiner, L. P. 1973. Pathogenesis of demyelination induced by a mouse hepatitis. *Arch. Neurol.* **28:**298–303.

175. Weiner, L. P., R. T. Johnson, and R. M. Herndon. 1973. Viral infections and demyelinating diseases. *N. Engl. J. Med.* **288:**1103–1110.

176. Weiss, S. R., P. W. Zoltick, and J. L. Leibowitz. 1993. The ns 4 gene of mouse hepatitis virus (MHV), strain A 59 contains two orfs and thus differs from ns 4 of the JHM and S strains. *Arch. Virol.* **129:**301–309.

177. **Wilson, L., P. Gage, and G. Ewart.** 2006. Hexamethylene amiloride blocks E protein ion channels and inhibits coronavirus replication. *Virology* **353:**294–306.

178. **Wu, G. F., A. A. Dandekar, L. Pewe, and S. Perlman.** 2000. CD4 and CD8 T cells have redundant but not identical roles in virus-induced demyelination. *J. Immunol.* **165:**2278–2286.

179. **Wu, G. F., and S. Perlman.** 1999. Macrophage infiltration, but not apoptosis, is correlated with immune-mediated demyelination following murine infection with a neurotropic coronavirus. *J. Virol.* **73:**8771–8780.

180. **Wurm, T., H. Chen, T. Hodgson, P. Britton, G. Brooks, and J. A. Hiscox.** 2001. Localization to the nucleolus is a common feature of coronavirus nucleoproteins, and the protein may disrupt host cell division. *J. Virol.* **75:**9345–9356.

181. **Yamada, A., F. Taguchi, and K. Fujiwara.** 1979. T lymphocyte-dependent difference in susceptibility between DDD and C3H mice to mouse hepatitis virus, MHV-3. *Jpn. J. Exp. Med.* **49:**413–421.

182. **Yokomori, K., M. Asanaka, S. A. Stohlman, S. Makino, R. A. Shubin, W. Gilmore, L. P. Weiner, F. I. Wang, and M. M. Lai.** 1995. Neuropathogenicity of mouse hepatitis virus JHM isolates differing in hemagglutinin-esterase protein expression. *J. Neurovirol.* **1:**330–339.

183. **Yokomori, K., S. C. Baker, S. A. Stohlman, and M. M. Lai.** 1992. Hemagglutinin-esterase-specific monoclonal antibodies alter the neuropathogenicity of mouse hepatitis virus. *J. Virol.* **66:**2865–2874.

184. **Yokomori, K., L. R. Banner, and M. M. Lai.** 1991. Heterogeneity of gene expression of the hemagglutinin-esterase (HE) protein of murine coronaviruses. *Virology* **183:**647–657.

185. **Yokomori, K., and M. M. Lai.** 1991. Mouse hepatitis virus S RNA sequence reveals that nonstructural proteins ns4 and ns5a are not essential for murine coronavirus replication. *J. Virol.* **65:**5605–5608.

186. **Yokomori, K., N. La Monica, S. Makino, C. K. Shieh, and M. M. Lai.** 1989. Biosynthesis, structure, and biological activities of envelope protein gp65 of murine coronavirus. *Virology* **173:**683–691.

187. **Yokomori, K., S. A. Stohlman, and M. M. Lai.** 1993. The detection and characterization of multiple hemagglutinin-esterase (HE)-defective viruses in the mouse brain during subacute demyelination induced by mouse hepatitis virus. *Virology* **192:**170–178.

188. **Yount, B., K. M. Curtis, E. A. Fritz, L. E. Hensley, P. B. Jahrling, E. Prentice, M. R. Denison, T. W. Geisbert, and R. S. Baric.** 2003. Reverse genetics with a full-length infectious cDNA of severe acute respiratory syndrome coronavirus. *Proc. Natl. Acad. Sci. USA* **100:**12995–13000.

189. **Yount, B., M. R. Denison, S. R. Weiss, and R. S. Baric.** 2002. Systematic assembly of a full-length infectious cDNA of mouse hepatitis virus strain A59. *J. Virol.* **76:**11065–11078.

190. **Yu, X., W. Bi, S. R. Weiss, and J. L. Leibowitz.** 1994. Mouse hepatitis virus gene 5b protein is a new virion envelope protein. *Virology* **202:**1018–1023.

191. **Yuwaraj, S., J. Ding, M. Liu, P. A. Marsden, and G. A. Levy.** 2001. Genomic characterization, localization, and functional expression of fgl2, the human gene encoding fibroleukin: a novel human procoagulant. *Genomics* **71:**330–338.

*Nidoviruses*
Edited by S. Perlman, T. Gallagher, and E. J. Snijder
© 2008 ASM Press, Washington, DC

Chapter 18

# Coronaviruses of Domestic Livestock and Poultry: Interspecies Transmission, Pathogenesis, and Immunity

LINDA J. SAIF

In 2002–2003, severe acute respiratory syndrome (SARS), a new fatal respiratory disease of humans, appeared in China and rapidly spread globally (24, 55, 76, 77, 83). It was caused by a previously unrecognized coronavirus (CoV), SARS-CoV, that was likely of zoonotic origin from a wildlife reservoir (bats or civet cats) (33, 58, 62). The emergence of SARS-CoV stunned the medical community, but animal coronavirologists had previously documented the propensity of CoVs to cause fatal respiratory and enteric disease in animals, their interspecies transmission, and the existence of wildlife reservoirs (90, 91). Although there was compelling evidence for emergence of new CoV strains and genetic changes in existing strains leading to new tissue tropisms or disease syndromes in animals, the extensive diversity and disease impact of CoVs were not widely appreciated before the SARS epidemic.

Like SARS-CoV, the CoVs of domestic livestock and poultry cause primarily respiratory and/or enteric disease (Table 1). These animal CoVs belong to each of the three established CoV groups, with two subgroups recognized for groups 1 (1a and 1b) and 2 (2a and 2b) (Table 1). The swine enteric CoVs, porcine epidemic diarrhea virus (PEDV) and transmissible gastroenteritis virus (TGEV), and the spike protein (S protein) gene deletion respiratory mutant of TGEV, the porcine respiratory CoV (PRCV), belong to group 1. The latter two CoVs (group 1a) are closely related genetically (98 and 97.6% nucleotide identity between the complete genomes of PRCV ISU-1 and Miller and Purdue TGEV strains, respectively) (122) and antigenically (60, 95), with the major immunodominant neutralizing antigenic site (A) conserved on PRCV and TGEV. PEDV is more distantly related and is

in subgroup 1b with human CoVs 229E and NL63 and bat CoV. Antibodies to PEDV do not neutralize TGEV or PRCV, although a shared antigen was shown by immunoblotting analysis (80). A further unexplained observation is the antigenic cross-reactivity between the group 1a CoVs and SARS CoV, likely at the level of the N protein (34a, 55, 105).

Bovine CoV (BCoV) (which causes pneumoenteric infections in cattle), wild-ruminant CoVs, and swine hemagglutinating encephalomyelitis virus (HEV) belong to CoV subgroup 2a along with canine respiratory CoV and human CoVs OC43 and HKU1. With the exception of HEV, which also infects the central nervous system, causing a wasting disease (79), the viruses cause enteric and/or respiratory disease (Table 1). Similarly, the recently discovered SARS-CoVs that are associated with both respiratory and enteric infections in humans and animals (civet cats, raccoon dogs, and bats) belong to a new CoV subgroup, 2b. An important difference between group 1 and 3 CoVs and group 2 CoVs is the presence of a hemagglutinin-esterase (HE) glycoprotein in a subset of group 2 CoVs, including BCoV and wild-ruminant CoVs. HE forms a second dense layer of short surface projections, in contrast to the longer surface S glycoproteins present on all CoVs, as illustrated in Fig. 1.

Avian CoVs are the exclusive members of CoV group 3. They cause respiratory and enteric infections, but some strains of the chicken CoV, infectious bronchitis virus (IBV), also cause nephritis and infections of the reproductive tract (10, 19).

The focus of this chapter is on representative CoVs of livestock and poultry from each of these three groups, with emphasis on the respiratory and enteric CoV infections and analogies to SARS-CoV.

Linda J. Saif • Food Animal Health Research Program, Ohio Agricultural Research and Development Center, and Department of Veterinary Preventive Medicine, College of Veterinary Medicine, The Ohio State University, Wooster, OH 44691.

**Table 1.** Reference animal coronaviruses: groups, target tissues, and types of diseases

| Group | Virus | Host | Disease or infected tissue | | |
|-------|-------|------|------------|--------|-------|
| | | | Respiratory | Enteric[a] | Other |
| 1a | Transmissible gastrointestinal virus (TGEV) | Pig | X (upper) | X(SI) | |
| | Porcine respiratory coronavirus (PRCV) | Pig | X (upper/lower) | | Viremia |
| | Canine enteric CoV (CECoV) | Dog | | X | |
| | Feline coronavirus (FCoV) | Cat | X | X | Systemic (FIPV) |
| 1b | Human coronaviruses 229E and NL63 | Human | X (upper/lower) | | |
| | Porcine epidemic diarrhea virus (PEDV) | Pig | | X (SI, colon) | |
| | Bat *(Miniopterus)* CoV | Bat | X (upper) | X | Subclinical? |
| 2a | Human coronaviruses OC43 and HKU1 | Human | X (upper) | ?? (BCoV?) | |
| | Hemagglutinating encephalitis virus (HEV) | Pig | X | | CNS[b] |
| | Bovine coronavirus (BCoV) | Cattle | X (lung) | X (SI, colon) | |
| | Wild ruminant CoVs[c] | Multiple | ? | X | |
| | Canine respiratory CoV (CRCoV) | Dog | X | ? | |
| 2b | Severe acute respiratory syndrome (SARS) CoV | Human | X (lung) | X | Viremia, kidney? |
| | Civet cat *(Paguma larvata)* CoV | Palm civet | X | X | Subclinical? |
| | Raccoon dog *(Nyctereutes procyonoides)* CoV | Raccoon dog | ? | X | Subclinical? |
| | Horseshoe bat *(Rhinolophus sinicus)* CoV | Bat | ? | X | Subclinical? |
| 3 | Infectious bronchitis virus (IBV) | Chicken | X (upper) | X (no diarrhea) | Viremia, kidney, oviduct |
| | Turkey coronavirus (TCoV) | Turkey | | X (SI) | |

[a] SI, small intestine; ??, BCoV-like CoV from a child (123).
[b] CNS, central nervous system.
[c] Wild-ruminant CoVs include isolates from sambar deer *(Cervus unicolor),* white-tailed deer *(Odocoileus virginianus),* waterbuck *(Kobus ellipsiprymnus)* (108), giraffe *(Giraffa camelopardalis)* (36a), and elk *(Cervus elaphus)* (65).

The goal is to provide insights into comparative aspects of transmission, pathogenesis, and immunity for these animal CoVs.

## EPIDEMIOLOGY, INTERSPECIES TRANSMISSION, AND WILDLIFE RESERVOIRS

The likelihood that SARS-CoV is a zoonotic infection transmitted from wild animals to humans is not unprecedented based on previous veterinary research on interspecies transmission and wildlife reservoirs for animal CoVs. In this section, the initial descriptions, epidemiology, interspecies transmission, and possible wildlife reservoirs for selected group 1, 2, and 3 animal CoVs are reviewed.

### Group 1 CoVs

#### Subgroup 1a: TGEV and PRCV epidemiology

Transmissible gastroenteritis (TGE) has been recognized in swine since 1946 and occurs worldwide (95). Both epidemic and endemic forms of TGE occur, especially in North America; however, endemic TGEV is more common in Europe and Asia due to the widespread presence in pigs of the respiratory variant PRCV, which induces at least partial immunity to TGEV (95). Epidemic TGEV occurs primarily during winter in TGEV/PRCV-seronegative herds, infecting pigs of all ages but producing severe diarrhea and dehydration in suckling pigs under 2 to 3 weeks of age. Mortality is high in this population (often 100%). Endemic TGEV occurs in partially immune herds, including PRCV-seropositive herds. It is especially common in herds with continuous farrowing due to the presence of susceptible pigs postweaning, after loss of maternal antibodies. Morbidity may be high, but mortality is low (10 to 20%) and related to the age when infected. Interestingly, the seroprevalence of TGEV in Europe has declined significantly coincident with the spread of PRCV. Besides the small intestine, TGEV also infects the upper respiratory tract and is transiently shed nasally; nevertheless, the major transmission route appears to be fecal-oral (53, 117).

PRCV, a mutant of TGEV with S protein gene deletions of various sizes (621 to 681 nucleotides [nt]), altered tissue tropism (respiratory), and reduced virulence, emerged independently in the 1980s in Europe (78) and the United States (118). Smaller deletions also occurred proximal to or in open reading frame 3a (ORF3a) (encoding an undefined nonstructural protein), resulting in its lack of expression (54, 60, 75). Based on the S protein gene deletion with loss of an antigenic site (D), TGEV and PRCV strains in clinical specimens (nasal secretions/tissues, gut tissues, or feces) or antibodies in serum can be differentiated genetically by nested reverse transcriptase

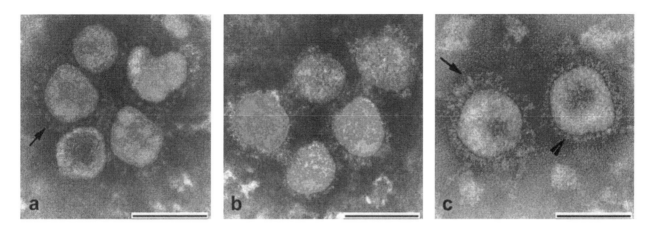

Figure 1. Immuno-EM of tissue culture-adapted animal CoVs. Particles were reacted with antisera to TGEV (a) or BCoV (b and c). (a) PRCV showing single layer of surface spikes (arrow); (b and c) group 2 CoVs (WD strain of BCoV [b] and sambar deer CoV [c] showing shorter surface HE (arrowhead) and longer spikes (arrow) resulting in a dense outer fringe. Bar = 100 μm.

PCR (RT-PCR) assays (54, 74) or antigenically by use of monoclonal antibodies (MAbs) to site D in blocking enzyme-linked immunosorbent assay (ELISA) (95), respectively.

PRCV infections are often subclinical or associated with mild respiratory disease, although lung lesions are almost invariably present. The virus has become endemic in many European swine herds, and PRCV infections also occur in Asia (60, 95). A small serologic survey in the United States of asymptomatic swine herds in Iowa reported that many were seropositive for PRCV antibodies (119). Swine population density, distances between farms, and season influence the epidemiology of PRCV. The virus spreads long distances (several kilometers) by airborne transmission or directly by contact. Although PRCV-seronegative pigs of all ages are susceptible to infection, PRCV persists in closed herds by infecting newly weaned pigs, after passive maternal antibodies have declined. PRCV, like TGEV, can disappear from herds in summer and reemerge in older pigs in winter (60, 78, 95) potentially persisting as subclinical infections in pigs in summer or perhaps in other animal reservoirs (see Interspecies Transmission). It is notable that in Europe (but less so in North America) the more virulent enteric TGEV infections have been displaced following the widespread dissemination of PRCV.

## Subgroup 1b: PEDV epidemiology

In the late 1970s through the 1980s a new porcine CoV, PEDV, appeared first in Europe and then throughout Asia (80). However, to date there are no reports of PEDV in North or South America. The initial PEDV outbreaks in Europe resembled TGE, with fecal-oral transmission and severe diarrhea, but with

slower spread, lower overall mortality in baby pigs (average, 50%), and more marked variation in morbidity and mortality in breeding herds. Such acute outbreaks with high piglet mortality are now uncommon in Europe, but until recently they accounted for enormous losses (thousands of pigs) among suckling pigs in Asia. Currently PEDV appears to have become endemic in several Asian countries, unlike in some European countries where PEDV outbreaks are rare and the prevalence has declined markedly. However, recent wide-scale serologic surveys are lacking.

## Subgroup 1a: TGE/PRCV interspecies transmission and wildlife reservoirs

Interspecies transmission has been documented experimentally for the various subgroup 1a CoVs most closely related to the TGEV/PRCV cluster, including canine enteric CoV (CECoV) and feline CoV (FCoV). These viruses share close biologic, antigenic, and genetic relationships and may represent host range mutants of an ancestral CoV (46, 69, 95). They cross-react in virus neutralization tests and with MAbs to the S, nucleocapsid (N), or membrane (M) protein, and all share antigenic subsite Ac on the S protein. Interestingly, neutralizing immunoglobulin G (IgG) MAbs to the S protein of TGEV effectively mediate antibody-dependent enhancement of FCoV (feline infectious peritonitis virus [FIPV] strains) infection of macrophages in vitro, demonstrating the functional cross-reactivities of the S antibodies (72). The type II FCoV and CECoV and TGEV share >90% amino acid identities in the M and N proteins and >80% overall amino acid identities in the S protein, with >94% identity from amino acids (aa) 275 to 1447 (31). TGEV, PRCV, and FCoV also share a common receptor, aminopeptidase N. They cross-infect pigs, dogs, and cats with variable levels of disease expression and cross-protection in the heterologous host (92, 95).

Possible wild and domestic animal reservoirs for TGEV were recognized prior to their postulated role in the SARS-CoV outbreak. Wild and domestic carnivores (foxes, dogs, and, possibly, mink) seroconvert to TGEV positivity and are suggested as potential subclinical carriers of TGEV, serving as reservoirs between seasonal (winter) epidemics, but only virus excreted by dogs has been confirmed as infectious for pigs (95). Wild birds *(Sturnus vulgaris)* and flies *(Musca domestica)* have been proposed as mechanical vectors for TGEV.

### Subgroup 1b: PEDV interspecies transmission and wildlife reservoirs

The emergence and origin of PEDV in European swine described in the late 1970s and subsequently in Asia remain an enigma. Less cross-reactivity has been reported between the TGEV-related CoVs and PEDV using polyclonal antisera or MAbs, except for one-way reactivity with the N protein (80, 95). Also, unlike the other animal group 1 CoVs, PEDV grows in Vero cells (African green monkey kidney), as do SARS-CoVs. Of interest, a group 1 CoV was recently discovered in fecal and respiratory samples of bats *(Miniopterus* spp.) in Hong Kong with the nucleotide sequences of the RNA-dependent RNA polymerase and S protein gene fragments most closely related to those of PEDV (82). More full-length genomic sequence data for multiple group 1 CoV isolates, including additional ones from wildlife, may provide further insight into group 1 CoV genetic relationships, origin, and common ancestors.

### Group 2 CoVs

### Subgroup 2a: BCoV epidemiology

Bovine CoV is a pneumoenteric virus that is shed in both feces and upper respiratory tract secretions. It is ubiquitous in cattle worldwide, based on BCoV antibody seroprevalence data (18, 86, 92). The past three decades have witnessed dramatic breakthroughs in our understanding of the role of BCoV in three distinct clinical syndromes in cattle (Table 2): calf diarrhea (18, 92); winter dysentery (WD)with hemorrhagic diarrhea in adults (4, 13, 86, 92, 107, 109, 110, 114); and respiratory infections in cattle of various ages, including the bovine respiratory disease complex (BRDC) or shipping fever of feedlot cattle (15, 18, 29, 37–39, 42, 43, 56, 57, 102–104, 106).

Calf diarrhea associated with BCoV infection is most common in calves under 3 weeks of age, when passively acquired colostral and milk antibody levels have declined, but clinical disease may occur in calves up to 3 months of age (Table 2) (18, 42, 43, 92). The occurrence of severe diarrhea, resulting in dehydration and death, depends on BCoV dose, calf age, and calf immune status. Enteric infections with BCoV have been reported for calves, with prevalence rates of 8 to 69% in diarrheic calves and 0 to 24% in subclinically infected calves. Mixed infections with other enteric pathogens, such as rotavirus, calicivirus, and *Cryptosporidium,* are common, and the additive effect of multiple pathogens on calf disease severity is also recognized (85). Disease is more prevalent in winter, probably due to greater viral stability in the cold, and outbreaks often occur yearly on the same farm.

BCoV is also implicated as a cause of mild respiratory disease (coughing and rhinitis) or pneumonia in 2- to 6-month-old calves and is detected in nasal secretions, the lungs, and often the intestine and feces (Table 2) (18, 42, 43, 68, 84, 92). In studies of calves from birth to 20 weeks of age, Heckert et al. (42, 43) documented both fecal and nasal shedding of BCoV, but with diarrhea most prominent upon initial infection of calves with BCoV. Subsequently repeated or intermittent respiratory shedding episodes occurred in the same animal, with or without respiratory disease, but with subsequent transient increases in serum antibody titers consistent with these reinfections. These findings further suggest a lack of long-term mucosal immunity in the upper respiratory tract after natural BCoV infection, confirming similar observations for human respiratory CoV (7) and PRCV (6). Consequently, within a herd, reservoirs for BCoV infection may be virus cycling in clinically or subclinically infected calves, young adult cattle in which sporadic nasal shedding prevails, or clinically or subclinically infected adults. BCoV is transmitted via both fecal-oral and potentially respiratory (aerosol) routes.

WD occurs in adult dairy and beef cattle and in captive wild ruminants during the winter months and is characterized by hemorrhagic diarrhea, frequent respiratory signs, anorexia, and a marked reduction in milk production in dairy cattle (Table 2) (13, 86, 92, 110, 114). WD occurs most commonly from November to March in the northern United States. It has also been reported in Europe, Australia, and Asia (86, 92, 114). The morbidity rate ranges from 20 to 100%, but the mortality rate is usually low (1 to 2%), although longer-term reduced milk production has been reported. BCoV has been implicated as a cause of WD both in epidemiological studies (99) and in experimental transmission studies in seropositive nonlactating (110) or seronegative lactating dairy cows (107). Although BCoV is the major etiologic agent associated with WD, other host, environmental, or viral factors and interactions related to disease

Table 2. Summary of disease syndromes associated with BCoV infections

| Disease syndrome | Clinical signs | Cells infected | Lesions[a] | | Shedding[b] | | |
| --- | --- | --- | --- | --- | --- | --- | --- |
| | | | Respiratory | Enteric | Nasal | Fecal | Ages affected |
| **Calf disease syndromes** | | | | | | | |
| Calf diarrhea | Diarrhea<br>Dehydration<br>Fever, anorexia | Intestinal, nasal, ± lung epithelial cells | +/−<br>Lung emphysema | ++<br>J, I, colon<br>Villous atrophy | 2–8 days | 2–8 days | Birth–4 wk |
| Calf pneumonia | Cough<br>Rhinitis<br>± Pneumonia<br>± Diarrhea<br>Fever, anorexia | Nasal ± lung Tracheal ±Intestinal epithelial cells | +/−<br>Pneumonia | +/−<br>J, I, colon<br>Villous atrophy | 5 days | NR | 2 wk–6 mo |
| **Young adult/ adult disease syndromes** | | | | | | | |
| WD | Hemorrhagic diarrhea<br>Dehydration<br>±Rhinitis, dry cough<br>Fever, anorexia | Intestinal, nasal ± lung epithelial cells? | NR | ++<br>J, I, colon<br>Enterocolitis | +/− | 1–4 days | 6 mo–adult |
| Shipping fever or BRDC | Cough, dyspnea<br>± Rhinitis<br>± Pneumonia<br>± Diarrhea<br>Fever, anorexia | Nasal, trachea Bronchi, alveoli ± Intestinal epithelial cells | Interstitial emphysema Bronchiolitis Alveolitis ± Bacteria | +/−<br>NR | 5–10 days (17 days) | 4–8 days (17 days) | 6–10 mo |

[a] J, jejunum; I, ileum; NR, not reported; +/−, mild or no lesions; ++, moderate to severe lesions.
[b] Shedding detected by infectivity or antigen assays; parentheses denote shedding detected by RT-PCR. In experimental challenge studies, the incubation periods for disease onset and shedding both ranged from 2 to 8 days.

manifestation, especially the severe bloody diarrhea and winter prevalence, remain unknown.

Since 1995, BCoV has been increasingly implicated in the BRDC associated with respiratory disease and reduced growth performance in feedlot cattle (Table 2) (15, 37, 56, 57, 102–104, 106). BCoV was detected from nasal secretions and lungs of cattle with pneumonia and from feces (37, 39, 56, 57, 102–104, 106). In a subsequent study, a high percentage of feedlot cattle (45%) shed BCoV both nasally and in feces as determined by ELISA (15). Application of nested RT-PCR detected higher BCoV nasal and fecal shedding rates, 84 and 96%, respectively (37). Storz et al. (103) reported that 25 of 26 Texas feedlot cattle that died had a BCoV infection and that both BCoV and *Pasteurella* were isolated from lungs of the cattle with necrotizing pneumonia.

Some investigators have shown an association between nasal shedding of BCoV and respiratory disease. In a large feedlot study (*n* = 1,074 cattle), Lathrop et al. (56) noted that feedlot calves shedding BCoV nasally and seroconverting to BCoV positivity (>4-fold) were 1.6 times more likely to have respiratory disease and 2.2 times more likely to have pulmonary lesions at slaughter than animals that did not shed BCoV. Similarly, in studies by Hasoksuz et al. (37) and

Thomas et al. (106), calves shedding BCoV nasally were 2.7 and 1.5 times, respectively, more likely to have respiratory disease than calves that were not shedding. In another study, nasal shedding of BCoV increased the risk of requiring treatment for respiratory disease (81). Intranasal vaccination of such calves using a commercial modified live BCoV calf vaccine on entry to a feedlot reduced the risk of calves developing the BRDC.

From these studies, we conclude that both respiratory and enteric shedding of BCoV are common in feedlot cattle, with peak shedding at 0 to 4 days after arrival at feedlots. In one study, in which 3-day-prearrival specimens were tested, nasal shedding consistently preceded fecal shedding (106). Additionally, many cattle (61 to 74%) shed BCoV at the buyer-order barn prior to shipping to feedlots (104). A high percentage (91 to 95%) of feedlot cattle seroconverted (2 to 4-fold-increased titers) to BCoV positivity by 3 weeks postarrival. An important observation from several studies was that cattle arriving with relatively high BCoV antibody ELISA titers or neutralizing antibodies in serum were less likely to shed BCoV, seroconvert, or develop the BRDC (15, 57, 64, 66, 106). Furthermore, some investigators have shown that BCoV infections had a negative impact on weight gains in feedlot cattle (15, 37), which suggests that

BCoV may have an impact on herd health and performance. Similarly, higher titers in serum of antibody against BCoV have been associated with increased weight gains (66, 106).

In spite of their association with distinct disease syndromes, all BCoV isolates tested to date from both enteric and respiratory infections are antigenically similar, comprising a single serotype, but with two or three subtypes identified by neutralization tests or using MAbs (18, 38, 39, 92, 109). Although genetic differences (point mutations but not deletions) have been detected in the S protein gene between enteric and respiratory isolates, including ones from the same animal (16, 40), in vivo studies revealed a high level of cross-protection between such isolates (14, 26). Inoculation of gnotobiotic or colostrum-deprived calves with calf diarrhea, WD, or respiratory BCoV strains led to both nasal and fecal CoV shedding followed by complete cross-protection against diarrhea after challenge with a calf diarrhea strain (14, 26). However, subclinical nasal and fecal virus shedding (detected only by RT-PCR) in calves challenged with the heterologous BCoV strains (14, 26) confirmed field studies suggesting that subclinically infected animals may be a reservoir for BCoV in infected herds (42, 43). Cross-protection against BCoV-induced respiratory disease has not been evaluated.

## Subgroup 2a: BCoV interspecies transmission and wildlife reservoirs

The likelihood that SARS-CoV of humans is a zoonotic infection potentially transmitted from wild animals is not surprising in light of the previous identification of possible wildlife reservoirs for BCoV. Captive wild ruminants from the United States, including sambar deer *(Cervus unicolor)*, white-tailed deer *(Odocoileus virginianus)*, waterbucks *(Kobus ellipsiprymnus)*, elk *(Cervus elaphus)*, and, more recently, giraffes (36a), harbor CoVs biologically (growth in HRT-18 cells and hemagglutinin of mouse and chicken erythrocytes) and antigenically (cross-neutralizing) closely related to BCoV (65, 108). The deer and waterbuck isolates were from animals with bloody diarrhea resembling WD in cattle (108). Although CoVs were previously detected by electron microscopy (EM) and ELISA (BCoV antigen specific) in diarrheic feces of sitatungas *(Tragelaphus spekei)* and musk oxen *(Ovibos moschatus)* from a wildlife park in England, they failed to replicate in vitro (HRT-18 cells) or in vivo (gnotobiotic calves) (11).

Serologically, 6.6 and 8.7% of sera from white-tailed deer in Ohio and mule deer in Wyoming, respectively, were positive for antibodies to BCoV by indirect immunofluorescence tests (108). Caribou *(Rangifer tarandus)* were also BCoV seropositive (25). These studies confirm the existence of CoVs in captive and native wild ruminants that are antigenically closely related to BCoV. Thus, the possibility exists that native wild ruminants may transmit bovine-like CoVs to cattle (see below) or visa versa. Unfortunately, few serologic surveys of wild ruminants in native habitats have been done. Moreover, most of the CoVs from wild ruminants have not yet been sequenced to assess their genetic similarity to BCoV. An exception is the recent full-length genomic sequence for an antigenically related giraffe CoV (GiCoV-OH3) that shares 99.3 to 99.6% amino acid identity with two enteric BCoV strains (36a).

Although many CoVs have restricted host ranges, some, such as the subgroup 2a BCoV and, more recently, the subgroup 2b SARS-CoV, appear to be promiscuous (90, 91). Coronaviruses genetically (>95% nucleotide identity) and/or antigenically similar to BCoV have been detected from respiratory samples of dogs with respiratory disease (27) and also from humans (123) and wild ruminants (see prior section). A human enteric CoV isolate from a child with acute diarrhea (HECoV-4408) was genetically (99% nucleotide identity in the S protein and HE genes with BCoV) and antigenically more closely related to BCoV than to human CoV OC43, suggesting that this isolate is a BCoV variant. More evidence for this likelihood was the recent report that the HECoV-4408 strain infects (upper respiratory tract and intestine) and causes diarrhea and intestinal lesions in gnotobiotic calves (36). It also induces complete cross-protective immunity against the virulent BCoV-DB2 enteric strain. Notably, the wild-ruminant CoV isolates from sambar and white-tailed deer, giraffe, and waterbuck also infected the upper respiratory and intestinal tracts of gnotobiotic calves and caused diarrhea (36a, 108), affirming experimentally that wild ruminants may serve as a reservoir for CoV strains transmissible to cattle.

Bovine CoV can also experimentally infect and cause mild disease (diarrhea) in phylogenetically diverse species such as avian hosts, including baby turkeys but not baby chickens (48). It is notable that in the latter study, the BCoV-DB2 calf-virulent strain infected baby turkeys, causing diarrhea and reduced weight gain, and the virus was transmitted to unexposed contact control birds. However, in an earlier study (22) using cell culture-adapted BCoV strains as an inoculum in turkey poults, intestinal infectivity was seen but without lesions or clinical disease, suggesting that BCoV strain or virulence differences (after cell culture adaptation) can influence BCoV pathogenicity for turkey poults. These data raise intriguing questions of whether wild birds (such as wild turkeys) could also be a reservoir for bovine-like CoVs transmissible to cattle or wild ruminants or, conversely, if cattle (or ruminants) can transmit CoVs to wild birds or poultry. There are few, if any, seroprevalence surveys for bovine-like CoVs in avian species and only limited data for wild ruminants (25, 108). The reasons for the broad host range of BCoV are unknown but may relate to the use of acetylated neuraminic acid as a host cell receptor or the presence of a hemagglutinin on BCoV. Both factors may have a role in binding to diverse cell types.

## Group 3 CoVs

### IBV and TCoV epidemiology

Infectious bronchitis is a highly contagious, ubiquitous respiratory disease of chickens that is endemic worldwide (10, 19). It is caused by the CoV IBV, first isolated in the 1930s. Like SARS-CoV, it is spread by aerosol or, possibly, fecal-oral transmission. Genetically and antigenically closely related CoVs have been isolated from pheasants and turkeys (9, 10, 32, 34, 47), but in young turkeys, turkey CoV (TCoV) causes mainly enteritis. Recently, other galliform birds (peafowl, guinea fowl, and partridge) were found to be infected by CoVs genetically similar, if not identical, to IBV strains (9). CoVs representing potential new species within group 3, based on partial genomic sequence data, were identified from a graylag goose *(Anser anser)*, a mallard duck *(Anas platyrhynchos)*, and a pigeon *(Columbia livia)* using pan-CoV RT-PCR (9). Unfortunately, these CoVs could not be isolated by inoculation into embryonated domestic fowl eggs for further studies.

IBV is heterogeneous, having multiple serotypes with extensive antigenic variation and broad tissue tropisms and pathogenicity. IBV strains differ in their virulence, but the host genetic background can also influence infection outcome (2, 9, 19). Respiratory infections of chickens with IBV are characterized by tracheal rales, coughing, and snicking (sneezing), but not pneumonia. The disease is most severe in chicks (10, 19). IBV also replicates in the oviduct, causing decreased egg production or quality. Nephropathogenic strains infect the kidneys, causing mortality in young birds, whereas in broilers, death ensues from systemic *Escherichia coli* infections after IBV damage to the respiratory tract. Interestingly, the genetically closely related pheasant CoV (PhCoV) causes disease (respiratory and kidney) similar to that of IBV in chickens (9, 32).

TCoV has been identified in North America, Australia, the United Kingdom, Italy, and Brazil (9, 34). Although able to infect birds of all ages, TCoV (also referred to as bluecomb virus) causes diarrhea accompanied by anorexia and decreased weight gain in young turkeys (34). More recently, TCoV has also been associated with the poult enteritis and mortality syndrome characterized by high mortality, severe growth retardation, and immune dysfunction. TCoV is shed in feces and transmitted within and between flocks by the fecal-oral route, including mechanical transmission of feces. Infection of turkey flocks with TCoV results in decreased growth rates in poults and decreased egg production in breeder hens. Increased mortality is dependent upon age, concurrent or secondary infections, and management practices.

### IBV and TCoV interspecies transmission and wild bird reservoirs

A high degree of sequence identity (85 to 90%) is present between the polymerase (ORF1b) and M and N proteins of TCoV, PhCoV, and IBV (9, 34), and IBV and TCoV are antigenically related as well (34, 47). The exception is in the S protein. IBV and PhCoV share about 90% identity in the S protein and induce similar disease syndromes in chickens and pheasants (9). In contrast, only about 34% identity exists in the S protein between IBV and the enteric TCoV strains; three TCoV strains examined shared 91% amino acid identity (63). Whether these dramatic genetic differences between the S proteins of TCoV and IBV reflect the altered enteric tropism or adaptation to a new host species for TCoV is unclear.

The close antigenic and genetic similarities between these three avian CoVs raise the possibility that they represent host range mutants as described for the group 1a CoVs (TGEV/PRCV, FCoV, and CECoV); if so, they might exhibit interspecies transmission and disease induction in heterologous hosts. However, when TCoV or PhCoV was experimentally inoculated into chickens, only asymptomatic infections were observed (32, 47). A caveat is that, as with group 1 CoVs, strain differences may influence their virulence for heterologous hosts (9, 95). In contrast, when CoVs closely related to IBV isolated from guinea fowl or teal were inoculated into chickens, disease occurred (9). Although confirming that IBV-like CoVs can replicate in nonchicken hosts, conclusions must be considered tentative because avian CoV was isolated from birds that were located in the vicinity of chickens. Thus, it is unclear if they merely represented IBV field strains acquired from nearby chickens. There is clearly a need to screen other nongallinaceous birds, including wild birds, for IBV-like or other group 3 CoVs that are infectious or emerging disease threats for domestic poultry.

## PATHOGENESIS

Research on respiratory and enteric CoV infections in natural animal hosts (swine, cattle, and poultry) has provided important information on CoV disease pathogenesis, possible potentiators for increased disease severity, and vaccine strategies. In animals, CoV infections are generally most severe in the young. A notable difference between SARS-CoV and most fatal animal CoV infections is the unexplained propensity of SARS-CoV to cause more severe disease in adults than in children. However, in adult animals, respiratory CoV infections are more severe or often fatal when combined with other factors, including stress and transport of animals (shipping fever of cattle), high exposure doses, aerosols, treatment with corticosteroids, and coinfections with other respiratory pathogens (viruses, bacteria, and bacterial lipolysaccharides [LPS]). Likewise, such variables, by accentuating viral shedding or increasing the titers shed, may contribute to the phenomenon of superspreaders (a major factor in the spread of SARS) (97). The following sections provide a perspective on the pathogenesis of selected group 1, 2, and 3 enteric and respiratory CoV infections of livestock and poultry and the role of various cofactors in disease potentiation.

## Group 1 CoVs

### Subgroup 1a: TGEV and PRCV pathogenesis

The emergence of a naturally occurring S protein gene deletion mutant of TGEV, PRCV with an altered (respiratory) tissue tropism, has provided a unique opportunity for comparative studies of these two CoVs in the same host species (pigs). TGEV and PRCV exemplify localized enteric (TGEV) and respiratory (PRCV) infections most severe in neonatal (less than 2 weeks) and young adult (1 to 3 months) pigs, respectively (60, 95).

After exposure, presumably mainly by the fecal-oral route, TGEV quickly targets small intestinal villous enterocytes, infecting virtually 100% of the small intestine, excluding the proximal duodenum (95). This rapid loss of most functional villous enterocytes leads to pronounced villous atrophy, resulting in severe malabsorptive diarrhea and potentially fatal disease in neonates (Table 1). After a short incubation period (18 to 48 h), typical clinical signs of TGE in neonates include transient vomiting and yellow, watery diarrhea. Fecal shedding of TGEV normally persists for up to 2 weeks, but in a few studies, chronic or intermittent fecal shedding by sows was detected (95). In adults, TGEV is mild, with transient diarrhea or inappetence, but curiously, pregnant or lactating animals develop more severe clinical signs, with elevated temperatures and agalactia.

Extraintestinal infections by TGEV are recognized, including infection of the mammary gland of lactating sows after natural infection or experimental injection or infusion of virus (53, 95). TGEV also infects the upper respiratory tract, with transient nasal shedding (53, 95), but infection and lesions in the lung are uncommon. Especially noteworthy, highly attenuated strains of TGEV replicate more extensively in the upper respiratory tract than in the intestine of neonatal pigs (28, 113); such attenuated strains might represent temperature-sensitive mutants selected by serial passage in cell culture. A reverse correlation was also observed between the level of attenuation of TGEV and the extent of intestinal infection. Interestingly, two nucleotide changes (at nt 214 and 655) were detected in the S protein gene between enteric (PUR46-MAD) and respiratory/enteric (PTV) TGEV strains, with the mutation in aa 219 (nt 655) most critical for altered respiratory tropism (Table 3) (3, 96). Point mutations in the S protein gene leading to a shift from an enteric to respiratory tropism were also noted in the TGEV-TOY56 strain after multiple passages in cell culture (96).

Comparisons of the entire genomic sequences of two pairs of virulent (parental) and attenuated (serial cell culture-passaged parental strain) TGEV strains

---

Table 3. Tissues infected by respiratory/enteric coronaviruses in animal hosts and changes in the S protein gene[a]

| Infected tissue or condition | Group 1 CoV, pigs | | | Group 2 CoV, cattle | |
| --- | --- | --- | --- | --- | --- |
| | TGEV-V | TGEV-A (vaccine) | PRCV | BCoV-E | BCoV-R |
| Viremia | − | − | + | NR | NR |
| Upper respiratory tract | + | ++ | ++ | + | ++ |
| Lower respiratory tract | +/− | + | +++ | + | +++ |
| Intestine | +++ | + | +/− | +++ (colon) | ++ (colon) |

[a]TGEV-V, virulent TGEV; TGEV-A, attenuated TGEV; BCoV-E, enteric BCoV; BCoV-R, respiratory BCoV; NR, not reported; −, no infection; +/−, variable infection; +, low level of infection; ++, moderate level of infection; +++, high level of infection. In TGEV-V the S protein gene is intact. In TGEV-A, the S protein gene has point mutations at nt 214, 665, and 1753 (3, 122); in PRCV the S protein gene has a deletion of 621 to 681 nt in size; and in BCoV-E and BCoV-R the S protein gene has point mutations (16, 40), including 42 aa changes at 38 sites (40).

(Miller and Purdue) revealed a common change in nt 1753 of the S protein gene resulting in a serine-to-alanine mutation at position 585 of the attenuated strains: alanine was also present in this position for the less pathogenic and respiratory PRCV-ISU-1 strain and for the attenuated TGEV-TOY56 strain (Table 3) (122). The role of this change in TGEV tissue tropism or virulence is unknown, but it resides in the major antigenic site A/B (aa 506 to 706) and the cell receptor binding domain (aa 522 to 744) of TGEV.

Like SARS-CoV, PRCV, an S protein gene deletion mutant of TGEV, spreads by droplets and has a pronounced tropism for the lungs, replicating to titers of $10^7$ to $10^8$ 50% tissue culture infective doses ($TCID_{50}$) and producing interstitial pneumonia affecting from 5% to as much as 60% of the lung (21, 35, 41, 60, 95). Although many uncomplicated PRCV infections are mild or subclinical, such lung lesions are almost invariably present. Furthermore, the severity of clinical signs and the degree of pathology appear to be PRCV strain dependent. Vaughn et al. (117) suggested that PRCV strains with larger deletions in the S protein gene (PRCV-1894) had reduced pathogenicity compared to PRCV strains with smaller deletions (AR310 and LEPP).

Clinical signs of PRCV infection, like SARS, include fever with variable degrees of dyspnea, polypnea, anorexia, and lethargy and less coughing and rhinitis. Also, like for SARS-CoV (17, 70), PRCV replicates in lung epithelial cells and antigen is detected in type I and II pneumocytes and alveolar macrophages. In lungs, bronchiolar infiltration by mononuclear cells, lymphohistiocytic exudates, and epithelial cell necrosis lead to interstitial pneumonia. PRCV induces transient viremia with virus also detected from nasal swabs and in the tonsils and trachea, similar to SARS-CoV (24, 55, 76, 77). PRCV further replicates in a few undefined cells in the intestinal lamina propria, but without inducing villous atrophy or diarrhea and with limited fecal shedding. Recently, however, fecal isolates of PRCV were detected with consistent, minor (point mutations) in the S protein gene compared to nasal isolates from the same pig (20). No diarrhea and limited fecal shedding were observed in pigs inoculated with the fecal PRCV isolates, suggesting their possible lack of intestinal stability. Such observations suggest the presence of CoV quasispecies in the host (23), with some strains more adapted to the intestine, a potential corollary for the intestinal infection and fecal shedding of SARS-CoV (12, 24, 55, 61, 76, 77).

It is widely thought that the 5′ deletion (621 to 681 nt in size) in the S protein gene of PRCV plays a major role in the altered tissue tropism and reduced virulence of PRCV. Recombinant TGEV strains from infectious clones and MAb neutralization-resistant mutants have been used to try to pinpoint the molecular basis for the difference in pathogenicity and tissue tropism between TGEV and PRCV strains (3, 5, 96). Attenuated mutants of TGEV (Purdue-115 strain) selected with MAbs to S-protein site D (absent on PRCV) exhibited reduced enteropathogenicity that correlated with a point mutation or small deletion in the S protein gene encoding the N-terminal subregion (region deleted in PRCV) (5). Ballesteros et al. (3) concluded that a substitution in aa 219 of the S protein of a PUR46-MAD recombinant generated between enteric/respiratory (attenuated PUR46-MAD) and attenuated respiratory PTV (formerly NEB72) strains of TGEV resulted in the loss of enteric tropism. They speculated that this mutation affected virus binding to an intestinal coreceptor.

Use of infectious clones of TGEV and PRCV may further assist in identifying other genes that influence CoV tropism and virulence. Amino acid changes in the M protein affect alpha interferon (IFN-α) induction by the attenuated Purdue-P115 strain, implying a potential role in altered host response and virulence (59). The deletions or mutations observed in nonstructural proteins 3a and 3b of all PRCV strains may lead to nonexpression or may render these proteins nonfunctional (75). An infectious clone of PUR46-MAD with ORF3 gene deletions showed a slightly reduced pathogenicity in vivo (but the initial strain used was already attenuated) but normal replication in cell culture (100). Using IBV infectious clones, similar effects of ORF3 deletion were reported (45). Although a TGEV strain (96-1933) with an ORF3a deletion maintained pig virulence, the virus isolated and sequenced was not plaque purified and tested in pigs to confirm the presence of a single strain of TGEV (67). This is important because of previously reported mixtures of virulent and attenuated TGEV strains in an early in vivo passage of the virulent Purdue strain of TGEV (96).

## Subgroup 1b: PEDV pathogenesis

The pathogenesis (including clinical signs, lesions and disease) of PEDV in the small intestine of piglets closely resembles that of TGEV (80), but with a lower rate of replication and longer incubation period. However, unlike with TGEV, colonic villi were also infected, with cellular changes in colonic enterocytes containing PEDV particles in older swine. Features of PEDV infection not seen in TGE are acute back muscle necrosis and, occasionally, sudden death in finishing and adult pigs.

## Group 2 CoVs

### Subgroup 2a: BCoV pathogenesis

Besides severe pneumonia (70), shedding of SARS-CoV in feces and the occurrence of diarrhea in many patients (12, 61, 76) suggest that SARS-CoV may be pneumoenteric like BCoV. Enteric and/or respiratory shedding of virus was also detected in wild animals harboring SARS-CoV (Table 1) (33, 58, 62). Thus, a review of the pathogenesis of BCoV in cattle in the context of each of the three clinical syndromes (Table 2) provides comparative data on another group 2 CoV with dual respiratory and enteric tropism.

Calf diarrhea BCoV strains infect the epithelial cells of the distal small and large intestine and superficial and crypt enterocytes of the colon, leading to villous atrophy and crypt hyperplasia (Table 2) (92, 114). As summarized in Table 2, after an incubation period of 3 to 4 days, calves develop a severe, malabsorptive diarrhea persisting for 2 to 8 days, resulting in dehydration and often death. Concurrent fecal and nasal shedding often occur, and most diarrheic calves necropsied have BCoV antigen in both intestinal and respiratory (turbinate, nasal, and tracheal) epithelial cells. These results were also confirmed by experimental BCoV challenge studies of calves (84, 94). Saif et al. (94) reported intestinal lesions in all calves inoculated with an enteric BCoV calf isolate (DB2), but lesions (focal emphysema) and BCoV antigen in the lung were less frequent (20 to 30% of calves). Thus, enteric strains of BCoV induce diarrhea and are potentially pneumoenteric, but respiratory disease is variable.

BCoV is also implicated as a cause of mild respiratory disease (coughing and rhinitis) or pneumonia in 2- to 6-month-old calves, and viral antigen is detected in nasal secretions, the lungs, and often the intestines (68, 84). Experimental calf challenge studies using calf respiratory BCoV isolates confirmed both fecal and nasal shedding and diarrhea but only variable respiratory disease (68, 84). However, in the field, as described below, respiratory BCoV infections are likely exacerbated by stress or respiratory coinfections.

A plausible scenario for the pathogenesis of BCoV and its transit to the intestine has been proposed based on the time course of BCoV nasal and fecal shedding in natural and experimental BCoV infections (42, 94, 106). Following initial and extensive replication in the nasal mucosa, BCoV may spread to the gastrointestinal tract after the swallowing of large quantities of virus coated in mucous secretions. This initial respiratory amplification of BCoV and its protective coating by mucus may allow larger amounts of this labile, enveloped, but infectious virus to transit to the gut after swallowing. A similar scenario may prevail for the SARS-CoV to explain its pneumoenteropathogenicity with prominent fecal shedding and diarrhea in some patients (12, 61, 76).

For WD, intestinal lesions and BCoV-infected cells in the colonic crypts of dairy and beef (feedlot) cattle resemble those described for calf diarrhea (Table 2) (13, 114). The disease is acute, with only transient BCoV shedding detected in feces (1 to 4 days) by immuno-EM or ELISA (13, 86). BCoV isolates from WD outbreaks at least partially reproduced the disease (diarrhea) in BCoV-seropositive nonlactating dairy cows (110) and more authentically (bloody diarrhea and decreased milk production) in BCoV-seronegative lactating dairy cows (107). Interestingly, in the latter study, older cattle were more severely affected than similarly exposed calves, mimicking the more severe SARS cases seen in adults versus children (76).

In these two experimental studies, the incubation period ranged from 3 to 8 days and diarrhea persisted for 1 to 6 days. Fecal shedding of BCoV was coincident with or preceded diarrhea and persisted for 1 to 4 days. No respiratory disease or fever was evident in the BCoV-seropositive cows, but nasal shedding of BCoV was detected in 1 of 5 cows (110). In contrast, BCoV-seronegative cows directly exposed to calves experimentally infected with a WD strain of BCoV developed transient fevers, mild cough, and serous mucopurulent discharge (107). These data are consistent with field outbreak reports indicating variable signs of respiratory disease in cattle with WD (13, 86). They further document the very short shedding window (1 to 4 days) for detection of BCoV in feces, showing the need for acute-phase samples for definitive BCoV diagnosis or the testing of seroresponses to BCoV on a herd basis (86). As reviewed in the BCoV epidemiology section, WD isolates of BCoV are antigenically closely related to calf enteric and respiratory isolates, and the various strains, regardless of clinical origin, elicit cross-protection against one another in calf challenge studies (4, 14, 26, 38).

The BRDC of feedlot calves is most pronounced during the first weeks after arrival at feedlots. This overlaps with a high prevalence of respiratory viral and secondary bacterial coinfections and various environmental or host stress factors during this period (see below). During the past decade a growing number of reports have provided epidemiological or experimental evidence suggesting that BCoV infection contributes substantially to the BRDC. Multiple previous studies (reviewed earlier) have documented both nasal and fecal shedding of BCoV by calves shortly after arrival in feedlots and subsequent seroconversion to BCoV (Table 2). Storz et al. (102) showed a progression in development of the BRDC for natural cases, initiated by BCoV infection (nasal shedding) upon arrival followed by dual infections with BCoV and respiratory bacteria *(Mannheimia haemolytica* and *Pasteurella multocida)*. This led to pneumonia and deaths in 26 cases, most of which involved concurrent high titers of BCoV and bacteria in the lungs. The authors concluded that these data supported a role for BCoV in the BRDC as defined by Evans' criteria for causation. In this and another study (103), researchers confirmed the presence of BCoV antigen in respiratory epithelial cells or isolated BCoV from nasal secretions, trachea, bronchi, or lung aveoli and documented the presence of interstitial emphysema, bronchiolitis, and aveolitis in concert with bacterial infection (Table 2). Thus, the BRDC appears to be a multifactorial disease, with BCoV playing an early role in inciting the disease. Although multifactorial/multiagent experiments describing interactions among respiratory viruses, bacteria, and stress have highlighted their synergistic effects in the BRDC (51), no such experiments have been reported for BCoV. Such studies of BCoV-seronegative, stressed calves of feedlot age are needed to further elucidate the role of BCoV in the BRDC and the mechanisms involved in predisposing calves to development of fatal pneumonia.

Unlike the scenario for the almost exclusive respiratory tropism of PRCV, no deletions have been detected in the S protein gene of respiratory BCoV strains, most of which also possess an enteric tropism as revealed by calf challenge studies (14). Several groups have compared the S (or S1) protein gene sequences of WD or respiratory and enteric BCoV isolates, including isolates from the same animal (16, 29, 40, 52, 121). Focusing on the hypervariable region (aa 452 to 593) containing the neutralizing epitope (S1B) of the S1 subunit, four groups (16, 29, 40, 121) reported that respiratory strains (or respiratory and enteric isolates from the same feedlot calf) had changes in aa 510 and 531 compared to the reference enteric Mebus and a WD strain (DBA). One of the polymorphic positions (aa 531) discriminated between enteric (aspartic acid or asparagine) and respiratory (glycine) BCoV strains in two studies (16, 121), but not in another (40). Others (52) reported that the S protein gene sequences of Korean WD BCoV isolates were similar to those of respiratory and enteric BCoV strains. Nevertheless, all investigators showed the greatest amino acid sequence divergence (42 aa changes at 38 distinct sites [40]) and most differences by phylogenetic analysis between the historic (1972) reference Mebus enteric BCoV and more recent BCoV isolates, regardless of clinical

origin. The relevance of the observed genetic changes to viral pathogenesis in vivo is unknown. Although Hasoksuz et al. (38) observed antigenic and biological differences among BCoV isolates, variability was not necessarily related to the clinical origin of the isolates. Because BCoV, like other RNA viruses, represents a quasispecies (23), some viruses within the quasispecies may be more suitable for respiratory than intestinal replication, contributing to sequence changes reported for such isolates from the same host (20).

## Group 3 CoVs

### IBV pathogenesis

IBV replicates at multiple epithelial surfaces of chickens, including ones not associated with pathology (alimentary tract and gonads) and those associated with pathology (respiratory tract [nose, trachea, lungs, and air sacs], kidney [tubes and ducts], and oviduct) (8, 10, 19). IBV replicates mainly in epithelial cells, causing necrosis and edema with small areas of pneumonia near large bronchi in the respiratory tract and interstitial nephritis in the kidney (8, 10, 19). In these infected tissues, there is a loss of cilia from epithelial cells, edema, and various degrees of mononuclear cell or heterophil infiltration. IBV strains differ in virulence, and only a small percentage of IBV strains are highly nephropathogenic. Of interest for SARS is the persistence of IBV in the kidney and its prolonged fecal shedding, because SARS-CoV is also detected in urine and shed longer term in feces (76, 77). However, it is unclear if SARS-CoV shedding in urine is a consequence of viremia or a kidney infection like with IBV. The genetic basis for these differences in IBV strains is unclear, but serial passage of a respiratory IBV strain via the cloacal route resulted in an altered kidney tropism (111). The extent of mortality from IBV infection is age dependent (greatest in chicks) and influenced by the chickens' genetic background (2).

IBV is recovered intermittently from the respiratory tract for about 28 days after infection and from the feces after clinical recovery (20 weeks postinoculation) (8, 10, 19). The cecal tonsil and the kidney are possible reservoirs for IBV persistence, similar to the persistence of FCoV in the intestine of cats (44). IBV was recovered from both tracheal and cloacal swabs from chickens at onset of egg production, suggesting reexcretion of IBV from chronically infected, stressed (coming into lay) birds, as also demonstrated for fecal shedding of FCoV or BCoV after induction of immunosuppression (71, 110). The ability of IBV strains to persist in the host provides a longer opportunity for new mutants to be selected with altered tissue tropisms and virulence from among the viral RNA quasispecies (23). The persistence of IBV and its replication in multiple tissues may contribute to the sequence diversity in the IBV S protein and explain the vast array of IBV serotypes, a notable difference compared to only one or two serotypes for most group 1 or 2 CoVs.

## TCoV pathogenesis

TCoV infection is associated mainly with diarrhea and weight loss in young poults or a drop in egg production in breeder hens (34, 49). Replication of TCoV is confined to the apical enterocytes of the intestinal villi and the epithelium of the bursa of Fabricius. Like other enteric CoVs, TCoV causes a malabsorptive, maldigestive diarrhea presumably due to viral destruction or functional alterations in infected enterocytes. Severe disease and high mortality were features of early TCoV infections (bluecomb) and experimental studies using crude fecal or intestinal homogenates; recent studies using embryo-propagated TCoV strains indicate negligible mortality and moderate growth depression (49). Similar to the role of BCoV in the BRDC, interactions between TCoV and other agents (E. coli, astrovirus, etc.) in the development of more severe enteric disease have been described (34, 49). TCoV is shed in feces of turkeys for several weeks after recovery from clinical disease and was detected in intestinal contents for 6 and 7 weeks postinoculation by virus isolation and RT-PCR, respectively.

## COFACTORS THAT EXACERBATE CoV INFECTIONS, DISEASE, OR SHEDDING

Underlying disease or respiratory coinfections, dose and route of infection, and immunosuppression (corticosteroids) are all potential cofactors that can exacerbate the severity of group 1 (TGEV or PRCV), group 2 (BCoV), and group 3 (IBV or TCoV) CoV infections. In addition, similar cofactors may enhance the severity of SARS-CoV or play a role in the superspreader cases seen in the SARS epidemic (97) by enhancing virus transmission or host susceptibility.

### Impact of Respiratory Coinfections on CoV Infections, Disease, and Shedding

The BRDC (shipping fever) is recognized as a multifactorial, polymicrobial respiratory disease complex in young adult feedlot cattle, with several factors exacerbating respiratory disease, including BCoV infections (15, 37, 56, 57, 102–104, 106). The BRDC can be precipitated by several viruses, alone or in combination (BCoV, bovine respiratory syncytial virus, parainfluenza 3 virus, and bovine herpesvirus), including viruses similar to common human respiratory viruses and viruses capable of mediating immunosuppression (bovine viral diarrhea virus, etc.). The shipping of cattle long distances to feedlots and the comingling of cattle from multiple farms create physical stresses that overwhelm the animal's defense mechanisms and provide close contact for exposure to high concentrations of new pathogens or strains not previously encountered. Such factors are analogous to the physical stress of long airplane trips with close contact among individuals from diverse regions of the world, both of which may play a role in enhancing an individual's susceptibility to SARS or the transmission of SARS-CoV (73, 120). For the BRDC, various predisposing factors (viruses and stress) allow commensal bacteria of the nasal cavity (Mannheimia haemolytica, Pasteurella, Mycoplasma, etc.) to infect the lungs, leading to a fatal fibrinous pneumonia (56, 102–104) like that seen in SARS patients (17, 70, 77).

In broiler chickens, severe disease or death ensues from systemic E. coli coinfections after IBV damage to the respiratory tract or Mycoplasma coinfections with IBV (10, 19). Similarly for the enteric TCoV, coinfection with either enteropathogenic E. coli or astrovirus led to enhanced disease severity compared to that caused by each agent alone (34, 49).

It is also possible that antibiotic treatment of such animals (or SARS patients) coinfected with CoVs and bacteria, with massive release of bacterial LPS, could precipitate induction of proinflammatory cytokines, which could further enhance lung damage. For example, Van Reeth et al. (115) showed that pigs infected with PRCV followed by a subclinical dose of E. coli LPS within 24 h developed enhanced fever and more severe respiratory disease compared to those obtained with each agent alone. They concluded that the effects were likely mediated by the significantly enhanced levels of proinflammatory cytokines induced by the bacterial LPS. Thus, there is a need to examine both LPS and lung cytokine levels in SARS patients as possible mediators of the severity of SARS. Bacteria (Chlamydia spp.) have been isolated from SARS patients, but their role in enhancing the severity of SARS is undefined (83).

Interactions between PRCV and other respiratory viruses may also parallel the potential for concurrent or preexisting respiratory viral infections to interact with SARS-CoV (such as metapneumoviruses, influenza viruses, reoviruses, respiratory syncytial virus, or OC43 or 229E CoV). Hayes (41) showed that sequential dual infections of pigs with the arterivirus porcine respiratory and reproductive syndrome virus, followed in 10 days by PRCV, significantly enhanced lung lesions and reduced weight gains compared to those obtained with each virus alone. The dual infections also led to more pigs shedding PRCV nasally for a prolonged period and, surprisingly, to fecal shedding of PRCV. The lung lesions observed resembled those in SARS victims (17, 70).

In another study, Van Reeth and Pensaert (116) inoculated pigs with PRCV followed in 2 to 3 days by swine influenza A virus (SIV). They found that SIV lung titers were reduced in the dually infected compared to the singly infected pigs, but paradoxically the lung lesions were more severe in the dually infected pigs. They postulated that the high levels of IFN-α induced by PRCV may mediate interference with SIV replication, but might also contribute to the enhanced lung lesions. Such studies are highly relevant to possible dual infections by SARS-CoV and influenza virus and the potential treatment of SARS patients with IFN-α.

## Impact of Route (Aerosols) and Dose on CoV Infections

Experimental inoculation of pigs showed that administration of PRCV by aerosol compared to the oronasal route, or in higher doses, resulted in shedding of higher virus titers for longer times (112, 113). In other studies, high PRCV doses induced more severe respiratory disease. Pigs given $10^{8.5}$ $TCID_{50}$ of PRCV had more severe pneumonia and a higher mortality rate than pigs exposed by contact (50), and higher intranasal doses of another PRCV strain (AR310) induced moderate respiratory disease, whereas lower doses produced subclinical infections (35). By analogy, hospital procedures that could potentially generate aerosols, or exposure to higher initial doses of SARS-CoV, may enhance SARS transmission or lead to enhanced respiratory disease (101).

## Impact of Treatment with Corticosteroids on CoV Infections of Animals

Corticosteroids are known to induce immuno-suppression and reduce the numbers of CD4 and CD8 T cells and certain cytokine levels (30). Many hospitalized SARS patients were treated with steroids to reduce lung inflammation, but there are no data to assess the outcome of this treatment on virus shedding or respiratory disease. A recrudescence of BCoV fecal shedding was observed in one of four WD BCoV-infected cows treated with dexamethasone (110). Similarly, treatment of older pigs with dexamethasone prior to TGEV challenge led to profuse diarrhea and reduced lymphoproliferative responses in the treated pigs (98). These data raise issues related to corticosteroid treatment of SARS patients and possible secondary immunosuppression and increased

and prolonged CoV shedding. Alternatively, corticosteroid treatment may be beneficial in reducing proinflammatory cytokines if found to play a major role in lung immunopathology (30).

## IMMUNITY AND VACCINES

As reviewed in the preceding section, an understanding of the pathogenesis of CoV infections, including the target organs infected and how virus is disseminated to these organs, has assisted in development of vaccine strategies. The realization that these animal CoVs cause the most severe disease in young animals and primarily infect epithelial cells lining the respiratory and/or intestinal tracts has necessitated development of mucosal vaccines effective at the local site of infection in neonates or young birds (TGEV, BCoV, and IBV) as well as in juveniles or adults (BCoV).

Development of safe and efficacious and new bioengineered vaccines for animal CoV infections has been problematic and only partially successful (see reviews in references 87 to 89 and 93). Problems encountered often relate to a lack of understanding of basic mechanisms of induction of mucosal immunity. Stimulation of protective mucosal immunity, especially priming of seronegative vaccinees, often requires use of live replicating vaccines or vectors as opposed to nonreplicating killed viruses or subunit vaccines (unless applied with effective mucosal delivery systems or adjuvants), to provide optimal mucosal antigenic stimulation and to avoid tolerance induction (87–89). In addition, most vaccines for mucosal pathogens may fail to induce sterilizing immunity or to prevent respiratory reinfections, as commonly observed for natural respiratory CoV infections (PRCV, IBV, BCoV, and human CoV); consequently, the major vaccine focus is often to prevent severe disease.

### Enteric CoV Vaccines

Because CoV-induced diarrheal disease is most severe in young animals, the major target for TGEV and BCoV vaccines is the suckling animal (reviewed in references 87 to 89, 93, and 95). These CoV vaccines are designed to immunize dams, with passive transfer of antibodies in milk to nursing offspring to prevent intestinal infections.

### Passive immunity to TGEV

Key new concepts related to mucosal immunity have originated from previous studies of passive immunity to TGEV infections in pigs (see reviews in references 87 to 89 and 95). Early studies revealed that sows that recovered from natural TGEV infections provided protective lactogenic immunity to their suckling pigs via neutralizing secretory IgA (sIgA) antibodies in milk. These protective sIgA antibodies were stimulated in milk only after an intestinal TGEV infection of the mother (sow), leading to the initial concept of a gut-mammary-sIgA immunologic axis (specific trafficking of IgA immunoblasts from the gut to the mammary gland) and an interconnected common mucosal immune system linking distant mucosal tissues.

In monogastric animals (pigs and humans) which secrete sIgA antibodies in milk, passive immunization against enteric pathogens is accomplished by exploiting the common mucosal immune system. Because neutralizing TGEV sIgA antibodies in milk are a correlate of protection in neonatal pigs, the strategy is to evoke the gut-mammary IgA axis by administering attenuated TGEV (TGEV-A) vaccines orally to induce sIgA antibodies in milk via intestinal stimulation of the mother. Problems encountered in the field application of this strategy were as follows (see reviews in references 87 to 89 and 95). First, the commercial TGEV-A vaccines given intranasally or orally were of low titer ($>10^6$ PFU) and replicated poorly in the adult intestine, so few IgA precursor B cells were induced in the intestine (112, 113) for subsequent migration to the mammary glands, leading to low IgA antibody titers in milk and only partial passive protection. Use of less attenuated TGEV strains or the antigenically related FIPV caused disease in baby pigs. These studies further illustrate the difficulty in priming for protective sIgA mucosal immune responses, even using live vaccines in naïve seronegative adult animals. However, in comparison, killed TGEV vaccines given parenterally (intramuscularly) induced only IgG antibodies in milk and no passive protection of suckling pigs against TGEV.

The emergence of PRCV also permitted comparative immunologic studies of immune responses and protection against enteric TGEV versus respiratory PRCV in the porcine host. Both maternal vaccination to provide passive antibodies in milk to suckling pigs and active immunity have been evaluated (6, 89, 95, 112, 113). The finding from the PRCV/TGEV pig studies that stimulation at one mucosal site (respiratory tract) does not necessarily evoke complete reciprocity in immune responses or protection at a distant mucosal site (intestine) led to a second important concept: compartmentalization exists within the common mucosal immune system. A single infection of the respiratory tract of pigs or sows with PRCV induced only partial active or passive immunity to TGEV, respectively (95, 112). This finding and results of other studies (reviewed in reference 95) suggest that repeated PRCV exposure is needed to stimulate adequate numbers of IgA memory cells in the intestine, for local gut protection, and for their subsequent transit from intestine to the mammary gland, with secretion of protective levels of IgA antibodies in milk.

For young pigs, VanCott et al. (112, 113) found that a single PRCV infection of the respiratory tract induced a few IgA antibody-secreting cells in the intestine but higher numbers of IgG antibody-secreting cells in the lower respiratory tract (bronchial lymph nodes). Importantly, PRCV infection primed for anamnestic IgG and IgA intestinal antibody responses after TGEV challenge, leading to partial protection. In the field, pigs experience multiple respiratory infections with PRCV, providing sufficient immunity to TGEV such that TGE has largely disappeared from European swine herds (60, 95). The relevance of these vaccine studies to SARS is that if SARS-CoV frequently causes primary intestinal infections, besides pneumonia, neither killed parenteral nor respiratory vaccines may prevent diarrheal disease or fecal shedding, or respiratory vaccines may require high and repeated doses to elicit intestinal immunity.

Use of parenteral TGEV subunit vaccines (baculovirus-expressed S glycoproteins) to induce active immunity to TGEV-induced diarrhea in weaned pigs elicited neutralizing antibodies in serum but failed to induce protection against TGEV-induced diarrhea (87–89, 95). The data confirm earlier findings using killed TGEV vaccines parenterally that indicated that serum neutralizing antibodies (in contrast to intestinal or milk sIgA antibodies) do not correlate with a high degree of protection against TGEV infection. However, in a subsequent study, partial protection against TGEV infection (fecal shedding) was induced in pigs vaccinated intraperitoneally with the S glycoprotein mixed with the N and M proteins. Other studies of TGEV also suggested that both recombinant N proteins (T-cell epitopes) and S proteins were required for maximal antibody responses to TGEV (1). Thus, in spite of long-term research efforts, effective TGEV enteric vaccines have remained elusive, but with the emergence of PRCV, nature appears to have generated its own highly effective vaccine to moderate the more virulent TGEV infections.

## Respiratory CoV Vaccines

In spite of its economic impact, no respiratory CoV vaccines have been developed to prevent BCoV-associated pneumonia in calves or in cattle with the BRDC. The correlates of immunity to respiratory BCoV infections remain undefined. Limited data from epidemiological studies of BCoV infections in cattle suggest that serum antibody titers to BCoV may be a marker for respiratory protection. Antibody isotype (IgG1, IgG2, and IgA), neutralizing antibody titer, and magnitude of antibody titer in serum of naturally infected calves or in cattle on arrival in feedlots were correlated in multiple studies with protection against respiratory disease, pneumonia, or BCoV respiratory shedding (15, 43, 64, 66, 106). However, whether the serum antibodies are themselves correlates of respiratory protection or only reflect prior enteric or respiratory exposure to BCoV is uncertain. In a recent study, intranasal vaccination of feedlot calves with a modified live BCoV calf vaccine on entry to a feedlot reduced the risk of the BRDC in calves (81).

The only available animal CoV vaccines targeted to prevent respiratory CoV infections (bronchi) are IBV vaccines for chickens. Both live attenuated and killed commercial IBV vaccines are used (8, 10, 19). Attenuated vaccines are used in broilers, usually at 1 day of age and 10 days later, because only short-term (6 to 7 weeks) protection is needed. Attenuated vaccines are administered by eyedrop or intranasally or, for mass application, by aerosol or in drinking water. For layers or breeders for which longer protection is needed (~18 months), attenuated vaccines are used for priming at 2 to 3 weeks of age followed by injection of killed oil emulsion booster vaccines, often at 8- to 10-week intervals throughout the laying cycle. The correlates and mechanisms of protection against IBV clinical disease are uncertain. High levels of neutralizing antibodies are thought to prevent viral dissemination from the respiratory tract, thus blocking secondary virus infection of the reproductive tract and kidneys (19). Also, high levels of maternal antibodies (yolk derived) prevented IBV infection of chicks for the first 2 weeks of life. These data suggest that neutralizing antibodies play a role in mediating protection against IBV. However cell-mediated immunity also plays a role in protection to IBV, as shown by the ability of adoptively transferred α/β CD8 T cells to protect chicks against IBV challenge (reviewed in references 8 and 10). Evidence suggests that the S1 glycoprotein and N protein (expressed in vectored or DNA plasmid vaccines) of IBV can induce variable levels of protection. The S1, N, and M proteins also induced cell-mediated immune responses to IBV. Problems encountered in vaccine protection against IBV include the existence of multiple serotypes or subtypes of IBV which may fail to cross-protect, variation in virulence among IBV field strains, and the possible increase in virulence of some live vaccines after back-passage in chickens, with the suggestion that point mutations in the genomes of attenuated vaccines may generate new epidemic strains of IBV (8, 10).

## SUMMARY AND CONCLUSIONS

In summary, as highlighted in this chapter, much progress has been made in the topics addressed, encompassing the comparative biology of animal CoVs. As documented, enteric coronaviruses alone can cause fatal infections in seronegative young animals. However, in adults respiratory CoV infections are more often fatal or more severe when combined with other factors, including high exposure doses, aerosols, treatment with corticosteroids, and respiratory coinfections (viruses, bacteria, and LPS). These variables may also influence the severity of disease or contribute to the phenomenon of superspreaders. Long-term and recent studies of animal CoVs have highlighted the potential for new CoV strains to emerge as deletion mutants or recombinants from existing strains or for new strains to appear from unknown or perhaps wildlife reservoirs; the latter is a likely origin for SARS-CoV. A number of CoV strains, particularly ones from wild animals, remain to be characterized, and the full genomic sequence is available for only a relatively small number of human and animal CoVs outside of SARS-CoVs. In addition, interspecies transmission of certain CoVs may not be uncommon, although the determinants of host range specificity among CoVs are undefined.

An understanding of CoV disease pathogenesis is critical for the design of effective vaccine strategies, yet many unanswered questions related to CoV disease mechanisms remain, including factors that exacerbate CoV respiratory disease or shedding. Consequently, development of safe and efficacious vaccines for animal CoV infections has been problematic and only partially successful. Problems encountered also often relate to a lack of understanding of basic mechanisms to induce mucosal immunity by vaccines targeted at preventing enteric or respiratory mucosal infections. Stimulation of protective mucosal immunity, especially priming of seronegative vaccinees, often requires use of live replicating vaccines or vectors as opposed to nonreplicating killed viruses or subunit vaccines (unless applied with effective mucosal delivery systems or adjuvants). These approaches mimic natural CoV infections and provide optimal mucosal antigenic stimulation while avoiding tolerance induction (87–89, 95). In addition, vaccines for mucosal pathogens may fail to induce sterilizing immunity or prevent reinfections, as commonly observed for natural CoV respiratory infections; therefore, the major vaccine focus may be to prevent severe disease. For both TGEV and IBV infections, live vaccines alone (TGEV) or for priming, followed by killed vaccines for boosting (IBV), provided at least partial protection against enteric and respiratory disease, respectively (8, 89, 93, 95). But as illustrated for IBV, live vaccines may revert to virulent if inadequately attenuated, raising safety issues.

We are embarking on a new era in CoV research attributable to both new discoveries and technological advances. First is the recent discovery and characterization of new CoV strains, including SARS-CoVs from humans and wildlife species. In parallel, the increasing availability of full length CoV genomic sequence data (30 kb), including data for virulent and attenuated CoV pairs or for original and adoptive host strains, presents new opportunities for comprehensive genomic and phylogenetic analyses. Finally, the recent development and application of reverse-genetics systems for CoVs should yield further breakthroughs in understanding the genetic basis for CoV pathogenicity and targets for the rational design of attenuated CoV vaccines.

What is lagging for further advancements in CoV research are appropriate animal models to study respiratory and/or enteric human CoV infections, including SARS-CoV, and a more comprehensive and in-depth understanding of the comparative pathogenesis and disease mechanisms related to CoV infections in natural or adoptive hosts. For example, the basic mechanisms of how CoVs induce a broad spectrum of respiratory disease (ranging from mild to fatal), age-related factors in disease susceptibility, and cofactors that exacerbate disease or lead to enhanced shedding and transmission (superspreaders) are unclear, and these difficult in vivo animal studies have been undertaken by only a few investigators. Also unknown is why some CoVs cause severe disease in neonates or in adoptive hosts but mild disease in adults or natural hosts, or vice versa.

Relatively little is known about the basis for interspecies transmission of CoVs or why some CoVs (group 2 BCoVs and SARS-CoVs) have broad host ranges. Although CoVs have been and continue to be recovered from wildlife reservoirs, with some strains closely related to human (SARS-CoV) and animal (BCoV) CoVs, we understand little about their ecology in the wildlife reservoir (including apparently health animals) or their potential to emerge as either public or animal health threats.

Finally, although we have successfully bioengineered CoV subunit and live vectored vaccines, with CoV vaccines based on infectious clones on the horizon, a basic lack of understanding of the induction of immunity at mucosal surfaces, the attributes of effective mucosal vaccines, and the immune correlates of protection for CoV infections remains a major obstacle to development of effective CoV and other mucosal vaccines.

## REFERENCES

1. **Anton, I. M., S. Gonzalez, M. J. Bullido, M. Corsin, C. Risco, J. P. Langeveld, and L. Enjuanes.** 1996. Cooperation between transmissible gastroenteritis coronavirus (TGEV) structural proteins in the in vitro induction of virus-specific antibodies. *Virus Res.* **46**:111–124.

2. **Bacon, L. D., D. B. Hunter, H. M. Zhang, K. Brand, and R. Etches.** 2004. Retrospective evidence that the MHC (B haplotype) of chickens influences genetic resistance to attenuated infectious bronchitis vaccine strains in chickens. *Avian Pathol.* **33**:605–609.

3. **Ballesteros, M. L., C. M. Sanchez, and L. Enjuanes.** 1997. Two amino acid changes at the N-terminus of transmissible gastroenteritis coronavirus spike protein result in the loss of enteric tropism. *Virology* **227**:378–388.

4. **Benfield, D. A., and L. J. Saif.** 1990. Cell culture propagation of a coronavirus isolated from cows with winter dysentery. *J. Clin. Microbiol.* **28**:1454–1457.

5. **Bernard, S., and H. Laude.** 1995. Site-specific alteration of transmissible gastroenteritis virus spike protein results in markedly reduced pathogenicity. *J. Gen. Virol.* **76**:2235–2241.

6. **Callebaut, P., E. Cox, M. Pensaert, and K. Van Deun.** 1990. Induction of milk IgA antibodies by porcine respiratory coronavirus infection. *Adv. Exp. Med. Biol.* **276**:421–428.

7. **Callow, K. A., H. F. Parry, M. Sergeant, and D. A. Tyrrell.** 1990. The time course of the immune response to experimental coronavirus infection of man. *Epidemiol. Infect.* **105**:435–446.

8. **Cavanagh, D.** 2003. Severe acute respiratory syndrome vaccine development: experiences of vaccination against avian infectious bronchitis coronavirus. *Avian Pathol.* **32**:567–582.

9. **Cavanagh, D.** 2005. Coronaviruses in poultry and others birds. *Avian Pathol.* **34**:439–448.

10. **Cavanagh, D., and S. Naqi.** 2003. Infectious bronchitis, p. 101–119. *In* Y. M. Saif, H. J. Barnes, J. R. Glisson, A. M. Fadly, L. R. McDougald, and D. E. Swayne (ed.), *Diseases of Poultry.* Iowa State Press, Ames.

11. **Chasey, D., D. J. Reynolds, J. C. Bridger, T. G. Debney, and A. C. Scott.** 1984. Identification of coronaviruses in exotic species of Bovidae. *Vet. Rec.* **115**:602–603.

12. **Chim, S. S., S. K. Tsui, K. C. Chan, T. C. Au, E. C. Hung, Y. K. Tong, R. W. Chiu, E. K. Ng, P. K. Chan, C. M. Chu, J. J. Sung, J. S. Tam, K. P. Fung, M. M. Waye, C. Y. Lee, K. Y. Yuen, Y. M. Lo, and CUHK Molecular SARS Research Group.** 2003. Genomic characterisation of the severe acute respiratory syndrome coronavirus of Amoy Gardens outbreak in Hong Kong. *Lancet* **362**:1807–1808.

13. **Cho, K. O., P. G. Halbur, J. D. Bruna, S. D. Sorden, K. J. Yoon, B. H. Janke, K. O. Chang, and L. J. Saif.** 2000. Detection and isolation of coronavirus from feces of three herds of feedlot cattle during outbreaks of winter dysentery-like disease. *J. Am. Vet. Med. Assoc.* **217**:1191–1194.

14. **Cho, K. O., M. Hasoksuz, P. R. Nielsen, K. O. Chang, S. Lathrop, and L. J. Saif.** 2001. Cross-protection studies between respiratory and calf diarrhea and winter dysentery coronavirus strains in calves and RT-PCR and nested PCR for their detection. *Arch. Virol.* **146**:2401–2419.

15. **Cho, K. O., A. E. Hoet, S. C. Loerch, T. E. Wittum, and L. J. Saif.** 2001. Evaluation of concurrent shedding of bovine coronavirus via the respiratory tract and enteric route in feedlot cattle. *Am. J. Vet. Res.* **62**:1436–1441.

16. **Chouljenko, V. N., K. G. Kousoulas, X. Lin, and J. Storz.** 1998. Nucleotide and predicted amino acid sequences of all genes encoded by the 3′ genomic portion (9.5 kb) of respiratory bovine coronaviruses and comparisons among respiratory and enteric coronaviruses. *Virus Genes* **17**:33–42.

17. Chow, K. C., C. H. Hsiao, T. Y. Lin, C. L. Chen, and S. H. Chiou. 2004. Detection of severe acute respiratory syndrome-associated coronavirus in pneumocytes of the lung. Am. J. Clin. Pathol. 121:574–580.

18. Clark, M. A. 1993. Bovine coronavirus. Br. Vet. J. 149:51–70.

19. Cook, M. A., and A. P. A. Mockett. 1995. Epidemiology of infectious bronchitis virus, p. 317–335. In S. Siddell (ed.), The Coronaviridae. Plenum Press, New York, NY.

20. Costantini, V., P. Lewis, J. Alsop, C. Templeton, and L. J. Saif. 2004. Respiratory and fecal shedding of porcine respiratory coronavirus (PRCV) in sentinel weaned pigs and sequence of the partial S-gene of the PRCV isolates. Arch. Virol. 149:957–974.

21. Cox, E., M. Pensaert, J. Hooyberghs, and K. Van Deun. 1990. Sites of replication of a porcine respiratory coronavirus in 5-week-old pigs with or without maternal antibodies. Adv. Exp. Med. Biol. 276:429–433.

22. Dea, S., A. Verbeek, and P. Tijssen. 1991. Transmissible enteritis of turkeys: experimental inoculation studies with tissue-culture-adapted turkey and bovine coronaviruses. Avian Dis. 35:767–777.

23. Domingo, E., E. Baranowski, C. M. Ruiz-Jarabo, A. M. Martin-Hernandez, J. C. Saiz, and C. Escarmis. 1998. Quasispecies structure and persistence of RNA viruses. Emerg. Infect. Dis. 4:521–527.

24. Drosten, C., S. Gunther, W. Preiser, S. van der Werf, H. R. Brodt, S. Becker, H. Rabenau, M. Panning, L. Kolesnikova, R. A. Fouchier, A. Berger, A. M. Burguiere, J. Cinatl, M. Eickmann, N. Escriou, K. Grywna, S. Kramme, J. C. Manuguerra, S. Muller, V. Rickerts, M. Sturmer, S. Vieth, H. D. Klenk, A. D. Osterhaus, H. Schmitz, and H. W. Doerr. 2003. Identification of a novel coronavirus in patients with severe acute respiratory syndrome. N. Engl. J. Med. 348:1967–1976.

25. Elazhary, M. A., J. L. Frechette, S. Silim, and R. S. Roy. 1981. Serological evidence of some bovine viruses in the caribou (Rangifer tarandus caribou) in Quebec. J. Wildl. Dis. 17:609–612.

26. El-Kanawati, Z. R., H. Tsunemitsu, D. R. Smith, and L. J. Saif. 1996. Infection and cross-protection studies of winter dysentery and calf diarrhea bovine coronavirus strains in colostrum-deprived and gnotobiotic calves. Am. J. Vet. Res. 57:48–53.

27. Erles, K., C. Toomey, H. W. Brooks, and J. Brownlie. 2003. Detection of a group 2 coronavirus in dogs with canine infectious respiratory disease. Virology 310:216–223.

28. Furuuchi, S., Y. Shimizu, and T. Kumagai. 1979. Multiplication of low and high cell culture passaged strains of transmissible gastroenteritis virus in organs of newborn piglets. Vet. Microbiol. 3:169–178.

29. Gelinas, A. M., A. M. Sasseville, and S. Dea. 2001. Identification of specific variations within the HE, S1, and ORF4 genes of bovine coronaviruses associated with enteric and respiratory diseases in dairy cattle. Adv. Exp. Med. Biol. 494:63–67.

30. Giomarelli, P., S. Scolletta, E. Borrelli, and B. Biagioli. 2003. Myocardial and lung injury after cardiopulmonary bypass: role of interleukin (IL)-10. Ann. Thorac. Surg. 76:117–123.

31. González, J. M., P. Gomez-Puertas, D. Cavanagh, A. E. Gorbalenya, and L. Enjuanes. 2003. A comparative sequence analysis to revise the current taxonomy of the family Coronaviridae. Arch. Virol. 148:2207–2235.

32. Gough, R. E., W. J. Cox, C. E. Winkler, M. W. Sharp, and D. Spackman. 1996. Isolation and identification of infectious bronchitis virus from pheasants. Vet. Rec. 138:208–209.

33. Guan, Y., B. J. Zheng, Y. Q. He, X. L. Liu, Z. X. Zhuang, C. L. Cheung, S. W. Luo, P. H. Li, L. J. Zhang, Y. J. Guan, K. M. Butt, K. L. Wong, K. W. Chan, W. Lim, K. F. Shortridge, K. Y. Yuen, J. S. Peiris, and L. L. Poon. 2003. Isolation and characterization of viruses related to the SARS coronavirus from animals in southern China. Science 302:276–278.

34. Guy, J. R. 2003. Turkey coronavirus enteritis, p. 300–307. In J. H. Barnes, J. R. Glisson, A. M. Fadly, L. R. McDougald, and D. E. Swayne (ed.), Diseases of Poultry, 11th ed. Iowa State Press, Ames.

34a. Hadya, N. S., et al. 2004. Antigenic relationships between human severe acute respiratory syndrome (SARS) and animal coronaviruses, abstr. W7-4. 23rd Annual Meeting of the American Society for Virology. American Society for Virology, Toledo, OH.

35. Halbur, P. G., P. S. Paul, E. M. Vaughn, and J. J. Andrews. 1993. Experimental reproduction of pneumonia in gnotobiotic pigs with porcine respiratory coronavirus isolate AR310. J. Vet. Diagn. Investig. 5:184–188.

36. Han, M. G., D.-S. Cheon, X. Zhang, and L. J. Saif. 2006. Cross-protection against a human enteric coronavirus and a virulent bovine enteric coronavirus in gnotobiotic calves. J. Virol. 80:12350–12356.

36a. Hasoksuz, M., K. Alekseev, A. Vlasova, X. Zhang, D. Spiro, R. Halpin, S. Wang, E. Ghedin, and L. J. Saif. 2007. Biologic, antigenic, and full-length genomic characterization of a bovine-like coronavirus isolated from a giraffe. J. Virol. 81:4981–4990.

37. Hasoksuz, M., A. E. Hoet, S. C. Loerch, T. E. Wittum, P. R. Nielsen, and L. J. Saif. 2002. Detection of respiratory and enteric shedding of bovine coronaviruses in cattle in an Ohio feedlot. J. Vet. Diagn. Investig. 14:308–313.

38. Hasoksuz, M., S. Lathrop, M. A. Al-dubaib, P. Lewis, and L. J. Saif. 1999. Antigenic variation among bovine enteric coronaviruses (BECV) and bovine respiratory coronaviruses (BRCV) detected using monoclonal antibodies. Arch. Virol. 144:2441–2447.

39. Hasoksuz, M., S. L. Lathrop, K. L. Gadfield, and L. J. Saif. 1999. Isolation of bovine respiratory coronaviruses from feedlot cattle and comparison of their biological and antigenic properties with bovine enteric coronaviruses. Am. J. Vet. Res. 60:1227–1233.

40. Hasoksuz, M., S. Sreevatsan, K. O. Cho, A. E. Hoet, and L. J. Saif. 2002. Molecular analysis of the S1 subunit of the spike glycoprotein of respiratory and enteric bovine coronavirus isolates. Virus Res. 84:101–109.

41. Hayes, J. R. 2000. Evaluation of dual infection of nursery pigs with U.S. strains of porcine reproductive and respiratory syndrome virus and porcine respiratory coronavirus. M.S. thesis. The Ohio State University, Columbus.

42. Heckert, R. A., L. J. Saif, K. H. Hoblet, and A. G. Agnes. 1990. A longitudinal study of bovine coronavirus enteric and respiratory infections in dairy calves in two herds in Ohio. Vet. Microbiol. 22:187–201.

43. Heckert, R. A., L. J. Saif, G. W. Myers, and A. G. Agnes. 1991. Bovine coronavirus respiratory and enteric infections in conventional dairy calves: epidemiology and isotype antibody responses in serum and mucosal secretions. Am. J. Vet. Res. 52:845–851.

44. Herrewegh, A. A., M. Mahler, H. J. Hedrich, B. L. Haagmans, H. F. Egberink, M. C. Horzinek, P. J. Rottier, and R. J. de Groot. 1997. Persistence and evolution of feline coronavirus in a closed cat-breeding colony. Virology 234:349–363.

45. Hodgson, T., P. Britton, and D. Cavanagh. 2006. Neither the RNA nor the proteins of open reading frames 3a and 3b of the coronavirus infectious bronchitis virus are essential for replication. J. Virol. 80:296–305.

46. Horzinek, M. C., H. Lutz, and N. C. Pedersen. 1982. Antigenic relationships among homologous structural polypeptides of porcine, feline, and canine coronaviruses. Infect. Immun. 37:1148–1155.

47. **Ismail, M. M., K. O. Cho, M. Hasoksuz, L. J. Saif, and Y. M. Saif.** 2001. Antigenic and genomic relatedness of turkey-origin coronaviruses, bovine coronaviruses, and infectious bronchitis virus of chickens. *Avian Dis.* **45:**978–984.

48. **Ismail, M. M., K. O. Cho, L. A. Ward, L. J. Saif, and Y. M. Saif.** 2001. Experimental bovine coronavirus in turkey poults and young chickens. *Avian Dis.* **45:**157–163.

49. **Ismail, M. M., A. Y. Tang, and Y. M. Saif.** 2003. Pathogenicity of turkey coronavirus in turkeys and chickens. *Avian Dis.* **47:**515–522.

50. **Jabrane, A., C. Girard, and Y. Elazhary.** 1994. Pathogenicity of porcine respiratory coronavirus isolated in Quebec. *Can. Vet. J.* **35:**86–92.

51. **Jakab, G. J.** 1982. Viral-bacterial interactions in pulmonary infection. *Adv. Vet. Sci. Comp. Med.* **26:**155–171.

52. **Jeong, J. H., G. Y. Kim, and S. S. Yoon.** 2005. Molecular analysis of S gene of spike glycoprotein of winter dysentery bovine coronavirus circulating in Korea during 2002–2003. *Virus Res.* **108:**207–212.

53. **Kemeny, L. J., V. L. Wiltsey, and J. L. Riley.** 1975. Upper respiratory infection of lactating sows with transmissible gastroenteritis virus following contact exposure to infected piglets. *Cornell Vet.* **65:**352–362.

54. **Kim, L., J. Hayes, P. Lewis, A. V. Parwani, K. O. Chang, and L. J. Saif.** 2000. Molecular characterization and pathogenesis of transmissible gastroenteritis coronavirus (TGEV) and porcine respiratory coronavirus (PRCV) field isolates co-circulating in a swine herd. *Arch. Virol.* **145:**1133–1147.

55. **Ksiazek, T. G., D. Erdman, C. S. Goldsmith, S. R. Zaki, T. Peret, S. Emery, S. Tong, C. Urbani, J. A. Comer, W. Lim, P. E. Rollin, S. F. Dowell, A. E. Ling, C. D. Humphrey, W. J. Shieh, J. Guarner, C. D. Paddock, P. Rota, B. Fields, J. DeRisi, J. Y. Yang, N. Cox, J. M. Hughes, J. W. LeDuc, W. J. Bellini, L. J. Anderson, and SARS Working Group.** 2003. A novel coronavirus associated with severe acute respiratory syndrome. *N. Engl. J. Med.* **348:**1953–1966.

56. **Lathrop, S. L., T. E. Wittum, K. V. Brock, S. C. Loerch, L. J. Perino, H. R. Bingham, F. T. McCollum, and L. J. Saif.** 2000. Association between infection of the respiratory tract attributable to bovine coronavirus and health and growth performance of cattle in feedlots. *Am. J. Vet. Res.* **61:**1062–1066.

57. **Lathrop, S. L., T. E. Wittum, S. C. Loerch, L. J. Perino, and L. J. Saif.** 2000. Antibody titers against bovine coronavirus and shedding of the virus via the respiratory tract in feedlot cattle. *Am. J. Vet. Res.* **61:**1057–1061.

58. **Lau, S. K., P. C. Woo, K. S. Li, Y. Huang, H. W. Tsoi, B. H. Wong, S. S. Wong, S. Y. Leung, K. H. Chan, and K. Y. Yuen.** 2005. Severe acute respiratory syndrome coronavirus-like virus in Chinese horseshoe bats. *Proc. Natl. Acad. Sci. USA* **102:**14040–14045.

59. **Laude, H., J. Gelfi, L. Lavenant, and B. Charley.** 1992. Single amino acid changes in the viral glycoprotein M affect induction of alpha interferon by the coronavirus transmissible gastroenteritis virus. *J. Virol.* **66:**743–749.

60. **Laude, H., K. Van Reeth, and M. Pensaert.** 1993. Porcine respiratory coronavirus: molecular features and virus-host interactions. *Vet. Res.* **24:**125–150.

61. **Leung, W. K., K. F. To, P. K. Chan, H. L. Chan, A. K. Wu, N. Lee, K. Y. Yuen, and J. J. Sung.** 2003. Enteric involvement of severe acute respiratory syndrome-associated coronavirus infection. *Gastroenterology* **125:**1011–1017.

62. **Li, W., Z. Shi, M. Yu, W. Ren, C. Smith, J. H. Epstein, H. Wang, G. Crameri, Z. Hu, H. Zhang, J. Zhang, J. McEachern, H. Field, P. Daszak, B. T. Eaton, S. Zhang, and L. F. Wang.** 2005. Bats are natural reservoirs of SARS-like coronaviruses. *Science* **310:**676–679.

63. **Lin, T. L., C. C. Loa, and C. C. Wu.** 2004. Complete sequences of 3′ end coding region for structural protein genes of turkey coronavirus. *Virus Res.* **106:**61–70.

64. **Lin, X., K. L. O'Reilly, M. L. Burrell, and J. Storz.** 2001. Infectivity-neutralizing and hemagglutinin-inhibiting antibody responses to respiratory coronavirus infections of cattle in pathogenesis of shipping fever pneumonia. *Clin. Diagn. Lab. Immunol.* **8:**357–362.

65. **Majhdi, F., H. C. Minocha, and S. Kapil.** 1997. Isolation and characterization of a coronavirus from elk calves with diarrhea. *J. Clin. Microbiol.* **35:**2937–2942.

66. **Martin, S. W., E. Nagy, P. E. Shewen, and R. J. Harland.** 1998. The association of titers to bovine coronavirus with treatment for bovine respiratory disease and weight gain in feedlot calves. *Can. J. Vet. Res.* **62:**257–261.

67. **McGoldrick, A., J. P. Lowings, and D. J. Paton.** 1999. Characterisation of a recent virulent transmissible gastroenteritis virus from Britain with a deleted ORF 3a. *Arch. Virol.* **144:**763–770.

68. **McNulty, M. S., D. G. Bryson, G. M. Allan, and E. F. Logan.** 1984. Coronavirus infection of the bovine respiratory tract. *Vet. Microbiol.* **9:**425–434.

69. **Motokawa, K., T. Hohdatsu, H. Hashimoto, and H. Koyama.** 1996. Comparison of the amino acid sequence and phylogenetic analysis of the peplomer, integral membrane and nucleocapsid proteins of feline, canine and porcine coronaviruses. *Microbiol. Immunol.* **40:**425–433.

70. **Nicholls, J. M., L. L. Poon, K. C. Lee, W. F. Ng, S. T. Lai, C. Y. Leung, C. M. Chu, P. K. Hui, K. L. Mak, W. Lim, K. W. Yan, K. H. Chan, N. C. Tsang, Y. Guan, K. Y. Yuen, and J. S. Peiris.** 2003. Lung pathology of fatal severe acute respiratory syndrome. *Lancet* **361:**1773–1778.

71. **Olsen, C. W.** 1993. A review of feline infectious peritonitis virus: molecular biology, immunopathogenesis, clinical aspects, and vaccination. *Vet. Microbiol.* **36:**1–37.

72. **Olsen, C. W., W. V. Corapi, R. H. Jacobson, R. A. Simkins, L. J. Saif, and F. W. Scott.** 1993. Identification of antigenic sites mediating antibody-dependent enhancement of feline infectious peritonitis virus infectivity. *J. Gen. Virol.* **74:**745–749.

73. **Olsen, S. J., H. L. Chang, T. Y. Cheung, A. F. Tang, T. L. Fisk, S. P. Ooi, H. W. Kuo, D. D. Jiang, K. T. Chen, J. Lando, K. H. Hsu, T. J. Chen, and S. F. Dowell.** 2003. Transmission of the severe acute respiratory syndrome on aircraft. *N. Engl. J. Med.* **349:**2381–2382.

74. **Paton, D., G. Ibata, J. Sands, and A. McGoldrick.** 1997. Detection of transmissible gastroenteritis virus by RT-PCR and differentiation from porcine respiratory coronavirus. *J. Virol. Methods* **66:**303–309.

75. **Paul, P. S., E. M. Vaughn, and P. G. Halbur.** 1997. Pathogenicity and sequence analysis studies suggest potential role of gene 3 in virulence of swine enteric and respiratory coronaviruses. *Adv. Exp. Med. Biol.* **412:**317–321.

76. **Peiris, J. M. S., Y. Guan, and K. Y. Yuen.** 2004. Severe acute respiratory syndrome. *Nat. Med.* **10:**588–597.

77. **Peiris, J. S., C. M. Chu, V. C. Cheng, K. S. Chan, I. F. Hung, L. L. Poon, K. I. Law, B. S. Tang, T. Y. Hon, C. S. Chan, K. H. Chan, J. S. Ng, B. J. Zheng, W. L. Ng, R. W. Lai, Y. Guan, K. Y. Yuen, and HKU/UCH SARS Study Group.** 2003. Clinical progression and viral load in a community outbreak of coronavirus-associated SARS pneumonia: a prospective study. *Lancet* **361:**1767–1772.

78. **Pensaert, M., P. Callebaut, and J. Vergote.** 1986. Isolation of a porcine respiratory, non-enteric coronavirus related to transmissible gastroenteritis. *Vet. Q.* **8:**257–261.

79. **Pensaert, M. B.** 2006. Hemagglutinating encephalomyelitis virus, p. 353. *In* B. Straw, J. J. Zimmerman, S. D'Allrire, and

D. J. Taylor (ed.), *Diseases of Swine*, 9th ed. Blackwell Publishing, Ames, IA.

80. Pensaert, M. B., and S.-G. Yeo. 2006. Porcine epidemic diarrhea, p. 367. *In* B. Straw, J. J. Zimmerman, S. D'Allrire, and D. J. Taylor (ed.), *Diseases of Swine*, 9th ed. Blackwell Publishing, Ames, Iowa.

81. Plummer, P. J., B. W. Rohrbach, R. A. Daugherty, R. A. Daugherty, K. V. Thomas, R. P. Wilkes, F. E. Duggan, and M. A. Kennedy. 2004. Effect of intranasal vaccination against bovine enteric coronavirus on the occurrence of respiratory tract disease in a commercial backgrounding feedlot. *J. Am. Vet. Med. Assoc.* **225:**726–731.

82. Poon, L. L., D. K. Chu, K. H. Chan, O. K. Wong, T. M. Ellis, Y. H. Leung, S. K. Lau, P. C. Woo, K. Y. Suen, K. Y. Yuen, Y. Guan, and J. S. Peiris. 2005. Identification of a novel coronavirus in bats. *J. Virol.* **79:**2001–2009.

83. Poutanen, S. M., D. E. Low, B. Henry, S. Finkelstein, D. Rose, K. Green, R. Tellier, R. Draker, D. Adachi, M. Ayers, A. K. Chan, D. M. Skowronski, I. Salit, A. E. Simor, A. S. Slutsky, P. W. Doyle, M. Krajden, M. Petric, R. C. Brunham, A. J. McGeer, National Microbiology Laboratory, Canada, and Canadian Severe Acute Respiratory Syndrome Study Team. 2003. Identification of severe acute respiratory syndrome in Canada. *N. Engl. J. Med.* **348:**1995–2005.

84. Reynolds, D. J., T. G. Debney, G. A. Hall, L. H. Thomas, and K. R. Parsons. 1985. Studies on the relationship between coronaviruses from the intestinal and respiratory tracts of calves. *Arch. Virol.* **85:**71–83.

85. Reynolds, D. J., J. H. Morgan, N. Chanter, P. W. Jones, J. C. Bridger, T. G. Debney, and K. J. Bunch. 1986. Microbiology of calf diarrhoea in southern Britain. *Vet. Rec.* **119:**34–39.

86. Saif, L. J. 1990. A review of evidence implicating bovine coronavirus in the etiology of winter dysentery in cows: an enigma resolved? *Cornell. Vet.* **80:**303–311.

87. Saif, L. J. 1996. Mucosal immunity: an overview and studies of enteric and respiratory coronavirus infections in a swine model of enteric disease. *Vet. Immunol. Immunopathol.* **54:**163–169.

88. Saif, L. J. 1999. Enteric viral infections of pigs and strategies for induction of mucosal immunity. *Adv. Vet. Med.* **41:**429–446.

89. Saif, L. J. 2004. Animal coronaviruses vaccines: lessons for SARS. *Dev. Biol.* **119:**129–140.

90. Saif, L. J. 2004. Animal coronaviruses: what can they teach us about the severe acute respiratory syndrome? *Rev. Sci. Tech. Off. Int. Epizoot.* **23:**643–660.

91. Saif, L. J. 2005. Comparative biology of coronaviruses: lessons for SARS, p. 84–99. *In* M. Peiris, L. J. Anderson, A. D. Osterhaus, K. Stohr, and K. Y. Yuen (ed.), *Severe Acute Respiratory Syndrome*. Blackwell Pub., Oxford, United Kingdom.

92. Saif, L. J., and R. A. Heckert. 1990. Enteric coronaviruses, p. 185–252. *In* L. J. Saif and K. W. Theil (ed.), *Viral Diarrheas of Man and Animals*. CRC Press, Boca Raton, FL.

93. Saif, L. J., and D. J. Jackwood. 1990. Enteric virus vaccines, p. 313. *In* L. J. Saif and K. W. Theil (ed.), *Viral Diarrheas of Man and Animals*. CRC Press, Boca Raton, FL.

94. Saif, L. J., D. R. Redman, P. D. Moorhead, and K. W. Theil. 1986. Experimentally induced coronavirus infections in calves: viral replication in the respiratory and intestinal tracts. *Am. J. Vet. Res.* **47:**1426–1432.

95. Saif, L. J., and K. Sestak. 2006. Transmissible gastroenteritis and porcine respiratory coronavirus, p. 489. *In* B. Straw, J. J. Zimmerman, S. D'Allaire, and D. J. Taylor (ed.), *Diseases of Swine*, 9th ed. Blackwell Publishing, Ames, IA.

96. Sanchez, C. M., A. Izeta, J. M. Sanchez-Morgado, S. Alonso, I. Sola, M. Balasch, J. Plana-Duran, and L. Enjuanes. 1999.

Targeted recombination demonstrates that the spike gene of transmissible gastroenteritis coronavirus is a determinant of its enteric tropism and virulence. *J. Virol.* **73:**7607–7618.

97. Shen, Z., F. Ning, W. Zhou, X. He, C. Lin, D. P. Chin, Z. Zhu, and A. Schuchat. 2004. Super-spreading SARS events in Beijing, 2003. *Emerg. Infect. Dis.* **10:**256–260.

98. Shimizu, M., and Y. Shimizu. 1979. Effects of ambient temperatures on clinical and immune responses of pigs infected with transmissible gastroenteritis virus. *Vet. Microbiol.* **4:**109–116.

99. Smith, D. R., P. J. Fedorka-Cray, R. Mohan, K. V. Brock, T. E. Wittum, P. S. Morley, K. H. Hoblet, and L. J. Saif. 1998. Epidemiologic herd-level assessment of causative agents and risk factors for winter dysentery in dairy cattle. *Am. J. Vet. Res.* **59:**994–1001.

100. Sola, I., S. Alonso, S. Zuniga, M. Balasch, J. Plana-Duran, and L. Enjuanes. 2003. Engineering the transmissible gastroenteritis virus genome as an expression vector inducing lactogenic immunity. *J. Virol.* **77:**4357–4369.

101. Somogyi, R., A. E. Vesely, T. Azami, D. Preiss, J. Fisher, J. Correia, and R. A. Fowler. 2004. Dispersal of respiratory droplets with open vs. closed oxygen delivery masks: implications for the transmission of severe acute respiratory syndrome. *Chest* **125:**1155–1157.

102. Storz, J., X. Lin, C. W. Purdy, V. N. Chouljenko, K. G. Kousoulas, F. M. Enright, W. C. Gilmore, R. E. Briggs, and R. W. Loan. 2000. Coronavirus and *Pasteurella* infections in bovine shipping fever pneumonia and Evans' criteria for causation. *J. Clin. Microbiol.* **38:**3291–3298.

103. Storz, J., C. W. Purdy, X. Lin, M. Burrell, R. E. Truax, R. E. Briggs, G. H. Frank, and R. W. Loan. 2000. Isolation of respiratory bovine coronavirus, other cytocidal viruses, and Pasteurella spp. from cattle involved in two natural outbreaks of shipping fever. *J. Am. Vet. Med. Assoc.* **216:**1599–1604.

104. Storz, J., L. Stine, A. Liem, and G. A. Anderson. 1996. Coronavirus isolation from nasal swab samples in cattle with signs of respiratory tract disease after shipping. *J. Am. Vet. Med. Assoc.* **208:**1452–1455.

105. Sun, Z. F., and X. J. Meng. 2004. Antigenic cross-reactivity between the nucleocapsid protein of severe acute respiratory syndrome (SARS) coronavirus and polyclonal antisera of antigenic group I animal coronaviruses: implication for SARS diagnosis. *J. Clin. Microbiol.* **42:**2351–2352.

106. Thomas, C., A. Hoet, S. Sreevatsan, T. Wittum, R. Briggs, G. Duff, and L. J. Saif. 2006. Transmission of bovine coronavirus and serologic responses in feedlot calves under field conditions. *Am. J. Vet. Res.* **67:**1412–1420.

107. Traven, M., K. Naslund, N. Linde, B. Linde, A. Silvan, C. Fossum, K. O. Hedlund, and B. Larsson. 2001. Experimental reproduction of winter dysentery in lactating cows using BCV—comparison with BCV infection in milk-fed calves. *Vet. Microbiol.* **81:**127–151.

108. Tsunemitsu, H., Z. R. el-Kanawati, D. R. Smith, H. H. Reed, and L. J. Saif. 1995. Isolation of coronaviruses antigenically indistinguishable from bovine coronavirus from wild ruminants with diarrhea. *J. Clin. Microbiol.* **33:**3264–3269.

109. Tsunemitsu, H., and L. J. Saif. 1995. Antigenic and biological comparisons of bovine coronaviruses derived from neonatal calf diarrhea and winter dysentery of adult cattle. *Arch. Virol.* **140:**1303–1311.

110. Tsunemitsu, H., D. R. Smith, and L. J. Saif. 1999. Experimental inoculation of adult dairy cows with bovine coronavirus and detection of coronavirus in feces by RT-PCR. *Arch. Virol.* **144:**167–175.

111. Uenaka, T., I. Kishimoto, T. Uemura, T. Ito, T. Umemura, and K. Otsuki. 1998. Cloacal inoculation with the Connecticut strain of avian infectious bronchitis virus: an attempt to produce nephropathogenic virus by in vivo passage using cloacal inoculation. *J. Vet. Med. Sci.* **60:**495–502.

112. VanCott, J. L., T. A. Brim, J. K. Lunney, and L. J. Saif. 1994. Contribution of antibody-secreting cells induced in mucosal lymphoid tissues of pigs inoculated with respiratory or enteric strains of coronavirus to immunity against enteric coronavirus challenge. *J. Immunol.* **152:**3980–3990.

113. VanCott, J. L., T. A. Brim, R. A. Simkins, and L. J. Saif. 1993. Isotype-specific antibody-secreting cells to transmissible gastroenteritis virus and porcine respiratory coronavirus in gut- and bronchus-associated lymphoid tissues of suckling pigs. *J. Immunol.* **150:**3990–4000.

114. Van Kruiningen, H. J., L. H. Khairallah, V. G. Sasseville, M. S. Wyand, and J. E. Post. 1987. Calfhood coronavirus enterocolitis: a clue to the etiology of winter dysentery. *Vet. Pathol.* **24:**564–567.

115. Van Reeth, K., H. Nauwynck, and M. Pensaert. 2000. A potential role for tumour necrosis factor-alpha in synergy between porcine respiratory coronavirus and bacterial lipopolysaccharide in the induction of respiratory disease in pigs. *J. Med. Microbiol.* **49:**613–620.

116. Van Reeth, K., and M. B. Pensaert. 1994. Porcine respiratory coronavirus-mediated interference against influenza virus replication in the respiratory tract of feeder pigs. *Am. J. Vet. Res.* **55:**1275–1281.

117. Vaughn, E. M., P. G. Halbur, and P. S. Paul. 1994. Three new isolates of porcine respiratory coronavirus with various pathogenicities and spike (S) gene deletions. *J. Clin. Microbiol.* **32:**1809–1812.

118. Wesley, R. D., R. D. Woods, H. T. Hill, and J. D. Biwer. 1990. Evidence for a porcine respiratory coronavirus, antigenically similar to transmissible gastroenteritis virus, in the United States. *J. Vet. Diagn. Investig.* **2:**312–317.

119. Wesley, R. D., R. D. Woods, J. D. McKean, M. K. Senn, and Y. Elazhary. 1997. Prevalence of coronavirus antibodies in Iowa swine. *Can. J. Vet. Res.* **61:**305–308.

120. Wilder-Smith, A., N. I. Paton, and K. T. Goh. 2003. Low risk of transmission of severe acute respiratory syndrome on airplanes: the Singapore experience. *Trop. Med. Int. Health* **8:**1035–1037.

121. Yoo, D., and D. Deregt. 2001. A single amino acid change within antigenic domain II of the spike protein of bovine coronavirus confers resistance to virus neutralization. *Clin. Diagn. Lab. Immunol.* **8:**297–302.

122. Zhang, X., M. Hasoksuz, D. Spiro, R. Halpin, S. Wang, S. Stollar, D. Janies, N. Hadya, Y. Tang, E. Ghedin, and L. J. Saif. 2007. Complete genomic sequences, a key residue in the spike protein and deletions in non-structural protein 3b of US strains of the virulent and attenuated coronaviruses, transmissible gastroenteritis virus and porcine respiratory coronavirus. *Virology* **358:**424–435.

123. Zhang, X. M., W. Herbst, K. G. Kousoulas, and J. Storz. 1994. Biological and genetic characterization of a hemagglutinating coronavirus isolated from a diarrhoeic child. *J. Med. Virol.* **44:**152–161.

*Nidoviruses*
Edited by S. Perlman, T. Gallagher, and E. J. Snijder
© 2008 ASM Press, Washington, DC

Chapter 19

# Severe Acute Respiratory Syndrome: Epidemiology, Pathogenesis, and Animal Models

JOHN NICHOLLS, J. S. MALIK PEIRIS, AND STANLEY PERLMAN

In November 2002, cases of atypical pneumonia were reported in the news media in southern China. The first major outbreak of disease outside of mainland China was reported from Hanoi, Vietnam. Carlo Urbani, an infectious diseases specialist working with the World Health Organization (WHO) in Vietnam, was one of the first to recognize that these patients had a novel illness and organized initial efforts to contain the outbreak. Unfortunately, Urbani himself contracted the disease and died from SARS. Days later, health care workers at a teaching hospital in the New Territories in Hong Kong came down with symptoms of a severe atypical pneumonia that subsequently became known as SARS (severe acute respiratory syndrome). During the early stages of the outbreak of SARS in 2002–2003, the WHO initiated and coordinated a virtual network of laboratories in the search for the cause of this rapidly spreading outbreak. A number of possible agents were detected in the course of investigating patients with suspected SARS, including human metapneumovirus and *Chlamydia* (87). In mid-March 2003, a novel coronavirus was isolated in culture independently by different research groups using FRhK-4 and Vero-E6 cells. Molecular tests consistently confirmed the presence of this new virus in patients with SARS in many parts of the world (17, 33, 35, 60). To fulfill Koch's postulates for disease etiology, experimental infection of cynomolgus macaques in The Netherlands provided evidence of virus replication and significant, but not identical, lung pathology associated with this novel coronavirus (20). The sharing of information and viruses within the WHO laboratory network allowed a consensus to be reached that this coronavirus was the etiologic agent of SARS.

Prior to SARS, there were only two human coronaviruses, strains 229E and OC43, belonging to groups 1 and 2, respectively, that were known to infect humans (84). These two viruses were associated with mild upper respiratory disease and the common cold, but they were rarely associated with severe human disease. It was therefore unexpected that this severe new human disease was caused by a novel coronavirus. What was the cellular tropism of SARS-coronavirus (SARS-CoV), and was the severity due to a direct viral effect or to the host immune response to this novel virus? The genetic sequence of SARS-CoV was fully determined within weeks of the virus being isolated (51, 97), and this confirmed that SARS-CoV was a novel coronavirus, distinct from all other human and animal coronaviruses but distantly related to the group 2 coronaviruses (73). It is now designated as a group 2b coronavirus.

## EPIDEMIOLOGY

### Zoonotic Spread

Patients with SARS invariably seroconverted to positivity for this novel virus in immunofluorescence assays, enzyme-linked immunosorbent assays, and neutralization tests (33, 60, 69). However, when the general population was examined, there was little evidence of preexisting antibody to SARS-CoV (44), suggesting that this was indeed a novel virus that recently emerged in the human population, very likely from an animal reservoir. In initial attempts to understand the pathophysiology of this new disease, monoclonal and polyclonal antibodies raised to previously identified animal coronaviruses were tested

**John Nicholls** • Department of Pathology, The University of Hong Kong, Hong Kong Special Administrative Region, China. **J. S. Malik Peiris** • Department of Microbiology, The University of Hong Kong, Hong Kong Special Administrative Region, China. **Stanley Perlman** • Department of Microbiology, University of Iowa, Iowa City, IA 52242.

on autopsy cases of two of the index patients who died of SARS. There was consistently no reaction, a finding that was interpreted at the time as pointing to the distinctive nature of SARS-CoV (55).

Studies after the 2003 outbreak showed that some of the patients with SARS-like disease in the early stages of the outbreak had occupational exposure to live game animals held within markets in Guangdong Province, China (90). Testing of animals in these live markets in Guangdong led to the detection of a SARS-like coronavirus in a number of small mammal species, including Himalayan palm civets (*Paguma larvata*) and raccoon dogs (*Nyctereutes procyonoides*) (24, 82). In addition, those handlers directly involved in the live-animal trade within these markets had a high seroprevalence for SARS-like viruses, although they gave no history of SARS-like disease (24). These findings suggested that the animal markets could be the interface at which interspecies transmission to humans occurred. In such markets, animals are continually removed for consumption while new animals are added, providing a continued supply of susceptible animals. Civets are susceptible to experimental infection with human SARS-CoV (88). However, SARS-CoV (virus RNA as detected by reverse transcriptase PCR [RT-PCR] or antibody) has not been consistently detected in the farms that supply civets to the live-animal markets. There are few data from wild-caught civets, but from the limited studies it does not appear that these animals are endemically infected in the wild. From these observations, it was proposed that the civets and raccoon dogs amplify and perpetuate the circulation of the virus within the live-animal market setting but are not the natural reservoir of the virus. In subsequent studies, viruses closely related to SARS-CoV were isolated from Chinese horseshoe bats (37, 47), indicating that these animals serve as a natural reservoir for the virus. Additionally, multiple other coronaviruses were isolated from several bat species, suggesting that coronaviruses are endemic within bat populations (13, 63, 78, 86).

Studies on the molecular evolution of SARS-CoV revealed that viruses in the early phase of the human SARS outbreak were more closely related to viruses detected in palm civets and other small mammals in the live-animal markets. The molecular evolution of the viruses in these markets has been elegantly detailed (32). These studies indicate that the virus was under strong positive selection in the early phase of outbreak, suggesting a process of adaptation to the new human host (23, 71, 94). Specific changes were detected in three genes within the SARS-CoV genome, as the virus adapted to the human host. Changes in the spike protein (S protein) occurred sequentially and likely represented adaptation to the host cell receptor (angiotensin-converting enzyme 2 [ACE2]). Mutations were also noted in the accessory protein 3a. Since 3a protein interacts with the S protein, these changes may reflect adaptation to changes in the S protein. Finally, deletions in an open reading frame (ORF) encoding another accessory protein, the ORF8 protein, were also detected in nearly all isolates; these deletions resulted in two novel ORFs, ORF8a and -8b (74). The biological significance of this deletion is not known at present, although recent data indicate that civets are equally susceptible to SARS-CoVs with and without the 29-nucleotide deletion (88). Interestingly, the virus was also evolving rapidly in palm civets, an observation that is compatible with the idea that civets may not be the natural reservoir of the virus. In the second episode of SARS in December 2003 and January 2004, the virus detected in the four patients with SARS-CoV infection was phylogenetically more closely related to SARS-CoV-like viruses identified in civets than to the viruses associated with the global outbreak in 2003, suggesting that the patients with these infections represented new introductions from the animal reservoir.

## Human-to-Human Transmission

SARS-CoV spread within exposed populations was bimodal. Most infected patients were not very contagious and spread virus to susceptible contacts by large droplets. Most of these individuals infected no one or only one to five contacts. In contrast, a larger number of contacts were infected in a few superspreading events (61). While the mechanism of superspreading events is not well understood, individuals involved in this mode of transmission appeared to have large virus burdens and to spread virus via aerosolization (small droplets). An analysis of the Amoy Gardens outbreak in Hong Kong found a high nasopharyngeal viral load in patients close to the index patient. The viral load decreased with decreasing distance from the index patient, consistent with a role for airborne transmission in the spread of infection in this instance (12).

Quantitative studies on viral load in the upper respiratory tract and the feces of patients infected with SARS-CoV revealed a progressive increase in viral load, peaking around day 10 after onset of disease symptoms (9, 50, 58). This explains the epidemiological observation that transmission mainly occurs after the fifth day of illness and is less common in the early stage of the illness (49, 67). This unusual feature of SARS allowed public health measures to be so dramatically successful in interrupting disease transmission. Although viral RNA was detectable by RT-PCR for many weeks into convalescence, virus isolation after the third week of illness was rare. Identification of SARS-CoV RNA in these patients may therefore represent either neutralized virus or residual viral genome rather than active viral replication.

## SARS-CoV ENTRY AND REPLICATION

The molecular biology of the coronaviruses is discussed elsewhere in this monograph, but of the various proteins produced by the virus, the S protein mediates virus attachment and entry into susceptible cells, and attention has focused on the interaction of S protein with human cells. A receptor for SARS-CoV has been identified as ACE2 (46). The structure of the SARS-CoV S protein/human ACE2 complex has been solved and indicates that the S protein does not bind to the catalytic site of ACE2 (45). Also, ACE2 lacking catalytic activity is able to efficiently bind the S protein. At present, human ACE2 is considered the primary host cell receptor for SARS-CoV. Evidence for this is that SARS-CoV replication in the lungs of ACE2-null mice is markedly suppressed, proving the importance of this receptor in vivo, at least in mice (34). Furthermore, ACE2 expression is detectable on pneumocytes, enterocytes, vascular endothelial cells, and smooth muscle cells (26, 79), and this finding of ACE2 on respiratory and intestinal epithelium is compatible with the known tropism of the virus (66). By immunofluorescence staining, Jia et al. and Sims et al. were able to show that ACE2 was expressed more on the apical than the basal surface and increased with the degree of differentiation of the animal cells (30, 72). Despite these interesting findings, immunohistochemical and in situ hybridization studies (54) of fatal human cases failed to show widespread involvement of the tracheobronchial tree compared to pneumocytes. The investigations by Jia and colleagues have shown that poorly differentiated primary human tracheobronchial cells or A549 cells grown on tissue culture plates express little ACE2 mRNA, which might limit their usefulness as models of SARS-CoV infection (30). It should also be borne in mind that not all the ACE2 antibodies that are available work reliably in archival tissue, and this may lead to discrepant findings between immunohistochemical results (26) and PCR findings. For instance, not all cells that express ACE2 are susceptible to virus infection (e.g., endothelial cells), and the presence of ACE2 in cell lines does not correlate with pathogenicity. Yamashita

and colleagues show that the colon carcinoma cell line CaCo-2 and Vero-E6 cells both express ACE2, yet only the latter show a cytopathic effect after SARS-CoV infection, implying that downsteam mechanisms are related to cytotoxicity (see below) (91). A number of other molecules, such as L-SIGN and DC-SIGN, have been demonstrated to bind SARS CoV (6, 29, 92), and at least one of these molecules, L-SIGN, mediates entry of SARS-CoV into cells. In general, these C-type lectins serve as binding receptors for viruses and may be relevant in transferring infectious virus bound to the surface of dendritic cells from one site to another. Of note, the binding site for L-SIGN on the SARS-CoV S protein has been identified and differs from the site that is responsible for binding to ACE2 (70). While L-SIGN may serve as a binding receptor under some circumstances, homozygosity for the neck repeat region of L-SIGN confers relative resistance to infection with SARS-CoV, perhaps by enhancing virus binding and degradation, thereby diminishing the ability of the molecule to mediate infection in *trans* (6).

The S protein of SARS-CoV also displays a degree of species specificity. For instance, the S protein of SARS-CoV strain Tor 2, a virus from the later phase of the outbreak in 2003, interacts efficiently with ACE2 of human and civet cat origin (48), allowing infection of both species. In contrast, the SARS-CoV S protein of civet origin binds well to ACE2 of civets but poorly to human ACE2. These differences were explored by Li et al., and in an elegant set of studies, it was shown that relatively small changes in the human ACE2 molecule converted it into a high-avidity binder for the palm civet S protein (48). Together, these results suggest that without prior adaptation, the civet virus is not well adapted to replicate in human cells. They also explain why the SARS-CoV-like virus found in civet cannot be maintained in culture in vitro in primate cell lines that effectively support the replication of human SARS-CoV. These results may also provide an explanation for the mild disease and low transmissibility observed when SARS-CoV reemerged from its animal reservoir to infect humans in December 2003 and January 2004. Furthermore, asymptomatic infections with SARS-CoV were uncommon during the outbreak of SARS in 2003 (40). Most persons at high risk through family or health care exposure either developed overt disease or did not seroconvert at all. This is in marked contrast to exposure to the precursor animal virus, in which asymptomatic infections were common (23). Since a potential source of a future reemergence of SARS is the bat-SARS-like CoV, comparable studies on the receptor binding of its S protein would be of interest.

## CLINICAL FEATURES

The clinical features of SARS have been reviewed in other reports (5, 11, 61) and are mentioned briefly. As befits its name, SARS typically presents as an illness with acute onset, fever, myalgia, malaise, and chills or rigor, without the rhinorrhea and sore throat that are commonly observed in patients with influenza (3, 60, 64, 80). A dry cough is common, but shortness of breath, tachypnea, or pleurisy is only prominent later in the course of the illness. About one-third of patients improve with resolution of radiographic changes. Others progress to have increasing shortness of breath, tachypnea, oxygen desaturation, worsening of chest signs on physical examination, and onset of diarrhea. In one study, tachycardia, unrelated to hypotension or fever, was present in 72% of patients (96). About 20 to 30% of all patients are admitted to intensive care units, and most of these require mechanical ventilation. The overall case fatality rate in the 2003 epidemic was 9.6%, and the terminal events were severe respiratory failure, multiple organ failure, sepsis, and intercurrent medical illness such as an acute myocardial infarction. Residual impairment of lung function persists in convalescence in over 20% of patients (57).

A watery diarrhea occurs in some patients, typically associated with clinical deterioration in the second week of the illness. This may result from direct infection of the gastrointestinal tract because ACE2 is expressed at high levels in the small intestine (26). Consistent with this, SARS-CoV infection of the gastrointestinal tract has been described (7, 15), although minimal cellular infiltrate or disruption of the intestinal architecture is detected. The reasons for this and the mechanism underlying the pathogenesis of diarrhea remain unclear, but it is worthy of note that clinical signs and histological findings are similar to those observed in cows infected with bovine coronavirus. It may be relevant that some human intestinal epithelial cell lines induce antiapoptotic cellular responses and support the persistent replication of SARs-CoV in vitro (14). Other extrapulmonary findings are less common but include hepatic dysfunction and central nervous system manifestations (15, 22, 89). Some of the latter may be related to therapies instituted for the treatment of SARS (see below).

Children have a much milder clinical course than adults (42). During the SARS outbreak in 2003, few children with SARS required intensive care, mortality was exceedingly rare, and it was rare for children to transmit infection to others. The basis for attenuated disease in children is not understood and may provide insight into factors important in SARS pathogenesis. Atypical presentations of SARS can occur in the elderly and in the immunocompromised. Patients may be afebrile and may present with nonspecific clinical symptoms such as decreased appetite or a general deterioration in their clinical condition. Such cases have led to nosocomial disease outbreaks with devastating consequences: transmission in the 2003 epidemic occurred disproportionately in hospital and health care settings (61).

The initial chest radiograph is abnormal in 60 to 100% of cases at initial presentation, depending on the duration of illness. It typically shows ground glass opacities and focal consolidation over the periphery and in the subpleural regions of the lower zones of the lung. As SARS progresses, abnormalities on chest radiographs are observed for all patients; the findings are consistent with severe lung disease and are not pathognomonic for SARS.

Retrospective studies have now identified a number of clinical and laboratory findings that predict outcome after SARS. Age, the presence of comorbidities, more extensive lung involvement, and abnormal lymphocyte subsets are poor prognostic indicators (8, 58). High viral loads in nasopharynx and serum early in the illness are an independent risk factor for mortality (12). Similarly, viral load in the nasopharynx and serum between days 10 and 15 of clinical illness also correlated with clinical outcome, including the need for mechanical ventilation and death (27). These findings suggest that the ultimate disease outcome is determined early in the course of the illness. Thus, the dose of the infecting virus inoculum, the early innate defenses of the host, or both are critical in determining the disease prognosis.

While there have been a number of attempts to try and predict SARS in the patients who present to accident and emergency departments, there is, unfortunately, no group of clinical or laboratory parameters that is unique for SARS (18). Therefore, identification of SARS-CoV or viral product in infected tissue or evidence of an antibody response to the virus is critical for diagnosis. Lymphopenia involving both CD4 and CD8 T cells is a common finding during the acute phase of SARS and is associated with an adverse outcome (85). This lymphopenia is rapidly reversed during convalescence. Some patients also have other hematological abnormalities, such as neutrophilia, a low platelet count, and an elevated plasma thromboplastin time.

## PATHOLOGICAL FINDINGS

The signs and symptoms of SARS in the early phase indicated that infection of the lower respiratory tract, and in particular the lung, rather than the upper respiratory tract was responsible for the severity of the disease. Within the acinus of the lung are a respiratory bronchiole, its distal alveolar duct, and alveolar sacs. Two types of epithelial cells line the alveoli: the flattened type 1 pneumocytes and the more cuboidal type 2. The type 1 pneumocytes are less numerous than the type 2 pneumocytes but have a large surface area. The epithelial cells are connected by tight junctions, but the underlying endothelial cells have leaky junctions that allow the extravasation of fluid. The type 1 cells are regarded as nonreplicating, whereas the type 2 cells are progenitor cells and replicate after injury to replace injured type 1 cells. This type 2 hyperplasia is interpreted as a nonspecific marker of alveolar injury and repair. In addition to the epithelial cells, alveolar macrophages are identified attached to the wall of the alveolus. These are nonspecific scavenger cells that are derived from monocytes that have emigrated from the blood and differ in function from the interstitial macrophages.

Autopsy findings in patients dying within the first 10 days of illness revealed diffuse alveolar damage, desquamation of pneumocytes, an inflammatory infiltrate, edema, and hyaline membrane formation (Color Plate 5A [see color insert]). From a pathogenic perspective this can be explained by damage to type 1 pneumocytes allowing the leakage of plasma proteins and inflammatory cells to produce the hyaline membranes. Patients dying later in the illness had an organizing diffuse alveolar damage (Color Plate 5B) together with squamous metaplasia and multinucleated giant cells of either macrophage or epithelial cell origin (16, 21, 41, 55). Focal thrombosis of pulmonary vessels was seen. When immunohistochemistry and in situ hybridization for SARS-CoV were used, virus-infected cells in the lung were identified by both techniques to be primarily flattened pneumocytes, i.e., those of type 1 morphology (Color Plate 5C), and macrophages (Color Plate 5D). Scanty positive bronchial epithelial cells have also been detected (54), and this has also been seen in a bronchial culture model (30, 72). Unlike with nonavian influenza virus infection, there is little histological evidence of bronchial epithelial cell necrosis. Viral antigen and RNA were detected by immunohistochemistry and in situ hybridization in lung biopsy or autopsy tissue of patients within the first 10 days of illness but rarely after then (Color Plate 5E) (54). We were, however, unable to detect virus antigen in lymph nodes draining the lung (unpublished observations). Although SARS-CoV could be detected in nasopharyngeal aspirates by PCR and culture, there have been no reports of the distribution of infected cells within the upper respiratory tract.

Although critical clinical symptoms relate to the respiratory tract, there have been contrasting reports on the extent of extrapulmonary virus dissemination. Evidence of SARS-CoV replication in the lungs and intestine is provided by detection of virus particles by electron microscopy, by virus isolation, and by the detection of viral antigens and nucleic acid by immunohistochemistry and in situ hybridization, respectively (4, 15, 33, 60). Viral RNA has also been detected using RT-PCR in lymph nodes, spleen, liver, heart, kidney, and skeletal muscle, suggesting multiorgan dissemination of the disease (19, 22), but in situ hybridization studies and immunohistochemistry do not fully support these findings (54). Lymphopenia is commonly detected in SARS, and necrosis and atrophy of the lymphoid tissue of lymph nodes and the white pulp of the spleen are observed at autopsy. Numbers of B and T lymphocytes, including both $CD4^+$ and $CD8^+$ T-lymphocyte subsets, natural killer cells, and dendritic cells, appear decreased during the acute stage of SARS. The mechanism underlying these findings remains obscure. Reductions in the white pulp of the spleen may reflect the endogenous stress response present in patients with severe illness; additionally, many SARS patients were treated with high-dose steroids, which also contribute to splenic atrophy. Lymphocytes do not carry ACE2 on their surface and appear to be refractory to virus infection. However, virus particles in lymphocytes were identified by electron microscopy in one study (22), although this has not been found by other investigators. Direct infection of lymphocytes, if confirmed, raises the possibility that destruction of lymphocytes by virus has a major role in pathogenesis. Independent of any direct infection of lymphocytes, apoptosis of bystander uninfected lymphocytes, as happens with other viral infections, may have contributed to the lymphopenia that was observed.

Viral RNA and antigen were also detected by RT-PCR and by immunohistochemistry in the brains of patients with SARS (22, 89); direct virus infection of the central nervous system may have contributed to long-term neurological or psychiatric sequelae in some patients.

The unique role that ACE2 has in lung protection may also contribute to severe disease in patients with SARS. It has been previously mentioned that ACE2 is likely to be the primary receptor for SARS-CoV. This enzyme is involved in the renin-angiotensin system, and it may have a protective effect in acute lung injury through its counterbalance of the effects of the stimulatory ACE1 and angiotensin (34). Downregulation of ACE2 may play a role in the pathogenesis of SARS and other infectious agents associated with acute lung injury leading to acute respiratory distress syndrome (ARDS); in the case of SARS, virus binding to ACE2 may directly cause its disappearance from the cell surface. In mouse models, treatment with recombinant human ACE2, or with inhibitors of the renin-angiotensin system, appears to mitigate the effects of acute lung injury. These may provide promising novel approaches for the management of SARS and ARDS in general (34).

## ANIMAL MODELS

Mice, ferrets, hamsters, and several species of nonhuman primates can be infected with SARS-CoV (reviewed in reference 77). Infection of cynomolgus macaques was used in the initial studies to fulfill Koch's postulates (20); however, others have had variable success in reproducing severe clinical illness in macaques. A recent study has found that SARS-CoV infection in cynomolgus macaques was associated with a pulmonary illness that was manifested as unifocal or multifocal pneumonia. However, the illness was more akin to the mild disease observed in children than the severe disease observed in adults (39). Immunocompetent mice and hamsters develop reproducible but clinically insignificant disease. Of note, aged mice or mice with defects in innate immunity develop more severe disease and may be useful for some studies. Thus far, the closest histological correlate for cellular tropism and lung damage is in nonhuman primates. Upper respiratory tract involvement was not reported in initial studies, but studies of African green monkeys do suggest that infection begins in airway cells, with subsequent spread to the alveoli (52). Laboratory infection of golden Syrian hamsters also shows a similar cellular pattern of infection, though hyaline membrane formation is not a conspicuous finding (68). However, it should be noted that occasional squamous cells and columnar cells of the upper respiratory tract in these hamsters did show the presence of SARS-CoV by immunohistochemistry. The next generation of animal models for SARS will involve the engineering of mice transgenic for expression of human ACE2, either under the control of a heterologous promoter or in place of murine ACE2 ("knock-in"). The latter approach, while more difficult, is advantageous because human ACE2 is expressed in the same cells as the endogenous protein.

## HOST RESPONSE TO SARS-CoV

Genetic polymorphisms associated with susceptibility to and disease severity of SARS have been identified. HLA-B*4601 was reported to associate with both disease susceptibility and severity in a Chinese population in Taiwan, but this association was not found in Hong Kong Chinese patients (53). In contrast, among Hong Kong Chinese, HLA-B*0703 rather than HLA-B*4601 was found to be associated with increased susceptibility to SARS. A number of polymorphisms in proteins involved in the innate immune response have been studied, including in L-selectin and mannose-binding lectin (6, 28). These polymorphisms show a statistically significant, but modest, effect on susceptibility to severe disease.

As described elsewhere in this volume, antiviral humoral and cellular immune responses are required for protective immunity against coronaviruses in general. The absence of significant human disease since 2003 and the absence of a reproducible animal model have hindered efforts to determine the components of an anti-SARS-CoV immune response. However, studies of patients from the 2003 epidemic showed that an anti-SARS-CoV antibody response developed 14 to 21 days postinfection. Antibodies against the SARS-CoV nucleocapsid and S proteins were detected in patients (43, 56). T-cell responses against the same two proteins have also been detected, and HLA-A-2-restricted epitopes have been identified in some cases (83, 98). Identification of SARS-CoV-specific T-cell epitopes will be useful in vaccine development.

Since one of the goals of characterizing the immune response is vaccine development, efforts were made to develop anti-SARS-CoV neutralizing antibodies that could be used either prophylactically or therapeutically. These antibodies would need to recognize both human and animal isolates of SARS-CoV, in order to prevent propagation and adaptation of animal isolates within human populations. As virus isolates from the earliest patients in the course of the outbreak in Guangdong or isolates of the animal precursor virus detected in civet are not available and have not yet been engineered using reverse-genetics methodology, virus neutralization of these animal-precursor-like viruses has been explored by generating lentivirus pseudotypes. These particles incorporate the S proteins from virus detected in civet (SZ3 and SZ16), early-phase human isolates (GD03, a civet-like virus isolated from humans following the reemergence of SARS in December 2003), or human strains isolated during the major SARS outbreak during early 2003 (e.g., Urbani) (93). The prototype Urbani virus isolated from a patient from the major human outbreak in 2003 was neutralized efficiently with homologous antibody as well as antibody to the animal-like SARS-CoV GD03. Surprisingly, the animal-precursor-like virus pseudotypes were refractory to neutralization both with homologous antibody and with antibody to the prototype Urbani virus. Indeed, the antibody to the Urbani virus enhanced virus entry of the civet SARS-CoV SZ3 and SZ16. The evasion of neutralization exhibited by the animal-precursor-like SARS-CoV was correlated with poor binding to the human ACE2 receptor. Neutralizing antibodies are usually directed against the receptor-binding domain of the S protein. Since this domain of the S protein is the one that is most likely to mutate during the process of adaptation to human ACE2, it is not surprising that antibodies could neutralize human but not animal isolates. Alternatively, it is possible that the animal precursor SARS-CoV uses a different receptor for viral entry and is thus able to evade neutralization by host antibody; however, there is no evidence for use of such a receptor.

A key component of the initial innate immune response to any virus infection is a type I interferon (IFN) response. The type I IFNs are potent antivirus cytokines that are produced by most cells in response to infection and activate the immune system. SARS interferes with the initiation of the innate response by inhibiting the expression of type I IFNs released by transformed cell lines, dendritic cells, and macrophages (10, 38, 75, 81). With other viral infections, IFN-β is initially produced in infected cells and its production requires phosphorylation and dimerization of a constitutively expressed protein, IFN-regulatory factor 3. However, IFN-regulatory factor 3 is not activated in SARS-CoV-infected cells in vitro (75). In contrast, a range of proinflammatory and macrophage-tropic chemokines are produced in SARS-CoV-infected macrophages.

Elevated levels of proinflammatory cytokines (interleukin 1 [IL-1], IL-6, and IL-12) and chemokines (CXCL8 [IL-8], CCL2 [MCP-1], and CXCL10 [IP-10]) are detected in the lungs and sera of patients with SARS in most, but not all, studies (10, 30a, 84a; reviewed in reference 62) and may also contribute to clinical disease and pathogenesis. CXCL8 is an attractant for neutrophils and may contribute to the neutrophilia that is observed in patients. Prolonged dysregulation of cytokine production has also been demonstrated by enzyme-linked immunospot assays in vitro (31, 38).

Collectively, these data suggest a model to explain the pathogenesis of SARS. The primary mechanism of pathogenesis in the lung is likely to be direct virus damage to primarily type 1 and, to a lesser extent, type 2 pneumocytes (54) (Fig. 1). SARS-CoV infection of primary human macrophages, dendritic cells, and tissue culture cells does not result in induction of a type I IFN response. Thus, a failure of the innate antiviral immune defenses of the host in the early stages of the disease may explain the progressive increase in viral load observed until day 10 postinfection. At this stage of illness, the adaptive immune responses become activated, presumably controlling further virus replication. Infiltration of macrophages into the lung is a prominent early manifestation of disease, perhaps contributing to immunopathological disease. By extension from in vitro analyses, SARS-CoV infection of these cells may result in the release of monocyte chemoattractants such as CCL2 and CXCL10, which are elevated in the sera of SARS patients. High SARS-CoV load, coupled with consequent expression of elevated levels of proinflammatory chemokines and cytokines, may result in the disease manifestations of SARS. While this model suggests that disease in SARS patients is partly immunopathological, this has not been confirmed either in infected patients or in any animal model. It is also not established that levels of proinflammatory cytokines or chemokines are higher in patients with SARS than in those with severe disease caused by other infectious agents. Baas and colleagues, using tissue profiling studies of patients who have died of ARDS with and without SARS, found no genes that could be attributed directly to SARS (2). These results further suggest that the pattern of cytokine dysregulation present in SARS patients is not unique and may reflect more the individual host immune response to severe pulmonary infection or the presence of preexisting pulmonary disease.

## THERAPY

No effective anti-SARS-CoV therapy is yet available. Many patients were treated with ribavirin and corticosteroids during the 2002–2003 SARS outbreak, based on the assumption that SARS-CoV would be susceptible to ribavirin and steroids would dampen an exuberant immune response. However, there is no evidence that the combination therapy improved outcomes. Treatment with type I IFN was also used in patients, but too few were treated to determine if this improved outcome. In support of the use of this therapy, treatment of experimentally infected macaques with pegylated IFN-α diminished clinical disease (25).

Several other approaches to therapy have been undertaken since 2003 (reviewed in references 59, 76, and 77). Fully human anti-SARS-CoV neutralizing antibodies have been developed and shown to be useful prophylactically in infected mice and hamsters. The SARS S protein has been expressed using heterologous vectors or by DNA immunization and shown

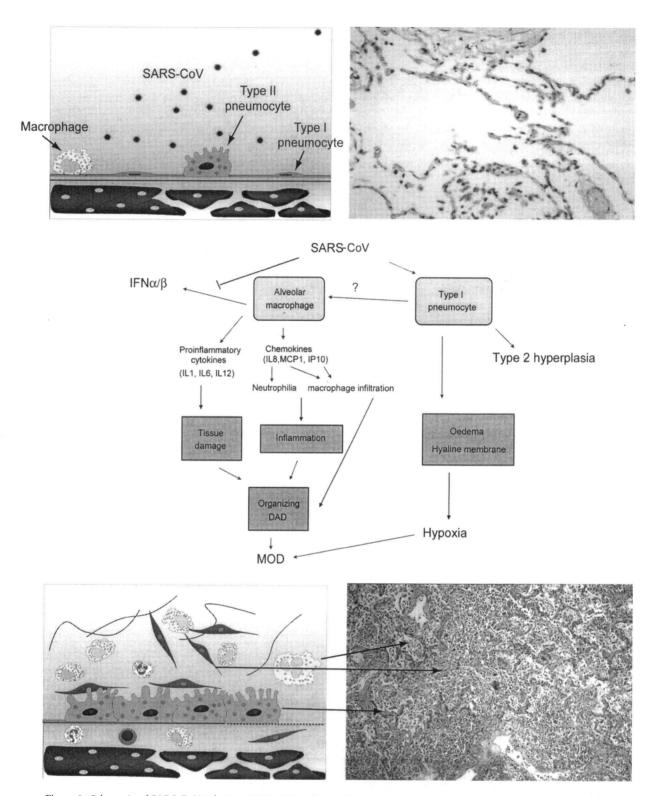

**Figure 1.** Schematic of SARS-CoV infection. SARS-CoV is detected in pneumocytes and in alveolar macrophages (upper left panel). Infection of macrophages results in the secretion of proinflammatory cytokines and chemokines but not IFN-β. Expression of these factors results in tissue damage, increased inflammation, and lung damage, resulting in the nonspecific pulmonary findings observed in patients with SARS (middle panel). As part of the disease process, infected type 1 pneumocytes slough into alveolar spaces and airways; regeneration is evidenced by proliferation of type 2 pneumocytes. Multinucleated giant cells are also observed in SARS-CoV-infected lungs (lower panels). Normal lung tissue is also shown (upper right panel).

to induce protective levels of anti-SARS-CoV antibody. Although vaccination with live attenuated SARS-CoV is likely to induce a potent protective immune response, the high rate of recombination exhibited by coronaviruses makes this approach less appealing. However, recent work suggests that it is possible to rewire the SARS-CoV genome, to attenuate the virus but also prevent recombination with wild-type SARS-CoV (95). If the rewired virus is immunogenic, this might be a very useful strategy for vaccine development. Finally, the structures of several SARS-CoV proteins, including the virus-encoded proteases (1, 65), have been determined and will be useful for the development of antiviral therapy. Because these proteins are virally encoded, molecules that inhibit their function should not inhibit host cell function.

## CONCLUSIONS

Clinical and pathological studies of SARS cases indicate that cells in the lower respiratory tract, particularly type 1 pneumocytes, are the prime targets of SARS, with macrophages subsequently being infected. Although ACE2 is the primary receptor for SARS, other receptors such as L-SIGN and DC-SIGN may facilitate virus infection, even under circumstances when the virus has not fully adapted to a new host. Epithelial lung damage together with macrophage activation results in increased levels of proinflammatory cytokines, which may result in additional tissue damage. The initial phase of lung disease exists for 10 to 14 days, after which many of the changes present can be attributed to the sequelae of diffuse lung damage, including the effects of mechanical ventilation. As with many other newly emerging infections, SARS had zoonotic origins, highlighting the need for a better understanding of the virus ecology of both wild and domestic animals. As many of these zoonoses do not cause disease in their natural host, surveillance needs to encompass viruses causing unobvious infections as well as those causing overt disease and will require the cooperation of multiple agencies, including those dealing with public health, veterinary medicine, and wildlife or the environment (36).

**Acknowledgments.** We thank Y. Guan, L. L. M. Poon, V. C. C. Cheng, and K. Y. Yuen for providing valuable references into the still rapidly evolving field of SARS pathogenesis and Kevin Fung for technical assistance in the SARS in situ hybridization and immunohistochemistry.

This work was supported in part by grants from the National Institutes of Health (PO1 AI060699).

## REFERENCES

1. Anand, K., J. Ziebuhr, P. Wadhwani, J. R. Mesters, and R. Hilgenfeld. 2003. Coronavirus main proteinase (3CLpro) structure: basis for design of anti-SARS drugs. *Science* 300:1763–1767.
2. Baas, T., J. K. Taubenberger, P. Y. Chong, P. Chui, and M. G. Katze. 2006. SARS-CoV virus-host interactions and comparative etiologies of acute respiratory distress syndrome as determined by transcriptional and cytokine profiling of formalin-fixed paraffin-embedded tissues. *J. Interferon Cytokine Res.* 26:309–317.
3. Booth, C. M., L. M. Matukas, G. A. Tomlinson, A. R. Rachlis, D. B. Rose, H. A. Dwosh, S. L. Walmsley, T. Mazzulli, M. Avendano, P. Derkach, I. E. Ephtimios, I. Kitai, B. D. Mederski, S. B. Shadowitz, W. L. Gold, L. A. Hawryluck, E. Rea, J. S. Chenkin, D. W. Cescon, S. M. Poutanen, and A. S. Detsky. 2003. Clinical features and short-term outcomes of 144 patients with SARS in the greater Toronto area. *JAMA* 289:2801–2809.
4. Chan, K. H., L. L. Poon, V. C. Cheng, Y. Guan, I. F. Hung, J. Kong, L. Y. Yam, W. H. Seto, K. Y. Yuen, and J. S. Peiris. 2004. Detection of SARS coronavirus in patients with suspected SARS. *Emerg. Infect. Dis.* 10:294–249.
5. Chan, P. K., J. W. Tang, and D. S. Hui. 2006. SARS: clinical presentation, transmission, pathogenesis and treatment options. *Clin. Sci. (London)* 110:193–204.
6. Chan, V. S., K. Y. Chan, Y. Chen, L. L. Poon, A. N. Cheung, B. Zheng, K. H. Chan, W. Mak, H. Y. Ngan, X. Xu, G. Screaton, P. K. Tam, J. M. Austyn, L. C. Chan, S. P. Yip, M. Peiris, U. S. Khoo, and C. L. Lin. 2006. Homozygous L-SIGN (CLEC4M) plays a protective role in SARS coronavirus infection. *Nat. Genet.* 38:38–46.
7. Chan, W. S., C. Wu, S. C. Chow, T. Cheung, K. F. To, W. K. Leung, P. K. Chan, K. C. Lee, H. K. Ng, D. M. Au, and A. W. Lo. 2005. Coronaviral hypothetical and structural proteins were found in the intestinal surface enterocytes and pneumocytes of severe acute respiratory syndrome (SARS). *Mod. Pathol.* 18:1432–1439.
8. Chau, T. N., P. O. Lee, K. W. Choi, C. M. Lee, K. F. Ma, T. Y. Tsang, Y. K. Tso, M. C. Chiu, W. L. Tong, W. C. Yu, and S. T. Lai. 2004. Value of initial chest radiographs for predicting clinical outcomes in patients with severe acute respiratory syndrome. *Am. J. Med.* 117:249–254.
9. Cheng, P. K., D. A. Wong, L. K. Tong, S. M. Ip, A. C. Lo, C. S. Lau, E. Y. Yeung, and W. W. Lim. 2004. Viral shedding patterns of coronavirus in patients with probable severe acute respiratory syndrome. *Lancet* 363:1699–1700.
10. Cheung, C. Y., L. L. M. Poon, I. H. Y. Ng, W. Luk, S.-F. Sia, M. H. S. Wu, K.-H. Chan, K.-Y. Yuen, S. Gordon, Y. Guan, and J. S. M. Peiris. 2005. Cytokine responses in severe acute respiratory syndrome coronavirus-infected macrophages in vitro: possible relevance to pathogenesis. *J. Virol.* 79:7819–7826.
11. Christian, M. D., S. M. Poutanen, M. R. Loutfy, M. P. Muller, and D. E. Low. 2004. Severe acute respiratory syndrome. *Clin. Infect. Dis.* 38:1420–1427.
12. Chu, C. M., V. C. Cheng, I. F. Hung, K. S. Chan, B. S. Tang, T. H. Tsang, K. H. Chan, and K. Y. Yuen. 2005. Viral load distribution in SARS outbreak. *Emerg. Infect. Dis.* 11:1882–1886.
13. Chu, D. K., L. L. Poon, K. H. Chan, H. Chen, Y. Guan, K. Y. Yuen, and J. S. Peiris. 2006. Coronaviruses in bent-winged bats (Miniopterus spp.). *J. Gen. Virol.* 87:2461–2466.
14. Cinatl, J., Jr., G. Hoever, B. Morgenstern, W. Preiser, J. U. Vogel, W. K. Hofmann, G. Bauer, M. Michaelis, H. F. Rabenau,

and H. W. Doerr. 2004. Infection of cultured intestinal epithelial cells with severe acute respiratory syndrome coronavirus. *Cell. Mol. Life Sci.* **61**:2100–2112.

15. Ding, Y., L. He, Q. Zhang, Z. Huang, X. Che, J. Hou, H. Wang, H. Shen, L. Qiu, Z. Li, J. Geng, J. Cai, H. Han, X. Li, W. Kang, D. Weng, P. Liang, and S. Jiang. 2004. Organ distribution of severe acute respiratory syndrome (SARS) associated coronavirus (SARS-CoV) in SARS patients: implications for pathogenesis and virus transmission pathways. *J. Pathol.* **203**:622–630.

16. Ding, Y., H. Wang, H. Shen, Z. Li, J. Geng, H. Han, J. Cai, X. Li, W. Kang, D. Weng, Y. Lu, D. Wu, L. He, and K. Yao. 2003. The clinical pathology of severe acute respiratory syndrome (SARS): a report from China. *J. Pathol.* **200**:282–289.

17. Drosten, C., S. Gunther, W. Preiser, S. van der Werf, H. R. Brodt, S. Becker, H. Rabenau, M. Panning, L. Kolesnikova, R. A. Fouchier, A. Berger, A. M. Burguiere, J. Cinatl, M. Eickmann, N. Escriou, K. Grywna, S. Kramme, J. C. Manuguerra, S. Muller, V. Rickerts, M. Sturmer, S. Vieth, H. D. Klenk, A. D. Osterhaus, H. Schmitz, and H. W. Doerr. 2003. Identification of a novel coronavirus in patients with severe acute respiratory syndrome. *N. Engl. J. Med.* **348**:1967–1976.

18. Fan, C. K., K. M. Yieh, M. Y. Peng, J. C. Lin, N. C. Wang, and F. Y. Chang. 2006. Clinical and laboratory features in the early stage of severe acute respiratory syndrome. *J. Microbiol. Immunol. Infect.* **39**:45–53.

19. Farcas, G. A., S. M. Poutanen, T. Mazzulli, B. M. Willey, J. Butany, S. L. Asa, P. Faure, P. Akhavan, D. E. Low, and K. C. Kain. 2005. Fatal severe acute respiratory syndrome is associated with multiorgan involvement by coronavirus. *J. Infect. Dis.* **191**:193–197.

20. Fouchier, R. A., T. Kuiken, M. Schutten, G. van Amerongen, G. J. van Doornum, B. G. van den Hoogen, M. Peiris, W. Lim, K. Stohr, and A. D. Osterhaus. 2003. Aetiology: Koch's postulates fulfilled for SARS virus. *Nature* **423**:240.

21. Franks, T. J., P. Y. Chong, P. Chui, J. R. Galvin, R. M. Lourens, A. H. Reid, E. Selbs, C. P. McEvoy, C. D. Hayden, J. Fukuoka, J. K. Taubenberger, and W. D. Travis. 2003. Lung pathology of severe acute respiratory syndrome (SARS): a study of 8 autopsy cases from Singapore. *Hum. Pathol.* **34**:743–748.

22. Gu, J., E. Gong, B. Zhang, J. Zheng, Z. Gao, Y. Zhong, W. Zou, J. Zhan, S. Wang, Z. Xie, H. Zhuang, B. Wu, H. Zhong, H. Shao, W. Fang, D. Gao, F. Pei, X. Li, Z. He, D. Xu, X. Shi, V. M. Anderson, and A. S. Leong. 2005. Multiple organ infection and the pathogenesis of SARS. *J. Exp. Med.* **202**:415–424.

23. Guan, Y., J. S. Peiris, B. Zheng, L. L. Poon, K. H. Chan, F. Y. Zeng, C. W. Chan, M. N. Chan, J. D. Chen, K. Y. Chow, C. C. Hon, K. H. Hui, J. Li, V. Y. Li, Y. Wang, S. W. Leung, K. Y. Yuen, and F. C. Leung. 2004. Molecular epidemiology of the novel coronavirus that causes severe acute respiratory syndrome. *Lancet* **363**:99–104.

24. Guan, Y., B. J. Zheng, Y. Q. He, X. L. Liu, Z. X. Zhuang, C. L. Cheung, S. W. Luo, P. H. Li, L. J. Zhang, Y. J. Guan, K. M. Butt, K. L. Wong, K. W. Chan, W. Lim, K. F. Shortridge, K. Y. Yuen, J. S. Peiris, and L. L. Poon. 2003. Isolation and characterization of viruses related to the SARS coronavirus from animals in southern China. *Science* **302**:276–278.

25. Haagmans, B. L., T. Kuiken, B. E. Martina, R. A. Fouchier, G. F. Rimmelzwaan, G. van Amerongen, D. van Riel, T. de Jong, S. Itamura, K. H. Chan, M. Tashiro, and A. D. Osterhaus. 2004. Pegylated interferon-alpha protects type 1 pneumocytes against SARS coronavirus infection in macaques. *Nat. Med.* **10**:290–293.

26. Hamming, I., W. Timens, M. L. Bulthuis, A. T. Lely, G. J. Navis, and H. van Goor. 2004. Tissue distribution of ACE2

protein, the functional receptor for SARS coronavirus. A first step in understanding SARS pathogenesis. *J. Pathol.* **203**:631–637.

27. Hung, I. F., V. C. Cheng, A. K. Wu, B. S. Tang, K. H. Chan, C. M. Chu, M. M. Wong, W. T. Hui, L. L. Poon, D. M. Tse, K. S. Chan, P. C. Woo, S. K. Lau, J. S. Peiris, and K. Y. Yuen. 2004. Viral loads in clinical specimens and SARS manifestations. *Emerg. Infect. Dis.* **10**:1550–1557.

28. Ip, W. K., K. H. Chan, H. K. Law, G. H. Tso, E. K. Kong, W. H. Wong, Y. F. To, R. W. Yung, E. Y. Chow, K. L. Au, E. Y. Chan, W. Lim, J. C. Jensenius, M. W. Turner, J. S. Peiris, and Y. L. Lau. 2005. Mannose-binding lectin in severe acute respiratory syndrome coronavirus infection. *J. Infect. Dis.* **191**:1697–1704.

29. Jeffers, S. A., S. M. Tusell, L. Gillim-Ross, E. M. Hemmila, J. E. Achenbach, G. J. Babcock, W. D. Thomas, Jr., L. B. Thackray, M. D. Young, R. J. Mason, D. M. Ambrosino, D. E. Wentworth, J. C. Demartini, and K. V. Holmes. 2004. CD209L (L-SIGN) is a receptor for severe acute respiratory syndrome coronavirus. *Proc. Natl. Acad. Sci. USA* **101**:15748–15753.

30. Jia, H. P., D. C. Look, L. Shi, M. Hickey, L. Pewe, J. Netland, M. Farzan, C. Wohlford-Lenane, S. Perlman, and P. B. McCray, Jr. 2005. ACE2 receptor expression and severe acute respiratory syndrome coronavirus infection depend on differentiation of human airway epithelia. *J. Virol.* **79**:14614–14621.

30a. Jiang, Y., J. Xu, C. Zhou, Z. Wu, S. Zhong, J. Liu, W. Luo, T. Chen, Q. Qin, and P. Deng. 2005. Characterization of cytokine and chemokine profiles of severe acute respiratory syndrome. *Am. J. Respir. Crit. Care Med.* **171**:850–857.

31. Jones, B. M., E. S. Ma, J. S. Peiris, P. C. Wong, J. C. Ho, B. Lam, K. N. Lai, and K. W. Tsang. 2004. Prolonged disturbances of in vitro cytokine production in patients with severe acute respiratory syndrome (SARS) treated with ribavirin and steroids. *Clin. Exp. Immunol.* **135**:467–473.

32. Kan, B., M. Wang, H. Jing, H. Xu, X. Jiang, M. Yan, W. Liang, H. Zheng, K. Wan, Q. Liu, B. Cui, Y. Xu, E. Zhang, H. Wang, J. Ye, G. Li, M. Li, Z. Cui, X. Qi, K. Chen, L. Du, K. Gao, Y. T. Zhao, X. Z. Zou, Y. J. Feng, Y. F. Gao, R. Hai, D. Yu, Y. Guan, and J. Xu. 2005. Molecular evolution analysis and geographic investigation of severe acute respiratory syndrome coronavirus-like virus in palm civets at an animal market and on farms. *J. Virol.* **79**:11892–11900.

33. Ksiazek, T. G., D. Erdman, C. S. Goldsmith, S. R. Zaki, T. Peret, S. Emery, S. Tong, C. Urbani, J. A. Comer, W. Lim, P. E. Rollin, S. F. Dowell, A. E. Ling, C. D. Humphrey, W. J. Shieh, J. Guarner, C. D. Paddock, P. Rota, B. Fields, J. DeRisi, J. Y. Yang, N. Cox, J. M. Hughes, J. W. LeDuc, W. J. Bellini, and L. J. Anderson. 2003. A novel coronavirus associated with severe acute respiratory syndrome. *N. Engl. J. Med.* **348**:1953–1966.

34. Kuba, K., Y. Imai, S. Rao, H. Gao, F. Guo, B. Guan, Y. Huan, P. Yang, Y. Zhang, W. Deng, L. Bao, B. Zhang, G. Liu, Z. Wang, M. Chappell, Y. Liu, D. Zheng, A. Leibbrandt, T. Wada, A. S. Slutsky, D. Liu, C. Qin, C. Jiang, and J. M. Penninger. 2005. A crucial role of angiotensin converting enzyme 2 (ACE2) in SARS coronavirus-induced lung injury. *Nat. Med.* **11**:875–879.

35. Kuiken, T., R. A. Fouchier, M. Schutten, G. F. Rimmelzwaan, G. van Amerongen, D. van Riel, J. D. Laman, T. de Jong, G. van Doornum, W. Lim, A. E. Ling, P. K. Chan, J. S. Tam, M. C. Zambon, R. Gopal, C. Drosten, S. van der Werf, N. Escriou, J. C. Manuguerra, K. Stohr, J. S. Peiris, and A. D. Osterhaus. 2003. Newly discovered coronavirus as the primary cause of severe acute respiratory syndrome. *Lancet* **362**:263–270.

36. Kuiken, T., F. A. Leighton, R. A. Fouchier, J. W. LeDuc, J. S. Peiris, A. Schudel, K. Stohr, and A. D. Osterhaus. 2005. Public

health. Pathogen surveillance in animals. *Science* 309:1680–1681.

37. Lau, S. K., P. C. Woo, K. S. Li, Y. Huang, H. W. Tsoi, B. H. Wong, S. S. Wong, S. Y. Leung, K. H. Chan, and K. Y. Yuen. 2005. Severe acute respiratory syndrome coronavirus-like virus in Chinese horseshoe bats. *Proc. Natl. Acad. Sci. USA* 102:14040–14045.

38. Law, H. K., C. Y. Cheung, H. Y. Ng, S. F. Sia, Y. O. Chan, W. Luk, J. M. Nicholls, J. S. Peiris, and Y. L. Lau. 2005. Chemokine upregulation in SARS coronavirus infected human monocyte derived dendritic cells. *Blood* 106:2366–2376.

39. Lawler, J. V., T. P. Endy, L. E. Hensley, A. Garrison, E. A. Fritz, M. Lesar, R. S. Baric, D. A. Kulesh, D. A. Norwood, L. P. Wasieloski, M. P. Ulrich, T. R. Slezak, E. Vitalis, J. W. Huggins, P. B. Jahrling, and J. Paragas. 2006. Cynomolgus macaque as an animal model for severe acute respiratory syndrome. *PLoS Med.* 3:e149.

40. Lee, H. K., E. Y. Tso, T. N. Chau, O. T. Tsang, K. W. Choi, and T. S. Lai. 2003. Asymptomatic severe acute respiratory syndrome-associated coronavirus infection. *Emerg. Infect. Dis.* 9:1491–1492.

41. Lee, N., D. Hui, A. Wu, P. Chan, P. Cameron, G. M. Joynt, A. Ahuja, M. Y. Yung, C. B. Leung, K. F. To, S. F. Lui, C. C. Szeto, S. Chung, and J. J. Sung. 2003. A major outbreak of severe acute respiratory syndrome in Hong Kong. *N. Engl. J. Med.* 348:1986–1994.

42. Leung, C. W., Y. W. Kwan, P. W. Ko, S. S. Chiu, P. Y. Loung, N. C. Fong, L. P. Lee, Y. W. Hui, H. K. Law, W. H. Wong, K. H. Chan, J. S. Peiris, W. W. Lim, Y. L. Lau, and M. C. Chiu. 2004. Severe acute respiratory syndrome among children. *Pediatrics* 113:e535–e543.

43. Leung, D. T., F. C. Tam, C. H. Ma, P. K. Chan, J. L. Cheung, H. Niu, J. S. Tam, and P. L. Lim. 2004. Antibody response of patients with severe acute respiratory syndrome (SARS) targets the viral nucleocapsid. *J. Infect. Dis.* 190:379–386.

44. Leung, D. T., W. W. van Maren, F. K. Chan, W. S. Chan, A. W. Lo, C. H. Ma, F. C. Tam, K. F. To, P. K. Chan, J. J. Sung, and P. L. Lim. 2006. Extremely low exposure of a community to severe acute respiratory syndrome coronavirus: false seropositivity due to use of bacterially derived antigens. *J. Virol.* 80:8920–8928.

45. Li, F., W. Li, M. Farzan, and S. C. Harrison. 2005. Structure of SARS coronavirus spike receptor-binding domain complexed with receptor. *Science* 309:1864–1868.

46. Li, W., M. J. Moore, N. Vasilieva, J. Sui, S. K. Wong, M. A. Berne, M. Somasundaran, J. L. Sullivan, K. Luzuriaga, T. C. Greenough, H. Choe, and M. Farzan. 2003. Angiotensin-converting enzyme 2 is a functional receptor for the SARS coronavirus. *Nature* 426:450–454.

47. Li, W., Z. Shi, M. Yu, W. Ren, C. Smith, J. H. Epstein, H. Wang, G. Crameri, Z. Hu, H. Zhang, J. Zhang, J. McEachern, H. Field, P. Daszak, B. T. Eaton, S. Zhang, and L. F. Wang. 2005. Bats are natural reservoirs of SARS-like coronaviruses. *Science* 310:676–679.

48. Li, W., C. Zhang, J. Sui, J. H. Kuhn, M. J. Moore, S. Luo, S. K. Wong, I. C. Huang, K. Xu, N. Vasilieva, A. Murakami, Y. He, W. A. Marasco, Y. Guan, H. Choe, and M. Farzan. 2005. Receptor and viral determinants of SARS-coronavirus adaptation to human ACE2. *EMBO J.* 24:1634–1643.

49. Lipsitch, M., T. Cohen, B. Cooper, J. M. Robins, S. Ma, L. James, G. Gopalakrishna, S. K. Chew, C. C. Tan, M. H. Samore, D. Fisman, and M. Murray. 2003. Transmission dynamics and control of severe acute respiratory syndrome. *Science* 300:1966–1970.

50. Lu, Y. T., P. J. Chen, C. Y. Sheu, and C. L. Liu. 2006. Viral load and outcome in SARS infection: the role of personal protective equipment in the emergency department. *J. Emerg. Med.* 30:7–15.

51. Marra, M. A., S. J. Jones, C. R. Astell, R. A. Holt, A. Brooks-Wilson, Y. S. Butterfield, J. Khattra, J. K. Asano, S. A. Barber, S. Y. Chan, A. Cloutier, S. M. Coughlin, D. Freeman, N. Girn, O. L. Griffith, S. R. Leach, M. Mayo, H. McDonald, S. B. Montgomery, P. K. Pandoh, A. S. Petrescu, A. G. Robertson, J. E. Schein, A. Siddiqui, D. E. Smailus, J. M. Stott, G. S. Yang, F. Plummer, A. Andonov, H. Artsob, N. Bastien, K. Bernard, T. F. Booth, D. Bowness, M. Czub, M. Drebot, L. Fernando, R. Flick, M. Garbutt, M. Gray, A. Grolla, S. Jones, H. Feldmann, A. Meyers, A. Kabani, Y. Li, S. Normand, U. Stroher, G. A. Tipples, S. Tyler, R. Vogrig, D. Ward, B. Watson, R. C. Brunham, M. Krajden, M. Petric, D. M. Skowronski, C. Upton, and R. L. Roper. 2003. The genome sequence of the SARS-associated coronavirus. *Science* 300:1399–1404.

52. McAuliffe, J., L. Vogel, A. Roberts, G. Fahle, S. Fischer, W. J. Shieh, E. Butler, S. Zaki, M. St.-Claire, B. Murphy, and K. Subbarao. 2004. Replication of SARS coronavirus administered into the respiratory tract of African green, rhesus and cynomolgus monkeys. *Virology* 330:8–15.

53. Ng, M. H., K. M. Lau, L. Li, S. H. Cheng, W. Y. Chan, P. K. Hui, B. Zee, C. B. Leung, and J. J. Sung. 2004. Association of human-leukocyte-antigen class I (B*0703) and class II (DRB1*0301) genotypes with susceptibility and resistance to the development of severe acute respiratory syndrome. *J. Infect. Dis.* 190:515–518.

54. Nicholls, J. M., J. Butany, L. L. Poon, K. H. Chan, S. L. Beh, S. Poutanen, J. S. Peiris, and M. Wong. 2006. Time course and cellular localization of SARS-CoV nucleoprotein and RNA in lungs from fatal cases of SARS. *PLoS Med.* 3:e27.

55. Nicholls, J. M., L. L. Poon, K. C. Lee, W. F. Ng, S. T. Lai, C. Y. Leung, C. M. Chu, P. K. Hui, K. L. Mak, W. Lim, K. W. Yan, K. H. Chan, N. C. Tsang, Y. Guan, K. Y. Yuen, and J. S. Peiris. 2003. Lung pathology of fatal severe acute respiratory syndrome. *Lancet* 361:1773–1778.

56. Nie, Y., G. Wang, X. Shi, H. Zhang, Y. Qiu, Z. He, W. Wang, G. Lian, X. Yin, L. Du, L. Ren, J. Wang, X. He, T. Li, H. Deng, and M. Ding. 2004. Neutralizing antibodies in patients with severe acute respiratory syndrome-associated coronavirus infection. *J. Infect. Dis.* 190:1119–1126.

57. Ong, K. C., A. W. Ng, L. S. Lee, G. Kaw, S. K. Kwek, M. K. Leow, and A. Earnest. 2004. Pulmonary function and exercise capacity in survivors of severe acute respiratory syndrome. *Eur. Respir. J.* 24:436–442.

58. Peiris, J. S., C. M. Chu, V. C. Cheng, K. S. Chan, I. F. Hung, L. L. Poon, K. I. Law, B. S. Tang, T. Y. Hon, C. S. Chan, K. H. Chan, J. S. Ng, B. J. Zheng, W. L. Ng, R. W. Lai, Y. Guan, and K. Y. Yuen. 2003. Clinical progression and viral load in a community outbreak of coronavirus-associated SARS pneumonia: a prospective study. *Lancet* 361:1767–1772.

59. Peiris, J. S., Y. Guan, and K. Y. Yuen. 2004. Severe acute respiratory syndrome. *Nat. Med.* 10:S88–S97.

60. Peiris, J. S., S. T. Lai, L. L. Poon, Y. Guan, L. Y. Yam, W. Lim, J. Nicholls, W. K. Yee, W. W. Yan, M. T. Cheung, V. C. Cheng, K. H. Chan, D. N. Tsang, R. W. Yung, T. K. Ng, and K. Y. Yuen. 2003. Coronavirus as a possible cause of severe acute respiratory syndrome. *Lancet* 361:1319–1325.

61. Peiris, J. S., K. Y. Yuen, A. D. Osterhaus, and K. Stohr. 2003. The severe acute respiratory syndrome. *N. Engl. J. Med.* 349:2431–2441.

62. Perlman, S., and A. A. Dandekar. 2005. Immunopathogenesis of coronavirus infections: implications for SARS. *Nat. Rev. Immunol.* 5:917–927.

63. Poon, L. L., D. K. Chu, K. H. Chan, O. K. Wong, T. M. Ellis, Y. H. Leung, S. K. Lau, P. C. Woo, K. Y. Suen, K. Y. Yuen,

Y. Guan, and J. S. Peiris. 2005. Identification of a novel coronavirus in bats. *J. Virol.* 79:2001–2009.

64. Poutanen, S. M., D. E. Low, B. Henry, S. Finkelstein, D. Rose, K. Green, R. Tellier, R. Draker, D. Adachi, M. Ayers, A. K. Chan, D. M. Skowronski, I. Salit, A. E. Simor, A. S. Slutsky, P. W. Doyle, M. Krajden, M. Petric, R. C. Brunham, and A. J. McGeer. 2003. Identification of severe acute respiratory syndrome in Canada. *N. Engl. J. Med.* 348:1995–2005.

65. Ratia, K., K. S. Saikatendu, B. D. Santarsiero, N. Barretto, S. C. Baker, R. C. Stevens, and A. D. Mesecar. 2006. Severe acute respiratory syndrome coronavirus papain-like protease: structure of a viral deubiquitinating enzyme. *Proc. Natl. Acad. Sci. USA* 103:5717–5722.

66. Ren, X., J. Glende, M. Al-Falah, V. de Vries, C. Schwegmann-Wessels, X. Qu, L. Tan, T. Tschernig, H. Deng, H. Y. Naim, and G. Herrler. 2006. Analysis of ACE2 in polarized epithelial cells: surface expression and function as receptor for severe acute respiratory syndrome-associated coronavirus. *J. Gen. Virol.* 87:1691–1965.

67. Riley, S., C. Fraser, C. A. Donnelly, A. C. Ghani, L. J. Abu-Raddad, A. J. Hedley, G. M. Leung, L. M. Ho, T. H. Lam, T. Q. Thach, P. Chau, K. P. Chan, S. V. Lo, P. Y. Leung, T. Tsang, W. Ho, K. H. Lee, E. M. Lau, N. M. Ferguson, and R. M. Anderson. 2003. Transmission dynamics of the etiological agent of SARS in Hong Kong: impact of public health interventions. *Science* 300:1961–1966.

68. Roberts, A., L. Vogel, J. Guarner, N. Hayes, B. Murphy, S. Zaki, and K. Subbarao. 2005. Severe acute respiratory syndrome coronavirus infection of golden Syrian hamsters. *J. Virol.* 79:503–511.

69. Rota, P. A., M. S. Oberste, S. S. Monroe, W. A. Nix, R. Campagnoli, J. P. Icenogle, S. Penaranda, B. Bankamp, K. Maher, M. H. Chen, S. Tong, A. Tamin, L. Lowe, M. Frace, J. L. DeRisi, Q. Chen, D. Wang, D. D. Erdman, T. C. Peret, C. Burns, T. G. Ksiazek, P. E. Rollin, A. Sanchez, S. Liffick, B. Holloway, J. Limor, K. McCaustland, M. Olsen-Rasmussen, R. Fouchier, S. Gunther, A. D. Osterhaus, C. Drosten, M. A. Pallansch, L. J. Anderson, and W. J. Bellini. 2003. Characterization of a novel coronavirus associated with severe acute respiratory syndrome. *Science* 300:1394–1399.

70. Shih, Y. P., C. Y. Chen, S. J. Liu, K. H. Chen, Y. M. Lee, Y. C. Chao, and Y. M. Chen. 2006. Identifying epitopes responsible for neutralizing antibody and DC-SIGN binding on the spike glycoprotein of the severe acute respiratory syndrome coronavirus. *J. Virol.* 80:10315–10324.

71. Simmons, G., J. D. Reeves, A. J. Rennekamp, S. M. Amberg, A. J. Piefer, and P. Bates. 2004. Characterization of severe acute respiratory syndrome-associated coronavirus (SARS-CoV) spike glycoprotein-mediated viral entry. *Proc. Natl. Acad. Sci. USA* 101:4240–4250.

72. Sims, A. C., R. S. Baric, B. Yount, S. E. Burkett, P. L. Collins, and R. J. Pickles. 2005. Severe acute respiratory syndrome coronavirus infection of human ciliated airway epithelia: role of ciliated cells in viral spread in the conducting airways of the lungs. *J. Virol.* 79:15511–15524.

73. Snijder, E. J., P. J. Bredenbeek, J. C. Dobbe, V. Thiel, J. Ziebuhr, L. L. Poon, Y. Guan, M. Rozanov, W. J. Spaan, and A. E. Gorbalenya. 2003. Unique and conserved features of genome and proteome of SARS-coronavirus, an early split-off from the coronavirus group 2 lineage. *J. Mol. Biol.* 331:991–1004.

74. Song, H. D., C. C. Tu, G. W. Zhang, S. Y. Wang, K. Zheng, L. C. Lei, Q. X. Chen, Y. W. Gao, H. Q. Zhou, H. Xiang, H. J. Zheng, S. W. Chern, F. Cheng, C. M. Pan, H. Xuan, S. J. Chen, H. M. Luo, D. H. Zhou, Y. F. Liu, J. F. He, P. Z. Qin, L. H. Li, Y. Q. Ren, W. J. Liang, Y. D. Yu, L. Anderson, M. Wang, R. H.

Xu, X. W. Wu, H. Y. Zheng, J. D. Chen, G. Liang, Y. Gao, M. Liao, L. Fang, L. Y. Jiang, H. Li, F. Chen, B. Di, L. J. He, J. Y. Lin, S. Tong, X. Kong, L. Du, P. Hao, H. Tang, A. Bernini, X. J. Yu, O. Spiga, Z. M. Guo, H. Y. Pan, W. Z. He, J. C. Manuguerra, A. Fontanet, A. Danchin, N. Niccolai, Y. X. Li, C. I. Wu, and G. P. Zhao. 2005. Cross-host evolution of severe acute respiratory syndrome coronavirus in palm civet and human. *Proc. Natl. Acad. Sci. USA* 102:2430–2435.

75. Spiegel, M., A. Pichlmair, L. Martinez-Sobrido, J. Cros, A. Garcia-Sastre, O. Haller, and F. Weber. 2005. Inhibition of beta interferon induction by severe acute respiratory syndrome coronavirus suggests a two-step model for activation of interferon regulatory factor 3. *J. Virol.* 79:2079–2086.

76. Stockman, L. J., R. Bellamy, and P. Garner. 2006. SARS: systematic review of treatment effects. *PLoS Med.* 3:e343.

77. Subbarao, K., and A. Roberts. 2006. Is there an ideal animal model for SARS? *Trends Microbiol.* 14:299–303.

78. Tang, X. C., J. X. Zhang, S. Y. Zhang, P. Wang, X. H. Fan, L. F. Li, G. Li, B. Q. Dong, W. Liu, C. L. Cheung, K. M. Xu, W. J. Song, D. Vijaykrishna, L. L. Poon, J. S. Peiris, G. J. Smith, H. Chen, and Y. Guan. 2006. Prevalence and genetic diversity of coronaviruses in bats from China. *J. Virol.* 80:7481–7490.

79. To, K. F., and A. W. Lo. 2004. Exploring the pathogenesis of severe acute respiratory syndrome (SARS): the tissue distribution of the coronavirus (SARS-CoV) and its putative receptor, angiotensin-converting enzyme 2 (ACE2). *J. Pathol.* 203:740–743.

80. Tsang, K. W., P. L. Ho, G. C. Ooi, W. K. Yee, T. Wang, M. Chan-Yeung, W. K. Lam, W. H. Seto, L. Y. Yam, T. M. Cheung, P. C. Wong, B. Lam, M. S. Ip, J. Chan, K. Y. Yuen, and K. N. Lai. 2003. A cluster of cases of severe acute respiratory syndrome in Hong Kong. *N. Engl. J. Med.* 348:1977–1985.

81. Tseng, C. T., L. A. Perrone, H. Zhu, S. Makino, and C. J. Peters. 2005. Severe acute respiratory syndrome and the innate immune responses: Modulation of effector cell function without productive infection. *J. Immunol.* 174:7977–7985.

82. Tu, C., G. Crameri, X. Kong, J. Chen, Y. Sun, M. Yu, H. Xiang, X. Xia, S. Liu, T. Ren, Y. Yu, B. T. Eaton, H. Xuan, and L. F. Wang. 2004. Antibodies to SARS coronavirus in civets. *Emerg. Infect. Dis.* 10:2244–2248.

83. Wang, Y. D., W. Y. Sin, G. B. Xu, H. H. Yang, T. Y. Wong, X. W. Pang, X. Y. He, H. G. Zhang, J. N. Ng, C. S. Cheng, J. Yu, L. Meng, R. F. Yang, S. T. Lai, Z. H. Guo, Y. Xie, and W. F. Chen. 2004. T-cell epitopes in severe acute respiratory syndrome (SARS) coronavirus spike protein elicit a specific T-cell immune response in patients who recover from SARS. *J. Virol.* 78:5612–5618.

84. Weiss, S. R., and S. Navas-Martin. 2005. Coronavirus pathogenesis and the emerging pathogen severe acute respiratory syndrome coronavirus. *Microbiol. Mol. Biol. Rev.* 69:635–664.

84a. Wong, C. K., C. W. Lam, A. K. Wu, W. K. Ip, N. L. Lee, I. H. Chan, L. C. Lit, D. S. Hui, M. H. Chan, S. S. Chung, and J. J. Sung. 2004. Plasma inflammatory cytokines and chemokines in severe respiratory syndrome. *Clin. Exp. Immunol.* 136:95–103.

85. Wong, R. S., A. Wu, K. F. To, N. Lee, C. W. Lam, C. K. Wong, P. K. Chan, M. H. Ng, L. M. Yu, D. S. Hui, J. S. Tam, G. Cheng, and J. J. Sung. 2003. Haematological manifestations in patients with severe acute respiratory syndrome: retrospective analysis. *BMJ* 326:1358–1362.

86. Woo, P. C., S. K. Lau, K. S. Li, R. W. Poon, B. H. Wong, H. W. Tsoi, B. C. Yip, Y. Huang, K. H. Chan, and K. Y. Yuen. 2006. Molecular diversity of coronaviruses in bats. *Virology* 351:180–187.

87. World Health Organization Multicentre Collaborative Network for Severe Acute Respiratory Syndrome Diagnosis.

2003. A multicentre collaboration to investigate the cause of severe acute respiratory syndrome. *Lancet* **361:**1730–1733.

88. Wu, D., C. Tu, C. Xin, H. Xuan, Q. Meng, Y. Liu, Y. Yu, Y. Guan, Y. Jiang, X. Yin, G. Crameri, M. Wang, C. Li, S. Liu, M. Liao, L. Feng, H. Xiang, J. Sun, J. Chen, Y. Sun, S. Gu, N. Liu, D. Fu, B. T. Eaton, L. F. Wang, and X. Kong. 2005. Civets are equally susceptible to experimental infection by two different severe acute respiratory syndrome coronavirus isolates. *J. Virol.* **79:**2620–2625.

89. Xu, J., S. Zhong, J. Liu, L. Li, Y. Li, X. Wu, Z. Li, P. Deng, J. Zhang, N. Zhong, Y. Ding, and Y. Jiang. 2005. Detection of severe acute respiratory syndrome coronavirus in the brain: potential role of the chemokine Mig in pathogenesis. *Clin. Infect. Dis.* **41:**1089–1096.

90. Xu, R. H., J. F. He, M. R. Evans, G. W. Peng, H. E. Field, D. W. Yu, C. K. Lee, H. M. Luo, W. S. Lin, P. Lin, L. H. Li, W. J. Liang, J. Y. Lin, and A. Schnur. 2004. Epidemiologic clues to SARS origin in China. *Emerg. Infect. Dis.* **10:**1030–1037.

91. Yamashita, M., M. Yamate, G. M. Li, and K. Ikuta. 2005. Susceptibility of human and rat neural cell lines to infection by SARS-coronavirus. *Biochem. Biophys. Res. Commun.* **334:**79–85.

92. Yang, Z. Y., Y. Huang, L. Ganesh, K. Leung, W. P. Kong, O. Schwartz, K. Subbarao, and G. J. Nabel. 2004. pH-dependent entry of severe acute respiratory syndrome coronavirus is mediated by the spike glycoprotein and enhanced by dendritic cell transfer through DC-SIGN. *J. Virol.* **78:**5642–5650.

93. Yang, Z. Y., H. C. Werner, W. P. Kong, K. Leung, E. Traggiai, A. Lanzavecchia, and G. J. Nabel. 2005. Evasion of antibody neutralization in emerging severe acute respiratory syndrome coronaviruses. *Proc. Natl. Acad. Sci. USA* **102:**797–801.

94. Yeh, S. H., H. Y. Wang, C. Y. Tsai, C. L. Kao, J. Y. Yang, H. W. Liu, I. J. Su, S. F. Tsai, D. S. Chen, and P. J. Chen. 2004. Characterization of severe acute respiratory syndrome coronavirus genomes in Taiwan: molecular epidemiology and genome evolution. *Proc. Natl. Acad. Sci. USA* **101:**2542–2547.

95. Yount, B., R. S. Roberts, L. Lindesmith, and R. S. Baric. 2006. Rewiring the severe acute respiratory syndrome coronavirus (SARS-CoV) transcription circuit: engineering a recombination-resistant genome. *Proc. Natl. Acad. Sci. USA* **103:**12546–12551.

96. Yu, C. M., R. S. Wong, E. B. Wu, S. L. Kong, J. Wong, G. W. Yip, Y. O. Soo, M. L. Chiu, Y. S. Chan, D. Hui, N. Lee, A. Wu, C. B. Leung, and J. J. Sung. 2006. Cardiovascular complications of severe acute respiratory syndrome. *Postgrad. Med. J.* **82:**140–144.

97. Zeng, F. Y., C. W. Chan, M. N. Chan, J. D. Chen, K. Y. Chow, C. C. Hon, K. H. Hui, J. Li, V. Y. Li, C. Y. Wang, P. Y. Wang, Y. Guan, B. Zheng, L. L. Poon, K. H. Chan, K. Y. Yuen, J. S. Peiris, and F. C. Leung. 2003. The complete genome sequence of severe acute respiratory syndrome coronavirus strain HKU-39849 (HK-39). *Exp. Biol. Med.* (Maywood) **228:**866–873.

98. Zhou, M., D. Xu, X. Li, H. Li, M. Shan, J. Tang, M. Wang, F. S. Wang, X. Zhu, H. Tao, W. He, P. Tien, and G. F. Gao. 2006. Screening and identification of severe acute respiratory syndrome-associated coronavirus-specific CTL epitopes. *J. Immunol.* **177:**2138–2145.

*Nidoviruses*
Edited by S. Perlman, T. Gallagher, and E. J. Snijder
© 2008 ASM Press, Washington, DC

Chapter 20

# Pathogenesis of Human Coronaviruses Other than Severe Acute Respiratory Syndrome Coronavirus

PIERRE J. TALBOT, HÉLÈNE JACOMY, AND MARC DESFORGES

Human coronavirus (HCoV) was first isolated in the mid-1960s from patients with upper respiratory tract disease. Indeed, as soon as 1965, Tyrrell and Bynoe propagated a new infectious agent on human embryonic tracheal organ culture, and intranasal inoculation of the original specimen caused common colds in human volunteers (99). Even though it was not possible to grow the infectious agent in cell lines, electron microscopy revealed virus-like particles similar to infectious bronchitis virus, which had been identified almost 20 years before (11). This new coronavirus was named the B814 strain (99). Shortly thereafter, Hamre and Procknow (43) passaged clinical samples on human embryonic kidney cells, leading to the discovery and isolation of the prototype HCoV-229E strain. At around the same time, McIntosh and collaborators (64), also using organ cultures, identified different viruses, which were designated OC, for organ cultures. The now-recognized prototype HCoV-OC43 strain was among these OC viruses and was adapted to grow in established cell lines. The characteristic "crown-like" ("*corona*" in Latin) morphological appearance of coronaviruses was established by Almeida and Tyrrell (1), from studies of infectious bronchitis virus and the B814 and 229E viruses, and the name coronavirus was born (1); the creation of the new *Coronaviridae* family took place shortly thereafter (97, 98).

Before severe acute respiratory syndrome (SARS) appeared in China in the fall of 2002 and was associated with SARS coronavirus (SARS-CoV) (25, 38, 54), serological studies only distinguished between two groups of HCoV, namely, HCoV-229E (group 1) and HCoV-OC43 (group 2). These viruses were considered responsible for 10 to 35% of common colds in humans (70). Since the SARS outbreak of 2002–2003, research on coronaviruses has entered into a new era and other HCoVs have been identified. These newly described HCoVs are the three highly related group 1 strains NL63 (103), NL (37), and New Haven (NH) (31), probably representing three different strains of the same virus (53), and the group 2 strain HKU1 (114). All known HCoV strains have a worldwide distribution and are recognized pathogens of the upper and lower respiratory tract. Even though no clear and direct association has ever been made between HCoV and other types of pathology, epidemiological studies have suggested a possible association between the presence of these ubiquitous and "innocuous" human viruses and the establishment and/or the exarcerbation of enteric and neurological disease.

## EPIDEMIOLOGY

HCoVs are endemic, and infections mainly occur in the winter and early spring (57, 70). The most probable route of entry of HCoV appears to be the nasal mucosa, and horizontal transmission via small aerosols is possible, at least for HCoV-229E (87).

Although HCoVs other than SARS-CoV are primarily associated with mild upper and lower respiratory tract disease, with the common cold the typical HCoV-induced pathology (70), HCoV was regularly associated with severe respiratory distress in newborns (39, 85, 86) and recognized as an important trigger of acute asthma exacerbations (29, 52, 71). More recently, both previously (229E and OC43) and newly (NL63 and HKU1) described HCoVs have

Pierre J. Talbot, Hélène Jacomy, and Marc Desforges • Laboratoire de neuroimmunovirologie, INRS-Institut Armand-Frappier, Laval, Québec H7V 1B7, Canada.

been associated with more severe acute lower respiratory tract infection, including pneumonia, in both infants and immunocompromised patients (40, 114). Moreover, various reports have implicated the 229E and OC43 groups in other pathologies, such as myocardites and meningites (80) and severe diarrhea (41, 78). Over the years, several reports have also suggested a possible link between the presence of HCoV within the human central nervous system (CNS) and various neurological disorders such as multiple sclerosis (MS), Parkinson's disease (PD), and encephalitis (5, 23, 34, 35, 45, 119).

### The Pre-SARS Era: HCoV-229E and HCoV-OC43

Together, HCoV-229E and HCoV-OC43 are responsible for up to one-third of common colds (70). Epidemiological surveys from the 1970s showed that these viruses have a worldwide distribution and that they circulate during seasonal outbreaks of respiratory infections (102). Nosocomial (hospital-acquired) upper respiratory tract infections with these two HCoVs were reported for premature newborns with apnea and bradycardia (85). Moreover, HCoV-229E was also found to be a common cause of nosocomial lower respiratory tract infection in a day care center for elderly people (33), and HCoV-229E-related pneumonia was also described for immunocompromised patients (40, 75).

Recent phylogenetic analysis based on the spike (S) and nucleocapsid (N) protein genes of HCoV-229E revealed that several different variants, causing different types of respiratory tract infections, were isolated from patients in Australia between 1979 and 2004. The sequencing and analysis of these HCoV-229E variants strongly suggested that genetic drift had occurred. However, the similarity among these variants circulating in Australia and other strains identified in other geographical locations during the same period revealed that HCoV-229E has not undergone major recombination since its isolation in 1967 (20). Even though the genetic stability of HCoV-OC43 was reported (92), sequencing of the HCoV-OC43 S gene isolated from a collection of respiratory tract specimens from neonates and infants at the University Hospital in Leuven, Belgium, revealed variability among field isolates. Unlike for HCoV-229E, the high degree of variability raised the possibility that several genetically distinct HCoV-OC43 strains with different temporal and possible geographical patterns circulated between January 2003 and March 2004 in Belgium (106).

Most coronaviruses exhibit a strict host species specificity, but as suggested by Butler and colleagues (18), HCoV-OC43 may represent a special case.

Indeed, sialic acid in the form of N-acetyl-9-O-acetylneuraminic acid was identified as a ligand for the S protein of HCoV-OC43 (55). The use of such a ubiquitous sugar moiety as a receptor at the cell surface may enable the virus to infect a broader range of species (18). Furthermore, a molecular clock analysis of the S gene sequences of bovine coronavirus (BCoV) and HCoV-OC43 suggests that a zoonotic transmission could have occurred in the late 19th century. Indeed, it is tempting to speculate that a worldwide human "influenza" epidemic that probably originated in Asia between 1889 and 1890 may have resulted from interspecies transmission of BCoV to humans. Thus, HCoV-OC43 could be a human-adapted strain of BCoV (108). The same report suggests that the most recent common ancestor of BCoV and HCoV-OC43 would have evolved in 1890 and that the "influenza-associated" epidemic induced pronounced CNS symptoms (108). A more recent report from the same authors even suggests that porcine hemagglutinating encephalomyelitis virus, a respiratory pathogen in piglets with neuroinvasive properties causing motor disorders, could have diverged from the common ancestor of BCoV and HCoV-OC43 around 1848 (105). These facts are interesting, considering that neuroinvasive properties were previously described for HCoV-OC43 in humans (5).

### Neuroinvasiveness and Neurotropism of HCoV-OC43 and HCoV-229E

The presence of viruses in the human CNS is now a recognized fact; the concept of a viral flora of the brain is emerging, with unpredictable consequences, be they detrimental (neurological disease) or beneficial (as for the bacterial flora in the intestine). Viral detection in the cerebrospinal fluid (CSF) of patients is seen as one indication of the ability of viruses to cross the blood-brain barrier. Viral infection of the human CNS may lead to acute encephalitis, which can even lead to death, depending on the cellular and anatomic tropism of different viruses (112). However, it has been more difficult to prove a causal role for any given virus in several chronic human neurological diseases, in part due to the difficulty in determining the relationship between the time of viral infection and the onset of disease. It has been suggested that certain childhood infections may increase the risk of age-related neurodegenerative disorders, although the evidence that supports these hypotheses is largely circumstantial (63). The close structural and biological relatedness of HCoV to the neurotropic coronaviruses of mice and pigs has led to speculation about the possible involvement of HCoV in neurological diseases (93, 94). Even though no clear specific association has been demonstrated for any known human neuropathology, HCoV-229E and HCoV-OC43 were clearly shown to be neuroinvasive and neurotropic (4–6, 13).

### Circumstantial Association of HCoV and Human Neuropathologies

The presence of HCoV has been detected in different neurological diseases in humans (although its presence obviously does not necessarily mean an etiologic association).

#### PD

An association with PD was based on the localization of mouse hepatitis virus antigens in basal ganglia; this was postulated to contribute to the eventual development of postencephalitic parkinsonism (35). This linkage was strengthened by a report of antiviral antibodies (34) and HCoV RNAs (23) in the CSF of PD patients. Moreover, detection of viral RNA in PD patient brains revealed that three out of three patients were positive for HCoV-229E and one was also positive for HCoV-OC43 (5). Genetic and environmental factors seem to be involved in the etiology of PD (72), and an increased percentage of health care workers and teachers with PD was reported, suggesting the possibility that a high level of exposure to viral or other respiratory infections was a risk factor for PD (96).

#### MS

MS represents another human neurological disease in which a virus likely plays a triggering role in genetically predisposed individuals (56). Many investigators believe that several viruses could be involved in triggering MS but that they may do so through similar direct and/or indirect mechanisms. Indeed, various, mostly neurotropic, viruses have been implicated in MS pathogenesis over the years (42, 51, 93). However, research has not led to the isolation of any specific virus with a direct link to MS. Association of coronaviruses with MS was suggested by their isolation from the CNS of two patients (17). These viruses were initially isolated by passage in mice, raising the concern that they were actually murine in origin (36, 110). However, reports by the same group appear to strengthen their possible relevance: preferential association of murine-like coronavirus genes with brain tissues from MS patients was observed (67), and primates were shown to be susceptible to murine coronavirus-induced demyelinating disease after intracerebral (68, 69) or peripheral (19) inoculation. Thus, isolates

from MS patients may have derived from infection by "murine-like" viruses. Other reports describe intrathecal antibody synthesis (81) and coronaviral RNA in the CSF (23) and in brain tissue (90) of patients. One study showed a significant association of colds with MS exacerbations, and a significant association of HCoV-229E infection with MS (45). Interestingly, the first report on the association of viral infections and MS (84) commented that seasonal HCoV infection patterns do fit the observed occurrence of MS exacerbations.

### Other neurological diseases

Acute disseminated encephalomyelitis is a neurological disorder characterized by inflammation of the brain and spinal cord and damage to the myelin sheath. It occurs most frequently after upper respiratory tract infections. Even though the etiologic agent remains unknown, HCoV-OC43 was detected in the CNS of a child with acute disseminated encephalomyelitis (119).

Although any possible association between HCoV and specific neuropathology remains to be confirmed and characterized, the detection of RNA by reverse transcriptase PCR and in situ hybridization in human brains does confirm that HCoVs are neuroinvasive (5).

### The Post-SARS Era

#### The HCoV-NL63 group

During the 2002–2003 winter season, a new HCoV, strain NL63, was isolated in The Netherlands (103). Initially isolated from a young child with lower respiratory tract disease, NL63 represents a group of newly described group 1 coronaviruses which are associated with both upper and lower respiratory tract disease, particularly in young children. Even though its discovery was published only in 2004, HCoV-NL63 has now been detected in clinical samples from patients with acute respiratory tract infection worldwide. Indeed, in the year following its description, the presence of the virus was associated with acute respiratory tract infection, mainly in children and young adults, in The Netherlands (104), Belgium (66), France (101), Canada (9, 10), Australia (7), Japan (26), and China (21). Therefore, HCoV-NL63 now has to be considered an important etiologic agent of upper and lower respiratory tract infections in humans.

Shortly after the publication of the discovery of HCoV-NL63 at the Amsterdam Medical Center (103), a report from the Rotterdam Erasmus Medical Center described a newly identified HCoV (named

HCoV-NL) from a clinical sample obtained in 1988 (37). Furthermore, less than a year later, the discovery of the New Haven coronavirus (HCoV-NH) in the United States was described at Yale University (31). An association was suggested between HCoV-NH and Kawasaki disease (30), a systemic inflammatory disease of unknown etiology, but this possible association is controversial, as two reports have failed to show any link between this disease and HCoV-NH (12, 27). As mentioned above, HCoV-NL63, -NL, and -NH probably represent three strains of the same viral species.

## HCoV-HKU1

Recently, the discovery of a novel HCoV in the nasopharyngeal aspirates of a 71-year-old man and a 35-year-old woman, both with pneumonia, was reported. The sequence of the entire genome revealed that this newly discovered HCoV (named HKU1 for Hong Kong University 1) was a distant member of group 2 coronaviruses (114). Since the publication of its discovery in January 2005, two different genotypes of HCoV-HKU1 have been detected in Hong Kong in a "cohort" of 10 patients who suffered from pneumonia (115). Sequence analysis performed on the polymerase and S and N genes demonstrated that the 10 isolates did not come from a single outbreak, and analysis of the S and N genes also revealed that two different genotypes (A and B) of HCoV-HKU1 were circulating in Hong Kong between 22 March 2003 and 21 March 2004 (115). Shortly thereafter, HCoV-HKU1 was detected in 10 patients (mainly young children) with upper or lower respiratory tract infection in Australia (89). Other studies have now identified strains of HKU1 circulating in New Haven, CT, using nasopharyngeal swabs and aspirates from children with either upper or lower respiratory tract infection (32) and at the Caen University Hospital in Caen, France, in respiratory and stool samples from either children or young adults (100). Recently, it was shown that a third HKU1 genotype (type C) has emerged from recombination between types A and B (116).

### Lessons for the future

As mentioned earlier, based mainly on serological data, HCoV-229E and HCoV-OC43 were the only known representatives of HCoV until very recently. As other strains were also detected during the 1960s, including the B814 strain, the existence of other serologically unrelated HCoVs was already considered highly probable in the mid-1990s (70). Therefore, the discovery of previously unknown members of the HCoVs in recent years was not surprising.

The medical importance of coronaviruses was suspected by some investigators for years, but it was not taken seriously until the SARS pandemic (88) showed that these ubiquitous "benign" viruses caused the first pandemic of the 21st century. International interest in coronaviruses has transformed the field and will surely lead to breakthroughs in the future. Moreover, this event emphasizes the need for research on a wide variety of viruses, not only the "virus du jour."

## PATHOGENESIS

### Cellular Receptors and Target Cells in the Respiratory Tract

HCoVs are recognized endemic human respiratory pathogens. Infections mostly occur during winter and spring within all age groups, and reinfections are common. However, even though they have been associated with pathology of the upper and lower respiratory tract for about 40 years now, the mechanisms underlying HCoV pathogenesis are still poorly understood.

One of the factors that influences a virus-induced pathogenesis is distribution of susceptible cells in the host, since virus binding to its target cell through a specific receptor is a critical early step in the infectious process. HCoV-229E uses aminopeptidase N, also called CD13 (118). SARS-CoV (60) and HCoV-NL63 (44) use angiotensin-converting enzyme 2 (ACE2); SARS-CoV can also use L-SIGN (CD209L), although L-SIGN is likely to function primarily to enhance infection rather than serve as a primary receptor (48). However, the cellular receptor for HCoV-HKU1 and HCoV-OC43 remains to be identified, even though sialic acid in the form of N-acetyl-9-O-acetylneuraminic acid was identified as a ligand for the S protein of HCoV-OC43 (55). All of the known receptors mentioned above have been shown to be expressed in different cell types within the respiratory tract and other tissues.

HCoVs other than SARS-CoV have been associated with different types of human pathology, but most often, these viruses cause diseases which are limited to the respiratory tract. A report on HCoV-229E infection of differentiated human airway epithelia revealed a polarized infection and a release of virions from the apical side of the cells towards the lumen in the airways (109). This could facilitate the following rounds of infection while limiting exposure of viral antigens to the immune system and the likelihood of systemic infection (109). ACE2, the cellular receptor for both SARS-CoV and HCoV-NL63, is also expressed on the apical surface of well-differentiated polarized airway epithelia, with the strongest expression on ciliated cells. These are the main target cells of SARS-CoV and, most probably, of HCoV-NL63 (50). Moreover, SARS-CoV particles are also preferentially released through the apical side of the target cells, but no such data are available for HCoV-NL63 (50). The main target cell in the respiratory tract for infection by HCoV-HKU1 and HCoV-OC43 is currently not known.

### Monocytes/Macrophages and Dendritic Cells as Targets of Infection

Even though HCoVs are recognized respiratory pathogens in humans, viral material, in the form of infectious particles, antigens, or RNA, was detected in tissues other than the respiratory tract. For example, infection of human monocytic cell lines and of primary monocytes/macrophages by HCoV-229E was reported (22, 24). Infection of peritoneal macrophages (74) and murine dendritic cells expressing human aminopeptidase N by HCoV-229E (111) suggests that HCoVs may use cells from the myeloid lineage to disseminate to other tissues, including the CNS (Fig. 1), where it could be associated with other types of pathologies.

Moreover, HCoV-229E-infected monocytes/macrophages eventually die by apoptosis in vitro when infection is performed at a high multiplicity of infection (22, 24). As previously suggested for the Theiler's murine encephalomyelitis virus, apoptosis might represent a mechanism by which HCoV-229E, which is cytolytic, is partially restricted in its replication in monocytic cells (82). Even though apoptosis is often presented as a potent defense mechanism for the host because it limits viral propagation (8), it could also help the virus to propagate from monocytes to monocytes or to macrophages, since phagocytosis of apoptotic cells by uninfected neighboring cells could contribute to the propagation and perpetuation of the infection, without extensive extracellular exposure of virus to the immune system (49).

Interestingly, the human monocytic cell line THP-1 is activated to produce tumor necrosis factor alpha (TNF-α) and matrix metalloproteinase 9 (MMP-9) following infection by HCoV-229E (24). Since monocytes mature into macrophages prior to tissue invasion, this activation of THP-1 cells suggests that HCoV-229E-infected monocytes would become activated in vivo. This maturation would facilitate their migration to additional tissues, especially in immunocompromised individuals, as was observed in mice infected with murine cytomegalovirus (79). The fact that HCoV-229E could only infect immunocompromised human aminopeptidase N (hAPN)-transgenic mice (58) raises the possibility that HCoV-229E could take advantage of an immunosuppressed environment to disseminate to different organs within susceptible individuals. The establishment of a persistent infection in a human

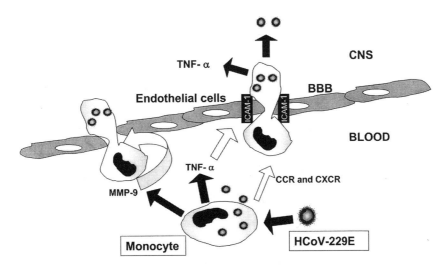

Figure 1. Human monocytic cells are susceptible to productive HCoV-229E infection, are activated following infection, and could serve as a viral reservoir for access to the CNS. Infected monocytic cells are activated and can produce TNF-α, which can induce the up-regulation of the adhesion molecule ICAM-1 on endothelial cells forming the blood-brain barrier (BBB), facilitating adhesion and passage of monocytes into the CNS. Infected and activated monocytic cells can also produce MMP-9. This metalloproteinase can induce an increased permeabilization of the BBB, also facilitating the passage of leukocytes into the CNS. Infection may also induce an up-regulation of chemokine receptors at the cell surface, also facilitating the passage of leukocytes into the CNS.

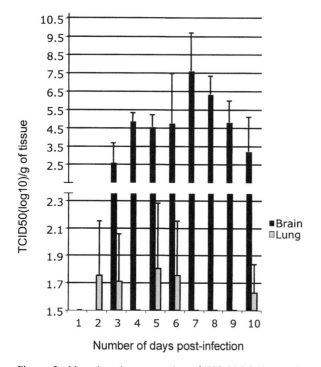

**Figure 2.** Neuroinvasive properties of HCoV-OC43 in mice. Fourteen-day-old C57BL/6 mice were infected intranasally with HCoV-OC43 (5,000 50% tissue culture infective doses [TCID$_{50}$]). Five animals were sacrificed every 24 h, and virus titers were measured in the CNS and lung. Infectious HCoV-OC43 was detectable in the brain as soon as 3 days postinfection and reached its maximum titer a few days later. Virus was also detected in the lungs. The detection limit of the assay was $10^{1.5}$ TCID$_{50}$/g. Inhalation of virus led to a generalized infection of the CNS and 90% mortality from encephalitis, demonstrating the neuroinvasiveness and neurovirulence of HCoV-OC43.

leukocytic cell line (24) is also consistent with the possibility that monocytes/macrophages serve as a reservoirs and vectors for HCoV-229E spread to tissues, including the CNS (5). Moreover, HCoV-OC43 was shown to infect the lungs in infected mice (47) (Fig. 2) and to be neuroinvasive after intranasal infection (18, 92) (Fig. 2). The latter suggests that virus may enter the CNS through the olfactory nerve and subsequent transneuronal spread.

Using nucleic acid amplification tests, identification of viral infections in respiratory tract samples is now much easier to perform (59, 107). The increased sensitivity of these techniques may lead to the discovery of new sites of viral replication within previously unsuspected targeted organs. This would have implications for virus-related human diseases, including those of the CNS.

## HCoVs and Human Neuropathologies

Even though the link between the presence of the virus and neurological diseases remains uncertain,

data from studies with both human material and animal models suggest that HCoVs could contribute to neurological diseases by direct or indirect mechanisms. Direct virus-induced neuronal death is one mechanism that may contribute to neuropathogenesis following CNS infection (3). On the other hand, various indirect causes of neuronal death leading to neurological disease exist. First, neuronal death or dysfunction could result from a bystander effect, since adjacent infected or inflamed glial cells have the potential to produce neurotoxic factors. Other indirect mechanisms involve the activation or reactivation of autoreactive T cells by epitope (determinant) spreading resulting from collateral inflammation and the release of autoantigens not cross-reactive with the disease-inducing epitope (65). Alternatively, determinants shared between microbes and self-peptides may also result in indirect tissue destruction, in a process known as molecular mimicry (73) (Fig. 3).

The development of an animal model of HCoV-OC43-induced CNS disease (47) has allowed the identification of molecular and cellular processes associated with neurological disease. Indeed, data obtained from this animal model indicate that neurons are the main target cells for HCoV-OC43 (47) and that they undergo nuclear fragmentation associated with activated caspase 3 positive staining, suggesting that infection can directly induce neuronal death (46). Apoptosis of neurons also occurs in the CNS of mice with acute encephalitis, suggesting that this mechanism could play a role in HCoV-OC43-induced neuropathogenesis (46).

On the other hand, HCoV-OC43 infection of mixed primary cultures of neural cells resulted in activation and release of proinflammatory molecules, including high levels of TNF-α, which, in turn, could contribute to apoptosis and neuronal degeneration. HCoV-OC43 can also infect primary cultures of human astrocytic and microglial cells (13) and activate human microglial and astrocytic cell lines to produce proinflammatory molecules that could be deleterious to neurons or myelin-producing oligodendrocytes (28).

HCoV-induced activation of autoreactive T cells may also be associated with neuropathology. Indeed, HCoV-229E and HCoV-OC43 can activate T cells cross-reactive for viral and myelin antigens in MS patients but not controls, presumably by molecular mimicry (15, 95). On the other hand, treatment of infected mice with the immunosuppressive drug cyclosporine results in a more rapid onset of encephalitis and an increased mortality rate, suggesting an important role for T cells in virus clearance and animal survival, without associated immunopathology (47). By contrast, the observed

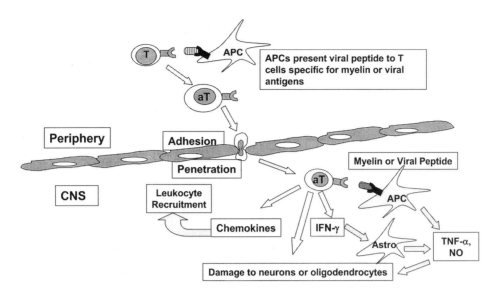

**Figure 3.** HCoVs and the molecular mimicry hypothesis in human neuropathology. Following infection by an HCoV, viral peptides are presented by antigen-presenting cells (APC) to T cells (T) specific for viral or myelin antigens. T cells become activated (aT) and can up-regulate adhesion molecules, which will promote interaction with cells from the blood-brain barrier (BBB) and facilitate penetration into the CNS. These activated T cells can then interact with the CNS-resident APC, microglia, which can present peptides derived from myelin components that can be recognized by virus-specific T cells, or vice versa, on the basis of shared similar sequences or conformations. Such myelin-virus cross-reactive T cells may therefore generate an autoimmune response with possible downstream immunopathological consequences. Chemokine secretion by activated T cells increases leukocyte recruitment, with potential amplification of the immune response. Gamma interferon (IFN-γ) production by activated T cells can increase cytokine (TNF-α) and nitric oxide (NO) production by glial cells (astrocytes and microglia), with potential damage to neurons and myelin-producing oligodendrocytes. Activated T cells may also cause direct cytotoxicity to neurons or oligodendrocytes.

delay in virus-induced death in RAG1$^{-/-}$ mice suggests that HCoV-OC43-induced encephalitis is in part mediated by the antiviral T-cell response (18), possibly via the activation of autoreactive T cells. These cells could contribute to possible demyelination in chronically infected animals or humans. Furthermore, some HCoV-OC43 mutants with expanded tropism were isolated from persistent infections. These variants harbored mutations in the S protein (91) and induced demyelination in susceptible mice (H. Jacomy and P. J. Talbot, unpublished data). Interestingly, as previously shown for mouse hepatitis virus (76), the S protein of HCoV-OC43 appears to be correlated with neurovirulence in mice (18).

A vacuolating encephalitis, associated with a strong inflammatory reaction, was induced after intracerebral (47) or intranasal (18) infection of susceptible mice. During the acute phase of encephalitis, when the virus was widely distributed throughout the CNS, neuronophagia, perivascular lymphocytic infiltrates, and activated microglial cells (Fig. 4) were present, even after complete clearance of the viral particles (47). Although histological analysis of mouse brain performed 1 year postinfection failed to detect HCoV-OC43 antigens, some of the animals showed

neuronal cell loss, especially in the hippocampal region, and sometimes clusters of gliosis were disseminated in the CNS (46).

Viral persistence in the CNS, confirmed by the presence of viral RNA, could be associated with increased neuronal degeneration leading to neuropathology in mice (46). Therefore, a respiratory pathogen, like the neurotropic and neuroinvasive HCoV, could be associated with neurodegenerative disease in susceptible individuals.

## THERAPY

As for virus infections in general, the development of vaccines against HCoVs is the best way to prevent infection and disease. However, as this topic is reviewed elsewhere, this chapter deals with recent advances in research and development on inhibitors that act at various steps of the virus replication cycle, from receptor binding to release of progeny infectious particles.

Most of the recent research on the development of therapeutic agents that could influence the outcome of HCoV infection has focused on SARS-CoV. However, as the coronaviruses are closely related in

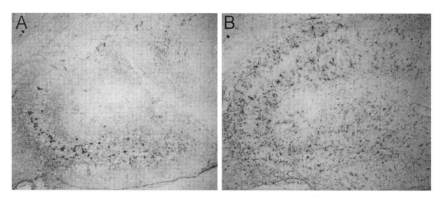

**Figure 4.** Inflammatory response following intracerebral HCoV-OC43 inoculation. Immunohistological staining of the brains of 21-day-old HCoV-OC43-infected BALB/c mice. At 6 days postinfection, infected hippocampal neurons (stained in black) (A) and microglial activation (revealed by Mac-2 staining) (B) are evident in the same region, demonstrating the strong inflammatory reaction in infected regions.

structure and mode of replication (16), several inhibitors that have been designed to control SARS-CoV infections might be valuable against other HCoVs. The identification and characterization of the different proteins encoded by the replicase gene and of virus-encoded proteases, which cleave the corresponding polyprotein, are becoming more and more important as specific inhibitors are developed and tested to measure their effect on HCoV replication. Therefore, enzymes that are essential in this replicative cycle provide possible targets for drug therapies against HCoVs. The coronavirus main protease ($M^{pro}$) represents one of the first targets to be studied (2). Because of a highly conserved substrate recognition pocket, $M^{pro}$ appears to be a particularly interesting target for the design of wide-spectrum inhibitors of coronavirus. Consistent with this possibility, a very promising molecule that inhibited $M^{pro}$ was recently described. This molecule inhibited the replication of coronaviruses belonging to all the genetic groups and exhibited very low cellular toxicity (117). Other viral enzymes encoded by the replicase gene that represent eventual potential drug targets are helicase (83) and the papain-like proteases (61).

Peptides derived from heptad repeat 2 of the S protein block membrane fusion and were shown to be effective in inhibiting SARS-CoV infection (14). The effectiveness of these peptides against HCoV-229E infection should be tested in the near future (62), and HCoV-NL63 infectivity has recently been shown to be reduced by these peptides (77). RNA interference against the S gene, pyrimidine nucleoside analogues, and intravenous immunoglobulin were also shown to be effective in inhibiting NL63 infection at different stages of the replication cycle (77). Inhibitors of HCoV-229E envelope protein, which

forms ion channels, also block the replication of the virus (113). Therefore, the envelope protein ion channel activity appears to be important for coronavirus replication, and inhibitors of this function could serve as potential anticoronaviral drugs.

## REFERENCES

1. **Almeida, J. D., and D. A. Tyrrell.** 1967. The morphology of three previously uncharacterized human respiratory viruses that grow in organ culture. *J. Gen. Virol.* **1**:175–178.
2. **Anand, K., J. Ziebuhr, P. Wadhwani, J. R. Mesters, and R. Hilgenfeld.** 2003. Coronavirus main protease (3CLpro) structure: basis for design of anti-SARS drugs. *Science* **300**:1763–1767.
3. **Anderson, J. R.** 2001. The mechanisms of direct, virus-induced destruction of neurons. *Curr. Top. Microbiol. Immunol.* **253**:15–33.
4. **Arbour, N., G. Côté, C. Lachance, M. Tardieu, N. R. Cashman, and P. J. Talbot.** 1999. Acute and persistent infection of human neural cell lines by human coronavirus OC43. *J. Virol.* **73**:3338–3350.
5. **Arbour, N., R. Day, J. Newcombe, and P. J. Talbot.** 2000. Neuroinvasion by human respiratory coronaviruses and association with multiple sclerosis. *J. Virol.* **74**:8913–8921.
6. **Arbour, N., S. Ekandé, G. Côté, C. Lachance, F. Chagnon, M. Tardieu, N. R. Cashman, and P. J. Talbot.** 1999. Persistent infection of human oligodendrocytic and neuroglial cell lines by human coronavirus 229E. *J. Virol.* **73**:3326–3337.
7. **Arden, K., M. D. Nissen, T. P. Sloots, and I. M. MacKay.** 2005. New human coronavirus, HCoV-NL63, associated with severe lower respiratory tract disease in Australia. *J. Med. Virol.* **75**:455–462.
8. **Barber, G. N.** 2001. Host defense, viruses and apoptosis. *Cell Death Differ.* **8**:113–126.
9. **Bastien, N., K. Anderson, L. Hart, P. Van Caeseele, K. Brandt, D. Milley, T. Hatchette, E. C. Weiss, and Y. Li.** 2005. Human coronavirus NL63 infection in Canada. *J. Infect. Dis.* **191**:503–506.
10. **Bastien, N., J. L. Robinson, A. Tse, B. E. Lee, L. Hart, and Y. Li.** 2005. Human coronavirus NL-63 infections in children: a 1-year study. *J. Clin. Microbiol.* **43**:4567–4573.

11. Beaudette, F. R., and C. B. Hudson. 1937. Cultivation of the virus of infectious bronchitis. *J. Am. Vet. Med. Assoc.* **90**:51–60.

12. Belay, E. D., D. D. Erdman, L. J. Anderson, T. C. Peret, S. J. Schrag, B. S. Fields, J. C. Burns, and L. B. Schonberger. 2005. Kawasaki disease and human coronavirus. *J. Infect. Dis.* **192**:352–353.

13. Bonavia, A., N. Arbour, V. W. Yong, and P. J. Talbot. 1997. Infection of primary cultures of human neural cells by human coronaviruses 229E and OC43. *J. Virol.* **71**:800–806.

14. Bosch, B. J., B. E. Martina, R. Van Der Zee, J. Lepault, B. J. Haijema, C. Versluis, A. J. Heck, R. De Groot, A. D. Osterhaus, and P. J. Rottier. 2004. Severe acute respiratory syndrome coronavirus (SARS-CoV) infection inhibition using spike protein heptad repeat-derived peptides. *Proc. Natl. Acad. Sci. USA* **101**:8455–8460.

15. Boucher, A., M. Desforges, P. Duquette, and P. J. Talbot. 2007. Long-term human coronavirus-myelin cross-reactive T-cell clones derived from multiple sclerosis patients. *Clin. Immunol.* **123**:258–267.

16. Brian, D. A., and R. S. Baric. 2005. Coronavirus genome structure and replication. *Curr. Top. Microbiol. Immunol.* **287**:1–30.

17. Burks, J. S., B. L. DeVald, L. D. Jankovsky, and J. C. Gerdes. 1980. Two coronaviruses isolated from central nervous system tissue of two multiple sclerosis patients. *Science* **209**:933–934.

18. Butler, N., L. Pewe, K. Trandem, and S. Perlman. 2006. Murine encephalitis caused by HCoV-OC43, a human coronavirus with broad species specificity, is partly immune-mediated. *Virology* **347**:410–421.

19. Cabirac, G. F., K. F. Soike, J. Y. Zhang, K. Hoel, C. Butunoi, G. Y. Cai, S. Johnson, and R. S. Murray. 1994. Entry of coronavirus into primate CNS following peripheral infection. *Microb. Pathog.* **16**:349–357.

20. Chibo, D., and C. Birch. 2006. Analysis of human coronavirus 229E spike and nucleoprotein genes demonstrates genetic drift between chronologically distinct strains. *J. Gen. Virol.* **87**:1203–1208.

21. Chiu, S. S., K. H. Chan, K. W. Chu, S. W. Kwan, Y. Guan, L. L. Poon, and J. S. Peiris. 2005. Human coronavirus NL63 infection and other coronavirus infections in children hospitalized with acute respiratory disease in Hong Kong, China. *Clin. Infect. Dis.* **40**:1721–1729.

22. Collins, A. R. 2002. In vitro detection of apoptosis in monocytes/macrophages infected with human coronavirus. *Clin. Diagn. Lab. Immunol.* **9**:1392–1395.

23. Cristallo, A., F. Gambaro, G. Biamonti, P. Ferrante, M. Battaglia, and P. M. Cereda. 1997. Human coronavirus polyadenylated RNA sequences in cerebrospinal fluid from multiple sclerosis patients. *New Microbiol.* **20**:105–114.

24. Desforges, M., T. C. Miletti, M. Gagnon, and P. J. Talbot. 2007. Activation of human monocytes after infection by human coronavirus 229E. *Virus Res.*, in press. E-pub ahead of print: doi:10.1016/j.virusres.2007.06.016.

25. Drosten, C., S. Gunther, W. Preiser, S. van der Werf, H. R. Brodt, S. Becker, H. Rabenau, M. Panning, L. Kolesnikova, R. A. Fouchier, A. Berger, A. M. Burguiere, J. Cinatl, M. Eickmann, N. Escriou, K. Grywna, S. Kramme, J. C. Manuguerra, S. Muller, V. Rickerts, M. Sturmer, S. Vieth, H. D. Klenk, A. D. Osterhaus, H. Schmitz, and H. W. Doerr. 2003. Identification of a novel coronavirus in patients with severe acute respiratory syndrome. *N. Engl. J. Med.* **348**:1967–1976.

26. Ebihara, T., R. Endo, X. Ma, N. Ishiguro, and H. Kikuta. 2005. Detection of human coronavirus NL63 in young children with bronchiolitis. *J. Med. Virol.* **75**:463–465.

27. Ebihara, T., R. Endo, X. Ma, N. Ishiguro, and H. Kikuta. 2005. Lack of association between New Haven coronavirus and Kawasaki disease. *J. Infect. Dis.* **192**:351–352.

28. Edwards, J. A., F. Denis, and P. J. Talbot. 2000. Activation of glial cells by human coronavirus OC43 infection. *J. Neuroimmunol.* **108**:73–81.

29. El-Sahly, H. M., R. L. Atmar, W. P. Glezen, and S. B. Greenberg. 2000. Spectrum of clinical illness in hospitalized patients with "common cold" virus infections. *Clin. Infect. Dis.* **31**:96–100.

30. Esper, F., E. D. Shapiro, C. Weibel, D. Ferguson, M. L. Landry, and J. S. Kahn. 2005. Association between a novel human coronavirus and Kawasaki disease. *J. Infect. Dis.* **191**:499–502.

31. Esper, F., C. Weibel, D. Ferguson, M. L. Landry, and J. S. Kahn. 2005. Evidence of a novel human coronavirus that is associated with respiratory tract disease in infants and young children. *J. Infect. Dis.* **191**:492–498.

32. Esper, F., C. Weibel, D. Ferguson, M. L. Landry, and J. S. Kahn. 2006. Coronavirus HKU1 infection in the United States. *Emerg. Infect. Dis.* **12**:775–779.

33. Falsey, A. R., R. M. McCann, W. J. Hall, M. M. Criddle, M. A. Formica, D. Wycoff, and J. E. Kolassa. 1997. The 'common cold' in frail older persons: impact of rhinovirus and coronavirus in a senior daycare center. *J. Am. Geriatr. Soc.* **45**:706–711.

34. Fazzini, E., J. Fleming, and S. Fahn. 1992. Cerebrospinal fluid antibodies to coronavirus in patients with Parkinson's disease. *Mov. Disord.* **7**:153–158.

35. Fishman, P. S., J. S. Gass, P. T. Swoveland, E. Lavi, M. K. Highkin, and S. Weiss. 1985. Infection of the basal ganglia by a murine coronavirus. *Science* **229**:877–879.

36. Fleming, J. O., A. K. El Zaatari, W. Gilmore, J. D. Berne, J. S. Burks, S. A. Stohlman, W. W. Tourtelotte, and L. P. Weiner. 1988. Antigenic assessment of coronaviruses isolated from patients with multiple sclerosis. *Arch. Neurol.* **45**:629–633.

37. Fouchier, R. A., N. G. Hartwig, T. M. Bestebroer, B. Niemeyer, J. C. de Jong, J. H. Simon, and A. D. Osterhaus. 2004. A previously undescribed coronavirus associated with respiratory disease in humans. *Proc. Natl. Acad. Sci. USA* **101**:6212–6216.

38. Fouchier, R. A., T. Kuiken, M. Schutten, G. van Amerongen, G. J. van Doornum, B. G. van der Hoogen, M. Peiris, W. Lim, K. Stohr, A. D. Osterhaus. 2003. Aetiology: Koch's postulates fulfilled for SARS virus. *Nature* **423**:240.

39. Gagneur, A., J. Sizun, S. Vallet, M. C. Legrand, B. Picard, and P. J. Talbot. 2002. Coronavirus-related nosocomial viral respiratory infections in a neonatal and paediatric intensive care unit: a prospective study. *J. Hosp. Infect.* **51**:59–64.

40. Gerna, G., G. Campanini, F. Rovida, E. Percivalle, A. Sarasini, A. Marchi, and F. Baldanti. 2006. Genetic variability of human coronavirus OC43-, 229E-, and NL63-like strains and their association with lower respiratory tract infections of hospitalized infants and immunocompromised patients. *J. Med. Virol.* **78**:938–949.

41. Gerna, G., N. Passarini, M. Battaglia, and E. G. Rondanelli. 1985. Human enteric coronaviruses: antigenic relatedness to human coronavirus OC43 and possible etiologic role in viral gastroenteritis. *J. Infect. Dis.* **151**:796–803.

42. Gilden, D. H. 2005. Infectious causes of multiple sclerosis. *Lancet Neurol.* **4**:195–202.

43. Hamre, D., and J. J. Procknow. 1966. A new virus isolated from the human respiratory tract. *Proc. Soc. Exp. Biol. Med.* **121**:190–193.

44. Hofmann, H., K. Pyrc, L. van der Hoek, M. Geier, B. Berkhout, and S. Pohlmann. 2005. Human coronavirus NL63 employs

the severe acute respiratory syndrome coronavirus receptor for cellular entry. *Proc. Natl. Acad. Sci. USA* **102:**7988–7993.

45. **Hovanec, D. L., and T. D. Flanagan.** 1983. Detection of antibodies to human coronaviruses 229E and OC43 in the sera of multiple sclerosis patients and normal subjects. *Infect. Immun.* **41:**426–429.

46. **Jacomy, H., G. Fragoso, G. Almazan, W. E. Mushynski, and P. J. Talbot.** 2006. Human coronavirus OC43 infection induces chronic encephalitis leading to disabilities in BALB/C mice. *Virology* **349:**335–346.

47. **Jacomy, H., and P. J. Talbot.** 2003. Vacuolating encephalitis in mice infected by human coronavirus OC43. *Virology* **315:**20–33.

48. **Jeffers, S. A., S. M. Tusell, L. Gillim-Ross, E. M. Hemmila, J. E. Achenbach, G. J. Babcock, W. D. Thomas, Jr., L. B. Thackray, M. D. Young, R. J. Mason, D. M. Ambrosino, D. E. Wentworth, J. C. Demartini, and K. V. Holmes.** 2004. CD209L (L-SIGN) is a receptor for severe acute respiratory syndrome coronavirus. *Proc. Natl. Acad. Sci. USA* **101:**15748–15753.

49. **Jelachich, M. L., and H. L. Lipton.** 1999. Restricted Theiler's murine encephalomyelitis virus infection in murine macrophages induces apoptosis. *J. Gen. Virol.* **80:**1701–1705.

50. **Jia, H. P., D. C. Look, L. Shi, M. Hickey, L. Pewe, J. Netland, M. Farzan, C. Wohlford-Lenane, S. Perlman, and P. B. McCray, Jr.** 2005. ACE2 receptor expression and severe acute respiratory syndrome coronavirus infection depend on differentiation of human airway epithelia. *J. Virol.* **79:**14614–14621.

51. **Johnson, R. T.** 1985. Viral aspects of multiple sclerosis, p. 319–336. *In* J. C. Koetsier (ed.), *Handbook of Clinical Neurology Demyelinating Diseases.* Elsevier, Amsterdam, The Netherlands.

52. **Johnston, S. L., P. K. Pattemore, G. Sanderson, S. Smith, F. Lampe, L. Josephs, P. Symington, S. O'Toole, S. H. Myint, D. A. J. Tyrrell, and S. T. Holgate.** 1995. Community study of role of viral infections in exacerbations of asthma in 9–11 year old children. *Br. Med. J.* **310:**1225–1228.

53. **Kahn, J. S.** 2006. The widening scope of coronaviruses. *Curr. Opin. Pediatr.* **18:**42–47.

54. **Ksiazek, T. G., D. Erdman, C. S. Goldsmith, S. R. Zaki, T. Peret, S. Emery, S. Tong, C. Urbani, J. A. Comer, W. Lim, P. E. Rollin, S. F. Dowell, A. E. Ling, C. D. Humphrey, W. J. Shieh, J. Guarner, C. D. Paddock, P. Rota, B. Fields, J. DeRisi, J. Y. Yang, N. Cox, J. M. Hughes, J. W. LeDuc, W. J. Bellini, L. J. Anderson, and the SARS Working Group.** 2003. A novel coronavirus associated with severe acute respiratory syndrome. *N. Engl. J. Med.* **348:**1953–1966.

55. **Kunkel, F., and G. Herrler.** 1993. Structural and functional analysis of the surface protein of human coronavirus OC43. *Virology* **195:**195–202.

56. **Kurtzke, J. F.** 1993. Epidemiologic evidence for multiple sclerosis as an infection. *Clin. Microbiol. Rev.* **6:**382–427.

57. **Larson, H. E., S. E. Reed, and D. A. J. Tyrell.** 1980. Isolation of rhinoviruses and coronaviruses from 38 colds in adults. *J. Med. Virol.* **5:**221–229.

58. **Lassnig, C., C. M. Sanchez, M. Egerbacher, I. Walter, S. Majer, T. Kolbe, P. Pallares, L. Enjuanes, and M. Muller.** 2005. Development of a transgenic mouse model susceptible to human coronavirus 229E. *Proc. Natl. Acad. Sci. USA* **102:**8275–8280.

59. **Lee, B. E., J. L. Robinson, V. Khurana, X. L. Pang, J. K. Preiksaitis, and J. D. Fox.** 2006. Enhanced identification of viral and atypical bacterial pathogens in lower respiratory tract samples with nucleic acid amplification tests. *J. Med. Virol.* **78:**702–710.

60. **Li, W., M. J. Moore, N. Vasilieva, J. Sui, S. K. Wong, M. A. Berne, M. Somasundaran, J. L. Sullivan, K. Luzuriaga, T. C.**

Greenough, H. Choe, and M. Farzan. 2003. Angiotensin-converting enzyme 2 is a functional receptor for the SARS coronavirus. *Nature* **426:**450–454.

61. **Lindner, H. A., N. Fotouhi-Ardakani, V. Lytvyn, P. Lachance, T. Sulea, and R. Ménard.** 2005. The papain-like protease from the severe acute respiratory syndrome coronavirus is a deubiquitinating enzyme. *J. Virol.* **79:**15199–15208.

62. **Liu, C., Y. Feng, F. Gao, Q. Zhang, and M. Wang.** 2006. Characterization of HCoV-229E fusion core: implications for structure basis of coronavirus membrane fusion. *Biochem. Biophys. Res. Commun.* **345:**1108–1115.

63. **Martyn, C. N.** 1997. Infection of childhood and neurological diseases in adult life. *Br. Med. Bull.* **53:**24–39.

64. **McIntosh, K., W. B. Becker, and R. M. Chanock.** 1967. Growth in suckling mouse brain of "IBV-like" viruses from patients with upper respiratory tract disease. *Proc. Natl. Acad. Sci. USA* **58:**2268–2273.

65. **McMahon, E. J., S. L. Bailey, C. Vanderlugt Castenada, H. Waldner, and S. D. Miller.** 2005. Epitope spreading initiates in the CNS in two mouse models of multiple sclerosis. *Nat. Med.* **11:**335–339.

66. **Moës, E., L. Vijgen, E. Keyaerts, K. Zlateva, S. Li, P. Maes, K. Pyrc, B. Berkhout, L. van der Hoek, and M. Van Ranst.** 2005. A novel pancoronavirus RT-PCR assay: frequent detection of human coronavirus NL63 in children hospitalized with respiratory tract infections in Belgium. *BMC Infect. Dis.* **5:**6.

67. **Murray, R. S., B. Brown, D. Brian, and G. F. Cabirac.** 1992. Detection of coronavirus RNA and antigen in multiple sclerosis brain. *Ann. Neurol.* **31:**525–533.

68. **Murray, R. S., G. Y. Cai, K. Hoel, J. Y. Zhang, K. F. Soike, and G. F. Cabirac.** 1992. Coronavirus infects and causes demyelination in primate central nervous system. *Virology* **188:**274–284.

69. **Murray, R. S., G. Y. Cai, K. F. Soike, and G. F. Cabirac.** 1997. Further observations on coronavirus infection of primate CNS. *J. Neurovirol.* **3:**71–75.

70. **Myint, S. H.** 1995. Human coronavirus infections, p. 389–401. *In* S. G. Siddell (ed.), *The Coronaviridae.* Plenum Press, New York, NY.

71. **Nicholson, K. G., J. Kent, and D. C. Ireland.** 1993. Respiratory viruses and exacerbations of asthma in adults. *Br. Med. J.* **307:**982–986.

72. **Olanow, C. W., and W. G. Tatton.** 1999. Etiology and pathogenesis of Parkinson's disease. *Annu. Rev. Neurosci.* **22:**123–144.

73. **Oldstone, M. B. A.** 2005. Molecular mimicry, microbial infection, and autoimmune disease: evolution of the concept. *Curr. Top. Microbiol. Immunol.* **296:**1–17.

74. **Patterson, S., and M. R. Macnaughton.** 1982. Replication of human respiratory coronavirus strain 229E in human macrophages. *J. Gen. Virol.* **60:**307–314.

75. **Pene, F., A. Merlat, A. Vabret, F. Rozenberg, A. Buzyn, F. Dreyfus, A. Cariou, F. Freymuth, and P. Lebon.** 2003. Coronavirus-229E-related pneumonia in immunocompromised patients. *Clin. Infect. Dis.* **37:**929–932.

76. **Phillips, J. J., M. M. Chua, E. Lavi, and S. R. Weiss.** 1999. Pathogenesis of chimeric MHV4/MHVA59 recombinant viruses: the murine coronavirus spike protein is a major determinant of neurovirulence. *J. Virol.* **73:**7752–7760.

77. **Pyrc, K., B. J. Bosch, B. Berkhout, M. F. Jebbink, R. Dijkman, P. Rottier, and L. van der Hoek.** 2006. Inhibition of human coronavirus NL63 infection at early stages of the replication cycle. *Antimicrob. Agents Chemother.* **50:**2000–2008.

78. **Resta, S., J. P. Luby, C. R. Rosenfeld, and J. D. Siegel.** 1985. Isolation and propagation of a human enteric coronavirus. *Science* **229:**978–981.

79. Reuter, J. D., D. L. Gomez, J. H. Wilson, and A. N. van den Pol. 2004. Systemic immune deficiency necessary for cytomegalovirus invasion of the mature brain. *J. Virol.* **78:**1473–1487.

80. Riski, H., and T. Hovi. 1980. Coronavirus infections of man associated with diseases other than the common cold. *J. Med. Virol.* **6:**259–265.

81. Salmi, A., B. Ziola, T. Hovi, and M. Reunanen. 1982. Antibodies to coronaviruses OC43 and 229E in multiple sclerosis patients. *Neurology* **32:**292–295.

82. Schlitt, B. P., M. Felrice, M. L. Jelachich, and H. L. Lipton. 2003. Apoptotic cells, including macrophages, are prominent in Theiler's virus-induced inflammatory, demyelinating lesions. *J. Virol.* **77:**4383–4388.

83. Seybert, A., C. C. Posthuma, L. C. van Dinten, E. J. Snijder, A. E. Gorbalenya, and J. Ziebuhr. 2005. A complex zinc finger controls the enzymatic activities of nidovirus helicases. *J. Virol.* **79:**696–704.

84. Sibley, W. A., C. R. Bamford, and K. Clark. 1985. Clinical viral infections and multiple sclerosis. *Lancet* **i:**1313–1315.

85. Sizun, J., D. Soupre, J. D. Giroux, D. Alix, D. Parscau, M. C. Legrand, M. Demazure, and C. Chastel. 1993. Nasal colonization with coronavirus and apnea of the premature newborn. *Acta Paediatr.* **82:**238.

86. Sizun, J., D. Soupre, M. C. Legrand, J. D. Giroux, S. Rubio, J. M. Cauvin, C. Chastel, D. Alix, and L. Deparscau. 1995. Neonatal nosocomial respiratory infection with coronavirus: a prospective study in a neonatal intensive care unit. *Acta Paediatr.* **84:**617–620.

87. Sizun, J., M. W. N. Yu, and P. J. Talbot. 2000. Survival of human coronaviruses 229E and OC43 in suspension and after frying on surfaces: a possible source of hospital-acquired infections. *J. Hosp. Infect.* **46:**55–60.

88. Skowronski, D. M., C. Astell, R. C. Brunham, D. E. Low, M. Petric, R. Roper, P. J. Talbot, T. Tam, and L. Babiuk. 2005. Severe acute respiratory syndrome (SARS): a year in review. *Annu. Rev. Med.* **56:**357–381.

89. Sloots, T. P., P. McErlean, D. J. Speicher, K. E. Arden, M. D. Nissen, and I. M. MacKay. 2006. Evidence of human coronavirus HKU1 and human bocavirus in Australian children. *J. Clin. Virol.* **35:**99–102.

90. Stewart, J. N., S. Mounir, and P. J. Talbot. 1992. Human coronavirus gene expression in the brains of multiple sclerosis patients. *Virology* **191:**502–505.

91. St.-Jean, J. R., M. Desforges, and P. J. Talbot. 2006. Genetic evolution of human coronavirus OC43 in neural cell culture. *Adv. Exp. Biol. Med.* **581:**499–502.

92. St.-Jean, J. R., H. Jacomy, M. Desforges, A. Vabret, F. Freymuth, and P. J. Talbot. 2004. Human respiratory coronavirus OC43: genetic stability and neuroinvasion. *J. Virol.* **78:**8824–8834.

93. Talbot, P. J., D. Arnold, and J. P. Antel. 2001. Virus-induced autoimmune reactions in the nervous system. *Curr. Top. Microbiol. Immunol.* **253:**247–271.

94. Talbot, P. J., and P. Jouvenne. 1992. Neurotropic potential of coronaviruses. *Med. Sci.* **8:**119–125.

95. Talbot, P. J., J. S. Paquette, C. Ciurli, J. P. Antel, and F. Ouellet. 1996. Myelin basic protein and human coronavirus 229E cross-reactive T cells in multiple sclerosis. *Ann. Neurol.* **39:**233–240.

96. Tsui, J. K., D. B. Calne, Y. Wang, M. Schulzer, and S. A. Marion. 1999. Occupational risk factors in Parkinson's disease. *Can. J. Public Health* **90:**334–337.

97. Tyrrell, D. A. J., J. D. Almeida, D. M. Berry, and K. McIntosh. 1968. Coronaviruses. *Nature* **220:**650.

98. Tyrrell, D. A., J. D. Almeida, C. H. Cunningham, W. R. Dowdle, M. S. Hofstad, K. McIntosh, M. Tajima, L. Y. Zakstelskaya, B. C. Easterday, A. Kapikian, and R. W. Bingham. 1975. Coronaviridae. *Intervirology* **5:**76–82.

99. Tyrrell, D. A. J., and M. L. Bynoe. 1965. Cultivation of a novel type of common-cold virus in organ cultures. *Br. Med. J.* **1:**1467–1470.

100. Vabret, A., J. Dina, J. Gouarin, J. Petitjean, S. Corbet, and F. Freymuth. 2006. Detection of the new human coronavirus HKU1: a report of 6 cases. *Clin. Infect. Dis.* **42:**634–639.

101. Vabret, A., T. Mourez, J. Dina, L. van der Hoek, S. Gouarin, J. Petitjean, J. Brouard, and F. Freymuth. 2005. Human coronavirus NL63, France. *Emerg. Infect. Dis.* **11:**1225–1229.

102. Vabret, A., T. Mourez, S. Gouarin, J. Petitjean, and F. Freymuth. 2003. An outbreak of coronavirus OC43 respiratory infection in Normandy, France. *Clin. Infect. Dis.* **36:**985–989.

103. van der Hoek, L., K. Pyrc, M. F. Jebbink, W. Vermeulen-Oost, R. J. Berkhout, K. C. Wolthers, P. M. Wertheim-van Dillen, J. Kaandorp, J. Spaargaren, and B. Berkhout. 2004. Identification of a new human coronavirus. *Nat. Med.* **10:**368–373.

104. van der Hoek, L., K. Sure, G. Ihorst, A. Stang, K. Pyrc, M. F. Jebbink, G. Petersen, J. Forster, B. Berkhout, and K. Uberla. 2005. Croup is associated with the novel coronavirus NL63. *PLoS Med.* **2:**764–770.

105. Vijgen, L., E. Keyaerts, P. Lemey, P. Maes, K. Van Reeth, H. Nauwynck, M. Pensaert, and M. Van Ranst. 2006. Evolutionary history of the closely related group 2 coronaviruses: porcine hemagglutinating encephalomyelitis virus, bovine coronavirus, and human cornavirus OC43. *J. Virol.* **80:**7270–7274.

106. Vijgen, L., E. Keyaerts, P. Lemey, E. Moës, S. Li, A. M. Vandamme, and M. Van Ranst. 2005. Circulation of genetically distinct contemporary human coronavirus OC43 strains. *Virology* **337:**85–92.

107. Vijgen, L., E. Keyaerts, E. Moes, P. Maes, G. Duson, and M. Van Ranst. 2005. Development of one-step, real-time, quantitative reverse transcriptase PCR assays for absolute quantitation of human coronaviruses OC43 and 229E. *J. Clin. Microbiol.* **43:**5452–5456.

108. Vijgen, L., P. Lemey, E. Keyaerts, and M. Van Ranst. 2005. Complete genomic sequence of human coronavirus OC43: molecular clock analysis suggests a relatively recent zoonotic coronavirus transmission event. *J. Virol.* **79:**1595–1604.

109. Wang, G., C. Deering, M. Macke, J. Shao, R. Burns, D. M. Blau, K. V. Holmes, B. L. Davidson, S. Perlman, and P. B. MacCray, Jr. 2000. Human coronavirus 229E infects polarized airway epithelia from the apical surface. *J. Virol.* **74:**9234–9239.

110. Weiss, S. R. 1983. Coronaviruses SD and SK share extensive nucleotide homology with murine coronavirus MHV-A59, more than that shared between human and murine coronaviruses. *Virology* **126:**669–677.

111. Wentworth, D. E., D. B. Tresnan, B. C. Turner, I. R. Lerman, B. Bullis, E. M. Hemmila, R. Levis, L. H. Shapiro, and K. V. Holmes. 2005. Cells of human aminopeptidase N (CD13) transgenic mice are infected by human coronavirus-229E in vitro, but not in vivo. *Virology* **335:**185–197.

112. Whitley, R. J., and J. W. Gnann. 2002. Viral encephalitis: familiar infections and emerging pathogens. *Lancet* **359:**507–513.

113. Wilson, L., P. Gage, and G. Ewart. 2006. Hexamethylene amiloride blocks E protein ion channels and inhibits coronavirus replication. *Virology* **353:**294–306.

114. Woo, P. C., S. K. Lau, C. M. Chu, K. H. Chan, H. W. Tsoi, Y. Huang, B. H. Wong, R. W. Poon, J. J. Cai, W. K. Luk, L. L. Poon, S. S. Wong, Y. Guan, J. S. Peiris, and K. Y. Yuen. 2005. Characterization and complete genome sequence of a novel coronavirus, coronavirus HKU1, from patients with pneumonia. *J. Virol.* **79:**884–895.

115. Woo, P. C., S. K. Lau, H. W. Tsoi, Y. Huang, R. W. Poon, C. M. Chu, R. A. Lee, W. K. Luk, G. K. Wong, B. H. Wong, V. C. Cheng, B. S. Tang, A. K. Wu, R. W. Yung, H. Chen, Y. Guan, K. H. Chan, and K. Y. Yuen. 2005. Clinical and molecular epidemiological features of coronavirus HKU1-associated community-acquired pneumonia. *J. Infect. Dis.* **192:**1898–1907.

116. Woo, P. C., S. K. P. Lau, C. C. Y. Yip, Y. Huang, H.-W. Tsoi, K.-H. Chan, and K. Y. Yuen. 2006. Comparative analysis of 22 coronavirus HKU1 genomes reveals a novel genotype and evidence of natural recombination in coronavirus HKU1. *J. Virol.* **80:**7136–7145.

117. Yang, H., W. Xie, X. Xue, K. Yang, J. Ma, W. Liang, Q. Zhao, Z. Zhou, D. Pei, J. Ziebuhr, R. Hilgenfeld, K. Y. Yuen, L. Wong, G. Gao, S. Chen, Z. Chen, D. Ma, M. Bartlam, and Z. Rao. 2005. Design of wide-spectrum inhibitors targeting coronavirus main proteases. *PLoS Biol.* **3:**1742–1752.

118. Yeager, C. L., R. A. Ashmun, R. K. Williams, C. B. Cardellichio, L. H. Shapiro, A. T. Look, and K. V. Holmes. 1992. Human aminopeptidase N is a receptor for human coronavirus 229E. *Nature* **357:**420–422.

119. Yeh, E. A., A. Collins, M. E. Cohen, P. K. Duffner, and H. Faden. 2004. Detection of coronavirus in the central nervous system of a child with acute disseminated encephalitis. *Pediatrics* **113:**73–76.

*Nidoviruses*
Edited by S. Perlman, T. Gallagher, and E. J. Snijder
© 2008 ASM Press, Washington, DC

# Chapter 21

# Arterivirus Pathogenesis and Immune Response

N. James MacLachlan, Udeni B. Balasuriya, Michael P. Murtaugh,
Stephen W. Barthold, and Linda J. Lowenstine

The family *Arteriviridae* within the order *Nidovirales* includes a single genus, *Arterivirus*. Equine arteritis virus (EAV) is the type species of the genus, and the three other currently known members are lactate dehydrogenase-elevating virus (LDV), porcine reproductive and respiratory syndrome virus (PRRSV), and simian hemorrhagic fever virus (SHFV). The family *Arteriviridae* was not established until 1996. However, the four viruses included in the family all were recognized prior to that time. EAV was first isolated in 1953, LDV in 1960, and SHF in 1968; PRRSV was not isolated until 1991. These viruses form a distinct phylogenetic group and share a common replication strategy, but LDV, PRRSV, and SHFV are more closely related to one another than they are to EAV. Although the arteriviruses share many common biological and molecular features, the epidemiology and pathogenesis of the infections caused by each virus are distinct, as are the diseases they cause. The host range of individual arteriviruses is also highly restricted; however, all four viruses share the ability to cause prolonged or truly persistent infections in their natural hosts, and the humoral immune response to LDV, PRRSV, and SHFV in naturally infected animals is frequently weak and ineffectual. This review presents aspects of the epidemiology, pathogenesis, immune response, and, where appropriate, the treatment and prevention of EAV, PRRSV, LDV, and SHFV infections of their respective hosts.

## EQUINE VIRAL ARTERITIS (EVA)

EAV causes reproductive and respiratory infections in equines (horses, donkeys, and mules), and some infected animals develop clinical manifestations referred to as equine viral arteritis (EVA) because of the characteristic injury to muscular arteries that occurs in severely affected horses (50). Although EAV was not isolated until 1953 (15), descriptions of a disease that very likely was EVA were first published in the late 18th and early 19th centuries, being referred to as "pinkeye," "infectious or epizootic cellulites," "influenza erysipelatosa," "Pferdestaupe," "Rotlaufseuche," and "equine influenza." Early investigators also recognized that apparently healthy stallions could transmit the disease to susceptible mares at breeding, and that these "carrier" stallions could be a source of infection for many years (9).

EAV infection of equines currently occurs worldwide, although the incidences of both EAV infection and overt EVA vary markedly among countries and among horses of different breeds (reviewed in references 17, 29, and 50). The vast majority of EAV infections are inapparent or subclinical, but occasional outbreaks of EVA occur that are characterized by any combination of influenza-like illness in adult horses, abortion in pregnant mares, and fatal interstitial pneumonia in young foals. Concern over EVA peaked following an extensive outbreak of the disease in Thoroughbred horses in Kentucky in 1984, and additional outbreaks subsequently have since been reported from several countries. Infection also recently has been reported in countries, such as Australia, New Zealand, and South Africa, that were previously thought to be free of the virus. This apparent global dissemination of EAV and rising incidence of EVA likely reflect the rapid national and international movement of

N. James MacLachlan, Stephen W. Barthold, and Linda J. Lowenstine • Department of Pathology, Microbiology and Immunology, School of Veterinary Medicine, University of California, Davis, CA 95616.   Udeni B. Balasuriya • Department of Veterinary Science, Gluck Equine Research Center, University of Kentucky, Lexington, KY 40546.   Michael P. Murtaugh • Department of Veterinary and Biomedical Sciences, University of Minnesota, St. Paul, MN 55108.

horses for competition and breeding, as well as heightened diagnostic scrutiny that stems from increasing concern over the potential importance of EAV infection.

## Epidemiology

EAV infection is spread by both the respiratory and venereal routes, and the persistently infected carrier stallion is the essential natural virus reservoir (17, 29, 50) (Fig. 1). Although the EAV carrier state in stallions had been recognized for many years, pioneering work to characterize this state was done by Peter Timoney and William McCollum in the course of their investigations of the 1984 outbreak of EVA in Kentucky (51). The carrier state occurs in some 30 to 50% of exposed stallions and persists for variable periods (weeks to lifelong infection). EAV is confined to the reproductive tract during persistence, and persistent infection does not occur in mares, geldings, or prepubertal colts. Not only is the carrier stallion the essential natural reservoir of EAV, but also genetic and antigenic variation is generated in the course of persistence; thus, an increasingly diverse population of related viral variants (quasispecies) is present in the semen of individual stallions (22). Outbreaks of EVA occur when one of

these variants is transmitted to a susceptible cohort, which typically is a mare bred to the stallion, although the virus also can be spread from carrier stallions by fomites (including semen-contaminated bedding). EAV can be efficiently transmitted by aerosol in populations of susceptible horses to cause explosive outbreaks. In marked contrast to the quasispecies evolution of EAV in the reproductive tract of carrier stallions, there is minimal genetic change in EAV during outbreaks of EVA, and the virus strains that cause individual outbreaks are genetically distinct (5).

The seroprevalence of EAV infection varies not only among countries but also among horses of different breeds and ages, with especially marked disparity between the prevalence of infection of Standardbred (up to 85%) and Thoroughbred horses (<5%) in the United States (23). EAV infection also is common in many European Warmblood breeds. There is no evidence of any breed-specific variation in susceptibility to EAV infection or in establishment of the carrier state; thus, the number of actively shedding carrier stallions likely determines the prevalence of EAV infection in individual horse breeds. The virulence of the strains of EAV associated with individual horse breeds may differ, and the strains shed by carrier Standardbred stallions are typically highly attenuated.

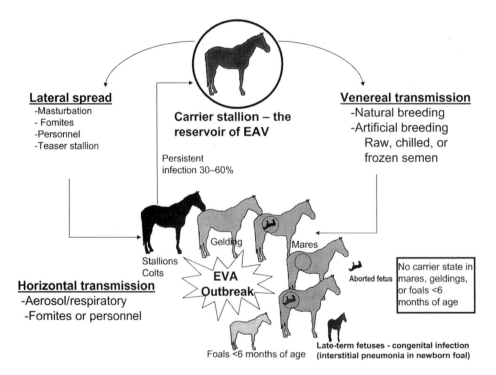

**Figure 1.** Epidemiology of EAV infection of horses, depicting the central role of the carrier stallion in maintenance and dissemination of the virus.

## Pathogenesis and Pathology

EAV replicates in pulmonary macrophages and endothelial cells following aerosol respiratory infection, and it rapidly spreads first to the draining lymph nodes and then systemically (13, 29). Although endothelial cells and macrophages are the principal sites of virus replication, selected epithelia, mesothelium, and smooth muscle cells of the media of arteries and the myometrium also may be infected. The clinical manifestations of EVA reflect endothelial injury and increased vascular permeability. However, the relative roles and importance of direct virus-mediated endothelial cell injury and virus-induced vasoactive and inflammatory cytokines in the pathogenesis of EAV-induced vascular injury are not yet clearly defined (32).

Clinical cases of EVA are characterized by an incubation period of 2 to 14 days followed by pyrexia, depression, anorexia, conjunctivitis and rhinitis, peripheral edema (periorbital and supraorbital, limbs, and ventral body, involving the scrotum and prepuce or mammary glands), urticaria, and abortion (17, 29, 50). Abortion rates differ between outbreaks but can be up to 50% of susceptible pregnant mares. Individual strains of EAV differ in their abortigenic potential, as they do in their virulence characteristics.

It is to be stressed that with the notable exception of fetal and neonatal infections, EAV infection of horses is very seldom fatal. The numerous publications describing lesions caused by the highly virulent horse-adapted Bucyrus strain of EAV reflect a severe infection that is not representative of the disease caused by field strains of the virus. Fetuses aborted after EAV infection usually do not show any obvious gross or histopathological lesions; they typically are autolyzed and may have increased peritoneal and pleural fluid, as well as petechial hemorrhages in the mucosal linings of the respiratory and digestive tracts and on the serosal lining of peritoneal and pleural cavities. Gross lesions in foals with fatal EVA include severe pulmonary edema, pleural and pericardial effusion, and petechial and ecchymotic serosal and mucosal hemorrhages in the small intestine. Microscopic lesions include interstitial pneumonia with hypertrophic type 2 pneumocytes containing intracytoplasmic EAV antigen, pulmonary edema, and fibrinoid necrosis of the tunica media of small muscular arteries (13).

## Immune Response

The innate immune response of the mucosa lining the respiratory and genital tracts provides the initial defense following venereal or aerosol EAV infection (reviewed in reference 6). The innate response includes the release of various antiviral and proinflammatory cytokines (e.g., interferons [IFNs], tumor necrosis factor [TNF], and interleukins [IL] such as IL-12) from virus-infected cells in the mucosa, infiltrating macrophages and natural killer (NK) cells. The precise role of innate immunity in the protective response of horses to EAV infection is yet to be adequately characterized. EAV infects alveolar macrophages (AMΦ) after respiratory infection of horses, but recent in vitro studies using cultured equine AMΦ confirmed that although these cells were susceptible to infection, they were refractory to productive replication of EAV, whereas productive replication occurred following EAV infection of cultured equine blood-derived macrophages (BMΦ). EAV infection of both equine AMΦ and BMΦ resulted in their activation with increased transcription of genes encoding proinflammatory mediators, including IL-1β, IL-6, IL-8, and TNF-α, with substantial production of TNF-α. Furthermore, virulent and avirulent strains of EAV induced different quantities of TNF-α and other proinflammatory cytokines (IL-1β, IL-6, and IL-8), and the magnitude of the cytokine response of equine AMΦ and BMΦ to EAV infection reflected the virulence of the infecting virus strain. These studies clearly show that cytokine mediators are produced by EAV-infected equine cells, and presumably, these are critical in determining the outcome of infection and severity of disease.

EAV infection induces long-lasting immunity in horses against reinfection with all strains of the virus. Resistance to reinfection is assumed to be mediated by neutralizing antibody (6). The antibody response of horses to individual EAV proteins differs markedly depending on the interval after infection, the infecting virus strain, the individual horse, and the specific serological assay used. Immunoblotting studies confirm that infected horses respond to a variety of structural viral proteins, and that sera from horses other than carrier stallions most consistently recognized the conserved carboxy-terminal region of the membrane (M) envelope protein. In contrast, sera from EAV carrier stallions most consistently reacted with the nucleocapsid (N) protein. The serum neutralization test, which principally detects antibodies to glycoprotein 5 (GP5), remains the most sensitive in detecting EAV-specific antibodies in horse serum. Neutralizing antibodies are detected within 1 to 2 weeks following infection, peak at 2 to 4 months, and persist for years thereafter.

There is only one serotype of EAV; however, field strains differ in both their neutralization and virulence phenotypes. The N-terminal region of GP5 (major envelope glycoprotein encoded by open reading frame 5 [ORF5]) expresses major neutralization determinants of EAV, and three distinct variable regions within GP5 are responsible for the heterogeneity in neutralization phenotype among field strains of the virus (4). GP5 and the M protein associate as a disulfide-linked heterodimer in the mature EAV virion, and authentic posttranslational modification (glycosylation) and conformational maturation of GP5 occur only in the presence of the M protein. Thus, this interaction is necessary for induction of EAV-neutralizing antibodies.

The appearance of neutralizing antibodies at 7 to 14 days after infection of horses with EAV typically coincides with the disappearance of virus from the circulation. However, virus does persist in the reproductive tract of carrier stallions for long periods despite the presence of high titers of virus-specific neutralizing antibodies in their serum. Novel genetic variants with distinct neutralization phenotypes arise during persistent infection of carrier stallions, and the altered neutralization phenotypes of these variants correlate with amino acid changes in distinct portions of GP5 (5, 22). However, all of these variants are neutralized by high-titered polyclonal equine sera, which strongly suggests that immune evasion is unlikely to be responsible for the establishment of persistent EAV infection of carrier stallions. Furthermore, the ratio of nonsynonymous substitutions per nonsynonymous site and synonymous substitutions per synonymous site for ORF5 of different EAV strains present in carrier stallions consistently is less than 1.0, which indicates that this variation is not the result of positive selection.

Antibodies clearly are important in preventing reinfection with viruses, but removal of virus-infected cells during acute infections typically is mediated by the cellular arm of the immune system. CD8$^+$ cytotoxic T lymphocytes play an important role in the control and clearance of many viral infections, including EAV infection of horses, although the specific viral protein(s) that is targeted by the cytotoxic T-lymphocyte response of EAV-infected horses remains to be thoroughly characterized (7).

## Vaccines and Therapy

As with other animal viral diseases, there is no specific antiviral treatment for horses infected with EAV, and naturally infected horses virtually always recover uneventfully. There currently also is no consistently effective treatment to eliminate the carrier state in stallions persistently infected with EAV other than castration; however, the EAV carrier state is testosterone dependent, and transient suppression of testosterone production in carrier stallions may offer therapeutic promise for the elimination of EAV infection (17).

Horses infected with EAV develop long-lasting immunity against reinfection with all strains of the virus, including the most virulent strains. Thus, vaccination is a logical and practical strategy for the control of EVA. There currently are two commercial vaccines that are widely used for protective immunization of horses against EAV infection, one a live attenuated (modified live virus [MLV]) and the other inactivated (killed). Experimental EAV vaccines also recently have been developed using recombinant DNA technology.

The MLV vaccine is administered intramuscularly to horses. A small minority of vaccinated horses develop mild febrile reactions and transient lymphopenia following vaccination, and virus may be sporadically isolated from the nasopharynx and buffy coat, but vaccinated stallions do not shed virus in either their semen or urine. The MLV vaccine is not recommended for use in pregnant mares, especially during the last 2 months of gestation, or in foals less than 6 weeks of age. Apparent fetal infections with MLV following vaccination of pregnant mares have been documented, albeit rarely. Maternal antibodies to EAV disappear between 2 and 6 months of age; thus, it is recommended that foals be vaccinated at 6 months of age. Colts should be vaccinated prior to the onset of puberty, as this prevents them from becoming persistently infected carriers. Thus, protective immunization of prepubertal colts is central to control of the spread of EAV infection.

An adjuvant-containing, inactivated EAV vaccine was formulated for use in the United Kingdom following an outbreak of EVA in 1993. This vaccine is also administered intramuscularly, and a booster immunization is recommended after 3 to 4 weeks and annually thereafter. Although this vaccine induces high titers of neutralizing antibodies, its ability to prevent EVA and persistent infection of stallions is less characterized than that of the MLV vaccine.

Several EAV subunit vaccines have been developed recently (reviewed in reference 6). Their potential benefits include lack of replication and the ability to distinguish vaccinated and naturally infected horses. They include a GP5-specific oligopeptide (amino acids [aa] 75 to 97) and a bacterial fusion protein containing aa 55 to 98, both of which include the key neutralizing domain of GP5; a Venezuelan equine encephalitis virus replicon particle-based vaccine that coexpresses GP5 and M protein; a live marker vaccine that lacks the major neutralization domain (aa 66 to 112) in GP5; and a DNA vaccine expressing ORF2b, -5, and -7. It is unlikely, however, that any subunit EAV vaccine will be widely used in the near future, at least in the United States, given the proven safety and reliability of the existing MLV.

## PRRS

A previously unrecognized disease characterized by severe reproductive losses, postweaning pneumonia, reduced growth performance, and increased mortality rate appeared in North American swine herds in the 1980s and was termed "mystery swine disease." A clinically similar disease spread rapidly throughout Europe in the early 1990s. A virus identified as "Lelystad virus" was first isolated and proven to reproduce the disease in 1991, and isolation of a North American strain of PRRSV followed shortly thereafter (10, 54). Retrospective serological studies indicate that PRRSV first appeared in North America in 1979, in Asia in 1985, and in Europe in 1987, and the virus was subsequently disseminated to swine populations throughout the world.

PRRSV is most similar genetically to LDV. The initial isolates of PRRSV from North America and Europe were very different; indeed, the European viruses were almost as distinct from the North American PRRSV isolates as they were from LDV (33). PRRSV isolates from other regions of the world were similar to the North American genotypes. The marked continental divergence of PRRSV suggests an earlier geographic separation followed by independent evolutionary trajectories. The near simultaneous appearance of similar diseases on different continents caused by genetically disparate virus strains may reflect recent changes in swine husbandry. Specifically, whereas swine formerly were raised outdoors in relatively small groups, swine production now occurs in densely populated operations housed in confinement.

### Epidemiology

PRRSV infects only domestic and feral pigs (*Sus scrofa*). It is spread by direct contact though saliva, nasal secretions, pugilism, semen, mammary secretions, and transplacental transmission in late gestation (reviewed in reference 58). The virus also is shed in urine and feces. The recent rapid global dissemination of PRRSV likely has occurred as a result of international trade and movement of infected pigs and semen. Spread within herds is due primarily to direct contact between infected and naïve swine, as separation of pens by a meter of airspace markedly reduces the rate of transmission. Endemic infection is perpetuated by a cycle of transmission from sows to piglets in utero or through colostrum and milk, by the regular introduction of breeding-age animals into a sow herd, and by comingling of susceptible and infected animals. Thus, once present in a herd, PRRSV is difficult to eliminate.

PRRSV principally is spread between herds by movement of infected pigs or use of infective semen for artificial insemination, but it also can be mechanically spread by fomites such as vehicles, needles, garments, and contaminated food and water. Blood-feeding insects also can function as mechanical vectors but are not considered significant. Airborne transmission is often implicated in the spread of PRRSV between premises, but experimental confirmation is lacking, and the role of airborne transmission in the epidemiology of PRRSV infection may require a better definition of the relative importance of factors such as viral excretion rates, strain variation, and the impact of environmental influences on virus infectivity.

PRRSV is readily transmitted to susceptible sows via the semen of infected boars. Virus is shed in the semen of infected boars for as long as 43 days, and viral RNA can be detected up to approximately 100 days (8). Venereal infection of gilts and sows usually results only in transient anorexia, inappetence, and lethargy, but not reproductive disease, whereas subsequent spread of the virus from these animals to susceptible sows in late gestation can result in reproductive failure and sow mortality.

### Pathogenesis and Pathology

PRRSV grows primarily in macrophages in the lungs and lymph nodes of infected swine (reviewed in references 45 and 58). Viremia begins as early as 12 to 24 h after infection, peaks within a week, and then declines until virus no longer is detected in blood at 4 to 6 weeks after infection. Viral antigens and nucleic acids are present in macrophages throughout the body, and inconsistently in respiratory epithelium, endothelium, fibroblasts, spermatids, and spermatocytes. Prolonged (4 to 6 months) infection of lymphoid tissues and the male reproductive tract occurs after resolution of clinical signs and viremia. Persistent infection can occur in pigs infected in utero, as young animals, or as adults. Viral antigen is localized to macrophages and/or dendritic cells during persistence, but there is no convincing evidence of viremia in this phase of the infection. There also is no evidence of immune evasion through selection of neutralization-resistant viruses during virus persistence.

Other than porcine macrophages, PRRSV replicates in vitro only in MA-104 African green monkey kidney cells and cotton rat lung cells. Infection of macrophages is cytolytic and leads to apoptotic destruction of bystander cells. The ability to grow in MA-104 cells is characteristic of North American isolates of PRRSV, whereas European strains grow extremely poorly or not at all in these cells. Biochemical and immunological studies suggest that GP5 either alone or complexed as a heterodimer with the M protein mediates cellular infection. CD163 expression is required for infection of permissive cells (53). However, the precise mechanism of cellular infection may be more complex and involve additional viral proteins, as substitution of PRRSV GP5 into an infectious cDNA clone of EAV did not alter tropism of the recombinant virus to include porcine macrophages (14). Furthermore, viral particles lacking the minor structural proteins GP2a, GP2b (envelope protein), GP3, and GP4 are not infectious (55).

The incidence of other infectious diseases is increased in PRRSV-infected swine herds, and mortality of up to 12 to 20% can occur (58). Diseases that commonly occur in PRRSV-infected swine include streptococcal meningitis, septicemic salmonellosis, Glasser's disease (*Haemophilus parasuis*), exudative dermatitis, sarcoptic mange (*Sarcoptes scabiei*), and bacterial bronchopneumonia. Although it is suspected that PRRSV infection of macrophages suppresses immunity and facilitates opportunistic infection of swine, innate host defense in the lungs of PRRSV-infected animals appears to be unaffected, and experimental coinfection studies with PRRSV and other pathogens have been inconclusive. Thus, the mechanism that is responsible for the increased incidence of other infectious diseases in PRRSV-infected swine herds remains to be adequately characterized.

Acute PRRS initially manifests as anorexia and lethargy in affected pigs (58). Clinically, affected animals are transiently lymphopenic, pyretic, hyperpneic, and dyspneic and can exhibit transient hyperemia or cyanosis of the extremities. Nursery and young growing pigs develop rough hair coats and their growth is slowed. PRRSV infection of sows that are either nonpregnant or in early to mid-gestation often is uncomplicated, whereas infection of sows in late gestation causes reproductive failure characterized by abortion and the birth of weak pigs. The mortality rate in infected sows varies markedly depending on the virulence of the infecting virus strain and can range anywhere from 1 to 50%. Severely affected sows can develop pulmonary edema, cystitis, nephritis, and nervous signs, including ataxia, circling, and paresis. Importantly, surviving sows often have delayed return to estrus and low conception rates at subsequent breeding. Piglets that survive in utero infection are born weak, frequently are viremic, and rarely survive to weaning. Affected piglets are listless and emaciated and display splay-legged posture, hyperpnea, dyspnea, and chemosis; they may develop neurological signs. Infected boars can exhibit anorexia, lethargy, and respiratory signs, with variable reduction in libido and semen quality.

The characteristic gross lesions of acute PRRS include enlarged lymph nodes, particularly the inguinal lymph nodes, and interstitial pneumonia. The severity and distribution of lesions reflect the virulence of the infecting viral strain. Microscopic lesions are inconsistently present by 10 days after infection. Germinal centers in affected lymph nodes exhibit either lympholysis or lymphoid depletion early in infection, and reactive hyperplasia subsequently. Fetuses and stillborn pigs rarely exhibit any characteristic lesions.

## Immune Response

Anti-PRRSV immunity is variable and weak, although infections are typically resolved and recovered pigs largely are resistant to reinfection (reviewed in reference 34). In contrast to the robust innate response of horse macrophages to EAV infection, PRRSV infection of pig AMΦ failed to elicit any significant expression of genes encoding proinflammatory cytokines. Similarly, production of type I IFNs after in vivo infection of swine apparently differs depending on the infecting strain of PRRSV, and PRRSV infection inhibits the production of type I IFN production that is induced by transmissible gastroenteritis virus infection; transmissible gastroenteritis virus is a strong inducer of IFN.

Neutralizing antibodies to PRRSV principally are directed against GP5 and to a lesser extent GP4 (6). The predicted ectodomain region of GP5 is approximately 30 aa in length, and there is marked variation in the glycosylation of this region of GP5 among field strains of the virus. The extent of glycosylation, or lack thereof, may affect accessibility of the linear neutralizing epitope in GP5 to neutralizing antibodies, thus delaying specific antibody production. Anti-GP5 and neutralizing antibodies appear considerably later in the course of PRRSV infection of swine than do those to the N and nonstructural viral proteins.

Antibodies to the nonstructural, N, and M proteins and GP5 appear within 7 to 14 days of infection, whereas those to the GP5 ectodomain and neutralizing antibodies do not appear until 21 to 28 days, when viral titers in blood are low or absent (36). The neutralizing antibody response varies significantly between swine but is typically weak (titers of 4 to 32), and it is not detected in some animals following PRRSV infection. Pigs that recover from natural or experimental PRRSV infection are usually resistant to homologous reinfection regardless of their neutralizing antibody status, and they do not demonstrate anamnestic antibody responses after reinfection. Thus, the role of antibodies in conferring protective immunity to PRRSV may differ from the role of antibodies to EAV, but the potential role of neutralizing antibodies has been established by passive transfer of PRRSV-specific antibodies to protect pigs against acute, viremic infection.

The cellular immune response to PRRSV includes virus-specific T-cell proliferation (both CD4$^+$ and CD8$^+$) that occurs 4 to 12 weeks after infection. The M protein may be an important target of the cell-mediated immunity response to PRRSV. As with other arteriviruses, PRRSV-specific T-cell responses are difficult to measure, and IFN-$\gamma$ production is not a reliable indicator of an immune response. Specifically, IFN-$\gamma$ responses vary markedly among infected animals that resolve acute infections, ranging from no obvious response to high-level but transient production of this cytokine following stimulation (56). Thus, the precise mechanisms whereby resolution of acute viremic infection occurs in PRRSV-infected swine remain to be adequately characterized. Furthermore, even after cessation of viremia, PRRSV persists in lung and lymph nodes despite host humoral and cellular immune responses, suggesting that other factors, such as macrophage permissiveness and innate immunity, may be important in mediating antiviral immunity. Thus, it has been proposed that the availability of permissive macrophages rather than acquired immunity determines the outcome of PRRSV infection, as occurs in LDV infection of mice (see below).

### Therapy and Vaccines

Spontaneous elimination of PRRSV from infected herds is rare; thus, control usually is achieved through a combination of management practices and vaccination. There are no effective treatments for PRRS in swine, and type I IFN or IFN-inducing agents are not beneficial. Rigorous biosecurity measures are required to prevent the introduction of PRRSV into susceptible herds through semen, movement of infected pigs, or fomites. Regular testing of breeding stock and daily testing of boars used for artificial insemination are necessary to ensure freedom from infection. Even when high-risk sources of infection such as semen, infected animals, and contaminated transportation vehicles are stringently controlled, reintroductions are common, particularly in regions of intensive pig production. Identification of the precise route of reintroduction is often difficult, and the role of airborne transmission of PRRSV remains controversial. Whereas experimental demonstration of airborne spread of PRRSV is difficult, the use of facilities with positive-pressure, HEPA-filtered air has maintained PRRS-free herds in swine-dense regions in which nearby farms have become infected.

Elimination of endemic PRRSV infection also is challenging. Total depopulation of a farm, followed by thorough disinfection with heat, chlorine, iodine, or quaternary ammonium compounds and drying, is an extreme but effective method. Modified procedures that identify and remove infected pigs can be effective but are dependent on imperfect diagnostic procedures. An alternative strategy is to close (quarantine) the herd to introduction of new animals, and then allow herd immunity to eliminate the virus from the population over the subsequent 6 to 12 months. However, breeding herds typically turn over 50% of their animals each year, so herd closure necessitates drastic changes to management practices.

Vaccination and controlled exposure (intentional infection) are used for immunological control of PRRSV infection in swine. Controlled exposure is the practice whereby incoming gilts are intentionally infected with serum containing the strain of PRRSV currently circulating on the premises. This practice assumes that the deleterious manifestations of acute infection in exposed gilts will be minor compared to the benefits of protecting these animals against economically devastating reproductive manifestations of PRRS.

Both live attenuated (MLV) and inactivated vaccines are available for prevention of PRRSV infection of swine. MLV PRRSV vaccines provide complete protection against PRRSV infection and PRRS in experimental studies, especially against closely related virus strains. In marked contrast, however, outbreaks of PRRS continue to occur in well-vaccinated herds, suggesting that vaccine-based immunity is not always effective. The extensive genetic variation that occurs among field strains of PRRSV might account for some instances of vaccine failure. However, there is no definitive evidence of true immunological escape. Furthermore, outbreaks of PRRS have occurred in intentionally infected herds in which the virus recovered from sick pigs is very similar to the inoculating strain used for controlled exposure. The controversy surrounding the use of MLV vaccines in protection against PRRS likely will continue until the mechanisms of immunological protection are better characterized. Specifically, the mechanism(s) by which MLV vaccines induce protective immunity is uncertain, as resistance is not reliably correlated to titers of neutralizing antibody or to correlates of PRRSV-specific cellular immune responses.

The potential transmission, circulation, and reversion to virulence of MLV PRRSV vaccines have further fueled the controversy surrounding their use. Vaccines based on inactivated viral preparations or recombinant proteins offer potential benefits in terms of their safety, but their efficacy is less certain.

Expression constructs that coexpress only GP5 and M protein of PRRSV recently have been developed, and initial studies with these constructs indicate that they can induce protective responses in immunized swine (25). In summary, although inactivated or recombinant subunit PRRSV vaccines have substantial theoretical advantage in terms of their safety, their protective efficacy remains to be adequately proven.

## LDV INFECTION OF MICE

LDV now is the generally accepted moniker for this virus, but it previously has been designated as lactate dehydrogenase virus, lactic dehydrogenase agent, lactic dehydrogenase-elevating virus, lactic dehydrogenase virus, the Riley agent, etc. The natural host of LDV is the house mouse, *Mus musculus domesticus,* and domesticated derivatives thereof, namely, the laboratory mouse. It has been isolated from feral *M. m. domesticus* from Australia, Europe, and the United States (28, 47). It is uncertain, but likely, that LDV is also indigenous among other subspecies of *M. musculus.* In keeping with the biological behavior of arteriviruses, it has extreme host and cellular (macrophage) specificity, but unlike other arteriviruses, it is generally nonpathogenic. It has been speculated that LDV crossed over from mice to wild boars in Europe, giving rise to PRRSV (38). Comprehensive reviews of the biology of LDV infection are published (11, 41, 47).

The initial discovery of LDV arose within a few years in three different laboratories. The circumstances of discovery in these initial reports revealed the essential characteristics of LDV biology. In the first study, a massive increase in the level of lactate dehydrogenase was observed in the plasma of mice injected with 26 different transplantable tumors (44). In the second study, a moderate degree of splenomegaly and lymph node enlargement was noted in otherwise subclinically affected mice inoculated with material from wild mice (42). The third report noted interference with replication of vesicular stomatitis virus in infected mice (46). These characteristics—enzyme elevation, contamination of transplantable tumors, clinically silent infection with mild pathology, and immunomodulation—represent the primary reasons why LDV is a significant adventitious agent in the laboratory mouse.

## Epidemiology

Direct contact between mice is required for transmission of LDV to occur, with pugilism as the primary means of transmission through bite wounds. Transmission by indirect contact can, rarely, occur. Dermal application of the virus has been shown to result in infection, probably through abrasions. Transmission can be curtailed by amputation of the incisors, emphasizing the importance of biting behavior in virus transmission. Virus is excreted in feces, urine, saliva, and milk, and can also be experimentally transmitted orally and intranasally. All strains of laboratory mice are susceptible to infection. Feces contain the highest titers of virus, and the coprophagic (eating of feces) behavior of mice, possibly more than salivary secretion, probably plays an important role in transmission through bite wounds. Notably, LDV is abundant in testicular tissue during the persistent phase of infection. Sexual transmission is therefore possible, but it has not been studied. Sexual transmission through semen occurs with both EAV and PRRSV (see respective sections in this chapter). Transmission of infection from parents to young is not frequent, and although transplacental transmission has been documented, it is strongly inhibited by maternal immunity. Thus, acutely infected, nonimmune dams efficiently transmit virus to their fetuses, but during persistent infection, maternal immunity prevents fetal infection. Although the placenta is readily infected, there is a strong concentration gradient of placental and umbilical cord trapping of maternal LDV antibody, which inhibits fetal infection. Furthermore, infection of the fetus is highly dependent upon gestational stage, with susceptibility arising at about 12 to 15 days of gestation, which coincides with macrophage maturation and expression of F4/80 on macrophages (59). Thus, the likelihood of natural maternal-fetal transmission in the context of an enzootically infected mouse population is remote. In laboratory mouse colonies, the most likely source of infection is iatrogenic inoculation of contaminated biological material, particularly transplantable tumors. LDV remains one of the most common murine pathogens to contaminate transplantable tumor lines.

LDVs that have been isolated from transplantable tumors are closely related to the quasispecies virus population present in wild mice. Experimental studies with LDV emphasize the fact that most virus pools contain both neuropathogenic (LDV-C and LDV-v) and nonneuropathogenic (LDV-P and LDV-vx) variants (28). LDV-P and LDV-vx variants invariably establish persistent infections in mice, which are maintained by selective cytocidal replication in a renewable subpopulation of macrophages (41, 47). These variants also resist serum neutralization due to three large N-linked polylactosaminoglycan chains on the short ectodomain of the VP-3P envelope glycoprotein (39). This region of VP-3P is involved in host receptor binding and contains the neutralization epitope. Neuropathogenic LDV-C and LDV-v variants lack the two N-terminal N glycosylation sites on their VP-3Ps, which permits them to interact with an alternate receptor on motor neurons but also enhances their immunogenicity and sensitivity to neutralization. Neuropathogenic variants are strongly suppressed in immunocompetent mice because of their sensitivity to neutralization. Thus, the nonneuropathogenic, neutralizing antibody-resistant variants predominate in persistently infected mice (40).

## Pathogenesis and Pathology

LDV replicates selectively in tissue macrophages. LDV is present in very high titers in peripheral blood. Titers in the spleen, liver, lymph nodes, and thymus are equivalent to those in blood, whereas titers in the kidneys, brain, lungs intestine, and pancreas are lower. Virus attains extremely high titer in serum within 12 to 14 h after inoculation due to rapid cytolysis of target macrophages, thereby releasing massive numbers of infectious virions into the circulation. Exhaustion of target cell populations subsequently attenuates the level of viremia, which persists at a lower level throughout the life of the mouse (47). The distribution of target cells varies with the interval of infection. During the first 24 h, numerous antigen- and RNA-positive cells are present in many tissues, including the peritoneum, bone marrow, thymus, spleen, lymph nodes, liver, pancreas, kidneys, adipose tissue, skeletal muscle, leptomeninges, reticular dermis, and testes. In lymphoid tissues, marginal zones are preferentially affected. During subsequent intervals, coinciding with the persistent phase of infection, there are few or no infected cells in most tissues, with the exception of the liver, spleen, lymph nodes, and testes. Persistent infection is maintained by selective infection of a continually renewable subpopulation of mature macrophages. A major component of this subpopulation expresses F4/80 cell surface antigen, which is present only on mature macrophages, and not progenitor stages. LDV-mediated depletion of macrophages results in impaired clearance of plasma enzymes, including lactate dehydrogenase, with 5- to 10-fold elevations. This phenomenon is not specific to lactate dehydrogenase, as the levels of several other enzymes are also significantly elevated (reviewed in references 11 and 47).

LDV induces a unique syndrome known as age-dependent poliomyelitis (ADPM), which has been touted as a model for human amyotrophic lateral sclerosis (48). ADPM with progressive paralysis was initially noted in C58 mice following injection of LDV-contaminated leukemia cells. Disease developed only in aged animals that became spontaneously immunosuppressed at 6 to 12 months of age, or in younger mice that were experimentally immmunosuppressed (3). The LDV that was isolated from these mice replicated in several different strains of mice but induced neurological disease only in C58 and AKR mice. Following infection of the leptomeninges, LDV spreads to motor neurons of the spinal cord and causes apoptotic cell death, with resulting progressive paralysis, respiratory failure, and death. ADPM is unique to C58 and AKR (and probably HRS) mice. These specific mouse strains possess multiple genomic proviral copies of endogenous N-ecotropic retroviruses that are expressed in high titers in multiple tissues. As these mice age, they develop thymic lymphoma and lymphoma-associated immunosuppression, but they also express retrovirus in ventral horn neurons. This unique combination of specific mouse strains that carry endogenous N-ecotropic murine leukemia virus, immunosuppression due to lymphoma, and neuronal coinfection with leukemia virus and LDV results in LDV-mediated neuronolysis. Furthermore, neuropathogenic LDV variants which possess altered cell tropism (neurotropism) are required. These variants, as noted above, are antibody neutralization sensitive and thus require host immunosuppression for their outgrowth within the infecting virus population. The mechanisms for neuronal susceptibility to LDV are not fully understood, but it is noteworthy that the strict species and cell tropism of LDV can be circumvented by infecting cell lines derived from other species with dual-, ampho-, and xenotropic murine leukemia viruses (viruses capable of infecting cells of species other than the mouse [24]).

## Immune Response

LDV successfully evades host immunity, thereby favoring persistence in a number of ways. Infection elicits a strong and specific immune response (11), but serum antibody and T-cell responses are not elicited in time to clear the high titers of replicating virus during the acute stage of infection, largely because virus replicates so rapidly within the first few hours following infection. The major factor in reducing virus titers in plasma during the early phase of infection is exhaustion of the target cell population, rather than any virus-specific immune response. Cytotoxic T cells disappear during persistent infection, apparently through clonal exhaustion. In addition, there is inhibition of IL-4 production with suppression of helper T cells (31). Virus isolated during early infection is efficiently neutralized, whereas virus isolated from persistently infected mice is neutralization resistant, suggesting selection for neutralization escape variants within the quasispecies population. Infection of immunocompetent mice triggers polyclonal B-cell activation, with enhanced specific and nonspecific immunoglobulin G2a (IgG2a)-restricted antibody responses. As infection proceeds, germinal centers expand, resulting in the only visible lesions, splenomegaly and lymphadenomegaly. In infected mice, viremia occurs in the form of infectious virus-IgG complexes. NK cells mediate minimal control of virus in infected mice. Notably, athymic nude mice or chemically immunosuppressed mice manifest kinetics of viremia similar to those of fully immunocompetent mice.

LDV-induced polyclonal B-cell activation stimulates the formation of hydrophobic IgG-containing immune complexes that do not contain viral antigens. These immune complexes peak at about 1 month and then persist throughout the course of infection. Similar nonspecific immune complexes are found in non-LDV-infected, autoimmune MRL/lpr mice. However, LDV infection suppresses the induction of autoimmunity in NZB × NZWF1 hybrid mice, suppresses the induction of experimental allergic encephalomyelitis in SJL mice, and prevents the onset of diabetes in NOD mice. LDV infection modulates a variety of immune responses through a number of direct and indirect effects, including depression of cellular immunity, cytokine perturbations, and macrophage function (11). Modulation of the immune response is the major concern for adventitious infection of laboratory mice with LDV.

The major neutralizing epitope of LDV mapped to the middle of the GP5 ectodomain (aa 37 to 44), where it is flanked by two glycosylation sites (reviewed in reference 6). The GP5 of strains of LDV (e.g., LDV-P and LDV-vx) that establish persistent infections in mice contain three N-glycans, which reduce the immunogenicity of the major neutralization epitope and render these strains highly resistant to in vivo neutralization by antibodies. In contrast, laboratory mutant strains of LDV (e.g., LDV-C and LDV-v) are highly susceptible to antibody neutralization and are incapable of establishing persistent infection of mice; rather, they are neurovirulent in immunosuppressed C58 and AKR mice. The GP5 ectodomain of these mutant viruses lacks the two N-terminal glycans (Asn-36 and Asn-45) flanking the major neutralization epitope, and the loss of these two glycosylation sites apparently makes the neutralization epitope both highly immunogenic and susceptible to in vivo neutralization by antibodies. The loss of these glycosylation sites also alters cellular tropism of LDV, leading to infection of spinal cord anterior horn neurons and subsequent paralysis of the infected mice.

## Therapy and Vaccines

Vaccines are not available and there is no need for them, as control of LDV infection in laboratory mice is by exclusion. LDV can be eliminated from contaminated cell lines and tumors by in vitro culture or passage through athymic nude rats. In such culture or passage the mouse macrophage subpopulation that is essential for virus replication is eliminated, with subsequent clearance of virus (11). An oft-held misconception is that LDV antibodies cannot be effectively detected due to the high-affinity virus-antibody complexes present in serum and the high level of nonspecific immune complexes that bind to enzyme-linked immunosorbent assay (ELISA) plates. Antibody can indeed be effectively detected in mice by 1 to 3 weeks of infection by ELISA or immunofluorescence, using purified LDV virions or infected cells as the antigen. A traditional approach for LDV infection has been a bioassay in which mice are inoculated with suspect material and then tested for 8- to 11-fold elevations in plasma lactate dehydrogenase, which rise within 24 h, peak at 72 to 96 h, and persist thereafter (47). This approach is being replaced with more sensitive, specific, and rapid nucleic acid PCR assays (52). LDV can be isolated from infected mice using primary peritoneal exudate cultures, but other cell lines, including macrophage lines, do not support LDV growth in vitro (11).

## SHF

SHF was first recognized in 1964 in primate centers in both the United States and Soviet Union in several species of recently imported macaques (*Macaca mulatta, Macaca speciosa, Macaca cynomolgus,* and *Macaca assamensis*) originating from a single supplier in India (26, 43, 49). Outbreaks subsequently occurred in 1967 in macaques at a facility in Sussex, England, and at the California Regional Primate Center (16, 35). Since that time there have been remarkably few reported outbreaks of SHF, the most notable of which was a combined outbreak of SHF and Ebola fever (Reston virus) in cynomolgus macaques that were recently imported into the United States from the Philippines (12, 43). Asymptomatic seroconversion of animal handlers during that Reston outbreak suggested that SHFV is zoonotic.

## Epidemiology

After the initial descriptions of SHF in the 1960s, studies of both African and Asian cercopithecine monkeys revealed that many species of African monkeys, including patas monkeys *(Erythrocebus patas)*, African green monkeys *(Chlorocebus aethiops)*, and baboons *(Papio* spp.), have been exposed to SHFV and that these species may be inapparent carriers of the virus (20, 37). Serological evidence also suggests that subclinical or asymptomatic SHFV infection occurs in Asian macaques in China, the Philippines, and Southeast Asia, perhaps with attenuated strains of the virus (57). Transmission of SHFV from African monkeys to any of three species of Asian macaque monkeys *(Macaca mulatta, Macaca arctoides,* and *Macaca fascicularis)* results in an acute, often fatal hemorrhagic fever. Transmission from African monkeys to macaques may be by direct contact, aerosol, or fomites or may occur iatrogenically through contaminated needles. The disease can easily spread between adjacent cages and rooms.

### Pathogenesis and Pathology

Like the other three arteriviruses, SHFV principally replicates in macrophages, although there is considerable variation in the cellular tropism, virulence, and immunogenicity of individual strains of SHFV in African monkeys (21). SHFVs of African origin are highly infectious and fatal in macaques. Patas monkeys are a probable reservoir, since perhaps 50% of these animals have antibodies to SHFV. Similarly, baboons and African green monkeys typically develop only mild disease, and they too may be reservoirs. Long-term viremia in these African species can occur without disease and without antibody formation. Identification of asymptomatic carriers through culture of peritoneal macrophages has been described. Patas monkeys can be cleared of persistent infection by superinfection with more virulent strains of African SHFV, and although monkeys thus treated may become ill, fatalities have not been reported (20).

Asian monkeys infected with African SHFV develop fever, facial petechiae, subcutaneous and retrobulbar hemorrhages, dehydration, melena, and splenomegaly (1, 2, 12, 37, 43). Histologically, there is hemorrhage in the marginal zones of the periarteriolar lymphoid sheaths and striking fibrin deposition in the splenic red pulp. Vascular damage and disseminated intravascular coagulation are likely central to the pathogenesis of SHF. Hemorrhagic necrosis of the proximal 5 to 10 cm of the duodenum is pathognomonic for hemorrhagic fever (occurring in both SHF and Ebola) but is not always present.

### Immune Response

There are few published studies on characterization of the molecular biology, pathogenesis, and immune response to SHFV. All known isolates of SHFV are antigenically related, and infected monkeys produce complement-fixing, ELISA, and neutralizing antibodies (18, 30). The humoral immune response of persistently infected patas monkeys varies with the infecting strain of SHFV. Thus, those patas monkeys infected with low-virulence strains (P-248 and P-741) had a minimal or no antibody response and a persistent low level of viremia, whereas a more virulent strain (LVR) induced antibodies within 7 days after infection, and the appearance of these antibodies was associated with rapid clearance of the virus (19). Neutralizing antibodies against one strain of SHFV do not completely neutralize other strains, suggesting that there is variation in the neutralization determinants of individual strains of SHFV. However, the neutralization determinants of SHFV are yet to be characterized. GP7 (p54) encoded by ORF7 of SHFV is homologous to GP5 of other arteriviruses, and preliminary analysis of the membrane topology and hydrophobicity of GP7 of SHFV predicted a short N-terminal ecotodomain (aa 37 to 58) as in LDV and PRRSV GP5 (6).

### Therapy and Vaccines

Vaccines have not been developed to prevent SHFV infection. Repeated administration of an IFN inducer prevented fatalities in rhesus macaques that were experimentally infected with SHFV (27). Supportive cares, including administration of heparin to treat disseminated intravascular coagulation, has been suggested, but euthanasia is more often elected.

### SUMMARY

In summary, although the biological characteristics of natural EAV, PRRSV, LDV, and SHFV infections of their respective animal hosts are very different, the viruses share common features, including their cellular tropism (macrophages) and potential to establish prolonged or persistent infections. The GP5s of EAV, PRRSV, and LDV are all of similar size (199 to 255 aa) and membrane topology, and major neutralization determinants of all three viruses are included in the N-terminal ectodomain of each protein. The equivalent protein of SHFV is not yet well characterized. The extent of GP5 glycosylation appears to significantly influence the neutralization phenotype and biological behavior of individual strains of both LDV and PRRSV but not EAV. Thus, inherent differences in the properties of the GP5s of EAV, PRRSV, and LDV may contribute to unique aspects of the biology of each virus during infection of its respective host.

**Acknowledgments.** This work was supported in part by grant number RR14905 from the National Center for Research Resources, a component of the National Institutes of Health (NIH), and by the Center for Equine Health, University of California—Davis, with funds provided by the Harriet E. Pfleger Foundation.

## REFERENCES

1. **Abildgaard, C., J. Harrison, C. Espana, W. Spangler, and D. Gribble.** 1975. Simian hemorrhagic fever: studies of coagulation and pathology. *Am. J. Trop. Med. Hyg.* **24**:537–544.

2. **Allen, A. M., A. E. Palmer, N. M. Tauraso, and A. Shelokov.** 1968. Simian hemorrhagic fever. II. Studies in pathology. *Am. J. Trop. Med. Hyg.* **17**:413–421.

3. **Anderson, G. W., C. Even, R. R. Rowland, G. A. Palmer, J. T. Harty, and P. G. Plagemann.** 1995. C58 and AKR mice of all ages develop motor neuron disease after lactate dehydrogenase-elevating virus infection but only if antiviral immune responses are blocked by chemical or genetic means or as a result of old age. *J. Neurovirol.* **1**:244–252.

4. **Balasuriya, U. B., J. C. Dobbe, H. W. Heidner, V. L. Smalley, A. Navarette, E. J. Snijder, and N. J. MacLachlan.** 2004. Characterization of the neutralization determinants of equine arteritis virus using recombinant chimeric viruses and site-specific mutagenesis of an infectious cDNA clone. *Virology* **321**:235–246.

5. **Balasuriya, U. B., J. F. Hedges, P. J. Timoney, W. H. McCollum, and N. J. MacLachlan.** 1999. Genetic stability of equine arteritis virus during horizontal and vertical transmission in an outbreak of equine viral arteritis. *J. Gen. Virol.* **85**:379–390.

6. **Balasuriya, U. B., and N. J. MacLachlan.** 2004. The immune response to equine arteritis virus: potential lessons for other arteriviruses. *Vet. Immunol. Immunopathol.* **102**:107–129.

7. **Castillo-Olivares, J., J. P. Tearle, F. Montesso, D. Westcott, J. H. Kydd, N. J. Davis-Poynter, and D. Hannant.** 2003. Detection of equine arteritis virus (EAV)-specific cytotoxic CD8+ T lymphocyte precursors from EAV-infected ponies. *J. Gen. Virol.* **84**:2745–2753.

8. **Chrisopher-Hennings, J., E. A. Nelson, R. J. Hines, J. K. Nelson, S. L. Swenson, J. J. Zimmerman, C. C. Chase, M. J. Yaeger, and D. A. Benfield.** 1995. Persistence of porcine reproductive and respiratory syndrome virus in serum and semen of adult boars. *J. Vet. Diagn. Investig.* **7**:456–464.

9. **Clark, I.** 1892. Transmission of pink-eye from apparently healthy stallions to mares. *J. Comp. Pathol.* **5**:261–264.

10. **Collins, J. E., D. A. Benfield, W. T. Christianson, L. Harris, J. C. Hennings, D. P. Shaw, S. M. Goyal, S. McCullough, R. B. Morrison, H. S. Joo, D. Gorcyca, and D. Chladek.** 1992. Isolation of swine infertility and respiratory syndrome virus (isolate ATCC VR-2332) in North America and experimental reproduction of disease in gnotobiotic pigs. *J. Vet. Diagn. Investig.* **4**:117–126.

11. **Coutelier, J.-P., and M. A. Brinton.** 2006. Lactate dehydrogenase-elevating virus, p. 215–234. *In* J. G. Fox, C. Newcomer, A. Smith, S. Barthold, F. Quimby, and M. Davisson (ed.), *The Mouse in Biomedical Research*, 2nd ed., vol II. Elsevier, San Diego, CA.

12. **Dalgard, D. W., R. J. Hardy, S. L. Pearson, G. J. Pucak, R. V. Quander, P. M. Zack, C. J. Peters, and P. B. Jahrling.** 1992. Combined simian hemorrhagic fever and Ebola virus infection in cynomolgus monkeys. *Lab. Anim. Sci.* **42**:152–157.

13. **Del Piero, F.** 2000. Equine viral arteritis. *Vet. Pathol.* **37**:287–296.

14. **Dobbe, J. C., Y. van der Meer, W. J. Spaan, and E. J. Snijder.** 2001. Construction of chimeric arteriviruses reveals that the ectodomain of the major glycoprotein is not the main determinant of equine arteritis virus tropism in cell culture. *Virology* **288**:283–294.

15. **Doll, E. R., J. T. Bryans, W. H. McCollum, and M. E. Crowe.** 1957. Isolation of a filterable agent causing arteritis of horses and abortion by mares: its differentiation from the equine abortion (influenza) virus. *Cornell Vet.* **47**:3–41.

16. **Espana, C.** 1974. Viral epizootics in captive nonhuman primates. *Lab. Anim. Sci.* **24**:167–176.

17. **Glaser, A. L., P. J. Rottier, M. C. Horzinek, and B. Colenbrander.** 1996. Equine arteritis virus: a review of clinical features and management aspects. *Vet. Q.* **18**:95–99.

18. **Godeny, E. K.** 2002. Enzyme-linked immunosorbent assay for detection of antibodies against simian hemorrhagic fever virus. *Comp. Med.* **52**:229–232.

19. **Gravell, M., W. T. London, M. E. Leon, A. E. Palmer, and R. S. Hamilton.** 1986. Differences among isolates of simian hemorrhagic fever (SHF) virus. *Proc. Soc. Exp. Biol. Med.* **181**:112–119.

20. **Gravell, M., W. T. London, M. E. Leon, A. E. Palmer, and R. S. Hamilton.** 1986. Elimination of persistent simian hemorrhagic fever (SHF) virus infection in patas monkeys. *Proc. Soc. Exp. Biol. Med.* **181**:219–225.

21. **Gravell, M., A. E. Palmer, M. Rodriguez, W. T. London, and R. S. Hamilton.** 1980. Method to detect asymptomatic carriers of simian hemorrhagic fever virus. *Lab. Anim. Sci.* **30**:988–991.

22. **Hedges, J. F., U. B. Balasuriya, P. J. Timoney, W. H. McCollum, and N. J. MacLachlan.** 1999. Genetic divergence with emergence of novel phenotypic variants of equine arteritis virus during persistent infection of stallions. *J. Virol.* **73**:3672–3681.

23. **Hullinger, P. J., I. A. Gardner, S. K. Hietala, G. L. Ferraro, and N. J. MacLachlan.** 2001. Seroprevalence of antibodies against equine arteritis virus in horses residing in the United States and imported horses. *J. Am. Vet. Med. Assoc.* **219**:946–949.

24. **Inada, T.** 1993. Replication of lactate dehydrogenase-elevating virus in various species cell lines infected with dual-, ampho- and xenotropic murine leukemia viruses in vitro. *Virus Res* **27**:267–281.

25. **Jiang, Y., L. Fang, S. Xiao, H. Zhang, Y. Pan, R. Luo, B. Li, and H. Chen.** 2007. Immunogenicity and protective efficacy of recombinant pseudorabies virus expressing the two major membrane-associated proteins of porcine reproductive and respiratory syndrome virus. *Vaccine* **25**:547–560.

26. **Lapin, B. A., and Z. V. Shevtsova.** 1971. On the identity of two simian hemorrhagic fever virus strains (Sukhumi and NIH). *Z. Versierkd.* **13**:21–23.

27. **Levy, H. B., W. London, D. A. Fuccillo, S. Baron, and J. Rice.** 1976. Prophylactic control of simian hemorrhagic fever in monkeys by an interferon inducer, polyriboinosinic-polyribocytidylic acid-poly-L-lysine. *J. Infect. Dis.* **133**(Suppl.):A256–A259.

28. **Li, K., T. Schuler, Z. Chen, G. E. Glass, J. E. Childs, and P. G. Plagemann.** 2000. Isolation of lactate dehydrogenase-elevating viruses from wild house mice and their biological and molecular characterization. *Virus Res.* **67**:153–162.

29. **MacLachlan, N. J., and U. B. Balasuriya.** 2007. Equine viral arteritis, p. 153–163. *In* M. Long and D. Sellon (ed.), *Equine Infectious Diseases*. Elsevier, St. Louis, MO.

30. **Madden, D. L., D. A. Fuccillo, J. A. Dorosz, W. T. London, A. E. Palmer, and G. A. Castellano.** 1978. Antigenic relationship of two strains of simian hemorrhagic fever virus. *Lab. Anim. Sci.* **28**:422–427.

31. Monteyne, P., J. Van Broeck, J. Van Snick, and J.-P. Coutelier. 1993. Inhibition by lactate dehydrogenase-elevating virus of in vivo interleukin 4 production during immunization with keyhole limpet haemocyanin. *Cytokine* **5:**394–397.

32. Moore, B. D., U. B. Balsuriya, J. L. Watson, C. M. Bosio, R. J. MacKay, and N. J. MacLachlan. 2003. Virulent and avirulent strains of equine arteritis virus induce different quantities of TNF-alpha and other proinflammatory cytokines in alveolar and blood-derived equine macrophages. *Virology* **314:**662–670.

33. Murtaugh, M. P., M. R. Elam, and L. T. Kakach. 1995. Comparison of the structural protein coding sequences of the VR-2332 and Lelystad virus strains of the PRRS virus. *Arch. Virol.* **140:**1451–1460.

34. Murtaugh, M. P., Z. Xiao, and F. Zuckermann. 2002. Immunological responses of swine to porcine reproductive and respiratory syndrome virus infection. *Viral Immunol.* **15:**533–547.

35. Myers, M. G., M. M. Vincent, S. A. Hensen, and N. M. Tauraso. 1972. Problems in the laboratory isolation of simian hemorrhagic fever viruses and isolation of the agent responsible for the Sussex-69 epizootic. *Appl. Microbiol.* **24:**62–69.

36. Nilubol, D., K. B. Platt, P. G. Halbur, M. Torremorell, and D. L. Harris. 2004. The effect of a killed porcine reproductive and respiratory syndrome virus (PRRSV) vaccine treatment on virus shedding in previously PRRSV infected pigs. *Vet. Microbiol.* **102:**11–18.

37. Palmer, A. E., A. M. Allen, N. M. Tauraso, and A. Shelokov. 1968. Simian hemorrhagic fever. I. Clinical and epizootiologic aspects of an outbreak among quarantined monkeys. *Am. J. Trop. Med. Hyg.* **17:**404–412.

38. Plagemann, P. G. 2003. Porcine reproductive and respiratory syndrome virus: origin hypothesis. *Emerg. Infect. Dis.* **9:**903–908.

39. Plagemann, P. G., Z. Chen, and K. Li. 1999. Polylactosaminoglycan chains on the ectodomain of the primary envelope glycoprotein of an arterivirus determine its neuropathogenicity, sensitivity to antibody neutralization and immunogenicity of the neutralization epitope. *Curr. Top. Virol.* **1:**27–43.

40. Plagemann, P. G., Z. Chen, and K. Li. 2001. Replication competition between lactate dehydrogenase-elevating virus quasispecies in mice. Implications for quasispecies selection and evolution. *Arch. Virol.* **146:**1283–1296.

41. Plagemann, P. G., and V. Moennig. 1992. Lactate dehydrogenase-elevating virus, equine arteritis virus, and simian hemorrhagic fever virus: a new group of positive-strand RNA viruses. *Adv. Virus. Res.* **41:**99–192.

42. Pope, J. H. 1961. Studies of a virus isolated from a wild house mouse, Mus musculus, and producing splenomegaly and lymph node enlargement in mice. *Aust. J. Exp. Biol. Med. Sci.* **39:**521–536.

43. Renquist, D. 1990. Outbreak of simian hemorrhagic fever. *J. Med. Primatol.* **19:**77–79.

44. Riley, V., F. Lilly, E. Huerto, and D. Bardell. 1960. Transmissible agent associated with 26 types of experimental mouse neoplasms. *Science* **132:**545–547.

45. Rossow, K. D. 1998. Porcine reproductive and respiratory syndrome. *Vet. Pathol.* **35:**1–20.

46. Rowe, W. P., J. W. Hartley, and R. J. Huebner. 1962. Polyoma and other indigenous mouse viruses, p. 131–142. *In* R. J. C. Harris (ed.), *The Problems of Laboratory Animal Diseases.* Academic Press, New York, NY.

47. Rowson, K. E., and B. W. Mahy. 1975. Lactic dehydrogenase virus. *Virology Monographs*, Vol. **13**. Springer-Verlag, New York, NY.

48. Sillevis Smitt, P. A., and J. M. de Jong. 1989. Animal models of amyotrophic lateral sclerosis and the spinal muscular atrophies. *J. Neurol. Sci.* **91:**231–258.

49. Tauraso, N. M., A. Shelokov, A. E. Palmer, and A. M. Allen. 1968. Simian hemorrhagic fever. 3. Isolation and characterization of a viral agent. *Am. J. Trop. Med. Hyg.* **17:**422–431.

50. Timoney, P. J., and W. H. McCollum. 1993. Equine viral arteritis. *Vet. Clin. N. Am. Equine Pract.* **9:**295–309.

51. Timoney, P. J., W. H. McCollum, A. W. Roberts, and T. W. Murphy. 1986. Demonstration of the carrier state in naturally acquired equine arteritis virus infection in the stallion. *Res. Vet. Sci.* **41:**279–280.

52. Wagner, A. M., J. K. Loganbill, and D. G. Besselsen. 2004. Detection of lactate dehydrogenase-elevating virus by use of a fluorogenic nuclease transcriptase-polymerase chain reaction assay. *Comp. Med.* **54:**288–292.

53. Welch, S.-K. W., J. G. Calvert, S. E. Slade, and S. L. Shields. 2005. Scavenger receptor CD163 is a cell permissive factor for infection with porcine reproductive and respiratory syndrome viruses. UniProtKB/Swiss-Prot entry Q2VL90.

54. Wensvoort, G., C. Terpstra, J. M. Pol, E. A. ter Laak, M. Bloemraad, E. P. de Kluyver, C. Kragten, L. van Buiten, A. den Besten, F. Wagenaar, J. M. Broekhuijsen, P. L. Moonen, T. Zetstra, E. A. de Boer, H. J. Tibben, M. F. de Jong, P. van't Veld, G. J. Groenland, J. A. van Gennep, M. T. Voets, J. H. Verheijden, and J. Braamskamp. 1991. Mystery swine disease in the Netherlands: the isolation of Lelystad virus. *Vet. Q.* **13:**121–130.

55. Wissink, E. H., M. V. Kroese, H. A. van Wijk, F. A. Rijsewijk, J. J. Meulenberg, and P. J. Rottier. 2005. Envelope protein requirements for the assembly of infectious virions of porcine reproductive and respiratory syndrome virus. *J. Virol.* **79:**12495–12506.

56. Xiao, Z., L. Batista, S. Dee, P. Halbur, and M. P. Murtaugh. 2004. The level of virus-specific T-cell and macrophage recruitment in porcine reproductive and respiratory syndrome virus infection in pigs is independent of the virus load. *J. Virol.* **78:**5923–5933.

57. Zhao, M., M. Ye, G. X. Luo, S. F. Chen, J. G. Xu, and P. Song. 1990. Virological survey of rhesus monkeys in China. *Lab. Anim. Sci.* **40:**29–32.

58. Zimmerman, J., D. A. Benfield, M. P. Murtaugh, F. Osorio, G. Stevenson, and M. Torremorell. 2005. Porcine reproductive and respiratory syndrome virus (porcine Arterivirus), p. 387–417. *In* B. J. Straw, S. D'Allair, W. L. Mengeling, and D. J. Taylor (ed.), *Diseases of Swine*, 9th ed. Iowa State University Press, Ames.

59. Zitterkopf, N. L., T. R. Haven, M. Huela, D. S. Bradley, and W. A. Cafruny. 2002. Placental lactate dehydrogenase-elevating virus (LDV) transmission: immune inhibition of umbilical cord infection, and correlation of fetal virus susceptibility with development of F4/80 antigen expression. *Placenta* **23:**438–446.

*Nidoviruses*
Edited by S. Perlman, T. Gallagher, and E. J. Snijder
© 2008 ASM Press, Washington, DC

Chapter 22

# The Immune Response to Coronaviruses

CORNELIA C. BERGMANN, THOMAS E. LANE, AND STEPHEN A. STOHLMAN

Coronaviruses (CoV) infect a variety of organs, including the liver, respiratory and enteric tracts, and the central nervous system (CNS). The resulting disease phenotypes comprise a vast spectrum ranging from acute life-threatening disease to chronic, inapparent infections. Host genetic background and age, in addition to the specific virus and route of entry, contribute to disease severity. Viral cellular and tissue tropism affects both the quality and quantity of the immune response, which ultimately determine viral control and pathogenesis. The pathogenesis of human CoV and that of animal CoV are discussed in other chapters and are included to supplement or enforce mechanistic insights driving immune responses to these viruses. This chapter focuses primarily on the in vivo interactions between the immune system and the infected CNS as a target of neurotropic mouse hepatitis virus (MHV) infection because these interactions have been examined in the greatest detail. Immune responses to additional viruses, e.g., transmissible gastroenteritis virus (TGEV), infectious bronchitis virus (IBV), and feline infectious peritonitis virus (FIPV), associated with diseases in other tissues are included, as well as the various MHV strains with distinct tissue tropisms; however, the reader is encouraged to consult other chapters for more detailed information.

## INNATE RESPONSES REGULATE ADAPTIVE RESPONSES

Induction of innate factors by viral replication provides the first line of antiviral defense and a milieu for induction of adaptive immunity (28, 77). MHV infection induces rapid, coordinated expression of proinflammatory cytokines, chemokines, matrix metalloproteinases (MMPs), and the tissue inhibitors of MMPs (TIMP) (5) (Color Plate 6A [see color insert]). In addition to soluble components, these early responses are associated with activation and recruitment of cellular components associated with innate immunity, e.g., neutrophils, NK cells, and monocytes/macrophages. The most rapidly induced proinflammatory cytokines within the MHV-infected CNS are alpha/beta interferon (IFN-α/β), tumor necrosis factor alpha (TNF-α), interleukin 1α (IL-1α), IL-1β, IL-6, and IL-12 (52, 55, 69, 71). Cytokine production is predominant in astrocytes and microglia. IL-6 up-regulation is a prominent response to many CNS infections and might enhance inflammatory cell passage across the blood-brain barrier (BBB) in conjunction with up-regulation of adhesion molecules on CNS endothelium (27). Distinct MHV strains generally induce similar cytokine patterns in mixed glial cultures and in vivo; however, mRNA encoding individual genes can be expressed at various relative ratios (38, 69, 70). For example, lethal neurotropic MHV-JHM induces higher IL-6, IFN-β, IL-1α, and IL-1β mRNA levels, but no differences in TNF-α levels, compared to the more benign dual liver- and CNS-tropic MHV-A59 (69, 70). IL-6 induction segregates to MHV-JHM background genes and not the spike (S) protein gene, as demonstrated by JHM/A59 recombinants (70). Furthermore, MHV-A59 prominently induces IFN-γ, but less IFN-β mRNA, than MHV-JHM in vivo (69, 70). By contrast, MHV-JHM variants differing only in the S protein exhibit no significant differences in cytokine induction, except in overall magnitude (52). Not surprisingly, in vitro analysis of MHV-inducible genes revealed that the expression patterns are vastly distinct in different cell types. L cells infected with MHV-A59 show no evidence for induction of IL-6, TNF-α,

Cornelia C. Bergmann and Stephen A. Stohlman • Department of Neurosciences, Cleveland Clinic, Cleveland, OH 44195. Thomas E. Lane • Department of Molecular Biology and Biochemistry, University of California, Irvine, CA 92697.

IFN-α/β mRNA, or IFN-inducible genes (93), supporting studies which failed to detect IFN-α/β protein in supernatants of L cells infected with MHV-1, -3, -S, -A59, or -JHM (16). By contrast, primary conventional dendritic cells (DCs) respond with low, and plasmacytoid DCs respond with high, levels of type I IFN mRNA and protein secretion following MHV infection (8, 104, 105). IFN-β mRNA is also induced following infection of mixed glial cultures by MHV-2, -A59, and -JHM in vitro (38, 71) and in CNS and lung tissues infected with neurotropic MHV-JHM and MHV-1, respectively (12, 70). Although IFN-α/β protein detection has been elusive following MHV-JHM infection in vivo (83), IFN-α/β is present in both the tissues and serum of IBV- and TGEV-infected animals (32, 51). In TGEV-infected cells, this property is associated with membrane (M) and envelope (E) proteins (2, 9). Although many MHV strains are poor inducers of IFN-α/β (16, 83, 93, 94), CoV are clearly sensitive to the antiviral effects of IFN-α/β (12, 56). While MHV-A59 and -JHM have sensitivities higher than those observed for vesicular stomatitis virus, hepatotropic strains MHV-2 and MHV-3 are most resistant to type I IFN (16). However, the modest effects of IFN-β treatment on MHV-JHM replication in bone marrow-derived DCs in vitro (104) suggests that the infected cell type, in addition to virus strain, determines IFN-α/β sensitivity. Finally, in contrast to the IFN antagonists uncovered in severe acute respiratory syndrome CoV (SARS-CoV) (76), gene products of other CoV antagonizing IFN-α/β function have yet to be identified.

There is also substantial evidence that IFN-α/β provides protection against MHV infection in vivo. Administration of recombinant IFN-β prior to infection suppresses viral replication and liver pathology following MHV-2 infection as well as pulmonary pathology following MHV-1 infection and respiratory diseases induced by IBV (12, 46, 56). Similarly, intranasal IFN-α/β prevented spread of MHV-JHM into the CNS but did not inhibit visceral dissemination (74). Enhanced virulence following inhibition of type I IFN (37) and the rapid mortality of MHV-A59-infected IFN-α/β receptor-deficient mice (8) further demonstrate a vital protective role for type I IFN. The crucial source of IFN-α/β secretion following peripheral MHV-A59 infection was identified as plasmacytoid DCs, and protection correlated with prevention of dissemination to nonlymphoid tissue (8). However, despite functional IFN-α/β responsiveness and recruitment of neutrophils, macrophages, and NK cells in SCID, RAG$^{-/-}$, and nude mice, these immune deficient mice fail to control neurotropic MHV, implying that innate responses alone are insufficient to combat infection (7, 26, 101).

In addition to direct antiviral effects, type I IFNs also modulate both innate and adaptive immune function (28, 62, 77). The pleiotropic effects of type I IFNs are especially difficult to dissect in the CNS, as IFN-α/β acts on cells in lymphoid tissue, resident CNS cells, and cells trafficking into the CNS. Gene profiling of MHV-JHM-infected neuronal cultures revealed up-regulation of transcription factors IRF7, STAT-1, and ISGF3, as well as induction of major histocompatibility complex (MHC) class I heavy chains, multiple cofactors involved in class I antigen processing, and nonclassical MHC class I molecules (71). Functional expression of IFN-α/β within the CNS in vivo is indicated by MHC class I surface expression on microglia following sublethal MHV-JHM infection of IFN-γ-deficient mice (6, 7). As MHC surface expression is undetectable in the noninflamed CNS, IFN-γ-independent virus-induced up-regulation of selected antigen presentation molecules potentially enhances both innate and adaptive lymphocyte function within the CNS. Furthermore, as both MHV-A59 and -JHM infect DCs in vitro (8, 90, 104, 105), very early events may affect DC antigen presentation function in lymphoid tissue and thus modulate the adaptive response prior to CNS recruitment. Indeed, MHV-JHM-infected DCs are impaired in supporting T-cell proliferation in vitro (104). However, as yet viral infection of DCs in vivo, as well as the triggering of adaptive immune responses by antigen-presenting cells (APC), remains elusive. Similarly, effects of IFN-α/β on adaptive responses during other CoV infections have not been analyzed.

Despite the induction of nitric oxide synthase 2 (the inducible NOS isoform) by neurotropic MHV, it exerts no detectable host antiviral or immune modulatory functions (35, 36, 100). Similarly, TNF-α is prominently produced by resident CNS cells (52). Although TNF-α translation is inhibited in MHV-infected cells (84), neither replication in vivo nor pathology is altered in the absence of TNF-α (60, 84). A minor, if any, role for TNF-α is supported by the inability to correlate the induction of TNF-α mRNA with enhanced virulence (52, 69, 70). Chemokines represent a large family of proteins that primarily function in recruitment and retention of immune cells during infection. MHV infection of the CNS results in an orchestrated expression of chemokines, including CCL2, CCL3, CCL4, CCL5, CXCL9, CXCL10, and CXCL11 (34, 78). Temporal expression of chemokine transcripts reveals that CCL3 and CXCL10 are most rapidly induced, with CCL2, CCL3, CCL4, CCL5 CCL7, CXCL9, and CXCL11 induction somewhat delayed during acute infection. CXCL10 is the prominent chemokine detected during both acute and chronic disease. Infection of CCL3$^{-/-}$ mice results in deficient activation and accumulation of myeloid DCs in cervical lymph nodes (CLN) and consequently muted activation of virus-specific T cells (86, 87). This is evident by the inability of virus-specific CD8 T cells to undergo egress from lymphatic tissue and migrate into the CNS due to impaired expression of tissue-specific chemokine homing receptors CXCR3 and CCR5 (86). In addition, virus-specific CD4 T cells produce an altered cytokine profile with an increase in the anti-inflammatory cytokine IL-10 and diminished secretion of the proinflammatory cytokine IFN-γ (87). This indicates that early expression of chemokines plays an important role in linking innate and adaptive immune responses. Blocking CXCL9 or CXCL10 during acute disease increases virus replication and mortality while reducing CNS infiltration by CXCR3$^+$ T cells, consistent with a crucial role for chemokines in host defense via attracting T cells to the site of infection (40, 41). By contrast, blocking CXCL10 during chronic disease, after infectious virus has been eliminated, proves to be beneficial to the resolution of residual clinical and pathological disease (40, 41, 78). Therefore, early CXCL10 expression is protective by recruiting antiviral T cells, but prolonged expression is detrimental via sustaining inflammation and pathology. In addition to CXCL10, CCL5 also promotes protection during acute disease as well as amplifying disease severity during chronic disease (17, 18). CCL5 recognizes the CCR1 and CCR5 receptors present on activated macrophages and T cells. MHV infection of CCR5$^{-/-}$ mice does not significantly impact host defense; however, virus-induced pathology is reduced due to reduced macrophage recruitment (18). Therefore, chemokines participate in modulating both protective innate and adaptive immunity but also influence the extent of tissue damage.

MMP activation is associated with several physiological processes, including the influx of inflammatory cells into tissues, activation of cytokines, and pathology (103). Compared to autoimmune mediated demyelinating disease of the CNS, MHV-JHM infection induces only a small subset of potential MMPs in the infected CNS, i.e., MMP-3, -9, and -12 (107, 108). Neutrophils, macrophages, and NK cells are the initial inflammatory cells recruited to the CNS during infection (5). MMP-9, which is prepackaged in neutrophils, contributes to loss of the tight junctions of the BBB, facilitating entry of inflammatory cells into the infected CNS (109). Although neutrophils are rapidly recruited into other anatomical sites of viral infection and MMPs are expected to be induced and/or activated, their participation in CoV infections other than MHV have not been studied. Unlike MMP-9 expression in innate infiltrates, MMP-3 and -12 expression is prominent in resident CNS cells.

However, their roles in migration of inflammatory cells, cytokine activation, and pathology are unclear. A potential mechanism for counteracting MMP-mediated tissue damage during MHV-JHM immune responses may reside in the sustained elevation of mRNA encoding the MMP inhibitor TIMP-1 (107, 108). Increased virulence by MHV-JHM variants is associated with increased MMP-9 activity and MMP-3, MMP-12, and TIMP-1 mRNA levels, albeit without affecting inflammation (108). This suggests that virulence may directly correlate with enhanced proteolytic activity at the site of infection. In addition to the CNS, the liver, lung, and enteric tract are primary targets of many MHV infections. Another protease, the prothrombinase fgl2, secreted by macrophages in MHV-3-susceptible, but not MHV-3-resistant, mice, contributes to fatal acute hepatic damage. This proteinase, induced by the MHV-3 nucleocapsid (N) protein (50), triggers the coagulation pathway, resulting in disseminated intravascular coagulation, severe liver damage, and death (42). fgl2 expression is also associated with diseased lung tissue in the murine MHV-1 model of SARS (12).

In addition to neutrophils and bone marrow-derived monocytes, NK cells constitute an early innate component of the inflammatory response. Infection of both T-cell-deficient rats and mice with MHV suggests that NK cells are not primary effectors of viral clearance (26, 75), although they may provide an integral component of overall immunity via local IFN-γ secretion. Nevertheless, despite peak accumulation of NK cells prior to T cells within the CNS of immune competent mice, there is little evidence for either a direct or indirect NK cell-dependent IFN-γ or perforin antiviral function (7, 110). Infection with a recombinant MHV expressing CXCL10 leads to extensive CNS accumulation of NK cells with antiviral activity in immunodeficient RAG1$^{-/-}$ mice (87). By stark contrast, IL-15-deficient mice, which lack NK cells, control MHV infection with kinetics similar to those in wild-type mice and exhibit no delays in either IFN-γ-dependent MHC class I or class II expression on microglia (110). Therefore, antiviral function of NK cells can be forced under targeted conditions; however, NK cells do not appear to contribute to either direct viral clearance or amplification of the immune response in immune competent mice.

### Cellular Immunity

Control of infections by enveloped viruses involves a coordinated immune response that is initiated and subsequently orchestrated by innate immune mediators such as macrophages, DCs, IFN-α/β, and chemokines.

These factors provide both an initial antiviral response and the appropriate milieu for activation of both cellular and humoral immune responses. For CoV, as well as other enveloped viruses, CD4 and CD8 T-cell responses generally precede induction of humoral immunity. This may reflect the coordinated shift from proinflammatory cytokines such as IFN-γ to the more anti-inflammatory cytokines such as IL-4, which provides "help" to the humoral response.

Even in the case of neurotropic MHV-JHM infection, during which replication is undetectable at peripheral sites, virus-specific T cells are detected in the CLN and spleen prior to the CNS (45). The early detection of primed T cells in lymphoid tissues and the observation that MHV-A59 and -JHM can both productively infect DCs in vitro (8, 90, 104, 105) support direct T-cell activation by infected APC in lymphoid tissue. Alternatively, viral antigen can be taken up by APC following drainage from cerebrospinal fluid or acquired by cells with a DC-like phenotype within the CNS, which subsequently migrate to CLN. Detection of DCs in the CNS as early as 2 days postinfection supports the possibility that viral-antigen-carrying DCs migrate to the CLN (87); however, the mechanisms and precise site(s) of T-cell priming during CoV infections, including the CNS, still require further validation.

Following peripheral expansion, T-cell numbers in the CNS increase to peak levels by 1 week postinfection, with a concomitant decline in the periphery (Color Plate 6B). Increasing T-cell infiltration coincides with reductions in infectious virus and a decline in CXCL9, CCL2, CCL3, and CCL7 as well as IL-1α, IL-1β, IL-6, IL-12, and IFN-β mRNA and leads to a decline in neutrophils and NK cells, while macrophages persist within the CNS (5). Peak T-cell infiltration is associated with peak antiviral function, as evidenced by maximal IFN-γ mRNA and cytolytic activity. Functional IFN-γ is evident by maximal MHC class I and II expression by 6 to 7 days postinfection (6). In the absence of IFN-γ, MHC class I expression is reduced and MHC class II remains undetectable on microglia and most CNS macrophages (6, 7). Both perforin-mediated cytolysis and IFN-γ contribute to antiviral effector functions and viral control within the CNS. An absence of IFN-γ results in enhanced mortality compared to that of perforin-deficient mice, although both mechanisms are required for efficient control of infectious virus (39, 53). The requirement of MHC molecule/T-cell receptor contact for secretion of IFN-γ and perforin-mediated cytolysis makes it difficult to distinguish the direct antiviral function of IFN-γ from the indirect effects mediated via enhanced target recognition and T-cell function. Nevertheless, the tightly controlled

regulation of MHC molecules is most pronounced in the CNS and less likely to play a role in other organs such as the liver. In addition to its critical role in controlling MHV replication in the CNS, IFN-γ is also critical for noncytolytic control of MHV replication in the retina (25). Another consequence of IFN-γ signaling in addition to direct antiviral activity appears to be regulation of MHV receptor expression. Receptor expression, and therefore susceptibility to infection of activated macrophages, correlates with resistance and susceptibility to MHV-3-induced hepatitis (48, 57). By contrast, reduced receptor expression by CNS resident macrophages was independent of IFN-γ (65).

## CD4 T cells

Virus-specific-CD4 T cells are activated rapidly after infection. CD4 T cells initially provide a source of IFN-γ, which, among its other activities (62), increases activation and expression of MHC molecules on infected target cells as well as macrophages and DCs, which function as APC to further amplify the cellular immune response. Macrophage activation is a prominent component of the immune response to MHV-induced hepatitis; however, there is only sparse information on the identity and activation of APC. Activation and accumulation of CD4 T cells within infected target organs have been well described for both IBV in the trachea and MHV within the CNS (5, 31).

Depletion of either CD4 or CD8 T cells prevents MHV clearance. CD4 T cells protect against acute disease without reducing virus replication (30, 85, 102). Interestingly, S-protein-specific CD4 T cells, which might be expected to facilitate protection by facilitating neutralizing anti-S protein antibodies (Ab), were less effective than N-protein-specific cells in this process. By contrast, N-protein-specific CD4 T cells facilitate induction of TGEV-specific Ab, including neutralizing anti-S Ab (1). Similar to the overall inability to affect virus replication, adoptive transfers of CD4 T cells from MHV-infected mice into immunodeficient recipients exhibited little antiviral activity (100). These data suggested an important role for CD4 T cells in protection but not as direct antiviral mediators. A clue to their potential role came from analysis of MHV-induced encephalitis. CD4 T cells cross the BBB but accumulate in the perivascular and subarachnoid spaces instead of trafficking to sites of virus replication (80). By contrast, CD8 T cells enter the parenchyma after migrating through the BBB. In the absence of CD4 T cells, CD8 T-cell survival and effector function are compromised (80). The differential abilities of CD4 T cells and CD8 T cells to traffic through infected tissue is associated with expression of the MMP inhibitor (TIMP-1) by CD4 T cells but not CD8 T cells (107). These data suggest that rather than expression of a protease to promote migration, expression of a protease inhibitor prevents migration of CD4 T cells. These data suggest that during CNS infection, CD4 T cells appear to exhibit little or no direct antiviral activity; however, either directly or indirectly they provide "factors" required for both CD8 T-cell migration and survival (106). In contrast to this limited role for CD4 T cells during CNS infection, class II-restricted CD4 T cells which exhibit cytotoxicity are critical for recovery from hepatitis following infection with the dually tropic MHV-A59 strain (22, 99).

## CD8 T cells

As in infections with other enveloped viruses, CD8 T cells are the primary effectors of CoV clearance. Vaccination with a recombinant virus expressing the S protein conferred complete protection from MHV challenge, including protection from persistent infection (15, 30). However, similar approaches, using the N protein as an immunogen or using minigenes encoding MHV-specific CD8 T-cell epitopes, resulted in variable outcomes (62, 82, 98). A recent comparative study of MHV-specific primary versus vaccination-induced memory CD8 T cells in response to infection revealed that a loss of cytolytic function reflects distinct differentiation states of primary and memory CD8 T cells (66). Importantly, reactivated memory CD8 T cells retained cytolytic function for prolonged periods with no evidence for increased pathology. However, although reactivated CD8 T cells were more effective at virus control, they were unable to prevent the virus reactivation that occurs in the absence of anti-MHV Ab (63). These data suggest that vaccination inducing only T cells may be beneficial in limiting acute CoV infection but might not suffice to prevent viral persistence. In the absence of CD8 T cells, clearance of infectious MHV is prevented or delayed (5). Transferred memory CD8 T cells control virus replication in immunodeficient hosts, confirming their role as primary effectors of virus clearance (6, 7). However, protection may be dependent on the mouse strain and T-cell specificity or activation state, as highly activated T cells are ineffective at controlling replication (100). To date, all MHV-derived CD8 and CD4 T-cell epitopes are localized within the structural N, S, and E proteins (58). Mice of the H-2$^d$ haplotype mount an immunodominant CD8 T-cell response to an epitope within the N protein conserved in most MHV strains. Mice of the H-2$^b$ haplotype respond to two epitopes within the S protein. The immunodominant epitope (S510) resides in a hypervariable domain, while the subdominant epitope (S598) is more conserved. At least 40 to 50% of CNS CD8 T cells are virus specific during and following resolution of acute infection (3, 44, 66). During acute disease, virus-specific CD8 T cells accumulate to at least 10-fold-higher frequencies in the CNS than in the periphery; numbers drop dramatically in lymphoid tissues during persistence (4, 44, 45). Virus-specific CD8 T cells in the tissue remain remarkably stable throughout infection; however, in contrast to acute infection, there is no evidence that T cells exert antiviral function during persistence (5) (Color Plate 6C). CD8 T-cell cytolytic activity is lost concomitant with virus clearance (4), and IFN-γ mRNA levels decline (52). Loss of cytolytic function is independent of demyelination (43) and viral load (66, 67). By contrast, there is no impairment in IFN-γ secretion upon antigen reexposure (4, 66, 67).

In the CNS, the vast majority of CD8 T cells express the CD44$^{hi}$, CD62L$^{-/lo}$, CD11a$^{hi}$, and CD49d (VLA-4) activation/memory phenotypic markers (4). Virus-specific CD8 T cells recruited into the CNS further retain CD69 expression, similar to other CNS inflammation models (4). By contrast, the early activation marker CD69 is only transiently up-regulated early during priming and expansion of T cells in secondary lymphoid organs. Virus-specific CD8 T cells can be distinguished from nonspecifically recruited bystander T cells by a CD43$^{hi}$ CD127$^{-/lo}$ phenotype contrasting with the CD43$^{int}$ CD127$^+$ phenotype of nonactivated memory T cells (10). Virus-specific CD8 T cells from the acutely inflamed CNS express granzyme B, exert ex vivo cytolytic effector function, and produce IFN-γ and, to a lesser degree, TNF-α (4, 63, 66). The critical role of IFN-γ, compared to perforin-mediated cytolysis, is evident by diminished virus control and enhanced mortality in infected IFN-γ-deficient, compared to perforin-deficient, mice (5, 39, 53). Mice lacking both antiviral functions exhibit a more severe phenotype, with uncontrolled virus CNS replication and mortality (6). These data support a concerted mode of action by IFN-γ and perforin-mediated cytolysis. By contrast, Fas/FasL interactions do not appear to play a role in MHV clearance from the CNS or pathology (54).

Analysis of the mechanisms of MHV control highlighted the differential use of T-cell effector mechanisms to clear infectious virus from the CNS (5, 39, 53). Perforin-mediated cytolysis controls replication in astrocytes and microglia in the absence of IFN-γ, but not in oligodendrocytes. By contrast, IFN-γ in the absence of perforin controls replication in oligodendrocytes, but not astrocytes or microglia. Adoptive transfer of virus-specific memory CD8 T cells deficient in either perforin or IFN-γ secretion into infected immunodeficient hosts confirmed glial-cell-type-dependent susceptibility to T-cell effector functions (6, 7). Direct proof for IFN-γ action specifically on oligodendrocytes was provided by studies using mice with an IFN-γ signaling defect selectively in oligodendroglia (19, 20). While inflammation was similar to that in wild-type mice and virus was cleared from other glial cells, virus specifically persisted in oligodendrocytes. These data have several implications for antiviral CD8 T-cell function in the CNS. First, perforin-mediated control of virus in microglia and astrocytes suggests sufficient MHC class I engagement to trigger effector function, even in the absence of IFN-γ. This may depend on the virus, since detection of class I expression on astrocytes has been elusive (68). Second, oligodendrocytes may be inherently resistant to cytolysis due to distinct thresholds of class I antigen presentation and up-regulation of antiapoptotic factors or inhibitory molecules. As class I expression on oligodendrocytes has been demonstrated in two independent models of MHV-JHM infection (63, 68), inhibitory ligands blocking CD8 function might protect against oligodendrocyte damage. The applicability of this concept to other target organs involving persistent CoV infections is not clear.

Despite potent antiviral activity, T cells are unable to prevent MHV persistence. After infectious virus is eliminated, viral mRNA persists and persistent virus sustains T cells within the target organ (5). Mechanisms underlying ineffective T-cell control are unclear, but it may result from a loss of function or emergence of epitope escape variants. However, the H-2$^b$-restricted immunodominant epitope is deleted in several commonly used MHV strains, including the avirulent MHV-JHM 2.2/7.2v-2 and the dually tropic MHV-A59. Furthermore, progressive accumulation of quasispecies with deletions and point mutations in this epitope have been observed in infected mice (72, 73). These alterations reside in a stem-loop structure susceptible to RNA recombination (73), suggesting that both immune pressure and replication strategies may contribute to the preferential emergence of mutants. The inability to clear infectious virus in the CNS following infection of neonatal mice protected by maternal antibody is associated with mutations within the immunodominant S510 epitope (61). Immune escape is also implicated in T-cell-preimmune mice challenged with an MHV-A59 recombinant virus expressing a foreign epitope expressed from the accessory gene 4 locus (11). However, following infection of adult mice there is no convincing evidence for a contribution of epitope escape variants in viral persistence (3, 39, 63). These findings suggest that T-cell escape variants play a minor role in primary infection

of naïve adult mice, but readily emerge in the presence of preexisting antibody or T-cell memory, especially in genome regions not affecting viral fitness.

## Humoral Immunity

Neutralizing and total antiviral Ab are present in the sera during acute and persistent CoV infections (29, 81). Although neutralizing Ab have been implicated in both protection and a reduced incidence of persistent CoV infection, clearance of infectious virus is complete or nearly complete before neutralizing Ab are detected. Passive transfer of nonneutralizing Ab protects infected recipients, although reductions in virus are not a constant finding (81). The MHV M and N proteins are detected on the surface of infected cells; however, is not clear whether this represents de novo synthesis or adsorbed virions. A nonneutralizing M protein-specific monoclonal Ab neutralized virus in vitro in the presence of complement; however, analysis of complement-deficient mice indicated that complement is not required for its in vivo effectiveness. It has been suggested, by analogy with other infections, that protection may involve Ab-dependent cellular cytotoxicity; however, in vitro analysis suggests that this may not be the principal mechanism. Similar to the role of CD4 T cells, the mechanism by which nonneutralizing Ab provide protection to mice during acute infection is not clear. Passive transfer of neutralizing Ab specific for the S glycoprotein at the time of infection protects mice from acute infection. Virus replication was reduced; however, persistent infection was not prevented. These findings question a strategy relying solely on neutralizing Ab for immune protection. In animals with chronic infection there is no apparent correlation between the level of Ab and degree of tissue destruction or protection from neurological disease. In fact, it has been postulated that Ab may contribute to the pathogenesis of chronic tissue destruction (81). These data, in addition to the well-established role of maternal Ab in fostering persistent infection (61), suggest a limited efficacy of vaccination strategies designed to induce only neutralizing Ab (81).

Furthermore, vaccine strategies that induce only neutralizing Ab may be deleterious. This is best illustrated in the case of FIPV. Administration of anti-S protein Ab or immunization with recombinant vaccine virus constructs expressing the S protein results in a robust neutralizing Ab response in domestic cats. However, these immune cats develop an accelerated, fatal disease after FIPV infection (92, 97). Disease enhancement compared to that in naïve cats is a consequence of increased uptake into, and infection of, macrophages. Importantly, this phenomenon of enhanced virulence in immune individuals has not been detected in naturally infected cats and has not been reported in other animal CoV infections.

B cells themselves were initially considered to be possible contributors to MHV clearance via the lysis of infected targets mediated through interactions of viral receptors on B cells with S proteins expressed on the surface of adjacent infected cells (24). However, viral clearance from B-cell-deficient mice suggests that neither this mechanism nor the secretion of Ab during acute infection participates in the control of infectious MHV (5, 67). By contrast, viral recrudescence in mice devoid of B cells suggests that T cells are ineffectual during viral persistence (64, 67). Interestingly, MHV-A59, which infects both the liver and the CNS, fails to reactivate in the liver in the absence of humoral immunity (47). Whether this reflects the absence of viral persistence in the liver or a fundamental difference in immune control in these two organs is unclear. Although virus recrudescence in Ab-deficient mice is prevented by passive transfer of neutralizing Ab, antiviral control waned as Ab decayed (64). This suggested that sustained Ab secretion is crucial to maintain viral persistence. Accumulation and retention of virus-specific Ab-secreting cells (ASC) within the CNS confirmed a role for intrathecal Ab synthesis in controlling persistence (88, 89). Similar to T cells, virus-specific ASC peak in secondary lymphoid tissue prior to appearing in the CNS, suggesting that maturation in secondary lymphoid organs precedes migration into the CNS. However, in distinct contrast to T cells, B cells accumulate in the CNS after clearance of infectious virus (Color Plate 6C). The kinetics of ASC accumulation, in addition to a phenotype consistent with progressively increasing differentiation during viral persistence, suggests ongoing maturation within the site of persistence. Retention of CNS ASC at high frequencies may be supported by induction and sustained expression of the B-cell survival factor BAFF during viral persistence (89). The CNS as a survival niche for ASC has previously been observed following other virus-induced CNS infections and chronic diseases (21, 91); however, these insights obtained via analysis of MHV infection provide the first evidence that local Ab secretion controls a persistent infection.

## IMMUNOPATHOGENIC MECHANISMS OF DISEASE

An underappreciated aspect of CoV infections is that both inapparent and acute symptomatic infections result in a myriad of immunological abnormalities, the bases of which are unclear (59). Importing naïve mice into MHV-contaminated colonies resulted in abnormal immune responses, including changes in susceptibility to pathogens and tumors, loss of lymphoid cellularity, reduced APC function and cytokine secretion, and altered macrophage function (81). Following acute infection, cytokine levels in the blood remained increased for at least 2 months postinfection. No increase in alloreactive T cells was detected at 1 month postinfection; however, an increase in self-reactive T cells was detected. Indeed, adoptive transfer of T cells from MHV-infected rats into naïve recipients results in inflammatory lesions in the CNS consistent with induction of autoimmune disease (95). Depressed T-cell proliferation was found at 1 month postinfection that returned to normal by 4 months. Interestingly, the ability to reject skin grafts was profoundly affected for at least 4 months following MHV infection. These data suggest that acute CoV infection, even in the absence of viral persistence, can induce profound and long-lasting changes in all compartments of the immune response.

In addition to causing an acute encephalomyelitis, the persistence of many MHV strains within the CNS is associated with chronic ongoing demyelination. Although these lesions have been well characterized for more than 30 years (33, 96), identification of a mechanism remains elusive. Electron microscopy initially suggested that demyelination was the result of virus-induced lysis of oligodendrocytes (23). More recently it became clear that tissue destruction requires not only infection of oligodendroglia but also an immune component in addition to macrophages. For example, immunodeficient mice are unable to control viral replication within the CNS, including the infection of oligodendroglia, yet demyelination is absent or very limited (7, 26, 100). Macrophages are the end mediators of myelin loss; however, inhibition of macrophage infiltration into the CNS during MHV infection suggested that microglia, the CNS resident macrophage, may also contribute to demyelination (101). By contrast, activation of microglia during MHV infection is insufficient to induce myelin loss in the absence of a balanced inflammatory response (7). TNF-α, a mediator of myelin loss in autoimmune models, plays no role in MHV-induced demyelination (60, 84). IFN-γ, which plays a dual role in CNS autoimmune disease, initially as a mediator of destruction and then to limit immune destruction, appears to be a requirement for myelin loss (6, 60). A unifying mechanism by which T cells amplify disease has yet to be defined. In addition, although the requirement for viral infection of oligodendroglia is not in dispute, recent data showing that a dramatic increase in the number of individual oligodendroglia infected does not increase the extent of acute or chronic demyelination (20) suggest that the overall regulation of tissue destruction in the CNS is complex. Evaluating the underlying molecular and cellular mechanisms of virus-induced demyelination has provided important insight into disease pathogenesis; however, the repair process, or remyelination, is often overlooked. Newly generated oligodendrocytes are associated with remyelination (23, 49). Platelet-derived growth factor and fibroblast growth factor 2 are increased during remyelination, suggesting that these signaling pathways are important in the repair process. These studies are limited but suggest that remyelination following virus-induced demyelination may provide unique insights into CNS repair processes.

Disease in felines infected with FIPV is also partly immunopathogenic. Cats are often persistently infected with feline enteric CoV (FECV). In rare instances, mutations in the virus result in the outgrowth of a more virulent virus, FIPV. FIPV is macrophage tropic and replicates more efficiently in these cells than do the more avirulent forms of FECV (79). Infected macrophages traffic to distal sites, resulting in pyogranulomatous vasculitis, serositis, fever, and weight loss (14). Another consequence of macrophage (and most likely, DC) infection is lymphocyte depletion and increased production of the anti-inflammatory cytokine IL-10 (13). FIPV-induced lymphopenia does not result from direct viral infection but is probably mediated by cytokines, e.g., TNF-α (29). By analogy with MHV, a robust CD8 T-cell response is probably required for FIPV clearance, and the infection of macrophage and DC APC is likely to inhibit this response.

## REFERENCES

1. Antón, I. M., C. Suñé, R. H. Meloen, F. Borrás-Cuesta, and L. Enjuanes. 1995. A transmissible gastroenteritis coronavirus nucleoprotein epitope elicits T helper cells that collaborate in the in vitro antibody synthesis to the three major structural viral proteins. *Virology* **212**:746–751.
2. Baudoux, P., C. Carrat, L. Besnardeau, B. Charley, and H. Laude. 1998. Coronavirus pseudoparticles formed with recombinant M and E proteins induce alpha interferon synthesis by leukocytes. *J. Virol.* **72**:8636–8643.
3. Bergmann, C., E. Dimacali, S. Stohl, W. Wei, M. M. Lai, S. Tahara, and N. Marten. 1998. Variability of persisting MHV RNA sequences constituting immune and replication-relevant domains. *Virology* **244**:563–572.
4. Bergmann, C. C., J. D. Altman, D. Hinton, and S. A. Stohlman. 1999. Inverted immunodominance and impaired cytolytic function of CD8+ T cells during viral persistence in the central nervous system. *J. Immunol.* **163**:3379–3387.
5. Bergmann, C. C., T. E. Lane, and S. A. Stohlman. 2006. Coronavirus infection of the central nervous system: host-virus stand-off. *Nat. Rev. Microbiol.* **4**:121–132.
6. Bergmann, C. C., B. Parra, D. R. Hinton, R. Chandran, M. Morrison, and S. A. Stohlman. 2003. Perforin-mediated effector function within the central nervous system requires IFN-gamma-mediated MHC up-regulation. *J. Immunol.* **170**:3204–3213.

7. Bergmann, C. C., B. Parra, D. R. Hinton, C. Ramakrishna, K. C. Dowdell, and S. A. Stohlman. 2004. Perforin and gamma interferon-mediated control of coronavirus central nervous system infection by CD8 T cells in the absence of CD4 T cells. *J. Virol.* **78**:1739–1750.
8. Cervantes-Barragan, L., R. Züst, F. Weber, M. Spiegel, K. S. Lang, S. Akira, V. Thiel, and B. Ludewig. 2007. Control of coronavirus infection through plasmacytoid dendritic-cell-derived type I interferon. *Blood* **109**:1131–1137.
9. Charley, B., and H. Laude. 1988. Induction of alpha interferon by transmissible gastroenteritis coronavirus: role of transmembrane glycoprotein E1. *J. Virol.* **62**:8–11.
10. Chen, A. M., N. Khanna, S. A. Stohlman, and C. C. Bergmann. 2005. Virus-specific and bystander CD8 T cells recruited during virus-induced encephalomyelitis. *J. Virol.* **79**:4700–4708.
11. Chua, M. M., K. C. MacNamara, L. San Mateo, H. Shen, and S. R. Weiss. 2004. Effects of an epitope-specific CD8+ T-cell response on murine coronavirus central nervous system disease: protection from virus replication and antigen spread and selection of epitope escape mutants. *J. Virol.* **78**:1150–1159.
12. De, A. N., E. Baig, X. Ma, J. Zhang, W. He, A. Rowe, M. Habal, M. Liu, I. Shalev, G. P. Downey, R. Gorczynski, J. Butany, J. Leibowitz, S. R. Weiss, I. D. McGilvray, M. J. Phillips, E. N. Fish, and G. A. Levy. 2006. Murine hepatitis virus strain 1 produces a clinically relevant model of severe acute respiratory syndrome in A/J mice. *J. Virol.* **80**:10382–10394.
13. Dean, G. A., T. Olivry, C. Stanton, and N. C. Pedersen. 2003. In vivo cytokine response to experimental feline infectious peritonitis virus infection. *Vet. Microbiol.* **97**:1–12.
14. de Groot-Mijnes, J. D., J. M. van Dun, R. G. van der Most, and R. J. de Groot. 2005. Natural history of a recurrent feline coronavirus infection and the role of cellular immunity in survival and disease. *J. Virol.* **79**:1036–1044.
15. Flory, E., M. Pfleiderer, A. Stuhler, and H. Wege. 1993. Induction of protective immunity against coronavirus-induced encephalomyelitis: evidence for an important role of CD8+ T cells in vivo. *Eur. J. Immunol.* **23**:1757–1761.
16. Garlinghouse, L. E., Jr., A. L. Smith, and T. Holford. 1984. The biological relationship of mouse hepatitis virus (MHV) strains and interferon: in vitro induction and sensitivities. *Arch. Virol.* **82**:19–29.
17. Glass, W. G., M. J. Hickey, J. L. Hardison, M. T. Liu, J. E. Manning, and T. E. Lane. 2004. Antibody targeting of the CC chemokine ligand 5 results in diminished leukocyte infiltration into the central nervous system and reduced neurologic disease in a viral model of multiple sclerosis. *J. Immunol.* **172**:4018–4025.
18. Glass, W. G., M. T. Liu, W. A. Kuziel, and T. E. Lane. 2001. Reduced macrophage infiltration and demyelination in mice lacking the chemokine receptor CCR5 following infection with a neurotropic coronavirus. *Virology* **288**:8–17.
19. Gonzalez, J. M., C. C. Bergmann, B. Fuss, D. R. Hinton, C. Kangas, W. B. Macklin, and S. A. Stohlman. 2005. Expression of a dominant negative IFN-gamma receptor on mouse oligodendrocytes. *Glia* **51**:22–34.
20. Gonzalez, J. M., C. C. Bergmann, C. Ramakrishna, D. R. Hinton, R. Atkinson, J. Hoskin, W. B. Macklin, and S. A. Stohlman. 2006. Inhibition of interferon-gamma signaling in oligodendroglia delays coronavirus clearance without altering demyelination. *Am. J. Pathol.* **168**:796–804.
21. Griffin, D. E. 2003. Immune responses to RNA-virus infections of the CNS. *Nat. Rev. Immunol.* **3**:493–502.
22. Heemskerk, M. H., H. M. Schoemaker, W. J. Spaan, and C. J. Boog. 1995. Predominance of MHC class II-restricted CD4+ cytotoxic T cells against mouse hepatitis virus A59. *Immunology* **84**:521–527.

23. Herndon, R. M., D. L. Price, and L. P. Weiner. 1977. Regeneration of oligodendroglia during recovery from demyelinating disease. *Science* 195:693–694.

24. Holmes, K. V., R. M. Welsh, and M. V. Haspel. 1986. Natural cytotoxicity against mouse hepatitis virus-infected target cells. I. Correlation of cytotoxicity with virus binding to leukocytes. *J. Immunol.* 136:1446–1453.

25. Hooks, J. J., Y. Wang, and B. Detrick. 2003. The critical role of IFN-gamma in experimental coronavirus retinopathy. *Investig. Ophthalmol. Vis. Sci.* 44:3402–3408.

26. Houtman, J. J., and J. O. Fleming. 1996. Dissociation of demyelination and viral clearance in congenitally immunodeficient mice infected with murine coronavirus JHM. *J. Neurovirol.* 2:101–110.

27. Ishihara, K., and T. Hirano. 2002. IL-6 in autoimmune disease and chronic inflammatory proliferative disease. *Cytokine Growth Factor Rev.* 13:357–368.

28. Kawai, T., and S. Akira. 2006. Innate immune recognition of viral infection. *Nat. Immunol.* 7:131–137.

29. Kiss, I., A. M. Poland, and N. C. Pedersen. 2004. Disease outcome and cytokine responses in cats immunized with an avirulent feline infectious peritonitis virus (FIPV)-UCD1 and challenge-exposed with virulent FIPV-UCD8. *J. Feline Med. Surg.* 6:89–97.

30. Korner, H., A. Schliephake, J. Winter, F. Zimprich, H. Lassmann, J. Sedgwick, S. Siddell, and H. Wege. 1991. Nucleocapsid or spike protein-specific CD4+ T lymphocytes protect against coronavirus-induced encephalomyelitis in the absence of CD8+ T cells. *J. Immunol.* 147:2317–2323.

31. Kotani, T., S. Wada, Y. Tsukamoto, M. Kuwamura, J. Yamate, and S. Sakuma. 2000. Kinetics of lymphocytic subsets in chicken tracheal lesions infected with infectious bronchitis virus. *J. Vet. Med. Sci.* 62:397–401.

32. La, B. C., and H. Laude. 1981. High interferon titer in newborn pig intestine during experimentally induced viral enteritis. *Infect. Immun.* 32:28–31.

33. Lampert, P. W., J. K. Sims, and A. J. Kniazeff. 1973. Mechanism of demyelination in JHM virus encephalomyelitis. Electron microscopic studies. *Acta Neuropathol.* 24:76–85.

34. Lane, T. E., V. C. Asensio, N. Yu, A. D. Paoletti, I. L. Campbell, and M. J. Buchmeier. 1998. Dynamic regulation of alpha- and beta-chemokine expression in the central nervous system during mouse hepatitis virus-induced demyelinating disease. *J. Immunol.* 160:970–978.

35. Lane, T. E., H. S. Fox, and M. J. Buchmeier. 1999. Inhibition of nitric oxide synthase-2 reduces the severity of mouse hepatitis virus-induced demyelination: implications for NOS2/NO regulation of chemokine expression and inflammation. *J. Neurovirol.* 5:48–54.

36. Lane, T. E., A. D. Paoletti, and M. J. Buchmeier. 1997. Disassociation between the in vitro and in vivo effects of nitric oxide on a neurotropic murine coronavirus. *J. Virol.* 71:2202–2210.

37. Lavi, E., and Q. Wang. 1995. The protective role of cytotoxic T cells and interferon against coronavirus invasion of the brain. *Adv. Exp. Med. Biol.* 380:145–149.

38. Li, Y., L. Fu, D. M. Gonzales, and E. Lavi. 2004. Coronavirus neurovirulence correlates with the ability of the virus to induce proinflammatory cytokine signals from astrocytes and microglia. *J. Virol.* 78:3398–3406.

39. Lin, M. T., S. A. Stohlman, and D. R. Hinton. 1997. Mouse hepatitis virus is cleared from the central nervous systems of mice lacking perforin-mediated cytolysis. *J. Virol.* 71:383–391.

40. Liu, M. T., B. P. Chen, P. Oertel, M. J. Buchmeier, D. Armstrong, T. A. Hamilton, and T. E. Lane. 2000. The T cell chemoattractant IFN-inducible protein 10 is essential in host defense against viral-induced neurologic disease. *J. Immunol.* 165:2327–2330.

41. Liu, M. T., H. S. Keirstead, and T. E. Lane. 2001. Neutralization of the chemokine CXCL10 reduces inflammatory cell invasion and demyelination and improves neurological function in a viral model of multiple sclerosis. *J. Immunol.* 167:4091–4097.

42. Marsden, P. A., Q. Ning, L. S. Fung, X. Luo, Y. Chen, M. Mendicino, A. Ghanekar, J. A. Scott, T. Miller, C. W. Chan, M. W. Chan, W. He, R. M. Gorczynski, D. R. Grant, D. A. Clark, M. J. Phillips, and G. A. Levy. 2003. The Fgl2/fibroleukin prothrombinase contributes to immunologically mediated thrombosis in experimental and human viral hepatitis. *J. Clin. Investig.* 112:58–66.

43. Marten, N. W., S. A. Stohlman, R. D. Atkinson, D. R. Hinton, J. O. Fleming, and C. C. Bergmann. 2000. Contributions of CD8+ T cells and viral spread to demyelinating disease. *J. Immunol.* 164:4080–4088.

44. Marten, N. W., S. A. Stohlman, and C. C. Bergmann. 2000. Role of viral persistence in retaining CD8$^+$ T cells within the central nervous system. *J. Virol.* 74:7903–7910.

45. Marten, N. W., S. A. Stohlman, J. Zhou, and C. C. Bergmann. 2003. Kinetics of virus-specific CD8$^+$-T-cell expansion and trafficking following central nervous system infection. *J. Virol.* 77:2775–2778.

46. Matsuyama, S., S. Henmi, N. Ichihara, S. Sone, T. Kikuchi, T. Ariga, and F. Taguchi. 2000. Protective effects of murine recombinant interferon-beta administered by intravenous, intramuscular or subcutaneous route on mouse hepatitis virus infection. *Antivir. Res.* 47:131–137.

47. Matthews, A. E., S. R. Weiss, M. J. Shlomchik, L. G. Hannum, J. L. Gombold, and Y. Paterson. 2001. Antibody is required for clearance of infectious murine hepatitis virus A59 from the central nervous system, but not the liver. *J. Immunol.* 167:5254–5263.

48. Mello, I. G., R. C. Vassao, and C. A. Pereira. 1993. Virus specificity of the antiviral state induced by IFN gamma correlates with resistance to MHV 3 infection. *Arch. Virol.* 132:281–289.

49. Messersmith, D. J., J. C. Murtie, T. Q. Le, E. E. Frost, and R. C. Armstrong. 2000. Fibroblast growth factor 2 (FGF2) and FGF receptor expression in an experimental demyelinating disease with extensive remyelination. *J. Neurosci. Res.* 62:241–256.

50. Ning, Q., S. Lakatoo, M. Liu, W. Yang, Z. Wang, M. J. Phillips, and G. A. Levy. 2003. Induction of prothrombinase fgl2 by the nucleocapsid protein of virulent mouse hepatitis virus is dependent on host hepatic nuclear factor-4 alpha. *J. Biol. Chem.* 278:15541–15549.

51. Otsuki, K., T. Nakamura, N. Kubota, Y. Kawaoka, and M. Tsubokura. 1987. Comparison of two strains of avian infectious bronchitis virus for their interferon induction, viral growth and development of virus-neutralizing antibody in experimentally-infected chickens. *Vet. Microbiol.* 15:31–40.

52. Parra, B., D. R. Hinton, M. T. Lin, D. J. Cua, and S. A. Stohlman. 1997. Kinetics of cytokine mRNA expression in the central nervous system following lethal and nonlethal coronavirus-induced acute encephalomyelitis. *Virology* 233:260–270.

53. Parra, B., D. R. Hinton, N. W. Marten, C. C. Bergmann, M. T. Lin, C. S. Yang, and S. A. Stohlman. 1999. IFN-gamma is required for viral clearance from central nervous system oligodendroglia. *J. Immunol.* 162:1641–1647.

54. Parra, B., M. T. Lin, S. A. Stohlman, C. C. Bergmann, R. Atkinson, and D. R. Hinton. 2000. Contributions of Fas-Fas ligand interactions to the pathogenesis of mouse hepatitis virus in the central nervous system. *J. Virol.* 74:2447–2450.

55. Pearce, B. D., M. V. Hobbs, T. S. McGraw, and M. J. Buchmeier. 1994. Cytokine induction during T-cell-mediated clearance of mouse hepatitis virus from neurons in vivo. *J. Virol.* **68:**5483–5495.

56. Pei, J., M. J. Sekellick, P. I. Marcus, I. S. Choi, and E. W. Collisson. 2001. Chicken interferon type I inhibits infectious bronchitis virus replication and associated respiratory illness. *J. Interferon Cytokine Res.* **21:**1071–1077.

57. Pereira, C. A., C. Moreira, M. H. Tsuhako, and M. T. de Franco. 2005. Mouse hepatitis virus 3 binding to macrophages correlates with resistance to experimental infection. *Scand. J. Immunol.* **62**(Suppl. 1):95–99.

58. Perlman, S. 1998. Pathogenesis of coronavirus-induced infections. Review of pathological and immunological aspects. *Adv. Exp. Med. Biol.* **440:**503–513.

59. Perlman, S., and A. A. Dandekar. 2005. Immunopathogenesis of coronavirus infections: implications for SARS. *Nat. Rev. Immunol.* **5:**917–927.

60. Pewe, L., and S. Perlman. 2002. Cutting edge: CD8 T cell-mediated demyelination is IFN-gamma dependent in mice infected with a neurotropic coronavirus. *J. Immunol.* **168:**1547–1551.

61. Pewe, L., G. F. Wu, E. M. Barnett, R. F. Castro, and S. Perlman. 1996. Cytotoxic T cell-resistant variants are selected in a virus-induced demyelinating disease. *Immunity* **5:**253–262.

62. Platanias, L. C. 2005. Mechanisms of type-I- and type-II-interferon-mediated signalling. *Nat. Rev. Immunol.* **5:**375–386.

63. Ramakrishna, C., R. A. Atkinson, S. A. Stohlman, and C. C. Bergmann. 2006. Vaccine-induced memory CD8+ T cells cannot prevent central nervous system virus reactivation. *J. Immunol.* **176:**3062–3069.

64. Ramakrishna, C., C. C. Bergmann, R. Atkinson, and S. A. Stohlman. 2003. Control of central nervous system viral persistence by neutralizing antibody. *J. Virol.* **77:**4670–4678.

65. Ramakrishna, C., C. C. Bergmann, K. V. Holmes, and S. A. Stohlman. 2004. Expression of the mouse hepatitis virus receptor by central nervous system microglia. *J. Virol.* **78:**7828–7832.

66. Ramakrishna, C., S. A. Stohlman, R. A. Atkinson, D. R. Hinton, and C. C. Bergmann. 2004. Differential regulation of primary and secondary CD8+ T cells in the central nervous system. *J. Immunol.* **173:**6265–6273.

67. Ramakrishna, C., S. A. Stohlman, R. D. Atkinson, M. J. Shlomchik, and C. C. Bergmann. 2002. Mechanisms of central nervous system viral persistence: the critical role of antibody and B cells. *J. Immunol.* **168:**1204–1211.

68. Redwine, J. M., M. J. Buchmeier, and C. F. Evans. 2001. In vivo expression of major histocompatibility complex molecules on oligodendrocytes and neurons during viral infection. *Am. J. Pathol.* **159:**1219–1224.

69. Rempel, J. D., S. J. Murray, J. Meisner, and M. J. Buchmeier. 2004. Differential regulation of innate and adaptive immune responses in viral encephalitis. *Virology* **318:**381–392.

70. Rempel, J. D., S. J. Murray, J. Meisner, and M. J. Buchmeier. 2004. Mouse hepatitis virus neurovirulence: evidence of a linkage between S glycoprotein expression and immunopathology. *Virology* **318:**45–54.

71. Rempel, J. D., L. A. Quina, P. K. Blakely-Gonzales, M. J. Buchmeier, and D. L. Gruol. 2005. Viral induction of central nervous system innate immune responses. *J. Virol.* **79:**4369–4381.

72. Rowe, C. L., S. C. Baker, M. J. Nathan, and J. O. Fleming. 1997. Evolution of mouse hepatitis virus: detection and characterization of spike deletion variants during persistent infection. *J. Virol.* **71:**2959–2969.

73. Rowe, C. L., J. O. Fleming, M. J. Nathan, J. Y. Sgro, A. C. Palmenberg, and S. C. Baker. 1997. Generation of coronavirus spike deletion variants by high-frequency recombination at regions of predicted RNA secondary structure. *J. Virol.* **71:**6183–6190.

74. Smith, A. L., S. W. Barthold, and D. S. Beck. 1987. Intranasally administered alpha/beta interferon prevents extension of mouse hepatitis virus, strain JHM, into the brains of BALB/cByJ mice. *Antivir. Res.* **8:**239–245.

75. Sorensen, O., A. Saravani, and S. Dales. 1987. In vivo and in vitro models of demyelinating disease. XVII. The infectious process in athymic rats inoculated with JHM virus. *Microb. Pathog.* **2:**79–90.

76. Spiegel, M., A. Pichlmair, L. Martínez-Sobrido, J. Cros, A. García-Sastre, O. Haller, and F. Weber. 2005. Inhibition of beta interferon induction by severe acute respiratory syndrome coronavirus suggests a two-step model for activation of interferon regulatory factor. *J. Virol.* **79:**2079–2086.

77. Stetson, D. B., and R. Medzhitov. 2006. Type I interferons in host defense. *Immunity* **25:**373–381.

78. Stiles, L. N., M. P. Hosking, R. A. Edwards, R. M. Strieter, and T. E. Lane. 2006. Differential roles for CXCR3 in CD4+ and CD8+ T cell trafficking following viral infection of the CNS. *Eur. J. Immunol.* **36:**613–622.

79. Stoddart, C. A., and F. W. Scott. 1989. Intrinsic resistance of feline peritoneal macrophages to coronavirus infection correlates with in vivo virulence. *J. Virol.* **63:**436–440.

80. Stohlman, S. A., C. C. Bergmann, M. T. Lin, D. J. Cua, and D. R. Hinton. 1998. CTL effector function within the central nervous system requires CD4+ T cells. *J. Immunol.* **160:**2896–2904.

81. Stohlman, S. A., C. C. Bergmann, and S. Perlman. 1999. Persistent mouse hepatitis viral infections, p. 537–557. *In* R. Ahmed and I. Chen (ed.), *Persistent Viral Infections.* John Wiley and Sons, New York, NY.

82. Stohlman, S. A., C. C. Bergmann, R. C. van der Veen, and D. R. Hinton. 1995. Mouse hepatitis virus-specific cytotoxic T lymphocytes protect from lethal infection without eliminating virus from the central nervous system. *J. Virol.* **69:**684–694.

83. Stohlman, S. A., P. R. Brayton, R. C. Harmon, D. Stevenson, R. G. Ganges, and G. K. Matsushima. 1983. Natural killer cell activity during mouse hepatitis virus infection: response in the absence of interferon. *Int. J. Cancer* **31:**309–314.

84. Stohlman, S. A., D. R. Hinton, D. Cua, E. Dimacali, J. Sensintaffar, F. M. Hofman, S. M. Tahara, and Q. Yao. 1995. Tumor necrosis factor expression during mouse hepatitis virus-induced demyelinating encephalomyelitis. *J. Virol.* **69:**5898–5903.

85. Stohlman, S. A., G. K. Matsushima, N. Casteel, and L. P. Weiner. 1986. In vivo effects of coronavirus-specific T cell clones: DTH inducer cells prevent a lethal infection but do not inhibit virus replication. *J. Immunol.* **136:**3052–3056.

86. Trifilo, M. J., C. C. Bergmann, W. A. Kuziel, and T. E. Lane. 2003. CC chemokine ligand 3 (CCL3) regulates CD8+-T-cell effector function and migration following viral infection. *J. Virol.* **77:**4004–4014.

87. Trifilo, M. J., C. Montalto-Morrison, L. N. Stiles, K. R. Hurst, J. L. Hardison, J. E. Manning, P. S. Masters, and T. E. Lane. 2004. CXC chemokine ligand 10 controls viral infection in the central nervous system: evidence for a role in innate immune response through recruitment and activation of natural killer cells. *J. Virol.* **78:**585–594.

88. Tschen, S. I., C. C. Bergmann, C. Ramakrishna, S. Morales, R. Atkinson, and S. A. Stohlman. 2002. Recruitment kinetics and composition of antibody-secreting cells within the central nervous system following viral encephalomyelitis. *J. Immunol.* **168:**2922–2929.

89. Tschen, S. I., S. A. Stohlman, C. Ramakrishna, D. R. Hinton, R. D. Atkinson, and C. C. Bergmann. 2006. CNS viral infection diverts homing of antibody-secreting cells from lymphoid organs to the CNS. *Eur. J. Immunol.* **36:**603–612.

90. Turner, B. C., E. M. Hemmila, N. Beauchemin, and K. V. Holmes. 2004. Receptor-dependent coronavirus infection of dendritic cells. *J. Virol.* **78:**5486–5490.

91. Uccelli, A., F. Aloisi, and V. Pistoia. 2005. Unveiling the enigma of the CNS as a B-cell fostering environment. *Trends Immunol.* **26:**254–259.

92. Vennema, H., R. J. de Groot, D. A. Harbour, M. Dalderup, T. Gruffydd-Jones, M. C. Horzinek, and W. J. Spaan. 1990. Early death after feline infectious peritonitis virus challenge due to recombinant vaccinia virus immunization. *J. Virol.* **64:**1407–1409.

93. Versteeg, G. A., O. Slobodskaya, and W. J. Spaan. 2006. Transcriptional profiling of acute cytopathic murine hepatitis virus infection in fibroblast-like cells. *J. Gen. Virol.* **87:**1961–1975.

94. Virelizier, J. L., A. D. Dayan, and A. C. Allison. 1975. Neuropathological effects of persistent infection of mice by mouse hepatitis virus. *Infect. Immun.* **12:**1127–1140.

95. Watanabe, R., H. Wege, and V. ter Meulen. 1983. Adoptive transfer of EAE-like lesions from rats with coronavirus-induced demyelinating encephalomyelitis. *Nature* **305:**150–153.

96. Weiner, L. P. 1973. Pathogenesis of demyelination induced by a mouse hepatitis. *Arch. Neurol.* **28:**298–303.

97. Weiss, R. C., and F. W. Scott. 1981. Antibody-mediated enhancement of disease in feline infectious peritonitis: comparisons with dengue hemorrhagic fever. *Comp. Immunol. Microbiol. Infect. Dis.* **4:**175–189.

98. Wesseling, J. G., G. J. Godeke, V. E. Schijns, L. Prevec, F. L. Graham, M. C. Horzinek, and P. J. Rottier. 1993. Mouse hepatitis virus spike and nucleocapsid proteins expressed by adenovirus vectors protect mice against a lethal infection. *J. Gen. Virol.* **74:**2061–2069.

99. Wijburg, O. L., M. H. Heemskerk, A. Sanders, C. J. Boog, and N. Van Rooijen. 1996. Role of virus-specific CD4+ cytotoxic T cells in recovery from mouse hepatitis virus infection. *Immunology* **87:**34–41.

100. Wu, G. F., A. A. Dandekar, L. Pewe, and S. Perlman. 2000. CD4 and CD8 T cells have redundant but not identical roles in virus-induced demyelination. *J. Immunol.* **165:**2278–2286.

101. Wu, G. F., and S. Perlman. 1999. Macrophage infiltration, but not apoptosis, is correlated with immune-mediated demyelination following murine infection with a neurotropic coronavirus. *J. Virol.* **73:**8771–8780.

102. Yamaguchi, K., N. Goto, S. Kyuwa, M. Hayami, and Y. Toyoda. 1991. Protection of mice from a lethal coronavirus infection in the central nervous system by adoptive transfer of virus-specific T cell clones. *J. Neuroimmunol.* **32:**1–9.

103. Yong, V. W., C. Power, P. Forsyth, and D. R. Edwards. 2001. Metalloproteinases in biology and pathology of the nervous system. *Nat. Rev. Neurosci.* **2:**502–511.

104. Zhou, H., and S. Perlman. 2006. Mouse hepatitis virus does not induce beta interferon synthesis and does not inhibit its induction by double-stranded RNA. *J. Virol.* **81:**568–574.

105. Zhou, H., and S. Perlman. 2006. Preferential infection of mature dendritic cells by mouse hepatitis virus strain JHM. *J. Virol.* **80:**2506–2514.

106. Zhou, J., D. R. Hinton, S. A. Stohlman, C. P. Liu, L. Zhong, and N. W. Marten. 2005. Maintenance of CD8+ T cells during acute viral infection of the central nervous system requires CD4+ T cells but not interleukin-2. *Viral Immunol.* **18:**162–169.

107. Zhou, J., N. W. Marten, C. C. Bergmann, W. B. Macklin, D. R. Hinton, and S. A. Stohlman. 2005. Expression of matrix metalloproteinases and their tissue inhibitor during viral encephalitis. *J. Virol.* **79:**4764–4773.

108. Zhou, J., S. A. Stohlman, R. Atkinson, D. R. Hinton, and N. W. Marten. 2002. Matrix metalloproteinase expression correlates with virulence following neurotropic mouse hepatitis virus infection. *J. Virol.* **76:**7374–7384.

109. Zhou, J., S. A. Stohlman, D. R. Hinton, and N. W. Marten. 2003. Neutrophils promote mononuclear cell infiltration during viral-induced encephalitis. *J. Immunol.* **170:**3331–3336.

110. Zuo, J., S. A. Stohlman, J. B. Hoskin, D. R. Hinton, R. Atkinson, and C. C. Bergmann. 2006. Mouse hepatitis virus pathogenesis in the central nervous system is independent of IL-15 and natural killer cells. *Virology* **350:**206–215.

*Nidoviruses*
Edited by S. Perlman, T. Gallagher, and E. J. Snijder
© 2008 ASM Press, Washington, DC

Chapter 23

# Torovirus Pathogenesis and Immune Responses

ARMANDO E. HOET AND LINDA J. SAIF

Toroviruses are pleomorphic viruses with a peplomer-bearing envelope containing an elongated tubular nucleocapsid with helical symmetry. They contain a linear, nonsegmented, positive- and single-stranded polyadenylated RNA genome (33, 35, 69, 86). A schematic representation of the typical extracellular morphology of torovirus and particles as visualized by electron microscopy (EM) is shown in Color Plate 7 (see color insert). Toroviruses resemble an open "torus" (Latin word for circular convex molding in the form of a doughnut shape that some columns have in their bases) (32, 72, 82, 86). After the initial report of toroviruses in horses and cattle (83, 90), torovirus-like (TVL) particles were detected using EM in feces from human patients with gastroenteritis (5). Subsequently, based on numerous reports highlighting the presence of toroviruses in humans (4–7, 15, 36, 40, 41, 43, 44, 48, 50, 59, 76), the term human torovirus was used to describe the TVL particles detected in human fecal samples (15, 42).

Currently only four species are recognized as members of the *Torovirus* genus in the *Coronaviridae* family: equine torovirus (EToV), initially known as Berne virus (8, 10); bovine torovirus (BToV), originally known as Breda virus (8, 9); human torovirus (HToV) (4, 5, 31, 36); and porcine torovirus (31, 49, 67). TVL particles have been detected in feces from other animal species, such as turkeys (1–3), dogs (19), and cats (60). In addition, antibodies against toroviruses are frequently detected in ungulates such as horses, sheep, goats, and pigs (33–35, 84, 86).

Toroviruses have been identified as a potential pathogen inducing diarrhea in humans. During recent years evidence has accumulated implicating HToV as a cause of diarrhea in young and/or immunocompromised individuals, in many cases as a nosocomial agent (4–7, 15, 36, 40, 41, 43, 44, 48, 50, 55, 59, 76). An interesting aspect of these findings is the reported cross-reactivity between HToV and BToV that was demonstrated by enzyme-linked immunosorbent assay (ELISA), immuno-EM, hemagglutination inhibition (HI), immunoblotting, and nucleic acid hybridization (cDNA probe) assays (4, 5, 15, 44, 45, 48, 86). Several researchers have used BToV reagents or genetic sequences from this virus to identify HToV in human samples, indicating a close antigenic and genetic relatedness between these two viruses (4, 40, 44, 86). Therefore, understanding the epidemiology of BToV in cattle populations may have relevance for future studies to address the zoonotic potential of BToV. In addition, BToV infections of cattle may serve as an animal model potentially applicable to human strains of torovirus. Furthermore, if HToVs are confirmed to cause diarrhea in humans, this raises the possibility of using the antigenically related BToV to develop diagnostic assays, as well as a future vaccine candidate for humans.

The main objective of this chapter is to provide a comprehensive review of torovirus pathogenesis and immune responses. A brief epidemiological background highlighting HToVs is also provided. A comprehensive review of BToV emphasizing epidemiology and disease association was recently published (29).

## EPIDEMIOLOGY

### Distribution

The geographic distribution of toroviruses in humans and animals is worldwide, with the virus identified in countries such as Brazil, Belgium, Canada, Costa Rica, France, Germany, Great Britain,

**Armando E. Hoet** • Department of Veterinary Preventive Medicine, College of Veterinary Medicine, The Ohio State University, Columbus, OH 43210. **Linda J. Saif** • Food Animal Health Research Program, Ohio Agricultural Research and Development Center, and Department of Veterinary Preventive Medicine, College of Veterinary Medicine, The Ohio State University, Wooster, OH 44691.

Hungary, India, The Netherlands, New Zealand, South Africa, the United States, and, most recently, Austria (6, 16, 17, 21, 28, 36, 38, 40, 43, 47, 48, 51, 53, 57, 61, 78–81). In the United States, BToV appears to be widespread in regions where examined, but a lack of routine or commercially available diagnostic tests has hampered its wider detection and prevalence studies. In our study in Ohio, BToV was detected using ELISA and/or reverse transcriptase PCR in 9.7% of fecal samples from cattle of different ages with diarrhea, with 56% of total BToV-positive samples detected from young calves less than 3 weeks of age. The BToV-positive calves represented 26.4% of all the calves tested (28). In other studies, we detected BToV in veal calves (6.5%) and in feedlot calves (12.3%) at their arrival to the farm and feedlot, respectively, after transport from multiple states such as Ohio, West Virginia, Pennsylvania, and New York. These findings indicate that BToV is present as a minimum in the limited numbers of states surveyed to date (27, 30).

## Hosts

As indicated in the introduction, toroviruses are found in several animal species, including humans. However, toroviruses have been association with disease only in cattle, humans, and turkeys (2, 15, 30, 36, 55).

## Disease Association

Most reports associating HToV and disease involve children with acute diarrhea, persistent (chronic) diarrhea, or necrotizing enterocolitis (NEC) (4, 5, 36, 40, 44, 48, 50, 51, 55). Several investigators using ELISA and/or EM to analyze human fecal samples found toroviruses as the sole pathogen in children with acute or persistent diarrhea, or they detected toroviruses in higher proportions in clinically affected children (prevalence between 22 and 35%) than in healthy individuals (prevalence from 0 to 14.5%) (36, 40, 44). Most recently, toroviruses were identified by direct EM in stool samples from 48% of infants with NEC that had been admitted to intensive care units, compared with only 17% of non-NEC controls (55). Furthermore, children shedding HToV were 3.1 times more likely to manifest gastroenteritis than the asymptomatic control group (36). In general, the affected children were afebrile and exhibited watery diarrhea and dehydration, with vomiting three or four times a day. No other pathogens were detected in the feces of these patients (48).

In addition to the above reports, other findings suggest that HToV may be a causal agent of human enteric infections. First, seroconversion occurred in many patients shedding HToV, whereby the affected individual developed a specific antibody response (fourfold or more) as measured using an HI test with purified HToV (36). Second, toroviruses are frequently the only enteropathogen identified in the fecal samples from ill individuals (36, 48), or they are more prevalent in fecal samples from affected individuals than other enteric pathogens (such as rotavirus) (40). Based on such findings, Jamieson et al. (36) concluded that "toroviruses were the principal identifiable cause of nosocomial diarrhea in immunocompromised and older children" in the Hospital for Sick Children, Toronto, Canada.

In cattle, the clinical manifestations of a torovirus infection (mainly diarrhea) occur within 24 to 72 h postexposure, without a requirement for a viremic phase (18, 20, 62, 63, 66, 86, 89, 91). The affected animals often develop brilliant yellow, profuse watery diarrheic feces that persist for 2 to 6 days, with simultaneous fever, depression, various degrees of anorexia, dehydration, and weakness. Extremely large numbers of torovirus particles are shed for 4 to 6 days after the onset of the diarrhea, with peak shedding on day 3 or 4 (63, 66, 85, 86, 90, 91). As has been observed in humans, young calves from a few days up to 4 months old appear to be the most susceptible to clinical cases of diarrhea after torovirus infections; however, such clinical infections are more frequently observed in calves 2 to 5 days of age (17, 30, 39, 47, 86, 90). There is little information on torovirus morbidity and mortality in the literature; however, in the first reported outbreak of BToV, the morbidity rate was 56.5%, with a mortality rate of 8.7% and a fatality rate of 15.4% (90).

## PATHOGENESIS AND PATHOLOGY

EToV, the prototype torovirus, is the only torovirus to grow in cell culture, permitting detailed characterization of the replication mechanisms and genome of toroviruses (70, 71) (see also chapter 11). However, EToV reportedly produces only subclinical infections in the equine species (84); consequently, EToV has not been useful to study the pathogenesis of this group of viruses. In contrast, the majority of the studies describing the pathogenesis and pathology of toroviruses has been based on experimental studies of BToV, which consistently produces diarrhea in orally or intranasally inoculated colostrum-deprived and gnotobiotic calves 3 to 50 days old (18, 63, 66, 86, 89, 91). BToV has also been identified as an enteric pathogen that causes mild to profuse diarrhea in cattle under field conditions (16, 30, 39, 47, 51, 68, 90). Therefore, although BToV does not replicate in vitro, the majority of published pathogenesis and epidemiological studies have focused on BToV.

## Longitudinal Intestinal Tropism

In experimental studies, BToV virions and antigen have been observed by EM and immunofluorescence (IF), respectively, in epithelial cells from the mid-jejunum through the ileum and from the surface of the large intestine to within its deep folds (specially in the colon) (18, 20, 62, 63, 86, 89, 91). The torovirus-infected areas appear to be randomly scattered or patchy throughout the affected intestine, with villous atrophy and focal necrosis of epithelial cells observed (18, 62, 63, 90). Mild to moderate inflammatory responses have also been observed histologically in the affected areas, principally in the small intestine (18, 62, 63, 90). No major macroscopic changes or gross lesions have been observed upon necropsy of BToV-infected animals, which mainly show signs of dehydration together with reddening and loss of tone of the thin-walled lower small intestine (42, 62, 86).

## Vertical Intestinal Tropism

In the mid-jejunum, BToV infects epithelial cells from the lower half of the villi extending deep into the crypts. Likewise, in the lower jejunum and ileum, the entire villi can be positive for torovirus antigen by IF, as can the majority of the crypt enterocytes (18, 90). Interestingly, Woode et al. (90) suggested that the first site for viral replication was the immature epithelial cells of the crypts, from which the infection could migrate up the villi; however, this possible vertical spread of toroviruses in the villi has not yet been proven. Dome epithelial cells and M cells have been also reported to contain viral antigen detected by IF, leading to cytopathic changes (63, 89). Although torovirus virions in several stages of degradation have been observed inside macrophages, it is believed that BToV infects only enterocytes, suggesting that macrophages have ingested virus or cellular debris (18). Torovirus particles or antigen have not been identified in other cell types or organs.

BToV has been observed attached to the apical surface of enterocytes, but it has not been seen attached to the microvilli of goblet cells or to the microfolds of M cells associated with Peyer's patches (86). Based on EM and IF studies, in vivo entry or penetration of BToV into the enterocytes is believed to be by a receptor-mediated endocytosis-like mechanism (18, 63).

Detailed descriptions of cytopathic effects produced by BToV on epithelial cells have been given elsewhere (18, 20, 63, 90, 91). Briefly, severe vacuolar degeneration, necrosis, and exfoliation have been observed in BToV-infected enterocytes just a few hours postinfection. As the infection progresses, a change in the enteroabsorptive cells from columnar to squamous or cuboidal is observed (90); infected cells exhibited ultrastructural changes, including rounded shape, vacuolated cytoplasm, and separation from each other (86). Villous atrophy and crypt hyperplasia are also detected. Likewise, fusion of the villi or folds, in which a "bridge" is frequently made with virus-infected cells, has been seen (86).

Several patches of denuded and multifocal necrotic areas are found throughout the distal small intestine, where the crypts are dilated, containing a large amount of cell debris and abundant infiltration of the lamina propria by macrophages and neutrophils (18, 20, 63, 66, 89–91). Similar lesions have been observed in the colon (principally spiral colon) and cecum, where BToV-infected epithelial cells cover the intestine surface and the crypts (63, 89). In addition, cytopathic effects similar to those observed in the enterocytes were seen in dome epithelial cells and M cells over the Peyer's patches (63, 89). Damage of these cells could influence the immune responses, as proposed by Koopmans and Horzinek (43), delaying antibody responses and affecting mucosal memory.

The characteristic torus shape of the toroviruses is observed only in extracellular viral particles or in vacuoles near the cell surface and never in the cytoplasm of the cell, where the virus nucleocapsid shows a straight or "bacillary" shape (also described as a brick-shaped or elongated virion with rounded ends) similar to that of the rhabdoviruses (18, 63, 86, 90). Virus maturation apparently occurs intracellularly during the egress process, whereby the appearance of the virus nucleocapsid changes from a straight shape (intracellular) into a torus shape (extracellular). The release of the virion into the intestinal lumen has been suggested to occur through reverse pinocytosis, which explains the presence of virus-containing vesicles seen near the cell surface (13, 18, 35, 86).

An unexplained aspect of BToV pathology is the presence of free torovirus particles in the intestinal lumen before any cytopathic changes are observed in enterocytes. This raises the possibility that more than one viral replicative cycle occurs before visible damage to the host cell is observed (18, 86). Virus release via exocytotic fusion of virion-containing vesicles with the plasma membrane could allow several waves of virus release without inducing cytolysis of enterocytes. This characteristic of BToV egress could also explain why the diarrhea induced by this microorganism is mild to moderate but the number of virions shed is so high, a phenomenon we have observed in BToV-inoculated colostrum-deprived and gnotobiotic calves in our laboratory. This mechanism may also explain why the virus can be detected in feces without the presence of diarrhea (18).

In general, the lesions reported for BToV infections are very similar to the ones described for bovine rotavirus and bovine coronavirus (BCoV), making it impossible to provide a differential diagnosis based only on histopathology (90). Nonetheless, BCoV may not infect the crypt enterocytes as frequently as BToV, which can infect and destroy both crypt and villous enterocytes of the small intestine as well as surface and crypt enterocytes in the large intestine; this may be a unique characteristic of BToV infections (18, 20, 63, 90). On the other hand, bovine rotavirus infects the epithelial cells of the villous tips in the proximal small intestine; in contrast, BToV does not generally infect the duodenum or proximal small intestine (90).

## Diarrhea Causation

The mechanisms whereby toroviruses induce diarrhea have not been fully determined. Nevertheless, it has been speculated that the extensive colonic lesions produced by BToV could reduce the ability of the intestinal tract to absorb water, resulting in watery diarrhea (90). Woode and others also suggest that damage to the villous and crypt enterocytes of the small intestine could produce malabsorption (90). In support of these suggestions, BToV reduced the absorption of D-xylose by the intestine by 15 to 65%, indicating that BToV-mediated epithelial cell damage produced intestinal malabsorption (85, 91). The mild to moderate diarrhea can be explained by the finding that although BToV produces significant cell damage, such damage occurs over 50 to 70% of the surface only in the caudal portion of the small intestine (85, 91).

Animals with mixed infections of BToV and other enteric pathogens (e.g., rotavirus and astroviruses) develop more severe watery diarrhea than the clinical disease induced by either pathogen alone, suggesting an additive effect among pathogens (89, 91). A similar association was observed in one of our field studies, in which veal calves shedding more than two pathogens at a time were six times more likely to manifest clinical disease than those shedding a single pathogen (30).

## Respiratory Disease

BToV antigen and viral RNA have been detected in nasal samples (27), and during BToV outbreaks, calves with respiratory disease signs have also been described (46). However, there is little information about the distribution of BToV infection in the respiratory tract and the cytopathological changes that the virus produces in the respiratory epithelia. In 1992, respiratory toroviral infections detected by IF were reported for young calves from 4 days up to 6 months of age, as well as in a Belgian calf that died of pneumonia (78, 79). However, the reagents used in these studies were apparently contaminated with BCoV antibodies (14), making the validity of these conclusions uncertain.

## Mode of Transmission

Transmission of BToV has been suggested to occur through the oral/nasal route by direct contact with contaminated feces or nasopharyngeal secretions (13, 82, 86, 88, 90). The oral pathway has already been proven experimentally, since oral inoculation of calves with BToV induces diarrhea with viral shedding in feces (89–91). On the other hand, based on our detection of BToV antigen and viral RNA in nasal secretions of almost all calves by day 3 after their arrival to the feedlot (27), BToV may also be transmitted via the nasal route, as has been reported for other coronaviruses such as BCoV, a virus previously associated with the bovine respiratory disease complex, or shipping fever (12, 37, 52, 54, 56, 58, 73–75). Intranasal inoculation of BToV has been shown under experimental conditions to induce infection and disease in young colostrum-deprived or gnotobiotic calves (86), and nasal shedding of BToV has been detected in both types of BToV-inoculated calves (62, 63; L. J. Saif, unpublished data).

In a recent field study of BCoV in feedlot calves, we observed that nasal viral shedding clearly preceded fecal shedding (77), confirming previous reports suggesting that respiratory tract infections by BCoV generally preceded enteric infections (11, 22, 23, 26, 64, 65). It is conceivable that a similar scenario may occur for the enveloped BToV, and like with the enveloped BCoV, initial replication may occur in nasal epithelial cells, increasing the titers of these labile enveloped viruses and coating them in nasal mucus before they are swallowed. This would enhance and protect the virus and aid transit though the rumen and the intestinal tract. Thus, initial replication of these enveloped viruses in the upper respiratory tract could increase their opportunity for survival during passage through the rumen and into the gastrointestinal tract, helping to ensure that enough viable viral particles infect the intestine, with subsequent large amounts of virus excreted in the feces (65). Although BToV antigen and viral RNA have been detected in nasal samples (27), there are no published reports confirming the nasal replication of BToV and its contribution to the pathogenesis of BToV. Therefore, further studies are needed not only to confirm nasal replication but also to determine the extent of damage (if any) to the upper or lower respiratory epithelia, its possible association with respiratory illness alone or in concert with other respiratory pathogens, and the possibility of aerosol transmission.

## IMMUNE RESPONSES

There is little information about the immune response to torovirus infections, and the majority of studies have focused mainly on the humoral immune response to BToV infections in cattle. Nevertheless, in torovirus infections, as in many other enteric viral diseases, the presence of circulating maternal antibodies (such as colostrum-passive immunity) and the immune status of the individual affect the clinical outcome and/or severity of the diarrhea produced by these viruses.

In the United States, a very high seroprevalence of BToV antibodies in cattle as measured by ELISA has been reported and ranges from 88.5 to 89.7% (85, 88, 91). This high seroprevalence can only be explained by the widespread presence of BToV in the cattle population and active infections among animals of different ages, as we described in our epidemiological studies (27, 28, 30). The high seroprevalence of BToV antibodies in the adult cattle population can also account for the titers of antibody to BToV found in neonatal calves (7 days old) in our veal study, in which 82% of the calves had antibodies to BToV when tested on their arrival at the farm (30). A similar high seropositivity rate (90%) was also reported for calves less than 1 month old (46). Such a high seroprevalence in young calves is believed to be related to intake of colostrum containing maternal antibodies to BToV, which, as described earlier, affect the course of BToV infection in neonatal calves.

For example, newborn and young calves deprived of maternal antibodies (or with very low antibody titers to BToV due to limited colostrum intake) develop moderate to severe diarrhea, with high viral shedding, after exposure to or inoculation with BToV (30, 82). We observed that BToV-seronegative calves (<10 HI units) were up to 7.4 times as likely to shed BToV in feces during their first month of life as calves that had moderate to high (≥1:20 to 80 and ≥1:160 to 1:640 HI units, respectively) circulating maternally derived antibodies to BToV (30). The calves shedding BToV were 6.95 times more likely to have diarrhea than calves not shedding BToV (30). In any case, after a primary infection of such seronegative calves, an active immune response is induced, reflected by the

development of BToV-specific immunoglobulin M (IgM) and IgG antibodies in serum, reaching peak titers 1 to 2 and 3 to 4 weeks after infection, respectively. Interestingly, no IgA seroconversion was observed in this group of animals (39, 42, 86). In some cases only a few calves actively seroconverted with persisting titers of IgG1 antibody to BToV (39, 42). The detailed time course of IgG1, IgM, and IgA antibody responses to BToV after natural exposure or contact has been described previously (39).

In contrast, we have observed that calves with moderate to high circulating maternal antibodies (as indicated above) are partially protected against disease, developing no diarrhea or milder diarrhea than calves with little or no passive maternal antibodies against BToV (30). Although maternal antibodies can affect the clinical manifestations of the disease, they apparently do not protect the calf against infection; therefore, infected calves may still be subclinically infected and shed small amounts of BToV in feces without developing diarrhea (30). Interestingly, in some cases, no increased antibody titers were detected by HI assays in these asymptomatic, seropositive calves up to 21 days after the initial detection of virus, suggesting delayed antibody responses due to the presence of maternal antibodies (30). Several investigators studying BToV and other *Coronaviridae*, such as BCoV, have described how the presence of passive (IgG1) serum antibodies may not block viral shedding in calves up to 4 months of age, but affects the calves' immune responses by decreasing or delaying their active immune responses (24, 25, 39, 43, 47, 82, 86, 91). The production of IgM antibodies to BToV in colostrum-fed (seropositive) neonatal calves is relatively late, occurring 3 to 5 weeks after infection, and there is no measurable IgG seroconversion to BToV positivity (39, 42, 43, 47, 86, 91).

A natural decline in circulating maternal antibodies to BToV has been observed in calves that have acquired colostral maternal antibodies against BToV, with calves becoming seronegative by 2 to 6 months of age (39, 46). Decrease of passive antibody titers has been observed as early as 8 weeks after birth, accordingly to Van de Boom (cited by Weiss and Horzinek [82]). Koopmans et al. (46) also reported a similar finding, indicating that up to 90% of the young calves that previously had titers of maternal antibody to BToV became totally seronegative at 3 to 4 months of age. In our feedlot study, the vast majority (93%) of the feedlot calves at 5 to 7 months of age were already seronegative to BToV at their arrival at the feedlot, which provides additional evidence of the natural decline of maternally derived immunity to BToV and the potential increased susceptibility of this group of animals to new BToV infections (27). In support of this increased susceptibility, we found that 100% of seronegative calves arriving at the feedlot were infected at arrival or shortly thereafter, shedding BToV fecally and/or nasally, and actively seroconverting (as measured by HI). In contrast, only 57% of the arriving calves that were seropositive to BToV seroconverted (27).

A deficient or lack of anti-BToV mucosal immunologic memory may also be present in calves previously infected with this virus. This statement is based on the observation that after the introduction into the adult herd of seronegative young calves that previously shed BToV, the calves again developed BToV infections with mild diarrhea, followed by seroconversion to all antibody isotypes (39). Several authors have suggested that there are two possible explanations for such an apparent lack of or deficient immunological memory response to BToV infections. First, BToV may interfere with an active immune response in young calves by infecting and damaging M cells, thereby affecting or delaying the active immune response (42). Second, the lack of or deficient active antibody responses to BToV may be due to maternal antibody interference (39, 42, 46) as observed in BCoV-infected bovids. In this instance, the presence of maternal antibodies decreased or delayed systemic and mucosal anti-BCoV antibody responses in calves (25).

The transient immune response, the loss of circulating maternal antibodies, the presence of stressful conditions (e.g., transport, change of diet, new environment, or commingling), and/or contact with infected adult individuals shedding BToV are important risk factors that can predispose an incoming seronegative calf entering an adult herd or feedlot to new BToV infections (27, 39, 42, 46). Such exposures could lead to BToV-associated diarrhea and production losses in these types of animals. Nevertheless, if an older calf is infected upon arrival at the feedlot (or the herd), it will develop an immune response that will clear the BToV 2 to 3 weeks after the initial infection, with no BToV shedding detected by ELISA or reverse transcriptase PCR in those animals by day 21 postarrival (27).

## CONCLUDING REMARKS

In conclusion, toroviruses have been detected in cattle in several states in the United States and in other countries worldwide. They infect many animal species, including humans. In cattle, BToV is a pathogen capable of producing cytolytic infection of enterocytes throughout the distal small and entire large intestine and of inducing diarrhea. Furthermore,

BToV is antigenically and genetically closely related to HToV, indicating a potential zoonotic link for this pathogen. In addition, there has been an increasing number of reports associating torovirus infections with clinical illness in humans, especially in young and/or immunocompromised individuals. This suggests that toroviruses are emerging as a potential public health concern that needs to be studied further. Consequently, additional questions about torovirus epidemiology and ecology, pathogenesis (e.g., nasal replication and effect of mixed infections), disease association and impact on cattle health and performance, and the zoonotic potential of BToV, need to be addressed by the scientific community in the near future.

## REFERENCES

1. Ali, A., and D. L. Reynolds. 1997. Stunting syndrome in Turkey poults: isolation and identification of the etiologic agent. *Avian Dis.* **41**:870–881.
2. Ali, A., and D. L. Reynolds. 2000. Characterization of the stunting syndrome agent: relatedness to known viruses. *Avian Dis.* **44**:45–50.
3. Ali, A., and D. L. Reynolds. 2003. Turkey torovirus infection, p. 332–336. *In* Y. Saif, H. J. Barnes, J. R. Glisson, A. M. Fadly, L. R. McDougald, and D. E. Sawyne (ed.), *Disease of Poultry*, 11th ed. Blackwell Publishing, Ames, IA.
4. Beards, G. M., D. W. G. Brown, J. Green, and T. H. Flewett. 1986. Preliminary characterization of torovirus-like particles of humans: comparison with Berne virus of horses and Breda virus of Calves. *J. Med. Virol.* **20**:67–78.
5. Beards, G. M., J. Green, C. Hall, T. H. Flewett, F. Lamouliatte, and P. Du Pasquier. 1984. An enveloped virus in stools of children and adults with gastroenteritis that resembles the Breda virus of calves. *Lancet* **i**:1050–1052.
6. Brown, D. W. G., G. M. Beards, and T. H. Flewett. 1987. Detection of Breda virus antigen and antibody in humans and animals by enzyme immunoassay. *J. Clin. Microbiol.* **25**:637–640.
7. Brown, D. W. G., R. Selvakumar, D. J. Daniel, and V. I. Mathan. 1988. Prevalence of neutralizing antibodies to Berne virus in animals and humans in Vellore, South India. *Arch. Virol.* **98**:267–269.
8. Cavanagh, D. 1997. *Nidovirales*: a new order comprising *Coronaviridae* and *Arteriviridae*. *Arch. Virol.* **143**:629–633.
9. Cavanagh, D., D. A. Brian, M. A. Brinton, L. Enjuanes, K. V. Holmes, M. C. Horzinek, M. M. C. Lai, H. Laude, P. G. W. Plagemann, S. G. Siddell, W. J. M. Spaan, F. Taguchi, and P. J. Talbot. 1994. The *Coronaviridae* now comprises two genera, *Coronavirus* and *Torovirus*: report of the *Coronaviridae* Study Group, p. 255–257. *In* H. Laude and J. F. Vautherot (ed.), *Coronaviruses: Molecular Biology and Virus-Host Interactions*. Plenum Press, New York, NY.
10. Cavanagh, D., and D. Brown. 1990. *Coronaviruses and Their Diseases*. Plenum Press, New York, NY.
11. Cho, K. J., A. E. Hoet, S. C. Loerch, T. E. Wittum, and L. J. Saif. 2001. Evaluation of concurrent shedding of bovine coronavirus via the respiratory tract and enteric route in feedlot cattle. *Am. J. Vet. Res.* **62**:1436–1441.
12. Chouljenko, V. N., X. Q. Lin, J. Storz, K. G. Kousoulas, and A. E. Gorbalenya. 2001. Comparison of genomic and predicted

amino acid sequences of respiratory and enteric bovine coronaviruses isolated from the same animal with fatal shipping pneumonia. *J. Gen. Virol.* **82:**2927–2933.

13. **Cornelissen, L. A. H. M.** 1999. What are toroviruses? p. 7–20. *In* L. A. H. M. Cornelissen (ed.), *Molecular Characterization of Ungulate Toroviruses.* Universiteit Utrecht, Utrecht, The Netherlands.

14. **Cornelissen, L. A. H. M., P. A. M. van Woensel, R. J. de Groot, M. C. Horzinek, N. Visser, and H. F. Egberink.** 1998. Cell culture-grown putative bovine respiratory torovirus identified as a coronavirus. *Vet. Rec.* **142:**683–686.

15. **Duckmanton, L., B. Luan, J. Devenish, R. Tellier, and M. Petric.** 1997. Characterization of torovirus from human fecal specimens. *Virology* **239:**158–168

16. **Duckmanton, L. M., S. Carman, E. Nagy, and M. Petric.** 1998. Detection of bovine torovirus in fecal specimens of calves with diarrhea from Ontario farms. *J. Clin. Microbiol.* **36:**1266–1270.

17. **Durham, P. J. K., L. E. Hassard, G. R. Norman, and R. L. Yemen.** 1989. Viruses and virus-like particles detected during examination of feces from calves and piglets with diarrhea. *Can. Vet. J.* **30:**876–881.

18. **Fagerland, J. A., J. F. L. Pohlenz, and G. N. Woode.** 1986. A morphological study of the replication of Breda virus (proposed family Toroviridae) in bovine intestinal cells. *J. Gen. Virol.* **67:**1293–1304.

19. **Finlaison, D. S.** 1995. Faecal viruses of dogs—an electron microscope study. *Vet. Microbiol.* **46:**295–305.

20. **Hall, G. A.** 1987. Comparative pathology of infection by novel diarrhoea viruses. *Ciba Found. Symp.* **128:**192–217.

21. **Haschek, B., D. Klein, V. Benetka, C. Herrera, I. Sommerfeld-Stur, S. Vilcek, K. Moestl, and G. M. Beards.** 2006. Detection of bovine torovirus in neonatal calf diarrhea in Lower Austria and Styria (Austria). *J. Vet. Med. B* **53:**160–165.

22. **Hasoksuz, M. H., S. L. Lathrop, K. L. Gadfield, and L. J. Saif.** 1999. Isolation of bovine respiratory coronaviruses from feedlot cattle and comparison of their biological and antigenic properties with bovine enteric coronaviruses. *Am. J. Vet. Res.* **60:**1227–1233.

23. **Heckert, R. A., L. J. Saif, K. H. Hoblet, and A. G. Agnes.** 1990. A longitudinal study of bovine coronavirus enteric and respiratory infections in dairy calves in two herds in Ohio. *Vet. Microbiol.* **22:**187–201.

24. **Heckert, R. A., L. J. Saif, J. P. Mengel, and G. W. Myers.** 1991. Mucosal and systemic antibody responses to bovine coronavirus structural proteins in experimentally challenge-exposed calves fed low or high amounts of colostral antibodies. *Am. J. Vet. Res.* **52:**700–708.

25. **Heckert, R. A., L. J. Saif, and G. W. Myers.** 1991. Mucosal and systemic isotype specific antibody responses to bovine coronavirus structural proteins in naturally infected dairy calves. *Am. J. Vet. Res.* **52:**852–857.

26. **Heckert, R. A., L. J. Saif, G. W. Myers, and A. G. Agnes.** 1991. Epidemiologic factors and isotype-specific antibody responses in serum and mucosal secretions of dairy calves with bovine coronavirus respiratory tract and enteric tract infections. *Am. J. Vet. Res.* **52:**845–851.

27. **Hoet, A. E., K. O. Cho, K. O. Chang, S. C. Loerch, T. E. Wittum, and L. J. Saif.** 2002. Enteric and nasal shedding of bovine torovirus (Breda virus) in feedlot cattle. *Am. J. Vet. Res.* **63:**342–348.

28. **Hoet, A. E., P. R. Nielsen, M. Hasoksuz, C. Thomas, T. E. Wittum, and L. J. Saif.** 2003. Detection of bovine torovirus and other enteric pathogens in feces from diarrhea cases in cattle. *J. Vet. Diagn. Investig.* **15:**205–212.

29. **Hoet, A. E., and L. J. Saif.** 2004. Bovine torovirus (Breda virus) revisited. *Anim. Health Res. Rev.* **5:**157–171.

30. **Hoet, A. E., J. Smiley, C. Thomas, P. R. Nielsen, T. E. Wittum, and L. J. Saif.** 2003. Association of enteric shedding of bovine torovirus (Breda virus) and other enteropathogens with diarrhea in veal calves. *Am. J. Vet. Res.* **64:**485–490.

31. **Holmes, K. V.** 2001. Enteric infections with coronaviruses and toroviruses. *Novartis Found. Symp.* **238:**258–275.

32. **Horzinek, M. C.** 1999. Toroviruses (Coronaviridae), p. 1798–1803. *In* A. Granoff and R. Webster (ed.), *Encyclopedia of Virology,* 2nd ed. Academic Press, San Diego, CA.

33. **Horzinek, M. C., T. H. Flewett, L. J. Saif, W. J. M. Spaan, M. Weiss, and G. N. Woode.** 1987. A new family of vertebrate viruses: *Toroviridae. Intervirology* **27:**17–24.

34. **Horzinek, M. C., and M. Weiss.** 1984. Toroviridae: a taxonomic proposal. *Zentbl. Vetmed. Reihe B* **31:**649–659.

35. **Horzinek, M. C., and M. Weiss.** 1990. Toroviruses, p. 253–262. *In* L. J. Saif and K. W. Theil (ed.), *Viral Diarrheas of Man and Animals.* CRC Press, Boca Raton, FL.

36. **Jamieson, F. B., E. E. L. Wang, C. Bain, J. Good, L. M. Duckmanton, and M. Petric.** 1998. Human torovirus: a new nosocomial gastrointestinal pathogen. *J. Infect. Dis.* **178:**1263–1269.

37. **Kapil, S., and S. M. Goyal.** 1995. Bovine coronavirus-associated respiratory disease. *Compend. Continuing Educ. Practi. Vet.* **17:**1179–1181.

38. **Kluver, S.** 1991. Electron microscopical and serological study of the occurrence of Breda torovirus, a cause of calf diarrhoea. Ph.D. thesis. Tierärztliche Hochschule, Hannover, Germany.

39. **Koopmans, M., H. Cremers, G. N. Woode, and M. C. Horzinek.** 1990. Breda virus (Toroviridae) infection and systemic antibody response in sentinel calves. *Am. J. Vet. Res.* **51:**1443–1448.

40. **Koopmans, M., S. Goosen, A. Lima, I. Mcauliffe, J. Nataro, L. Barret, R. I. Glass, and R. Guerrant.** 1997. Association of torovirus with acute and persistent diarrhea in children. *Pediatr. Infect. Dis. J.* **16:**504–507.

41. **Koopmans, M., A. Herrewegh, and M. C. Horzinek.** 1991. Diagnosis of torovirus infection. *Lancet* **337:**859. (Letter.)

42. **Koopmans, M., and M. C. Horzinek.** 1994. Toroviruses of animals and humans: a review. *Adv. Virus Res.* **43:**233–273.

43. **Koopmans, M., and M. C. Horzinek.** 1995. The pathogenesis of torovirus infections in animals and humans, p. 403–413. *In* S. G. Siddell (ed.), *The Coronaviridae.* Plenum Press, New York, NY.

44. **Koopmans, M., M. Petric, R. I. Glass, and S. S. Monroe.** 1993. Enzyme-linked immunosorbent assay reactivity of torovirus-like particles in fecal specimens from humans with diarrhea. *J. Clin. Microbiol.* **31:**2738–2744.

45. **Koopmans, M., E. J. Snijder, and M. C. Horzinek.** 1991. cDNA probes for the diagnosis of bovine torovirus (Breda virus) infection. *J. Clin. Microbiol.* **29:**493–497.

46. **Koopmans, M., U. Van Den Boom, G. N. Woode, and M. C. Horzinek.** 1989. Seroepidemiology of Breda virus in cattle using ELISA. *Vet. Microbiol.* **19:**233–243.

47. **Koopmans, M., L. van Wuijckhuise-Sjouke, Y. H. Schukken, H. Cremers, and M. C. Horzinek.** 1991. Association of diarrhea in cattle with torovirus infections on farms. *Am. J. Vet. Res.* **52:**1769–1773.

48. **Krishnan, T., and T. N. Naik.** 1997. Electronmicroscopic evidence of torovirus like particles in children with diarrhoea. *Indian J. Med. Res.* **105:**108–110.

49. **Kroneman, A., L. A. H. M. Cornelissen, M. C. Horzinek, R. J. de Groot, and H. F. Egberink.** 1998. Identification and characterization of a porcine torovirus. *J. Virol.* **72:**3507–3511.

50. **Lacombe, D., F. Lamouliatte, C. Billeaud, and B. Sandler.** 1988. Virus Breda et entéropathie hémorragique, Rappel á propos d'une observation. *Arch. Fr. Pediatr.* **45:**442.

51. Lamouliatte, F., P. Du Pasquier, F. Rossi, J. Laporte, and J. P. Loze. 1987. Studies on bovine Breda virus. *Vet. Microbiol.* **15**:261–278.

52. Lathrop, S. L., T. E. Wittum, K. V. Brock, S. C. Loerch, L. J. Perino, H. R. Bingham, F. T. McCollum, and L. J. Saif. 2000. Association between infection of the respiratory tract attributed to bovine coronavirus and health and growth performance of cattle in feedlots. *Am. J. Vet. Res.* **61**:1062–1066.

53. Liebler, E. M., S. Kluver, J. F. Pohlenz, and M. Koopmans. 1992. The significance of bredavirus as a diarrhea agent in calf herds in Lower Saxony. *Dtsch. Tieraerztl. Wochenschr.* **99**:195–200.

54. Lin, X. Q., K. L. O'Reilly, J. Storz, C. W. Purdy, and R. W. Loan. 2000. Antibody responses to respiratory coronavirus infections of cattle during shipping fever pathogenesis. *Arch. Virol.* **145**:2335–2349.

55. Lodha, A., N. De Silva, M. Petric, and A. M. Moore. 2005. Human torovirus: a new virus associated with neonatal necrotizing enterocolitis. *Acta Paediatr.* **94**:1085–1088.

56. Martin, S. W., E. Nagy, P. E. Shewen, and R. J. Harland. 1998. The association of titers to bovine coronavirus with treatment for bovine respiratory disease and weight gain in feedlot calves. *Can. J. Vet. Res.* **62**:257–261.

57. Matiz, K., S. Kecskeméti, I. Kiss, Z. Adám, J. Tanyi, and B. Nagy. 2002. Torovirus detection in faecal specimens of calves and pigs in Hungary: short communication. *Acta Vet. Hung.* **50**:293–296.

58. McNulty, M. S., D. G. Bryson, G. M. Allan, and E. F. Logan. 1984. Coronavirus infection of the bovine respiratory tract. *Vet. Microbiol.* **9**:425–434.

59. Middleton, P. J. 1996. Viruses that multiply in the gut and cause endemic and epidemic gastroenteritis. *Clin. Diagn. Virol.* **6**:93–101.

60. Muir, P., D. A. Harbour, T. J. Gruffydd-Jones, P. E. Howard, C. D. Hopper, E. A. D. Gruffydd-Jones, H. M. Broadhead, C. M. Clarke, and M. E. Jones. 1990. A clinical and microbiological study of cats with protruding nictitating membranes and diarrhoea: isolation of a novel virus. *Vet. Rec.* **127**:324–330.

61. Pérez, E., A. Kummeling, M. M. H. Janssen, C. Jiménez, R. Alvarado, M. Caballero, P. Donado, and R. H. Dwinger. 1998. Infectious agents associated with diarrhoea of calves in the canton of Tilarán, Costa Rica. *Prev. Vet. Med.* **33**:195–205.

62. Pohlenz, J. F., G. N. Woode, N. F. Cheville, A. H. Mokresh, and K. A. Mohammed. 1982. Morphologic lesions in the intestinal mucosa of newborn calves reproduced by unclassified virus ("Breda-virus"), p. 252–254. *In Proceedings of 12th World Congress on Cattle Diseases.*

63. Pohlenz, J. F. L., N. F. Cheville, G. N. Woode, and A. H. Mokresh. 1984. Cellular lesions in intestinal mucosa of gnotobiotic calves experimentally infected with a new unclassified bovine virus (Breda virus). *Vet. Pathol.* **21**:407–417.

64. Reynolds, D. J., T. G. Debney, G. A. Hall, L. H. Thomas, and K. R. Parsons. 1985. Studies on the relationship between coronaviruses from the intestinal and respiratory tracts of calves. *Arch. Virol.* **85**:71–83.

65. Saif, L. J., D. R. Redman, P. D. Moorhead, and K. W. Theil. 1986. Experimentally induced coronavirus infections in calves: viral replication in the respiratory and intestinal tract. *Am. J. Vet. Res.* **47**:1426–1432.

66. Saif, L. J., D. R. Redman, K. W. Theil, P. D. Moorhead, and C. K. Smith. 1981. Studies on an enteric "Breda" virus in calves, abstr. 62, p. 42. *In 62nd Annu. Meet. Conf. Res. Workers Anim. Diagn.*

67. Scott, A. C., M. J. Chaplin, M. J. Stack, and L. J. Lund. 1987. Porcine torovirus? *Vet. Rec.* **120**:583.

68. Scott, F. M. M., A. Holliman, G. W. Jones, E. W. Gray, and J. Fitton. 1996. Evidence of torovirus infection in diarrhoeic cattle. *Vet. Rec.* **138**:284–285.

69. Snijder, E. J., J. Ederveen, W. J. M. Spaan, M. Weis, and M. C. Horzinek. 1988. Characterization of Berne virus genomic and messenger RNAs. *J. Gen. Virol.* **69**:2135–2144.

70. Snijder, E. J., and M. C. Horzinek. 1993. Toroviruses: replication, evolution and comparison with other members of the coronavirus-like superfamily. *J. Gen. Virol.* **74**:2305–2316.

71. Snijder, E. J., and M. C. Horzinek. 1995. The molecular biology of toroviruses, p. 219–238. *In* S. G. Siddell (ed.), *The Coronaviridae.* Plenum Press, New York, NY.

72. Snijder, E. J., M. C. Horzinek, and W. J. M. Spaan. 1994. The coronaviruslike superfamily, p. 235–244. *In* H. Laude and J. F. Vautherot (ed.), *Coronaviruses: Molecular Biology and Virus-Host Interactions.* Plenum Press, New York, NY.

73. Storz, J., C. W. Purdy, L.-X. Qing, M. Burrell, R. E. Truax, R. E. Briggs, G. H. Frank, and R. W. Loan. 2000. Isolation of respiratory bovine coronavirus, other cytocidal viruses, and *Pasteurella* spp. from cattle involved in two natural outbreaks of shipping fever. *J. Am. Vet. Med. Assoc.* **216**:1599–1604.

74. Storz, J., L.-X. Qing, C. W. Purdy, V. N. Chouljenko, K. G. Kousoulas, F. M. Enright, W. C. Gilmore, R. E. Briggs, and R. W. Loan. 2000. Coronavirus and *Pasteurella* infections in bovine shipping fever pneumonia and Evans' criteria for causation. *J. Clin. Microbiol.* **38**:3291–3297.

75. Storz, J., L. Stine, A. Liem, and G. A. Anderson. 1996. Coronavirus isolation from nasal swab samples in cattle with signs of respiratory tract disease after shipping. *J. Am. Vet. Med. Assoc.* **208**:1452–1455.

76. Tellier, R., and M. Petric. 1993. Human torovirus—purification from faeces, abstr. W24-4, p. 47. *In IXth International Congress of Virology.*

77. Thomas, C. J., A. E. Hoet, S. Sreevatsan, T. E. Wittum, R. E. Briggs, and L. J. Saif. 2006. Transmission of bovine coronavirus and serologic responses in feedlot calves under field conditions. *Am. J. Vet. Res.* **67**:1412–1420.

78. Vanopdenbosch, E., G. Wellemans, G. Charlier, and K. Petroff. 1992. Bovine torovirus: cell culture propagation of a respiratory isolate and some epidemiological data. *Vlaams Diergeneeskd. Tijdschr.* **61**:45–49.

79. Vanopdenbosch, E., G. Wellemans, J. Oudewater, and K. Petroff. 1992. Prevalence of torovirus infections in Belgian cattle and their role in respiratory, digestive and reproductive disorders. *Vlaams Diergeneeskd. Tijdschr.* **61**:187–191.

80. Vanopdenbosch, E., G. Wellemans, and K. Petroff. 1991. Breda virus associated with respiratory disease in calves. *Vet. Rec.* **129**:203.

81. Vorster, J. H., and G. H. Gerdes. 1993. Breda virus-like particles in calves in South Africa. *J. S. Afr. Vet. Assoc.* **64**:58.

82. Weiss, M., and M. C. Horzinek. 1987. The proposed family Toroviridae: agents of enteric infections. *Arch. Virol.* **92**:1–15.

83. Weiss, M., F. Steck, and M. C. Horzinek. 1983. Purification and partial characterization of a new enveloped RNA virus (Berne virus). *J. Gen. Virol.* **64**:1849–1858.

84. Weiss, M., F. Steck, R. Kaderli, and M. C. Horzinek. 1984. Antibodies to Berne virus in horses and other animals. *Vet. Microbiol.* **9**:523–531.

85. Woode, G. N. 1987. Breda and Breda-like viruses: diagnosis, pathology and epidemiology. *Ciba Found. Symp.* **128**:175–191.

86. **Woode, G. N.** 1990. Breda virus, p. 311–316. *In* Z. Dinter and B. Morein (ed.), *Virus Infections of Ruminants*, 3rd ed. Elsevier Science Publishers B.V., Amsterdam, The Netherlands.

87. **Woode, G. N.** 1982. Etiology of enteric viral infections of calves: pathological and clinical aspects, p. 201–208. *In Proceedings of 12th World Congress on Cattle Diseases*.

88. **Woode, G. N.** 1994. The Toroviruses: bovine (Breda virus) and equine (Berne virus) and the Torovirus-like agents of humans and animals, p. 581–602. *In* A. Z. Kapikian (ed.), *Viral Infections of the Gastrointestinal Tract*, 2nd ed. Marcel Dekker, New York, NY.

89. **Woode, G. N., J. F. L. Pohlenz, N. E. Kelso-Gourley, and J. A. Fagerland.** 1984. Astrovirus and Breda virus infections of dome cell epithelium of bovine ileum. *J. Clin. Microbiol.* **19:**623–630.

90. **Woode, G. N., D. E. Reed, P. L. Runnels, M. A. Herrig, and H. T. Hill.** 1982. Studies with an unclassified virus isolated from diarrheic calves. *Vet. Microbiol.* **7:**221–240.

91. **Woode, G. N., L. J. Saif, M. Quesada, N. J. Winand, J. F. L. Pohlenz, and N. K. Gourley.** 1985. Comparative studies on three isolates of Breda virus of calves. *Am. J. Vet. Res.* **46:**1003–1010.

*Nidoviruses*
Edited by S. Perlman, T. Gallagher, and E. J. Snijder
© 2008 ASM Press, Washington, DC

Chapter 24

# Molecular Biology and Pathogenesis of Roniviruses

JEFF A. COWLEY AND PETER J. WALKER

Currently all available information on the *Roniviridae* has come from studies of yellow head virus (YHV), gill-associated virus (GAV), and genotypic variants of these viruses detected in disparate populations of the black tiger shrimp species, *Penaeus monodon*. These viruses are very closely related and are currently classified as the type species *Gill-associated virus* of the genus *Okavirus*, the only recognized genus in the family. This review covers what is known of the biology of okaviruses as well as molecular characteristics that place these viruses within the order *Nidovirales* and distinguish them from the coronaviruses, toroviruses, and arteriviruses. The term okavirus is used to describe common properties shared by YHV and GAV. Individual virus names are used only when data relate to the specific characteristics of each virus. Additional information on the biology and molecular structure of YHV and GAV can be found in a recent review (26).

The black tiger shrimp is indigenous to costal habitats throughout much of the Indo-Pacific region, from the east coast of Africa, throughout South, Southeast, and East Asia, to Australia and islands of the southwest Pacific basin. Sequence information from okaviruses collected from various locations indicates that the viruses reported as YHV and GAV represent but two genotypes of several that have evolved in the various geographically segregated populations of shrimp (119; P. M. Wijegoonawardane et al., unpublished data). These genotypic variants, including YHV and GAV, are collectively referred to as the YHV complex (119). The natural distribution of *P. monodon* and the genetic relationships of YHV complex viruses from different geographic locations suggest an association that may predate the tectonic drift that dispersed the Gondwanaland supercontinent some 260 million years ago.

This is consistent with the ancient origins and evolutionary conservation of penaeid shrimp, for which Triassic fossils have been discovered in Madagascar; examples of the genus *Penaeus* have been reported to date to the late Cretaceous period (32). Moreover, the okavirus genome organization and RNA transcription strategy are relatively simple compared to those of vertebrate nidoviruses, which appear to have evolved in increasing complexity to adapt to higher-order vertebrate hosts. Thus, the okaviruses might be regarded as primitive time capsules that provide unique insights into aspects of nidovirus evolution (see also chapter 2).

## ORIGIN, HOST RANGE, AND TRANSMISSION MODES

### Origin

The term "yellow head," or "hua leung" in Thai, was first used to describe a disease that caused mass mortalities in black tiger shrimp on farms in central Thailand in 1990 (64). Typically, shrimp displayed a generalized pale or bleached appearance and accompanying yellow-brownish discoloration of the cephalothorax and gills (Color Plate 8 [see color insert]). Electron microscopy of various tissues from shrimp with naturally acquired (12) and experimentally induced (5) yellow head disease (YHD) identified the causative agent as a previously undescribed bacilliform-shaped, enveloped virus (Fig. 1). Virions were observed to mature within the cytoplasm by budding of filamentous helical nucleocapsids through endoplasmic membranes and to be present in large arrays in cytoplasmic vesicles within necrotic lymphoid organ (LO) and gill cells, in masses underlying the

**Jeff A. Cowley** • CSIRO Livestock Industries, Queensland Bioscience Precinct, St. Lucia, Queensland 4067, Australia. **Peter J. Walker** • CSIRO Livestock Industries, Australian Animal Health Laboratory, Geelong, Victoria 3220, Australia.

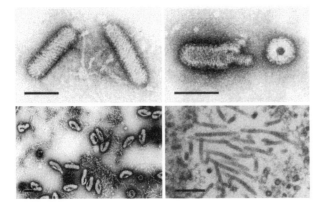

**Figure 1.** Transmission electron micrographs of negative-stained YHV particles. (Top left) Enveloped virions showing diffuse surface projections; (top right) virion in which the envelope has been damaged, exposing the internal helical nucleocapsid; (bottom left) virions with envelope extensions allowing them to assume circular structures similar to those of toroviruses; (bottom right) ultra-thin section showing the cytoplasm of a gill cell of an infected shrimp with nonenveloped nucleocapsid filaments displaying striations due to their helical symmetry. Scale bars =100 nm. The first three images are reproduced with permission from reference 74.

cuticle of secondary gill filaments, and in intercellular spaces (5). Injection of naïve *P. monodon* with filtrates of gill, LO, muscle, and hepatopancreas from YHD-affected shrimp resulted in rapid morbidity, onset of mortalities within 24 h and 100% cumulative mortality within 3 to 5 days (5). Based on the gross signs of disease, this new virulent pathogen was named YHV (36, 37, 126).

A virus morphologically indistinguishable from YHV was subsequently observed in healthy wild and farmed *P. monodon* in eastern Australia in 1993–1994 (106). However, there were no apparent signs of disease, and virions and filamentous helical nucleocapsids were observed only within the LO in partitioned clusters of cells with hypertrophied nuclei, termed "spheroids" (106). To distinguish this virus from the highly virulent YHV reported from Thailand, it was named lymphoid organ virus (LOV). In the summer grow-out season of 1995–1996, mass mortalities of *P. monodon* occurred at some farms in eastern Australia. Lethargic, moribund shrimp congregated and died at pond edges. Gross signs of disease included generalized reddening of the body, particularly at appendage extremities, and a brownish-pink discoloration of the gills (103). LOV-like nucleocapsids and virions were observed in abundance. However, as nucleocapsids and virions accumulated at high levels in the gills as well as LO cells, the virus was named gill-associated virus (103). Following intramuscular injection of filtered, whole cephalothorax, LO, or gill extracts from moribund shrimp, *P. monodon* ceased feeding and

became lethargic, and mortalities commenced within 3 to 4 days, reaching 100% cumulative mortality within 10 to 14 days (103, 116, 118, 119). The tissue distribution of the virus and histopathology caused in LO and other tissues were similar to YHD, but the typical gross signs, including pale-yellowish coloration of the carapace, were not evident. The markedly slower accumulation of mortalities, both during outbreaks in ponds and following experimental infection, suggested that GAV was a new pathogen that was related to but less virulent than YHV.

Subsequent nucleotide sequence analysis confirmed that YHV and GAV are closely related but distinct viruses, sharing approximately 80 to 85% nucleotide sequence identity (86 to 96% amino acid sequence identity) in relatively highly conserved regions of the replicase (open reading frame 1b [ORF1b]) gene (18, 91) and more distant relationships in intergenic regions (IGRs) and structural protein genes (51, 92). However, comparison of isolates of GAV from moribund shrimp and LOV from healthy shrimp indicated that they did not represent distinct genetic lineages but formed a single genetic cluster with relatively low nucleotide sequence divergence (<2.8% identity). It was also observed that injection of a filtered LO extract from LOV-infected *P. monodon* can induce an acute GAV-like disease (119; K. M. Spann et al., unpublished data) and that dilution of a GAV inoculum prepared from moribund shrimp results in an asymptomatic, chronic LOV-like infection which is primarily restricted to LO spheroid cells. This suggests that the outcome of infection is dose dependent, and at the same dose, there is no evidence that LOV and GAV differ in virulence or pathology. Rather, they appear to be isolates of the same virus recovered from chronic and acute infection states (15, 119). To avoid confusion, and recognizing the significance of its association with disease, it was thus recommended that GAV be adopted as the name for the yellow head-like virus detected in Australian shrimp (119).

Following the initial peak of YHD, YHV-like particles were also detected commonly in healthy farmed *P. monodon* in Thailand (33, 36, 78). Moreover, retrospective examination of earlier electron micrographs revealed the existence of virus in healthy broodstock prior to the emergence of YHD in the region (35, 37). By the late 1990s, there were also reports of YHD and/or YHV-like viruses in farmed *P. monodon* in China and several countries throughout Southeast Asia and the Indo-Pacific region. In eastern Australia, screening over consecutive seasons from 1997 to 1999 by reverse transcription-nested PCR indicated that the prevalence of GAV infection was 98% in wild and farmed *P. monodon* (15, 119). In the Philippines, a survey using immunoblot analysis

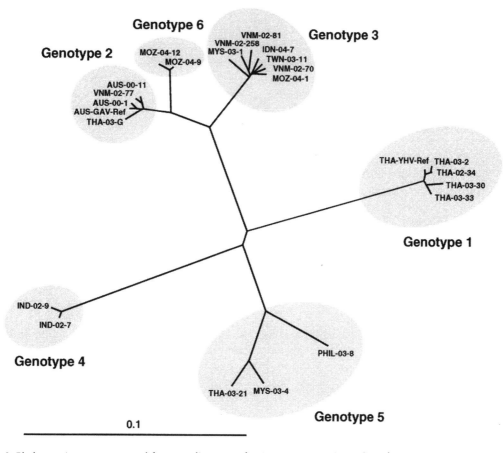

**Figure 2.** Phylogenetic tree constructed from an alignment of a 671-nt sequence in an ORF1b gene region encompassing part a of the helicase domain obtained from 26 viruses detected in *P. monodon* from the Indo-Pacific region. Viruses clustered into the six described yellow head complex genotypes, including YHV (genotype 1), GAV (genotype 2) and four other genotypes (genotypes 3, 4, 5, and 6) detected only in healthy shrimp. The viruses were detected in shrimp collected in Australia (AUS), India (IND), Indonesia (IDN), Malaysia (MYS), Mozambique (MOZ), the Philippines (PHL), Taiwan (TWN), Thailand (THA), and Vietnam (VNM) between 1997 and 2004 (Wijegoonawardane et al., unpublished).

of tissue samples collected in 1996 and 1997 indicated that there was a prevalence of infection of 17% in wild broodstock and 55% in postlarvae sampled from hatcheries, and a prevalence range of 0 to 67% in juvenile *P. monodon* from selected farms (75). As new genotypic variants were subsequently identified in healthy *P. monodon* from Vietnam and Thailand (80, 101, 119), it was suggested that the yellow head-related viruses be considered as a viral complex (119), with variants having evolved independently in isolated populations of shrimp. This concept has been supported by a recent study of *P. monodon* collected from throughout the Indo-Pacific region that has indicated the existence of at least six distinct genotypes in the complex (Fig. 2), most of which have been detected only in healthy shrimp (Wijegoonawardane et al., unpublished).

The reason for the sudden emergence of a highly virulent YHV genotype in intensive *P. monodon* aquaculture in Thailand in the early 1990s remains

unknown. A review of particle morphology, morphogenesis, and histopathology has suggested that YHV may have been responsible for the crash of the shrimp farming industry in Taiwan in the mid-1980s (12), and there is genetic evidence that YHV isolates from Thailand and Taiwan are virtually indistinguishable (119). Whatever the source of the initial outbreak, it is clear that a previously unknown pathogen struck the shrimp farming industry at the time of prolific expansion in Asia. YHD may have emerged from the background of asymptomatic chronic infections in *P. monodon* as a result of a chance mutation or recombination event. It is also possible that another crustacean is the natural host of YHV and that the practice of farming this marine shrimp species in terrestrial ponds has provided the opportunity for exposure to a new exogenous pathogen. However, a species jump appears unlikely, as available evidence indicates that viruses in the YHV complex display a strong natural host preference for *P. monodon*. Without question, pond densities and stock distribution networks in the intensive coastal aquaculture regions of Asia played a role in perpetuating outbreaks once YHD had emerged. Moreover, as for GAV, there is evidence that shrimp exposed to a low dose of YHV can escape disease and develop a chronic persistent infection (37, 119). It is also known that changes in water pH or reduced dissolved oxygen can induce acute YHV infection in asymptomatic carriers (37). It is most probable that YHV, like other genotypes, is a natural infection of *P. monodon* that occurs at relatively low prevalence as a chronic infection in wild populations. Environmental stress factors linked to aquaculture practices may compromise the innate pathogen defenses of shrimp, leading to elevated virus replication and unleashing its pathogenic potential.

## Host Range

The primary natural shrimp host of YHV and GAV is *P. monodon* (34, 37, 118, 119). However, there is evidence of natural infection in other species, including Kuruma shrimp *(Penaeus japonicus)* and white shrimp *(Penaeus setiferus)* (63, 65, 120) and mysid shrimp *(Palaemon styliferus)*, as well as krill *(Euphausia* spp.), paste shrimp *(Acetes* spp.), and other small shrimp species collected from outbreak ponds can transmit infections and thus might serve as carriers (34, 36). In Australia, GAV has been detected by reverse transcription-nested PCR in brown tiger shrimp *(Penaeus esculentus)* cocultivated with *P. monodon* (119) and in white banana prawns *(Penaeus merguiensis)* (J. A. Cowley et al., unpublished data).

Although natural YHV or GAV infection in species other than *P. monodon* appears to be uncommon, infection and/or disease has been established experimentally in many marine and freshwater shrimp. For YHV, susceptible species indigenous to the Indo-Pacific region include *P. merguiensis*, Antarctic krill *(Euphasia superba)*, barred estuarine shrimp *(Palaemon setiferus)*, mysid shrimp *(Palaemon styliferus)*, northern white shrimp *(Palaemon serrifer)*, king prawns *(Metapenaeus affinis)*, yellow prawns *(Metapenaeus brevicornis)*, red endeavor prawns *(Metapenaeus ensis)*, Sunda River prawns *(Macrobrachium sintangense)*, and riceland prawns *(Macrobrachium lanchesteri)* (12, 34, 36, 66, 67). Susceptible species indigenous to the Americas include Pacific white shrimp *(Penaeus vannamei)*, Pacific blue shrimp *(Penaeus stylirostris)*, white shrimp *(Penaeus setiferus)*, brown shrimp *(Penaeus aztecus)*, and brown-spotted prawns *(Penaeus duorarum)* (62, 68, 69). For GAV, *P. japonicus*, *P. esculentus*, and *P. merguiensis* have been infected experimentally (104, 105). Although the species above are susceptible to YHV and/or GAV, the

severity of disease can vary significantly according to the species and age at challenge.

Certain species of crabs and freshwater shrimp, as well as artemia, have been reported to be refractory to YHV infection (34). Longyant et al. (66) recently reported that none of 16 crab species commonly found in *P. monodon* farming areas in Thailand were susceptible to YHV infection in bioassays. Even so, YHV appears to have a relatively wide range of susceptible hosts among penaeid and palaemonid shrimp, and its natural host range is likely to be restricted by behavioral, environmental, and geographic factors that may well have been disrupted by aquaculture practices. Genetic and biological reasons for age- and species-related differences in infection and disease susceptibility have yet to be determined but would be a fertile field for future study.

## Transmission Modes

Horizontal transmission of YHV in *P. monodon* occurs readily following cannibalism of infected carcasses, following segregated cohabitation of uninfected and diseased shrimp, and via exposure to seawater containing filtered extracts of infected shrimp tissue (37, 62). Ingestion is the likely natural route of entry of virions shed into seawater, but the possibility of infection via the exposed mucosal surfaces of the gills cannot be excluded. GAV transmitted by ingestion of tissue from moribund *P. monodon* can also result in acute infection and disease, and ingestion of tissues from healthy, chronically infected shrimp can transmit infection to naïve *P. esculentus* (119). In high-density aquaculture systems, the cannibalization of weak or diseased shrimp is a common behavior and would account for the rapid escalation of disease and mortalities that can occur during YHD and GAV outbreaks (116). YHV has also been transmitted to *P. monodon* by feeding *Acetes* spp. and *Palaemon styliferus* collected from ponds affected by YHD (34, 36), implicating other crustacean species as potential sources of infection.

Vertical transmission of GAV in *P. monodon* has been demonstrated experimentally (19). Virus can exist within both spermatophores of males and mature ovarian tissue of females (21, 119). In spermatophores, clusters of virus particles have been observed in seminal fluid but not in sperm cells (19). The parental source of transmitted virus has been investigated by exploiting nucleotide sequence variations in GAV strains infecting each parent in a mating pair and associated with newly spawned eggs. The evidence suggests that transseminal transmission is the primary route of infection but that transovarian transmission can also occur when viral loads are sufficiently high in the female (19). Following hatching, GAV is difficult to detect in larval stages (nauplius and protozoea) but can often be detected as shrimp reach the early postlarva stages. Therefore, it appears that the virus present in seminal fluid or ovarian tissues is associated with the egg casing rather than the germ plasm (19, 119). However, additional studies are required to identify more definitively the location of egg-associated virus and to identify how larvae become infected.

## VIRUS-HOST INTERACTIONS

Physiological stress induced in *P. monodon* by reduced water quality and intensive farming practices appears to have contributed to the original YHD outbreaks in Thailand (12). Although this is impossible to prove, factors such as reduced dissolved oxygen or changes in water pH can induce acute YHD in shrimp with asymptomatic infections established by injecting a low dose of YHV (34). Consistent with this, handling stress associated with repeated bleeding can sufficiently compromise immune function in *P. monodon* with naturally acquired asymptomatic GAV infections to allow viral loads in hemocytes and other tissues to increase in the order of 1,000-fold over a 9-day period (21).

Asymptomatic infection by okaviruses is invariably associated with the sequestration of infected hemocytes within the LO in the form of partitioned aggregates of cells with hypertrophied nuclei referred to as spheroids (1, 106). Spheroids also form in response to infection with other shrimp viruses, including the dicistrovirus Taura syndrome virus. Evidence suggests that spheroids are an integral component of the innate defense system of crustaceans and are involved in the containment and clearing of viral infection (26, 45, 46). However, as for all virus-host interactions, the ability of shrimp to contain potentially pathogenic okavirus infections is influenced by variations in virulence and dose of exposure, the presence of other coinfecting pathogens, and environmental stressors that may compromise the defense response. As shrimp are poikilothermic, the progression of infection is also susceptible to variations in ambient temperature, which influence the rate of viral replication.

In the acute stage of infection, okaviruses become systemically distributed throughout all tissues of mesodermal and ectodermal origin, including the LO, gill, hemocytes, cuticular epithelium, hematopoietic tissue, and the spongy connective tissues of many organs as well as fixed phagocytes in the heart, gill, and hepatopancreas (5, 12, 71, 103, 105, 109, 110).

For Taura syndrome virus, which also establishes an acute systemic infection, changes in spheroid morphology during the transitions from early to acute-stage infection, and through to convalescence, indicated that apoptotic cell death might contribute to viral clearance (45, 46). For YHV and GAV, the transition from chronic to acute infection is accompanied by the systemic spread of virus replication from LO spheroids to neighboring stromal matrix cells of LO tubules and to all tissues of mesodermal and ectodermal origin. Once disease occurs, severe necrosis is evident in the LO and other organs, and aggregations of fixed phagocytes/hemocytes (referred to as ectopic spheroids) accumulate within the haemal spaces of receptive tissues (5, 12, 103, 105, 109, 110). The progression of YHD is also accompanied by widespread apoptosis, and it has been suggested that this could ultimately contribute to multiple organ dysfunctions (56). Apoptosis also occurs in shrimp infected with a highly virulent nimavirus, white spot syndrome virus (86), and is believed to be a primary contributor to shrimp death (124).

No continuous crustacean cells lines are yet available to study okavirus replication in vitro. However, primary cell cultures derived from explants of *P. monodon* LO tissue support YHV replication, with associated cytopathology typified by cell rounding and detachment (13, 65, 70). Use of an end point infectivity assay using primary LO cells (70) has confirmed transmission electron microscopic observations that LO and gill tissues are the primary sites of YHV replication and virion accumulation (71) and shown that mature virions are released into culture medium well before the appearance of cytopathology (2). Virion maturation and envelope acquisition by okaviruses primarily occur at smooth endoplasmic membranes (5, 12, 106). The detection of virions in cell culture supernatants prior to cytopathology is consistent with observations of virions occasionally budding directly at the plasma membrane prior to cell lysis.

## VIRION MORPHOLOGY, ASSEMBLY, AND STRUCTURE

Okavirus particles are enveloped rod-shaped (bacilliform) structures ∼45 nm in diameter and ∼150 to 200 nm in length (Fig. 1) (5, 12, 68, 74, 94, 103, 106, 120, 121, 126). The lipid envelope is studded with regularly spaced projections ∼8 nm thick and up to 11 nm long. In some purified YHV preparations, narrowed envelopes extending from the ends of virions allow particles to assume a doughnut-shaped appearance (Fig. 1) (74, 121) somewhat

## Okavirus

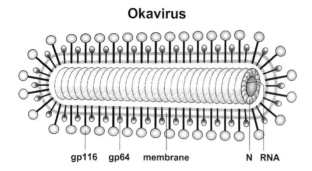

gp116   gp64   membrane        N   RNA

**Figure 3.** Schematic representation of the rod-shaped virions of okaviruses highlighting the positioning of the p20 protein in the helical nucleocapsid and the gp116 and gp64 surface glycoproteins forming the envelope protrusions. Reproduced with permission from reference 100a.

similar to the bent and spherical torovirus particles (122). The internal nucleocapsid is a tightly coiled structure with a diameter of ~25 nm and a 5- to 7-nm helical periodicity. In infected cells, unassembled nucleocapsids, which appear slightly smaller in diameter (14 to 18 nm), can vary substantially in length, from ~80 nm to over 800 nm (Fig. 1) (12, 106). Nucleocapsids bud at endoplasmic reticulum/Golgi membranes into cytoplasmic vesicles that often contain densely packed or paracrystalline arrays of mature enveloped virions. Less frequently, virions also appear to bud at the plasma membrane (5) or nuclear envelope (12). Release of mature virions into intercellular space appears to occur primarily by the fusion of vesicles with the plasma membrane. Budding of elongated nucleocapsids can generate similarly elongated assemblages of mature virions butted end to end, which subsequently appear to fragment into discrete units (12, 14, 106, 120, 126). The mechanism by which multiple nucleocapsids become tethered without apparent demarcation of their ends is not known. However, the seamless nature of the elongated nucleocapsids suggests that they are assembled at the time of genomic RNA replication and nucleocapsid protein (N protein) coating.

As shown in the schematic diagram in Fig. 3, okavirus particles are comprised of two envelope glycoproteins, gp116 and gp64, and a p20 structural N protein that associates with the genomic RNA to form the helical viral nucleocapsids (51, 74, 121).

## GENOME ORGANIZATION

### Genome Size and Structure

Complete nucleotide sequences have been determined for the plus-strand single-stranded RNA (ssRNA) genomes of GAV (26,235 nucleotides [nt])

and YHV (26,662 nt) (14, 16, 20, 51, 91, 92; N. Sittidilokratna, personal communication). As shown in Fig. 4, the GAV genome contains five long ORFs arranged in the order 5'-ORF1a/ORF1b-ORF2-ORF3-ORF4-3' and is polyadenylated at the 3' terminus (20). The YHV genome has a similar organization, but the ORF4 gene of GAV (corresponding to 83 aa) is severely truncated (22 aa) due to a nucleotide insertion near the 5' end of the gene (26; N. Sittidilokratna, personal communication). The ORF4 genes of three other known genotypic variants in the YHV complex are also truncated by a nucleotide deletion in the same codon that introduces a premature stop codon resulting in ORF4 polypeptides 37 aa in length (P. M. Wijegoonawardane, personal communication).

### Ribosomal Frameshift Element

As in all nidoviruses, the 5' two-thirds of the okavirus genome comprises two long overlapping ORFs (ORF1a and ORF1b) that encode the replicase, the complex of nonstructural proteins utilized in viral replication (16, 91). ORF1b is expressed via the use of a −1 ribosomal frameshift that extends translation of ORF1a. The frameshift is mediated by a "slippery" heptanucleotide sequence (5'-AAAUUUU-3') and RNA pseudoknot structure existent in the overlap region (Fig. 4) (16, 91). A slippery sequence with this motif and accompanying complex pseudoknot structure is known to facilitate −1 ribosomal frameshifting at the *gag/pol* gene junction in some retroviruses (7, 50; see also chapter 3). However, coronaviruses, toroviruses, and arteriviruses employ a different slippery (G/UUUAAAC) motif and generally use H-type RNA pseudoknot structures that are more compact in sequence utilization than that used by okaviruses (6, 7, 22, 60, 96, 111).

In GAV, ORF1a translation generates an ~460-kDa polyprotein (pp1a). Functional analysis of the ORF1a/1b overlap sequence has identified −1 slippage at the $F^{4051}$ codon of the AAAUUUU slippery sequence that results in read-through sequence ORF1a-EANFSDK-ORF1b in the full-length ~758-kDa pp1ab polyprotein (16, 91). The efficiency (~24%) of the frameshift element determined using an in vitro translation system is comparable to that of coronavirus frameshift sites (7, 8, 16). Sequence comparison of GAV and YHV has shown the ORF1a/1b frameshift region to be highly conserved, with three of four nucleotide changes in predicted based-paired sequences being compensatory, presumably to retain structural requirements of the RNA pseudoknot critical for efficient translational slippage (26).

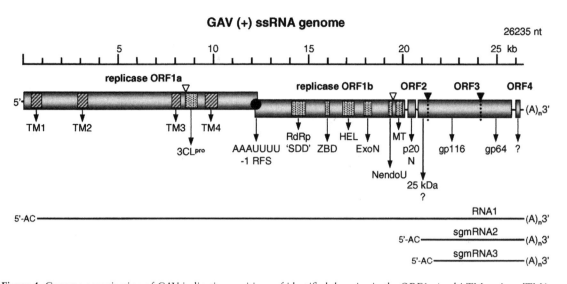

**Figure 4.** Genome organization of GAV indicating positions of identified domains in the ORF1a (multi-TM regions [TM1 to 4] and 3CL$^{pro}$) and ORF1b (SDD RdRp, zinc-binding domain [ZBD], helicase [HEL], 3'-to-5' exonuclease [ExoN], uridylate-specific endoribonuclease [NendoU], and C-terminal ribose-2'-O-methyltransferase [MT]) regions of the pp1a and pp1ab replicase polyproteins. Also indicated is the position of the AAAUUUU slippery sequence (•) of the −1 ribosomal frameshift site (RFS), the positions of the two identified 3CL$^{pro}$ cleavage sites (▽) in the pp1ab replicase polyprotein, and the positions of the two signal peptidase type 1-like cleavage sites (▼) used in the posttranslational release of the virion TM glycoproteins gp116 and gp64 from the ORF3 precursor protein. The start positions of the capped, non-leader-containing and 3'-polyade-nylated genomic RNA1 and two sg mRNAs (sg mRNA2 and -3) that initiate directly at TREs in the ORF1ab-ORF2 and ORF2-ORF3 IGRs are also shown. The YHV genome organization is similar to that of GAV except that ORF4 is severely truncated.

## Arrangement of the Structural Protein Genes

Other distinguishing features of okavirus genome organization are the number, order, and structure of genes encoding the structural proteins (Fig. 4). Oka-viruses contain only two structural protein genes. The ORF2 gene encodes the N protein (p20), and ORF3 encodes the two virion envelope glycoproteins (gp116 and gp64). The location of the N protein gene upstream of the glycoprotein gene is unique among nidoviruses, in which the N protein gene usually resides at a site near the 3' end of the genome (14, 41, 92). The okavirus ORF3 gene is also unique in that it encodes a polyprotein from which the two structural glycoproteins are released by posttranslational enzy-matic cleavage (20, 51) (Fig. 5). Proteolytic cleavage of ORF3 is also predicted to generate a small triple-membrane-spanning protein that is similar in size and structure to the integral membrane proteins (M and 3a proteins) of other nidoviruses. However, the nido-virus M and 3a proteins are encoded in discrete cis-trons, are structural components of the virion, and have a membrane topology in which the N terminus is external. The okavirus M-like protein is not a major component of virions and is predicted to have a mem-brane topology in which the C terminus is external (20, 51).

## MECHANISM OF SUBGENOMIC RNA (sgRNA) SYNTHESIS

Transcription of a 3'-coterminal nested set of sg mRNAs is a prerequisite for classification within the order *Nidovirales* (102). In GAV, Northern hybridization analysis has detected a genome-length RNA (RNA1) using ORF1a and -1b probes, RNA1 and an ~6-kb sg mRNA2 using probes within ORF2, and these two RNAs as well as an ~5.5-kb sg mRNA3 using probes within ORF3 and ORF4 (17). Primer extension and 5'-rapid amplification of cDNA ends (RACE) have also shown that RNA1,

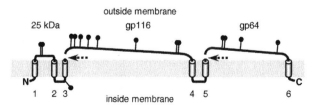

**Figure 5.** Schematic representation of the GAV ORF3 polyprotein membrane orientation indicating the relative positions of the six predicted TM domains, the 15 potential N-linked glycosylation sites (•), and the signal peptidase type 1 cleavage sites immediately preceding TM domains 3 and 5 used to generate the mature enve-lope glycoproteins gp116 and gp64.

sg mRNA2, and sg mRNA3 each possess 5′ ends initiating with AC dinucleotides (Fig. 4) (17). The 5′-terminal sg mRNA2 and -3 map to central regions of an identical 18-nt sequence in the 93-nt ORF1ab-ORF2 and 57-nt ORF2-ORF3 IGRs, respectively (17), which is also preserved in the corresponding YHV IGRs (26). Moreover, 5′-RACE has confirmed that, as in vertebrate nidoviruses, the 5′-AC termini of the GAV genomic RNA and sg mRNAs contain 7-methylguanosine triphosphate (m$^7$Gppp) caps (26). It appears likely that the conserved sequences in the IGRs of okaviruses function in a fashion similar to that of the transcription-regulating elements (TREs) used by toroviruses to transcribe non-leader-containing sg mRNAs (100, 114; see also chapter 9).

In both GAV and YHV, sequences in the region between ORF3 and ORF4 share a high level of homology with the highly conserved TREs in the ORF1ab-ORF2 and ORF2-ORF3 IGRs (20, 26). However, no corresponding sg mRNA is transcribed in abundance (17), and it has been suggested that an a A→G transition in this sequence at the position corresponding to the 5′ termini of sg mRNA2 and sg mRNA3 may render it ineffective as a TRE. In YHV and other genotypes in the complex, ORF4 is interrupted by insertions or deletions and expression of functional products from this region is highly unlikely. Nevertheless, in GAV, low-abundance sg mRNAs initiating at alternative sequences in the ORF3-ORF4 IGR have been detected using an m$^7$Gppp cap-dependent 5′-RACE method, and immunohistochemical analysis using a synthetic peptide antiserum suggests that an ORF4-encoded polypeptide might be expressed in infected cells at extremely low levels (Cowley et al., unpublished). The mechanisms by which nidovirus genomes have evolved to increasing complexity are yet to be resolved, but it is clear that, whether through loss or acquisition of function, this region of the okavirus genome is in the process of significant evolutionary development.

In GAV and YHV, ORF1a appears to commence at the first AUG codon, residing 68 to 71 nt downstream of the genome 5′ terminus, which occurs in a context favorable for translation initiation (16, 26, 58). Alignment of the YHV and GAV sequences indicates that there are 11 nucleotide substitutions in this 5′ untranslated region but the terminal 19 nt are identical. The preservation of this sequence may reflect a crucial role of the complementary sequence (i.e., the 3′ end of the full-length minus-strand RNA) in polymerase recognition and initiation of plus-strand synthesis. However, as only the 5′-terminal AC dinucleotide is shared between the genomic RNA and the sg mRNAs, the 3′-terminal UG dinucleotide might be sufficient to mediate recognition and transcription initiation by the polymerase. Moreover, the absence of a TRE-like

sequence in the 5′ untranslated region of genomic RNA may reflect the nonrequirement for signals to terminate minus-strand RNA synthesis.

No data are yet available on okavirus minus-strand RNA synthesis. However, double-stranded RNAs (dsRNAs) equivalent in length to the genomic RNA and two sg mRNAs of GAV have been identified in infected cells (17), and as in other nidoviruses, these appear to represent replicative intermediates (79, 88). It is plausible that the okavirus TRE sequences in the ORF1ab-ORF2 and ORF2-ORF3 IGRs act directly in attenuating minus-strand sgRNA synthesis at GU-3′ and/or initiating sg mRNA synthesis from this site to form these dsRNAs, without the need for acquisition of sequence derived from the genomic RNA 5′ terminus as occurs with coronaviruses and arteriviruses (79, 88; see also chapter 8).

In terms of the mechanism, an okavirus-like transcription strategy appears to be employed to produce all but the largest of the torovirus sg mRNAs (100, 114; see also chapter 9). However, while the TREs present in the torovirus IGRs are also highly conserved, and like in okaviruses direct the synthesis of sg mRNAs with 5′-AC dinucleotide termini (100, 114), no similarity between okaviruses and toroviruses exists in the TRE sequences surrounding the central AC dinucleotide. The development of a reverse-genetics system to rescue modified synthetic genomes, which in recent years has facilitated the detailed analysis of the transcriptional mechanisms used by arteriviruses and coronaviruses (see chapters 4 to 8), would greatly expedite exploration of the molecular mechanisms governing okavirus replication and transcription. However, such technology awaits establishment of a continuous cell line from shrimp or another crustacean that supports the replication of okaviruses.

## THE REPLICASE

GAV pp1a contains four hydrophobic regions that are predicted to form multiple transmembrane (TM) domains (Fig. 4) (15). A 3C-like cysteine proteinase (3CL$^{pro}$) motif sits between the two most C-terminal hydrophobic regions (15, 128). Apart from this motif, no other functional domains identified in the pp1a sequences of vertebrate nidoviruses have been identified in GAV (15, 41). However, in the ORF1b region of the replicase, functional motifs distantly related and all identified in the cognate proteins of coronaviruses, toroviruses, and arteriviruses are preserved in GAV and YHV (Fig. 4) (15, 39, 41, 91). The first of these domains is the the RNA-dependent RNA polymerase (RdRp). The okavirus RdRp contains all of the eight nidovirus active-site signature domains, including the catalytic SDD motif which characteristically distinguishes nidoviruses from all other plus-strand ssRNA viruses, which use the GDD motif (40, 53, 57). The downstream multinuclear zinc-binding domain (ZBD) comprises three blocks of four Cys/His residues with spacings and surrounding aromatic residues characteristic of TFIIIA-like zinc finger motifs (6, 22, 43). Further downstream is a helicase domain containing the characteristic NTP-binding motifs A (GppGtGKT) and B (DE) essential to dsRNA duplex unwinding during RNA synthesis (42, 89). Sequence alignments of the region downstream of the helicase indicate that the okavirus pp1ab also possesses 3′-to-5′ exonuclease (41, 95), uridylate-specific endoribonuclease (4, 49, 81, 95, 96) and C-terminal ribose-2′-O-methyltransferase (2′-O-MT) motifs (31, 95, 115), which, in coronaviruses, have been shown to be essential to RNA synthesis and progeny virus production (41).

Of the okavirus replicase motifs, only 3CL$^{pro}$ has been examined functionally (128). GAV 3CL$^{pro}$ displays greater sequence similarities to the NIa 3CL$^{pro}$ enzyme of tobacco etch virus and other plant potyviruses than to coronavirus 3CL$^{pro}$s (16, 128). As in coronaviruses, GAV 3CL$^{pro}$ is organized into three domains. However, while the motif containing the catalytic His$^{2879}$ residue is most similar to that of coronaviruses, the motif containing the catalytic Cys$^{2968}$ and the substrate-binding region is more closely related to those of potyviruses (128). GAV 3CL$^{pro}$ also shares with potyviruses several key residues (Thr$^{2963}$, His$^{2959}$, Ile$^{2961}$, and Gly$^{2981}$) which have roles in defining the NIa proteinase substrate binding pocket. These residues do not occur in coronavirus 3CL$^{pro}$, suggesting that the GAV proteinase has a substrate specificity (VAHQ↓S) more closely resembling that of the potyvirus enzyme (28, 54, 76).

Functional analysis of recombinant GAV 3CL$^{pro}$ expressed in *Escherichia coli* has shown that it cleaves autocatalytically in *cis* at the upstream $^{2827}$LVTHE ↓ VRTGN$^{2836}$ motif and in *trans* at the $^{6441}$KVNHE ↓ LYHVA$^{6450}$ motif in C-terminal region of the ORF1b product (128). Based on these data, a consensus cleavage motif, VxHE ↓ (L, V), has been proposed (128). However, scanning for potential pp1ab cleavage sites corresponding to those identified in vertebrate nidoviruses has indicated that GAV 3CL$^{pro}$ is also likely to function when T/S residues are in the P4 position and I/G/S/A residues are in position P1′ (128).

GAV 3CL$^{pro}$ appears to be unique among viral 3C-like proteinases in that its Cys-His catalytic core is combined with a canonical substrate binding pocket resembling that used by plant potyvirus NIa 3CL$^{pro}$s, rather than a noncanonical substrate pocket like that of coronavirus 3CL$^{pro}$s (128). These features of GAV 3CL$^{pro}$ link the evolution of proteinases in coronaviruses and potyviruses and provide insights into the evolutionary pathways that have led to differentiated structure and function in divergent plus-strand ssRNA viruses (128).

## STRUCTURAL PROTEINS

YHV particles contain three structural proteins. They are present in virions in relatively equal abundance and designated gp116, gp64, and p20 based on their glycosylation status and mass estimated by sodium dodecyl sulfate-polyacrylamide gel electrophoresis (51, 74, 90, 121). A larger protein (molecular mass, 170 kDa) reported in earlier studies (74) is likely to be a copurified host protein. Although initial work using sodium metaperiodate indicated only gp116 to be glycosylated (74), subsequent analyses using this and a thymol-staining method have clearly shown evidence of glycosylation for both gp116 and gp64 (51). This is consistent with the presence of multiple N-linked and O-linked glycosylation sites in the deduced amino acid sequence of each protein (20, 51).

### N Protein

Binding of a YHV monoclonal antibody (MAb) specific to the p20 protein (90) to free and virion encapsidated nucleocapsids provided tentative evidence that it was the viral N protein (101). This YHV MAb also cross-detected GAV-infected shrimp tissues, indicating that its epitope was conserved in the equivalent GAV protein (9). For GAV, antiserum to a synthetic peptide (T$^{97}$ to I$^{115}$) designed to an ORF2 gene coding sequence bound to nucleocapsids. Binding occurred preferentially at their ends or at internal regions exposed through lateral and transverse sectioning, indicating that the reactive epitope was embedded in rather than exposed on the nucleocapsid surface (14). As this antiserum also bound to GAV and YHV p20 protein, this conclusively showed the ORF2 gene to encode the okavirus N protein (14). As mentioned earlier, this structural gene arrangement differentiates the invertebrate okaviruses from all vertebrate nidoviruses, in which the N protein gene is positioned near the genome 3′-terminus downstream of genes encoding the other virion proteins.

The ORF2 genes of GAV and YHV encode N proteins that are 144 aa (15,998 Da) and 146 aa (16,326 Da) in length, respectively, and share 84% identity. They are highly basic proteins (pI = 9.75 to 9.90) that contain a high number (16.4 to 19.4%) of proline and glycine residues, suggesting a folded structure with many angular turns (14, 92).

The C-terminal halves of the okavirus N proteins also share four predicted phosphorylation sites, but it has yet to be determined whether any of these sites are utilized. Differences between the deduced molecular mass of the GAV and YHV ORF2 polypeptides and the size estimated by sodium dodecyl sulfate-polyacrylamide gel electrophoresis (molecular mass, 20 to 22 kDa) (14, 51, 74, 121) have been traced to a highly acidic C-terminal 9-aa sequence that retards N protein migration in gels (92).

Antigenic mapping of the YHV N protein indicates that linear epitopes reacting with polyclonal YHV antiserum are primarily located in the N-terminal ($M^1$ to $A^{36}$) and C-terminal regions ($Q^{74}$ to $X^{146}$). The study has also identified a highly antigenic linear site ($I^{116}$ to $E^{137}$) near the C-terminus that includes type-specific and cross-reactive epitopes (92). Similar analysis of recombinant GAV N proteins has supported the existence of highly antigenic linear epitopes in the near C-terminal region (14). There is also evidence that smaller forms of the native protein (molecular mass, ~17 kDa) detected in diseased shrimp tissue, and of recombinant N proteins expressed in *E. coli*, result from enzymatic degradation at a trypsin-sensitive ($KR^{109}$) motif (14). A KR motif exists in a comparable position in the torovirus N protein (29, 59, 97), and enzymatic degradation has been proposed as the source of two smaller N protein forms detected in cells infected with equine torovirus (47). While there is evidence that the smaller torovirus N proteins might arise from internal initiation of translation (97), the available data suggest that the smaller forms of the GAV N protein are generated by enzymatic cleavage (14).

### Envelope Glycoproteins

The two YHV TM glycoproteins (gp116 and gp64) appear to form the spikes visible on the surface of virions. The surface location of gp116 has been confirmed by immunoelectron microscopy (101). Although gp64 has also been assumed to protrude from the virion envelope, a gp64-specific MAb (Y18) does not bind to virions (101) and there is no direct evidence of its structural location. The mature envelope glycoproteins are generated by posttranslational cleavage of a polyprotein encoded in ORF3 in which the sequences of GAV (1,640 aa = 182 kDa) and YHV (1,666 aa = 186 kDa) possess six hydrophobic regions predicted to represent TM domains (20, 51). The third and fifth of the TM domains act as internal signal sequences to release gp116 and gp64, respectively (Fig. 5). Analysis of N-terminal amino acid sequences has indicated that gp116 is cleaved following TM domain 3 at the motif $AFA^{228}\downarrow$

and gp64 is cleaved following TM domain 5 at the motif $ASA^{1127}\downarrow$ (51). These sequences conform to the consensus Ala-X-Ala motif recognized by type 1 signal peptidases (10) and are conserved in the GAV ORF3 polypeptide (20). YHV gp116 contains seven potential N glycosylation sites (eight sites in GAV) and, based on predicted membrane topology, anchoring at its two C-terminal TM domains results in its C terminus also being exposed on the membrane surface. In YHV and GAV, gp64 has four potential N glycosylation sites and is a type 1 glycoprotein with a single C-terminal TM anchor.

The function and ultimate fate of the N-terminal ~25-kDa protein generated by cleavage of the precursor ORF3 polyprotein downstream of TM domain 3 are not yet known. In GAV, the predicted ectodomain between TM domains 1 and 2 possesses two potential N-linked glycosylation sites, one of which is conserved in YHV, and in each virus there are four conserved cysteine residues capable of forming disulfide bridges (20, 51). The predicted cleavage product contains three TM domains and is similar in size to the integral triple-membrane-spanning M proteins of coronaviruses (85), toroviruses (23, 99), and arteriviruses (24, 30). However, the predicted surface topology places the N terminus externally and C terminus internally, which is the reverse orientation to the nidovirus M proteins. Unlike the nidovirus M proteins, the okavirus triple-membrane-spanning protein is not a major structural component of virions and has not yet been identified in infected cells.

### THE OKAVIRUS CELL RECEPTOR

A virus overlay protein binding assay (VOPBA) using membrane proteins prepared from LO cells has recently been used to identify an ~65-kDa protein that is the putative cell receptor for YHV (3). Not surprisingly, the protein was detected in immunoblots of LO cell extracts using antiserum prepared to the VOPBA gel region. Preexposure of LO cells to this antiserum (1:2 dilution) reduced the YHV titer in culture medium by ~80% compared to naïve serum, which was taken as evidence of competitive exclusion of viral attachment to the receptor (3). Sequence analysis of a clone amplified following N-terminal amino acid sequencing of the 65-kDa protein identified a 512-aa sequence corresponding to an ORF (3). The C-terminal 117-aa portion possessed significant similarity to the L22 ribosomal protein consensus sequence (72), and the N-terminal 395-aa portion contained numerous perfect and imperfect repeated sequences, including six AAKGDAKPKA and two AAKPKPAKAEG motifs with no homologues identifiable in databases (3). The fusion of this unusual N-terminal extension to an L22 ribosomal protein sequence, and the presence of a K→Q shift in the KKYLQK$^{476}$ nucleolar localization-like sequence of the L22 domain (11), seemingly results in its trafficking to the plasma membrane rather than to the nucleolus, where it would normally function as an integral component of ribosomes. The 65-kDa protein appears to be expressed in a diverse range of tissues susceptible to YHV infection (3). Moreover, dsRNA corresponding to the identified coding sequence has been shown to markedly reduce expression levels in LO cells and YHV RNA levels detected following virus challenge. While this supports a role for protein in the intracellular transmission of YHV, it remains to be demonstrated that the C-terminal L22 ribosomal protein chimera is exposed on the cell plasma membrane and, if so, whether it indeed functions directly as the YHV cell surface receptor or indirectly via coassociation with heparin sulfate or glycosaminoglycans (3).

## INHIBITION OF YHV REPLICATION BY dsRNA

RNA interference (RNAi) is a dsRNA-induced gene silencing mechanism that is known to mediate antiviral responses in several terrestrial invertebrates, vertebrates, and plants (27, 48). In marine shrimp, dsRNA has been shown to induce silencing of homologous endogenous genes and to induce both nonspecific "innate" and sequence-specific inhibition of viral infection (83, 84). Synthetic dsRNAs corresponding to regions in the 3CL$^{pro}$, RdRp, and helicase domains of the YHV replicase gene have been shown to abrogate cytopathology and substantially reduce viral RNA and gp116 levels in YHV-infected LO cells (112). YHV replication is also inhibited with lower efficiency by dsRNAs targeted to sequences in the gp64 and gp116 coding regions of ORF3. RNAi-mediated inhibition of YHV replication has also been shown to occur in juvenile shrimp following tail muscle injection of a 3CL$^{pro}$-specific dsRNA (127). The dsRNA treatment completely abrogated mortalities following lethal YHV challenge, and the inhibitory effect was sustained for up to 5 days. Both in LO cell culture and in shrimp treated in vivo, the sequence-specific inhibitory effects of dsRNA are dose dependent (112, 127).

The identification of genes encoding Argonaute-1 (113) and the RNase III-like Dicer-1 protein (J. Su et al., unpublished data), and evidence that knockdown of Dicer-1 expression inhibits the sequence-specific antiviral effects of dsRNA (Su et al., unpublished), indicates that RNAi is active as an antiviral defense in shrimp. Nonspecific inhibition of infection with YHV and other shrimp viruses has also been observed following treatment with unrelated dsRNAs, poly(G·C) or small interfering RNAs (84, 112, 123, 127). This suggests that shrimp also possess an inducible innate antiviral pathway analogous to the Toll-like receptor 3-mediated pathway in mammals that results in the elimination of infected cells by apoptotic processes (55). There is no evidence of interferon or components of the vertebrate interferon pathway in shrimp or other invertebrates (82). Apoptosis has been reported for cells infected with okaviruses (56), but it is not yet known if apoptosis occurs in response to viral dsRNAs that accumulate during replication. Shrimp provide a useful model for the study of the response of invertebrates to virus infection, which remains largely uncharacterized. Moreover, it might be fruitful to examine whether okaviruses deploy strategies to evade RNAi and other host responses akin to those identified in several insect and vertebrate viruses (52, 61, 107, 108).

## TAXONOMY

The helical tubular nucleocapsids and rod-shaped enveloped virions of GAV and YHV detected in Australian and Thai *P. monodon* are morphologically indistinguishable (5, 12, 103, 106). Initial analyses of the YHV genome showed it to comprise a very long (at least 22-kb) ssRNA (126), and sequence comparisons with GAV showed the two viruses to be distinct genotypes or topotypes (18, 109, 125). Relative to a continuous ORF identified in a portion of the YHV genome amplified by PCR, the differential amplification of cDNA synthesized in either orientation from virion RNA indicated that it possessed mRNA (positive) polarity (109). Subsequent sequence determination of the 5'-terminal 20-kb region of the GAV genomic RNA identified a structural and functional organization that indisputably indicated a distant evolutionary relationship to vertebrate nidoviruses (16), rather than to rhabdoviruses as speculated earlier based on general particle resemblances, structural protein content, and flawed data on genomic RNA polarity (74).

Due to their origin from a marine invertebrate, rod-shaped virion architecture (5, 12, 103, 106), unique structural proteins (51, 74), distinct genome organizational features and distant phylogenetic relationships in pp1ab replicase domains (14, 16, 20, 38, 41, 91), and non-leader-requiring transcription strategy (17), it became apparent that GAV and YHV could not be accommodated in either of the established families, *Coronaviridae* and *Arteriviridae*, classified within the order *Nidovirales* (73, 102). The genus name *Okavirus* was proposed for the viruses (16), as the primary site of virus replication is the LO, which in Asian countries is commonly referred to as the Oka organ, in recognition of its structural and functional description in the late 1960s by the Japanese scientist M. Oka in his landmark studies on shrimp anatomy and physiology (77). *Roniviridae* (rod-shaped nidovirus) was subsequently accepted by the International Committee on Taxonomy of Viruses as a suitable family name (73, 117) in recognition of the strikingly different morphology of okavirus particles compared to the virion structures of coronaviruses, toroviruses, and arteriviruses (102).

## NIDOVIRUS EVOLUTIONARY CONSIDERATIONS LEARNED FROM OKAVIRUSES

It has been suggested that nidovirus genomes have evolved by modular evolution involving the exchange of complete genes or sets of genes (22, 41, 98). Gene or gene block transitions in ancestral nidoviruses may have led to differences in the gene number and ordering. Moreover, in vertebrate nidoviruses, the 3'-coterminal sg mRNAs are generally produced in decreasing abundance inversely related to their length. Thus, in the more complex vertebrate nidovirus genomes that transcribe four or more sg mRNAs, location of the N protein gene at a 3'-proximal site provides for high-level expression of a short sg mRNA. This allows abundant expression of the N protein, as is required for efficient nucleocapsid and virion assembly. In okaviruses, however, the two sg mRNAs are similar in size and transcribed in relatively similar abundances (17). Therefore, the N protein encoded in ORF2 in the slightly longer sg mRNA2 and the two envelope glycoproteins (gp116 and gp64) encoded in ORF3 are expressed in similar abundances from the two sg mRNAs. This simple transcription strategy may well eliminate the need for a 3'-proximal location of the N protein gene.

The transcription strategy of okaviruses that generates 3'-coterminal sg mRNAs without the acquisition of a 5' genomic leader sequence (16, 17) is also novel and of some interest to nidovirologists unraveling the complex discontinuous RNA transcription mechanism used by coronaviruses and arteriviruses (79, 87, 88). This okavirus strategy is similar to that of equine torovirus, for which sg mRNAs also possess common 5' AC termini that map to conserved intergenic sequences rather than 5' genomic leader sequences (99, 100). Interestingly, in equine torovirus a 5' genomic leader sequence was identified, but only

in the longest of the four sg mRNAs (114). Based on this finding, it has been hypothesized that toroviruses may be in evolutionary transition, employing alternative transcriptional strategies to facilitate efficient synthesis of all the sg mRNAs (79, 114). The okavirus genome organization and transcription strategy are the least complex among nidoviruses and utilize only two sg mRNAs. The torovirus genome has greater complexity, necessitating transcription of two additional sg mRNAs (100, 114), while in coronaviruses and arteriviruses the genome organization is more complex, requiring transcription of between five and nine sg mRNAs (25, 41, 79). It is possible that the simpler non-leader RNA transcription strategy was adopted early in nidovirus evolution, when genome complexity was low. With increased genome complexity to accommodate efficient replication in new hosts, the leader-dependent mechanism may have evolved to provide for efficient transcription of four or more genes. The establishment of reverse-genetics systems for okaviruses and/or toroviruses to allow the rescue of synthetic genomes should allow exploration of the fitness of recombinant viruses into which additional gene elements have been introduced.

Okaviruses have a high natural prevalence in disparate populations of the black tiger shrimp, *P. monodon*, and commonly exist as lifelong inapparent infections that may be transmitted vertically (15, 19, 106, 119). *P. monodon* appears, therefore, to be the primary natural host of okaviruses, and there is some genetic evidence to suggest that the evolution of individual genotypes has occurred over a geological time scale. Fossil records date penaeid shrimp species to the late Cretaceous period (32), and more primitive crustaceans have been dated to the Precambrian period, over 550 million years ago (93). Crustaceans are therefore ancient life forms that significantly predate the emergence of terrestrial vertebrates, and indeed the terrestrial arthropods, during the late Devonian period (~350 million years ago). Penaeid shrimp, in particular, appear to be well-adapted survivors that have changed little over a vast time span. It can be speculated, therefore, that okaviruses might be relatively primitive nidoviruses that have evolved slowly in a relatively stable biological environment and can be considered more ancient than their vertebrate nidovirus cousins. This appears to be reflected in their simpler genome organization (14, 16, 20, 51, 91) and less complex transcription strategy (17). It is also consistent with the extent of sequence divergence from other nidoviruses in the N-terminal ~2,000 aa of the replicase (16, 41) and phylogenetic distances determined for the polymerase, helicase, and other functional replicase motifs (16, 41, 44), including the 3C-like proteinase (128).

## REFERENCES

1. Anggraeni, M. S., and L. Owens. 2000. The haemocytic origin of lymphoid organ spheroid cells in the penaeid prawn *Penaeus monodon. Dis. Aquat. Org.* 40:85–92.

2. Assavalapsakul, W., D. R. Smith, and S. Panyim. 2003. Propagation of infectious yellow head virus particles prior to cytopathic effect in primary lymphoid cell cultures of *Penaeus monodon. Dis. Aquat. Org.* 55:253–258.

3. Assavalapsakul, W., D. R. Smith, and S. Panyim. 2006. Identification and characterisation of a *Penaeus monodon* lymphoid cell-expressed receptor for yellow head virus. *J. Virol.* 80:262–269.

4. Bhardwaj, K., L. Guarino, and C. C. Kao. 2004. The severe acute respiratory syndrome coronavirus Nsp15 protein is an endoribonuclease that prefers manganese as a cofactor. *J. Virol.* 78:12218–12224.

5. Boonyaratpalin, S., K. Supamattaya, J. Kasornchandra, S. Direkbusaracom, U. Ekpanithanpong, and C. Chantanachooklin. 1993. Non-occluded baculo-like virus, the causative agent of yellow head disease in the black tiger shrimp *(Penaeus monodon). Fish Pathol.* 28:103–109.

6. Bredenbeek, P. J., C. J. Pachuk, A. F. Noten, J. Charite, W. Luytjes, S. R. Weiss, and W. J. M. Spaan. 1990. The primary structure and expression of the second open reading frame of the polymerase gene of the coronavirus MHV-A59; a highly conserved polymerase is expressed by an efficient ribosomal frameshifting mechanism. *Nucleic Acids Res.* 18:1825–1832.

7. Brierley, I., P. Digard, and C. C. Inglis. 1989. Characterization of an efficient coronavirus ribosomal frameshifting signal: requirement for an RNA pseudoknot. *Cell* 57:537–547.

8. Brierley, I., A. J. Jenner, and S. C. Inglis. 1992. Mutational analysis of the "slippery-sequence" component of a coronavirus ribosomal frameshifting signal. *J. Mol. Biol.* 227:463–479.

9. Callinan, R. B., L. Jiang, P. T. Smith, and C. Soowannayan. 2003. Fatal, virus-associated peripheral neuropathy and retinopathy in farmed *Penaeus monodon* in eastern Australia. I. Pathology. *Dis. Aquat. Org.* 53:181–193.

10. Carlos, J. L., M. Paetzel, G. Brubaker, A. Karla, C. M. Ashwell, M. O. Lively, G. Cao, P. Bullinger, and R. E. Dalbey. 2000. The role of the membrane-spanning domain of type I signal peptidases in substrate cleavage site selection. *J. Biol. Chem.* 275:38813–38822.

11. Chang, S.-N., C-H. Lin, and A. Lin. 2000. An acidic amino acid cluster regulates the nucleolar localization and ribosome assembly of human ribosomal protein L22. *FEBS Lett.* 484:22–28.

12. Chantanachookin, C., S. Boonyaratpalin, J. Kasornchandra, S. Direkbusarakom, U. Aekpanithanpong, K. Supamattaya, S. Sriuraitana, and T. W. Flegel. 1993. Histology and ultrastructure reveal a new granulosis-like virus in *Penaeus monodon* affected by yellow-head disease. *Dis. Aquat. Org.* 17:145–157.

13. Chen, S. N., and C. S. Wang. 1999. Establishment of cell culture systems from penaeid shrimp and their susceptibility to white spot disease and yellow head viruses. *Methods Cell Sci.* 21:199–206.

14. Cowley, J. A., L. C. Cadogan, K. M. Spann, N. Sittidilokratna, and P. J. Walker. 2004. The gene encoding the nucleocapsid protein of gill-associated nidovirus of *Penaeus monodon* prawns is located upstream of the glycoprotein gene. *J. Virol.* 78:8935–8941.

15. Cowley, J. A., C. M. Dimmock, K. M. Spann, and P. J. Walker. 2000. Detection of Australian gill-associated virus (GAV) and lymphoid organ virus (LOV) of *Penaeus monodon* by RT-nested PCR. *Dis. Aquat. Org.* 39:159–167.

16. Cowley, J. A., C. M. Dimmock, K. M. Spann, and P. J. Walker. 2000. Gill-associated virus of *Penaeus monodon* prawns: an invertebrate virus with ORF1a and ORF1b genes related to arteri- and coronaviruses. *J. Gen. Virol.* 81:1473–1484.

17. Cowley, J. A., C. M. Dimmock, and P. J. Walker. 2002. Gill-associated nidovirus of *Penaeus monodon* prawns transcribes 3'-coterminal subgenomic mRNAs that do not possess 5'-leader sequences. *J. Gen. Virol.* 83:927–935.

18. Cowley, J. A., C. M. Dimmock, C. Wongteerasupaya, V. Boonsaeng, S. Panyim, and P .J. Walker. 1999. Yellow head virus from Thailand and gill-associated virus from Australia are closely related but distinct prawn viruses. *Dis. Aquat. Org.* 36:153–157.

19. Cowley, J. A., M. R. Hall, L. C. Cadogan, K. M. Spann, and P. J. Walker. 2002. Vertical transmission of gill-associated virus (GAV) in the black tiger prawn *Penaeus monodon. Dis. Aquat. Org.* 50:95–104.

20. Cowley, J. A., and P. J. Walker. 2002. The complete genome sequence of gill-associated virus of *Penaeus monodon* prawns indicates a gene organisation unique among nidoviruses. *Arch. Virol.* 147:1977–1987.

21. de la Vega, E., B. M. Degnan, M. R. Hall, J. A. Cowley, and K. J. Wilson. 2004. Quantitative real-time RT-PCR demonstrates that handling stress can lead to rapid increases of gill-associated virus (GAV) infection levels in *Penaeus monodon. Dis. Aquat. Org.* 59:195–203.

22. den Boon, J. A., E. J. Snijder, E. D. Chirnside, A. A. F. De Vries, M. C. Horzinek, and W. J. M. Spaan. 1991. Equine arterivirus is not a togavirus but belongs to the coronavirus-like superfamily. *J. Virol.* 65:2910–2920.

23. den Boon, J. A., E. J. Snijder, J. K. Locker, M. C. Horzinek, and P. J. Rottier. 1991. Another triple-spanning envelope protein among intracellularly budding RNA viruses: the torovirus E protein. *Virology* 182:655–663.

24. de Vries, A. A. F., E. D. Chirnside, M. C. Horzinek, and P. J. Rottier. 1992. Structural proteins of equine arteritis virus. *J. Virol.* 66:6294–6303.

25. de Vries, A. A. F., M. C. Horzinek, P. J. M. Rottier, and R. J. De Groot. 1997. The genome organization of the *Nidovirales*: similarities and differences between arteri-, toro-, and coronaviruses. *Semin. Virol.* 8:33–47.

26. Dhar, A. K., J. A. Cowley, K. W. Hasson, and P. J. Walker. 2004. Genomic organization, biology, and diagnosis of Taura syndrome virus and yellowhead virus of penaeid shrimp. *Adv. Virus Res.* 63:353–421.

27. Dong, Y., and M. Friedrich. 2005. Nymphal RNAi: systemic RNAi mediated gene knockdown in juvenile grasshopper. *BMC Biotechnol.* 5:25.

28. Dougherty, W. G., J. C. Carrington, S. M. Cary, and T. D. Parks. 1988. Biochemical and mutational analysis of a plant virus polyprotein cleavage site. *EMBO J.* 7:1281–1287.

29. Duckmanton, L. M., R. Tellier, P. Liu, and M. Petric. 1998. Bovine torovirus: sequencing of the structural genes and expression of the nucleocapsid protein of Breda virus. *Virus Res.* 58:83–96.

30. Faaberg, K, S., and P. G. Plagemann. 1995. The envelope proteins of lactate dehydrogenase-elevating virus and their membrane topography. *Virology* 212:512–525.

31. Feder, M., J. Pas, L. S. Wyrwicz, and J. M. Bujnicki. 2003. Molecular phylogenetics of the RrmJ/fibrillarin superfamily of ribose 2'-O-methyltransferases. *Gene* 302:129–138.

32. Feldmann, R. M., and C. E. Schweitzer. 2006. Paleobiogeography of Southern Hemisphere decapod Crustacea. *J. Paleontol.* 80:83–103.

33. Flegel, T. W. 1997. Special topic review: major viral diseases of the black tiger prawn *(Penaeus monodon)* in Thailand. *World J. Microbiol. Biotechnol.* **13**:433–442.

34. Flegel, T. W., S. Boonyaratpalin, and B. Withyachumnarnkul. 1997. Progress in research on yellow-head virus and white-spot virus in Thailand, p. 285–296. *In* T. W. Flegel and I. H. MacRae (ed.), *Diseases in Asian Aquaculture III.* Fish Health Section, Asian Fisheries Society, Manila, the Philippines.

35. Flegel, T. W., D. F. Fegan, S. Kongsom, S. Vuthikornudomkit, S. Sriurairatana, S. Boonyaratpalin, C. Chantanachookin, J. E. Vickers, and O. D. McDonald. 1992. Occurrence, diagnosis and treatment of shrimp diseases in Thailand, p. 57–112. *In* W. Fulks and K. L. Main (ed.), *Disease of Cultured Penaeid Shrimp in Asia and the United States.* Oceanic Institute, Honolulu, HI.

36. Flegel, T. W., D. F. Fegan, and S. Sriurairatana. 1995. Environmental control of infectious shrimp diseases in Thailand, p. 65–79. *In* M. Shariff, R. P. Subasinghe, and J. R. Arthur (ed.), *Diseases in Asian Aquaculture II.* Asian Fisheries Society, Manila, the Philippines.

37. Flegel, T. W., S. Sriurairatana, C. Wongterrasupaya, V. Boonsaeng, S. Panyim, and B. Withyachumnarnkul. 1995. Progress in characterization and control of yellow-head virus of *Penaeus monodon*, p. 76–83. *In* C. L. Browdy and J. S. Hopkins (ed.), *Swimming through Troubled Water: Proceedings of the Special Session on Shrimp Farming, Aquaculture '95.* World Aquaculture Society, Baton Rouge, LA.

38. Gonzalez, J. M., P. Gomez-Puertas, D. Cavanagh, A. E. Gorbalenya, and L. Enjuanes. 2003. A comparative sequence analysis to revise the current taxonomy of the family Coronaviridae. *Arch. Virol.* **148**:2207–2235.

39. Gorbalenya, A. E. 2001. Big nidovirus genome: when count and order of domains matter. *Adv. Exp. Med. Biol.* **494**:1–17.

40. Gorbalenya, A. E., V. M. Blinov, A. P. Donchenko, and E. V. Koonin. 1989. An NTP-binding motif is the most conserved sequence in a highly diverged monophyletic group of proteins involved in positive strand RNA viral replication. *J. Mol. Evol.* **28**:256–268.

41. Gorbalenya, A. E., L. Enjuanes, J. Ziebuhr, and E. J. Snijder. 2006. Nidovirales: evolving the largest RNA virus genome. *Virus Res.* **117**:17–37.

42. Gorbalenya, A. E., and E. V. Koonin. 1989. Viral proteins containing the purine NTP-binding sequence pattern. *Nucleic Acids Res.* **17**:8413–8440.

43. Gorbalenya, A. E., E. V. Koonin, A. P. Donchenko, and V. M. Blinov. 1989. Coronavirus genome: prediction of putative functional domains in the non-structural polyprotein by comparative amino acid sequence analysis. *Nucleic Acids Res.* **17**:4847–4861.

44. Gorbalenya, A. E., F. M. Pringle, J. L. Zeddam, B. T. Luke, C. E. Cameron, J. Kalmakoff, T. N. Hanzlik, K. H. Gordon, and V. K. Ward. 2002. The palm subdomain-based active site is internally permuted in viral RNA-dependent RNA polymerases of an ancient lineage. *J. Mol. Biol.* **324**:47–62.

45. Hasson, K. W., D. V. Lightner, J. Mari, J. R. Bonami, B. T. Poulos, L. L. Mohoney, R. M. Redman, B. L. White, and J. A. Brock. 1999. Taura syndrome virus (TSV) lesion development and the disease cycle in the Pacific white shrimp *Penaeus vannamei. Dis. Aquat. Org.* **36**:81–93.

46. Hasson, K. W., D. V. Lightner, J. Mari, J. R. Bonami, B. T. Poulos, L. L. Mohoney, R. M. Redman, B. L. White, and J. A. Brock. 1999. The geographic distribution of Taura syndrome virus (TSV) in the Americas: determination by histopathology and *in situ* hybridization using TSV-specific cDNA probes. *Aquaculture* **171**:13–26.

47. Horzinek, M. C., J. Ederveen, and M. Weiss. 1985. The nucleocapsid of Berne virus. *J. Gen. Virol.* **66**:1287–1296.

48. Isobe, R., K. Kojima, T. Matsuyama, G. X. Quan, T. Kanda, T. Tamura, K. Sahara, S. I. Asano, and H. Bando. 2004. Use of RNAi technology to confer enhanced resistance to BmNPV on transgenic silkworms. *Arch. Virol.* **149**:1931–1940.

49. Ivanov, K. A., T. Hertzig, M. Rozanov, S. Bayer, V. Thiel, A. E. Gorbalenya, and J. Ziebuhr. 2004. Major genetic marker of nidoviruses encodes a replicative endoribonuclease. *Proc. Natl. Acad. Sci. USA* **101**:12694–12699.

50. Jacks, T., H. D. Madhani, F. R. Masiarz, and H. E. Varmus. 1988. Signals for ribosomal frameshifting in the Rous sarcoma virus *gag-pol* region. *Cell* **55**:447–458.

51. Jitrapakdee, S., S. Unajak, N. Sittidilokratna, R. A. J. Hodgson, J. A. Cowley, P. J. Walker, S. Panyim, and V. Boonsaeng. 2003. Identification and analysis of gp116 and gp64 structural glycoproteins of yellow head nidovirus of *Penaeus monodon* shrimp. *J. Gen. Virol.* **84**:863–873.

52. Johnson, K. L., B. D. Price, L. D. Eckerle, and L. A. Ball. 2004. Nodamura virus nonstructural protein B2 can enhance viral RNA accumulation in both mammalian and insect cells. *J. Virol.* **78**:6698–6704.

53. Kamer, G., and P. Argos. 1984. Primary structural comparison of RNA-dependent polymerases from plant, animal and bacterial viruses. *Nucleic Acids Res.* **12**:7269–7282

54. Kang, H., Y. J. Lee, J. H. Goo, and W. J. Park. 2001. Determination of the substrate specificity of turnip mosaic virus NIa protease using a genetic method. *J. Gen. Virol.* **82**:3115–3117.

55. Karpala, A. J., T. J. Doran, and A. G. Bean. 2005. Immune responses to dsRNA: implications for gene silencing technologies. *Immunol. Cell Biol.* **83**:211–216.

56. Khanobdee, K., C. Soowannayan, T. W. Flegel, S. Ubol, and B. Withyachumnarnkul. 2002. Evidence for apoptosis correlated with mortality in the giant black tiger shrimp *Penaeus monodon* infected with yellow head virus. *Dis. Aquat. Org.* **48**:79–90.

57. Koonin, E. V. 1991. The phylogeny of RNA-dependent RNA polymerases of positive-strand RNA viruses. *J. Gen. Virol.* **72**:2197–2206.

58. Kozak, M. 1986. Point mutations define a sequence flanking the AUG initiator codon that modulates translation by eukaryotic ribosomes. *Cell* **44**:283–292.

59. Kroneman, A., L. A. Cornelissen, M. C. Horzinek, R. J. de Groot, and H. F. Egberink. 1998. Identification and characterization of a porcine torovirus. *J. Virol.* **72**:3507–3511.

60. Lee, H.-J., C.-K. Shieh, A. E. Gorbalenya, E. V. Koonin, N. La Monica, J. Tuler, A. Bagzhadzhyan, and M. M. C. Lai. 1991. The complete sequence (22 kilobases) of murine coronavirus gene 1 encoding the putative proteases and RNA polymerase. *Virology* **180**:567–582.

61. Li, H., W. X. Li, and S. W. Ding. 2002. Induction and suppression of RNA silencing by an animal virus. *Science* **296**:1319–1321.

62. Lightner, D. V., K. W. Hasson, B. L. White, and R. M. Redman. 1998. Experimental infection of Western Hemisphere penaeid shrimp with Asian white spot syndrome virus and Asian yellow head virus. *J. Aquat. Anim. Health* **10**:271–281.

63. Lightner, D. V., R. M. Redman, B. T. Poulos, L. M. Nunan, J. L. Mari, and K. W. Hasson. 1997. Risk of spread of penaeid shrimp viruses in the Americas by the international movement of live and frozen shrimp. *Rev. Sci. Tech. Off. Int. Epizoot.* **16**:146–160.

64. Limsuwan, C. 1991. *Handbook for Cultivation of Black Tiger Prawns.* Tansetakit, Bangkok, Thailand. (In Thai.)

65. Loh, P. C., E. C. B. Nadalan, Jr., L. M. Tapay, and Y. Lu. 1998. Recent developments in immunologically-based and cell culture protocols for the specific detection of shrimp viral pathogens, p. 255–259. *In* T. W. Flegel (ed.), *Advances in Shrimp Biotechnology*. National Center for Genetic Engineering and Biotechnology, Bangkok, Thailand.

66. Longyant, S., S. Sattaman, P. Chaivisuthangkura, S. Rukpratanporn, W. Sithigorngul, and P. Sithigorngul. 2006. Experimental infection of some penaeid shrimps and crabs by yellow head virus (YHV). *Aquaculture* 257:83–91.

67. Longyant, S., P. Sithigorngul, P. Chaivisuthangkura, S. Rukpratanporn, W. Sithigorngul, and P. Menasveta. 2005. Differences in susceptibility of palaemonid shrimp species to yellow head virus (YHV) infection. *Dis. Aquat. Org.* 64:5–12.

68. Lu, Y., L. M. Tapay, J. A. Brock, and P. C. Loh. 1994. Infection of the yellow head baculo-like virus (YBV) in two species of penaeid shrimp *Penaeus stylirostris* (Stimpson) and *Penaeus vannamei* (Boone) *J. Fish Dis.* 17:649–656.

69. Lu, Y., L. M. Tapay, R. B. Gose, J. A. Brock, and P. C. Loh. 1997. Infectivity of yellow head virus (YHV) and the Chinese baculo-like virus (CBV) in two species of penaeid shrimp *Penaeus stylirostris* (Stimpson) and *Penaeus vannamei* (Boone), p. 297–304. *In* T. W. Flegel and I. H. MacRae (ed.), *Diseases in Asian Aquaculture III*. Asian Fisheries Society, Manila, the Philippines.

70. Lu, Y., L. M. Tapay, P. C. Loh, J. A. Brock, and R. B. Gose. 1995. Development of a quantal assay in primary shrimp cell culture for yellow head baculovirus (YBV) of penaeid shrimp. *J. Virol. Methods* 52:231–236.

71. Lu, Y., L. M. Tapay, P. C. Loh, J. A. Brock, and R. B. Gose. 1995. Distribution of yellow-head virus in selected tissues and organs of penaeid shrimp *Penaeus vannamei*. *Dis. Aquat. Org.* 23:67–70.

72. Marchler-Bauer, A., J. B. Anderson, P. F. Cherukuri, C. DeWeese-Scott, L. Y. Geer, M. Gwadz, S. He, D. I. Hurwitz, J. D. Jackson, Z. Ke, C. J. Lanczycki, C. A. Liebert, C. Liu, F. Lu, G. H. Marchler, M. Mullokandov, B. A. Shoemaker, V. Simonyan, J. S. Song, P. A. Thiessen, R. A. Yamashita, J. J. Yin, D. Zhang, and S. H. Bryant. 2005. CDD: a conserved domain database for protein classification. *Nucleic Acids Res.* 33:D192–D196.

73. Mayo, M. A. 2002. A summary of taxonomic changes approved by ICTV. *Arch. Virol.* 147:1655–1656.

74. Nadala, E. C. B., Jr., L. M. Tapay, and P. C. Loh. 1997. Yellow-head virus: a rhabdovirus-like pathogen of penaeid shrimp. *Dis. Aquat. Org.* 31:141–146.

75. Natividad, K., F. O. Magbanua, V. P. Migo, C. G. Alfafara, J. D. Albaladejo, E. C. B. Nadala, Jr., P. C. Loh, and L. M. Tapay. 1999. Evidence of yellow head virus in cultured black tiger shrimp (*Penaeus monodon* Fabricius) from selected shrimp farms in the Philippines, p. 6. *In Book of Abstracts, Fourth Symposium on Diseases in Asian Aquaculture, Cebu City, Philippines, Nov. 1999.*

76. Nicolas, O., and J.-F. Laliberté. 1992. The complete nucleotide sequence of turnip mosaic potyvirus RNA. *J. Gen. Virol.* 73:2785–2793.

77. Oka, M. 1969. Studies on *Penaeus orientalis* Kishinouye. VIII. Structure of newly found lymphoid organ. *Bull. Jpn. Soc. Sci. Fish.* 35:245–250.

78. Pasharawipas, T., T. W. Flegel, S. Sriurairatana, and D. J. Morrison. 1997. Latent yellow-head infections in *Penaeus monodon* and implications regarding disease resistance or tolerance, p. 45–53. *In* T. W. Flegel, P. Menasveta, and S. Paisarnrat (ed.), *Shrimp Biotechnology in Thailand*. National Center for Biotechnology and Genetic Engineering, Bangkok, Thailand.

79. Pasternak, A. O., W. J. M. Spaan, and E. J. Snijder. 2006. Nidovirus transcription: how to make sense...? *J. Gen. Virol.* 87:1403–1421.

80. Phan, Y. T. N. 2001. Prevalence and co-prevalence of white spot syndrome virus (WSSV) and yellow head complex viruses (YHV-complex) in cultured giant tiger prawn (*Penaeus monodon*) in Vietnam. M.S. thesis. University of Queensland, Brisbane, Australia.

81. Posthuma, C. C., D. D. Nedialkova, J. C. Zevenhoven-Dobbe, J. H. Blokhuis, A. E. Gorbalenya, and E. J. Snijder. 2006. Site-directed mutagenesis of the nidovirus replicative endoribonuclease NendoU exerts pleiotropic effects on the arterivirus life cycle. *J. Virol.* 80:1653–1661.

82. Robalino, J., J. S. Almeida, D. McKillen, J. Colglazier, H. F. Trent III, Y. A. Chen, M. E. T. Peck, C. L. Browdy, R.W. Chapman, G. W. Warr, and P. S. Gross. 2007. Insights into the immune transcriptome of the shrimp *Litopenaeus vannamei*: tissue-specific expression profiles and transcriptomic responses to immune challenge. *Physiol. Genomics* 29:44–56.

83. Robalino, J., T. Bartlett, E. Shepard, S. Prior, G. Jaramillo, E. Scura, R. W. Chapman, P. S. Gross, C. L. Browdy, and G. W. Warr. 2005. Double-stranded RNA induces sequence-specific antiviral silencing in addition to nonspecific immunity in a marine shrimp: convergence of RNA interference and innate immunity in the invertebrate antiviral response? *J. Virol.* 79:13561–13571.

84. Robalino, J., C. L. Browdy, S. Prior, A. Metz, P. Parnell, P. S. Gross, and G. W. Warr. 2004. Induction of antiviral immunity by double-stranded RNA in a marine invertebrate. *J. Virol.* 78:10442–10448.

85. Rottier, P. J. M. 1995. The coronavirus membrane protein, p. 115–139. *In* S. G. Siddell (ed.), *The Coronaviridae*. Plenum Press, New York, NY.

86. Sahtout, A. H., M. D. Hassan, and M. Shariff. 2001. DNA fragmentation, an indicator of apoptosis, in cultured black tiger shrimp *Penaeus monodon* infected with white spot syndrome virus (WSSV). *Dis. Aquat. Org.* 44:155–159.

87. Sawicki, S. G., and D. L. Sawicki. 1999. A new model for coronavirus transcription. *Adv. Exp. Med. Biol.* 440:215–219.

88. Sawicki, S. G., D. L. Sawicki, and S. G. Siddell. 2007. A contemporary view of coronavirus transcription. *J. Virol.* 81:20–29.

89. Seybert, A., A. Hegyi, S. G. Siddell, and J. Ziebuhr. 2000. The human coronavirus 229E superfamily 1 helicase has RNA and DNA duplex-unwinding activities with 5′-to-3′ polarity. *RNA* 6:1056–1068.

90. Sithigorngul, P., S. Rukpratanporn, S. Longyant, P. Chaivisuthangkura, W. Sithigorngul, and P. Menasveta. 2002. Monoclonal antibodies specific to yellow-head virus (YHV) of *Penaeus monodon*. *Dis. Aquat. Org.* 49:71–76.

91. Sittidilokratna, N., R. A. J. Hodgson, J. A. Cowley, S. Jitrapakdee, V. Boonsaeng, S. Panyim, and P. J. Walker. 2002. Complete ORF1b-gene sequence indicates yellow head virus is an invertebrate nidovirus. *Dis. Aquat. Org.* 50:87–93.

92. Sittidilokratna, N., N. Phetchampai, V. Boonsaeng, and P. J. Walker. 2006. Structural and antigenic analysis of the yellow head virus nucleocapsid protein p20. *Virus Res.* 116:21–29.

93. Siveter, D. J., M. Williams, and D. Waloszek. 2001. A phosphatocopid crustacean with appendages from the Lower Cambrian. *Science* 293:479–481.

94. Smith, P. T. 2000. Diseases of the eye of farmed shrimp *Penaeus monodon*. *Dis. Aquat. Org.* 43:159–173.

95. Snijder, E. J., P. J. Bredenbeek, J. C. Dobbe, V. Thiel, J. Ziebuhr, L. L. Poon, Y. Guan, M. Rozanov, W. J. M. Spaan, and A. E. Gorbalenya. 2003. Unique and conserved features of genome and proteome of SARS-coronavirus, an early split-off from the coronavirus group 2 lineage. *J. Mol. Biol.* 331:991–1004.

96. Snijder, E. J., J. A. den Boon, P. J. Bredenbeek, M. C. Horzinek, R. Rijnbrand, and W. J. M. Spaan. 1990. The carboxyl-terminal part of the putative Berne virus polymerase is expressed by ribosomal frameshifting and contains sequence motifs which indicate that toro- and coronaviruses are evolutionarily related. *Nucleic Acids Res.* **18:**4535–4542.

97. Snijder, E. J., J. A. den Boon, W. J. M. Spaan, G. M. G. M. Verjans, and M. Horzinek. 1989. Identification and primary structure of the gene encoding the Berne virus nucleocapsid protein. *J. Gen. Virol.* **70:**3363–3370.

98. Snijder, E. J., and M. C. Horzinek. 1993. Toroviruses: replication, evolution and comparison with other members of the coronavirus-like superfamily. *J. Gen. Virol.* **74:**2305–2316.

99. Snijder, E. J., and M. C. Horzinek. 1995. The molecular biology of toroviruses, p. 219–238. *In* S. G. Siddell (ed.), *The Coronaviridae.* Plenum Press, New York, NY.

100. Snijder, E. J., M. C. Horzinek, and W. J. M. Spaan. 1990. A 3'-coterminal nested set of independently transcribed mRNAs is generated during Berne virus replication. *J. Virol.* **64:**331–338.

100a. Snijder, E. J., S. G. Siddell, and A. E. Gorbalenya. 2005. The order *Nidovirales*, p. 390–404. *In* B. W. Mahy and V. ter Meulen (ed.), *Topley and Wilson's Microbiology and Microbial Infections*, 10th ed, *Virology*, vol. 1. Hodder Arnold, London, United Kingdom.

101. Soowannayan, C., T. W. Flegel, P. Sithigorngul, J. Slater, A. Hyatt, S. Cramerri, T. Wise, M. S. Crane, J. A. Cowley, R. J. McCulloch, and P. J. Walker. 2003. Detection and differentiation of yellow head complex viruses using monoclonal antibodies. *Dis. Aquat. Org.* **57:**193–200.

102. Spaan, W. J. M., D. Cavanagh, R. J. de Groot, L. Enjuanes, A. E. Gorbalenya, E. J. Snijder, and P. J. Walker. 2005. Order *Nidovirales*, p. 937–945. *In* C. M. Fauquet, M. A. Mayo, J. Maniloff, U. Desselberger, and L. A. Ball (ed.), *Virus Taxonomy: Eighth Report of the International Committee on Taxonomy of Viruses.* Elsevier. Academic Press, San Diego, CA.

103. Spann, K. M., J. A. Cowley, P. J. Walker, and R. J. G. Lester. 1997. A yellow-head-like virus from *Penaeus monodon* cultured in Australia. *Dis. Aquat. Org.* **31:**169–179.

104. Spann, K. M., R. A. Donaldson, J. A. Cowley, and P. J. Walker. 2000. Differences in the susceptibility of some penaeid prawn species to gill-associated virus (GAV) infection. *Dis. Aquat. Org.* **42:**221–225.

105. Spann, K. M., R. J. McCulloch, J. A. Cowley, I. J. East, and P. J. Walker. 2003. Detection of gill-associated virus (GAV) by *in situ* hybridization during acute and chronic infections of *Penaeus monodon* and *P. esculentus. Dis. Aquat. Org.* **56:**1–10.

106. Spann, K. M., J. E. Vickers, and R. J. G. Lester. 1995. Lymphoid organ virus of *Penaeus monodon* from Australia. *Dis. Aquat. Org.* **23:**127–134.

107. Sullivan, C. S., and D. Ganem. 2005. A virus-encoded inhibitor that blocks RNA interference in mammalian cells. *J. Virol.* **79:**7371–7379.

108. Takeda, A., M. Tsukuda, H. Mizumoto, K. Okamoto, M. Kaido, K. Mise, and T. Okuno. 2005. A plant RNA virus suppresses RNA silencing through viral RNA replication. *EMBO J.* **24:**3147–3157.

109. Tang, K. F. J., and D. V. Lightner. 1999. A yellow head virus gene probe: nucleotide sequence and application for *in situ* hybridization. *Dis. Aquat. Org.* **35:**165–173.

110. Tang, K. F. J., K. M. Spann, L. Owens, and D. V. Lightner. 2002. *In situ* detection of Australian gill-associated virus with a yellow head virus gene probe. *Aquaculture* **205:**1–5.

111. ten Dam, E. B., C. W. A. Pleij, and L. Bosch. 1990. RNA pseudoknots: translational frameshifting and read through on viral RNAs. *Virus Genes* **4:**121–136.

112. Tirasophon, W., Y. Roshorm, and S. Panyim. 2005. Silencing of yellow head virus replication in penaeid shrimp cells by dsRNA. *Biochem. Biophys. Res. Commun.* **334:**102–107.

113. Unajak, S., V. Boonsaeng, and S. Jitrapakdee. 2006. Isolation and characterization of cDNA encoding Argonaute, a component of RNA silencing in shrimp (*Penaeus monodon*). *Comp. Biochem. Physiol.* **145:**179–187.

114. van Vliet, A. L., S. L. Smits, P. J. Rottier, and R. J. de Groot. 2002. Discontinuous and non-discontinuous subgenomic RNA transcription in a nidovirus. *EMBO J.* **21:**6571–6580.

115. von Grotthuss, M., L. S. Wyrwicz, and L. Rychlewski. 2003. mRNA cap-1 methyltransferase in the SARS genome. *Cell* **113:**701–702.

116. Walker, P. J. 2000. Australia, p. 39–44. *In* R. P. Subasinghe, J. R. Arthur, M. J. Phillips, and M. B. Reantaso (ed.), *Thematic Review on Management Strategies for Major Diseases in Shrimp Aquaculture.* Food and Agriculture Organization, Rome, Italy.

117. Walker, P. J., J. R. Bonami, V. Boonsaeng, P. S. Chang, J. A. Cowley, L. Enjuanes, T. W. Flegel, D. V. Lightner, P. C. Loh, E. J. Snijder, and K. Tang. 2005. Family *Roniviridae*, p. 975–979. *In* C. M. Fauquet, M. A. Mayo, J. Maniloff, U. Desselberger, and L. A. Ball (ed.), *Virus Taxonomy: Eighth Report of the International Committee on Taxonomy of Viruses.* Elsevier, Academic Press, San Diego, CA.

118. Walker, P. J., J. A. Cowley, K. M. Spann, and C. M. Dimmock. 1998. The emergence of yellow head-related viruses in Australia, p. 263–265. *In* T. W. Flegel (ed.), *Advances in Shrimp Biotechnology.* National Center for Genetic Engineering and Biotechnology, Bangkok, Thailand.

119. Walker, P. J., J. A. Cowley, K. M. Spann, R. A. J. Hodgson, M. R. Hall, and B. Withyachumnarnkul. 2001. Yellow head complex viruses: transmission cycles and topographical distribution in the Asia-Pacific region, p. 227–237. *In* C. L. Browdy and D. E. Jory (ed.), *The New Wave: Proceedings of the Special Session on Sustainable Shrimp Culture, Aquaculture 2001.* The World Aquaculture Society, Baton Rouge, LA.

120. Wang, C. S., K. J. Tang, G. H. Kuo, and S. N. Chen. 1996. Yellow head disease-like virus infection in the Kuruma shrimp *Penaeus japonicus* cultured in Taiwan. *Fish Pathol.* **31:**177–182.

121. Wang, Y.-C., and P.-S. Chang. 2000. Yellow head virus infection in the giant tiger prawn *Penaeus monodon* cultured in Taiwan. *Fish Pathol.* **35:**1–10.

122. Weiss, M., F. Steck, and M. C. Horzinek. 1983. Purification and partial characterization of a new enveloped RNA virus (Berne virus). *J. Gen. Virol.* **64:**1849–1858.

123. Westenberg, M., B. Heinhuis, D. Zuidema, and J. M. Vlak. 2005. siRNA injection induces sequence-independent protection in *Penaeus monodon* against white spot syndrome virus. *Virus Res.* **114:**133–139.

124. Wongprasert, K., K. Khanobdee, S. S. Glunukarn, P. Meeratana, and B. Withyachumnarnkul. 2003. Time-course and levels of apoptosis in various tissues of black tiger shrimp *Penaeus monodon* infected with white-spot syndrome virus. *Dis. Aquat. Org.* **55:**3–10.

125. Wongteerasupaya, C., V. Boonsaeng, S. Panyim, A. Tassanakajon, B. Withyachumnarnkul, and T. W. Flegel. 1997. Detection of yellow-head virus (YHV) of *Penaeus*

*monodon* by RT-PCR amplification. *Dis. Aquat. Org.* **31:** 181–186.

126. **Wongteerasupaya, C., S. Sriurairatana, J. E. Vickers, A. Anutara, V. Boonsaeng, S. Panyim, A. Tassanakajon, B. Withyachumnarnkul, and T. W. Flegel.** 1995. Yellow-head virus of *Penaeus monodon* is an RNA virus. *Dis. Aquat. Org.* **22:**45–50.

127. **Yodmuang, S., W. Tirasophon, Y. Roshorm, W. Chinnirunvong, and S. Panyim.** 2006. YHV-protease dsRNA inhibits YHV replication in *Penaeus monodon* and prevents mortality. *Biochem. Biophys. Res. Commun.* **341:**351–356.

128. **Ziebuhr, J., S. Bayer, J. A. Cowley, and A. E. Gorbalenya.** 2003. The 3C-like proteinase of an invertebrate nidovirus links coronavirus and potyvirus homologs. *J. Virol.* **77:**1415–1426.

*Nidoviruses*
Edited by S. Perlman, T. Gallagher, and E. J. Snijder
© 2008 ASM Press, Washington, DC

Chapter 25

# Vaccines for Severe Acute Respiratory Syndrome Virus and Other Coronaviruses

Luis Enjuanes, Marta L. DeDiego, Enrique Alvarez, Carmen Capiscol, and Ralph Baric

This chapter provides a brief overview of the state of the art on coronavirus (CoV) vaccines, with special attention paid to severe acute respiratory syndrome CoV (SARS-CoV), as this virus has had the largest impact on humans. First, we consider basic aspects affecting vaccine development, such as correlates of protection, antigenic variability, and role of B- and T-cell responses. Then we discuss different types of vaccines under development, including inactivated viruses, subunit vaccines, virus-like particles (VLPs), DNA vaccines, heterologous expression systems, and vaccines derived by reverse genetics. Finally, potential side effects of these vaccines are considered.

Both classical and recombinant vaccines have been produced to prevent CoV-induced diseases (72, 73, 209, 272). Nevertheless, the vaccines that are being applied today are classical vaccines. These vaccines provide protection against infectious bronchitis virus (IBV) (38, 119) and mouse hepatitis virus (MHV) (268) and, with variable results, against bovine coronavirus (BCoV) and TGEV (78, 216). For several CoVs (i.e., TGEV) and arteriviruses such as porcine reproductive and respiratory reproductive syndrome virus, currently administered vaccines are efficacious only when they are provided to previously infected animals, in order to burst their lactogenic immunity to protect newborn progeny (209).

In spite of long-term efforts, fully effective animal vaccines to prevent CoV infection of mucosal tissues remain elusive, and single-dose live but not killed vaccines induced the most consistent protection (209). Vaccines inducing mucosal immunity are the most effective, but unfortunately, these vaccines often are short-lived, a limitation observed even after natural infection. As a consequence, these vaccines may not prevent reinfection and effective immunization may require frequent boosting, factors complicating CoV vaccine design.

For this chapter we have used a previous review on SARS-CoV vaccines (74) as a starting point and included the advances in vaccine development for group 1, 2, and 3 CoVs. This chapter can be complemented by earlier reviews on CoV vaccines (38, 75, 77, 209) and more recent reviews on SARS-CoV (272, 294, 299, 304).

## CoV DISEASES

CoVs are classified in three groups on the basis of genetic analysis (97, 235). Group 1 includes CoVs infecting human, porcine, canine, and feline species, closely related in sequence and, in some cases, also antigenically (218). The prototype group 1 CoV is TGEV, an enteropathogenic CoV that replicates both in villus epithelial cells of the small intestine and in lung cells. A nonenteropathogenic virus related to TGEV, the porcine respiratory CoV (PRCV), replicates to high titers in the respiratory tract and undergoes limited replication in submucosal cells of the small intestine (51, 53). A TGEV-like disease was associated with porcine epidemic diarrhea virus (186). This virus, closely related to TGEV in sequence but antigenically distinct (218), also infects the enteric tract of swine. Canine coronavirus (CCoV) usually produces a mild gastroenteritis, although some virus strains cause a more severe and sometimes fatal diarrhea. Feline CoV causes a disease involving an antibody-dependent enhancement (ADE) of infection and immunocomplex-induced lesions (174). Epithelial

**Luis Enjuanes, Marta L. DeDiego, Enrique Alvarez, and Carmen Capiscol** • Centro Nacional de Biotecnología, CSIC, Campus Universidad Autónoma, Cantoblanco, Darwin 3, 28049 Madrid, Spain. **Ralph Baric** • Department of Microbiology and Immunology, University of North Carolina at Chapel Hill, 802 Mary Ellen Jones Building, Chapel Hill, NC 27599-7290.

cells are the main targets of porcine CoVs, although widely distributed cells such as macrophages are also infected.

Group 2 CoVs are associated mainly with respiratory, enteric, hepatic, and central nervous system diseases (272). Murine CoVs, included in group 2, display different tropisms and levels of virulence. The commonly used laboratory strains infect primarily the liver and the brain and thus provide animal models for encephalitis and hepatitis as well as the immune-mediated demyelinating disease that develops late after infection (188).

Group 3 CoVs, such as IBV, cause respiratory disease in chickens, infecting the ciliated epithelia of the nose and trachea. In addition, they may infect the alimentary tract, kidneys, and the oviduct, which may contribute to diminished egg production (38). In humans and fowl, CoVs primarily cause upper respiratory tract infections, while porcine CoVs and BCoVs establish enteric infections that result in severe economic loss (258).

Human CoVs (HCoVs) 229E and OC43 are members of groups 1 and 2, respectively. They are responsible for 10 to 20% of all common colds and have been implicated in gastroenteritis, upper and lower respiratory tract infections, and rare cases of encephalitis (68). HCoVs have also been associated with infant necrotizing enterocolitis (204) and are tentative candidates for association with multiple sclerosis (67). Recently, a new group 2 CoV causing SARS has emerged, infecting more than 8,000 people and causing more than 800 deaths in 5 months (70, 112, 158, 230, 250). SARS-CoV infection results in severe acute respiratory disease, pneumonia, diarrhea, and sometimes death (183). SARS-CoV is a zoonotic virus that crossed the species barrier, most likely originating from bats, and that has been amplified in other species, preferentially civets (150, 152, 276). SARS-CoV-induced diseases in these mammals, if any, have not yet been characterized.

## CORRELATES OF DISEASE PROTECTION IN CoV VACCINE DEVELOPMENT

Virion proteins comprise the principal vaccine immunogens. Therefore, it is important to note that in general, CoVs have a set of structural genes and proteins similar to that of group 1 viruses (187). SARS-CoV, by contrast, is more complex in both genetic structure and number of structural proteins (Fig. 1), and therefore, a greater constellation of potential vaccine proteins must be considered in protecting against SARS. The spike (S), envelope (E), and membrane (M) proteins and SARS-CoV protein 3a (122, 228) are viral membrane proteins with domains exposed to the external face of the virus that, in principle, could be involved in protection by inducing neutralizing antibodies. The requirements for protection against SARS-CoV may be different from those of previously known CoVs, as SARS-CoV has at least seven structural proteins (S, 3a, E, M, 7a, 7b, and nucleocapsid [N] proteins), three of which (3a, 7a, and 7b) have not been described for other CoVs (114, 115, 220). Hemagglutinin esterase (HE) is present only in group 2 CoVs and provides protection against BCoV in the murine system by eliciting both systemic and mucosal immunity (10). While all

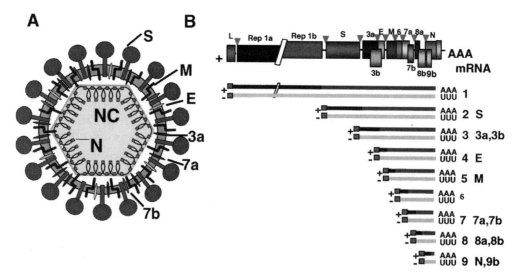

**Figure 1.** Structure and genome organization of CoVs. (A) Schematic diagram of SARS-CoV structure. 3a, 7a, and 7b are structural envelope SARS-CoV proteins. (B) Representation of a prototype SARS-CoV genome. AAA, poly(A) tail. Numbers and letters indicate viral genes.

virion proteins should be considered potential vaccine immunogens, the weight of current evidence argues that the S proteins typically elicit the strongest protection levels. Most likely this is due to the fact that antibodies binding to S proteins can prevent S protein interactions with cellular receptors (111) or S protein-mediated membrane fusion and other post-receptor binding steps essential for entry and infectivity. The role of S protein in protection and in CoV infection in general has been previously described (38, 75, 209). In this review special attention is paid to SARS-CoV S protein.

It has been shown that S and 3a proteins induce in vitro SARS-CoV neutralizing antibodies, S protein being the main component of protective immunity (200, 209). Although strong immune responses are elicited against both S and N proteins (32, 198, 240, 267, 305), passive-transfer studies illustrated that only S protein-specific antibodies confer protection from SARS-CoV replication in the mouse model (23, 240). Two domains have been defined in the CoV S protein, the amino-terminal (S1) and the carboxy-terminal (S2) halves. The S1 domain concentrates most of the epitopes involved in CoV neutralization (32, 38, 88, 106, 209, 210, 241, 243). The receptor-binding domain (RBD) located in the S1 subunit of S protein contains multiple conformational neutralizing epitopes. This suggests that recombinant proteins containing the RBD, and vectors encoding the RBD sequence, can be used to develop safe and effective SARS vaccines (126). Multiple neutralization domains and T-cell epitopes involved in protection also have been mapped in the amino-terminal half (S1) of the S protein (78, 175). Nevertheless, neutralization domains have also been described for the S2 domain (48, 138, 145, 157, 194, 208, 256). SARS-CoV neutralization by S2 protein-specific antibodies inhibits the interaction between heptad repeats 1 and 2, involved in coil-to-coil interactions, which are essential for S protein-mediated membrane fusion during virus entry (131, 301). The S1 protein epitopes are more effective immunogens than those in the S2 domain, at least with regard to generating virus-neutralizing antibodies (131). However, S2 epitopes may be more broadly conserved than those in S1. Interestingly, an identified S2 epitope critical in virus neutralization is highly conserved across different SARS-CoV isolates, a fact that is relevant for the development of effective vaccines against SARS-CoV (295).

The relevance of S protein in protection against SARS-CoV has been reinforced by the identification of neutralizing antibodies from convalescent patients. Continuous virus epitopes targeted by antibodies in plasma samples from convalescent SARS patients have been identified by biopanning with an M13 phage display dodecapeptide library (301). These epitopes converged to very short peptide fragments, mapping on the S, N, 3a, and 9b proteins and nonstructural protein 3 (nsp3). In addition, serum from most (82%) of the patients that recovered from SARS developed antibodies to the epitope-rich region on the spike S2 domain, indicating that this domain also may be an immunodominant site on the S protein (301).

Recent evidence has shown that SARS-CoV neutralization is sensitive to deglycosylation of the S protein, suggesting that conformational epitopes are important in antibody recognition (234). Although immunization with the S protein may provide the most effective protection against CoV infection, it also may induce ADE of diseases in the case of feline infectious peritonitis virus (FIPV). Attempts have been made to differentiate the antigenic epitopes inducing neutralizing antibodies from those inducing antibodies that cause ADE of disease (47).

SARS-CoV 3a protein consists of 274 amino acids (aa) and contains three putative transmembrane domains (122, 246). Protein 3a exposes in the cell surface the first 34 aa, located before the first transmembrane domain (2), and its C terminus, after the third transmembrane domain (aa 134 to 274), is facing the cytoplasm (246). Interestingly, in two separate cohorts of SARS patients, one from Taiwan (154) and the other from Hong Kong (301), B cells recognizing the N-terminal region of 3a protein were isolated. Moreover, a significant proportion (40%) of sera examined from convalescent SARS patients were positive in a dot blot assay against a synthetic peptide with a sequence corresponding to aa 12 to 27 of the N terminus of protein 3a (301). In addition, it was recently reported that the N-terminal domain of 3a protein elicits strong and potentially protective humoral responses in infected patients (300). Accordingly, rabbit polyclonal antibodies raised against a synthetic peptide corresponding to aa 15 to 28 of 3a protein inhibited SARS-CoV propagation in Vero-E6 cells, in contrast to antibodies specific for the C-terminal domain of the protein (2).

SARS-CoV E, M, and 7a proteins have shown low immunogenicity, as sera from three convalescent SARS patients did not recognize these proteins expressed in mammalian cells (200, 245). Immunization of hamsters with a parainfluenza virus vector has shown that SARS-CoV S protein alone provided complete protection, whereas expression of M, E, or N protein in the absence of S did not confer detectable protection (32).

The M protein of TGEV is required for virus assembly and budding, and M protein-specific antibodies significantly, but weakly, neutralize TGEV and mediate complement-dependent lysis of TGEV-infected cells (65, 205, 281). In addition, a mixture of S and M proteins showed a synergistic effect in the in vitro synthesis of TGEV neutralizing antibodies by immune leukocytes (7). Consistent with TGEV data, it has been described that SARS-CoV M protein also induced virus neutralizing antibodies in the absence of complement (32), and two major immunodominant epitopes on the M protein located in the N-terminal region have been identified by using sera from convalescent patients.

CoV N protein is an internal virus component, and antibodies specific for this protein do not neutralize virus infectivity (179). Nevertheless, N protein may play at least two main roles in protection against CoV infection. N protein may stimulate Th2 cells, which collaborate in the production of neutralizing antibodies specific for S protein (7). Analysis of the immune response to TGEV using an in vitro antibody synthesis system has shown that an optimum combination of viral proteins stimulating the production of TGEV neutralizing antibodies in vitro was a mixture of S and N proteins, or a combination of S protein oligomers (rosettes) and the N protein or peptides derived from it (6, 7). A second role of N protein could be the induction of T-cell responses specific for N protein fragments exposed on the surface of infected cells. These data suggest that N protein could be used in vaccines to promote the synthesis of S protein-specific neutralizing antibodies.

In the case of IBV, N protein expressed in bacteria induced protective immunity by activation of cytotoxic or helper T-cell responses (25, 224). A fragment of the N protein comprising the carboxy-terminal 120 aa residues was sufficient to induce homologous protection. The birds did not develop clinical signs, although some replication of the challenge virus was detected. Nevertheless, S protein must be superior to M and N proteins in protection in the IBV system, as chickens that had been immunized with immunoaffinity-purified S1 proteins developed tracheal and kidney immunity, while those chickens receiving purified N or M protein did not (119).

SARS-CoV N protein induces T-cell responses (87, 101, 304). In fact, the highest levels of humoral response and T-helper response in mice were induced by N protein (127). Patients who had recovered from SARS showed long-lived memory T-lymphocyte responses specific for epitopes located in the C-terminal region (aa 331 to 362) of N protein (185). These responses could persist for 2 years in the absence of antigen. Analysis of T-cell repertoires in health care workers who survived SARS-CoV infection revealed that their effector memory Vγ9Vδ2 T-cell populations were selectively expanded (191). In contrast, no such expansion of their αβ T-cell pools was detected. The expansion of the Vγ9Vδ2 T-cell population was associated with higher anti-SARS-CoV immunoglobulin G (IgG) titers. In addition, stimulated Vγ9Vδ2 T cells displayed gamma interferon (IFN-γ)-dependent anti-SARS-CoV activity and were able to directly kill SARS-CoV-infected targeted cells.

Protein 9b (98 aa), internal to N protein, elicits antibodies in 100% of SARS-CoV patients, indicating that it is expressed in natural disease and that it is immunogenic (200, 301).

## ANTIGENIC VARIATION AND EFFICACY OF CoV VACCINES

As described in previous sections, the most relevant antigen involved in CoV protection is the S protein (38, 44, 75, 125, 210, 272). The S protein also appears to be the most structurally diverse antigen among the various CoVs. The degrees of amino acid sequence homology among the S proteins of various CoVs differ for S1 and S2, with 39% homology over the first 274 aa and 93% homology for residues 275 to 1447 (124).

The information accumulated on the antigenic and functional structure of S protein in all CoVs indicates that it has a complex three-dimensional structure in the native state, with interactions between distant domains in the primary structure (75, 88, 106). Due to this antigenic complexity, the impact of antigenic variability on the development of CoV vaccines differs for each virus group. In viruses such as TGEV, due to the presence of a highly conserved, antigenically dominant epitope involved in TGEV neutralization, there is a cross-protection throughout all TGEV isolates (218).

Antigenic variability in S protein may be a more serious vaccine issue with the group 2 and 3 viruses. The HCoVs are quite diverse; in strains such as HCoV-229E, HCoV-OC43, HCoV-NL63, HCoV-HKU1, and SARS-CoV (19, 197, 265, 275, 278), there is a high degree of genetic and antigenic diversity among the S proteins (93, 264–266). Molecular clock analysis of the S protein gene sequences of BCoV and HCoV-OC43 shows an estimated evolutionary rate on the order of $4 \times 10^{-4}$ nucleotide substitutions per site per year (265). Antigenic variability seems to be a limited problem in the case of BCoV, as comparison of respiratory and enteric isolates has shown that most BCoV strains were similar and vaccines developed to protect against enteric strains also may protect against respiratory tract strains (105). S protein targets of cytotoxic T lymphocytes such as those of MHV (JHM strain) also may vary, leading to the evasion of cellular immune responses (133, 189).

In group 3 CoVs such as IBV, antigenic variability seems to be high (38). In the case of IBV, differences as little as 5% between S1 sequences can result in poor protection. Differences in S1 of 2 to 3% (10 to 15 aa) can change serotype, suggesting that a small number of epitopes are immunodominant with respect to neutralizing antibody (38). More than 20 IBV serotypes have been identified worldwide (39, 46, 58, 80, 120, 167). There has been an increasing number of new serotypic variants, possibly generated by the widespread use of live attenuated vaccines (89, 117, 123, 146, 153). IBV serotypes differ from each other by 20 to 50% of the S1 amino acids. In general, the immunity induced with one serotype protects poorly against infection by heterologous serotypes, with protection ranging from 0 to 70% (8, 38, 45, 163). Although vaccines have generally been used extensively, outbreaks of IBV occur frequently due to serotype differences.

Phylogenetic analysis of SARS-CoV isolates from animals and humans strongly suggests that the virus originated from bats (150, 152, 192), was amplified in palm civets, and was transmitted to the human population via live-animal markets (129). The neutralization of a set of eight pseudoviruses expressing the S glycoprotein of eight SARS-CoV strains, selected from the three phases of the SARS epidemic (early, middle, and late), plus another human isolate collected at the end of 2003 (GD03) and two civet cat isolates from 2003 (SZ16 and SZ3), has been studied (41, 284). Human monoclonal antibodies (MAbs) against the S protein of the Frankfurt (FRA-1) isolate were used, the antibodies being derived from Epstein-Barr virus-transformed B lymphocytes. The viruses tested in the neutralization assays included pseudotypes made with the S protein from members of the four main genetic clusters defined with the Bayesian analysis of the SARS-CoV glycoproteins (66, 74). Basically, all viruses pseudotyped with S proteins from different strains were neutralized to the same extent by MAbs specific for the FRA-1 isolate, except the human (GD03) and the two civet cat isolates (SZ16 and SZ3), indicating that there were at least two human SARS-CoV serotypes, which most likely originated from two independent transmissions of the virus from civet cats to humans (284). Recently, a recombinant virus bearing a GD03 zoonotic S glycoprotein was reported to display reduced neutralization kinetics using human convalescent-phase sera and murine sera from vaccinated animals (66). Although more recombinant viruses bearing zoonotic S glycoproteins are needed, these data suggest that the small amount of S heterogeneity reported in civet

and raccoon dog isolates is an important variable for consideration in SARS-CoV vaccine design.

The SARS-CoV-like virus isolated from bats of the *Rhinolophus* genus has higher than 92% nucleotide identity with the TOR-2 strain (150, 152). In addition, six novel CoVs from six different bat species have been described (276). Four of these CoVs belong to group 1, and two of them to group 2. Based on sequence data, Woo and colleagues have proposed the classification of bat CoVs into three subgroups (2a, 2b, and 2c). Subgroup 2b comprises both SARS-CoV and a bat SARS-CoV (Rp3 isolate). The sequences of these SARS-CoV isolates differ most in the S1 domain of the S protein, where identity fell to 64%. This sequence divergence in the S1 domain corroborated the serum neutralization studies, which indicate that although bat sera have a high level of cross-reactive antibodies, they failed to neutralize human or civet cat SARS-CoV when tested in Vero-E6 cells (152). In contrast, other authors (150) have reported that 42% of bat serum samples neutralized a human SARS-CoV isolate (HKU-39849) using FRhK-4 cells. The discrepancy could be due to the presence of a different SARS-CoV-like virus serotype in the bats studied by the two groups, or to the two test systems used in the evaluation. Vaccine design should take this SARS-CoV antigenic diversity into account.

A human MAb (80R), specific for the angiotensin-converting enzyme 2 (ACE2) RBD on S proteins, has been evaluated for immunoprophylaxis of SARS in an animal study. Epitope mapping, and analysis of spike variants, has shown that the vast majority of SARS-CoV strains, including the well-adapted and more pathogenic human strains from the 2002–2003 epidemic, are likely to be sensitive to neutralization by MAb 80R (242). These data suggest a limited variability of SARS-CoV S protein in terms of neutralization. In fact, Sui and colleagues suggest that in the case of an emergency, prophylaxis of SARS-CoV-exposed individuals with a single intravenous or intramuscular dose of MAb 80R (half-life of IgG1, around 21 days) may be sufficient to achieve a level in serum that would result in >99% reduction in the expected virus titers in the serum or tissue of humans or animals, based on previously published studies.

In the SARS-CoV S protein RBD, multiple conformational epitopes (I to VI) have been identified that confer the major target of neutralizing MAbs. Recombinant RBDs derived from the S protein sequences of TOR-2, GD03, and SZ3 viruses, the representative strains of human 2002–2003 and 2003–2004 SARS-CoV and palm civet SARS-CoV, respectively, induce high titers of cross-neutralizing antibodies in mice and rabbits that neutralize pseudoviruses expressing S proteins of TOR-2, GD03, and SZ3 viruses. Interestingly, epitope V, which may overlap the RBD and induce the most potent neutralizing antibodies, was conserved in these mutants. These data suggest that the major neutralization epitopes of SARS-CoV have been maintained during cross-species transmission (similar to what has been observed for TGEV; see above), and that RBD-based vaccines may induce broad protection against both human and animal SARS-CoV variants (107).

## TYPE OF IMMUNITY REQUIRED TO PREVENT CoV-INDUCED DISEASES

The relative degrees of importance of the humoral and cell responses vary among the different CoVs. For example, it has been demonstrated that passive administration of TGEV neutralizing polyvalent antibodies or MAbs provides full protection against challenge with virulent TGEV (22, 209, 253), with cell-mediated immune responses playing a more modest role in protection against TGEV challenge (28, 29, 259, 260). In contrast, in the case of FIPV, cellular immune responses appear to be the key to virus control (174). Minimizing the development of humoral antibodies may be valuable in avoiding ADE of disease and immune complex deposition (92, 108, 135).

The role of the immune response in clearance of MHV infection has been well characterized. Here, both antibody- and cell-mediated immune responses are required for protection. CD8$^+$ and CD4$^+$ T cells are primarily responsible for clearance of the virus during acute infections (272).

Many studies have shown that the presence or absence of antibodies to IBV does not correlate with protection. In fact, vaccinated chickens may be protected against respiratory disease caused by IBV, irrespective of the serum antibody titer (38, 119).

In the case of SARS-CoV, the humoral immune response induces full protection. In fact, S protein-specific virus neutralizing antibodies or immune serum provided passive protection (21, 240, 255, 295). In addition, human IgG MAbs neutralizing SARS-CoV, developed using phage display libraries, protected ferrets from lung disease and virus shedding in pharyngeal secretions (247). Immune responses to SARS-CoV, elicited by a DNA vaccine encoding a codon-optimized SARS S protein, or the S1 fragment, induced neutralizing antibodies as well as T-cell responses. Nevertheless, protection from SARS-CoV challenge was mediated by a humoral immune response but not by a T-cell-dependent mechanism (283, 293).

Surprisingly, immunodeficient mice can clear a SARS-CoV infection, revealing an important role for innate immune responses in the defenses against SARS-CoV. Mice that lack NK-T cells (CD1$^{-/-}$), NK cells, or both T and B cells (Ragl$^{-/-}$) cleared virus by day 9 after infection (95). The mice displayed high induction of proinflammatory cytokines, and possibly, interferon pathways were relevant in viral clearance. The importance of interferon has been reinforced by infecting Stat1-deficient mice with SARS-CoV (110). Stat1 is important to the regulation of interferons, and Stat1-deficient mice produced 100-fold increases in viral titer over the levels in control mice. Four SARS-CoV genes have been reported to encode antagonists of host innate immune responses, the nsp1 gene, open reading frame 3b (ORF3b), ORF6, and the N protein gene (128, 142). As ORF3b and ORF6 and parts of the nsp1 gene are nonessential for in vitro and in vivo replication, targeted mutations or deletions in these genes represent likely targets for attenuating SARS-CoV pathogenesis in vivo.

CoVs preferentially infect epithelial cells of the enteric and respiratory tract (212); therefore, induction of mucosal immunity is essential to protect against CoV-induced infections. A unique mucosal system has evolved to protect mucosal surfaces from pathogens (136, 173, 212). A characteristic of the mucosal immune system is the induction of B and T cells organized in gut-associated lymphoid tissue and bronchus-associated lymphoid tissue and their distribution to remote mucosal effector sites (i.e., lamina propia regions of the intestine, bronchi, genitourinary tract, and secretory glands) (212). Lactogenic immunity is of primary importance in providing newborn mammals immediate protection against CoV infections. Therefore, vaccination should be targeted to induce gut-mammary IgA (216). Similarly, mucosal immunity may be critical to prevent feline CoV infection and FIP (92). Notably, oral immunizations with nonreplicating or soluble antigens, or even after natural infection, induce poor secretory IgA responses of short duration (169, 172, 209) or lead to tolerance (172). Thus, protection of the respiratory tract following a single vaccination with live attenuated virus has been short-lived in chickens, showing declines 6 to 9 weeks after vaccination (57, 99). As a consequence, administration of several vaccine doses is required. Effective procedures to induce immunity at mucosal surfaces clearly need to be improved.

## INACTIVATED VERSUS LIVE VACCINES

Immunization with CoV group 1 inactivated TGEV or recombinant antigens induces only partial protection (148, 209, 216, 227). Thus, parenterally administered TGEV S glycoprotein vaccines elicit virus neutralizing antibodies to TGEV in serum and colostrum that provides only partial immunity in swine (229). Killed vaccines administered parenterally with adjuvant are also available to induce active or passive immunity to TGEV (213, 215), but the success of these vaccines in the field is limited due to a number of problems, such as the induction of low titers of local secretory IgA antibodies, poor cell-mediated immune responses, and the short duration of the immune response (209, 210). Only the repeated oral administration of S protein expressed in plants (corn) seems to provide protection to pigs against challenge with TGEV (149). The degree of protection is improved using two doses of attenuated virus boosted by a third administration of the attenuated virus or even by recombinant S protein. Still, only limited and variable protection (8 to 67% survival) is achieved (211).

Immunization of pigs with attenuated respiratory isolates derived from TGEV, such as PRCV, also induces partial (10 to 56% survival) protection against challenge with virulent virus. A single PRCV infection in the respiratory tract of pregnant swine induces partial passive immunity to TGEV (216), whereas repeated PRCV infections of the mother induce higher IgA antibody responses in milk and higher rates of protection against TGEV (226). In the field, pigs experience multiple respiratory infections with PRCV, providing a natural vaccine for TGEV such that TGE has largely disappeared from European swine herds (151).

Interestingly, immunization with an engineered, attenuated TGEV in which ORF3a has been partially replaced by a 636-nucleotide fragment of the replicase 1a gene protected >80% of pigs against challenge with virulent virus (279). This protection is higher than that conferred by any commercially available vaccine and is only slightly lower than the 87% protection observed in piglets nursing from sows exposed to virulent TGEV. This attenuated deletion mutant even protected young piglets, suggesting a vaccine potential.

Infection of pigs with virulent TGEV stimulates the most robust immunity and confers protection against subsequent TGEV challenge (28, 52, 259), although the duration of this immunity is unknown and probably is short-lived (209). Exposure of pregnant sows to a dose of virulent TGEV that may be lethal for newborn piglets but not for adult animals, 3 weeks before farrowing, provides 90 to 95% of protection to their nursing piglets after virulent TGEV challenge (214).

The value of CCoV vaccines in providing adequate immunity under field conditions is controversial (195), and in general, inactivated CCoV vaccines show low efficacy in reducing viral shedding in feces of dogs after CCoV infection (86, 195). Although the efficacy and duration of immunity elicited by inactivated CCoV vaccines have not been substantiated, killed CCoV vaccines have been licensed in the United States. A modified live CCoV vaccine was licensed in the United States in 1983 but was rapidly withdrawn due to a high rate (about 5%) of serious adverse reactions (160, 274). A modified live CCoV vaccine, available in California and licensed in the United States, appears to be safe, and 1-year immunity is claimed by the manufacturer. Unfortunately, the CCoV vaccine, when combined with canine cell-grown distemper vaccine, resulted in a high frequency of post-distemper encephalitis (35). In contrast, more recently, oronasal immunization with a modified live vaccine showed full protection against clinical signs, and virus shedding was not observed (196).

The development of vaccines against FIPV has been problematic (102). Vaccination with inactivated or subunit vaccines containing the M or N protein gene showed low and inconsistent protective efficacy (94, 262). In addition, immunization with recombinant vaccinia viruses expressing M protein was not protective against FIPV challenge (108). Furthermore, the immunization with a recombinant vaccinia virus expressing the S protein gene even showed an enhancement and accelerated progression of the disease upon challenge, leading to an early-death syndrome (261). A temperature-sensitive strain of FIPV available as a vaccine showed some protection against FIPV (12, 90, 91, 203), but its efficacy is under debate (81, 164, 222). The administration of closely related heterologous live CoVs fails to induce protection (17, 18, 239, 280). Vaccination with feline enteric CoV, low-virulence FIPV, or sublethal amounts of virulent FIPV occasionally provides some protection (180, 182). Unfortunately, in these cases results were too inconsistent to have clinical relevance (102). More recently, live attenuated viruses, obtained through the deletion of group-specific genes by targeted recombination, were used in vaccines against FIPV (60, 102).

Protection induced by inactivated or even live attenuated virus against group 2 CoVs resulted in better protection than in group 1 CoVs. Thus, vaccination against BCoV by the intranasal route reduced the risk of bovine respiratory tract disease (190). Neonatal diarrhea produced by BCoV can cause losses of up to 80% of calves. Passive protection can be provided by lactogenic immunity from immune adult cattle, but during milk production, antibody levels dramatically decrease. These antibody levels can be increased by immunization with inactivated virus plus oil adjuvants (54).

In experimental rodents, many different vaccines have proven effective in protecting against group 2 MHV. These vaccines include purified S protein (56) and synthetic peptides derived from the S2 protein (141, 244) or epitopes expressed in the tobacco mosaic virus system (140). The success of inactivated antigens in immune protection of mice may be due to the relatively higher ratio of antigen to body weight used in this small-animal model system. MHV produces several types of pathologies, and this system has been used for advanced studies on the role of the humoral and cellular immune responses in tissues not readily accessible to the immune system, such as the central nervous system and the eye, and to study the mechanism of virus persistence (133, 202).

Inactivated oil emulsion IBV vaccines were developed during the 1960s and 1970s. Chickens vaccinated with IBV S1 glycoprotein expressed by recombinant baculovirus have been partially (50%) protected (232). IBV immunization of chickens with inactivated virus is less efficient than that with live virus in spite of using a considerably larger amount of antigen, and single application of inactivated virus, in general, induces little or no protection against egg loss (38, 117). Two applications of inactivated IBV are much more efficacious than one. In the poultry industry, these inactivated viruses are not used alone. Because live vaccines are less expensive, and easier to apply, the approach commonly used in the poultry industry nowadays is to vaccinate young females two or more times with live vaccine, followed by one dose of inactivated vaccine as the birds come into lay. The live vaccines give protection to the young birds and prime the immune response to the later inactivated vaccine (38).

Although previous experiences with inactivated CoV vaccines were not very positive for the majority of *Coronaviridae* family members, inactivated SARS-CoV vaccines seem more promising. Many types of vaccines for SARS-CoV have been attempted, such as expression of recombinant proteins, or the use of virus vectors (27). Nevertheless, the classical approach using inactivated, cell culture-based SARS-CoV is likely to be the easiest way for SARS vaccine development, based on the well-established technologies for the development of such vaccines (237).

The fast spread of SARS initially prompted a Chinese company to develop a vaccine in collaboration with the Chinese Academy of Medical Sciences. A phase I clinical trial of SARS vaccine based on heat-inactivated virus was initiated in September 2004 in China. Inactivated SARS vaccine appeared to be safe in the volunteers. After the preliminary 56-day observation period, 11 out of 12 (91.6%) of the volunteers who received low-dosage vaccine and 12 out of 12 (100%) of the volunteers who received high-dosage vaccine showed blood serum conversion, with no obvious side effects (159, 299). However, the efficacy and long-term safety of this vaccine remain to be determined.

Approaches to chemically inactivate SARS-CoV involve somewhat variable methodologies. SARS-CoV was inactivated with propiolactone before (139) or after (223) being purified by centrifugation and administered to mice with or without adjuvant. The humoral immune response was more effective using inactivated virus with adjuvants than with the administration of recombinant adenoviruses expressing SARS-CoV S and N proteins. SARS-CoV has also been purified to up to 98% homogeneity by ultrafiltration, gel filtration, and exchange chromatography and then inactivated with β-propiolactone. Cynomolgus macaques were immunized with different amounts of the purified virus in the absence or in the presence of adjuvant. The monkeys were challenged by the nasal route 30 days postimmunization. High levels of neutralizing antibodies that prevented both the replication of SARS-CoV and interstitial pneumonia were elicited (199). Interestingly, no side effects were observed even in the presence of low-titer neutralizing antibodies, indicating that the purified SARS-CoV vaccine is safe in monkeys. In other approaches, SARS-CoV partially purified in sucrose cushions was completely inactivated with formaldehyde. This virus efficiently interfered with the binding of infectious virus to cells, indicating that the inactivated virus kept a functional receptor binding site (201). Polyethylene glycol-precipitated virus, alone or in the presence of cholera toxin B or CpG, elicited serum SARS-CoV-specific neutralizing antibodies in mice after intranasal administration, and IgA-specific antibodies accumulated in the trachea and lungs (201).

In another approach, formaldehyde-inactivated whole virus, prepared in Vero cells, was used in intramuscular immunization of 2- to 5-year-old rhesus monkeys (302). After 3 weeks, monkeys were challenged with SARS-CoV. Doses of 50 µg per animal conferred complete protection, whereas the control animals developed atypical SARS-CoV infection after challenge. The immunization preferentially induced Th1 responses but also enhanced other cellular immune responses, including the production of IFN-γ, which can increase the activity of natural killer cells and inhibit virus replication. No systematic side effects were observed in vaccinated animals postimmunization, even at the high dose (5,000 µg/monkey) and after two injections.

One vaccine manufactured to large scale, using fermenter cultures of Vero cells in serum-free medium, has been based on a double-inactivated, whole-virus vaccine (237). Culture supernatants were harvested and inactivated by formalin treatment and subsequent UV irradiation. This two-step inactivation procedure was utilized to ensure a high safety margin with respect to residual infectivity. Mice immunized twice with 1 μg of SARS-CoV vaccine using adjuvant (0.2% aluminum hydroxide) developed high titers of antibody against SARS-CoV S protein. The use of the adjuvant Al(OH)$_3$ had only a minor effect on the immunogenicity of the vaccine. In addition, cell-mediated immunity was elicited, as measured by the production of IFN-γ and interleukin 4 (IL-4) stimulation. A problem in SARS-CoV vaccine testing is with the robustness of the available animal models. Most vaccines have been tested in the murine model that measures virus replication 2 days postinfection. Infection produces little, if any, pathology or clinical disease, and measuring vaccine efficacy at 2 days postinfection minimizes the development of significant immune pathology that might be elicited by various SARS antigens. Moreover, primate and ferret models display variable disease outcomes and pathology and are not well characterized after day 4 of infection, suppressing the potential observation of adverse side effects associated with vaccine use. Better animal models are essential for truly evaluating the scope and functionality of the numerous candidate vaccine strains that have been developed in academic and commercial laboratories.

The antigenic and immunogenic properties of SARS-CoV S protein have been elucidated using recombinant S protein expressed in baculovirus vectors and insect cells (106). Four major antigenic domains have been defined, three of them located on the S1 and one on the S2 domain of S protein. Many MAbs showed potent neutralizing activity against SARS pseudoviruses constructed with the S proteins of TOR-2, GD03, and SZ3, prototype strains (see above). Of 38 MAbs, 32 bound to S1 and 6 bound to S2. Seventeen MAbs targeted the N-terminal region of S1 (aa 12 to 327), 9 MAbs recognized the RBD (aa 318 to 510), and 6 MAbs reacted with the C-terminal region of the S1 domain, which contains the major immunodominant site (aa 528 to 635). All of the RBD-specific MAbs had potent neutralization activity; six efficiently blocked virus-receptor interaction, confirming that the RBD contains the main neutralizing epitopes and that blockage of the receptor association is the major mechanism of SARS-CoV neutralization. Five MAbs for the S1 N-terminal region exhibited moderate neutralization activity, but none of the MAbs reacting with the S2 domain and the major immunodominant site in S1 showed neutralization activity. All the neutralizing antibodies

recognized conformational epitopes. These data show the relevance of the SARS-CoV S protein RBD for SARS inactivated vaccines.

A polypeptide containing aa 14 to 762 of the SARS-CoV S protein has been expressed using the baculovirus system, and affinity-purified protein was administered to mice with either saponin or Ribi as the adjuvant (24). Both regimens induced neutralizing MAbs, although the best results were obtained with saponin and polypeptide. After challenge, protective immunity was shown by the reduction of SARS-CoV titers in the upper and lower respiratory tract. This protein vaccine induced higher titers of neutralizing antibodies and more complete protection against an intranasal challenge than that achieved by inoculation of mice with live SARS-CoV (240), modified attenuated vaccinia virus Ankara strain (MVA) expressing the full-length S protein (23), or DNA expressing the full-length S protein or S protein lacking the transmembrane and cytoplasmic domains (283).

N protein plays a critical role in SARS-CoV pathogenesis, and high-level antinucleocapsid antibodies are detected in patients with SARS. N protein by itself does not provide protection against SARS-CoV infections. Still, a large number of studies using N protein as an antigen have been published. The immune response of mice vaccinated with a purified N protein fused to glutathione S-transferase elicited strong T-cell, IL-4, and antibody responses but a minimal IFN-γ response (101). SARS-CoV N protein expressed in *Escherichia coli* and then emulsified in Montanide ISA-51 containing the oligodeoxynucleotide CpG induced IgG2a N protein-specific antibodies in vaccinated BALB/c mice, suggesting a prevalence of the Th1 immune response (156). In contrast, mice immunized with N protein in phosphate-buffered saline produced mainly IgG1. Mice, monkeys, and humans recognized peptides between residues 156 and 175 of N protein.

## CoV VACCINES BASED ON VLPs

The formation of CoV VLPs requires the interaction of M and E proteins, at least for TGEV, FIPV, MHV, and IBV (20, 49, 50, 63, 96, 263). In contrast, in the case of SARS-CoV, the protein requirements for VLP formation vary in relation to the expression systems and cell types employed. Using baculovirus expression in insect cells, intracellular SARS-CoV VLPs were assembled from M and E proteins alone (109). Secretion of these VLPs to the extracellular media required the coexpression of S protein (168). These results are at variance with those obtained by expressing SARS-CoV proteins in human 293 renal epithelial cells under the control of cytomegalovirus promoters, using DNA plasmids (116). In this system, any combination of genes that expressed M and N proteins, with or without S or E protein, generated intracellular VLPs. These pseudoparticles did not form in the absence of the M and N proteins. The additional expression of the S protein allowed the formation of budding particles with morphology typical of SARS-CoV and related CoVs. One possibility is that different types of VLPs could be formed depending on the protein composition of these SARS-CoV VLPs, and additional studies are needed to clarify these findings. Protection by the administration of VLPs has not been reported.

## VACCINES PRODUCED IN PLANTS

The development of plant-based CoV vaccines has been reported (11, 148, 257, 303). The general methods involve the oral delivery of recombinant S proteins (TGEV, IBV, and porcine epidemic diarrhea virus) to elicit protective immunity. One of these studies includes an S protein plant-based vaccine candidate against TGEV that has advanced to early-phase farming trials (257). More recently, to develop safe, effective, and inexpensive vaccine candidates, the S1 domain of SARS-CoV S protein has been expressed in tomato and low-nicotine tobacco plants. High levels of expression of recombinant S1 protein (>0.1% total soluble protein) were observed in several transgenic lines by Western blot analysis. Plant-derived antigen induced systemic and mucosal immune responses in mice, with significantly increased levels of SARS-CoV-specific IgA after oral ingestion of tomato fruits expressing S1 protein. Sera of mice parenterally primed with tobacco-derived S1 protein revealed the presence of SARS-CoV-specific IgG. Protection studies are clearly needed.

## DNA VACCINES

In mouse models, DNA vaccines induce protective immunity against DNA and RNA viruses. In higher mammals, only some cases of DNA vaccination have proven efficacious (9, 69). Attempts to immunize with DNA expression systems against CoV-induced diseases were limited until SARS-CoV appeared. Immunization with DNA expressing N protein was partially protective for IBV (225). As immunization with S protein to prevent FIP leads to ADE of disease, the expression of N or M protein using DNA plasmids was attempted, but this did not protect against challenge infection with FIPV (94).

To elicit protection against SARS, several approaches based on DNA vaccination have been used. Some of them included prime-boost strategies and showed that the combination of the DNA vaccine expressing the S protein and the whole chemically inactivated virus can be used to enhance the magnitude of the immune response, and also to change the balance of humoral and cellular immune responses, at least in the murine model. A combination of the DNA and inactivated virus induced Th1 immune responses, while the whole killed virus vaccine induced Th2 immune responses (291). Mice immunized intramuscularly with a DNA vaccine expressing S protein and intraperitoneally boosted with *E. coli* expressing S peptides showed high neutralization titers. This vaccine might have a practical value for immunizing civet cats due to its low cost (277).

Other DNA vaccines express N protein alone or linked to calreticulin. The first ones preferentially induced responses of the IgG2a isotype, IFN-γ and IL-2, and CD8$^+$ cytotoxic T-lymphocyte responses to N protein, but produced strong delayed-type hypersensitivity that could have undesired side effects (296). The expression of N protein linked to calreticulin increases major histocompatibility complex class I presentation of linked antigen to CD8$^+$ T cells, in the absence of reported adverse effects (134). These vaccines led to the generation of strong N-specific humoral and T-cell-mediated immune responses in mice, but no protection experiments were shown. N protein has also been expressed linked to hLAMP, an approach that targets antigen to major histocompatibility class II, leading to a stronger memory cellular immune response (101).

Studies on DNA immunization to protect against SARS have been reported using DNAs encoding either full-length S protein or S proteins lacking C-terminal cytoplasmic or transmembrane domains (283). These vaccines induced neutralizing antibodies and T-cell responses resulting in protective immunity in mice. Viral replication was reduced more than six orders of magnitude in the lungs of mice vaccinated with these S protein plasmid DNA expression vectors. Protection was mediated by a humoral but not a T-cell-dependent immune mechanism, as shown by adoptive T-cell transfer in which donor T cells were unable to reduce pulmonary viral replication in recipient animals. By contrast, passive transfer of purified IgG from immunized mice provided immune protection against SARS-CoV (283). The vector expressing the S protein with the cytoplasmic domain partially deleted induced the most potent neutralizing antibody response.

## DEVELOPMENT OF CoV VACCINES BASED ON VIRAL EXPRESSION VECTORS

### Poxvirus Expression Vector-Based Vaccines

Group 1 and 3 CoV vaccines based on poxvirus expression vectors have shown little success. In fact, inoculation of pigs with highly attenuated MVA vaccine expressing the full-length S glycoprotein of TGEV failed to protect pigs against challenge (113). Furthermore, in the case of FIPV or feline enteric CoV, immunization with vaccinia virus vectors expressing S proteins led to ADE of disease and earlier death after FIPV challenge (108, 137). Also, immunization to protect against group 3 CoVs, such as IBV, with recombinant vaccinia virus expressing IBV S protein showed no protection in the natural host (252), although neutralizing antibodies were induced in inoculated mice.

In contrast, the use of poxvirus vectors has led to protection against SARS. Using the MVA vector, SARS-CoV S protein has been expressed by several groups (23, 40). Intranasal or intramuscular immunization of BALB/c mice elicited protective immunity, as shown by the reduction of SARS-CoV titers in the upper and lower respiratory tract of mice after challenge. Furthermore, passive transfer of serum from recombinant MVA-S protein-immunized mice to naïve mice also reduced the replication of SARS-CoV in the respiratory tract after challenge, demonstrating a role for S protein-specific antibodies in protection. One group (40) showed the induction of neutralizing antibodies in mice, ferrets, and monkeys, although protection experiments were not performed. The majority of the antibodies raised by the MVA recombinant expressing the full-length S protein were adsorbed by an S protein fragment including aa 400 to 600, a region containing the RBD, indicating the relevance of this S protein domain in protection.

Using another highly restricted host range mutant of the vaccinia virus (DI), derived from an authorized strain of smallpox vaccine used in Japan, SARS-CoV proteins alone (E, M, N, and S proteins) or in different combinations (E, M, and S proteins together or E, M, N, and S proteins together) have been expressed. The recombinant DI-poxvirus vaccines were administered to mice either subcutaneously or intranasally. Replication-deficient DI vaccines expressing S alone or in combination with other components, but not N protein alone, elicited strong protective immune responses against SARS-CoV infection (121).

### Ad Vector-Based Vaccines

Adenovirus (Ad) vectors inducing immunity to CoVs have been developed, but protection has only been shown in mice or in passive protection experiments with swine challenged with TGEV. The full-length TGEV S protein, or fragments of different amino acid lengths extended from the amino terminus, have been expressed using an Ad5 vector (254). The recombinant antigens included different sets of antigenic sites C, B, D, and A, previously defined in the TGEV S protein (88). These recombinants infect hamsters and swine (253) and induce TGEV neutralizing antibodies. Furthermore, hamsters immunized with these recombinants secrete TGEV neutralizing antibodies in the milk during lactation (253). Newborn piglets were protected against TGE mortality and partially protected against infection if they were given serum from the swine that were vaccinated with Ad5 vectors expressing S sites A to D. However, no direct challenge of the recombinant TGEV-Ad5-vaccinated pigs has been reported. PRCV S protein was also expressed using recombinant Ad5 vectors (34). Pigs oronasally inoculated with the Ad5-S protein vaccine were not protected against PRCV nasal shedding after PRCV challenge, but they had shorter shedding and rapid anamnestic neutralizing antibody responses to PRCV. MHV S, N, and M proteins have been expressed using human Ad5. Mice intraperitoneally inoculated with these recombinants elicit serum antibodies. Only antibodies to S protein neutralized MHV in vitro. After intracerebral challenge with a lethal dose of MHV, a significant fraction of animals vaccinated with Ad vectors expressing either the S or the N protein were protected. This protective effect was significantly stronger when the animals were immunized several times with recombinants expressing both S and N proteins (273).

BCoV HE has been expressed using Ad5. The recombinant HE polypeptide exists in monomeric (65 kDa) and dimeric (130 kDa) forms. Mice inoculated intraperitoneally with live recombinant Ad5-HE elicited a significant level of BcoV neutralizing antibodies. Systemic and mucosal immunities were elicited (10). Still, no respiratory BCoV vaccine has been developed to prevent BCoV-associated pneumonia in calves or in cattle with shipping fever (209).

SARS vaccines based on the use of Ad vectors have shown that expression of S protein alone, or in combination with N protein, led to the protection of mice against challenge with SARS-CoV. The efficacy of immunization with adenovirus vectors was compared with that of chemically inactivated virus. Whole killed virus vaccine was more effective in conferring protective immunity against live SARS-CoV (223). Other Ad vaccines tested in mice have expressed either the S (26) or the N (292) protein and shown that the S2 domain and the N protein contain strong T-cell epitopes, but no challenge experiments have been reported. In the monkey model, Ad-based vaccines induced strong SARS-CoV-specific immune responses, indicating that these vectors are promising vaccine candidates, but, again, no information on protection has been provided (87). Ad5 vectors with deletions in the E1 and E3 regions have also been used to express the S1 domain of the SARS-CoV S protein (490 aa) (155). Wistar rats immunized three times with these recombinant Ads produced antiserum capable of protecting against SARS-CoV infection in cell culture. Histopathological examination found no evident side effects in the immunized animals. Nevertheless, in vivo protection experiments were not performed. Therefore, additional work is required with the Ad-based SARS vaccines.

To circumvent interference by preexisting immunity to human Ad5, a chimpanzee Ad vector with different serotype (AdC7) was developed. Its efficacy was assessed after intramuscular injection of the vector into mice, and preexisting antibodies showed a minimal effect on the potency of the AdC7-based genetic vaccine (298).

Finally, a recombinant Ad has been used in boosting a SARS-CoV DNA vaccine, and this regimen generated enhanced humoral and cellular immune responses to SARS-CoV N protein (43).

## Adeno-Associated Virus

Immunization of mice with recombinant adeno-associated virus expressing the RBD of SARS-CoV S protein elicited virus neutralizing antibodies. The level of these antibodies was increased at least fivefold by boosting with the vector (71), suggesting that recombinant adeno-associated virus vectors are promising SARS candidate vaccines.

## Venezuelan Equine Encephalitis (VEE) Virus Vector-Based Vaccines

Severe disease and high death rates were noted in senescent human populations infected with SARS-CoV, while children under 12 years of age did not develop the severe disease that was seen in adults (66, 170). These data suggest that the quality of the immune response may play a role in the outcome of virus infection. The ability of vaccines to induce robust immune responses in senescent experimental animals has been evaluated to determine if protection can be elicited in elderly populations.

To evaluate vaccine efficacy against homologous and heterologous strains, the Urbani S glycoprotein and N protein genes were inserted into VEE virus replicon particles (VRP-S or VRP-N) (66). In addition, expression of the influenza A virus hemagglutinin

(HA) glycoprotein (VRP-HA) was used as a control. Using reverse genetics, synthetically resurrected recombinant viruses bearing the GD03 S glycoprotein, which replicated to high titers in Vero and human airway epithelial cells, have been obtained (15). Importantly, human convalescent-phase sera which had plaque reduction neutralization titer 50% ($PRNT_{50}$) values of about 1:1,600 against late-phase isolates like Urbani nevertheless reduced about 10- to 15-fold the heterologous icGD03 virus ($PRNT_{50}$, 1:150). Young and senescent BALB/c mice with ages exceeding 1 year at the time of challenge were vaccinated with VRP-HA, VRP-S, VRP-N, or a combination of VRP-S and VRP-N and challenged with recombinant SARS-CoV expressing the Urbani S protein or the antigenically different GD03 S protein. In vaccinated animals, VRP-S vaccines provided complete short- and long-term protection against homologous challenge, protecting both young and senescent mice from Urbani strain replication. After challenge, VRP-S-vaccinated mice and mice vaccinated with VRP-S plus VRP-N displayed few, if any, pathological lesions in the lung, whereas VRP-HA-vaccinated aged mice demonstrated pathological lesions in the lung similar to those reported in the literature (206). VRP-S vaccines also provided short-term protection in young mice challenged with the heterologous GD03 S protein, despite the significantly reduced ability of anti-Urbani S protein antibody to neutralize virus expressing GD03 S protein. In contrast, vaccination of senescent mice with VRP-S provided limited protection (~38%) and the combination of VRP-S and VRP-N vaccines provided little long-term protection against infection by the antigenically different SARS-CoV GD03, although virus titers were reduced about 10-fold compared with VRP-HA-vaccinated controls. The SARS-CoV GD03 challenge also produced pathological lesions in both the VRP-HA- and SARS-CoV-vaccinated animals. These lesions were virtually indistinguishable from those produced by infection with the SARS-CoV Urbani strain. Therefore, it is likely that declining immunity of senescent animals in combination with the reduced ability of antibody to neutralize heterologous challenge viruses resulted in vaccine failure in aged animals.

It seems that vaccine approaches that induce less robust neutralization responses, like DNA and killed vaccines, might completely fail in protecting senescent populations against SARS-CoV GD03 challenge. Vaccine efficacy is often attenuated in the elderly (83, 233, 297). Immune complications include a generalized decrease in the function of B and T cells and innate immune function; diminished macrophage and granulocyte function, cellular traffic, and cell growth and differentiation; and decreased NK cell numbers and activity. New vaccine protocols should be developed eliciting complete protection against antigenically heterologous forms of SARS-CoV, especially in the most vulnerable elderly populations. There is a need for further testing of vaccines that induce an anti-N protein response in more animal models, similar to what has been described with other viral systems (84, 166).

### Parainfluenza Virus-Based Vectors

A vector based in an existing live attenuated parainfluenza virus that is being developed for intranasal pediatric immunization against human parainfluenza virus type 3 was used to express SARS-CoV S protein (33). Vector administration by mucosal immunization to African green monkeys resulted in the production of a systemic immune response. After challenge with SARS-CoV, all monkeys in the control group shed SARS-CoV. In contrast, no viral shedding occurred in the group immunized with the parainfluenza virus vector expressing the S protein. Recombinant viruses expressing SARS-CoV S, M, and N proteins, individually or in combination, have been evaluated for immunogenicity and protection in hamsters, as these animals support the replication of both SARS-CoV and the parainfluenza virus vector (32). A single intranasal administration of the vector expressing the S glycoprotein induced a high titer of SARS-CoV neutralizing antibodies, only twofold lower than that induced by SARS-CoV infection. This response provided complete protection against SARS-CoV challenge in the lower respiratory tract and partial protection in the upper respiratory tract. In contrast, expression of M, N, or E protein did not induce detectable serum SARS-CoV neutralizing antibodies.

### Rhabdovirus-Based Vector

A recombinant rabies virus vector has been used to express the S protein of SARS-CoV (79). Immunogenicity studies in mice showed the induction of SARS-CoV neutralizing antibodies after a single dose, but no protection studies have been shown. Similarly, an attenuated vesicular stomatitis virus vector was used to express the S protein of SARS-CoV (130). Mice vaccinated with this vector developed SARS-CoV neutralizing antibodies that controlled challenge with SARS-CoV performed at 1 or 4 months after a single vaccination. In summary, immunization to prevent SARS using different live vector systems has shown that protection is mainly mediated by humoral immune responses to the S protein. In general, protection against SARS-CoV has proven to be much more efficient than for other CoVs.

### CoV VACCINE CANDIDATES ENGINEERED BY REVERSE GENETICS

CoVs have several advantages as vectors over other viral expression systems: (i) CoVs are single-stranded RNA viruses that replicate in the cytoplasm without a DNA intermediary, making integration of the virus genome into the host cell chromosome unlikely (147); (ii) these viruses have the largest RNA virus genome and, in principle, have room for the insertion of large foreign genes (76); (iii) these viruses in general infect the mucosal surfaces, both respiratory and enteric, and therefore, vectors may be used to target the antigen to the enteric and respiratory areas to stimulate gut-associated lymphoid tissues and induce a strong pleiotropic secretory immune response; (iv) the tropism of CoVs can be engineered by modifying the S protein gene (14, 143, 217); (v) nonpathogenic CoV strains infecting most species of interest (human, porcine, bovine, canine, feline, and avian) are available and therefore suitable to develop safe virus vectors; and (vi) infectious CoV cDNA clones are available to design expression systems.

Two types of CoV vectors have been developed by engineering CoV genomes. One is based on helper-dependent expression systems (77). The other one is based on single genomes engineered by targeted recombination or by the construction of a cDNA encoding an infectious RNA. In addition, CoV-derived replicons have also been used for expression of foreign genes (77).

Targeted recombination introduces specific changes into the CoV genome through recombination between a donor synthetic RNA and a recipient parent virus possessing some characteristic that allows its counterselection (162). This strategy has some features that are essential for the development of vectors for vaccination and therapy: (i) it allows the generation of attenuated viruses by deletion of some genes (62, 103); (ii) it permits rearrangement of CoV gene order, providing a safety guard due to the low probability of restoring virulent progeny through recombination with virulent field CoV (64); and (iii) it permits facile engineering of vector tropism by modification of the S protein. The first nonviral protein expressed using a CoV-derived vector was green fluorescent protein (GFP) (82). The GFP gene was inserted into the MHV genome by replacing the nonessential gene 4 by targeted recombination. Further studies have shown that expression of the enhanced GFP under the control of an optimized transcription-regulating sequence (TRS), replacing gene 4, led to high and stable protein expression levels both in vitro and in vivo (219). Multivalent expression vectors were also generated by targeted recombination of the

MHV genome (61). Two unrelated luciferase genes were expressed at distinct genomic positions. Expression levels were a function of gene identity and insertion site, with higher expression levels close to the genome 3' end. In this study, expression of foreign genes was also combined with the deletion of nonessential genes and the rearrangement of CoV gene order. Combining these two strategies, in vivo attenuated and safe vector viruses can be generated (62, 64).

The first infectious CoV cDNA clone was obtained for TGEV. This cDNA was propagated as a bacterial artificial chromosome (BAC) (5), and its stability in *E. coli* was improved by the insertion of an intron (98). Since then, several infectious cDNAs have been engineered as BACs, such as SARS-CoV (3) and HCoV-OC43 (238). The major advantage of this system is that CoV reverse genetics only involves standard recombinant DNA technologies performed within bacteria, with high efficiency in the rescue of recombinant viruses (77). Two alternative procedures have also been used for the generation of infectious CoV cDNAs. One of them involves the assembling of a full-length CoV cDNA by in vitro ligation of adjoining cDNA subclones spanning the entire genomic RNA. The cDNA is then in vitro transcribed to generate a full-length CoV RNA that is infectious. The advantage of this system is that it allows the assembly of RNA or DNA genomes which are too large or unstable in cloning vectors (16). This strategy was first used to obtain an infectious TGEV cDNA (286), and it was subsequently improved and used to generate infectious cDNAs for MHV (288), SARS-CoV (287), and IBV (285). Another strategy to obtain CoV infectious cDNAs was based on the in vitro transcription of infectious RNA from a cDNA copy of a CoV genome that has been cloned and propagated in vaccinia virus. This strategy has been used to generate infectious clones for HCoV-229E (248) and IBV (36). The advantages of this system are the high stability of cloned cDNAs in the vaccinia virus and the fact that modifications can be made using homologous recombination of the vaccinia virus genome (30).

Single CoV-derived vectors have been generated for members of CoV groups 1, 2, and 3 using the infectious cDNAs described above. Vectors based on group 1 viruses have been derived from TGEV and HCoV-229E. Using the TGEV infectious cDNA maintained as a BAC, the GFP gene was successfully expressed by replacing the nonessential 3a and 3b genes by sequences encoding GFP. The engineered genome with the GFP gene at the position of ORF3a and -3b was very stable (>30 passages in cultured cells) and led to the production of high protein levels (50 $\mu$g/10$^6$ cells) (231). Therefore, expression levels

using these vectors are similar to those described for vectors derived from other positive strand RNA viruses such as Sindbis virus (1, 85). Using TGEV-derived vectors expressing GFP, the induction of lactogenic immunity has been demonstrated (231). Recombinant TGEVs have also been assembled by in vitro junction of six cDNA fragments encoding a full-length genome, in which the GFP gene has replaced ORF3a, leading to the production of a TGEV that grew to titers of 10$^8$ PFU/ml and expressed GFP in a high proportion of cells (55).

Group 2 CoV-derived vectors have been constructed for MHV. The gene encoding GFP was inserted into MHV replacing ORF4, resulting in high GFP expression levels (16). Group 3 CoV vectors have been engineered using the IBV genome. GFP was expressed replacing the nonessential gene 5a. The recombinant virus grew to a titer 10-fold lower than that of the wild-type virus, and GFP expression was lost at a very early passage (285).

Noninfectious CoV-derived vectors have also been generated based on replicons derived from the group 1 CoVs TGEV and HCoV-229E. The advantages of these systems are that (i) there is increased room for the insertion of foreign genes in comparison with infectious cDNAs, (ii) multigene expression vectors can be engineered due to the transcriptional strategy of CoVs, and (iii) there is increased safety during vaccination, as the replicons are noninfectious. A set of TGEV-derived replicons has been generated from the infectious cDNA. GFP was successfully expressed from these replicons, with high expression levels in 80% of the transfected cells (4). A multigene RNA replicon based on HCoV-229E has been developed (251) containing the 5' and 3' ends of this virus, the entire human CoV replicase gene, and three reporter genes (chloramphenicol acetyltransferase, luciferase, and GFP). Each reporter gene is located downstream of a human CoV TRS, which is required for the synthesis of individual mRNAs. The transfection of the vector and human CoV N protein mRNA into BHK-21 cells resulted in the expression of chloramphenicol acetyltransferase, luciferase, and GFP at relatively low levels (0.46 ng/10$^6$ cells, 25 relative light units/10$^6$ cells, and 3% of cells, respectively) (221, 249, 251). A SARS-CoV-derived replicon that includes N protein has also been constructed and is highly stable (3). This replicon is being used to address basic questions on SARS-CoV replication and to select antivirals.

Replication-competent propagation-deficient virus vectors have been developed based on complementing TGEV genomes deficient in the essential E protein gene with E-gene-expressing packaging cell lines (177). Two types of cell lines were constructed, transiently or stably expressing TGEV E protein. Virus titers were directly related to E protein expression levels (177).

A second strategy for the construction of replication-competent propagation-deficient TGEV genomes expressing heterologous genes involves the assembly of an infectious cDNA from six cDNA fragments ligated in vitro (55). The defective virus with the essential E protein gene deleted was complemented by the expression of the E gene using the VEE virus replicon. However, titers of recombinant virus expressing GFP were at least 10- to 100-fold lower (around $10^4$ PFU/ml) than with the system that used stably transformed cells or the Sindbis virus vector to complement E protein gene deletion (177).

In addition, it has been shown that HCoV-based vector RNA can be encapsidated into propagation-deficient pseudovirions that, in turn, can be used to transduce immature and mature human dendritic cells (251).

The effect of the deletion of group-specific genes in different CoVs has been studied. Studies using MHV as a model have shown that deletion mutants removing ORF4, -5a, and -7a and the HE gene are attenuating in the natural host (62). Similarly, studies deleting ORF7 of TGEV (178) and ORF3abc and -7ab of FIPV (102) led to virus attenuation. However, SARS-CoV deletion mutants lacking ORF3a, -3b, -6, -7a, or -7b influenced the in vitro and in vivo replication efficiency in the mouse model very little (290). Only deletion of ORF3a has shown a minor decrease (less than 1 log unit) in virus growth (290). All recombinant viruses replicated close to wild-type levels in the murine model, suggesting either that the group-specific ORFs play a small role in in vivo replication efficiency or that the mouse model is not of sufficient quality for discerning the role of the group-specific ORFs in disease. In fact, it has been surprising that ORFs like ORF3a, -7a, and -7b, which encode structural virus proteins (114, 122, 220, 228), have little influence on in vivo virus replication in the mouse model. Furthermore, deletion of more than one gene, such as deletion of ORF3a and -3b, or a combination of ORF7a and -7b, showed little effect on virus growth in the murine model. Therefore, the effect of SARS-CoV gene deletions needs to be tested in more relevant animal models. Interestingly, the simultaneous deletion of combinations of group-specific genes such as 6, 7a, 7b, 8a, 8b, and 9b has led to the production of an infectious SARS-CoV deletion mutant that propagates in cell culture with a titer almost identical to that of the parental wild-type virus. The virulence of this deletion mutant is being tested in vivo to determine whether it is a promising vaccine candidate (M. L. DeDiego, S. Perlman, and L. Enjuanes, unpublished results).

A recombinant SARS-CoV (rSARS-CoV) that lacks the E protein gene was attenuated in vitro and in an animal model (59). The E gene was previously shown to be a nonessential gene for group 2 CoV MHV (144), although elimination of this gene reduced virus growth in cell culture more than 1,000-fold. Interestingly, viable SARS-CoVs with a deletion of the E gene (SARS-CoV-ΔE) were recovered in Vero-E6 cells with a relatively high titer (around $10^6$ PFU/ml) (Fig. 2A) and also from human Huh-7 and CaCo-2 cells with reduced titers. Electron microscopy of cells infected with wild-type SARS-CoV and cells infected with SARS-CoV-ΔE showed higher virus production in parental-virus-infected cells. In contrast, for group 1 CoV TGEV, expression of the E gene product was essential for virus release and spread. Propagation of TGEV with a deletion of the E gene (TGEV-ΔE) was restored by providing E protein in *trans* (55, 177).

The hamster model has been used to study SARS-CoV-ΔE pathogenicity, because it demonstrates elements present in human cases of SARS-CoV infections, including interstitial pneumonitis and consolidation (59). An ideal animal model that completely reproduces human clinical disease and pathological findings has not been identified, and problems associated with the murine and primate models have been reported. Nevertheless, the hamster model reproducibly supports SARS-CoV replication in the respiratory tract to a higher titer and for a longer duration than in mice or nonhuman primates. Virus replication in this model is accompanied by histological evidence of pneumonitis, and the animals develop viremia and extrapulmonary spread of virus (207). Although overt clinical disease is absent, the hamster model is useful for the evaluation of SARS-CoV infection. Titers of rSARS-CoV achieved in the respiratory tract of hamsters were 100- to 1,000-fold higher than titers of the rSARS-CoV-ΔE virus, suggesting that this mutant virus is attenuated (Fig. 2B). Histopathological examination of lungs from infected hamsters was performed at 2 and 5 days postinfection, because it has been shown that pulmonary disease is most notable at these time points. Detection of viral antigen was reduced in lungs from rSARS-CoV-ΔE-infected hamsters, and pulmonary inflammation was less prominent in these animals than in rSARS-CoV-infected animals, indicating that rSARS-CoV-ΔE is attenuated in vivo (59). In fact, reduction of SARS-CoV titers in patients has been associated with a considerable reduction in pathogenicity and with increased survival rates (42, 118). Therefore, SARS-CoV-ΔE attenuated virus is a promising vaccine candidate that is being evaluated in other animal models (mice, ferrets, and macaques).

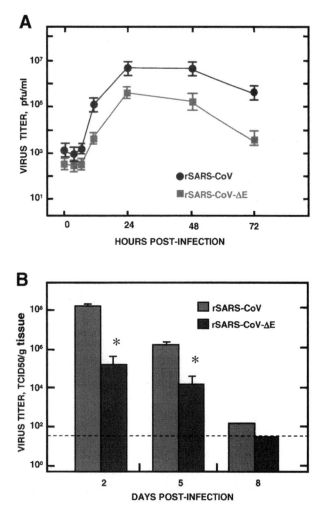

**Figure 2.** Growth kinetics of rSARS-CoV-ΔE in vitro and in vivo. (A) Vero-E6 cells were infected at a multiplicity of infection of 0.5 with either the rSARS-CoV-ΔE or the recombinant wild-type virus. At different times postinfection, virus titers were determined by plaque assay. Error bars represent standard deviations of the mean from three experiments. (B) Hamsters were inoculated with $10^3$ tissue culture infectious doses ($TCID_{50}$) of rSARS-CoV or rSARS-CoV-ΔE. Animals were sacrificed and tissues were harvested at different times postinfection. Viral titers in the lungs were determined in Vero-E6 cell monolayers. The nonparametric Mann-Whitney U statistical method was used for ascertaining the significance of observed differences. Statistical significance is indicated by an asterisk ($P < 0.05$). The dotted line indicates the lower limit of detection.

## FUTURE TRENDS IN SARS-CoV REVERSE-GENETICS VACCINES

Live attenuated virus vaccines face a series of potential concerns, including reversion to wild-type phenotype and recombination repair with circulating heterogeneous human CoVs or zoonotic SARS-CoV strains. Consequently, live virus vaccine formulations should include rational approaches for minimizing the potential for reversion to wild-type phenotype

and simultaneously resist recombination repair. It is clear that modifications of the SARS-CoV genome could lead to viruses with an attenuated phenotype that could be considered safe and effective vaccine candidates. The replicase as a target for attenuating CoVs is an unexplored territory, likely equipped with alleles that might influence replication efficiency and virulence. The SARS-CoV replicase represents a major target of future research endeavors.

CoVs have a characteristic, strictly conserved genome organization, with structural genes occurring in the order 5'-polymerase-S-E-M-N-3'. MHV mutants with the genes encoding the structural proteins located in different order were constructed (64). These recombinant viruses were tested for the ability to replicate in the natural host, the mouse. The results indicate that the canonical CoV genome organization is not essential for in vivo replication. Some of the mutants showed an attenuated phenotype, similar to what has been observed for vesicular stomatitis virus (13). Therefore, deliberate rearrangement of the viral genes may be useful in the generation of attenuated CoVs, which, due to their reduced risk of generating viable viruses by recombination with circulating field viruses, would make safer vaccines.

Vaccines based on modifications of the replicase gene could in principle be generated by mutagenesis, as modifications introduced in the MHV nsp1 coding regions have identified residues important for protein processing and viral RNA replication that may affect virus virulence and could be introduced in vaccine candidates (31). SARS-CoV nsp1 blocks host macromolecular synthesis and abrogates interferon signaling (128), providing further evidence that nsp1 coding regions represent potential virulence determinants. Alternatively, Tyr6398His substitution in ORF1b-nsp14 has been demonstrated that attenuates MHV replication in mice (236). Similarly, deletion of the nsp2 gene in MHV and SARS-CoV has been shown to yield viable attenuated mutant viruses that replicate about 1 log unit less efficiently than wild-type virus in cell culture and in animals, and may also provide a foundation for the design of live vaccines (100). As the nsp14 Tyr residue and nsp2 are highly conserved, it may be possible to engineer common *Coronaviridae* attenuating alleles via recombinant DNA techniques. Alternatively, changes in gene order within the replicase or even relocation to the 3' end of the genome, if tolerated, may lead to attenuated virus phenotypes.

Other options to include safeguards into the genetically engineered vaccines, particularly those that can prevent the recovery of the original virulent phenotype by recombination between the vaccine strain and viruses circulating in the field (such as

HCoV-229E, -OC43, or -NL63), have been developed. One of them is the construction of replication-competent, propagation-deficient viruses (pseudovirions) that are defective in one gene conferring an attenuated phenotype or even in virus propagation (74, 77). These viruses could be grown in packaging cell lines providing in *trans* the missing protein. In the case of SARS-CoV, vaccine candidates without the E protein gene have been constructed. In order to prevent the rescue of the virulent phenotype by recombination with a circulating HCoV, the deletion of an essential gene located in a position distant from gene E and the relocation of this gene to the position previously occupied by the E gene have been proposed. A potential recombination leading to the rescue of gene E would lead to the loss of the essential gene relocated to the position previously occupied by gene E.

An alternative approach for developing safer, recombination-resistant live CoV vaccines has been developed by modifying the TRS of a vaccine strain to a sequence incompatible with the TRS of any known circulating CoV. The idea here is that recombination events between wild-type CoVs and SARS-CoV with a remodeled TRS would result in genomes containing mixed regulatory sequences that block expression of subgenomic mRNAs and are therefore lethal (Fig. 3, top) (289). TRSs among CoVs are highly conserved and direct the expression of subgenomic RNAs. Using a molecular clone, the SARS-CoV TRS network was remodeled from ACGAAC to CCGGAT (Fig. 3, bottom). This rewiring of the genomic transcription network allows for efficient replication of the mutant virus. This recombinant virus replicated to titers equivalent to those of wild-type virus and expressed the typical ratios of subgenomic RNAs and proteins. Interestingly, some new transcripts were noted, initiating from the replicase gene, most of which could encode N-terminally truncated ORF1a polyproteins. It is not clear if these novel transcripts might influence pathogenic outcomes, although in some instances nsp3 is truncated, potentially allowing for the establishment of dominant negative phenotypes on replication in cell

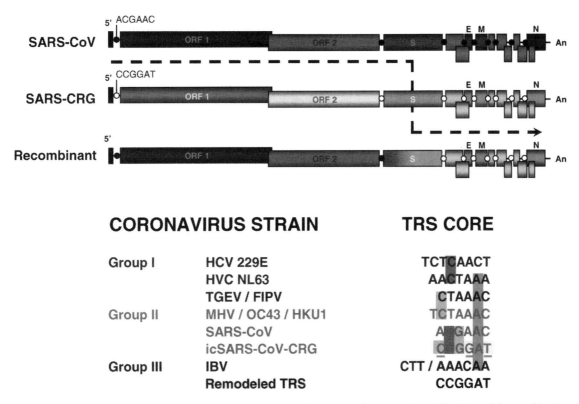

**CORONAVIRUS STRAIN**        **TRS CORE**

| | | |
|---|---|---|
| Group I | HCV 229E | TCTCAACT |
| | HVC NL63 | AACTAAA |
| | TGEV / FIPV | CTAAAC |
| Group II | MHV / OC43 / HKU1 | TCTAAAC |
| | SARS-CoV | ACGAAC |
| | icSARS-CoV-CRG | CCGGAT |
| Group III | IBV | CTT / AAACAA |
| | **Remodeled TRS** | CCGGAT |

Figure 3. Reorganization of the SARS-CoV genome to generate safe attenuated virus vaccines. (Top) Potential recombination between vaccine and field CoV strains leading to the generation of a recombinant SARS-CoV. The wild-type SARS-CoV TRS, ACGAAC (black circles), was changed to CCGGAT (white circles), leading to SARS-CRG virus. Since the wild-type and mutant TRS signals are not compatible in regulating subgenomic transcription (289), a recombination event resulting in a viral genome with mixed TRS signals is not viable. (Bottom) The icSARS-CoV TRS is unique from that of other described CoVs. TRSs for selected group 1, 2, and 3 CoVs are summarized. At the bottom, the TRS selected to generate a safe recombinant SARS-CoV is indicated.

culture and animals (289). An attractive SARS-CoV vaccine could further be modified by building attenuating mutations on the genetic template of the recombination-resistant TRS-rewired virus for use either as a safe, high-titer seed stock for making killed vaccines or as a live virus vaccine. One interesting refinement of this approach would be to include secondary traps that are activated in recombinant genomes. In this instance, wild-type TRSs can be designed into intragenic sites in essential ORFs like the S and M glycoprotein genes. In recombinant viruses encoding wild-type leader TRSs, subgenomic transcription might initiate within the essential structural genes and the resulting N-terminal deletions would likely be lethal or severely attenuating.

## POTENTIAL SIDE EFFECTS OF SARS-CoV VACCINES

Both humoral and T-cell-mediated responses to animal CoVs may exacerbate disease or cause new health problems (301). T-cell responses have been implicated in the demyelinization of the brain and spinal cord following infection with neurotropic MHV (37, 282). Adverse humoral responses to another group 2 CoV, BCoV, have also been linked to the development of shipping fever in cattle (171). Moreover, previous exposure to FIPV, or passive or active immunization against this virus, caused early-death syndrome instead of providing immune protection (181, 182, 270). This disease exacerbation was due to the virus-specific antibodies that facilitated and enhanced uptake and spread of the virus, causing ADE of infectivity (193, 261, 271), which is caused by S protein-specific antibodies (47, 48, 175, 176).

With this scenario of side effects caused by some CoV vaccines, a safety concern is that SARS-CoV could induce similar antibody- or cell-mediated immune pathologies. This concern was increased mainly by two reports. One study, utilizing lentivirus pseudotyped with various SARS-CoV S proteins (284), indicated that within the S protein, there are minor differences among eight strains transmitted during human outbreaks in early 2003, whereas substantial functional changes were detected in S protein derived from a case in late 2003 from Guandong Province, China (isolate GD03), and from two civet cats (SZ3 and SZ16). The GD03 S protein-pseudotyped virus is markedly resistant to antibody neutralization. Alternatively, antibodies that neutralized most human S glycoproteins enhanced virus entry mediated by two civet cat virus S glycoproteins related to the GD03 isolate (284). In a second study

(269), it has been shown that the administration of MVA-based SARS-CoV S vaccine, but not MVA alone, into ferrets followed by live SARS-CoV challenge resulted in enhanced hepatitis. Nevertheless, these side effects have not been reported in other studies with SARS-CoV in ferrets, in which it has been shown that ferrets are a useful model for SARS-CoV (161). Fortunately, ADE of disease has not been observed with any human SARS-CoV strain. Therefore, it will be important to assess vaccines in relevant animal models as they become available. Antibodies directed against SARS-CoV were found to be protective and not to enhance viral infectivity in the mouse or hamster models (23, 207, 240, 283) using inactivated SARS-CoV, or after immunization with recombinant Ad vectors expressing the S and N proteins of SARS-CoV (223). Nevertheless, the effect of these vaccines in humans remains unknown (301). Side effects have not been observed in other animal models, such as African green monkeys that, 2 months after administration of SARS-CoV into the respiratory tract, were challenged with SARS-CoV. No evidence of enhanced disease upon challenge was shown (165).

Consistent with these results, cynomolgus macaques immunized with different amounts of purified virus, in the absence or the presence of adjuvant, and challenged by the nasal route 30 days postimmunization showed no side effects even in the presence of low-titer neutralizing antibodies. Temperature, breathing, appetite, mental state, and all biochemical indexes were normal for immunized monkeys, and no abnormalities were observed in major organs such as the lungs, liver, and kidneys. All control nonvaccinated animals showed interstitial pneumonia. These results indicate that the purified SARS-CoV vaccine is safe in monkeys (199). In summary, immunization of mice using either S protein or whole inactivated virus (237), or of monkeys with whole inactivated SARS-CoV (199, 302), most frequently resulted in the absence of side effects after providing different types of SARS-CoV vaccines. However, these results should be interpreted with caution, as (i) the in vivo models are acute replication models that induce little, if any, disease pathology; (ii) most pathological examinations were conducted early after challenge, missing potential late manifestations of immune pathology that might be induced; and (iii) the impacts of host aging and virus heterologous challenge have not been well studied.

A different situation may be faced in immunization of elderly or senescent animal models. In fact, VEE virus expressing N protein failed to induce protection in either young or senescent mice, and resulted in enhanced immunopathology following viral challenge between days 4 and 14 postinfection. In young animals, N protein-induced pathology was also observed between 4 and 14 days postinfection, time points not evaluated in earlier studies. Therefore, caution has to be taken before including N protein in vaccine formulations by expressing N protein using DNA immunization, killed vaccines, or VEE virus vectors (66), as no protection was elicited in mice against homologous challenge, and no benefit to vaccination with a cocktail of both S and N proteins was observed. Rather, the coexpression of N protein in vaccine regimens which failed to simultaneously induce a strong neutralizing anti-S protein antibody response led to an increased number of lymphocytic and eosinophilic inflammatory infiltrates, which are also characteristic of the immune pathology observed with respiratory syncytial virus (RSV) infection, following vaccination with formalin-inactivated RSV (68, 104). Therefore, the concern has been raised that expression of N protein may result in vaccine-enhanced pulmonary disease, as previously described for viruses such as RSV (132). The data suggest that the presence of N protein in vaccines should be evaluated in each vaccine formulation (66). Although thus far, no human SARS-CoV S protein vaccine has been shown to be involved in ADE of disease, possible immunopathological complications of SARS vaccine candidates require rigorous clinical and immunological evaluation.

## CONCLUDING REMARKS

Whereas the production of effective and safe vaccines for animal CoVs previously reported has not been satisfactory (38, 75, 209), the production of inactivated, subunit, or vaccines based on DNA or recombinant vectors, or by reverse genetics using SARS-CoV genomes, seems more promising. An optimum animal model for SARS-CoV vaccine evaluation is still required. After preclinical trials in animal models, efficacy and safety evaluation of the most promising vaccine candidates described has to be performed in humans.

**Acknowledgments.** This work was supported by grants from the Comisión Interministerial de Ciencia y Tecnología (CICYT), the Consejería de Educación y Cultura de la Comunidad de Madrid, Fort Dodge Veterinaria, and the European Communities (Frame VI, DISSECT project SP22-CT-2004-511060). Marta L. DeDiego received a fellowship from the Department Education and Science of Spain. Enrique Alvarez received a contract from the National Institute of Health (ISCIII) of Spain. Carmen Capiscol received a fellowship from the Community of Madrid. This work was also supported by National Institutes of Health grants AI059136 and AI059443 to R.B.

## REFERENCES

1. Agapov, E. V., I. Frolov, B. D. Lindenbach, B. M. Pragai, S. Schlesinger, and C. M. Rice. 1998. Noncytopathic Sindbis virus RNA vectors for heterologous gene expression. *Proc. Natl. Acad. Sci. USA* **95:**12989–12994.

2. Akerström, S., Y. J. Tan, and A. Mirazimi. 2006. Amino acids 15–28 in the ectodomain of SARS coronavirus 3a protein induces [sic] neutralizing antibodies. *FEBS Lett.* **580:**3799–3803.

3. Almazán, F., M. L. DeDiego, C. Galán, D. Escors, E. Álvarez, J. Ortego, I. Sola, S. Zuñiga, S. Alonso, J. L. Moreno, A. Nogales, C. Capiscol, and L. Enjuanes. 2006. Construction of a severe acute respiratory syndrome coronavirus infectious cDNA clone and a replicon to study coronavirus RNA synthesis. *J. Virol.* **80:**10900–10906.

4. Almazan, F., C. Galan, and L. Enjuanes. 2004. The nucleoprotein is required for efficient coronavirus genome replication. *J. Virol.* **78:**12683–12688.

5. Almazán, F., J. M. González, Z. Pénzes, A. Izeta, E. Calvo, J. Plana-Durán, and L. Enjuanes. 2000. Engineering the largest RNA virus genome as an infectious bacterial artificial chromosome. *Proc. Natl. Acad. Sci. USA* **97:**5516–5521.

6. Anton, I. M., S. Gonzalez, M. J. Bullido, M. Corsin, C. Risco, J. P. Langeveld, and L. Enjuanes. 1996. Cooperation between transmissible gastroenteritis coronavirus (TGEV) structural proteins in the in vitro induction of virus-specific antibodies. *Virus Res.* **46:**111–124.

7. Anton, I. M., C. Sune, R. H. Meloen, F. Borras-Cuesta, and L. Enjuanes. 1995. A transmissible gastroenteritis coronavirus nucleoprotein epitope elicits T helper cells that collaborate in the in vitro antibody synthesis to the three major structural viral proteins. *Virology* **212:**746–751.

8. Arvidson, Y., G. A. Tannock, M. Zerbes, and J. Ignjatovic. 1991. Efficacy of Australian vaccines against recent isolates of avian infectious bronchitis viruses. *Aust. Vet. J.* **68:**211–212.

9. Arvin, A. M., and H. B. Greenberg. 2006. New viral vaccines. *Virology* **344:**240–249.

10. Baca-Estrada, M. E., X. Liang, L. A. Babiuk, and D. Yoo. 1995. Induction of mucosal immunity in cotton rats to haemagglutinin-esterase glycoprotein of bovine coronavirus by recombinant adenovirus. *Immunology* **86:**134–140.

11. Bae, J. L., J. G. Lee, T. J. Kang, H. S. Jang, Y. S. Jang, and M. S. Yang. 2003. Induction of antigen-specific systemic and mucosal immune responses by feeding animals transgenic plants expressing the antigen. *Vaccine* **21:**4052–4058.

12. Baldwin, C. W., and F. W. Scott. 1997. Attempted immunization of cats with feline infectious peritonitis virus propagated at reduced temperatures. *Am. J. Vet. Res.* **58:**251–256.

13. Ball, L. A., C. R. Pringle, B. Flanagan, V. P. Perepelitsa, and G. W. Wertz. 1999. Phenotypic consequences of rearranging the P, M, and, G genes of vesicular stomatis virus. *J. Virol.* **73:**4705–4712.

14. Ballesteros, M. L., C. M. Sanchez, and L. Enjuanes. 1997. Two amino acid changes at the N-terminus of transmissible gastroenteritis coronavirus spike protein result in the loss of enteric tropism. *Virology* **227:**378–388.

15. Baric, R. S., T. Sheahan, D. Deming, E. Donaldson, B. Yount, A. C. Sims, R. S. Roberts, M. Frieman, and B. Rockx. 2006. SARS coronavirus vaccine development. *Adv. Exp. Med. Biol.* **581:**553–560.

16. Baric, R. S., and A. C. Sims. 2005. Development of mouse hepatitis virus and SARS-CoV infectious cDNA constructs. *Curr. Top. Microbiol. Immunol.* **287:**229–252.

17. Barlough, J. E., C. M. Johnson-Lussenburg, C. A. Stoddart, R. H. Jacobson, and F. W. Scott. 1985. Experimental inoculation

of cats with human coronavirus 229E and subsequent challenge with feline infectious peritonitis virus. *Can. J. Comp. Med.* **49**:303–307.

18. Barlough, J. E., C. A. Stoddart, G. P. Soresso, R. H. Jacobson, and F. W. Scott. 1984. Experimental inoculation of cats with canine coronavirus and subsequent challenge with feline infectious peritonitis virus. *Lab. Anim. Sci.* **34**:592–597.

19. Bastien, N., K. Anderson, L. Hart, P. Van Caeseele, K. Brandt, D. Milley, T. Hatchette, E. C. Weiss, and Y. Li. 2005. Human coronavirus NL63 infection in Canada. *J. Infect. Dis.* **191**:503–506.

20. Baudoux, P., C. Carrat, L. Besnardeau, B. Charley, and H. Laude. 1998. Coronavirus pseudoparticles formed with recombinant M and E proteins induce alpha interferon synthesis by leukocytes. *J. Virol.* **72**:8636–8643.

21. Berry, J. D., S. Jones, M. A. Drebot, A. Andonov, M. Sabara, X. Y. Yuan, H. Weingartl, L. Fernando, P. Marszal, J. Gren, B. Nicolas, M. Andonova, F. Ranada, M. J. Gubbins, T. B. Ball, P. Kitching, Y. Li, A. Kabani, and F. Plummer. 2004. Development and characterization of neutralising monoclonal antibody to the SARS-coronavirus. *J. Virol. Methods* **120**:87–96.

22. Bestagno, M., I. Sola, E. Dallegno, P. Sabella, M. Poggianella, J. Plana-Duran, L. Enjuanes, and O. R. Burrone. 2007. Recombinant dimeric small immunoproteins neutralize transmissible gastroenteritis virus infectivity efficiently in vitro and confer passive immunity in vivo. *J. Gen. Virol.* **88**:187–195.

23. Bisht, H., A. Roberts, L. Vogel, A. Bukreyev, P. L. Collins, B. R. Murphy, K. Subbarao, and B. Moss. 2004. Severe acute respiratory syndrome coronavirus spike protein expressed by attenuated vaccinia virus protectively immunizes mice. *Proc. Natl. Acad. Sci. USA* **101**:6641–6646.

24. Bisht, H., A. Roberts, L. Vogel, K. Subbarao, and B. Moss. 2005. Neutralizing antibody and protective immunity to SARS coronavirus infection of mice induced by a soluble recombinant polypeptide containing an N-terminal segment of the spike glycoprotein. *Virology* **334**:160–165.

25. Boots, A. M. H., B. J. Benaissatrouw, W. Hesselink, E. Rijke, C. Schrier, and E. J. Hensen. 1992. Induction of anti-viral immune responses by immunization with recombinant-DNA encoded avian coronavirus nucleocapsid protein. *Vaccine* **10**:119–124.

26. Boyer, J., A. Krause, J. Qiu, N. Hackett, G. Kobinger, Y. Zhi, J. M. Wilson, and R. G. Crystal. 2004. Anti-SARS humoral and cellular immunity evoked by an adenovirus vector expressing spike glycoprotein from SARS coronavirus. *Mol. Ther.* **9**:210.

27. Bradbury, J. 2003. Custom-made vaccines at speed. *Drug Discov. Today* **8**:518–519.

28. Brim, T. A., J. L. Van Cott, J. K. Lunney, and L. J. Saif. 1995. Cellular immune responses of pigs after primary inoculation with porcine respiratory coronavirus or transmissible gastroenteritis virus and challenge with transmissible gastroenteritis virus. *Vet. Immunol. Immunopathol.* **48**:35–54.

29. Brim, T. A., J. L. Van Cott, J. K. Lunney, and L. J. Saif. 1994. Lymphocyte proliferation responses of pigs inoculated with transmissible gastroenteritis virus or porcine respiratory coronavirus. *Am. J. Vet. Res.* **55**:494–501.

30. Britton, P., S. Evans, B. Dove, M. Davies, R. Casais, and D. Cavanagh. 2005. Generation of a recombinant avian coronavirus infectious bronchitis virus using transient dominant selection. *J. Virol. Methods* **123**:203–211.

31. Brockway, S. M., and M. R. Denison. 2005. Mutagenesis of the murine hepatitis virus nsp1-coding region identifies residues important for protein processing, viral RNA synthesis, and viral replication. *Virology* **340**:209–223.

32. Buchholz, U. J., A. Bukreyev, L. Yang, E. W. Lamirande, B. R. Murphy, K. Subbarao, and P. L. Collins. 2004. Contributions of the structural proteins of severe acute respiratory syndrome coronavirus to protective immunity. *Proc. Natl. Acad. Sci. USA* **101**:9804–9809.

33. Bukreyev, A., E. W. Lamirande, U. J. Buchholz, L. N. Vogel, W. R. Elkins, M. St. Claire, B. R. Murphy, K. Subbarao, and P. L. Collins. 2004. Mucosal immunisation of African green monkeys (Cercopithecus aethiops) with an attenuated parainfluenza virus expressing the SARS coronavirus spike protein for the prevention of SARS. *Lancet* **363**:2122–2127.

34. Callebaut, P., L. Enjuanes, and M. Pensaert. 1996. An adenovirus recombinant expressing the spike glycoprotein of porcine respiratory coronavirus immunogenic in swine. *J. Gen. Virol.* **77**:309–313.

35. Carmichael, L. E. 1997. *Vaccine for Dogs.* Elsevier, New York, NY.

36. Casais, R., V. Thiel, S. G. Siddell, D. Cavanagh, and P. Britton. 2001. Reverse genetics system for the avian coronavirus infectious bronchitis virus. *J. Virol.* **75**:12359–12369.

37. Castro, R. F., and S. Perlman. 1995. CD8$^+$ T-cell epitopes within the surface glycoprotein of a neurotropic coronavirus and correlation with pathogenicity. *J. Virol.* **69**:8127–8131.

38. Cavanagh, D. 2003. Severe acute respiratory syndrome vaccine development: experiences of vaccination against avian infectious bronchitis coronavirus. *Avian Pathol.* **32**:567–582.

39. Cavanagh, D., K. Mawditt, M. Sharma, S. E. Drury, H. L. Ainsworth, P. Britton, and R. E. Gough. 2001. Detection of a coronavirus from turkey poults in Europe genetically related to infectious bronchitis virus of chickens. *Avian Pathol.* **30**:355–368.

40. Chen, Z., L. Zhang, C. Qin, L. Ba, C. E. Yi, F. Zhang, Q. Wei, T. He, W. Yu, J. Yu, H. Gao, X. Tu, A. Gettie, M. Farzan, K. Y. Yuen, and D. D. Ho. 2005. Recombinant modified vaccinia virus Ankara expressing the spike glycoprotein of severe acute respiratory syndrome coronavirus induces protective neutralizing antibodies primarily targeting the receptor binding region. *J. Virol.* **79**:2678–2688.

41. Chinese SARS Molecular Epidemiology Consortium. 2004. Molecular evolution of the SARS coronavirus during the course of the SARS epidemic in China. *Science* **303**:1666–1669.

42. Chu, C. M., L. L. Poon, V. C. Cheng, K. S. Chan, I. F. Hung, M. M. Wong, K. H. Chan, W. S. Leung, B. S. Tang, V. L. Chan, W. L. Ng, T. C. Sim, P. W. Ng, K. I. Law, D. M. Tse, J. S. Peiris, and K. Y. Yuen. 2004. Initial viral load and the outcomes of SARS. *Can. Med. Assoc. J.* **171**:1349–1352.

43. Chunling, M., Y. Kun, X. Jian, Q. Jian, S. Hua, and Z. Minsheng. 2006. Enhanced induction of SARS-CoV nucleocapsid protein-specific immune response using DNA vaccination followed by adenovirus boosting in BALB/c mice. *Intervirology* **49**:307–318.

44. Compton, S. R., C. B. Stephensen, S. W. Snyder, D. G. Weismiller, and K. V. Holmes. 1992. Coronavirus species specificity: murine coronavirus binds to a mouse-specific epitope on its carcinoembryonic antigen-related receptor glycoprotein. *J. Virol.* **66**:7420–7428.

45. Cook, J. K. A., J. Chesher, W. Baxendale, N. Greenwood, M. B. Huggins, and S. J. Orbell. 2001. Protection of chickens against renal damage caused by a nephropathogenic infectious bronchitis virus. *Avian Pathol.* **30**:423–426.

46. Cook, J. K. A., S. J. Orbell, M. A. Woods, and M. B. Huggins. 1999. Breadth of protection of the respiratory tract provided by different live-attenuated infectious bronchitis vaccines against challenge with infectious bronchitis viruses of heterologous types. *Avian Pathol.* **28**:471–479.

47. Corapi, W. V., R. J. Darteil, J.-C. Audonnet, and G. E. Chappuis. 1995. Localization of antigenic sites of the S glycoprotein of feline infectious peritonitis virus involved in neutralization and antibody-dependent enhancement. *J. Virol.* 69:2858–2862.

48. Corapi, W. V., C. W. Olsen, and F. W. Scott. 1992. Monoclonal antibody analysis of neutralization and antibody-dependent enhancement of feline infectious peritonitis virus. *J. Virol.* 66:6695–6705.

49. Corse, E., and C. E. Machamer. 2003. The cytoplasmic tails of infectious bronchitis virus E and M proteins mediate their interaction. *Virology* 312:25–34.

50. Corse, E., and C. E. Machamer. 2000. Infectious bronchitis virus E protein is targeted to the Golgi complex and directs release of virus-like particles. *J. Virol.* 74:4319–4326.

51. Cox, E., J. Hooyberghs, and M. B. Pensaert. 1990. Sites of replication of a porcine respiratory coronavirus related to transmissible gastroenteritis virus. *Res. Vet. Sci.* 48:165–169.

52. Cox, E., M. B. Pensaert, and P. Callebaut. 1993. Intestinal protection against challenge with transmissible gastroenteritis virus of pigs immune after infection with the porcine respiratory coronavirus. *Vaccine* 11:267–272.

53. Cox, E., M. B. Pensaert, P. Callebaut, and K. van Deun. 1990. Intestinal replication of a porcine respiratory coronavirus closely related antigenically to the enteric transmissible gastroenteritis virus. *Vet. Microbiol.* 23:237–243.

54. Crouch, C. F., S. Oliver, D. C. Hearle, A. Buckley, A. J. Chapman, and M. J. Francis. 2000. Lactogenic immunity following vaccination of cattle with bovine coronavirus. *Vaccine* 19:189–196.

55. Curtis, K. M., B. Yount, and R. S. Baric. 2002. Heterologous gene expression from transmissible gastroenteritis virus replicon particles. *J. Virol.* 76:1422–1434.

56. Daniel, C., and P. J. Talbot. 1990. Protection from lethal coronavirus infection by affinity-purified spike glycoprotein of murine hepatitis virus, strain A59. *Virology* 174:87–94.

57. Darbyshire, J. H., and R. W. Peters. 1984. Sequential development of humoral immunity and assessment of protection in chickens following vaccination and challenge with avian infectious bronchitis virus. *Res. Vet. Sci.* 37:77–86.

58. Darbyshire, J. H., J. G. Rowell, J. K. Cook, and R. W. Peters. 1979. Taxonomic studies on strains of avian infectious bronchitis virus using neutralisation tests in tracheal organ cultures. *Arch. Virol.* 61:227–238.

59. DeDiego, M. L., E. Alvarez, F. Almazan, M. T. Rejas, E. Lamirande, A. Roberts, W. J. Shieh, S. R. Zaki, K. Subbarao, and L. Enjuanes. 2007. A severe acute respiratory syndrome coronavirus that lacks the E gene is attenuated in vitro and in vivo. *J. Virol.* 81:1701–1713.

60. de Haan, C. A., B. J. Haijema, D. Boss, F. W. Heuts, and P. J. Rottier. 2005. Coronaviruses as vectors: stability of foreign gene expression. *J. Virol.* 79:12742–12751.

61. de Haan, C. A., L. van Genne, J. N. Stoop, H. Volders, and P. J. Rottier. 2003. Coronaviruses as vectors: position dependence of foreign gene expression. *J. Virol.* 77:11312–11323.

62. de Haan, C. A. M., P. S. Masters, S. Shen, S. Weiss, and P. J. M. Rottier. 2002. The group-specific murine coronavirus genes are not essential, but their deletion, by reverse genetics, is attenuating in the natural host. *Virology* 296:177–189.

63. de Haan, C. A. M., H. Vennema, and P. J. M. Rottier. 2000. Assembly of the coronavirus envelope: homotypic interactions between the M proteins. *J. Virol.* 74:4967–4978.

64. de Haan, C. A. M., H. Volders, C. A. Koetzner, P. S. Masters, and P. J. M. Rottier. 2002. Coronaviruses maintain viability despite dramatic rearrangements of the strictly conserved genome organization. *J. Virol.* 76:12491–12502.

65. Delmas, B., J. Gelfi, and H. Laude. 1986. Antigenic structure of transmissible gastroenteritis virus. II. Domains in the peplomer glycoprotein. *J. Gen. Virol.* 67:1405–1418.

66. Deming, D., T. Sheahan, M. Heise, B. Yount, N. Davis, A. Sims, M. Suthar, J. Harkema, A. Whitmore, R. Pickles, A. West, E. Donaldson, K. Curtis, R. Johnston, and R. Baric. 2006. Vaccine efficacy in senescent mice challenged with recombinant SARS-CoV bearing epidemic and zoonotic spike variants. *PLoS Med.* 3:2359–2375.

67. Denison, M. R. 1999. The common cold. Rhinoviruses and coronaviruses, p. 253–280. *In* R. Dolin and P. F. Wright (ed.), *Lung Biology in Health and Disease*, vol. 127. *Viral Infections of the Respiratory Tract*. Marcel Dekker, Inc., New York, NY.

68. De Swart, R. L., T. Kuiken, H. H. Timmerman, G. van Amerongen, B. G. Van Den Hoogen, H. W. Vos, H. J. Neijens, A. C. Andeweg, and A. D. Osterhaus. 2002. Immunization of macaques with formalin-inactivated respiratory syncytial virus (RSV) induces interleukin-13-associated hypersensitivity to subsequent RSV infection. *J. Virol.* 76:11561–11569.

69. Donnelly, J. J., B. Wahren, and M. A. Liu. 2005. DNA vaccines: progress and challenges. *J. Immunol.* 175:633–639.

70. Drosten, C., S. Günther, W. Preiser, S. van der Werf, H.-R. Brodt, S. Becker, H. Rabenau, M. Panning, L. Kolesnikova, R. A. M. Fouchier, A. Berger, A.-M. Burguière, J. Cinatl, M. Eickmann, N. Escriou, K. Grywna, S. Kramme, J.-C. Manuguerra, S. Müller, V. Rickerts, M. Stürmer, S. Vieth, H.-D. Klenk, A. D. M. E. Osterhaus, H. Schmitz, and H. W. Doerr. 2003. Identification of a novel coronavirus in patients with severe acute respiratory syndrome. *N. Engl. J. Med.* 348:1967–1976.

71. Du, L., Y. He, Y. Wang, H. Zhang, S. Ma, C. K. Wong, S. H. Wu, F. Ng, J. D. Huang, K. Y. Yuen, S. Jiang, Y. Zhou, and B. J. Zheng. 2006. Recombinant adeno-associated virus expressing the receptor-binding domain of severe acute respiratory syndrome coronavirus S protein elicits neutralizing antibodies: implication for developing SARS vaccines. *Virology* 353: 6–16.

72. Enjuanes, L. (ed.). 2005. *Current Topics in Microbiology and Immunology* vol. 287. *Coronavirus Replication and Reverse Genetics*. Springer, Berlin, Germany.

73. Enjuanes, L., F. Almazan, and J. Ortego. 2003. Virus-based vectors for gene expression in mammalian cells: coronavirus, p. 151–168. *In* S. C. Makrides (ed.), *Gene Transfer and Expression in Mammalian Cells*. Elsevier Science B.V., Boston, MA.

74. Enjuanes, L., M. L. DeDiego, E. Alvarez, D. Deming, T. Sheahan, and R. Baric. Vaccines to prevent severe acute respiratory syndrome coronavirus-induced disease. *Virus Res.*, in press. [Epub ahead of print.] doi:10.1016/j.virres.2007.01.010.

75. Enjuanes, L., C. Smerdou, J. Castilla, I. M. Anton, J. M. Torres, I. Sola, J. Golvano, J. M. Sanchez, and B. Pintado. 1995. Development of protection against coronavirus induced diseases. A review. *Adv. Exp. Med. Biol.* 380:197–211.

76. Enjuanes, L., I. Sola, F. Almazán, J. Ortego, A. Izeta, J. M. González, S. Alonso, J. M. Sánchez-Morgado, D. Escors, E. Calvo, C. Riquelme, and C. M. Sánchez. 2001. Coronavirus derived expression systems. *J. Biotechnol.* 88:183–204.

77. Enjuanes, L., I. Sola, S. Alonso, D. Escors, and S. Zúñiga. 2005. Coronavirus reverse genetics and development of vectors for gene expression. *Curr. Top. Microbiol. Immunol.* 287:161–197.

78. Enjuanes, L., and B. A. M. Van der Zeijst. 1995. Molecular basis of transmissible gastroenteritis coronavirus epidemiology, p. 337–376. *In* S. G. Siddell (ed.), The *Coronaviridae*. Plenum Press, New York, NY.

79. Faber, M., E. W. Lamirande, A. Roberts, A. B. Rice, H. Koprowski, B. Dietzschold, and M. J. Schnell. 2005. A single immunization with a rhabdovirus-based vector expressing severe acute respiratory syndrome coronavirus (SARS-CoV) S

protein results in the production of high levels of SARS-CoV-neutralizing antibodies. *J. Gen. Virol.* **86**:1435–1440.

80. Farsang, A., C. Ros, L. H. Renstrom, C. Baule, T. Soos, and S. Belak. 2002. Molecular epizootiology of infectious bronchitis virus in Sweden indicating the involvement of a vaccine strain. *Avian Pathol.* **31**:229–236.

81. Fehr, D., E. Holznagel, S. Bolla, B. Hauser, A. A. Herrewegh, M. C. Horzinek, and H. Lutz. 1997. Placebo-controlled evaluation of a modified live virus vaccine against feline infectious peritonitis: safety and efficacy under field conditions. *Vaccine* **15**:1101–1109.

82. Fischer, F., C. F. Stegen, C. A. Koetzner, and P. S. Masters. 1997. Analysis of a recombinant mouse hepatitis virus expressing a foreign gene reveals a novel aspect of coronavirus transcription. *J. Virol.* **71**:5148–5160.

83. Frasca, D., R. L. Riley, and B. B. Blomberg. 2005. Humoral immune response and B-cell functions including immunoglobulin class switch are downregulated in aged mice and humans. *Semin. Immunol.* **17**:378–384.

84. Frech, S. A., R. T. Kenney, C. A. Spyr, H. Lazar, J. F. Viret, C. Herzog, R. Gluck, and G. M. Glenn. 2005. Improved immune responses to influenza vaccination in the elderly using an immunostimulant patch. *Vaccine* **23**:946–950.

85. Frolov, I., T. A. Hoffman, B. M. Prágai, S. A. Dryga, H. V. Huang, S. Schlesinger, and C. M. Rice. 1996. Alphavirus-based expression vectors: strategies and applications. *Proc. Natl. Acad. Sci. USA* **93**:11371–11377.

86. Fulker, R., T. Wasmoen, R. Atchison, H. J. Chu, and W. Acree. 1995. Efficacy of an inactivated vaccine against clinical disease caused by canine coronavirus. *Adv. Exp. Med. Biol.* **380**:229–234.

87. Gao, W., A. Tamin, A. Soloff, L. D'Aiuto, E. Nwanegbo, P. D. Robbins, W. J. Bellini, S. Barratt-Boyes, and A. Gambotto. 2003. Effects of a SARS-associated coronavirus vaccine in monkeys. *Lancet* **362**:1895–1896.

88. Gebauer, F., W. A. P. Posthumus, I. Correa, C. Suñé, C. M. Sánchez, C. Smerdou, J. A. Lenstra, R. Meloen, and L. Enjuanes. 1991. Residues involved in the formation of the antigenic sites of the S protein of transmissible gastroenteritis coronavirus. *Virology* **183**:225–238.

89. Gelb, J., Jr., Y. Weisman, B. S. Ladman, and R. Meir. 2005. S1 gene characteristics and efficacy of vaccination against infectious bronchitis virus field isolates from the United States and Israel (1996 to 2000). *Avian Pathol.* **34**:194–203.

90. Gerber, J. D. 1995. Overview of the development of a modified live temperature sensitive FIPV vaccine. *Feline Pract.* **23**:62–66.

91. Gerber, J. D., J. D. Ingersoll, A. M. Gast, K. K. Christianson, N. L. Selzer, R. M. Landon, N. E. Pfeiffer, R. L. Sharpee, and W. H. Beckenhauer. 1990. Protection against feline infectious peritonitis by intranasal inoculation of a temperature-sensitive FIPV vaccine. *Vaccine* **8**:536–541.

92. German, A. C., C. R. Helps, and D. A. Harbour. 2004. FIP: a novel approach to vaccination. Proceedings from the 2nd International FCoV/FIP Symposium, Glasgow, 4–7 August 2002. *J. Feline Med. Surg.* **6**:119–124.

93. Gerna, G., G. Campanini, F. Rovida, E. Percivalle, A. Sarasini, A. Marchi, and F. Baldanti. 2006. Genetic variability of human coronavirus OC43-, 229E-, and NL63-like strains and their association with lower respiratory tract infections of hospitalized infants and immunocompromised patients. *J. Med. Virol.* **78**:938–949.

94. Glansbeek, H. L., B. L. Haagmans, E. G. te Lintelo, H. F. Egberink, V. Duquesne, A. Aubert, M. C. Horzinek, and P. J. Rottier. 2002. Adverse effects of feline IL-12 during DNA vaccination against feline infectious peritonitis virus. *J. Gen. Virol.* **83**:1–10.

95. Glass, W. G., K. Subbarao, B. Murphy, and P. M. Murphy. 2004. Mechanisms of host defense following severe acute respiratory syndrome-coronavirus (SARS-CoV) pulmonary infection of mice. *J. Immunol.* **173**:4030–4039.

96. Godeke, G. J., C. A. de Haan, J. W. Rossen, H. Vennema, and P. J. Rottier. 2000. Assembly of spikes into coronavirus particles is mediated by the carboxy-terminal domain of the spike protein. *J. Virol.* **74**:1566–1571.

97. Gonzalez, J. M., P. Gomez-Puertas, D. Cavanagh, A. E. Gorbalenya, and L. Enjuanes. 2003. A comparative sequence analysis to revise the current taxonomy of the family Coronaviridae. *Arch. Virol.* **148**:2207–2235.

98. Gonzalez, J. M., Z. Penzes, F. Almazan, E. Calvo, and L. Enjuanes. 2002. Stabilization of a full-length infectious cDNA clone of transmissible gastroenteritis coronavirus by the insertion of an intron. *J. Virol.* **76**:4655–4661.

99. Gough, R. E., and D. J. Alexander. 1979. Comparison of duration of immunity in chickens infected with a live infectious bronchitis vaccine by three different routes. *Res. Vet. Sci.* **26**:329–332.

100. Graham, R. L., A. C. Sims, S. M. Brockway, R. S. Baric, and M. R. Denison. 2005. The nsp2 replicase proteins of murine hepatitis virus and severe acute respiratory syndrome coronavirus are dispensable for viral replication. *J. Virol.* **79**:13399–13411.

101. Gupta, V., T. M. Tabiin, K. Sun, A. Chandrasekaran, A. Anwar, K. Yang, P. Chikhlikar, J. Salmon, V. Brusic, E. T. Marques, S. N. Kellathur, and T. J. August. 2006. SARS coronavirus nucleocapsid immunodominant T-cell epitope cluster is common to both exogenous recombinant and endogenous DNA-encoded immunogens. *Virology* **347**:127–139.

102. Haijema, B. J., H. Volders, and P. J. Rottier. 2004. Live, attenuated coronavirus vaccines through the directed deletion of group-specific genes provide protection against feline infectious peritonitis. *J. Virol.* **78**:3863–3871.

103. Haijema, B. J., H. Volders, and P. J. M. Rottier. 2003. Switching species tropism: an effective way to manipulate the feline coronavirus genome. *J. Virol.* **77**:4528–4538.

104. Hancock, G. E., D. J. Speelman, K. Heers, E. Bortell, J. Smith, and C. Cosco. 1996. Generation of atypical pulmonary inflammatory responses in BALB/c mice after immunization with the native attachment (G) glycoprotein of respiratory syncytial virus. *J. Virol.* **70**:7783–7791.

105. Hasoksuz, M., S. L. Lathrop, K. L. Gadfield, and L. J. Saif. 1999. Isolation of bovine respiratory coronaviruses from feedlot cattle and comparison of their biological and antigenic properties with bovine enteric coronaviruses. *Am. J. Vet. Res.* **60**:1227–1233.

106. He, Y., J. Li, S. Heck, S. Lustigman, and S. Jiang. 2006. Antigenic and immunogenic characterization of recombinant baculovirus-expressed severe acute respiratory syndrome coronavirus spike protein: implication for vaccine design. *J. Virol.* **80**:5757–5767.

107. He, Y., J. Li, W. Li, S. Lustigman, M. Farzan, and S. Jiang. 2006. Cross-neutralization of human and palm civet severe acute respiratory syndrome coronaviruses by antibodies targeting the receptor-binding domain of spike protein. *J. Immunol.* **176**:6085–6092.

108. Hebben, M., V. Duquesne, J. Cronier, B. Rossi, and A. Aubert. 2004. Modified vaccinia virus Ankara as a vaccine against feline coronavirus: immunogenicity and efficacy. *J. Feline Med. Surg.* **6**:111–118.

109. Ho, Y., P. H. Lin, C. Y. Liu, S. P. Lee, and Y. C. Chao. 2004. Assembly of human severe acute respiratory syndrome coronavirus-like particles. *Biochem. Biophys. Res. Commun.* **318**:833–838.

110. Hogan, R. J., G. Gao, T. Rowe, P. Bell, D. Flieder, J. Paragas, G. P. Kobinger, N. A. Wivel, R. G. Crystal, J. Boyer, H. Feldmann, T. G. Voss, and J. M. Wilson. 2004. Resolution of primary severe acute respiratory syndrome-associated coronavirus infection requires Stat1. *J. Virol.* **78:**11416–11421.

111. Holmes, K. V., and S. R. Compton. 1995. Coronavirus receptors, p. 55–72. *In* S. G. Siddell (ed.), *The Coronaviridae.* Plenum Press, New York, NY.

112. Holmes, K. V., and L. Enjuanes. 2003. The SARS coronavirus: a postgenomic era. *Science* **300:**1377–1378.

113. Hu, S., J. Bruszewski, R. Smallig, and J. K. Browne. 1987. Studies of TGEV spike protein GP195 expressed in *E. coli* and by a TGE-vaccinia virus recombinant, p. 63–82. *In* M. Zouhair Attasi and H. L. Bachrach (ed.), *Immunobiology of Proteins and Peptides—III. Viral and Bacterial Antigens.* Plenum Press, New York, NY.

114. Huang, C., N. Ito, C. T. Tseng, and S. Makino. 2006. Severe acute respiratory syndrome coronavirus 7a accessory protein is a viral structural protein. *J. Virol.* **80:**7287–7294.

115. Huang, C., K. Narayanan, N. Ito, C. J. Peters, and S. Makino. 2006. Severe acute respiratory syndrome coronavirus 3a protein is released in membranous structures from 3a protein-expressing cells and infected cells. *J. Virol.* **80:**210–217.

116. Huang, Y., Z. Y. Yang, W. P. Kong, and G. J. Nabel. 2004. Generation of synthetic severe acute respiratory syndrome coronavirus pseudoparticles: implications for assembly and vaccine production. *J. Virol.* **78:**12557–12565.

117. Huang, Y. P., and C. H. Wang. 2006. Development of attenuated vaccines from Taiwanese infectious bronchitis virus strains. *Vaccine* **24:**785–791.

118. Hung, I. F., V. C. Cheng, A. K. Wu, B. S. Tang, K. H. Chan, C. M. Chu, M. M. Wong, W. T. Hui, L. L. Poon, D. M. Tse, K. S. Chan, P. C. Woo, S. K. Lau, J. S. Peiris, and K. Y. Yuen. 2004. Viral loads in clinical specimens and SARS manifestations. *Emerg. Infect. Dis.* **10:**1550–1557.

119. Ignjatovic, J., and L. Galli. 1994. The S1 glycoprotein but not the N or M proteins of avian infectious bronchitis virus induces protection in vaccinated chickens. *Arch. Virol.* **138:**117–134.

120. Ignjatovic, J., and P. G. McWaters. 1991. Monoclonal antibodies to three structural proteins of avian infectious bronchitis virus: characterization of epitopes and antigenic differentiation of Australian strains. *J. Gen. Virol.* **72:**2915–2922.

121. Ishii, K., H. Hasegawa, N. Nagata, T. Mizutani, S. Morikawa, T. Suzuki, F. Taguchi, M. Tashiro, T. Takemori, T. Miyamura, and Y. Tsunetsugu-Yokota. 2006. Induction of protective immunity against severe acute respiratory syndrome coronavirus (SARS-CoV) infection using highly attenuated recombinant vaccinia virus DIs. *Virology* **351:**368–380.

122. Ito, N., E. C. Mossel, K. Narayanan, V. L. Popov, C. Huang, T. Inoue, C. J. Peters, and S. Makino. 2005. Severe acute respiratory syndrome coronavirus 3a protein is a viral structural protein. *J. Virol.* **79:**3182–3186.

123. Jackwood, M. W., D. A. Hilt, and T. P. Brown. 2003. Attenuation, safety, and efficacy of an infectious bronchitis virus GA98 serotype vaccine. *Avian Dis.* **47:**627–632.

124. Jacobs, L., R. De Groot, B. A. M. Van der Zeijst, M. C. Horzinek, and W. Spaan. 1987. The nucleotide sequence of the peplomer gene of porcine transmissible gastroenteritis virus (TGEV): comparison with the sequence of the peplomer protein of feline infectious peritonitis virus (FIPV). *Virus Res.* **8:**363–371.

125. Jeffers, S. A., S. M. Tusell, L. Gillim-Ross, E. M. Hemmila, J. E. Achenbach, G. J. Babcock, W. D. Thomas, Jr., L. B. Thackray, M. D. Young, R. J. Mason, D. M. Ambrosino, D. E. Wentworth, J. C. Demartini, and K. V. Holmes. 2004. CD209L (L-SIGN) is a receptor for severe acute respiratory syndrome coronavirus. *Proc. Natl. Acad. Sci. USA* **101:**15748–15753.

126. Jiang, S., Y. He, and S. Liu. 2005. SARS vaccine development. *Emerg. Infect. Dis.* **11:**1016–1020.

127. Jin, H., C. Xiao, Z. Chen, Y. Kang, Y. Ma, K. Zhu, Q. Xie, Y. Tu, Y. Yu, and B. Wang. 2005. Induction of Th1 type response by DNA vaccinations with N, M, and E genes against SARS-CoV in mice. *Biochem. Biophys. Res. Commun.* **328:**979–986.

128. Kamitani, W., K. Narayanan, C. Huang, K. Lokugamage, T. Ikegami, N. Ito, H. Kubo, and S. Makino. 2006. Severe acute respiratory syndrome coronavirus nsp1 protein suppresses host gene expression by promoting host mRNA degradation. *Proc. Natl. Acad. Sci. USA* **103:**12885–12890.

129. Kan, B., M. Wang, H. Jing, H. Xu, X. Jiang, M. Yan, W. Liang, H. Zheng, K. Wan, Q. Liu, B. Cui, Y. Xu, E. Zhang, H. Wang, J. Ye, G. Li, M. Li, Z. Cui, X. Qi, K. Chen, L. Du, K. Gao, Y. T. Zhao, X. Z. Zou, Y. J. Feng, Y. F. Gao, R. Hai, D. Yu, Y. Guan, and J. Xu. 2005. Molecular evolution analysis and geographic investigation of severe acute respiratory syndrome coronavirus-like virus in palm civets at an animal market and on farms. *J. Virol.* **79:**11892–11900.

130. Kapadia, S. U., J. K. Rose, E. Lamirande, L. Vogel, K. Subbarao, and A. Roberts. 2005. Long-term protection from SARS coronavirus infection conferred by a single immunization with an attenuated VSV-based vaccine. *Virology* **340:**174–182.

131. Keng, C. T., A. Zhang, S. Shen, K. M. Lip, B. C. Fielding, T. H. Tan, C. F. Chou, C. B. Loh, S. Wang, J. Fu, X. Yang, S. G. Lim, W. Hong, and Y. J. Tan. 2005. Amino acids 1055 to 1192 in the S2 region of severe acute respiratory syndrome coronavirus S protein induce neutralizing antibodies: implications for the development of vaccines and antiviral agents. *J. Virol.* **79:**3289–3296.

132. Kim, H. W., J. G. Canchola, C. D. Brandt, G. Pyles, R. M. Chanock, K. Jensen, and R. H. Parrott. 1969. Respiratory syncytial virus disease in infants despite prior administration of antigenic inactivated vaccine. *Am. J. Epidemiol.* **89:**422–434.

133. Kim, T. S., and S. Perlman. 2003. Protection against CTL escape and clinical disease in a murine model of virus persistence. *J. Immunol.* **171:**2006–2013.

134. Kim, T. W., J. H. Lee, C. F. Hung, S. Peng, R. Roden, M. C. Wang, R. Viscidi, Y. C. Tsai, L. He, P. J. Chen, D. A. Boyd, and T. C. Wu. 2004. Generation and characterization of DNA vaccines targeting the nucleocapsid protein of severe acute respiratory syndrome coronavirus. *J. Virol.* **78:**4638–4645.

135. Kiss, I., A. M. Poland, and N. C. Pedersen. 2004. Disease outcome and cytokine responses in cats immunized with an avirulent feline infectious peritonitis virus (FIPV)-UCD1 and challenge-exposed with virulent FIPV-UCD8. *J. Feline Med. Surg.* **6:**89–97.

136. Kiyono, H., P. L. Ogra, and J. R. McGhee. 1996. *Mucosal Vaccines.* Academic Press, Inc., San Diego, CA.

137. Klepfer, S., A. P. Reed, M. Martinez, B. Bhogal, E. Jones, and T. J. Miller. 1995. Cloning and expression of FECV spike gene in vaccinia virus. Immunization with FECV S causes early death after FIPV challenge. *Adv. Exp. Med. Biol.* **380:**235–241.

138. Koch, G., L. Hartog, A. Kant, and D. J. van Roozelaar. 1990. Antigenic domains on the peplomer protein of avian infectious bronchitis virus: correlation with biological functions. *J. Gen. Virol.* **71:**1929–1935.

139. Kong, W. P., L. Xu, K. Stadler, J. B. Ulmer, S. Abrignani, R. Rappuoli, and G. J. Nabel. 2005. Modulation of the immune response to the severe acute respiratory syndrome spike glycoprotein by gene-based and inactivated virus immunization. *J. Virol.* **79:**13915–13923.

140. Koo, M., M. Bendahmane, G. A. Lettieri, A. D. Paoletti, T. E. Lane, J. H. Fitchen, M. J. Buchmeier, and R. N. Beachy. 1999. Protective immunity against murine hepatitis virus (MHV) induced by intranasal or subcutaneous administration of hybrids of tobacco mosaic virus that carries an MHV epitope. *Proc. Natl. Acad. Sci. USA* **96:**7774–7779.

141. Koolen, M. J. M., M. A. J. Borst, M. C. Horzinek, and W. J. M. Spaan. 1990. Immunogenic peptide comprising a mouse hepatitis virus A59 B-cell epitope and an influenza virus T-cell epitope protects against lethal infection. *J. Virol.* **64:**6270–6273.

142. Kopecky-Bromberg, S. A., L. Martinez-Sobrido, M. Frieman, R. A. Baric, and P. Palese. 2007. Severe acute respiratory syndrome coronavirus open reading frame (ORF) 3b, ORF 6, and nucleocapsid proteins function as interferon antagonists. *J. Virol.* **81:**548–557.

143. Kuo, L., G.-J. Godeke, M. J. B. Raamsman, P. S. Masters, and P. J. M. Rottier. 2000. Retargeting of coronavirus by substitution of the spike glycoprotein ectodomain: crossing the host cell species barrier. *J. Virol.* **74:**1393–1406.

144. Kuo, L., and P. S. Masters. 2003. The small envelope protein E is not essential for murine coronavirus replication. *J. Virol.* **77:**4597–4608.

145. Kusters, J. G., E. J. Jager, H. G. Niesters, and B. A. Van der Zeijst. 1990. Sequence evidence for RNA recombination in field isolates of avian coronavirus infectious bronchitis virus. *Vaccine* **8:**605.

146. Ladman, B. S., C. R. Pope, A. F. Ziegler, T. Swieczkowski, C. J. Callahan, S. Davison, and J. Gelb, Jr. 2002. Protection of chickens after live and inactivated virus vaccination against challenge with nephropathogenic infectious bronchitis virus PA/Wolgemuth/98. *Avian Dis.* **46:**938–944.

147. Lai, M. M. C., and D. Cavanagh. 1997. The molecular biology of coronaviruses. *Adv. Virus Res.* **48:**1–100.

148. Lamphear, B. J., J. M. Jilka, L. Kesl, M. Welter, J. A. Howard, and S. J. Streatfield. 2004. A corn-based delivery system for animal vaccines: an oral transmissible gastroenteritis virus vaccine boosts lactogenic immunity in swine. *Vaccine* **22:**2420–2424.

149. Lamphear, B. J., S. J. Streatfield, J. M. Jilka, C. A. Brooks, D. K. Barker, D. D. Turner, D. E. Delaney, M. Garcia, B. Wiggins, S. L. Woodard, E. E. Hood, I. R. Tizard, B. Lawhorn, and J. A. Howard. 2002. Delivery of subunit vaccines in maize seed. *J. Control. Release* **85:**169–180.

150. Lau, S. K., P. C. Woo, K. S. Li, Y. Huang, H. W. Tsoi, B. H. Wong, S. S. Wong, S. Y. Leung, K. H. Chan, and K. Y. Yuen. 2005. Severe acute respiratory syndrome coronavirus-like virus in Chinese horseshoe bats. *Proc. Natl. Acad. Sci. USA* **102:**14040–14045.

151. Laude, H., K. Van Reeth, and M. Pensaert. 1993. Porcine respiratory coronavirus: molecular features and virus-host interactions. *Vet. Res.* **24:**125–150.

152. Li, W., Z. Shi, M. Yu, W. Ren, C. Smith, J. H. Epstein, H. Wang, G. Crameri, Z. Hu, H. Zhang, J. Zhang, J. McEachern, H. Field, P. Daszak, B. T. Eaton, S. Zhang, and L. F. Wang. 2005. Bats are natural reservoirs of SARS-like coronaviruses. *Science* **310:**676–679.

153. Lin, K. Y., H. C. Wang, and C. H. Wang. 2005. Protective effect of vaccination in chicks with local infectious bronchitis viruses against field virus challenge. *J. Microbiol. Immunol. Infect.* **38:**25–30.

154. Liu, I. J., P. R. Hsueh, C. T. Lin, C. Y. Chiu, C. L. Kao, M. Y. Liao, and H. C. Wu. 2004. Disease-specific B cell epitopes for serum antibodies from patients with severe acute respiratory syndrome (SARS) and serologic detection of SARS antibodies by epitope-based peptide antigens. *J. Infect. Dis.* **190:**797–809.

155. Liu, R. Y., L. Z. Wu, B. J. Huang, J. L. Huang, Y. L. Zhang, M. L. Ke, J. M. Wang, W. P. Tan, R. H. Zhang, H. K. Chen, Y. X. Zeng, and W. Huang. 2005. Adenoviral expression of a truncated S1 subunit of SARS-CoV spike protein results in specific humoral immune responses against SARS-CoV in rats. *Virus Res.* **112:**24–31.

156. Liu, S. J., C. H. Leng, S. P. Lien, H. Y. Chi, C. Y. Huang, C. L. Lin, W. C. Lian, C. J. Chen, S. L. Hsieh, and P. Chong. 2006. Immunological characterizations of the nucleocapsid protein based SARS vaccine candidates. *Vaccine* **24:**3100–3108.

157. Makino, S., J. O. Fleming, J. G. Keck, S. T. Stohlman, and M. M. C. Lai. 1987. RNA recombination of coronaviruses: localization of neutralizing epitopes and neuropathogenic determinants on the carboxyl terminus of peplomers. *Proc. Natl. Acad. Sci. USA* **84:**6567–6571.

158. Marra, M. A., S. J. M. Jones, C. R. Astell, R. A. Holt, A. Brooks-Wilson, Y. S. N. Butterfield, J. Khattra, J. K. Asano, S. A. Barber, S. Y. Chan, A. Cloutier, S. M. Coughlin, D. Freeman, N. Girn, O. L. Griffith, S. R. Leach, M. Mayo, H. McDonald, S. B. Montgomery, P. K. Pandoh, A. S. Petrescu, A. G. Robertson, J. E. Schein, A. Siddiqui, D. E. Smailus, J. M. Stott, G. S. Yang, F. Plummer, A. Andonov, H. Artsob, N. Bastien, K. Bernard, T. F. Booth, D. Bowness, M. Czub, M. Drebot, L. Fernando, R. Flick, M. Garbutt, M. Gray, A. Grolla, S. Jones, H. Feldmann, A. Meyers, A. Kabani, Y. Li, S. Normand, U. Stroher, G. A. Tipples, S. Tyler, R. Vogrig, D. Ward, B. Watson, R. C. Brunham, M. Krajden, M. Petric, D. M. Skowronski, C. Upton, and R. L. Roper. 2003. The genome sequence of the SARS-associated coronavirus. *Science* **300:**1399–1404.

159. Marshall, E., and M. Enserink. 2004. Medicine. Caution urged on SARS vaccines. *Science* **303:**944–946.

160. Martin, M. L. 1985. Canine coronavirus enteritis and a recent outbreak following modified-live virus vaccination. *Comp. Cont. Educ. Pract. Vet.* **7:**1013–1017.

161. Martina, B. E., B. L. Haagmans, T. Kuiken, R. A. Fouchier, G. F. Rimmelzwaan, G. Van Amerongen, J. S. Peiris, W. Lim, and A. D. Osterhaus. 2003. SARS virus infection of cats and ferrets. *Nature* **425:**915.

162. Masters, P. S., and P. J. Rottier. 2005. Coronavirus reverse genetics by targeted RNA recombination. *Curr. Top. Microbiol. Immunol.* **287:**133–159.

163. Matthijs, M. G., J. H. van Eck, J. J. de Wit, A. Bouma, and J. A. Stegeman. 2005. Effect of IBV-H120 vaccination in broilers on colibacillosis susceptibility after infection with a virulent Massachusetts-type IBV strain. *Avian Dis.* **49:**540–545.

164. McArdle, F., B. Tennant, M. Bennet, D. F. Kelly, C. J. Gaskell, and R. M. Gaskell. 1995. Independent evaluation of a modified live FIPV vaccine under experimental conditions (University of Liverpool experiences). *Feline Pract.* **23:**67–71.

165. McAuliffe, J., L. Vogel, A. Roberts, G. Fahle, S. Fischer, W. J. Shieh, E. Butler, S. Zaki, M. St. Claire, B. Murphy, and K. Subbarao. 2004. Replication of SARS coronavirus administered into the respiratory tract of African Green, rhesus and cynomolgus monkeys. *Virology* **330:**8–15.

166. McElhaney, J. E. 2005. The unmet need in the elderly: designing new influenza vaccines for older adults. *Vaccine* **23**(Suppl. 1):10–25.

167. Meulemans, M., M. Boschmans, T. P. Decaesstecker, P. van den Berg, D. Denis, and G. Cavanagh. 2001. Epidemiology of infectious bronchitis virus in Belgian broilers: a retrospective study, 1986 to 1995. *Avian Pathol.* **30:**411–421.

168. Mortola, E., and P. Roy. 2004. Efficient assembly and release of SARS coronavirus-like particles by a heterologous expression system. *FEBS Lett.* **576:**174–178.

169. Newby, T. J. 1984. Protective immune responses in the intestinal tract, p. 143–198. *In* T. J. Newby and C. R. Stokes (ed.), *Local Immune Responses of the Gut.* CRC Press, Boca Raton, FL.

170. Ng, P. C., C. W. Leung, W. K. Chiu, S. F. Wong, and E. K. Hon. 2004. SARS in newborns and children. *Biol. Neonate* **85:**293–298.

171. O'Connor, A., S. W. Martin, E. Nagy, P. Menzies, and R. Harland. 2001. The relationship between the occurrence of undifferentiated bovine respiratory disease and titer changes to bovine coronavirus and bovine viral diarrhea virus in 3 Ontario feedlots. *Can. J. Vet. Res.* **65:**137–142.

172. Ogra, P. L. 1996. Mucosal immunoprophylaxis: an introductory overview. *In* H. Kiyono, P. L. Ogra, and J. R. McGhee (ed.), *Mucosal Vaccine.* Academic Press., San Diego, CA.

173. Ogra, P. L., J. Mestechy, M. E. Lann, W. Strober, J. Bienenstock, and J. R. McGhee. 1999. *Mucosal Immunity*, 2nd ed. Academic Press, London, United Kingdom.

174. Olsen, C. W. 1993. A review of feline infectious peritonitis virus: molecular biology, immunopathogenesis, clinical aspects, and vaccination. *Vet. Microbiol.* **36:**1–37.

175. Olsen, C. W., W. V. Corapi, R. H. Jacobson, R. A. Simkins, L. J. Saif, and F. W. Scott. 1993. Identification of antigenic sites mediating antibody-dependent enhancement of feline infectious peritonitis virus infectivity. *J. Gen. Virol.* **74:**745–749.

176. Olsen, C. W., W. V. Corapi, C. K. Ngichabe, J. D. Baines, and F. W. Scott. 1992. Monoclonal antibodies to the spike protein of feline infectious peritonitis virus mediate antibody-dependent enhancement of infection of feline macrophages. *J. Virol.* **66:**956–965.

177. Ortego, J., D. Escors, H. Laude, and L. Enjuanes. 2002. Generation of a replication-competent, propagation-deficient virus vector based on the transmissible gastroenteritis coronavirus genome. *J. Virol.* **76:**11518–11529.

178. Ortego, J., I. Sola, F. Almazan, J. E. Ceriani, C. Riquelme, M. Balasch, J. Plana-Durán, and L. Enjuanes. 2003. Transmissible gastroenteritis coronavirus gene 7 is not essential but influences *in vivo* virus replication and virulence. *Virology* **308:**13–22.

179. Pang, H., Y. Liu, X. Han, Y. Xu, F. Jiang, D. Wu, X. Kong, M. Bartlam, and Z. Rao. 2004. Protective humoral responses to severe acute respiratory syndrome-associated coronavirus: implications for the design of an effective protein-based vaccine. *J. Gen. Virol.* **85:**3109–3113.

180. Pedersen, N. C. 1987. Virologic and immunologic aspects of feline infectious peritonitis virus infection. *Adv. Exp. Med. Biol.* **218:**529–550.

181. Pedersen, N. C., J. F. Boyle, K. Floyd, A. Fudge, and J. Barker. 1981. An enteric coronavirus infection of cats and its relationship to feline infectious peritonitis. *Am. J. Vet. Res.* **42:**368–377.

182. Pedersen, N. C., and K. Floyd. 1985. Experimental studies with three new strains of feline infectious peritonitis virus: FIPV-UCD2, FIPV-UCD3, and FIPV-UCD4. *Comp. Cont. Educ. Pract. Vet.* **7:**1001–1011.

183. Peiris, J. S., K. Y. Yuen, A. D. Osterhaus, and K. Stohr. 2003. The severe acute respiratory syndrome. *N. Engl. J. Med.* **349:**2431–2441.

184. Peiris, J. S. M., S. T. Lai, L. L. M. Poon, Y. Guan, L. Y. C. Yam, W. Lim, J. Nicholls, W. K. S. Yee, W. W. Yan, and M. T. Cheung. 2003. Coronavirus as a possible cause of severe acute respiratory syndrome. *Lancet* **361:**1319–1325.

185. Peng, H., L. T. Yang, L. Y. Wang, J. Li, J. Huang, Z. Q. Lu, R. A. Koup, R. T. Bailer, and C. Y. Wu. 2006. Long-lived memory T lymphocyte responses against SARS coronavirus nucleocapsid protein in SARS-recovered patients. *Virology* **351:**466–475.

186. Pensaert, M. B., and P. De Bouck. 1978. A new coronavirus-like particle associated with diarrhea in swine. *Arch. Virol.* **58:**243–247.

187. Penzes, Z., J. M. González, E. Calvo, A. Izeta, C. Smerdou, A. Mendez, C. M. Sánchez, I. Sola, F. Almazán, and L. Enjuanes. 2001. Complete genome sequence of transmissible gastroenteritis coronavirus PUR46-MAD clone and evolution of the Purdue virus cluster. *Virus Genes* **23:**105–118.

188. Perlman, S. 1998. Pathogenesis of coronavirus-induced infections: review of pathological and immunological aspects. *Adv. Exp. Med. Biol.* **440:**503–514.

189. Pewe, L., S. Xue, and S. Perlman. 1998. Infection with cytotoxic T-lymphocyte escape mutants results in increased mortality and growth retardation in mice infected with a neurotropic coronavirus. *J. Virol.* **72:**5912–5918.

190. Plummer, P. J., B. W. Rohrbach, R. A. Daugherty, R. A. Daugherty, K. V. Thomas, R. P. Wilkes, F. E. Duggan, and M. A. Kennedy. 2004. Effect of intranasal vaccination against bovine enteric coronavirus on the occurrence of respiratory tract disease in a commercial backgrounding feedlot. *J. Am. Vet. Med. Assoc.* **225:**726–731.

191. Poccia, F., C. Agrati, C. Castilletti, L. Bordi, C. Gioia, D. Horejsh, G. Ippolito, P. K. S. Chan, D. S. C. Hui, J. J. Y. Sung, M. R. Capobianchi, and M. Malkovsky. 2006. Anti-severe acute respiratory syndrome coronavirus immune responses: the role played by Vγ9Vδ2 T cells. *J. Infect. Dis.* **193:**1244–1249.

192. Poon, L. L., D. K. Chu, K. H. Chan, O. K. Wong, T. M. Ellis, Y. H. Leung, S. K. Lau, P. C. Woo, K. Y. Suen, K. Y. Yuen, Y. Guan, and J. S. Peiris. 2005. Identification of a novel coronavirus in bats. *J. Virol.* **79:**2001–2009.

193. Porterfield, J. S. 1986. Antibody-dependent enhancement of viral infectivity. *Adv. Virus Res.* **31:**335–355.

194. Posthumus, W. P. A., J. A. Lenstra, W. M. M. Schaaper, A. P. van Nieuwstadt, L. Enjuanes, and R. H. Meloen. 1990. Analysis and simulation of a neutralizing epitope of transmissible gastroenteritis virus. *J. Virol.* **64:**3304–3309.

195. Pratelli, A., A. Tinelli, N. Decaro, F. Cirone, G. Elia, S. Roperto, M. Tempesta, and C. Buonavoglia. 2003. Efficacy of an inactivated canine coronavirus vaccine in pups. *New Microbiol.* **26:**151–155.

196. Pratelli, A., A. Tinelli, N. Decaro, V. Martella, M. Camero, M. Tempesta, M. Martini, L. E. Carmichael, and C. Buonavoglia. 2004. Safety and efficacy of a modified-live canine coronavirus vaccine in dogs. *Vet. Microbiol.* **99:**43–49.

197. Pyrc, K., M. F. Jebbink, B. Berkhout, and L. van der Hoek. 2004. Genome structure and transcriptional regulation of human coronavirus NL63. *Virol. J.* **1:**1–7.

198. Qin, C., J. Wang, Q. Wei, M. She, W. A. Marasco, H. Jiang, X. Tu, H. Zhu, L. Ren, H. Gao, L. Guo, L. Huang, R. Yang, Z. Cong, Y. Wang, Y. Liu, Y. Sun, S. Duan, J. Qu, L. Chen, W. Tong, L. Ruan, P. Liu, H. Zhang, J. Zhang, D. Liu, Q. Liu, T. Hong, and W. He. 2005. An animal model of SARS produced by infection of Macaca mulatta with SARS coronavirus. *J. Pathol.* **206:**251–259.

199. Qin, E., H. Shi, L. Tang, C. Wang, G. Chang, Z. Ding, K. Zhao, J. Wang, Z. Chen, M. Yu, B. Si, J. Liu, D. Wu, X.

Cheng, B. Yang, W. Peng, Q. Meng, B. Liu, W. Han, X. Yin, H. Duan, D. Zhan, L. Tian, S. Li, J. Wu, G. Tan, Y. Li, Y. Liu, H. Liu, F. Lv, Y. Zhang, X. Kong, B. Fan, T. Jiang, S. Xu, X. Wang, C. Li, X. Wu, Y. Deng, M. Zhao, and Q. Zhu. 2006. Immunogenicity and protective efficacy in monkeys of purified inactivated Vero-cell SARS vaccine. *Vaccine* **24**:1028–1034.

200. Qiu, M., Y. Shi, Z. Guo, Z. Chen, R. He, R. Chen, D. Zhou, E. Dai, X. Wang, B. Si, Y. Song, J. Li, L. Yang, J. Wang, H. Wang, X. Pang, J. Zhai, Z. Du, Y. Liu, Y. Zhang, L. Li, B. Sun, and R. Yang. 2005. Antibody responses to individual proteins of SARS coronavirus and their neutralization activities. *Microbes Infect.* **7**:882–889.

201. Qu, D., B. Zheng, X. Yao, Y. Guan, Z. H. Yuan, N. S. Zhong, L. W. Lu, J. P. Xie, and Y. M. Wen. 2005. Intranasal immunization with inactivated SARS-CoV (SARS-associated coronavirus) induced local and serum antibodies in mice. *Vaccine* **23**:924–931.

202. Ramakrishna, C., R. A. Atkinson, S. A. Stohlman, and C. C. Bergmann. 2006. Vaccine-induced memory CD8+ T cells cannot prevent central nervous system virus reactivation. *J. Immunol.* **176**:3062–3069.

203. Reeves, N. C., R. V. Pollock, and E. T. Thurber. 1992. Long-term follow-up study of cats vaccinated with a temperature-sensitive feline infectious peritonitis vaccine. *Cornell Vet.* **82**:117–123.

204. Resta, S., J. P. Luby, C. D. Rosenfeld, and J. D. Siegel. 1985. Isolation and propagation of a human enteric coronavirus. *Science* **229**:978–981.

205. Risco, C., I. M. Antón, C. Suñé, A. M. Pedregosa, J. M. Martín-Alonso, F. Parra, J. L. Carrascosa, and L. Enjuanes. 1995. Membrane protein molecules of transmissible gastroenteritis coronavirus also expose the carboxy-terminal region on the external surface of the virion. *J. Virol.* **69**:5269–5277.

206. Roberts, A., C. Paddock, L. Vogel, E. Butler, S. Zaki, and K. Subbarao. 2005. Aged BALB/c mice as a model for increased severity of severe acute respiratory syndrome in elderly humans. *J. Virol.* **79**:5833–5838.

207. Roberts, A., L. Vogel, J. Guarner, N. Hayes, B. Murphy, S. Zaki, and K. Subbarao. 2005. Severe acute respiratory syndrome coronavirus infection of golden Syrian hamsters. *J. Virol.* **79**:503–511.

208. Routledge, E., R. Stauber, M. Pfleiderer, and S. G. Siddell. 1991. Analysis of murine coronavirus surface glycoprotein functions by using monoclonal antibodies. *J. Virol.* **65**:254–262.

209. Saif, L. J. 2004. Animal coronavirus vaccines: lessons for SARS. *Dev. Biol.* **119**:129–140.

210. Saif, L. J. 1993. Coronavirus immunogens. *Vet. Microbiol.* **37**:285–297.

211. Saif, L. J. 1999. Enteric viral infections of pigs and strategies for induction of mucosal immunity. *Adv. Vet. Med.* **41**:429–446.

212. Saif, L. J. 1996. Mucosal immunity: an overview and studies of enteric and respiratory coronavirus infections in a swine model of enteric disease. *Vet. Immunol. Immunopathol.* **54**:163–169.

213. Saif, L. J., and D. J. Jackwood. 1990. Enteric virus vaccines: theoretical considerations, current status and future approaches, p. 313–329. *In* L. J. Saif and K. W. Thiel (ed.), *Viral Diarrheas of Man and Animals.* CRC Press, Boca Raton, FL.

214. Saif, L. J., J. L. van Cott, and T. A. Brim. 1994. Immunity to transmissible gastroenteritis virus and porcine respiratory coronavirus infections in swine. *Vet. Immunol. Immmunopathol.* **43**:89–97.

215. Saif, L. J., and R. D. Wesley. 1992. Transmissible gastroenteritis, p. 362–386. *In* A. D. Leman, B. E. Straw, W. L. Mengeling, S. D'Allaire, and D. J. Taylor (ed.), *Diseases of Swine,* 7th ed. Wolfe Publishing Ltd., Ames, IA.

216. Saif, L. J., and R. D. Wesley. 1999. Transmissible gastroenteritis and porcine respiratory coronavirus, p. 295–325. *In* A. D. Leman, B. E. Straw, W. L. Mengeling, S. D'Allaire, and D. J. Taylor (ed.), *Diseases of Swine,* 7th ed. Wolfe Publishing Ltd., Ames, IA.

217. Sanchez, C. M., A. Izeta, J. M. Sánchez-Morgado, S. Alonso, I. Sola, M. Balasch, J. Plana-Duran, and L. Enjuanes. 1999. Targeted recombination demonstrates that the spike gene of transmissible gastroenteritis coronavirus is a determinant of its enteric tropism and virulence. *J. Virol.* **73**:7607–7618.

218. Sanchez, C. M., G. Jiménez, M. D. Laviada, I. Correa, C. Suñe, M. J. Bullido, F. Gebauer, C. Smerdou, P. Callebaut, J. M. Escribano, and L. Enjuanes. 1990. Antigenic homology among coronaviruses related to transmissible gastroenteritis virus. *Virology* **174**:410–417.

219. Sarma, J. D., E. Scheen, S. H. Seo, M. Koval, and S. R. Weiss. 2002. Enhanced green fluorescent protein expression may be used to monitor murine coronavirus spread in vitro and in the mouse central nervous system. *J. Neurovirol.* **8**:381–391.

220. Schaecher, S. R., J. M. Mackenzie, and A. Pekosz. 2006. The ORF7b protein of SARS-CoV is expressed in virus-infected cells and incorporated into SARS-CoV particles. *J. Virol.* **81**:718–731.

221. Schelle, B., N. Karl, B. Ludewig, S. G. Siddell, and V. Thiel. 2005. Selective replication of coronavirus genomes that express nucleocapsid protein. *J. Virol.* **79**:6620–6630.

222. Scott, F. W., W. V. Corapi, and C. W. Olsen. 1995. Independent evaluation of a modified live FIPV vaccine under experimental conditions (Cornell experience). *Feline Pract.* **23**:74–76.

223. See, R. H., A. N. Zakhartchouk, M. Petric, D. J. Lawrence, C. P. Mok, R. J. Hogan, T. Rowe, L. A. Zitzow, K. P. Karunakaran, M. M. Hitt, F. L. Graham, L. Prevec, J. B. Mahony, C. Sharon, T. C. Auperin, J. M. Rini, A. J. Tingle, D. W. Scheifele, D. M. Skowronski, D. M. Patrick, T. G. Voss, L. A. Babiuk, J. Gauldie, R. L. Roper, R. C. Brunham, and B. B. Finlay. 2006. Comparative evaluation of two severe acute respiratory syndrome (SARS) vaccine candidates in mice challenged with SARS coronavirus. *J. Gen. Virol.* **87**:641–650.

224. Seo, S. H., and E. W. Collisson. 1997. Specific cytotoxic T lymphocytes are involved in in vivo clearance of infectious brochitis virus. *J. Virol.* **71**:5173–5177.

225. Seo, S. H., L. Wang, R. Smith, and E. W. Collisson. 1997. The carboxyl-terminal 120-residue polypeptide of infectious bronchitis virus nucleocapsid induces cytotoxic T lymphocytes and protects chickens from acute infection. *J. Virol.* **71**:7889–7894.

226. Sestak, K., I. Lanza, S. K. Park, P. A. Weilnau, and L. J. Saif. 1996. Contribution of passive immunity to porcine respiratory coronavirus to protection against transmissible gastroenteritis virus challenge exposure in suckling pigs. *Am. J. Vet. Res.* **57**:664–671.

227. Sestak, K., R. K. Meister, J. R. Hayes, L. Kim, P. A. Lewis, G. Myers, and L. J. Saif. 1999. Active immunity and T-cell populations in pigs intraperitoneally inoculated with baculovirus-expressed transmissible gastroenteritis virus structural proteins. *Vet. Immunol. Immunopathol.* **70**:203–221.

228. Shen, S., P. S. Lin, Y. C. Chao, A. Zhang, X. Yang, S. G. Lim, W. Hong, and Y. J. Tan. 2005. The severe acute respiratory syndrome coronavirus 3a is a novel structural protein. *Biochem. Biophys. Res. Commun.* **330**:286-292.

229. Shoup, D. I., D. J. Jackwood, and L. J. Saif. 1997. Active and passive immune responses to transmissible gastroenteritis virus (TGEV) in swine inoculated with recombinant baculovirus-expressed TGEV spike glycoprotein vaccines. *Am. J. Vet. Res.* **58:**242–250.

230. Snijder, E. J., P. J. Bredenbeek, J. C. Dobbe, V. Thiel, J. Ziebuhr, L. L. M. Poon, Y. Guan, M. Rozanov, W. J. M. Spaan, and A. E. Gorbalenya. 2003. Unique and conserved features of genome and proteome of SARS-coronavirus, an early split-off from the coronavirus group 2 lineage. *J. Mol. Biol.* **331:**991–1004.

231. Sola, I., S. Alonso, S. Zúñiga, M. Balach, J. Plana-Durán, and L. Enjuanes. 2003. Engineering transmissible gastroenteritis virus genome as an expression vector inducing latogenic immunity. *J. Virol.* **77:**4357–4369.

232. Song, C. S., Y. J. Lee, C. W. Lee, H. W. Sung, J. H. Kim, I. P. Mo, Y. Izumiya, H. K. Jang, and T. Mikami. 1998. Induction of protective immunity in chickens vaccinated with infectious bronchitis virus S1 glycoprotein expressed by a recombinant baculovirus. *J. Gen. Virol.* **79:**719–723.

233. Song, H., P. W. Price, and J. Cerny. 1997. Age-related changes in antibody repertoire: contribution from T cells. *Immunol. Rev.* **160:**55–62.

234. Song, H. C., M. Y. Seo, K. Stadler, B. J. Yoo, Q. L. Choo, S. R. Coates, Y. Uematsu, T. Harada, C. E. Greer, J. M. Polo, P. Pileri, M. Eickmann, R. Rappuoli, S. Abrignani, M. Houghton, and J. H. Han. 2004. Synthesis and characterization of a native, oligomeric form of recombinant severe acute respiratory syndrome coronavirus spike glycoprotein. *J. Virol.* **78:**10328–10335.

235. Spaan, W. J. M., D. Brian, D. Cavanagh, R. J. de Groot, L. Enjuanes, A. E. Gorbalenya, K. V. Holmes, P. Masters, P. Rottier, F. Taguchi, and P. J. Talbot. 2005. *Coronaviridae*, p. 947–964. *In* C. M. Fauquet, M. A. Mayo, J. Maniloff, U. Desselberger, and L. A. Ball (ed.), *Virus Taxonomy: Eighth Report of the International Committee on Taxonomy of Viruses.* Academic Press, San Diego, CA.

236. Sperry, S. M., L. Kazi, R. L. Graham, R. S. Baric, S. R. Weiss, and M. R. Denison. 2005. Single-amino-acid substitutions in open reading frame (ORF) 1b-nsp14 and ORF 2a proteins of the coronavirus mouse hepatitis virus are attenuating in mice. *J. Virol.* **79:**3391–3400.

237. Spruth, M., O. Kistner, H. Savidis-Dacho, E. Hitter, B. Crowe, M. Gerencer, P. Bruhl, L. Grillberger, M. Reiter, C. Tauer, W. Mundt, and P. N. Barrett. 2006. A double-inactivated whole virus candidate SARS coronavirus vaccine stimulates neutralising and protective antibody responses. *Vaccine* **24:**652–661.

238. St-Jean, J. R., M. Desforges, F. Almazán, H. Jacomy, L. Enjuanes, and P. J. Talbot. 2006. Recovery of a neurovirulent human coronavirus OC43 from an infectious cDNA clone. *J. Virol.* **80:**3670–3674.

239. Stoddart, C. A., J. E. Barlough, C. A. Baldwin, and F. W. Scott. 1988. Attempted immunisation of cats against feline infectious peritonitis using canine coronavirus. *Res. Vet. Sci.* **45:**383–388.

240. Subbarao, K., J. McAuliffe, L. Vogel, G. Fahle, S. Fischer, K. Tatti, M. Packard, W. J. Shieh, S. Zaki, and B. Murphy. 2004. Prior infection and passive transfer of neutralizing antibody prevent replication of severe acute respiratory syndrome coronavirus in the respiratory tract of mice. *J. Virol.* **78:**3572–3577.

241. Sui, J., W. Li, A. Murakami, A. Tamin, L. J. Matthews, S. K. Wong, M. J. Moore, A. S. Tallarico, M. Olurinde, H. Choe, L. J. Anderson, W. J. Bellini, M. Farzan, and W. A. Marasco. 2004. Potent neutralization of severe acute respiratory syndrome (SARS) coronavirus by a human mAb to S1 protein that blocks receptor association. *Proc. Natl. Acad. Sci. USA* **101:**2536–2541.

242. Sui, J., W. Li, A. Roberts, L. J. Matthews, A. Murakami, L. Vogel, S. K. Wong, K. Subbarao, M. Farzan, and W. A. Marasco. 2005. Evaluation of human monoclonal antibody 80R for immunoprophylaxis of severe acute respiratory syndrome by an animal study, epitope mapping, and analysis of spike variants. *J. Virol.* **79:**5900–5906.

243. Suñe, C., G. Jiménez, I. Correa, M. J. Bullido, F. Gebauer, C. Smerdou, and L. Enjuanes. 1990. Mechanisms of transmissible gastroenteritis coronavirus neutralization. *Virology* **177:**559–569.

244. Talbot, P. J., G. Dionne, and M. Lacroix. 1988. Vaccination against lethal coronavirus-induced encephalitis with a synthetic decapeptide homologous to a domain in the predicted peplomer stalk. *J. Virol.* **62:**3032–3036.

245. Tan, Y. J., P. Y. Goh, B. C. Fielding, S. Shen, C. F. Chou, J. L. Fu, H. N. Leong, Y. S. Leo, E. E. Ooi, A. E. Ling, S. G. Lim, and W. Hong. 2004. Profiles of antibody responses against severe acute respiratory syndrome coronavirus recombinant proteins and their potential use as diagnostic markers. *Clin. Diagn. Lab. Immunol.* **11:**362–371.

246. Tan, Y. J., E. Teng, S. Shen, T. H. P. Tan, P. Y. Goh, B. C. Fielding, E. E. Ooi, H. C. Tan, S. G. Lim, and W. Hong. 2004. A novel severe acute respiratory syndrome coronavirus protein, U274, is transported to the cell surface and undergoes endocytosis. *J. Virol.* **78:**6723–6734.

247. ter Meulen, J., A. B. Bakker, E. N. van den Brink, G. J. Weverling, B. E. Martina, B. L. Haagmans, T. Kuiken, J. de Kruif, W. Preiser, W. Spaan, H. R. Gelderblom, J. Goudsmit, and A. D. Osterhaus. 2004. Human monoclonal antibody as prophylaxis for SARS coronavirus infection in ferrets. *Lancet* **363:**2139–2141.

248. Thiel, V., J. Herold, B. Schelle, and S. Siddell. 2001. Infectious RNA transcribed *in vitro* from a cDNA copy of the human coronavirus genome cloned in vaccinia virus. *J. Gen. Virol.* **82:**1273–1281.

249. Thiel, V., J. Herold, B. Schelle, and S. G. Siddell. 2001. Viral replicase gene products suffice for coronavirus discontinuous transcription. *J. Virol.* **75:**6676–6681.

250. Thiel, V., K. A. Ivanov, A. Putics, T. Hertzig, B. Schelle, S. Bayer, B. Wessbrich, E. J. Snijder, H. Rabenau, H. W. Doerr, A. E. Gorbalenya, and J. Ziebuhr. 2003. Mechanisms and enzymes involved in SARS coronavirus genome expression. *J. Gen. Virol.* **84:**2305–2315.

251. Thiel, V., N. Karl, B. Schelle, P. Disterer, I. Klagge, and S. G. Siddell. 2003. Multigene RNA vector based on coronavirus transcription. *J. Virol.* **77:**9790–9798.

252. Tomley, F. M., A. P. Mockett, M. E. Boursnell, M. M. Binns, J. K. Cook, T. D. Brown, and G. L. Smith. 1987. Expression of the infectious bronchitis virus spike protein by recombinant vaccinia virus and induction of neutralizing antibodies in vaccinated mice. *J. Gen. Virol.* **68:**2291–2298.

253. Torres, J. M., C. Alonso, A. Ortega, S. Mittal, F. Graham, and L. Enjuanes. 1996. Tropism of human adenovirus type 5-based vectors in swine and their ability to protect against transmissible gastroenteritis virus. *J. Virol.* **70:**3770–3780.

254. Torres, J. M., C. M. Sanchez, C. Suñe, C. Smerdou, L. Prevec, F. Graham, and L. Enjuanes. 1995. Induction of antibodies protecting against transmissible gastroenteritis coronavirus (TGEV) by recombinant adenovirus expressing TGEV spike protein. *Virology* **213:**503–516.

255. Traggiai, E., S. Becker, K. Subbarao, L. Kolesnikova, Y. Uematsu, M. R. Gismondo, B. R. Murphy, R. Rappuoli, and A. Lanzavecchia. 2004. An efficient method to make human

monoclonal antibodies from memory B cells: potent neutralization of SARS coronavirus. *Nat. Med.* **10**:871–875.

256. Tripet, B., D. J. Kao, S. A. Jeffers, K. V. Holmes, and R. S. Hodges. 2006. Template-based coiled-coil antigens elicit neutralizing antibodies to the SARS-coronavirus. *J. Struct. Biol.* **155**:176–194.

257. Tuboly, T., W. Yu, A. Bailey, S. Degrandis, S. Du, L. Erickson, and E. Nagy. 2000. Immunogenicity of porcine transmissible gastroenteritis virus spike protein expressed in plants. *Vaccine* **18**:2023–2028.

258. U.S. Department of Agriculture. 2002. *Part II: Reference of Swine Health and Health Management in the United States, 2000. National Animal Health Monitoring System.* U.S. Department of Agriculture, Washington, DC.

259. Van Cott, J. L., T. A. Brim, J. K. Lunney, and L. J. Saif. 1994. Contribution of antibody-secreting cells induced in mucosal lymphoid tissues of pigs inoculated with respiratory or enteric strains of coronavirus to immunity against enteric coronavirus challenge. *J. Immunol.* **152**:3980–3990.

260. Van Cott, J. L., T. A. Brim, R. A. Simkins, and L. J. Saif. 1993. Isotype-specific antibody-secreting cells to transmissible gastroenteritis virus and porcine respiratory coronavirus in gut- and bronchus-associated lymphoid tissues of suckling pigs. *J. Immunol.* **150**:3990–4000.

261. Vennema, H., R. J. de Groot, D. A. Harbour, M. Dalderup, T. Gruffydd-Jones, M. C. Horzinek, and W. J. Spaan. 1990. Early death after feline infectious peritonitis virus challenge due to recombinant vaccinia virus immunization. *J. Virol.* **64**:1407–1409.

262. Vennema, H., R. J. De Groot, D. A. Harbour, M. C. Horzinek, and W. J. M. Spaan. 1991. Primary structure of the membrane and nucleocapsid protein genes of feline infectious peritonitis virus and immunogenicity of recombinant vaccinia viruses in kittens. *Virology* **181**:327–335.

263. Vennema, H., G. J. Godeke, J. W. A. Rossen, W. F. Voorhout, M. C. Horzinek, D. J. Opstelten, and P. J. M. Rottier. 1996. Nucleocapsid-independent assembly of coronavirus-like particles by co-expression of viral envelope protein genes. *EMBO J.* **15**:2020–2028.

264. Vijgen, L., E. Keyaerts, P. Lemey, E. Moes, S. Li, A. M. Vandamme, and M. Van Ranst. 2005. Circulation of genetically distinct contemporary human coronavirus OC43 strains. *Virology* **337**:85–92.

265. Vijgen, L., E. Keyaerts, E. Moes, I. Thoelen, E. Wollants, P. Lemey, A. M. Vandamme, and M. Van Ranst. 2005. Complete genomic sequence of human coronavirus OC43: molecular clock analysis suggests a relatively recent zoonotic coronavirus transmission event. *J. Virol.* **79**:1595–1604.

266. Vijgen, L., P. Lemey, E. Keyaerts, M. Van Ranst, J. R. St-Jean, H. Jacomy, M. Desforges, P. J. Talbot, A. Vabret, and F. Freymuth. 2005. Genetic variability of human respiratory coronavirus OC43. *J. Virol.* **79**:3223–3225.

267. Wang, Z., Z. Yuan, M. Matsumoto, U. R. Hengge, and Y. F. Chang. 2005. Immune responses with DNA vaccines encoded different gene fragments of severe acute respiratory syndrome coronavirus in BALB/c mice. *Biochem. Biophys. Res. Commun.* **327**:130–135.

268. Wege, H., A. Schliephake, H. Korner, E. Flory, and H. Wege. 1993. An immunodominant CD4$^+$ T cell site on the nucleocapsid protein of murine coronavirus contributes to protection against encephalomyelitis. *J. Gen. Virol.* **74**:1287–1294.

269. Weingartl, H., M. Czub, S. Czub, J. Neufeld, P. Marszal, J. Gren, G. Smith, S. Jones, R. Proulx, Y. Deschambault, E. Grudeski, A. Andonov, R. He, Y. Li, J. Copps, A. Grolla, D. Dick, J. Berry, S. Ganske, L. Manning, and J. Cao. 2004. Immunization with modified vaccinia virus Ankara-based recombinant vaccine against severe acute respiratory syndrome is associated with enhanced hepatitis in ferrets. *J. Virol.* **78**:12672–12676.

270. Weiss, R. C., W. J. Dodds, and F. W. Scott. 1980. Disseminated intravascular coagulation in experimentally induced feline infectious peritonitis. *Am. J. Vet. Res.* **41**:663–671.

271. Weiss, R. C., and F. W. Scott. 1981. Antibody-mediated enhancement of disease in feline infectious peritonitis: comparisons with dengue hemorrhagic fever. *Comp. Immunol. Microbiol. Infect. Dis.* **4**:175–189.

272. Weiss, S. R., and S. Navas-Martin. 2005. Coronavirus pathogenesis and the emerging pathogen severe acute respiratory syndrome coronavirus. *Microbiol. Mol. Biol. Rev.* **69**: 635–664.

273. Wesseling, J. G., G. J. Godeke, V. E. C. J. Schijns, L. Prevec, F. L. Frank, M. C. Horzinek., and P. J. M. Rottier. 1993. Mouse hepatitis virus spike and nucleocapsid proteins expressed by adenovirus vector protect mice against a lethal infection. *J. Gen. Virol.* **74**:2061–2069.

274. Wilson, R. B., J. A. Holladay, and J. A. Cave. 1986. A neurologic syndrome associated with use of a canine coronavirus-parvovirus vaccine in dogs. *Comp. Cont. Educ. Pract. Vet.* **8**:117–122.

275. Woo, P. C., S. K. Lau, C. M. Chu, K. H. Chan, H. W. Tsoi, Y. Huang, B. H. Wong, R. W. Poon, J. J. Cai, W. K. Luk, L. L. Poon, S. S. Wong, Y. Guan, J. S. Peiris, and K. Y. Yuen. 2005. Characterization and complete genome sequence of a novel coronavirus, coronavirus HKU1, from patients with pneumonia. *J. Virol.* **79**:884–895.

276. Woo, P. C., S. K. Lau, K. S. Li, R. W. Poon, B. H. Wong, H. W. Tsoi, B. C. Yip, Y. Huang, K. H. Chan, and K. Y. Yuen. 2006. Molecular diversity of coronaviruses in bats. *Virology* **351**:180–187.

277. Woo, P. C., S. K. Lau, H. W. Tsoi, Z. W. Chen, B. H. Wong, L. Zhang, J. K. Chan, L. P. Wong, W. He, C. Ma, K. H. Chan, D. D. Ho, and K. Y. Yuen. 2005. SARS coronavirus spike polypeptide DNA vaccine priming with recombinant spike polypeptide from Escherichia coli as booster induces high titer of neutralizing antibody against SARS coronavirus. *Vaccine* **23**:4959–4968.

278. Woo, P. C., S. K. Lau, H. W. Tsoi, Y. Huang, R. W. Poon, C. M. Chu, R. A. Lee, W. K. Luk, G. K. Wong, B. H. Wong, V. C. Cheng, B. S. Tang, A. K. Wu, R. W. Yung, H. Chen, Y. Guan, K. H. Chan, and K. Y. Yuen. 2005. Clinical and molecular epidemiological features of coronavirus HKU1-associated community-acquired pneumonia. *J. Infect. Dis.* **192**:1898–1907.

279. Woods, R. D. 2001. Efficacy of a transmissible gastroenteritis coronavirus with an altered ORF-3 gene. *Can. J. Vet. Res.* **65**:28–32.

280. Woods, R. D., and N. C. Pedersen. 1979. Cross-protection studies between feline infectious peritonitis and porcine transmissible gastroenteritis viruses. *Vet. Microbiol.* **4**: 11–16.

281. Woods, R. D., R. D. Wesley, and P. A. Kapke. 1987. Complement-dependent neutralization of transmissible gastroenteritis virus by monoclonal antibodies. *Adv. Exp. Med. Biol.* **218**:493–500.

282. Wu, G. F., A. A. Dandekar, L. Pewe, and S. Perlman. 2001. The role of CD4 and CD8 T cells in MHV-JHM-induced demyelination. *Adv. Exp. Med. Biol.* **494**:341–347.

283. Yang, Z. Y., W. P. Kong, Y. Huang, A. Roberts, B. R. Murphy, K. Subbarao, and G. J. Nabel. 2004. A DNA vaccine induces SARS coronavirus neutralization and protective immunity in mice. *Nature* **428**:561–564.

284. Yang, Z. Y., H. C. Werner, W. P. Kong, K. Leung, E. Traggiai, A. Lanzavecchia, and G. J. Nabel. 2005. Evasion of antibody neutralization in emerging severe acute respiratory syndrome coronaviruses. *Proc. Natl. Acad. Sci. USA* **102:**797–801.

285. Youn, S., J. L. Leibowitz, and E. W. Collisson. 2005. In vitro assembled, recombinant infectious bronchitis viruses demonstrate that the 5a open reading frame is not essential for replication. *Virology* **332:**206–215.

286. Yount, B., K. M. Curtis, and R. S. Baric. 2000. Strategy for systematic assembly of large RNA and DNA genomes: the transmissible gastroenteritis virus model. *J. Virol.* **74:**10600–10611.

287. Yount, B., K. M. Curtis, E. A. Fritz, L. E. Hensley, P. B. Jahrling, E. Prentice, M. R. Denison, T. W. Geisbert, and R. S. Baric. 2003. Reverse genetics with a full-length infectious cDNA of severe acute respiratory syndrome coronavirus. *Proc. Natl. Acad. Sci. USA* **100:**12995–13000.

288. Yount, B., M. R. Denison, S. R. Weiss, and R. S. Baric. 2002. Systematic assembly of a full-length infectious cDNA of mouse hepatitis virus strain A59. *J. Virol.* **76:**11065–11078.

289. Yount, B., R. S. Roberts, L. Lindesmith, and R. S. Baric. 2006. Rewiring the severe acute respiratory syndrome coronavirus (SARS-CoV) transcription circuit: engineering a recombination-resistant genome. *Proc. Natl. Acad. Sci. USA* **103:**12546–12551.

290. Yount, B., R. S. Roberts, A. C. Sims, D. Deming, M. B. Frieman, J. Sparks, M. R. Denison, N. Davis, and R. S. Baric. 2005. Severe acute respiratory syndrome coronavirus group-specific open reading frames encode nonessential functions for replication in cell cultures and mice. *J. Virol.* **79:**14909–14922.

291. Zakhartchouk, A. N., Q. Liu, M. Petric, and L. A. Babiuk. 2005. Augmentation of immune responses to SARS coronavirus by a combination of DNA and whole killed virus vaccines. *Vaccine* **23:**4385–4391.

292. Zakhartchouk, A. N., S. Viswanathan, J. B. Mahony, J. Gauldie, and L. A. Babiuk. 2005. Severe acute respiratory syndrome coronavirus nucleocapsid protein expressed by an adenovirus vector is phosphorylated and immunogenic in mice. *J. Gen. Virol.* **86:**211–215.

293. Zeng, F., K. Y. Chow, C. C. Hon, K. M. Law, C. W. Yip, K. H. Chan, J. S. Peiris, and F. C. Leung. 2004. Characterization of humoral responses in mice immunized with plasmid DNAs encoding SARS-CoV spike gene fragments. *Biochem. Biophys. Res. Commun.* **315:**1134–1139.

294. Zhang, D. M., G. L. Wang, and J. H. Lu. 2005. Severe acute respiratory syndrome: vaccine on the way. *Chin. Med. J.* **118:**1468–1476.

295. Zhang, H., G. Wang, J. Li, Y. Nie, X. Shi, G. Lian, W. Wang, X. Yin, Y. Zhao, X. Qu, M. Ding, and H. Deng. 2004. Identification of an antigenic determinant on the S2 domain of the severe acute respiratory syndrome coronavirus spike glycoprotein capable of inducing neutralizing antibodies. *J. Virol.* **78:**6938–6945.

296. Zhao, P., J. Cao, L. J. Zhao, Z. L. Qin, J. S. Ke, W. Pan, H. Ren, J. G. Yu, and Z. T. Qi. 2005. Immune responses against SARS-coronavirus nucleocapsid protein induced by DNA vaccine. *Virology* **331:**128–135.

297. Zheng, B., S. Han, Y. Takahashi, and G. Kelsoe. 1997. Immunosenescence and germinal center reaction. *Immunol. Rev.* **160:**63–77.

298. Zhi, Y., J. Figueredo, G. P. Kobinger, H. Hagan, R. Calcedo, J. R. Miller, G. Gao, and J. M. Wilson. 2006. Efficacy of severe acute respiratory syndrome vaccine based on a nonhuman primate adenovirus in the presence of immunity against human adenovirus. *Hum. Gene Ther.* **17:**1–7.

299. Zhi, Y., J. M. Wilson, and H. Shen. 2005. SARS vaccine: progress and challenge. *Cell. Mol. Immunol.* **2:**101–105.

300. Zhong, X., Z. Guo, H. Yang, L. Peng, Y. Xie, T. Y. Wong, and S. T. Lai. 2006. Amino terminus of the SARS coronavirus protein 3a elicits strong, potentially protective humoral responses in infected patients. *J. Gen. Virol.* **87:**369–373.

301. Zhong, X., H. Yang, Z. F. Guo, W. Y. Sin, W. Chen, J. Xu, L. Fu, J. Wu, C. K. Mak, C. S. Cheng, Y. Yang, S. Cao, T. Y. Wong, S. T. Lai, Y. Xie, and Z. Guo. 2005. B-cell responses in patients who have recovered from severe acute respiratory syndrome target a dominant site in the S2 domain of the surface spike glycoprotein. *J. Virol.* **79:**3401–3408.

302. Zhou, J., W. Wang, Q. Zhong, W. Hou, Z. Yang, S. Y. Xiao, R. Zhu, Z. Tang, Y. Wang, Q. Xian, H. Tang, and L. Wen. 2005. Immunogenicity, safety, and protective efficacy of an inactivated SARS-associated coronavirus vaccine in rhesus monkeys. *Vaccine* **23:**3202–3209.

303. Zhou, J. Y., J. X. Wu, L. Q. Cheng, X. J. Zheng, H. Gong, S. B. Shang, and E. M. Zhou. 2003. Expression of immunogenic S1 glycoprotein of infectious bronchitis virus in transgenic potatoes. *J. Virol.* **77:**9090–9093.

304. Zhu, M. 2004. SARS immunity and vaccination. *Cell. Mol. Immunol.* **1:**193–198.

305. Zhu, M. S., Y. Pan, H. Q. Chen, Y. Shen, X. C. Wang, Y. J. Sun, and K. H. Tao. 2004. Induction of SARS-nucleoprotein-specific immune response by use of DNA vaccine. *Immunol. Lett.* **92:**237–243.

*Nidoviruses*
Edited by S. Perlman, T. Gallagher, and E. J. Snijder
© 2008 ASM Press, Washington, DC

Chapter 26

# Emerging Nidovirus Infections

LEO L. M. POON

## SARS OUTBREAKS

Severe acute respiratory syndrome (SARS) is the first novel infectious respiratory disease identified in this millennium. The first known case of SARS was identified in Foshan City, Guangdong Province, China, on 16 November 2002 (75). The disease was then reported in many cities in Guangdong Province and was officially recognized by the World Health Organization (WHO) in February 2003 (55). After its introduction to Hong Kong in mid-February 2003, the virus spread across Vietnam, Singapore, Canada, Taiwan, and elsewhere within weeks. Because avian H5N1 virus was isolated from two patients with viral pneumonia after they traveled to mainland China (40), it was initially postulated that the outbreak of atypical pneumonia was caused by a pandemic avian influenza virus. Early studies of small patient subsets also suggested that other human pathogens such as chlamydiae and paramyxoviruses might be the causative agent of the disease (41). These hypotheses, however, were soon discarded after subsequent investigations were performed (see below). On 15 March 2003, the WHO issued a travel advisory and officially named the mysterious atypical pneumonia "SARS." In addition, an international collaborative research network of laboratories around the world (11 laboratories in nine countries) was set up by the WHO to identify the etiology of SARS (55). By the end of March 2003, three research groups independently identified a novel coronavirus as the causative agent for the disease (4, 27, 39). An enormous multinational effort was initiated to contain spread of the disease. On 5 July 2003, all known chains of human-to-human transmission of the disease were broken and the WHO declared that the epidemic had been contained worldwide. Subsequent surveillance studies indicated that the virus was derived from animals (17) (see below). In this outbreak, over 8,000 patients with SARS were reported, with more than 20% of these patients identified as health care workers. Approximately 10% of all patients died from the disease (42).

After the 2002–2003 SARS outbreak was contained, sporadic human cases continued to be reported. Laboratory-acquired infections from three countries were reported in 2003–2004. In one instance, the index patient transmitted the virus to seven persons (35). Additionally, four community-acquired infections were identified in Guangdong Province (33). Although it is not clear how these patients was infected, further investigations suggested that at least two of them were likely exposed to animals carrying SARS-like coronaviruses (62). These findings, like those in the 2002–2003 epidemic, suggested that SARS resulted from zoonotic transmissions.

## IDENTIFICATION OF A NOVEL CORONAVIRUS AS THE CAUSE OF SARS

It is well known that some animal coronaviruses (e.g., feline infectious peritonitis virus and transmissible gastroenteritis virus) cause fatal infections in their hosts (48). However, relatively little attention had been focused on human coronaviruses (e.g., human coronavirus 229E [HCoV-229E] and HCoV-OC43) before the SARS era. This is partly explained by the fact that these human coronaviruses (and even recently identified human coronaviruses, with the exception of SARS coronavirus [SARS-CoV]) were associated primarily with mild enteric and respiratory diseases in healthy individuals. Thus, the identification of a coronavirus as the etiological cause of a fatal infection in humans was surprising. In order to

**Leo L. M. Poon** • Department of Microbiology, The University of Hong Kong, Hong Kong SAR, China.

conclusively demonstrate that this novel virus was the primary cause of SARS, researchers from the WHO collaborative network used several different approaches. At the mid-phase of the outbreak, isolation of SARS-CoV and determination of the sequence of its genome facilitated the development of diagnostic tools that could be used to probe for evidence of viral infection in patients with clinical signs and symptoms of SARS (4, 27, 39). Using these molecular and/or serological assays, several groups demonstrated that most SARS patients from different geographical regions were positive for infection with SARS-CoV. By contrast, there was no evidence of SARS-CoV infection in healthy controls. Fouchier et al. further demonstrated that cynomolgus macaques *(Macaca fascicularis)* infected with a purified SARS-CoV isolate developed diseases with pathological changes similar to those observed in human cases (12), although the virus was found to cause relatively mild clinical presentations in this animal model. Nonetheless, the above findings and the success in reisolating the virus from these experimentally infected animals demonstrated that this novel virus fulfilled Koch's postulates. On 15 April 2003, 2 days after releasing the first SARS-CoV genomic sequence to the public domain, the WHO announced that SARS-CoV had been confirmed as the primary cause of SARS (55).

## THE SARS-CoV GENOME AND ITS CLASSIFICATION

The genome of SARS-CoV is that of a typical coronavirus. The genome of coronavirus is a single, positive-stranded RNA, approximately 29.7 kb in length. The genomic RNA is capped and polyadenylated. Like all other coronaviruses, the SARS genomic RNA has several open reading frames (ORFs) which encode the replicase (ORF1a and ORF1ab), spike (S) (ORF2), envelope (ORF4), membrane (ORF5), and nucleocapsid (ORF9) proteins. The proteins encoded by these ORFs were extensively reviewed by others (37, 51), although the functions of some nonstructural proteins encoded by ORF1a and ORF1ab are not completely clear yet. Apart from these essential ORFs, the viral genome contains additional ORFs that encode "accessory" proteins (3a, 3b, 6, 7a, 7b, 8a, 8b, and 9b) (51). It was demonstrated that recombinant viruses without these accessory ORFs were viable in cell cultures, indicating that these accessory ORFs might encode luxury functions for virus replication (72). Indeed, studies on accessory proteins 3a, 3b, and 7a in transfected cells suggested that these proteins could induce apoptosis (29, 56, 73). There is also evidence suggesting that the 3a and

7a proteins are incorporated into the virions (20, 21). Recent data also suggest that the 3a protein forms homotetramers with ion channel activity (34). The protein encoded from ORF6 was shown to increase DNA synthesis in cells (13). Data from a crystal structure study of the 9b protein suggested that this protein might be a lipid binding protein (38). Overall, these accessory proteins might play critical roles in viral replication, and some of these proteins might be relevant to the pathogenesis of the infection.

Sequence analysis of SARS-CoV isolated from civets and humans showed that all animal isolates contained a 29-nucleotide (nt) sequence which is absent from most human isolates (17). As a result of this deletion, ORF8 in human isolates encodes 8a and 8b proteins, whereas the corresponding ORF in the animal viruses encodes for a single protein, known as 8ab protein. The 8ab protein has N and C termini that are identical to those of the 8a and 8b proteins, respectively. Studies on recombinant SARS-CoV indicated that this deletion in human isolates had little impact on in vitro virus replication or RNA synthesis (72). However, the 8b protein was recently shown to be distinct from its counterpart in the animal precursor virus. In that particular study, the 8a, 8b, and 8ab proteins were found to have differential affinities for various SARS-CoV structural proteins (26). Even more interesting, the expression of the envelope protein of SARS-CoV was found to be down-regulated by 8b but not 8a or 8ab in infected cells. In other coronaviral infections, the envelope protein was shown to induce apoptosis. Thus, these observations suggest that the 29-nt deletion might modulate the replication or pathogenesis of human SARS-CoV.

Coronaviruses have been subdivided into three groups (groups 1 to 3), and the classification of these viruses is primarily based on antigenic and genetic relationships. All previously known mammalian coronaviruses are classified as group 1 or 2 viruses. Interestingly, the classification of SARS-CoV was initially quite controversial because antigenic and genetic studies of SARS-CoV yielded inconsistent results. SARS-CoV is serologically cross-reactive with group 1 and group 2 coronaviruses (1, 27). However, partial viral sequences determined in initial studies suggested that the virus was genetically distinct from all previously established groups (4, 27, 39). Because this virus is genetically equidistant from other groups, one suggestion was to classify it as a group 4 virus (36, 47, 74). Others suggested that SARS-CoV was a recombinant between coronaviruses of different groups (45, 53, 54). It is now generally agreed that this virus is a distant member of the group 2 coronaviruses (7, 14, 51), and currently, SARS-CoV is classified as a group 2b coronavirus (15). However, one should note that the virus possesses several unique features which are absent from other classical group 2 viruses (renamed as group 2a viruses). For example, this virus has some regions which are highly similar to group 3 coronaviruses (46, 54). More strikingly, unlike other classical group 2 members, its viral genome does not contain a hemagglutinin esterase (HE) gene. In fact, none of the recently identified group 2 bat coronaviruses (see below) encode HE, indicating that the presence of this gene is a unique feature of group 2a viruses. These observations also suggest that the group 2a coronaviruses are descended from a common ancestor and are a sublineage that is distinct from other group 2 viruses.

## ISOLATION OF SARS-CoV IN PALM CIVETS AND OTHER ANIMALS PRESENT IN LIVE-ANIMAL MARKETS

In the early to middle phase of the SARS outbreak, several explanations for the appearance of this novel coronavirus were proposed. The virus was proposed to originate in human or animal populations. Other suggestions were that SARS-CoV was a recombinant between group 2 and group 3 coronaviruses or was developed in a laboratory for use as a biological weapon. Perhaps the most extreme speculation was that SARS-CoV originated in outer space (63). Fairly quickly, the zoonotic theory was supported by the isolation of SARS-like coronaviruses from Himalayan palm civets *(Paguma larvata)* in Guangdong Province (17).

The first SARS-CoV surveillance study in a wet market in Guangzhou was prompted by the realization that some early SARS patients had close associations with the wild animals sold in these locales for human consumption (75). In this study, evidence of SARS-like coronavirus infections was found in samples collected from civets, a raccoon dog *(Nyctereutes procyonoides),* and a Chinese ferret-badger *(Melogale moschata)* (17). In particular, SARS-like viral isolates were recovered from infected civets. Genetic analysis of these viral RNAs indicated that the human and animal isolates were almost identical (99.8% sequence identity). Serological studies revealed that a significant fraction of traders in wild live-animal markets in Guangdong Province had antibodies against SARS-CoV. Interestingly, none of these animal workers had developed SARS before or during the outbreak, suggesting that most animal SARS-like coronaviruses can only cause asymptomatic or mild infections in humans. This is further supported by the fact that none of the four cases of confirmed animal SARS-like coronavirus infections in 2003–2004 were

fatal or resulted in secondary transmission (33). The explanation for these differences between SARS-CoV and animal SARS-like coronavirus infections in humans is not known and remains an area of active investigation. These differences might partly reflect differences between the S proteins of the human and animal SARS viruses; the S protein from animal isolates does not have a high affinity for human angiotensin-converting enzyme 2 (ACE2), a receptor that is essential for the cellular entry of human SARS-CoV (32). It is possible that some of the animal SARS-CoV isolates acquired critical additional mutations that allow these viruses to be transmitted to humans.

Serological and molecular studies indicated that the prevalence of animal SARS-CoV in civets from civet farms was low (24, 58). Some of the studied farms were even found to be free of the virus. By contrast, a great majority of civets in wildlife markets were found to be infected. These observations suggest that the animals are more susceptible to infection with SARS-CoV under stressful conditions. Nonetheless, these data provide convincing evidence that spread of the virus from civets to humans most likely occurred in live-animal markets.

## SARS-LIKE CORONAVIRUS IN HORSESHOE BATS

Several lines of evidence hinted that palm civets might not be the natural carrier of the virus. First, sequence analyses revealed that SARS-CoV isolated from civets were under high selection pressure (24, 52), suggesting that the virus was not fully adapted to these animals. Experimental infections of civets also indicated that these animals might not be the natural host of the virus (70). In addition, the relative prevalence of the animal SARS-like coronaviruses in animal farms was much lower than in animal markets (24, 58). These results were also supported by findings that none of the palm civets captured from natural habitats were positive by serology or PCR for the virus (41). Overall, it seemed more likely that the civets might have acquired the virus from another animal species.

Soon after the discovery of the first coronaviruses in bats (41) (see below), a group of novel group 2b coronaviruses were identified in *Rhinolophus* spp. (horseshoe bats) (Fig. 1) (28, 31, 57), suggesting that SARS-CoV might originate from bats. Serological tests indicated that these coronaviruses were endemic in these bat species. In one of these studies, almost half of the serum samples collected from these bats were able to neutralize human SARS-CoV in tissue culture cells, demonstrating that this group of coronaviruses are antigenically similar (28). In

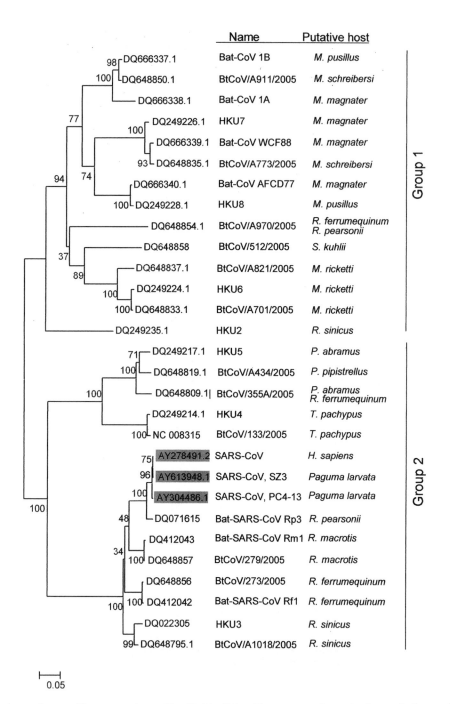

**Figure 1.** Phylogenetic tree of bat coronaviruses identified in China. The names and putative hosts of all recently found bat coronaviruses (3, 28, 31, 41, 67) are indicated. The tree was constructed by the neighbor-joining method based on partial RNA-dependent RNA polymerase sequences (402 nt) of bat coronaviruses, animal SARS-CoV isolated in 2003 (SZ3) and 2004 (PC4-13), and human SARS-CoV. The bootstrap values were determined by 1,000 replicates. The scale bar shows the estimated genetic distance of these viruses. The GenBank accession numbers of these sequences are shown in the tree. The accession numbers representing SARS-CoV and animal SARS-CoV are shaded.

addition, only fecal, and not respiratory, samples from bats were positive for these novel group 2b viruses, implying that these viruses might have an enteric tropism. No obvious signs of disease were reported.

Notably, these bat SARS-like coronaviruses have only about 90% nucleotide sequence identity to SARS-CoV (44). Phylogenetic studies of these group 2b viruses (i.e., SARS-CoV, animal SARS-CoV, and bat SARS-like coronaviruses) revealed that their S protein genes are clustered into two subgroups, one of bat coronaviruses and another of SARS viruses from humans and civets (44, 57). For example, the S1 domain of the S protein of the SARS-like coronaviruses is only about 64% identical to the corresponding region in SARS-CoV. In addition, the nonstructural protein 3 (nsp3) and S, 3a, and 8 protein amino acid sequences were found to be very different (44). Since coronaviruses usually have low mutation rates (30), it seems unlikely that these viruses diverged to this extent within a short time as a consequence of host adaptation. In addition, as the S1 domain is responsible for receptor binding, it is not clear whether these bat SARS-like coronaviruses can utilize civet ACE2 for zoonotic transmission. Collectively, these results suggest, given that there are several group 2b viruses circulating in horseshoe bats, that there are very likely bats in this genus that are infected with viruses with closer genetic relationships to SARS-CoV. Whether there is another intermediate host to transmit the virus from bats to civets is yet to be determined.

## NOVEL CORONAVIRUSES IDENTIFIED IN THE POST-SARS ERA

The isolation of a novel coronavirus as the etiological agent for SARS has led to a resurgence of interest in coronaviruses. The zoonotic transfer of SARS-CoV from civets to humans highlights the potential threats posed by coronaviruses endemic in wild animals. Before the SARS outbreak, most coronaviruses were identified in humans or domestic animals. This bias occurred because viral investigations are often driven by clinically and economically important disease outbreaks in human and animal populations. By contrast, relatively little is known about the prevalence of coronaviruses in wild animals. Since the SARS outbreak, greater efforts have been made to identify novel coronaviruses in wildlife, domestic animals, and humans. Over the last few years, several novel coronaviruses from groups 1 to 3 have been identified.

### Novel Group 1 and 2 Coronaviruses in Bats

The discovery of SARS-CoV in civets from wet markets prompted investigators to launch a survey of the prevalence of coronaviruses in wild animals in Hong Kong (41). In this surveillance study, wild mammalian, avian, and reptile species caught from natural reservoirs were sampled and about 300 samples were examined by PCR assays specific for coronaviruses. Of these samples, the first bat coronavirus was identified in three bent-winged bat species (*Miniopterus* spp.) (41). This virus was initially classified as group 1 coronavirus and was found to be phylogenetically close to porcine epidemic diarrhea virus. At first, based on a study of a small number of samples, viruses

from these bent-winged bats were classified as a single species. However, after long-term and more extensive surveillance on populations of these bats, these viruses were reclassified into two different coronavirus groups (named bat coronaviruses 1A and 1B) (3). Additionally, these two groups of viruses were found to have different host specificities (3).

The identification of these different coronaviruses in bats suggested that there might be multiple unrecognized coronaviruses in bats (41). Recent studies on other bat species have confirmed this hypothesis (28, 31, 57, 67). In these investigations, several novel group 1 and group 2 members were identified in different bat species circulating in a single geographical region. The names of these novel bat coronaviruses and their phylogenetic relations are summarized in Fig. 1. These bat coronaviruses were found to be host specific (Fig. 1). None of these studies reported possible recombination events between these bat viruses. However, the same bat virus could be occasionally detected in two different species, suggesting that interspecies transmission might occur (3). Thus, the possibility of recombination between these bat viruses cannot be excluded. In all of these studies, fecal samples were the predominant samples positive for these viruses, but respiratory samples were also positive in a fraction of cases (3, 41). These results imply that these viruses predominantly have an enteric tropism. Further investigation is required to elucidate the persistence of infection, the tissue tropism, and the pathogenicity of these viruses.

These newly identified bat coronaviruses are phylogenetically highly diverse (Fig. 1), suggesting that coronaviruses coevolved with bats or that they were established in bat populations for a time sufficiently long for a progenitor virus to evolve into several genetically distinct viruses. In addition, the phylogenetic tree of these viruses revealed two interesting observations. First, the group 1 bat coronaviruses were found to be highly divergent and to form clusters with other previously known group 1 coronaviruses (57). By contrast, the group 2 bat viruses were found to establish two separate lineages that are not related to all previously known group 2 viruses (57). Further surveillance of bat coronaviruses in different geographical regions might help to reveal a more comprehensive picture of how bat coronaviruses, or even coronaviruses in general, have evolved.

### A Novel Group 1 Coronavirus in Humans, HCoV-NL63

A novel human coronavirus, HCoV-NL63, was discovered in infants with respiratory illness by two independent groups soon after the identification of

SARS-CoV (11, 61). The virus was found to be closely related to HCoV-229E and was associated with mild respiratory illness (61). Some studies suggested that this virus might be associated with Kawasaki disease (9). However, this association were soon rejected by others (6, 49).

Among all the newly identified coronaviruses, HCoV-NL63 is the most well characterized. One of the most surprising findings about this virus is that, unlike all classical group 1 viruses, which use CD13 as the receptor for cellular entry, HCoV-NL63 uses ACE2 for virus entry (19). As SARS-CoV and HCoV-NL63 use the same receptor for entry, it will be of interest to identify the factors that modulate the pathogenesis and tissue tropism of these viruses. In addition, L-SIGN was reported to play a role in SARS-CoV infections by facilitating cell entry (2, 22). It will be interesting to investigate whether L-SIGN also has role in the life cycle of HCoV-NL63. Other details related to this virus, such as its epidemiology, genome organization, molecular biology, and tissue tropism, were recently reviewed by van der Hoek et al. (60) and are not covered in this chapter.

### A Novel Group 1 Coronavirus in Spotted Hyenas

East et al. reported a novel group 1 coronavirus in wild spotted hyenas (Crocuta crocuta) (5). The S protein gene of this virus was found to be phylogenetically related to group 1 canine and type II feline coronaviruses. Serological studies of spotted hyenas revealed that infection with this virus occurs commonly. From a limited number of specimens, viral RNA was only detected in fecal samples, suggesting the virus has an enteric tropism and is transmitted via the fecal-oral route. Diarrhea is the only observable clinical outcome that appears to be associated with the infection, after long-term observation.

### A Novel Group 1 Virus in Ferrets

Epizootic catarrhal enteritis in ferrets was first identified in 2003 (64). Using consensus primers for coronaviruses, Wise and colleagues confirmed that a novel group 1 coronavirus, ferret enteric coronavirus, is the etiological agent for the disease (65). The virus was found to be phylogenetically clustered with feline coronavirus, canine coronavirus, and transmissible gastroenteritis virus as a group 1 coronavirus. In agreement with the clinical presentation, virus RNA and antigen were primarily found in the small and large intestine of infected ferrets. As observed in other coronavirus infections, these results indicated that the fecal-oral route might be the major mode of transmission of the disease.

### A Novel Group 2 Virus in Dogs

In 2003, a novel group 2 coronavirus was identified by Erles et al. (8). This virus is genetically closely related to bovine coronavirus and HCoV-OC43. Unlike the group 1 canine enteric coronavirus, this new canine virus was found to be associated with respiratory diseases in dogs. In this study, 30% of the studied dogs were found to be seropositive for this virus, and more than half of the dogs with mild cough were positive for this virus in PCR assays. These findings indicated that this novel virus is a very common respiratory pathogen in dog populations. This was confirmed by subsequent investigations using canine samples from other geographical regions (25, 43). One should note that only respiratory and/or blood samples were studied in the above work. However, in another study, the virus was detected in a rectal sample from a dog with respiratory and gastrointestinal diseases (71). Further work is required to better understand the pathogenesis of this new canine virus.

### A Novel Group 2 Coronavirus in Humans, HCoV-HKU1

The SARS outbreak resulted in the initiation of multiple studies in which human respiratory specimens were retrospectively screened for coronaviruses (66). In one study, a novel human group 2 coronavirus (HCoV-HKU1) was detected using a pair of conserved primers for coronaviruses. The virus was first detected in a nasopharyngeal aspirate sample from a 71-year-old man with respiratory illness. This novel virus is genetically different from HCoV-OC43, the other known human group 2 coronavirus. Subsequent studies demonstrated that this virus is a common human pathogen (10, 50, 59). Epidemiological studies suggested that this virus is associated with respiratory illnesses, and in about 2.4% of patients with community-acquired pneumonia, disease is caused by this virus (68). In addition, this virus was detected in stool samples from patients with acute enteric disease, suggesting that this pathogen might also cause gastroenteritis (59). Further sequencing studies of this virus suggested that novel genotypes of HCoV-HKU1 might be generated by natural recombination events between HCoV-HKU1 from different genotypes (69).

### Novel Group 3 Coronaviruses in Birds

A surveillance study in Norway reported three novel coronaviruses in wild graylag geese (Anser anser), feral pigeons (Columbia livia), and mallards (Anas platyrhynchos) (23). Using degenerate primers that cross-reacted with coronaviruses from three different groups, only group 3 viruses were detected in the studied samples. These results suggested that group 3 coronaviruses are fundamentally different from members of the other two groups. These novel avian viruses were isolated from cloacal samples of these animals. A significant fraction of fecal samples (25%) from the geese in this study was positive for the goose coronavirus, suggesting that the virus might be spread by the fecal-oral transmission route. The infected graylag geese showed lower body weights than virus-negative birds, showing that the infection was clinically significant. Of note, only cloacal swabs were examined in this investigation. Thus, it is possible that some of these viruses might be transmitted by other routes.

## A Novel Parrot Coronavirus

A novel coronavirus was isolated from spleen, liver, and kidney of a dead green-cheeked Amazon parrot *(Amazona viridigenalis Cassin)* (16) and was likely associated with the psittacine proventricular dilatation disease observed in this bird. The virus was found to be antigenically different from infectious bronchitis virus, a well-characterized group 3 coronavirus. Strikingly, based on analysis of a 66-amino-acid sequence in the RNA-dependent RNA polymerase, this virus was found to be very distinct from all other coronaviruses. As the analyzed sequence was relatively short, further investigations will be required to determine whether this novel virus represents a novel group or subgroup of coronaviruses.

## FURTHER PERSPECTIVES

SARS was the first pandemic in this century. The disease had a severe impact on health care, the economy, and the tourist industry in many countries. The outbreak served as a useful warning that greater preparation was needed to deal with possible future pandemics, such as avian H5N1 influenza virus (18). The SARS outbreak highlighted the importance of multidisciplinary research and of cooperation between multiple laboratories in tackling emerging diseases. Much basic and clinical research on coronaviruses has been triggered by this outbreak. The SARS pandemic also led to the search for novel coronaviruses in humans and animals, resulting in the identification of at least two new human and several new animal coronaviruses within the last 4 years. In some instances, it has been difficult to fit these new viruses into the existing taxonomy. As more and more coronaviruses that are phylogenetically distinct from classical group 1 to 3 viruses are discovered, an alternative classification system of coronaviruses will need to be considered. Further, difficulties in culturing some of these novel viruses have inhibited efforts to better understand the basic biology of these viruses and to perform systematic studies of the antigens of these novel viruses. Another area of future research is determination of the pathogenesis of these novel coronaviruses that circulate in wildlife. Some infected wild animals do not even appear to develop signs of clinical disease. This may reflect, in part, a lack of understanding of the biology and epidemiology of these wild animal species. Prior to developing suitable in vitro or in vivo models for these novel viruses, long-term and systematic surveillance might be the most practical approach to further understand these viruses that circulate in wildlife. Nonetheless, these discoveries have opened up multiple new areas of research in this field and suggested that there are many novel coronaviruses that are yet to be identified. More importantly, some of these hitherto-unknown coronaviruses might have zoonotic potential. Given the catastrophic consequences of the SARS epidemic, further long-term investigations on viruses in wildlife and the ecology of their hosts should be encouraged.

**Acknowledgments.** The work is supported by funds from the Research Grant Council of Hong Kong (HKU 7343/04M), the VOC SARS Research funds from the University of Hong Kong, and European Research Project SARS-DTV (contract no. SP22-CT-2004).

## REFERENCES

1. Chan, K. H., V. C. Cheng, P. C. Woo, S. K. Lau, L. L. Poon, Y. Guan, W. H. Seto, K. Y. Yuen, and J. S. Peiris. 2005. Serological responses in patients with severe acute respiratory syndrome coronavirus infection and cross-reactivity with human coronaviruses 229E, OC43, and NL63. *Clin. Diagn. Lab. Immunol.* 12:1317–1321.
2. Chan, V. S., K. Y. Chan, Y. Chen, L. L. Poon, A. N. Cheung, B. Zheng, K. H. Chan, W. Mak, H. Y. Ngan, X. Xu, G. Screaton, P. K. Tam, J. M. Austyn, L. C. Chan, S. P. Yip, M. Peiris, U. S. Khoo, and C. L. Lin. 2006. Homozygous L-SIGN (CLEC4M) plays a protective role in SARS coronavirus infection. *Nat. Genet.* 38:38–46.
3. Chu, D. K., L. L. Poon, K. H. Chan, H. Chen, Y. Guan, K. Y. Yuen, and J. S. Peiris. 2006. Coronaviruses in bent-winged bats (Miniopterus spp.). *J. Gen. Virol.* 87:2461–2466.
4. Drosten, C., S. Gunther, W. Preiser, S. van der Werf, H. R. Brodt, S. Becker, H. Rabenau, M. Panning, L. Kolesnikova, R. A. Fouchier, A. Berger, A. M. Burguiere, J. Cinatl, M. Eickmann, N. Escriou, K. Grywna, S. Kramme, J. C. Manuguerra, S. Muller, V. Rickerts, M. Sturmer, S. Vieth, H. D. Klenk, A. D. Osterhaus, H. Schmitz, and H. W. Doerr. 2003. Identification of a novel coronavirus in patients with severe acute respiratory syndrome. *N. Engl. J. Med.* 348:1967–1976.
5. East, M. L., K. Moestl, V. Benetka, C. Pitra, O. P. Honer, B. Wachter, and H. Hofer. 2004. Coronavirus infection of spotted hyenas in the Serengeti ecosystem. *Vet. Microbiol.* 102:1–9.

6. **Ebihara, T., R. Endo, X. Ma, N. Ishiguro, and H. Kikuta.** 2005. Lack of association between New Haven coronavirus and Kawasaki disease. *J. Infect. Dis.* **192:**351–352. (Author reply, **192:**353.)

7. **Eickmann, M., S. Becker, H. D. Klenk, H. W. Doerr, K. Stadler, S. Censini, S. Guidotti, V. Masignani, M. Scarselli, M. Mora, C. Donati, J. H. Han, H. C. Song, A. Abrignani, A. Covacci, and R. Rappuoli.** 2003. Phylogeny of the SARS coronavirus. *Science* **302:**1504–1505.

8. **Erles, K., C. Toomey, H. W. Brooks, and J. Brownlie.** 2003. Detection of a group 2 coronavirus in dogs with canine infectious respiratory disease. *Virology* **310:**216–223.

9. **Esper, F., E. D. Shapiro, C. Weibel, D. Ferguson, M. L. Landry, and J. S. Kahn.** 2005. Association between a novel human coronavirus and Kawasaki disease. *J. Infect. Dis.* **191:**499–502.

10. **Esper, F., C. Weibel, D. Ferguson, M. L. Landry, and J. S. Kahn.** 2006. Coronavirus HKU1 infection in the United States. *Emerg. Infect. Dis.* **12:**775–779.

11. **Fouchier, R. A., N. G. Hartwig, T. M. Bestebroer, B. Niemeyer, J. C. de Jong, J. H. Simon, and A. D. Osterhaus.** 2004. A previously undescribed coronavirus associated with respiratory disease in humans. *Proc. Natl. Acad. Sci. USA* **101:**6212–6216.

12. **Fouchier, R. A., T. Kuiken, M. Schutten, G. van Amerongen, G. J. van Doornum, B. G. van den Hoogen, M. Peiris, W. Lim, K. Stohr, and A. D. Osterhaus.** 2003. Aetiology: Koch's postulates fulfilled for SARS virus. *Nature* **423:**240.

13. **Geng, H., Y. M. Liu, W. S. Chan, A. W. Lo, D. M. Au, M. M. Waye, and Y. Y. Ho.** 2005. The putative protein 6 of the severe acute respiratory syndrome-associated coronavirus: expression and functional characterization. *FEBS Lett.* **579:**6763–6768.

14. **Goebel, S. J., J. Taylor, and P. S. Masters.** 2004. The 3′ *cis*-acting genomic replication element of the severe acute respiratory syndrome coronavirus can function in the murine coronavirus genome. *J. Virol.* **78:**7846–7851.

15. **Gorbalenya, A. E., E. J. Snijder, and W. J. Spaan.** 2004. Severe acute respiratory syndrome coronavirus phylogeny: toward consensus. *J. Virol.* **78:**7863–7866.

16. **Gough, R. E., S. E. Drury, F. Culver, P. Britton, and D. Cavanagh.** 2006. Isolation of a coronavirus from a green-cheeked Amazon parrot (Amazon viridigenalis Cassin). *Avian Pathol.* **35:**122–126.

17. **Guan, Y., B. J. Zheng, Y. Q. He, X. L. Liu, Z. X. Zhuang, C. L. Cheung, S. W. Luo, P. H. Li, L. J. Zhang, Y. J. Guan, K. M. Butt, K. L. Wong, K. W. Chan, W. Lim, K. F. Shortridge, K. Y. Yuen, J. S. Peiris, and L. L. Poon.** 2003. Isolation and characterization of viruses related to the SARS coronavirus from animals in southern China. *Science* **302:**276–278.

18. **Ho, M. S., and I. J. Su.** 2004. Preparing to prevent severe acute respiratory syndrome and other respiratory infections. *Lancet Infect. Dis.* **4:**684–689.

19. **Hofmann, H., K. Pyrc, L. van der Hoek, M. Geier, B. Berkhout, and S. Pohlmann.** 2005. Human coronavirus NL63 employs the severe acute respiratory syndrome coronavirus receptor for cellular entry. *Proc. Natl. Acad. Sci. USA* **102:**7988–7993.

20. **Huang, C., N. Ito, C. T. Tseng, and S. Makino.** 2006. Severe acute respiratory syndrome coronavirus 7a accessory protein is a viral structural protein. *J. Virol.* **80:**7287–7294.

21. **Ito, N., E. C. Mossel, K. Narayanan, V. L. Popov, C. Huang, T. Inoue, C. J. Peters, and S. Makino.** 2005. Severe acute respiratory syndrome coronavirus 3a protein is a viral structural protein. *J. Virol.* **79:**3182–3186.

22. **Jeffers, S. A., S. M. Tusell, L. Gillim-Ross, E. M. Hemmila, J. E. Achenbach, G. J. Babcock, W. D. Thomas, Jr., L. B. Thackray, M. D. Young, R. J. Mason, D. M. Ambrosino, D. E. Wentworth, J. C. Demartini, and K. V. Holmes.** 2004. CD209L (L-SIGN) is a receptor for severe acute respiratory syndrome coronavirus. *Proc. Natl. Acad. Sci. USA* **101:**15748–15753.

23. **Jonassen, C. M., T. Kofstad, I. L. Larsen, A. Lovland, K. Handeland, A. Follestad, and A. Lillehaug.** 2005. Molecular identification and characterization of novel coronaviruses infecting graylag geese (Anser anser), feral pigeons (Columbia livia) and mallards (Anas platyrhynchos). *J. Gen. Virol.* **86:**1597–1607.

24. **Kan, B., M. Wang, H. Jing, H. Xu, X. Jiang, M. Yan, W. Liang, H. Zheng, K. Wan, Q. Liu, B. Cui, Y. Xu, E. Zhang, H. Wang, J. Ye, G. Li, M. Li, Z. Cui, X. Qi, K. Chen, L. Du, K. Gao, Y. T. Zhao, X. Z. Zou, Y. J. Feng, Y. F. Gao, R. Hai, D. Yu, Y. Guan, and J. Xu.** 2005. Molecular evolution analysis and geographic investigation of severe acute respiratory syndrome coronavirus-like virus in palm civets at an animal market and on farms. *J. Virol.* **79:**11892–11900.

25. **Kaneshima, T., T. Hohdatsu, K. Satoh, T. Takano, K. Motokawa, and H. Koyama.** 2006. The prevalence of a group 2 coronavirus in dogs in Japan. *J. Vet. Med. Sci.* **68:**21–25.

26. **Keng, C. T., Y. W. Choi, M. R. Welkers, D. Z. Chan, S. Shen, S. Gee Lim, W. Hong, and Y. J. Tan.** 2006. The human severe acute respiratory syndrome coronavirus (SARS-CoV) 8b protein is distinct from its counterpart in animal SARS-CoV and down-regulates the expression of the envelope protein in infected cells. *Virology* **354:**132–142.

27. **Ksiazek, T. G., D. Erdman, C. S. Goldsmith, S. R. Zaki, T. Peret, S. Emery, S. Tong, C. Urbani, J. A. Comer, W. Lim, P. E. Rollin, S. F. Dowell, A. E. Ling, C. D. Humphrey, W. J. Shieh, J. Guarner, C. D. Paddock, P. Rota, B. Fields, J. DeRisi, J. Y. Yang, N. Cox, J. M. Hughes, J. W. LeDuc, W. J. Bellini, and L. J. Anderson.** 2003. A novel coronavirus associated with severe acute respiratory syndrome. *N. Engl. J. Med.* **348:**1953–1966.

28. **Lau, S. K., P. C. Woo, K. S. Li, Y. Huang, H. W. Tsoi, B. H. Wong, S. S. Wong, S. Y. Leung, K. H. Chan, and K. Y. Yuen.** 2005. Severe acute respiratory syndrome coronavirus-like virus in Chinese horseshoe bats. *Proc. Natl. Acad. Sci. USA* **102:**14040–14045.

29. **Law, P. T., C. H. Wong, T. C. Au, C. P. Chuck, S. K. Kong, P. K. Chan, K. F. To, A. W. Lo, J. Y. Chan, Y. K. Suen, H. Y. Chan, K. P. Fung, M. M. Waye, J. J. Sung, Y. M. Lo, and S. K. Tsui.** 2005. The 3a protein of severe acute respiratory syndrome-associated coronavirus induces apoptosis in Vero E6 cells. *J. Gen. Virol.* **86:**1921–1930.

30. **Leparc-Goffart, I., S. T. Hingley, M. M. Chua, X. Jiang, E. Lavi, and S. R. Weiss.** 1997. Altered pathogenesis of a mutant of the murine coronavirus MHV-A59 is associated with a Q159L amino acid substitution in the spike protein. *Virology* **239:**1–10.

31. **Li, W., Z. Shi, M. Yu, W. Ren, C. Smith, J. H. Epstein, H. Wang, G. Crameri, Z. Hu, H. Zhang, J. Zhang, J. McEachern, H. Field, P. Daszak, B. T. Eaton, S. Zhang, and L. F. Wang.** 2005. Bats are natural reservoirs of SARS-like coronaviruses. *Science* **310:**676–679.

32. **Li, W., C. Zhang, J. Sui, J. H. Kuhn, M. J. Moore, S. Luo, S. K. Wong, I. C. Huang, K. Xu, N. Vasilieva, A. Murakami, Y. He, W. A. Marasco, Y. Guan, H. Choe, and M. Farzan.** 2005. Receptor and viral determinants of SARS-coronavirus adaptation to human ACE2. *EMBO J.* **24:**1634–1643.

33. **Liang, G., Q. Chen, J. Xu, Y. Liu, W. Lim, J. S. Peiris, L. J. Anderson, L. Ruan, H. Li, B. Kan, B. Di, P. Cheng, K. H. Chan, D. D. Erdman, S. Gu, X. Yan, W. Liang, D. Zhou, L. Haynes, S. Duan, X. Zhang, H. Zheng, Y. Gao, S. Tong, D. Li, L. Fang, P. Qin, and W. Xu.** 2004. Laboratory diagnosis of four recent sporadic cases of community-acquired SARS,

Guangdong Province, China. *Emerg. Infect. Dis.* **10:**1774–1781.

34. Lu, W., B. J. Zheng, K. Xu, W. Schwarz, L. Du, C. K. Wong, J. Chen, S. Duan, V. Deubel, and B. Sun. 2006. Severe acute respiratory syndrome-associated coronavirus 3a protein forms an ion channel and modulates virus release. *Proc. Natl. Acad. Sci. USA* **103:**12540–12545.

35. Mackenzie, J. S. 2006. *Biosafety and Biocontainment Issues.* WHO Press, Geneva, Switzerland.

36. Marra, M. A., S. J. Jones, C. R. Astell, R. A. Holt, A. Brooks-Wilson, Y. S. Butterfield, J. Khattra, J. K. Asano, S. A. Barber, S. Y. Chan, A. Cloutier, S. M. Coughlin, D. Freeman, N. Girn, O. L. Griffith, S. R. Leach, M. Mayo, H. McDonald, S. B. Montgomery, P. K. Pandoh, A. S. Petrescu, A. G. Robertson, J. E. Schein, A. Siddiqui, D. E. Smailus, J. M. Stott, G. S. Yang, F. Plummer, A. Andonov, H. Artsob, N. Bastien, K. Bernard, T. F. Booth, D. Bowness, M. Czub, M. Drebot, L. Fernando, R. Flick, M. Garbutt, M. Gray, A. Grolla, S. Jones, H. Feldmann, A. Meyers, A. Kabani, Y. Li, S. Normand, U. Stroher, G. A. Tipples, S. Tyler, R. Vogrig, D. Ward, B. Watson, R. C. Brunham, M. Krajden, M. Petric, D. M. Skowronski, C. Upton, and R. L. Roper. 2003. The genome sequence of the SARS-associated coronavirus. *Science* **300:**1399–1404.

37. Masters, P. S. 2006. The molecular biology of coronaviruses. *Adv. Virus Res.* **66:**193–292.

38. Meier, C., A. R. Aricescu, R. Assenberg, R. T. Aplin, R. J. Gilbert, J. M. Grimes, and D. I. Stuart. 2006. The crystal structure of ORF-9b, a lipid binding protein from the SARS coronavirus. *Structure* **14:**1157–1165.

39. Peiris, J. S., S. T. Lai, L. L. Poon, Y. Guan, L. Y. Yam, W. Lim, J. Nicholls, W. K. Yee, W. W. Yan, M. T. Cheung, V. C. Cheng, K. H. Chan, D. N. Tsang, R. W. Yung, T. K. Ng, and K. Y. Yuen. 2003. Coronavirus as a possible cause of severe acute respiratory syndrome. *Lancet* **361:**1319–1325.

40. Peiris, J. S., W. C. Yu, C. W. Leung, C. Y. Cheung, W. F. Ng, J. M. Nicholls, T. K. Ng, K. H. Chan, S. T. Lai, W. L. Lim, K. Y. Yuen, and Y. Guan. 2004. Re-emergence of fatal human influenza A subtype H5N1 disease. *Lancet* **363:**617–619.

41. Poon, L. L., D. K. Chu, K. H. Chan, O. K. Wong, T. M. Ellis, Y. H. Leung, S. K. Lau, P. C. Woo, K. Y. Suen, K. Y. Yuen, Y. Guan, and J. S. Peiris. 2005. Identification of a novel coronavirus in bats. *J. Virol.* **79:**2001–2009.

42. Poon, L. L., Y. Guan, J. M. Nicholls, K. Y. Yuen, and J. S. Peiris. 2004. The aetiology, origins, and diagnosis of severe acute respiratory syndrome. *Lancet Infect. Dis.* **4:**663–671.

43. Priestnall, S. L., J. Brownlie, E. J. Dubovi, and K. Erles. 2006. Serological prevalence of canine respiratory coronavirus. *Vet. Microbiol.* **115:**43–53.

44. Ren, W., W. Li, M. Yu, P. Hao, Y. Zhang, P. Zhou, S. Zhang, G. Zhao, Y. Zhong, S. Wang, L. F. Wang, and Z. Shi. 2006. Full-length genome sequences of two SARS-like coronaviruses in horseshoe bats and genetic variation analysis. *J. Gen. Virol.* **87:**3355–3359.

45. Rest, J. S., and D. P. Mindell. 2003. SARS associated coronavirus has a recombinant polymerase and coronaviruses have a history of host-shifting. *Infect. Genet. Evol.* **3:**219–225.

46. Robertson, M. P., H. Igel, R. Baertsch, D. Haussler, M. Ares, Jr., and W. G. Scott. 2005. The structure of a rigorously conserved RNA element within the SARS virus genome. *PLoS Biol.* **3:**e5.

47. Rota, P. A., M. S. Oberste, S. S. Monroe, W. A. Nix, R. Campagnoli, J. P. Icenogle, S. Penaranda, B. Bankamp, K. Maher, M. H. Chen, S. Tong, A. Tamin, L. Lowe, M. Frace, J. L. DeRisi, Q. Chen, D. Wang, D. D. Erdman, T. C. Peret, C. Burns, T. G. Ksiazek, P. E. Rollin, A. Sanchez, S. Liffick, B. Holloway, J. Limor, K. McCaustland, M. Olsen-Rasmussen, R. Fouchier, S. Gunther, A. D. Osterhaus, C. Drosten, M. A. Pallansch, L. J. Anderson, and W. J. Bellini. 2003. Characterization of a novel coronavirus associated with severe acute respiratory syndrome. *Science* **300:**1394–1399.

48. Saif, L. J. 2004. Animal coronavirus vaccines: lessons for SARS. *Dev. Biol.* **119:**129–140.

49. Shimizu, C., H. Shike, S. C. Baker, F. Garcia, L. van der Hoek, T. W. Kuijpers, S. L. Reed, A. H. Rowley, S. T. Shulman, H. K. Talbot, J. V. Williams, and J. C. Burns. 2005. Human coronavirus NL63 is not detected in the respiratory tracts of children with acute Kawasaki disease. *J. Infect. Dis.* **192:**1767–1771.

50. Sloots, T. P., P. McErlean, D. J. Speicher, K. E. Arden, M. D. Nissen, and I. M. Mackay. 2006. Evidence of human coronavirus HKU1 and human bocavirus in Australian children. *J. Clin. Virol.* **35:**99–102.

51. Snijder, E. J., P. J. Bredenbeek, J. C. Dobbe, V. Thiel, J. Ziebuhr, L. L. Poon, Y. Guan, M. Rozanov, W. J. Spaan, and A. E. Gorbalenya. 2003. Unique and conserved features of genome and proteome of SARS-coronavirus, an early split-off from the coronavirus group 2 lineage. *J. Mol. Biol.* **331:**991–1004.

52. Song, H. D., C. C. Tu, G. W. Zhang, S. Y. Wang, K. Zheng, L. C. Lei, Q. X. Chen, Y. W. Gao, H. Q. Zhou, H. Xiang, H. J. Zheng, S. W. Chern, F. Cheng, C. M. Pan, H. Xuan, S. J. Chen, H. M. Luo, D. H. Zhou, Y. F. Liu, J. F. He, P. Z. Qin, L. H. Li, Y. Q. Ren, W. J. Liang, Y. D. Yu, L. Anderson, M. Wang, R. H. Xu, X. W. Wu, H. Y. Zheng, J. D. Chen, G. Liang, Y. Gao, M. Liao, L. Fang, L. Y. Jiang, H. Li, F. Chen, B. Di, L. J. He, J. Y. Lin, S. Tong, X. Kong, L. Du, P. Hao, H. Tang, A. Bernini, X. J. Yu, O. Spiga, Z. M. Guo, H. Y. Pan, W. Z. He, J. C. Manuguerra, A. Fontanet, A. Danchin, N. Niccolai, Y. X. Li, C. I. Wu, and G. P. Zhao. 2005. Cross-host evolution of severe acute respiratory syndrome coronavirus in palm civet and human. *Proc. Natl. Acad. Sci. USA* **102:**2430–2435.

53. Stanhope, M. J., J. R. Brown, and H. Amrine-Madsen. 2004. Evidence from the evolutionary analysis of nucleotide sequences for a recombinant history of SARS-CoV. *Infect. Genet. Evol.* **4:**15–19.

54. Stavrinides, J., and D. S. Guttman. 2004. Mosaic evolution of the severe acute respiratory syndrome coronavirus. *J. Virol.* **78:**76–82.

55. Stöhr, K. 2003. A multicentre collaboration to investigate the cause of severe acute respiratory syndrome. *Lancet* **361:**1730–1733.

56. Tan, Y. J., B. C. Fielding, P. Y. Goh, S. Shen, T. H. Tan, S. G. Lim, and W. Hong. 2004. Overexpression of 7a, a protein specifically encoded by the severe acute respiratory syndrome coronavirus, induces apoptosis via a caspase-dependent pathway. *J. Virol.* **78:**14043–14047.

57. Tang, X. C., J. X. Zhang, S. Y. Zhang, P. Wang, X. H. Fan, L. F. Li, G. Li, B. Q. Dong, W. Liu, C. L. Cheung, K. M. Xu, W. J. Song, D. Vijaykrishna, L. L. Poon, J. S. Peiris, G. J. Smith, H. Chen, and Y. Guan. 2006. Prevalence and genetic diversity of coronaviruses in bats from China. *J. Virol.* **80:**7481–7490.

58. Tu, C., G. Crameri, X. Kong, J. Chen, Y. Sun, M. Yu, H. Xiang, X. Xia, S. Liu, T. Ren, Y. Yu, B. T. Eaton, H. Xuan, and L. F. Wang. 2004. Antibodies to SARS coronavirus in civets. *Emerg. Infect. Dis.* **10:**2244–2248.

59. Vabret, A., J. Dina, S. Gouarin, J. Petitjean, S. Corbet, and F. Freymuth. 2006. Detection of the new human coronavirus HKU1: a report of 6 cases. *Clin. Infect. Dis.* **42:**634–639.

60. van der Hoek, L., K. Pyrc, and B. Berkhout. 2006. Human coronavirus NL63, a new respiratory virus. *FEMS Microbiol. Rev.* **30:**760–773.

61. van der Hoek, L., K. Pyrc, M. F. Jebbink, W. Vermeulen-Oost, R. J. Berkhout, K. C. Wolthers, P. M. Wertheim-van Dillen, J. Kaandorp, J. Spaargaren, and B. Berkhout. 2004. Identification of a new human coronavirus. *Nat. Med.* **10:**368–373.

62. Wang, M., M. Yan, H. Xu, W. Liang, B. Kan, B. Zheng, H. Chen, H. Zheng, Y. Xu, E. Zhang, H. Wang, J. Ye, G. Li, M. Li, Z. Cui, Y. F. Liu, R. T. Guo, X. N. Liu, L. H. Zhan, D. H. Zhou, A. Zhao, R. Hai, D. Yu, Y. Guan, and J. Xu. 2005. SARS-CoV infection in a restaurant from palm civet. *Emerg. Infect. Dis.* **11:**1860–1865.

63. Wickramasinghe, C., M. Wainwright, and J. Narlikar. 2003. SARS—a clue to its origins? *Lancet* **361:**1832.

64. Williams, B. H., M. Kiupel, K. H. West, J. T. Raymond, C. K. Grant, and L. T. Glickman. 2000. Coronavirus-associated epizootic catarrhal enteritis in ferrets. *J. Am. Vet. Med. Assoc.* **217:**526–530.

65. Wise, A. G., M. Kiupel, and R. K. Maes. 2006. Molecular characterization of a novel coronavirus associated with epizootic catarrhal enteritis (ECE) in ferrets. *Virology* **349:**164–174.

66. Woo, P. C., S. K. Lau, C. M. Chu, K. H. Chan, H. W. Tsoi, Y. Huang, B. H. Wong, R. W. Poon, J. J. Cai, W. K. Luk, L. L. Poon, S. S. Wong, Y. Guan, J. S. Peiris, and K. Y. Yuen. 2005. Characterization and complete genome sequence of a novel coronavirus, coronavirus HKU1, from patients with pneumonia. *J. Virol.* **79:**884–895.

67. Woo, P. C., S. K. Lau, K. S. Li, R. W. Poon, B. H. Wong, H. W. Tsoi, B. C. Yip, Y. Huang, K. H. Chan, and K. Y. Yuen. 2006. Molecular diversity of coronaviruses in bats. *Virology* **351:** 180–187.

68. Woo, P. C., S. K. Lau, H. W. Tsoi, Y. Huang, R. W. Poon, C. M. Chu, R. A. Lee, W. K. Luk, G. K. Wong, B. H. Wong, V. C. Cheng, B. S. Tang, A. K. Wu, R. W. Yung, H. Chen, Y. Guan, K. H. Chan, and K. Y. Yuen. 2005. Clinical and molecular epidemiological features of coronavirus HKU1-associated community-acquired pneumonia. *J. Infect. Dis.* **192:**1898–1907.

69. Woo, P. C., S. K. Lau, C. C. Yip, Y. Huang, H. W. Tsoi, K. H. Chan, and K. Y. Yuen. 2006. Comparative analysis of 22 coronavirus HKU1 genomes reveals a novel genotype and evidence of natural recombination in coronavirus HKU1. *J. Virol.* **80:**7136–7145.

70. Wu, D., C. Tu, C. Xin, H. Xuan, Q. Meng, Y. Liu, Y. Yu, Y. Guan, Y. Jiang, X. Yin, G. Crameri, M. Wang, C. Li, S. Liu, M. Liao, L. Feng, H. Xiang, J. Sun, J. Chen, Y. Sun, S. Gu, N. Liu, D. Fu, B. T. Eaton, L. F. Wang, and X. Kong. 2005. Civets are equally susceptible to experimental infection by two different severe acute respiratory syndrome coronavirus isolates. *J. Virol.* **79:**2620–2625.

71. Yachi, A., and M. Mochizuki. 2006. Survey of dogs in Japan for group 2 canine coronavirus infection. *J. Clin. Microbiol.* **44:**2615–2618.

72. Yount, B., R. S. Roberts, A. C. Sims, D. Deming, M. B. Frieman, J. Sparks, M. R. Denison, N. Davis, and R. S. Baric. 2005. Severe acute respiratory syndrome coronavirus group-specific open reading frames encode nonessential functions for replication in cell cultures and mice. *J. Virol.* **79:**14909–14922.

73. Yuan, X., Y. Shan, Z. Zhao, J. Chen, and Y. Cong. 2005. G0/G1 arrest and apoptosis induced by SARS-CoV 3b protein in transfected cells. *Virol. J.* **2:**66.

74. Zeng, F. Y., C. W. Chan, M. N. Chan, J. D. Chen, K. Y. Chow, C. C. Hon, K. H. Hui, J. Li, V. Y. Li, C. Y. Wang, P. Y. Wang, Y. Guan, B. Zheng, L. L. Poon, K. H. Chan, K. Y. Yuen, J. S. Peiris, and F. C. Leung. 2003. The complete genome sequence of severe acute respiratory syndrome coronavirus strain HKU-39849 (HK-39). *Exp. Biol. Med.* (Maywood) **228:**866–873.

75. Zhong, N. S., B. J. Zheng, Y. M. Li, Poon, Z. H. Xie, K. H. Chan, P. H. Li, S. Y. Tan, Q. Chang, J. P. Xie, X. Q. Liu, J. Xu, D. X. Li, K. Y. Yuen, Peiris, and Y. Guan. 2003. Epidemiology and cause of severe acute respiratory syndrome (SARS) in Guangdong, People's Republic of China, in February, 2003. *Lancet* **362:**1353–1358.

# INDEX

Accessory proteins, 35, 40–41
  coronavirus, 186–187, 235–244
    group 1, 235–237
    group 2, 237–239
    group 3, 239–240
  murine hepatitis virus, 271–272
9-O-Acetylated sialic acids, as coronavirus receptors, 149
Acute disseminated encephalomyelitis, human coronavirus
    in, 315
Adeno-associated virus, in coronavirus vaccine
    development, 390
Adenovirus, in coronavirus vaccine development,
    389–390
ADP-ribose-1″-phosphatase, coronavirus, 71–72
Age-dependent poliomyelitis, in lactate dehydrogenase-
    elevating virus infections, 333
Alveoli, pathology of, in SARS, 303, Color Plate 5
Aminopeptidase N, coronavirus, 149, 316
Angiotensin-converting enzyme 2 receptors
  antibodies to, 383
  for coronaviruses, 149–151, 165, Color Plate 4
  for SARS-CoV, 301, 303–304
Animals, viruses of, *see specific viruses and animals*
Antibody(ies)
  bovine coronavirus, 292–293
  bovine torovirus, 355–356
  coronavirus, 344–345
  equine arteritis virus, 327–328
  feline coronavirus, 344–345
  infectious bronchitis virus, 384
  lactate dehydrogenase-elevating virus, 334
  porcine reproductive and respiratory syndrome virus,
    330–331
  SARS-CoV, 304–305
  simian hemorrhagic fever virus, 335
  torovirus, 355–356
  transmissible gastroenteritis virus, 291–292, 384
Antiviral agents, 11
Apoptosis, in coronavirus infections, 249–251, 317–318
Arteries, endothelial cells of, equine arteritis virus
    infection of, 327
Arteriviruses, *see also specific arteriviruses*
  cell entry by, 171
  discovery of, 325
  evolution of, 23–24
  genomes of, 29
    organization of, 34–35, 121
    regulation and expression of, 39–41, 121

  sizes of, 47, 48
  structures of, 15
  infections due to, 10, 47–49
  infectious clones of, 54
  phylogeny of, 16–17
  receptors for, 6
  replication of, 5–8, 83–101, Color Plate 2
    chymotrypsin-like protease in, 85, 89–91
    comparative sequence analysis of, 83–84
    cysteine proteases in, 87, 89
    nonstructural proteins in, 85, 91–98
    PCPα in, 85, 87, 88, 91–92
    PCPβ in, 85, 87, 88, 91–92
    proteolytic processing, 87–91
    RdRp in, 85
    replication complex structure in, 98
    ribosomal frameshifting in, 35–36, 86–87
    RNA signals for, 121
    zinc-binding domains in, 85–86
  RNA synthesis in, 123
  structural proteins of, 211–234
    in assembly, 227–229
    biosynthesis of, 211–213
    in cell entry, 226–227
    E proteins, 213–214, 227–228
    glycoprotein 2, 214–215
    glycoprotein 3, 215–216
    glycoprotein 4, 216–218
    glycoprotein 5, 218–223
    M proteins, 223, 227
    N proteins, 223–226, 227
  structures of, 5, Color Plate 1
  taxonomy of, 3, 325
Autophagy
  in coronavirus infections, 252–253
  in double-membrane vesicle formation, 107–108
Avian sarcoma and leukosis virus, cell entry by, 165

B cells
  in coronavirus infections, 344–345
  in lactate dehydrogenase-elevating virus infections,
    334
Bacterial artificial chromosome system, 54–56
Bafiniviruses, 134
Bat coronavirus (BtCoV), 411–413
  antigenic variation of, 383
  epidemiology of, 300
  evolution of, 22